Mosby's

Review Questions for the
NCLEX-RN®
Examination

Mosby's

Review Questions for the
NCLEX-RN®
Examination

FIFTH EDITION

Editor
†**Dolores F. Saxton,** R.N., B.S.Ed., M.A., M.P.S., Ed.D.

Associate Editors

Phyllis K. Pelikan, R.N., A.A.S., B.S., M.A.
Patricia M. Nugent, R.N., A.A.S., B.S., M.S., Ed.M., Ed.D.
Judith S. Green, R.N., B.A., A.A.S., M.A.

Content Editors

Jane K. Brody, R.N., B.S.N., M.S.N., Ph.D.
Phyllis Portnoy Cohen, R.N.C., B.S.N., M.S.
JoAnn Schmidt-Festa, R.N.C., B.S., M.S., Ph.D.
Colleen Glavinspiehs, R.N., B.S., M.S.N., D.N.Sc., F.N.P.
Christina Algiere Kasprisin, R.N., M.S., Ed.D.
Anita Throwe, R.N., B.S.N., M.S., C.S.
Barbara A. Vitale, R.N., A.A.S., B.S.N., M.A.

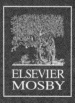

†Deceased

ELSEVIER
MOSBY

11830 Westline Industrial Drive
St. Louis, Missouri 63146

Mosby's Review Questions for the NCLEX-RN® Examination   ISBN 0-323-02468-8
Fifth Edition

Notice

Pharmacology is an ever-changing field. Standard safety precautions must be followed, but
as new research and clinical experience broaden our knowledge, changes in treatment and
drug therapy may become necessary or appropriate. Readers are advised to check the most
current product information provided by the manufacturer of each drug to be administered
to verify the recommended dose, the method and duration of administration, and
contraindications. It is the responsibility of the licensed health care provider, relying on
experience and knowledge of the patient, to determine dosages and the best treatment for
each individual patient. Neither the publisher nor the editor assumes any liability for any
injury and/or damage to persons or property arising from this publication.

Previous editions copyrighted 1991, 1995, 1998, 2001.

International Standard Book Number 0-323-02468-8

Executive Vice President: Sally Schrefer
Executive Publisher: Darlene Como
Executive Editor: Loren Wilson
Senior Developmental Editor: Nancy L. O'Brien
Publication Services Manager: Pat Joiner
Project Manager: Sarah E. Fike
Designer: Julia Dummitt

Printed in the United States of America

Last digit is the print number: 9   8   7   6   5   4   3   2   1

Contributors

Janet T. Ihlenfeld, R.N., B.S.N., M.S.N., Ph.D.
D'Youville College
Buffalo, New York

Laurie Gaspari Kaudewitz, R.N., R.N.C.,
B.S.N., M.S.N.
East Tennessee State University College of Nursing
Johnson City, Tennessee

Anita L. Throwe, R.N., B.S.N., M.S., C.S.
Durant Children's Center
Florence, South Carolina

Carol C. Genereux, R.N., B.S.N., M.S.N., A.N.P.
New England Baptist Hospital
Boston, Massachusetts

Jo Elberg, R.N., B.S., M.A.E.
Iowa Central Community College
Fort Dodge, Iowa

Judy E. White, R.N.C., B.S.N., M.A., M.S.N.
Sanford University, Ida V. Moffett School of Nursing
Birmingham, Alabama

Jeanne Millett, R.N., B.S., M.S., Ed.D., F.N.P.
Private practice
Slingerlands, New York

Deborah Williams, R.N., M.S.N., Ed.D.
Western Kentucky University
Bowling Green, Kentucky

Carol Flaugher, R.N., B.S.N., M.S.N.
State University of New York at Buffalo School of
Nursing
Buffalo, New York

This text was developed to meet the requests of students for "still more questions—with answers and rationales." This fifth edition has been increased to more than 4700 single-item questions, both multiple-choice and alternate format, that reflect the NCLEX-RN® examination. They are included in the written text as well as in the accompanying dual platform CD-ROM. To meet the requirements of students who have different study styles and learning needs, the questions are presented in four distinct formats:

- The questions in the clinical chapters are grouped according to categories of concern for a specific clinical area. The categories of concern reflect specific content areas within a broad clinical area from which the material in the question has been drawn. We have presented these questions in the traditional clinical groupings because we believe that, even when preparing for an integrated test similar to the NCLEX-RN examination, most students will need to study all the distinct parts before attempting to put them together.

- Fifty-item quizzes conclude each clinical nursing chapter. Two quizzes are included at the end of each of the following chapters: Childbearing and Women's Health Nursing (Chapter 2), Pediatric Nursing (Chapter 3), and Mental Health Nursing (Chapter 4). Three 50-item quizzes are included at the end of Medical-Surgical Nursing (Chapter 5). The quizzes integrate the content from the various categories of concern within a specific clinical area. These quizzes provide a bridge for moving from the clinical chapters to the comprehensive examinations.

- Two comprehensive examinations, consisting of 265 questions each, are provided to approximate the NCLEX-RN examination test plan. The first part of each test consists of 75 questions, the minimum number of questions required to receive a grade on the NCLEX-RN examination. The second part of each test consists of 190 questions, which when added to the previous 75 questions totals 265 questions. This is the maximum number of questions allowed on the NCLEX-RN examination.

- A dual-based CD-ROM contains all of the questions in the textbook and an additional 1048 bonus questions that are not contained in the textbook. Five additional 50-question quizzes not contained in the textbook can be found on the CD-ROM. The CD-ROM allows students to practice their test-taking skills on a computer and build confidence for taking the computerized NCLEX-RN examination

For each question in the textbook and on the CD-ROM there is a reason why the correct answer is correct, as well as why each of the other options is incorrect. Each question in the textbook is identified in relation to the level of difficulty. In addition, each question has been analyzed according to client needs, critical thinking/professional decision making, steps in the nursing process, the clinical area, and the category of concern (specific area of content). Questions incorporate material from the basic sciences, nutrition, and pharmacology, as well as current information relative to topics such as gerontology, rehabilitation, the DSM-IV, ethical/legal nursing practice, management responsibilities, and the delivery of health care.

All the questions in this textbook were developed by outstanding and experienced nursing educators and practitioners. The editorial panel reviewed questions initially submitted, selecting and editing the most pertinent for inclusion in a mass field-testing project. Students graduating from baccalaureate, associate degree, and diploma nursing programs in various locations in the United States and Canada provided a diverse testing group. The results were statistically analyzed, and this analysis was used to select the highest quality questions for inclusion in this text and to determine each question's level of difficulty.

We believe that *Mosby's Review Questions for the NCLEX-RN Examination*, along with our other publications, *Mosby's Comprehensive Review of Nursing* and *Mosby's AssessTest,* and our computer products, *Mosby's Comprehensive Review of Nursing* CD-ROM, *Mosby's Online AsessTest,* and *Mosby's Computer Adaptive Test (CAT) for the NCLEX-RN Examination,* provide the necessary tools for students to base their study and review for both coursework and the NCLEX-RN examination. It is our belief that if students study the material and develop a strong knowledge base, the method of testing should not have a major influence on their performance.

We offer our sincere appreciation to our many colleagues for their contributions: to Loren Wilson, Executive Editor, for her guidance, infinite patience, support, and friendship; to Nancy O'Brien, Senior Developmental Editor, for her ability to solve our problems quickly and efficiently and for her expert management of this project; to our content editors for their careful reading and thoughtful critique of our manuscript; to Dale Wolff, our typist and computer expert for her insightful queries; and to our families and friends for their love, understanding, and encouragement.

Phyllis K. Pelikan
Patricia M. Nugent
Judith S. Green

Contents

Illustration Credits

Chapter 2 (p. 21)
Dickason EJ, Schultz MO, Silverman BL: *Maternal-Infant Nursing Care,* 3rd ed, St. Louis, 1998, Mosby.

Chapter 3 (p. 158) and CD-ROM (Pediatric Questions, Figure 1)
Wong DL, Hockenberry-Eaton M, Wilson D, Winkelstein ML, Schwartz P: *Wong's Essentials of Pediatric Nursing,* 6th ed, St. Louis, 2001, Mosby.

Chapter 5 (pp. 413 and 461) and CD-ROM (Medical-Surgical Questions, Figures 1 and 2)

Lewis SM, Heitkemper MM, Dirksen SR: *Medical-Surgical Nursing: Assessment and Management of Clinical Problems,* 6th ed, St. Louis, 2004, Mosby.

Chapter 7 (pp. 696 and 724) and CD-ROM (Childbearing Questions, Figures 1 and 2)
Lowdermilk DL, Perry SE: *Maternity & Women's Health Care,* 8th ed, St. Louis, 2004, Mosby.

CD-ROM (Medical-Surgical Questions, Figures 3 and 4)
Potter PA, Perry AG: *Fundamentals of Nursing,* 5th ed, St. Louis, 2001, Mosby.

Chapter 1

Preparing for the Licensure Examination

INTRODUCTION

Licensure examinations in the United States and Canada have been integrated and comprehensive for many years. Both contain objective multiple-choice questions that historically comprised the entire test. In 2003 the National Council of State Boards of Nursing (NCSBN) added questions to the NCLEX-RN® examination that are alternatives to these traditional multiple-choice items. These questions require the candidate to fill in the blank, identify specific anatomic locations on a picture or diagram, or select more than one option as a correct answer. This edition of *Mosby's Review Questions for the NCLEX-RN® Examination* contains both multiple-choice questions and alternate item format questions.

To answer all questions appropriately, a candidate should understand and correlate certain aspects of anatomy and physiology, the behavioral sciences, basic nursing, medication administration, the client's attitude toward illness; the nurse's legal, ethical, and managerial responsibilities; and other pertinent factors that comprise nursing practice. Most questions are based on nursing situations similar to those with which candidates have had experience because both the United States and Canada emphasize the nursing care of clients with representative common national health problems. Some questions, however, require candidates to apply basic principles and techniques to clinical situations with which they have had little, if any, actual experience.

To adequately prepare for an integrated comprehensive examination, it is necessary to understand the discrete parts that comprise the universe under consideration. This is one of the major principles of learning on which this review and these study materials have been developed. Using this concept, this text first presents questions for each major clinical area that test the student's knowledge of principles and theories underlying nursing care in a variety of situations (acute, critical, and long term); in a variety of settings (acute-care hospitals, nursing homes, and the community); and with a variety of nursing approaches to promote health and prevent illness (including primary, secondary, and tertiary care).

The text concludes with two integrated comprehensive tests reflecting the licensure examinations. The questions in the integrated comprehensive tests require the student to cross clinical disciplines and respond to individual and specific needs associated with given health problems.

All of the questions have rationales supporting the correct answers. In addition, rationales are presented to document why each of the other choices is inappropriate. Reviewing the rationales enables the student to verify information and reinforce knowledge.

CLASSIFICATION OF QUESTIONS

Questions are classified according to level of difficulty, client needs, critical thinking/professional decision making, steps of the nursing process, clinical area, and category of concern. These appear after the rationale for each correct answer.

After the rationale for the correct answer there is a number **(1, 2, or 3)** in parentheses. This number indicates the level of difficulty of the question and reflects the percentage of tested students answering the question correctly.

1. The number 1 signifies that 75% or more of the students in the testing group answered the question correctly.
2. The number 2 signifies that between 50% and 75% of the students in the testing group answered the question correctly.
3. The number 3 signifies that fewer than 50% of the students in the testing group answered the question correctly.

In the clinical chapters (Chapters 2, 3, 4, and 5), the questions are from a specific clinical area and are grouped by their category of concern. The category of concern reflects the specific content area within the broad clinical area from which the material in the question has been drawn. After each correct rationale there are three sets of letters that classify the question by the following specific categories: Client Need, Critical Thinking/Professional Decision Making, and Step of the Nursing Process. Each clinical chapter concludes with multiple 50-item quizzes. These questions are from the specific clinical area but they are not grouped by category of concern. Therefore, the letters following the correct rationale classify each question by Client Need, Critical Thinking/Professional Decision Making, Step of the Nursing Process, and Category of Concern.

In the Comprehensive Examinations (Chapters 6 and 7), the clinical nursing content areas are integrated. Therefore, the letters after the correct rationale classify each question by Client Need, Critical Thinking/Professional Decision Making, Step of the Nursing Process, Clinical Area, and Category of Concern. The series of letters always appears in the same order for all questions.

The following are presented to assist the reader in understanding and reviewing these classifications.

Client Needs

Client Needs are those health care needs of the client that the nurse must address.

1. A safe and therapeutic environment **(SE).** These needs include but are not limited to:
   a. Coordination of care among the health team members, health teaching, and legal, ethical, and managerial responsibilities
   b. Promotion of safety and prevention of infection, accidents, and errors in care
2. Physiologic and anatomic equilibrium **(PB).** These needs include but are not limited to:
   a. Provision of care and comfort related to nutrition, hygiene, elimination, mobility, rest and sleep, and reduction of risks that interfere with psychologic, physiologic, or anatomic integrity
   b. Management of pharmacologic and parenteral therapies including purpose, route, range of dosages, interactions, expected side effects, and untoward effects
   c. Prevention of complications and iatrogenic problems, focusing on diagnostic testing, evaluation of test results, laboratory values, procedures, and treatments
   d. Direction and assistance with adaptations to physiologic problems based on acute, chronic, or life-threatening conditions which include imbalances in fluids and electrolytes, hemodynamics, pathologic responses to therapies, alterations in body systems
3. Health promotion throughout the life span **(PM).** This need includes but is not limited to providing for the achievement of the highest possible level of functioning by promotion and acceptance of physiologic and psychologic changes throughout the life cycle, supporting optimum family growth and development including reproduction and childrearing, facilitating self-care and health maintenance through assessment, education, health programs, and support services.
4. Psychosocial and emotional equilibrium **(PI).** This need includes but is not limited to supporting adaptation to and management of stress, recognizing sociocultural, religious, spiritual, and emotional influences on health, encouraging the use of support systems, employing mental health concepts and therapeutic communication, dealing with real or imagined threats to self-esteem using interventions to limit psychopathology, and creating an environment that supports, fosters, and promotes optimum emotional health.

Critical Thinking/Professional Decision Making

The Critical Thinking/Professional Decision Making classification addresses the professional nurse's ability to use scientific thinking and to delegate responsibilities to meet desired outcomes. It is an integral part of all client care situations.

1. Clinical judgment **(CJ).** This includes the organized identification of a problem, collection of data, implementation of a plan of action, and evaluation of the outcomes.
2. Legal and ethical accountability **(LE).** This includes the recognition of the laws and regulations governing the practice of nursing, the state laws, as well as the ethical obligations included in the American Nurses' Association Code for Nurses.
3. Managerial responsibilities **(MR).** This includes the delegation of duties, assignment, supervision, and evaluation of licensed and unlicensed assistive personnel, taking into consideration role expectations, level of competence, legal requirements, and institutional policies. Included are guidance and coordination of all those coming in contact with the client in the health care system, extending to the client and the client's significant others.

Step of the Nursing Process

Step of the Nursing Process includes the five components of the nursing process that represent the various types of nursing behaviors.

1. Assessment **(AS).** This involves gathering subjective and objective data about the client's health status from meaningful sources, grouping the data into categories,

and communicating the information to others. The database for making nursing decisions is determined through the assessment phase.

2. Analysis **(AN).** This involves interpreting the data obtained during the assessment phase to identify the client's actual or potential health care needs and to formulate nursing diagnoses.

3. Planning **(PL).** This involves designing strategies to correct, minimize, or prevent problems identified during the assessment and analysis steps, sets priorities for the problems diagnosed, develops both short- and long-term goals with the client and/or client's family, establishes outcome criteria for nursing interventions, and formulates the nursing care plan.

4. Implementation **(IM).** This involves initiating and completing the plan of care. The nurse may perform the care or assist, teach, counsel, or supervise the client, the client's significant others, or other health team members to perform specific interventions based on the client's identified needs, diagnoses, priorities, and goals.

5. Evaluation **(EV).** This involves determining the effectiveness of nursing intervention. The nurse compares the actual outcomes with the expected outcomes to determine client compliance with and response to the intervention or therapy. The nurse uses the evaluation phase to identify whether the health care need still exists, which would require modification of the plan, or whether new health care needs have developed, which would require new interventions.

Clinical Area
Clinical Area includes the basic areas of nursing clinical practice. Although the content of a test item may fall into more than one clinical area, the test item is classified according to the major problem involved.

1. Childbearing and women's health nursing **(CW)**
2. Pediatric nursing **(PE)**
3. Mental health nursing **(MH)**
4. Medical/surgical nursing **(MS)**

Category of Concern
Category of Concern reflects the specific content area within the broad clinical area from which the material in the question has been drawn.

1. Pediatric and Medical/Surgical Nursing
   a. Nursing practice **(NP)**
   b. Growth and development **(GD)**
   c. Blood and immunity **(BI)**
   d. Cardiovascular **(CV)**

    e. Endocrine **(EN)**
    f. Fluid and electrolyte **(FE)**
    g. Gastrointestinal **(GI)**
    h. Integumentary **(IT)**
    i. Neuromuscular **(NM)**
    j. Reproductive and genitourinary **(RG)**
    k. Respiratory **(RE)**
    l. Skeletal **(SK)**
    m. Drug-related responses **(DR)**
    n. Emotional needs related to health problems **(EH)**

2. Childbearing and Women's Health Nursing
   a. Nursing practice **(NP)**
   b. Emotional needs related to childbearing and women's health **(EC)**
   c. Reproductive choices **(RC)**
   d. Healthy childbearing **(HC)**
   e. High-risk pregnancy **(HP)**
   f. Normal neonate **(NN)**
   g. High-risk neonate **(HN)**
   h. Reproductive problems **(RP)**
   i. Women's health **(WH)**
   j. Drug-related responses **(DR)**

3. Mental Health
   a. Nursing practice **(NP)**
   b. Personality development **(PD)**
   c. Therapeutic relationships **(TR)**
   d. Emotional disorders related to physical health and childbearing **(ED)**
   e. Disorders first evident before adulthood **(BA)**
   f. Anxiety, somatoform, factitious, and dissociative disorders **(AX)**
   g. Crisis situations **(CS)**
   h. Dementia, delirium, and other cognitive disorders **(DD)**
   i. Eating and sleep disorders **(ES)**
   j. Disorders of mood **(MO)**
   k. Disorders of personality **(PR)**
   l. Schizophrenic disorders **(SD)**
   m. Substance abuse **(SA)**
   n. Drug-related responses **(DR)**

GUIDELINES FOR USING THIS BOOK

A. Start in one clinical area. Answer all of the questions in the area. Do not worry if you select the same numbered answer repeatedly.

B. As you answer each question, write a few words about why you think that answer was correct and justify why you selected the answer.

C. If you guess at an answer in this text, you should make a special mark to identify it as a guess. This will permit you to recognize areas that need further review. It also will help you to see how correct your guessing can be.

D. You may find it easier to tear out the sheets with answers and rationales for the area you are reviewing and compare your answers with those provided. If you answered the item correctly, check your reason for selecting the answer with the rationale presented. If you answered the item incorrectly, read the rationale to determine why the answer you selected was incorrect. In addition, you should review the correct answer and rationale for each item answered incorrectly. If you still do not understand your mistake, look up the theory pertaining to these questions. You should carefully review all questions and rationales for items you identified as guesses because you did not have mastery of the material being questioned.

E. Several days later, review the area again. If you miss the same question a second time, you need further study of the material.

F. After you have completed the clinical area questions, begin taking the comprehensive tests because they will assist you in applying knowledge and principles from the specific clinical area to any nursing situation. The following steps are suggested:
   1. Arrange for a quiet, uninterrupted time span for each of the comprehensive tests.
   2. Pace yourself during the testing period; allow about one minute per question.
   3. Do not rush.
   4. Answer every question.

G. Since most examinations have specified time limits, you will need to pace yourself during the practice testing period, working as quickly and accurately as possible. It is helpful to estimate the time that can be spent on each item and still complete the examination in the allotted time. You can obtain this figure by dividing the testing time by the number of items on the test. For example, with a one-hour (60-minute) testing period and approximately 60 items, an average of one minute per item will be the appropriate pace.

H. To help analyze your mistakes on the comprehensive examinations and to provide a database for making future study plans, two types of worksheets are included in this text. One is designed to aid you in identifying and recording errors in the way you process information. The other is to help you identify and record gaps in knowledge. These worksheets follow the Answers and Rationales for each test in the Comprehensive Test Section. Instructions for their use appear on each worksheet.

I. After completing your worksheets, do the following:
   1. Use Worksheet 1 to identify the frequency with which you made particular errors. As you review material in class notes or study

material such as *Mosby's Comprehensive Review of Nursing,* pay special attention to correcting your most common problems.
   2. Use Worksheet 2 to identify the topics you want to review. It might be helpful to set priorities; review the most difficult topics first so that you will have time to review them more than once.

J. Use this opportunity to learn from your mistakes.
   1. Because you receive immediate feedback on your performance, you have an excellent opportunity to learn from your mistakes. Answer every question. Do not leave any questions unanswered; use educated or pure guesses.
   2. The mistakes you make on the questions in this text will be as valuable to you as the confident feeling you get from answering correctly.

GUIDELINES FOR USING THE CD-ROM

Mosby's Review Questions for the NCLEX-RN Examination® includes a dual platform (PC and Macintosh) disk. The disk contains seven files. The first six files present all the questions that are included in the book and the seventh file contains more than 1275 additional questions that do not appear in the book.

The first four files are divided into Childbearing and Women's Health Nursing, Pediatric Nursing, Mental Health Nursing, and Medical/Surgical Nursing. These files contain all the questions that appear in Chapters 2 through 5 in the book. When in each file, questions can be selected by category codes according to specific specifications. This allows you to study content within a concentrated area of information selected by you. Also, questions can be selected randomly to cross the spectrum of content within a clinical nursing area. This allows you to prepare for a comprehensive examination at the end of a unit of study. All questions include the rationales for the correct and incorrect answers.

Files 5 and 6 include the Comprehensive Examinations 1 and 2 that appear in Chapters 6 and 7 in *Mosby's Review Questions for the NCLEX-RN Examination®*. When in one of these files, you can proceed from questions 1 through 265 at your own pace. These tests simulate a computerized examination that has content that crosses the nursing disciplines. All questions include rationales for correct and incorrect answers. At the completion of each comprehensive examination you will receive a personalized review of your performance that identifies your strengths and weaknesses. This information can be used to direct your future study.

File 7 consists of over 1275 questions that do not appear in *Mosby's Review Questions for the NCLEX-RN Examination®*. When in this file, you can access questions by category codes according to specific specifications selected by you. This allows you to review content guided by your personal study needs. Also, questions can be accessed randomly from all the clinical nursing areas. This simulates the NCLEX-RN® examination. All questions include rationales for correct and incorrect answers. At the completion of a self-constructed, individualized examination in this file, you will receive a personalized review of your performance. This personalized performance review identifies your strengths and weaknesses and should guide your future study. By studying those areas that need improvement, you can utilize your study time more productively and maximize your ability to pass the NCLEX-RN® examination.

READINESS FOR THE LICENSURE EXAMINATION

A few individuals can improve their scores significantly by a highly concentrated period of study immediately before taking an examination. Most, however, profit by spreading their review over a much longer period. Cramming usually does not help. Identification of your own specific strengths and weaknesses should eliminate much of the anxiety of deciding what material to study by giving you a sense of direction and a means of setting priorities.

Reduce Stress

Stress is a part of life. While there is no way to prevent it, it is possible to reduce it by diffusing your emotional responses before stress gets the better of you. Controlling stress allows you to use it instead of being abused by it. The following are tips to reduce and control stress:

1. Talk it out, but try to talk it out with someone who is not as stressed as you are. This relieves the burden of coping alone and helps put things in perspective. Try talking with people who have had the same experience and understand what you are going through.
2. Obtain as much information as you can. STUDY!!!
3. Keep fit. Good nutrition, regular exercise, and ample sleep help.
4. Try relaxation exercises. Relaxation is essential to reducing stress.
5. Sort out the important things. Take stock of your strengths. Set realistic deadlines. Drop the nonessentials.
6. Spend time on yourself and your needs outside of nursing.
7. Be greedy and put yourself first. Be flexible with yourself. Do not set rigid, unmanageable goals.
8. Discover your positive defenses and use them.
9. Become familiar with reading questions on a computer screen. Familiarity reduces anxiety and decreases errors.

Manage Test-Taking Time

The computerized NCLEX-RN® examination is not a timed test, but there is a maximum five-hour period. The computerized test reportedly has been designed to measure an individual's level of knowledge, skills, and abilities to determine that the competency level is achieved. The test length will vary depending on each candidate's performance but will contain 75 to 265 questions.

Although certain questions will be more difficult than others and will require more time, spending too much time on these difficult items may compromise your overall performance.

Do not be pressured into finishing early. Do not rush! Students who achieve higher scores on examinations are typically those who use all the time available.

Build Test-Taking Confidence

You should feel confident and competent if you have studied and reviewed the content to be tested and you are armed with methods for reading and answering questions. Your emotional state is vitally important when thinking about, preparing for, and taking any test. Think positively.

While you are taking the test, you may have problems with a question. On a written examination it is often best to move on to another question that you can answer and come back to the more difficult question. However, on the computerized NCLEX-RN® examination you must answer the question before you can go on to the next question, so remain calm. Anxiety can block the recall of familiar information required to answer questions, so control it early. Do not stop to think about gaps in your preparation or waste time and emotional energy building anxiety. Focus on the positive. You have the ability to make sound "educated guesses." Now is the time to use it. Questions that seem complicated at first glance often can be answered by just such guesses. Remain calm and confident.

You will find that practice test-taking experiences will give you confidence for the actual examination. After you have completed studying this book, you may wish to take a simulated examination such as *Mosby's AssessTest* before you take the licensure examination. The *AssessTest* is a computer-scored, multiple-choice and alternate format question examination designed to test nursing knowledge and evaluate your ability to apply that knowledge in clinical situations. The extensive computer analysis of your performance, which is the most outstanding feature of this test, will help you design effective and efficient plans for further study and review. The Online *AssessTest* is helpful if you need to build confidence in your computer skills.

TAKING THE LICENSURE EXAMINATION

On the NCLEX-RN® examination all of the client needs, five steps of the nursing process and clinical areas are represented. There is less emphasis in the areas of maternity (obstetric) nursing and severe mental illness, whereas there is a greater emphasis on medical-surgical principles, interpersonal skills, especially communication, and managerial, legal, and ethical responsibilities. The score on the examination is reported as pass or fail.

The most crucial requisite for doing well on the licensure examination is a sound understanding of the subject and a high level of reading comprehension. Determination to do well and a degree of confidence will further enhance your chance of passing and achieving the recognition deserved.

At least three other requirements must be met if your performance is to reflect accurately your professional competence. First, you must scrupulously follow the directions given by the examiner and those appearing at the beginning of the test. Second, you must read each question carefully before deciding how to answer it. Third, you must record the answers in the manner specified.

The computerized NCLEX-RN® examination is an individualized testing experience in which the computer chooses your next question based on the ability and competency you have demonstrated on previous questions. The minimum number of questions will be 75 and the maximum 265. You must answer each question before the computer will present the next question, and you cannot go back to any previously answered questions. There is no deduction for incorrect answers so you are not penalized for guessing. You cannot leave an answer blank, and since you have a one in four (25%) chance of guessing the correct answer, go for it. Remember: you do not have to get all the questions correct to pass.

You also should keep in mind that if you practice and learn the material, the method of testing (oral, written, or computer) should not significantly influence your performance.

GENERAL STRATEGIES

1. Develop a plan for study and stick to it. A good plan is to allow one week per clinical area.

2. As you study, identify your problem areas that need attention.
3. Avoid planning other activities that will add stress to your life between now and the time you take the NCLEX-RN® examination. Enough will happen spontaneously; do not plan to add to it.
4. Do not change your pattern of study. It obviously has contributed to your being here, so it worked. If you have studied alone, continue to study alone. If you have studied in a group, form a study group.
5. Practice timed tests and stay within their suggested time frames. You usually will have about one minute per question on most examinations.
6. Pace yourself during the testing period and work as accurately as possible. Do not rush. Excessive pressure on yourself early in the examination can result in early fade-out.
7. Although certain questions are more difficult and require more time, do not spend too much time on one question because it can compromise your overall performance.
8. If you find you tend to reread test answers and change the right ones to wrong ones, stop going back, even if you are taking tests that permit you to go back. If you find that going back helps you to correct wrong answers, by all means go back and review your answers, provided that the test permits you to go back. Remember: your first answer is usually correct and should not be changed without reason. You cannot go back on the NCLEX-RN® examination.
9. Do not read information into questions, and avoid speculating. Reading into questions creates errors in judgment.
10. Make certain that the answer you select is reasonable and obtainable under ordinary circumstances and that the action can be carried out in the given situation.
11. Avoid selecting answers that state hospital rules or regulations as a reason or rationale for action.
12. Look for answers that focus on the client or that are directed toward the client's feelings.
13. If the question asks for an immediate action or response, all the answers may be correct, so base your selection on identified priorities for action.
14. Do not select answers that contain exceptions to the general rule, controversial material, or responses that appear to be degrading.
15. Do not be pressured into finishing early. Use all the time necessary without pressuring yourself.

We wish you success on the NCLEX-RN® examination and as you pursue your career goals.

Chapter 2

Childbearing and Women's Health Nursing

REVIEW QUESTIONS

NURSING PRACTICE (NP)

1. A female client is scheduled for a hysterectomy. When discussing the preoperative preparation, the nurse identifies that the client has no understanding of the surgery. The nurse should:
   1. Describe the proposed surgery to the client
   2. Proceed with implementing the preoperative plan
   3. Notify the physician that the client needs information
   4. Explain to the client gently that she should have asked more questions

2. A client in labor is being prepared for a cesarean birth. The most important nursing intervention before the anesthesia is administered would be to:
   1. Prepare the abdomen
   2. Obtain an informed consent
   3. Initiate an intravenous infusion
   4. Insert an indwelling urinary catheter

3. New parents are asked to sign the consent for their son to be circumcised. They ask for the nurse's opinion of the procedure. The best response by the nurse would be:
   1. "You should talk to the physician about this if you have any questions."
   2. "It is absolutely safe, and it is best for all male infants to be circumcised."
   3. "There are advantages and disadvantages to circumcision. Let's talk about it."
   4. "Although it is a somewhat painful experience for the baby, I would allow it if I were you."

4. A new mother tells the nurse that her baby "spits up" after each formula feeding. The nurse teaches her how to position the baby after feedings. After the next feeding the nurse observes that the mother positions the baby correctly. The nurse evaluates this activity to:
   1. Prepare a basic teaching plan
   2. Validate that learning has occurred
   3. Ascertain the mother's knowledge base
   4. Determine the mother's readiness to learn

5. The parents do not want their newborn's eyes treated with a prophylactic agent. The nurse's best response to this would be:
   1. "This is really for the baby's good."
   2. "This is a legal requirement and must be done."
   3. "Have you discussed this with your pediatrician?"
   4. "You'll have to sign an informed consent to refuse the treatment."

6. When obtaining informed consent for sterilization from a developmentally challenged adult client, the nurse must be sure that the:
   1. Parent or guardian signs the consent
   2. Client comprehends the outcome of the procedure
   3. Client is fully able to explain what the procedure entails
   4. Parent or guardian has encouraged the client to make the decision

EMOTIONAL NEEDS RELATED TO CHILDBEARING AND WOMEN'S HEALTH (EC)

7. Because of the high discomfort level during the transition phase of labor, nursing care should be directed toward:
   1. Administering medication
   2. Helping the client maintain control
   3. Decreasing the rate of intravenous fluid
   4. Having the client breathe in uniform patterns

8. The nurse is aware that during the taking-in phase of the postpartum period, the area of health teaching that the client will be most responsive to would be:
   1. Perineal care
   2. Infant feeding
   3. Infant hygiene
   4. Family planning

9. A postpartum adolescent mother confides to the nurse that she hopes her baby will be good and sleep through the night. The nurse should plan to teach the mother to:
   1. Cuddle the baby and talk softly when crying occurs
   2. Put a soft, cuddly toy next to the baby at bedtime
   3. Add cereal to the bedtime bottle to ensure deep sleep
   4. Keep the baby awake for longer periods during the day

10. The husband of a woman who had her fourth child three weeks ago states she has been irritable and crying since coming home from the hospital. The nurse tries to assist him in understanding the situation by stating that:
    1. His wife probably has postpartum blues that will pass soon
    2. Having four children is tiring and assistance may be needed
    3. This behavior is common after birth and he should not be too concerned
    4. Often, women express themselves by crying and he should allow her to continue

11. A client with mild preeclampsia is told that she must remain on bed rest at home. The client starts to cry and tells the nurse that she has two small children at home who need her. The nurse's best response would be:
    1. "How do you plan to manage with getting child care help?"
    2. "Are you worried about how you will be able to handle this problem?"
    3. "You can get a neighbor to help out, and your husband can do the housework in the evening."
    4. "You'll be able to fix light meals, and the children can go to nursery school a few hours each day."

12. The best nursing intervention to achieve cooperation of an extremely anxious client during her first pelvic examination to confirm pregnancy would be to:
    1. Assist the physician so the examination can be finished quickly
    2. Distract the client by asking her preference as to the sex of the child
    3. Maintain eye contact, touch gently, and thoroughly explain the procedure
    4. Encourage the client to close her eyes and hold her breath during the pelvic examination

13. A pregnant client whose first child has Down syndrome is about to undergo an amniocentesis. The client tells the nurse that she does not know what she will do if this baby has the same diagnosis. The client asks the nurse, "Do you think abortion is the same as killing?" The nurse's best response would be:
    1. "Some people think this is what an abortion is."
    2. "No, I do not think so, but it is your decision to make."
    3. "I really can't answer that question. You seem ambivalent about abortion."
    4. "I don't want to answer that question at this time. How do you feel about it?"

14. A client who has just delivered an infant with Down syndrome tells the nurse that she could not possibly take a retarded child home and asks whether she should plan to place the child in an institution. An appropriate statement by the nurse at this time would be:
    1. "It must be difficult not to realize your vision of a perfect child."
    2. "I understand how you feel, and I will notify the nursery personnel of your decision."
    3. "Give yourself time to get acquainted, and you will see that your baby may not be retarded."
    4. "You should not make such a hasty decision, as your baby is like any other baby right now."

15. A neonate is born with exstrophy of the bladder and the parents are upset. They are told that corrective surgery will be done as soon as possible. At this time the nurse can best help the parents by:
    1. Keeping the infant clean to aid in decreasing the odor of urine
    2. Teaching the parents about preoperative and postoperative care
    3. Responding to the newborn in the same manner as to any other newborns
    4. Reassuring the parents that after surgery their baby will have a normal life

16. A 4-day-old male in the neonatal intensive care unit (NICU) was born with exstrophy of the bladder and ambiguous genitalia. The everted bladder is inflamed and there is continual leaking of urine onto the surrounding skin. His mother visits him daily in the intensive care unit. The nurse's initial concern when working with the mother would be to:
    1. Promote her acceptance of her baby as he is

2. Teach her how to care for her baby's urinary needs
3. Prepare her for the surgery her baby will eventually require
4. Instruct her in ways she can meet her baby's special emotional needs

17. A client with severe preeclampsia who has been admitted to the hospital anxiously asks the nurse, "Will my baby be all right?" The nurse's most appropriate response would be:
   1. "There is no way of telling at this time what the outcome will be."
   2. "The baby will probably be all right; it's protected by the amniotic fluid."
   3. "If you do what the doctor tells you to do, everything will progress normally."
   4. "We will be constantly monitoring your baby's condition. Would you like to listen to the baby's heartbeat?"

18. A client in active labor is rushed from the emergency service to the labor and birth suite screaming, "Knock me out." Examination reveals that her cervix is 9 cm dilated. While trying to calm her, the nurse should respond:
   1. "I'll rub your back which will help ease your pain."
   2. "You will get a shot when you reach the birthing room."
   3. "I'm sure you're in pain, but try to bear with it for the baby's sake."
   4. "Medication may interfere with the baby's first breaths; try to bear the pain."

19. A preterm male newborn will be in the neonatal intensive care unit (NICU) for several weeks. The parents live about 100 miles away and say they can visit only every two weeks or so. When planning care for this newborn and the family, it would be important for the nurse to:
   1. Focus on the infant's biophysical needs in view of his present critical condition
   2. Refer the infant's parents to the social worker to arrange housing close to the hospital
   3. Prepare a detailed teaching plan for the parents and administer it on the day of the infant's discharge
   4. Plan for some contact with the parents between visits by sending e-mail letters and pictures of the baby

20. The nurse should be aware of the stages of parental adjustment that follow birth of an infant at risk who is in the neonatal intensive care unit (NICU). To better plan nursing care, nursing observations and assessments should be based on the recognition that the:
   1. Mother should not see the infant until she has completed the necessary grief work
   2. Mother should be reunited with her infant as soon as possible to enhance adjustment
   3. Parents should be encouraged to visit the newborn within the first 24 hours after birth
   4. Nurse should wait until the parents request to see the newborn before suggesting a visit

21. When first seeing her preterm infant in the neonatal intensive care unit (NICU), the mother immediately starts to cry and refuses to touch the baby. The nurse understands that this behavior represents:
   1. A typical detachment behavior
   2. An incomplete bonding behavior
   3. An expected reaction to the situation
   4. A reaction to the NICU environment

22. The parents of a preterm newborn visit the neonatal intensive care unit for the first time. They are obviously overwhelmed by the amount of equipment and the tiny size of their baby. It would be most helpful at this time for the nurse to:
   1. Show the parents how they can touch the baby
   2. Place the baby in the mother's lap and stay close by
   3. Give a detailed explanation of the equipment and its purposes
   4. Discourage the parents from staying too long on this first visit

23. When seeing her preterm infant son in the neonatal intensive care unit for the first time, a mother exclaims, "My baby is so little. How will I ever care for him?" The nurse should explain to the mother that she:
   1. Can watch his care to assist her in becoming familiar with the specific routines
   2. Should find someone with preterm care training to help her at home the first week
   3. Will be able to care for him in a special nursery for a few days prior to his discharge
   4. Will be encouraged to participate in his care as much as possible from the beginning

24. On the third postpartum day, a client who had an unexpected cesarean birth is found crying during morning rounds. She says, "I know my baby is fine, but I can't help crying. I wanted natural childbirth so much. Why did this have to happen to me?" The nurse responds knowing that:
    1. The client's feelings will pass after she has bonded with her baby
    2. The client is probably suffering from a postpartum depression and needs special care
    3. A woman's self-concept is severely affected by a cesarean birth, and the client's statement reflects this
    4. A cesarean birth may be a traumatic psychologic experience in addition to an acute obstetric emergency

25. Before an amniocentesis, both parents express nervousness about the fetus's safety during the test. The nursing intervention that would best promote the parents' ability to cope is:
    1. Initiating a parent-physician conference
    2. Reassuring them that the procedure is safe
    3. Informing them about the procedure step by step
    4. Arranging for the father to be present during the test

26. The nurse recognizes that the husband of a client is reacting positively to his wife's pregnancy when, during the second trimester, he says:
    1. "I had to take a part-time job to cover the rent for a larger apartment."
    2. "I'm so proud of my wife. I'm already digging a baseball diamond in our backyard."
    3. "I get so excited when I feel the baby kicking. Maybe he will be a kicker for the Pittsburgh Steelers."
    4. "After the childbirth class last night, when I saw how bloody the delivery was, I hope I'll be able to stay for the birth."

27. During labor, a client tells the nurse that she and her husband are very concerned because the baby is coming two months early. The nurse's best response would be:
    1. "You should be concerned; I feel for you."
    2. "Your physician is very good; try not to worry about it now."
    3. "I can understand why you are concerned; let's talk about it."
    4. "Don't worry; the care of preterm babies has greatly improved."

28. A client who is at 28 weeks' gestation and in active labor is crying. She says, "I just know this baby will die. What's the use of doing all this to save it." The nurse should recognize that the client is:

1. Depressed and needs firm, positive handling
2. Is in need of sedation so that she can cope with the impending birth
3. Demonstrating difficulty in dealing with the birth by using the word "it"
4. Experiencing anticipatory grief by withdrawing from the bonding process

29. A neonate born at 32 weeks' gestation and weighing 3 pounds is admitted to the neonatal intensive care unit. The nurse plans to take the neonate's mother to visit the infant in the intensive care unit:
    1. As soon as possible after the birth
    2. When the infant's condition has stabilized
    3. When the infant is out of immediate danger
    4. After the physician writes an order permitting it

30. A common concern of the mother after an unexpected cesarean birth that the nurse should anticipate would be the:
    1. Postoperative pain and scarring
    2. Prolonged period of hospitalization
    3. Sense of failure in the birthing process
    4. Inability to assume her mothering role

31. A nurse is instructing a client to cough and deep breathe after an emergency cesarean birth. The client says, "Get out of here. Don't you know that I am in pain?" The most effective response would be:
    1. "I'm sure you are in pain; rest now and I'll come back later."
    2. "Your pain is to be expected, but you must exercise your lungs."
    3. "I'll give you something for your pain. We can start exercising tomorrow."
    4. "If you are unable to cough, I understand, but try to take five or six good deep breaths."

32. A client who has had a cesarean birth seems upset. She has been having difficulty breastfeeding for two days and now asks the nurse practitioner to bring her a bottle of formula. The nurse's best initial action would be to:
    1. Go to the nursery and get the requested formula
    2. Assess the client's positioning and breastfeeding technique
    3. Ask the primary nurse to administer a pain medication to the client
    4. Notify the pediatrician of the mother's request to switch feeding methods

33. On the first postpartum day, a client whose infant is rooming-in asks the nurse to return her baby to the nursery and bring the baby to her only at

feeding time. The best response by the nurse would be:
1. "I think you are having difficulty caring for the baby."
2. "All right, I will inform the other nurses of your decision."
3. "It seems that you have changed your mind about rooming-in."
4. "Oh, you must be tired. I'll bring the baby back at feeding time."

34. A 16-year-old at 24 weeks' gestation visits the prenatal clinic for the first time. After the physical examination she tells the nurse, "I can't believe how large I am; will I get much bigger?" The nurse responds knowing that:
1. Adolescents generally regain their figures two weeks after delivery, thus size is of moderate concern
2. Adolescents are in a high-risk category, and weight gain should be limited to prevent complications
3. Body image is important to adolescent development, thus pregnant teenagers are concerned about body size
4. The physiologic growth of the adolescent is more rapid than an adult's, thus the gravid size is larger than that of someone who is older

35. A client at 37 weeks' gestation delivers a healthy boy. When inspecting her newborn in the birthing room the client asks, "What's this sticky white stuff all over him?" The nurse's most appropriate response would be:
1. "It's a secretion from the baby's fat cells and is called milia."
2. "Your baby was born three weeks early and we expect to see this."
3. "This is vernix, which helps protect the baby while he's in the uterus."
4. "It's nothing to be concerned about. All newborn babies are covered with it."

36. The mother of a pregnant teenager asks the nurse how her daughter could have been so foolish since birth control had been discussed with her many times. The nurse's best response would be:
1. "Apparently your daughter was not listening to you."
2. "You should have made sure the boyfriend understood birth control too."
3. "Teenagers often fail to use birth control because they forget to discuss this with their sexual partner."
4. "Although teenagers can intellectually discuss birth control, they don't believe anything will happen to them."

37. The parents of a male newborn ask the nurse whether they should have their son circumcised. The nurse's most appropriate response would be:
1. "It would probably be a good idea because circumcision is known to prevent penile cancer."
2. "That's something you both will have to decide after you discuss it thoroughly with your doctor."
3. "The Academy of Pediatrics recommends that circumcision not be done routinely because of the risks associated with the procedure."
4. "I'm sure you have discussed this with your doctor, but let's review the benefits and risks of circumcision."

38. A 45-year-old woman, with large intramural leiomyomas that did not respond to medical therapies, has been advised to have an abdominal hysterectomy. She asks the nurse whether there is any surgery other than an abdominal hysterectomy available. The nurse should respond:
1. "You should ask your physician."
2. "Sorry, there are no other options."
3. "You seem uncertain about having the hysterectomy."
4. "A vaginal hysterectomy is a possible alternative for you."

39. A client in preterm labor does not respond to therapy and must be delivered. The client begins to cry and says, "I'm so worried about my baby." The nurse should respond:
1. "You're receiving the best medical care available."
2. "All of this must leave you very confused and frightened."
3. "Think positively; your anxiety will increase your contractions."
4. "This hospital has a neonatal unit and can handle emergencies."

40. A 28-year-old attorney is recovering from her third consecutive spontaneous abortion in two years. When planning care for this client, the nurse understands that the most therapeutic intervention would be to:
1. Focus on the client's physical needs
2. Encourage the client to verbalize her feelings about the loss
3. Remind the client that she will be able to become pregnant again
4. Encourage the client to think of herself, her husband, and their future

41. After a difficult labor a client gives birth to a 9-pound boy who dies shortly afterward. That evening the client tearfully describes to the nurse her projected image of her son and what his future would have been. The nurse's most therapeutic response would be:
    1. "It must be difficult to think of him now."
    2. "I am sure he would have been a wonderful child."
    3. "Don't dwell on this now. It only increases the pain."
    4. "I guess that both you and your husband wanted a son."

42. A client's newborn is neurologically impaired. The most important nursing action should be to:
    1. Assist the client and her family with the grieving process
    2. Perform neurological assessments of the newborn every four hours
    3. Arrange for social services to discuss possible placement of the newborn
    4. Obtain an order for an antidepressant to help the client cope with the depressing news

43. The nurse is obtaining the history of a client in the third trimester who is visiting the prenatal clinic for the first time. She tells nurse she has two toddlers at home and their father abandoned the family last month. The nurse recognizes that the client probably has:
    1. Lost weight during her pregnancy
    2. Ambivalence about her pregnancy
    3. Been denying the reality of her pregnancy
    4. Had nausea and vomiting throughout her pregnancy

44. When a client in the prenatal clinic is dressing at the completion of her pelvic examination, she states, "Why must I be pregnant now? It's the wrong time." It would be most therapeutic for the nurse to respond:
    1. "Why don't you want this pregnancy?"
    2. "This is a normal response to pregnancy."
    3. "No time is ever the right time to be pregnant."
    4. "You do not seem to be excited about this pregnancy."

45. A client had a mastectomy because of breast cancer. She has started taking chemotherapy, which caused hair loss. The client states, "I feel like I have lost my sense of power." The nurse's best response would be:
    1. "Hair does not empower a person."
    2. "Losing power seems important to you; let's talk about it."
    3. "Knowledge is power; would you like pamphlets to read?"
    4. "Losing hair is common; it will grow back so you should not worry."

46. A 49-year-old client is admitted with a diagnosis of cervical cancer. While obtaining her health history she tells the nurse, "I have not had a Pap smear for over five years. I probably wouldn't be in the hospital today if I'd had those tests more often." The nurse should respond:
    1. "Can you tell me why you haven't gone?"
    2. "You feel like you've neglected your health."
    3. "It's never too late to start taking care of yourself."
    4. "Most women hate to have Pap smears done, but it's really important."

47. While waiting for his 38-year-old wife to change clothes following an amniocentesis, the husband says to the nurse, "I sure hope that they don't find anything wrong. I don't know how we would deal with a retarded child. We have two small children at home." The nurse's best response would be:
    1. "Your other children are healthy, so chances are the third will be also."
    2. "It must be difficult worrying about whether or not your baby is healthy."
    3. "There are plenty of resources available to help families with retarded children."
    4. "The potential of Down syndrome children differs, making early decisions difficult."

48. A husband is sitting in the waiting room while his wife is getting her infertility prescription refilled by the clinic pharmacist. The nurse sits down beside him and he blurts out, "It's like there are three of us in bed—my wife, me, and the doctor." This is reflective of his feelings of:
    1. Guilt
    2. Anger
    3. Depression
    4. Unworthiness

REPRODUCTIVE CHOICES (RC)

49. The nurse, as part of a teaching plan about contraception, tells the client that:
    1. The rim of the condom must be held in place while withdrawing the penis from the vagina

2. Diaphragms are equally effective whether or not the partners choose to use a spermicidal cream
3. No sperm can reach the ovum if the man uses coitus interruptus and withdraws before ejaculation
4. Individuals using periodic abstinence should have intercourse on days when the woman has a rise in temperature

50. A 28-year-old married woman seeks advice from the nurse in her company health office about oral contraceptives. The nurse should advise her that if she smokes:
    1. Oral contraceptives can cause thrombophlebitis
    2. Some oral contraceptives are safe, others are not
    3. Some oral contraceptives can be used without concern
    4. Oral contraceptives can be used with other methods

51. A client is taking oral contraceptives. The nurse should inform the client to stop taking the contraceptive and report to the physician immediately if she experiences:
    1. Vertigo and nausea
    2. Weight loss and breast pain
    3. Hypotension and amenorrhea
    4. Headaches and visual disturbances

52. The nurse should instruct the client taking oral contraceptives to increase her dietary intake of:
    1. Calcium
    2. Potassium
    3. Vitamin E
    4. Vitamin B$_6$

53. Oral contraceptives are prescribed for a client in the family planning clinic. As part of teaching, the nurse plans to inform the client of the possibility of developing:
    1. Cervicitis
    2. Ovarian cysts
    3. Fibrocystic disease
    4. Breakthrough bleeding

54. The nurse at a women's health clinic knows that client teaching regarding use of an oral contraceptive is understood when the client states:
    1. "I can stop the pill and try to get pregnant right away."
    2. "I can miss two periods and not worry about being pregnant."
    3. "I will put a baby's picture on my bathroom mirror, so I'll see it every morning."
    4. "I am so glad we won't have to mess with condoms even if I miss just one pill during the month."

55. When counseling a client with diabetes mellitus who requests contraceptive information, it would be most therapeutic for the nurse to focus on:
    1. Rhythm
    2. The IUD
    3. A diaphragm
    4. Oral contraceptives

56. The nurse in a family planning center knows that a client understands the discussion about the use of diaphragm when the client states, "After intercourse, a diaphragm must be left in place for:
    1. 1 to 2 hours."
    2. 6 to 8 hours."
    3. 10 to 12 hours."
    4. 16 to 20 hours."

57. When teaching a client to use a diaphragm to prevent pregnancy, the nurse should tell the client that the diaphragm:
    1. May or may not be used with a spermicidal lubricant to be effective
    2. Must be inserted with the dome facing down to be maximally effective
    3. Often appears puckered, but this will not interfere with its effectiveness
    4. Should remain in place for at least six hours after intercourse to be effective

58. A couple tells the nurse that they wish to use the rhythm method of birth control. The wife tells the nurse that she menstruates every 32 days for 2 days. The nurse should teach the couple that, based on this cycle, ovulation probably occurs:
    1. On the 14th day of the cycle
    2. 10 days after the first day of bleeding
    3. 14 days before the start of the next menses
    4. 2 to 3 days after the last day of menstrual bleeding

59. The school nurse is teaching a group of 16-year-old girls about the female reproductive system. One student asks how long after ovulation it is possible for conception to occur. The nurse's most accurate response is based on the knowledge that an ovum is no longer viable after
    1. 12 hours
    2. 24 hours
    3. 48 hours
    4. 72 hours

60. A client states that she wishes to use the calendar method of birth control. The nurse is aware that the client understands how to calculate the beginning of the fertile period when she states, "I will:
    1. Subtract 11 days from the length of my longest cycle."
    2. Subtract 18 days from the length of my shortest cycle."
    3. Abstain from sexual intercourse after the 10th day of my cycle."
    4. Abstain from intercourse from the 10th day prior to the middle of my average cycle."

61. A client asks the nurse about the use of an intrauterine device (IUD) for contraception. When discussing this method with the client, the nurse includes that a possible problem with IUD use would be:
    1. Expulsion of the device
    2. Occasional dyspareunia
    3. Perforation of the uterus
    4. Frequent vaginal infections

62. The nurse informs a client contemplating implantable progestin (Norplant) as a means of contraception that the most common side effect is:
    1. Vertigo
    2. Dyspareunia
    3. An increase in breast size
    4. Irregular menstrual bleeding

63. A married client, 35 years old, who is to undergo a tubal ligation is assessed by the nurse to determine the client's possible emotional response to the procedure. A factor in the history that would contribute most to the healthy resolution of any emotional problem associated with sterilization would be that the client:
    1. Has a son and daughter and feels her family is complete
    2. Thinks the surgery will relieve her monthly dysmenorrhea
    3. Knows that her husband does not want her to have any more children
    4. Has just had a complicated birth and never wants to undergo another birth again

64. A female client, undergoing infertility testing, is taught how to examine her cervical mucus. After listening to the instructions the client says, "That sounds gross. I don't think I can do it." The nurse is aware that:
    1. Having a baby is not that important to this client
    2. It is possible that the client is being unduly fastidious

3. The client is afraid of finding out that the problem is her fault
4. Some women are uncomfortable touching their genitals and discharges

65. A couple in their late thirties, who wish to have a child, have been referred to the clinical genetics services. They have a family history of an inheritable problem but have some reservations about genetic counseling because they have heard that genetic clinics favor abortion when the studies reveal a defective fetus. The nurse can put them at ease by telling them that genetic counselors:
    1. Help families understand the diagnosis, the probable cause of the disorder, and how the condition can be managed
    2. Are able to predict which families are going to have defective children and then recommend contraception, not abortion
    3. Recommend abortion only if the fetus is diagnosed as having a condition that is not considered compatible with life
    4. Diagnose the probability of a defective fetus and then the family's own physician is responsible for taking the appropriate action.

66. A couple at the prenatal clinic for a first visit tells the nurse that their 2-year-old has just been diagnosed with cystic fibrosis. They state there is no family history of this disorder. They ask the nurse what the chances are for their having another child with cystic fibrosis. Based on the knowledge that this disorder has an autosomal-recessive mode of inheritance, the nurse should respond that:
    1. There is a 50% chance that this baby will also be affected
    2. If this baby is male, there is a 50% chance of his being affected
    3. If this baby is female, there is no chance of her being affected, but she will be a carrier
    4. There is a 25% chance the baby will be affected, and a 50% chance it will be a carrier

67. A newly married female client asks the nurse to explain the different methods of family planning. She decides to use the diaphragm. When teaching the client about using a diaphragm, the nurse should instruct her:
    1. To completely cover the outside of the dome of the diaphragm with spermicidal jelly or cream
    2. That a douche within an hour after intercourse enhances the effectiveness of the diaphragm

3. To insert the diaphragm before intercourse and leave it in at least six hours after intercourse
4. That correct placement of the diaphragm allows an inch between the diaphragm and the vaginal wall

68. A couple has been married for five years and would like to start a family. When talking with them regarding the timing and frequency of their sexual intercourse, the husband says, "Well, I guess we are going to have to jump into bed three or four times a day, every day until it works." The nurse's best response would be to:
   1. Tell them to continue relations as usual until conception occurs
   2. Instruct them on the frequency and timing of intercourse for conception
   3. Discourage this because sperm production decreases with frequent intercourse
   4. Agree that the frequency of intercourse must increase but twice daily is sufficient

69. A female client with Hodgkin's disease is to start total nodal irradiation. She and her husband have been trying to have a child and are quite concerned when they learn that radiation includes the pelvic nodal area. The nurse should refer them to the physician because the nurse should be aware that:
   1. Intense radiation to the area always causes permanent sterilization
   2. The radiation used is not radical enough to destroy ovarian function
   3. The ovaries can be surgically moved and placed in a shielded area
   4. Ovarian function will be temporarily destroyed but will return in time

70. A young client who has become sexually active asks the nurse, "What is the most effective way to prevent a pregnancy?" The nurse's best response would be:
   1. "Abstain from sex."
   2. "Use birth control pills."
   3. "Use a condom and foam."
   4. "Have an intrauterine device inserted."

71. A client asks the nurse what she should do if she forgets to take the pill one day. The nurse's best response would be:
   1. "Take your pills as instructed."
   2. "Call the physician immediately."
   3. "Continue as usual; missing one day is no problem."
   4. "The next day take one pill in the morning and one before bedtime."

HEALTHY CHILDBEARING (HC)

72. At a client's first visit to the prenatal clinic, the nurse asks the client when she had her last menstrual period so the estimated date of birth (EDB) can be evaluated. The client responds, "January 21st." Using Nägele's rule, the nurse calculates:
   1. October 14
   2. October 28
   3. November 21
   4. September 28

73. When discussing fetal development with a pregnant client, the nurse explains that:
   1. If a baby is to be left-handed after birth, the structures on the left side of the embryo's body develop before those on the right side
   2. Development proceeds from head to tail, so the embryo's brain, central nervous system, and heart are formed and functioning before limb buds appear
   3. Development of structures in the embryo proceeds from external to internal structures so the heart is formed and starts functioning after the limb buds appear
   4. The brain and central nervous system are formed early in the embryonic period, and the right side of the brain starts functioning much earlier than the left side

74. At a client's first prenatal visit the nurse midwife performs a pelvic examination. The nurse states that her cervix is bluish-purple, which is known as Chadwick's sign. The client becomes concerned and asks if something is wrong. The nurse's most appropriate response would be, "It is a normal finding and:
   1. Helps confirm your pregnancy."
   2. Occurs because the blood is trapped by the pregnant uterus."
   3. Is caused by increased blood flow to the uterus during pregnancy."
   4. Is nothing for you to worry about. We see it in lots of pregnant women."

75. A client at seven weeks' gestation tells the nurse in the prenatal clinic that she has been bothered by episodes of nausea, but no vomiting, throughout the day. The nurse should recommend:
   1. "Take low sodium antacids after meals."
   2. "Drink carbonated beverages with meals."
   3. "Eat small but frequent meals throughout the day."
   4. "Eat toast or dry crackers in the morning before rising."

76. A client visiting the prenatal clinic for the first time tells the nurse that she has heard conflicting stories about sex during pregnancy and asks about continuing sexual activity. The nurse's best response would be:
1. "Intercourse should be discontinued after the second trimester."
2. "Sexual activity should be avoided during the last four weeks of pregnancy."
3. "This information can only be given by your obstetrician or nurse midwife."
4. "With an uncomplicated pregnancy, there are no limitations on sexual activity."

77. An active 19-year-old primigravida attends prenatal clinic for the first time. She asks the nurse if she can continue playing tennis and go horseback riding while she is pregnant. The nurse should reply:
1. "Continue all usual activities as long as you are comfortable."
2. "Horseback riding is acceptable, but only until six months' gestation."
3. "Tennis is good exercise for you, but horseback riding is too strenuous."
4. "Tennis and horseback riding are really too strenuous for a pregnant woman."

78. A pregnant client is experiencing nausea and vomiting. The nurse is aware that this discomfort:
1. Is always present in early pregnancy
2. Will disappear when lightening occurs
3. Is a common response to an unwanted pregnancy
4. May be related to the human chorionic gonadotropin (hCG) level

79. The nurse is aware that absorption of drugs taken orally during pregnancy may be altered as the result of:
1. Delayed gastrointestinal emptying
2. Decreased glomerular filtration rates
3. Developing fetal-placental circulation
4. Increased secretion of hydrochloric acid

80. A client at her first visit to the prenatal clinic asks which immunization can be administered safely to a pregnant woman. The nurse should reply:
1. TOPV
2. Mumps
3. Rubella
4. Rubeola

81. The nurse instructs a pregnant client about the sources of protein that assist in meeting the daily requirements of:
1. 15 g
2. 30 g
3. 45 g
4. 60 g

82. A client who is eight weeks pregnant tells the nurse that she does not feel like making love to her husband and is concerned that her husband may not understand. The nurse could most appropriately respond:
1. "How long have you had this problem?"
2. "Why don't you feel like having intercourse?"
3. "I'm sure your husband eventually will understand your feelings are related to pregnancy."
4. "A decrease in libido is an expected occurrence in pregnant women during the first trimester."

83. At 12 weeks' gestation the nurse midwife examines a client and finds her uterus is enlarged and:
1. Just above the symphysis pubis
2. Buried deep in the pelvic cavity
3. Three fingers above the symphysis pubis
4. Causing noticeable bulging of the abdominal wall

84. A primigravida complains of morning sickness. The nurse should plan to teach her to:
1. Increase fluid intake
2. Eat three small meals a day
3. Increase calcium in her diet
4. Avoid long periods without food

85. The nurse discusses with a newly pregnant client, who is 5-feet, 3-inches tall and weighs 125 pounds, the recommended weight gain during pregnancy. The nurse is aware that, to fall within the recommended weight gain during pregnancy, at term, the client should weigh about:
1. 130 pounds
2. 135 pounds
3. 140 pounds
4. 150 pounds

86. A primigravida who is in her seventh week of gestation asks the nurse when she can expect to feel her baby move. The nurse should reply that quickening usually occurs in the:
1. 12th week
2. 16th week
3. 20th week
4. 24th week

87. A pregnant client asks the nurse for information about toxoplasmosis during pregnancy. The nurse teaches the client that:
1. Pork and beef should be properly cooked before eating
2. Toxoplasmosis is a disease that is prevalent just in foreign countries

3. Eating salads with mayonnaise should be avoided during the summer
4. Raw shellfish are intermediary hosts and should be avoided during pregnancy

88. A pregnant client tells the nurse that she thinks she has developed an allergy, since her nose is often very congested and she is unable to breathe. The nurse states:
   1. "Using a nasal decongestant once or twice a day will help."
   2. "It is common for women to develop allergies during pregnancy."
   3. "This is not normal; perhaps you have a chronic respiratory infection."
   4. "It is an expected occurrence; the increased hormones are responsible for the congestion."

89. The nurse should explain to the newly pregnant primigravida that the fetal heartbeat will first be heard with:
   1. A fetoscope around 8 weeks
   2. A fetoscope at 12 to 14 weeks
   3. An electronic Doppler after 17 weeks
   4. An electronic Doppler at 10 to 12 weeks

90. A client who is 10 weeks pregnant returns for her second prenatal visit. She asks why she has to urinate so often. The nurse tells her that urinary frequency in the first trimester is:
   1. Caused by the baby's head descending into the uterus
   2. Influenced by the enlarging uterus, which is still contained in the pelvis
   3. A result of the mother's kidneys filtering more waste products because of the growing fetus
   4. Mostly a psychologic phenomenon that results from knowing that the pregnancy has occurred

91. A client at 10 weeks' gestation tells the nurse that she voids often, without dysuria, and would like to know what to do. The nurse is aware that this client will have to:
   1. Decrease her fluid intake during the day
   2. Contact her physician as soon as possible
   3. Maintain increased fluid intake during the day
   4. Try to resist the urge to void as long as possible

92. Between 12 and 24 weeks' gestation, applicable prenatal teaching for a pregnant client should include information about:
   1. Preparation for the baby, travel to the hospital, signs of labor

2. Growth of the fetus, personal hygiene, and nutritional guidance
   3. Interventions for nausea and vomiting, growth of the fetus, expectations for care
   4. Danger signs of preeclampsia, relaxation breathing techniques, and signs of labor

93. A client in her second trimester is at the prenatal clinic for a routine visit. While listening to the fetal heart, the nurse hears a heartbeat at the rate of 136 in the right upper quadrant and also at the midline below the umbilicus. The sources of these sounds are:
   1. Heart rates of two fetuses
   2. Maternal and fetal heart rates
   3. Fetal heart rate and funic souffle
   4. Uterine souffle and fetal heart rate

94. A client, whose weight was average for her height before becoming pregnant, is concerned that she has gained 15 pounds after only 23 weeks of being pregnant. The most appropriate response by the nurse would be:
   1. "You have gained the amount recommended for someone at 23 weeks' gestation."
   2. "Do not be concerned. The doctor will discuss weight gain when you are examined."
   3. "You have actually gained less than what is recommended and could increase your calories by a small amount."
   4. "This is slightly more than what is recommended at this point, but we can refer you to a dietitian for counseling."

95. A client at 28 weeks' gestation has gained 13 pounds and tells the nurse in the prenatal clinic that she is glad she has not gained as much weight as her sister during pregnancy. An appropriate response by the nurse to the client's comment would be:
   1. "Do you think you are getting fat?"
   2. "Are you trying to watch your figure?"
   3. "You have to eat right during pregnancy."
   4. "Tell me what you have been eating lately."

96. A primigravida at 34 weeks' gestation tells the nurse that although she is wearing low-heeled shoes and avoiding heavy lifting, she is beginning to experience some lower backaches. After discussing proper body mechanics, the nurse should recommend that the client:
   1. Wear a maternity girdle while awake
   2. Do pelvic tilt exercises several times a day
   3. Sleep flat on her back with her feet elevated
   4. Take two acetaminophen (Tylenol) extended release caplets each morning

97. During a client's prenatal visit at 35 weeks' gestation, she reports that she feels she is unable to breathe comfortably. The nurse bases the response on the fact that the client probably:
    1. Has a fetus in the breech position, which is decreasing the intrathoracic space
    2. Has an elevated diaphragm, which is causing her to feel as though she is having difficulty breathing
    3. Is experiencing shortness of breath associated with pregnancy and there are no appropriate nursing interventions
    4. Is experiencing metabolic demands that are exceeding her oxygen consumption thus causing shortness of breath

98. The nurse tells a pregnant client that fetal weight gain during pregnancy is:
    1. Initiated in the second trimester
    2. Greatest during the first trimester
    3. Most marked in the third trimester
    4. Equally distributed throughout pregnancy

99. The nurse explains to a pregnant couple that in childbirth classes the emphasis is on:
    1. Birth as a family experience
    2. Labor without using analgesics
    3. Education, breathing, and exercise
    4. Nutrition, relaxation, and breathing

100. A pregnant client, interested in childbirth education, asks how the Lamaze method differs from the Read method. The nurse explains that the Lamaze method:
    1. Is a much easier method to teach and learn
    2. Requires a good deal of prenatal preparation
    3. Avoids the use of pain-relieving drugs during labor
    4. Is a calm, relaxed approach based on "childbirth without pain"

101. During a childbirth class the nurse evaluates that the clients understand how to use effleurage correctly when the clients are observed:
    1. Rocking gently back and forth on their knees
    2. Practicing panting to avoid pushing during labor
    3. Massaging their abdomens gently with their fingertips
    4. Taking deep breaths before simulated contractions

102. The need to improve pubococcygeal muscle tone is explored during a childbirth class. The nurse recognizes that a client understands the instructions about how to strengthen the muscle when she states she should do:
    1. Tailor sitting
    2. Pelvic rocking
    3. Forward tilting
    4. Kegel's exercises

103. The nurse recognizes that a pregnant client does not understand the teaching about fetal growth and development when the client states:
    1. "The mother must observe proper nutrition."
    2. "The fetus gets food from the amniotic fluid."
    3. "There are two umbilical arteries and one vein."
    4. "The baby's oxygen needs are provided for by the mother."

104. At a childbirth preparation class the nurse teaches the participants about the "spurt of energy" before labor and why the client should conserve this energy because during labor it:
    1. Helps to increase the progesterone level
    2. Is needed for pushing during the first stage of labor
    3. Will decrease the intensity of uterine contractions
    4. May limit fatigue which might influence the need for pain medication

105. During a prenatal class the nurse is discussing nutrition requirements throughout pregnancy. The nurse explains that caloric needs in the second and third trimesters increase daily by:
    1. 100 calories
    2. 300 calories
    3. 500 calories
    4. 700 calories

106. A client attending a prenatal class about nutrition tells the nurse that she is a pure vegetarian (vegan). The nurse, concerned that the client might not meet all her protein needs, encourages her to include in her diet:
    1. Macaroni with cheese
    2. Scrambled eggs and milk
    3. Whole grain cereals and nuts
    4. Brown rice and whole wheat bread

107. A pregnant client, who is a strict vegetarian, asks the nurse if there is anything special she should do in relation to her diet while pregnant. The nurse should teach the importance of:
    1. Taking a vitamin supplement daily
    2. Eating at least 40 g of protein a day
    3. Drinking at least 1 quart of milk per day
    4. Including a variety of specific vegetable proteins in her daily diet

108. Folic acid supplements are prescribed for a prenatal client. The nurse is aware that these are necessary to prevent:
1. Pernicious anemia
2. Anaphylactic shock
3. Erythroblastosis fetalis
4. Fetal neural tube defects

109. When discussing dietary needs during pregnancy, a client tells the nurse that milk constipates her at times. The nurse should explain that it is preferable to:
1. Substitute a variety of cheeses for the milk
2. Increase her prenatal capsules and omit the milk
3. Substitute skimmed or buttermilk for whole milk
4. Treat constipation in some way other than omitting milk

110. During a counseling discussion of nutrition, the nurse explains to a pregnant client that she will need additional calcium during pregnancy and that the best source is milk. The client states, "I never drink milk or eat milk products. They turn my stomach." The best reply by the nurse would be:
1. "How unfortunate; this may cause your teeth to loosen."
2. "Just make sure the rest of your diet is nutritionally sound."
3. "You will have to try and drink some milk so that your baby will have strong bones."
4. "There are many mineral and vitamin supplements the physician can prescribe."

111. The nurse explains to a pregnant client who does not like milk that there are other foods that are good sources of calcium and advises the client to eat:
1. Corn
2. Liver
3. Broccoli
4. Lean meat

112. The nurse teaches a client that the increased need for vitamin A to meet rapid tissue growth during pregnancy may be met by using increased amounts of food such as:
1. Carrots
2. Citrus fruits
3. Nonfat milk
4. Extra egg whites

113. The nurse knows that a client in early pregnancy understands the need to increase her intake of complete proteins during her pregnancy when she reports she is eating more:
1. Spinach and broccoli
2. Milk, eggs, and cheese
3. Beans, peas, and lentils
4. Whole grain cereals and breads

114. A newly married client visits the woman's health clinic because she has not been feeling well. The nurse suspects that the client is probably pregnant when:
1. Her menses is already seven days late
2. Her urine immunoassay test is positive
3. She relates that urinary frequency occurs every two to three hours
4. She complains of nausea and vomiting episodes every morning

115. A client who has type 1 diabetes had a nonstress test that was reactive. The nurse would recognize that the client understood what she was taught about the results when she is overheard telling her husband that the test was:
1. Normal, due to an increase in FHR with fetal movement
2. Abnormal, due to a decrease in FHR with fetal movement
3. Abnormal, due to an increase in FHR with maternal movement
4. Normal, due to the FHR remaining unchanged with maternal movement

116. At a routine monthly visit, while assessing a client who is in her 26th week of gestation, the nurse identifies the presence of striae gravidarum, which:
1. Are brownish blotches on the face
2. Is a bluish discoloration of the cervix
3. Are reddish streaks on the abdomen and breasts
4. Is a black line from the umbilicus to the mons veneris

117. The nurse understands that an ultrasound examination ordered for a pregnant client in the first trimester is used primarily to:
1. Estimate fetal age
2. Detect mental retardation
3. Rule out congenital defects
4. Approximate fetal linear growth

118. A pregnant client's blood test reveals an elevated alpha-fetoprotein (AFP). The nurse is aware that this test result may indicate the presence of:
1. Cystic fibrosis
2. Phenylketonuria
3. Down syndrome
4. Neural tube defects

119. A client in the 16th week of pregnancy is scheduled for ultrasonography. When preparing the client for the procedure, the nurse informs her that for this test it will be necessary to:
    1. Have an enema the night before the examination
    2. Fast for 12 hours to minimize the possibility of vomiting
    3. Monitor closely afterward for signs of precipitate labor
    4. Drink at least 1 L of water one to two hours before the test and avoid urinating during that time

120. The nurse understands that when a contraction stress test is interpreted as negative it means:
    1. The fetus at this time has oxygen reserves but the test should be repeated weekly
    2. The test should be repeated in 24 hours because examination results indicate hyperstimulation
    3. Immediate birth should be considered because there is no fetal heart acceleration with fetal movement
    4. A trial induction should be started because fetal heart rate acceleration with movement is indicative of a false result

121. Nursing care for a pregnant client who is to have an oxytocin stimulated-contraction test should include:
    1. Having the client empty her bladder
    2. Placing the client in a supine position
    3. Keeping the client on nothing by mouth
    4. Preparing the client for insertion of internal monitors

122. The nurse is aware that a client at 40 weeks' gestation is experiencing true labor if:
    1. Cervical dilation has occurred
    2. Her membranes have ruptured
    3. The pains become more noticeable
    4. The fetal heart rate baseline decreases

123. The nurse is assessing a primigravida who has been admitted in early labor because her membranes have ruptured. She is at 41 weeks' gestation. Her contractions are irregular and her cervix is 3 cm dilated. The fetal head is at station 0 and the fetal heart rate tracing is reactive. The nurse should encourage her to:
    1. Sit in a chair and watch TV
    2. Take a walk around the unit
    3. Maintain a left lateral position
    4. Do accelerated-decelerated breathing

124. A primigravida at 36 weeks' gestation is admitted to the birthing room with ruptured membranes and a cervix that is 2 cm dilated and 75% effaced. A priority question the nurse should ask would be:
    1. "What is the expected date of birth?"
    2. "Are you planning to breastfeed or formula-feed?"
    3. "What time was your last meal, and what did you eat?"
    4. "How frequent are your contractions and how long do they last?"

125. A client, who is admitted to the birthing room, is a Gravida III Para I. This means that the client:
    1. Had one premature baby
    2. Has had an induced abortion
    3. Had two previous pregnancies
    4. Has three living children at home

126. When a client at 39 weeks' gestation arrives in the birthing suite she says, "I think my membranes have ruptured." When confirming if the membranes have ruptured, the nurse should:
    1. Test the leaking fluid with nitrazine paper and observe the color changes
    2. Take the client's temperature because ruptured membranes predispose to infection
    3. Avoid performing a vaginal examination to prevent the introduction of microorganisms
    4. Have the client provide a clean catch urine specimen and send it to laboratory for a culture

127. During labor the nurse encourages the client to void. The nurse recognizes that an overdistended urinary bladder during labor can:
    1. Interfere with the delivery of the placenta
    2. Interfere with the assessment of cervical dilation
    3. Prevent the diagnosis of cephalopelvic disproportion
    4. Predispose to uterine hemorrhage immediately after birth

128. A client is admitted in active labor. During the assessment between contractions the nurse palpates her abdomen to determine the fetal presentation, which is the:
    1. Position of the fetal body parts
    2. Portion of the fetus that enters the pelvis first
    3. Relationship of the fetal presenting part to the mother's pelvis
    4. Relationship of the long axis of the fetus to the long axis of the mother

129. A client is admitted to the birthing room in active labor. The nurse determines that the fetus is in the left occipital posterior (LOP) position. The nurse is aware that in this position the fetal heart can best be heard at point:

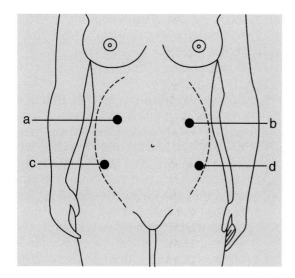

   1. a
   2. b
   3. c
   4. d

130. The nurse performs Leopold's maneuvers on a newly admitted client in labor. Palpation reveals a soft, firm mass in the fundus, a firm, smooth mass on the mother's left side, several knobs and protrusions on the mother's right side, and a hard, round moveable mass in the pubic area with the brow on the right. Based on these findings, the nurse recognizes that the fetal position is:
   1. LOA
   2. ROA
   3. LMP
   4. RMP

131. The fetus of a client in labor is in the LOP position. To alleviate some of the discomfort caused by this type of labor, the nurse should advise the client's partner to:
   1. Encourage the client to sleep between contractions
   2. Elevate the head of the client's bed to a 45-degree angle
   3. Instruct the client to take deeper breaths during contractions
   4. Apply pressure to the client's sacral area during a contraction

132. An expectant couple asks the nurse about the cause of low back pain in labor. The nurse replies that this pain occurs most often when the position of the baby is:
   1. Breech
   2. Transverse
   3. Occiput anterior
   4. Occiput posterior

133. The position that the nurse teaches the client to avoid when experiencing back pain during labor would be the:
   1. Sitting position
   2. Supine position
   3. Right lateral position
   4. Left side-lying position

134. A woman who is having contractions is concerned whether she is in true labor. She states, "How will you know if I am really in labor?" The nurse's response is based on the knowledge that:
   1. A bloody show is rare with false labor
   2. Fetal movement is decreased in true labor
   3. The cervix dilates and effaces in true labor
   4. The membranes rupture when true labor begins

135. The teaching plan for a father who is acting as a coach during labor would include the information that it would be best for him to:
   1. Leave his wife alone periodically so that she can rest between contractions
   2. Let his wife know the progress she is making and that she is doing a good job
   3. See that his wife remains supine so that the monitoring equipment is not disturbed
   4. Keep the conversation in the labor room to a minimum so that his wife can concentrate

136. The partner of a woman in labor is having difficulty timing the frequency of contractions and asks the nurse to review the procedure. The nurse instructs the partner to note the time from the:
   1. End of one contraction to the beginning of the next contraction
   2. Beginning of one contraction to the end of the next contraction
   3. Beginning of one contraction to the end of the same contraction
   4. Beginning of one contraction to the beginning of the next contraction

137. A husband who is coaching his wife during labor demonstrates an understanding of the transition phase of labor when with each contraction he instructs his wife to:
    1. Take cleansing breaths and push
    2. Take quick, shallow breaths and blow
    3. Use slow, rhythmic diaphragmatic breathing
    4. Switch from accelerated to decelerated breathing

138. After being in labor for six hours a client is admitted to the birthing room. The client is 5 cm dilated and at −1 station. In the next hour her contractions gradually become irregular but are more uncomfortable. When caring for her, the nurse should first check for:
    1. False labor
    2. A full bladder
    3. Uterine dysfunction
    4. A breech presentation

139. A nurse places a client on the bedpan to void several times during the first stage of labor. This is done because a full bladder:
    1. Is often injured during labor
    2. May inhibit the progress of labor
    3. Jeopardizes the status of the fetus
    4. Predisposes the client to urinary infection

140. A client in active labor is admitted to the birthing room. A vaginal examination reveals a 6- to 7-cm dilation. Based on this finding the nurse should expect that this client would:
    1. Have a profuse bloody show
    2. Appear unable to control her shaking legs
    3. Be uncomfortable because of nausea and vomiting
    4. Have contractions of 60-seconds duration every three to five minutes

141. As the nurse inspects the perineum of a client who has been admitted in active labor, the client suddenly turns pale and says she feels as if she is going to faint even though she is lying flat on her back. The nurse should:
    1. Elevate her feet
    2. Elevate her head
    3. Turn her on her left side
    4. Start oxygen and IV fluids

142. A client in labor is admitted to the birthing room. The nurse's assessment reveals that the fetus is at −1 station, which means the presenting part is:
    1. Visible at the vaginal opening
    2. One cm below the ischial spines

    3. One cm above the ischial spines
    4. At the level of the ischial spines

143. During the assessment of a client in labor the cervix is determined to be 4 cm dilated. The nurse understands that this client is in the stage of labor known as:
    1. First
    2. Second
    3. Prodromal
    4. Transitional

144. A vaginal examination reveals that a client's cervix is 50% effaced and 6 cm dilated. The head is at 0 station, and the fetus is in an ROA position. The contractions are occurring every three to four minutes, lasting 60 seconds and are of moderate intensity. From these data the nurse would assess that the client is:
    1. Early in the first stage of labor
    2. In the transitional phase of labor
    3. Beginning the second stage of labor
    4. Midway through the first stage of labor

145. A multipara is admitted to the birthing room in active labor. Her vital signs are: temperature, 98° F; pulse, 70 beats per minute; respirations, 18; and blood pressure, 126/76. A vaginal examination reveals a cervix 50% effaced and 6 cm dilated with the vertex presenting at +2 station. The client is complaining of pain and asks for medication. The nurse should be concerned about respiratory depression of the infant at birth if the client were given:
    1. Naloxone (Narcan)
    2. Lorazepam (Ativan)
    3. Midazolam (Versed)
    4. Meperidine HCl (Demerol)

146. During labor a client begins to experience dizziness and tingling of her hands. The nurse instructs the client to:
    1. Use a fast deep-breathing pattern
    2. Pant during the next three contractions
    3. Hold her breath with the next contraction
    4. Breathe into her cupped hands or a paper bag

147. A client in the active phase of labor states, "I feel all wet. I think I urinated." The nurse should first:
    1. Give her the bedpan
    2. Change the bed linens
    3. Inspect the perineal area
    4. Auscultate the fetal heart rate

148. After four hours of early labor a client's cervix remains 3 cm dilated. A prolonged latent phase

is probable. The nurse should be prepared to provide an explanation and assist primarily with:
1. Artificial rupture of membranes
2. Oxytocin stimulation of labor by infusion
3. Fluoroscopy for cephalopelvic disproportion
4. Electronic fetal heart and uterine activity monitoring

149. The nurse assesses a primigravida who had been in labor for five hours. The fetal heart rate tracing is reassuring. Contractions are of mild intensity lasting 30 seconds and are three to five minutes apart. An oxytocin infusion has been ordered. The priority nursing intervention at this time would be to:
1. Check cervical dilation every hour
2. Keep the labor environment dark and quiet
3. Infuse oxytocin by piggybacking into the primary line
4. Position the client on the left side throughout the infusion

150. The nurse is aware that when external fetal monitoring is compared to internal fetal monitoring, one advantage is that external fetal monitoring:
1. Is simpler to read
2. Allows the client freedom of movement
3. More accurately monitors the fetal heart
4. Does not introduce foreign materials into the uterus

151. When direct monitoring of the fetal heart rate during the first stage of labor shows an irregular baseline with variability, a nursing priority would be to:
1. Administer oxygen
2. Notify the physician
3. Change the client's position
4. Continue to monitor the client

152. During labor a client has an internal fetal monitor applied. The nurse should take action in response to a fetal heart rate that:
1. Does not drop during contractions
2. Fluctuates from 130 to 140 beats per minute
3. Uniformly drops to 120 beats per minute with each contraction
4. Repeatedly drops abruptly to 90 beats per minute unrelated to contractions

153. A client in labor is receiving oxytocin. When observing late decelerations in the fetal heart rate, the nurse should first:
1. Administer oxygen
2. Place her on her left side
3. Check the blood pressure
4. Discontinue the oxytocin infusion

154. Although a client in labor is prepared and plans to participate in the labor and birth process, she states that she is in severe discomfort. An order for butorphanol (Stadol) is given. The safest time during labor for the nurse to administer this medication would be during the:
1. Early phase
2. Active phase
3. Transition phase
4. Expulsion phase

155. A client's membranes rupture. The nurse, observing an abrupt deceleration in the fetal heart rate, inspects the vaginal area and notes a prolapsed cord. The nurse should immediately:
1. Elevate the presenting part of the cord until birth
2. Administer oxygen by face mask at 7 L/minute
3. Notify the physician of the findings of the examination
4. Instruct the client to assume a dorsal recumbent position

156. Priority nursing intervention for a laboring client with a sudden prolapse of the umbilical cord protruding from the vagina should focus on:
1. Gently replacing the cord in the vaginal vault
2. Covering the cord with a sterile moist dressing
3. Starting oxygen at 10 L/minute via a tight face mask
4. Checking the fetal heart rate every 15 minutes

157. A vaginal examination reveals that a client in labor is 7 cm dilated. Soon afterward she becomes nauseated, has the hiccups, and has an increase in bloody show. The nurse recognizes that these clinical manifestations indicate that the client is starting the:
1. Latent phase of labor
2. Active phase of labor
3. Transition phase of labor
4. Early active phase of labor

158. Observation of a client in labor reveals that she is entering the transition phase of the first stage of labor. The nurse would recognize this by identifying:
1. Redness of the face and an urge to push
2. A bulging perineum, crowning, and caput
3. Increased bloody show, irritability, and shaking
4. Contractions that are longer and more frequent

159. The nurse is aware that the management of a client in the transition phase of labor is primarily directed toward:
    1. Decreasing the client's fluid intake
    2. Helping the client maintain control
    3. Having the client breathe simple patterns
    4. Reducing the client's discomfort with opioid medication

160. While having contractions every two to three minutes that last from 60 to 90 seconds, a client complains of having rectal pressure. The nurse should:
    1. Attach an external fetal heart monitor
    2. Inspect the client's perineum for bulging
    3. Determine when the client's labor began
    4. Ask the client whether her membranes have ruptured

161. A client in labor states that she feels an urge to push. The nurse examines her and finds that the cervix is 7 cm dilated. The breathing pattern that the nurse advises the client to use would be:
    1. Expulsion breathing
    2. Rhythmic chest breathing
    3. Continuous blowing-breathing
    4. Accelerated-decelerated breathing

162. A primigravida at term is admitted to the birthing room in active labor. Later, when the client is 8 cm dilated, she tells the nurse that she has the urge to push. The nurse instructs her to pant-blow at this time because pushing can:
    1. Prolapse the cord
    2. Rupture the uterus
    3. Cause cervical edema
    4. Lead to a precipitous birth

163. A client's membranes rupture during the transition phase of labor and the amniotic fluid appears pale green. Because of this finding, after the birth the nurse should be prepared to:
    1. Stimulate the baby to cry
    2. Administer oxygen by face mask
    3. Put a moist saline dressing on the cord stump
    4. Provide for suctioning of the oropharynx when the head emerges

164. When doing her shallow breathing during transition, a laboring client experiences tingling and numbness of her fingertips. The nurse encourages her to breathe into:
    1. A paper bag
    2. An oxygen mask
    3. A compressed air mask
    4. An incentive spirometer

165. The nurse is observing the electronic fetal monitor as a client in labor enters the second stage. The nurse identifies early decelerations of the fetal heart rate with return to baseline at the end of each contraction. This usually indicates:
    1. Fetal acidosis
    2. Fetal cord prolapse
    3. Maternal hypotension
    4. Fetal head compression

166. The nurse is aware that when a local anesthetic is used for birth of a neonate:
    1. Labor is slowed after its administration
    2. Maternal respirations may be depressed
    3. There is a danger of maternal aspiration
    4. Reactions such as vertigo and tinnitus may occur

167. The cervix of a client in labor is fully dilated and 100% effaced. The fetal head is at +3 station, the fetal heart rate ranges from 140 to 150 beats per minute, and the contractions are two minutes apart lasting 60 seconds. When inspecting the perineum the nurse would expect to find:
    1. Small tears in the perineum
    2. Greenish-yellow amniotic fluid
    3. Increasing amounts of amniotic fluid
    4. A small amount of caput with each contraction

168. A pregnant woman arrives in the emergency department crying, "My baby is coming!" The nurse identifies that the baby's head is crowning and birth is imminent. The nurse should support the baby's head by:
    1. Applying suprapubic pressure
    2. Placing a hand firmly against the perineum
    3. Distributing the fingers evenly around the head
    4. Maintaining firm pressure against the anterior fontanel

169. A client gives birth to an 8-pound baby. Ten minutes after the birth, the placenta has not yet separated. The nurse should expect to:
    1. Administer a second dose of oxytocin
    2. Apply fundal pressure to stimulate separation
    3. Continue to assess the client for signs of separation
    4. Prepare a consent form because manual removal is indicated

170. Five minutes after the birth of a neonate, the nurse midwife assesses that the client's

placenta is separating when:
1. The fundus becomes completely relaxed
2. There is a lengthening of the umbilical cord
3. The client complains of unbearable abdominal pain
4. Bright red blood continually seeps out of the vaginal opening

171. One hour after delivery, the nurse palpates a client's fundus to determine if involution is taking place. The fundus is firm, in the midline, and two finger-breadths below the umbilicus. Based on these findings the nurse should:
1. Encourage the client to void
2. Notify the physician immediately
3. Massage the uterus vigorously and attempt to express clots
4. Identify this as expected and continue periodic assessments

172. The primary outcome for client care in the third stage of labor would be:
1. An absence of discomfort
2. A firmly contracted fundus
3. An efficient FH beat to beat variability
4. A maternal respiratory rate between 16 and 20

173. The nurse is evaluating uterine tone eight hours after a woman has delivered a healthy infant. The nurse would be able to determine that the uterus is involuting appropriately when:
1. Numerous clots are passed vaginally
2. Bleeding from the episiotomy has stopped
3. There is a moderate amount of lochia rubra
4. No uterine cramps occur during breast-feeding

174. A client is to receive an epidural anesthetic during labor. After the client is anesthetized, the nurse should monitor the client for:
1. Lightheadedness
2. Urinary retention
3. Decreased temperature
4. Decreased level of consciousness

175. After a cesarean birth, the nurse performs fundal checks every 15 minutes. During one check the nurse notes that the fundus is soft and boggy. The priority nursing action at this time is to:
1. Elevate the client's legs
2. Massage the client's fundus
3. Increase the oxytocin drip rate
4. Examine the client's perineum for bleeding

176. After the birth of an infant the mother's vital signs are T, 99.4° F; P, 80 regular and strong; R, 16 slow and even; and BP, 148/92 mm Hg. The assessment the nurse should monitor more frequently is the client's:
1. Pulse
2. Respiration
3. Temperature
4. Blood pressure

177. In the second hour after birth of a neonate a client's uterus is found to be firm, above the level of the umbilicus, and to the right of midline. The appropriate intervention would be to:
1. Observe for signs of retained secundines
2. Assist the client to the bathroom to empty her bladder
3. Massage her uterus vigorously to prevent hemorrhage
4. Tell the client that this is a sign of uterine stabilization

178. The nurse is aware that a client could be at increased risk for postpartum hemorrhage if the client:
1. Breastfed in the birthing room
2. Received a pudendal block for the birth
3. Delivered a baby who weighed 9 pounds, 8 ounces
4. Had a third stage of labor that lasted 10 minutes

179. During the fourth stage of labor, about one hour after giving birth, a client begins to shiver uncontrollably. The best nursing action would be to:
1. Check the vital signs since the client may be going into hypovolemic shock
2. Monitor the client's blood pressure because shivering may cause it to elevate
3. Obtain an order to increase the amount of IV fluids as the client is probably dehydrated
4. Cover the client with additional blankets to alleviate this typical postpartum sensation of feeling cold

180. A primipara gave birth to a 7-pound neonate 12 hours ago. Although an ice bag had been applied to her perineal area, the client continues to complain of rectal pressure causing excruciating pain in the area of the episiotomy. The nurse makes the nursing diagnosis "Acute pain related to:
1. Presence of multiple hemorrhoids."
2. Documented low pain tolerance of client."
3. Presence of infection in episiotomy area."
4. Development of a hematoma in the episiotomy area."

181. In the postpartum period, the nurse anticipates that a primipara with a second-degree laceration and repair is most likely to develop:
    1. Posterior vaginal varicosities
    2. Difficulty voiding spontaneously
    3. Delayed onset of milk production
    4. Maladaptive bonding and attachment

182. The nurse teaches a postpartum client how to care for her episiotomy at home. The nurse would know that the priority instruction was understood when the client states:
    1. "I should discontinue the sitz baths once I am in my own home."
    2. "I must not climb up or down stairs for at least three days after discharge."
    3. "I should continue the sitz baths three times a day if it makes me feel better."
    4. "I must continue perineal care after I go to the bathroom until everything is healed."

183. Twelve hours after a spontaneous birth, a client's temperature is 100.4° F. The nurse recognizes that this elevation probably is an indication of:
    1. Mastitis
    2. Dehydration
    3. Puerperal infection
    4. Urinary tract infection

184. Twenty-four hours after an uncomplicated labor and birth, a client's CBC reveals a WBC count of 17,000/mm^3. The nurse should interpret this WBC count as being indicative of:
    1. The usual decrease in white blood cells
    2. The expected response to the labor process
    3. An acute sexually transmitted viral disease
    4. A bacterial infection of the reproductive system

185. A primipara about to be discharged with her newborn asks the nurse many questions regarding her baby's care. Her questions demonstrate that she has started the phase known as:
    1. Let down
    2. Taking in
    3. Taking hold
    4. Early parenting

186. To help prevent postpartum infection, the most important discharge instruction given by the nurse would be:
    1. "Don't take tub baths for at least six weeks."
    2. "Wash your hands before and after changing your sanitary napkins."
    3. "Douche gently with Betadine solution twice a day for one week or more."

    4. "Tampons are better than sanitary napkins for inhibiting bacteria in the postpartum period."

187. Before discharge a postpartum client and the nurse discuss methods of birth control. The client asks the nurse, "When will I begin to ovulate again?" The nurse's most appropriate response would be:
    1. "I really can't tell you. Everyone is so different."
    2. "Ovulation may occur before you begin menstruation."
    3. "Ovulation will occur after your first menstrual period."
    4. "This is something you should discuss at your first clinic visit."

188. During the postpartum period, a client tells the nurse she was very uncomfortable during her pregnancy because of varicose veins. In light of this information, the nurse's assessment should include:
    1. A daily clotting time
    2. Tests for platelet fragility
    3. Frequent Hgb and Hct values
    4. Monitoring for signs of thrombophlebitis

189. The comment by a new mother of twins on the third postpartum day that indicates to the nurse the need for further assessment would be:
    1. "I hope I'll be a good mother to these sweet babies."
    2. "I've been urinating large amounts ever since I delivered."
    3. "My breasts feel full, heavy, and tingly before I feed the babies."
    4. "My lochia is bright red with small brown clots the size of my thumb."

190. When preparing a teaching plan about self-care during the postpartum period, the nurse understands that on the fourth postpartum day the lochia is known as:
    1. Alba
    2. Rubra
    3. Serosa
    4. Purpura

191. A client vaginally delivers a 7-pound, 2-ounce baby and has made the decision to breastfeed the infant. When instructing the client regarding breastfeeding, the nurse tells the client to expect that:
    1. Weight loss will occur rapidly
    2. Lochial flow will be increased
    3. Uterine involution will be delayed

4. Use of heat will be contraindicated

192. A new mother asks for assistance with removing the baby from her breast. The nurse should teach her to:
    1. Pinch the baby's nostrils gently to help release the nipple
    2. Break the suction with a finger in the corner of the baby's mouth
    3. Let the baby nurse as long as desired without interruption
    4. Pull the nipple out of the baby's mouth when the baby falls asleep

193. A statement by a breastfeeding mother that indicates that the nurse's teaching about stimulating the breastfeeding let-down reflex has been successful would be, "I will:
    1. Drink at least 2 quarts of low-fat milk a day."
    2. Wear a snug-fitting breast binder 24 hours a day."
    3. Take a cool shower before each breastfeeding."
    4. Apply warm moist packs and massage my breasts before each feeding."

194. As a result of her newborn's vigorous sucking, a client's nipples become sore and tender. The best nursing action would be to:
    1. Apply continuous ice packs
    2. Give analgesic medication as ordered
    3. Expose the nipples to air several times a day
    4. Remove the baby from the breast for a few days

195. A client who has been breastfeeding her newborn every three hours develops sore nipples. The nurse should plan to teach her how to decrease nipple soreness by:
    1. Using breast shields at each feeding
    2. Changing nursing positions during each feeding
    3. Washing the nipples with mild soap and rinsing with warm water
    4. Checking to see that only the edge of the nipple is in the baby's mouth

196. A new mother wishes to breastfeed her infant and asks the nurse whether she needs to alter her diet. The nurse can best respond:
    1. "Just eat as you have been doing during your pregnancy."
    2. "Just drink a lot of milk; you need the calcium to make your own milk."
    3. "Don't worry about it, your body will produce the amount of milk your baby needs."

4. "You'll need greater amounts of the same foods you've been eating and more fluids."

197. A client arrives at the clinic with swollen, tender breasts and "flu-like" symptoms. A diagnosis of mastitis is made. The nurse should first plan to:
    1. Assist her to wean the infant gradually
    2. Teach her to empty her breasts frequently
    3. Review breastfeeding techniques with her
    4. Send a sample of her milk for culture and sensitivity

198. Before discharge the nurse should teach the formula-feeding mother that if breast engorgement occurs, she should:
    1. Wear a tightly fitted brassiere
    2. Take two aspirin every four hours
    3. Cease drinking milk for two weeks
    4. Apply hot compresses to the breasts

199. A client who is formula feeding her infant is taught how to care for her engorged breasts. The nurse realizes that the client does not understand the teaching when the client states:
    1. "I'm wearing a well-fitting, tight brassiere."
    2. "I am drinking 2 quarts of fluid every 24 hours."
    3. "I'm expressing milk from my breasts every three or four hours."
    4. "I do not let warm water run over my breasts when I am showering."

HIGH-RISK PREGNANCY (HP)

200. A client, at her first visit to the prenatal clinic, states that she has missed three menstrual periods, thinks she has twins because her abdomen is so large, but has started to have a brownish vaginal discharge. Her blood pressure is elevated, indicating that she may have gestational hypertension. The nurse is aware that a further assessment is required because she may have:
    1. Renal failure
    2. A placenta previa
    3. Abruptio placentae
    4. A hydatidiform mole

201. The nurse determines the fundal height of a client at 16 weeks' gestation to be one fingerbreadth above the umbilicus. The nurse should:
    1. Assess for two distinct fetal heart rates
    2. Ascertain birth weights of children of any siblings
    3. Inform the client that she is mistaken about her dates
    4. Instruct the client about appropriate weight gain during pregnancy

202. The nurse understands that the postpartum client who is at the highest risk for developing a puerperal infection would be a:
    1. Woman who has lost 350 mL of blood during delivery
    2. Primipara who has delivered an infant weighing 8½ pounds
    3. Multipara who had a hemoglobin level of 11 g on admission to the hospital
    4. Woman who has been voiding in amounts of 75 to 80 mL and requires catheterization

203. A client, gravida VI, with a history of four preterm births with fetal deaths and diabetes mellitus in her family, smokes 1½ packs of cigarettes a day. Both she and her husband work full time. Based on an analysis of this client's risk status, the nurse should:
    1. Suggest to the client that she and her husband be seen by a geneticist
    2. Explain to the client that she must stop smoking immediately for the health of the baby
    3. Schedule this client for cerclage placement because of her history of multiple preterm births
    4. Suggest to the client that she see a physician who specializes in the care of women with high-risk pregnancies

204. A client who is having a difficult labor is diagnosed with cephalopelvic disproportion. The nurse would question the medical order that states:
    1. Maintain NPO status
    2. Start peripheral IV of D51/4 NS
    3. Record fetal heart tones every 15 minutes
    4. Add 10 units of oxytocin (Pitocin) to 1000 mL of IV solution

205. Priority nursing care for a client who has just delivered her fifth child should include:
    1. Palpating her fundus because she is at risk for uterine atony
    2. Offering her fluids because multiparas generally lose more fluid during labor
    3. Assessing her bladder tone because she is at increased risk for urinary tract infection
    4. Performing passive range-of-motion exercises on her extremities because she is at risk for thrombophlebitis

206. The nurse is caring for a group of postpartum clients. The one the nurse should observe most closely would be a:
    1. Primipara who has had an 8-pound baby
    2. Grand multipara who experienced a labor of only one hour
    3. Primipara who received 100 mg of Demerol during her labor
    4. Multipara whose placenta separated and who delivered in 10 minutes

207. During their first visit to the obstetrician, a young couple asks the nurse whether the wife should have an amniocentesis for genetic studies. The nurse responds that the indications for these studies include:
    1. A recent history of drug use
    2. Prior spontaneous abortions
    3. First pregnancies in women over 30
    4. A history of questionable genetic problems

208. The nurse should plan to teach a client who is to have an amniocentesis that ultrasonography will be performed just before the procedure to determine the:
    1. Fetal gestational age
    2. Location of the umbilical cord
    3. Amount of fluid in the amniotic sac
    4. Position of the fetus and the placenta

209. A 38-year-old client who is at 16 weeks' gestation is scheduled for an amniocentesis. The nurse is aware that an amniocentesis cannot determine the fetus':
    1. Sex
    2. Size
    3. Lung maturity
    4. Chromosomal make-up

210. During the third trimester a client has an amniocentesis to determine fetal lung maturity. To detect immediate complications, the nurse caring for the client should first:
    1. Assess the fetal heart rate (FHR)
    2. Position the client on her left side
    3. Apply pressure for five minutes at the puncture site
    4. Check the client for vaginal bleeding or discharge

211. A client is to have an amniocentesis at 38 weeks' gestation to determine fetal lung maturity. The nurse recognizes that lung maturity is adequate when the L/S ratio is:
    1. 1:1
    2. 1:2
    3. 2:1
    4. 1.5:1

212. After an amniocentesis, the priority nursing care should include:
1. Giving perineal care
2. Encouraging fluids every hour
3. Changing the abdominal dressing
4. Observing for signs of uterine contractions

213. A client with frank vaginal bleeding is admitted to the birthing unit at 30 weeks' gestation. The admission data indicate: BP, 110/70; P, 90; R, 22; FHR, 132 and regular; uterus nontender and no contractions, and membranes are intact. Based on this information, the nurse suspects that this client has:
1. Preterm labor
2. Uterine inertia
3. Placenta previa
4. Abruptio placentae

214. The nurse explains to a pregnant client undergoing a nonstress test that the test is a way of evaluating the condition of the fetus by comparing the fetal heart rate with:
1. Fetal lie
2. Fetal movement
3. Maternal blood pressure
4. Maternal uterine contractions

215. A client at 42 weeks' gestation has a contraction stress test (CST). The nurse understands that a positive test might indicate that the:
1. Placenta has stopped growing
2. Fetus is not ready to be delivered
3. Amniotic fluid is meconium stained
4. Function of the placenta has diminished

216. A client with a high-risk pregnancy is to undergo an oxytocin-stimulated contraction stress test. The nurse understands that this test would not be done if the client had:
1. Blurred vision
2. Vaginal bleeding
3. Sickle cell disease
4. Increasing hypertension

217. Laboratory studies reveal that a pregnant client's blood type is O and she is Rh positive. Problems related to incompatibility may develop in her infant if the infant is:
1. Rh negative
2. Type A or B
3. Born preterm
4. Type O, Rh positive

218. A 16-year-old primigravida, who appears to be at or close to term, arrives at the emergency department stating that she is in labor and is complaining of pain continuing between contractions. The nurse palpates the abdomen which is firm with no signs of relaxation. The nurse concludes that the:
1. Fetus' birth may be imminent
2. Client may have placenta previa
3. Client may have abruptio placentae
4. Fetus may be in the breech presentation

219. A client who is pregnant for the first time and is carrying twins is scheduled for a cesarean birth. Preoperative teaching should include telling the client to expect to:
1. Ambulate frequently within 24 hours of surgery
2. Need an enema to have an effective bowel movement
3. Be discharged between five to seven days postpartum
4. Take sponge baths until the incision is completely healed

220. The nurse is aware that a critical outcome that would facilitate an uncomplicated recovery after a multiple birth is the woman's:
1. Uterus being contracted and in midline
2. Capacity to breastfeed the babies immediately
3. Request for sources of information on parenting twins
4. Ability to rest comfortably and discuss the birth of the babies

221. On the first postpartum day, a major concern of nursing intervention for a client who had a cesarean birth would be:
1. Promoting dietary intake
2. Promoting bowel function
3. Relieving gaseous distention
4. Relieving postoperative pain

222. After the removal of an indwelling catheter, a client who has had a cesarean birth, has difficulty voiding. The nurse can best evaluate whether the client has emptied her bladder by:
1. Catheterizing the client for residual urine
2. Gently palpating the client's bladder for distention
3. Measuring the amount of urine the client has voided
4. Asking the client whether she still feels the urge to void

223. On her first visit to the prenatal clinic a client with rheumatic heart disease asks the nurse if she will have special nutritional needs. The nurse should respond that in addition to the regular pregnancy diet she probably will need supplemental:
    1. Vitamins C and D
    2. Iron and folic acid
    3. Vitamins B_2 and B_{12}
    4. Calcium and magnesium

224. The nursing action that has the highest priority for a client with Class 1 heart disease during the postpartum period would be:
    1. Promotion of aggressive ambulation
    2. Observation for cardiac decompensation
    3. Assessment of the mother's reaction to the birth
    4. Advisement about activity, diet, and discharge plans

225. The nursing plan of care for a client with Class 1 heart disease during her last weeks of pregnancy, should include:
    1. Maintaining bed rest, administering oxygen and penicillin, and observing for cardiac decompensation
    2. Instituting seizure precautions and instructing her to report dyspnea, coughing, palpitations, and increased fatigue
    3. Administering ordered prophylactic penicillin, promoting periods of rest, and checking urine for protein every four hours
    4. Advising her to limit stress, promoting rest after meals, and preparing her for the use of analgesia and anesthesia during labor

226. The position that the nurse should encourage a client with cardiac disease to assume during labor would be:
    1. Supine
    2. Semi-Fowler's
    3. High Fowler's
    4. Trendelenburg

227. The nurse is aware that placenta previa occurs when:
    1. There is premature separation of a normally implanted placenta
    2. The placenta is not implanted securely in place on the uterine wall
    3. There is premature aging of a placenta implanted in the uterine fundus
    4. The placenta is implanted in the lower uterine segment, covering part or all of the os

228. The nurse gently performs Leopold's maneuvers on a client with a suspected placenta previa and expects to find the:
    1. Fetal head firmly engaged
    2. Small fetal parts difficult to palpate
    3. Uterus hard and tetanically contracted
    4. Fetal presenting part high and floating

229. A client with heavy bleeding because of placenta previa is admitted to the hospital. The nurse places the client in a lateral Trendelenburg's position to:
    1. Prevent shock
    2. Control bleeding
    3. Keep pressure off the cervix
    4. Move the placenta off the cervix

230. If the physician plans to do a speculum examination on a client with a marginal placenta previa, the nurse should have available:
    1. One unit of freeze-dried plasma
    2. Vitamin K for intramuscular injection
    3. Two units of typed and screened blood
    4. Heparin sodium for intravenous injection

231. The husband of a client at 24 weeks' gestation, who has been admitted to the hospital for preeclampsia, screams to the nurse that his wife is having a seizure. The nurse's immediate action should be to:
    1. Turn the client's head to the side
    2. Place an airway into the client's mouth
    3. Check the client for a spontaneous birth
    4. Assess the fetal heart rate for decelerations

232. A pregnant client is admitted to the hospital with abdominal pain and severe vaginal bleeding. After assessment, the nurse makes a nursing diagnosis of decreased cardiac output related to hemorrhage. A priority nursing action should be to:
    1. Administer oxygen
    2. Elevate the head of the bed
    3. Draw blood for Hgb and Hct
    4. Give an opioid intramuscularly for pain

233. The nurse recognizes that stimulation of labor with an oxytocin infusion would be contraindicated if the client had:
    1. Diabetes mellitus
    2. Mild preeclampsia
    3. Total placenta previa
    4. Premature rupture of the membranes

234. When caring for a client in labor with a marginal placenta previa, it would be most important for the nurse to:
    1. Assess the fetal heart tones by fetoscope
    2. Frequently assess the height of the fundus
    3. Evaluate the external blood loss by pad count
    4. Perform frequent vaginal and rectal examinations

235. Dietary counseling for a pregnant client with sickle cell anemia should include supplemental folic acid. The nurse recognizes that this is important because it:
    1. Prevents sickle cell crises
    2. Decreases the sickling of RBCs
    3. Lessens the oxygen needs of cells
    4. Compensates for a rapid turnover of RBCs

236. The laboratory blood tests of a client at 10 weeks' gestation reveal that she has anemia. The client refuses to take an iron supplement. The nurse teaches her that the best sources of iron are liver and some seafood. In addition, the nurse encourages her to eat:
    1. Nuts and pasta
    2. Raisins and figs
    3. Cheese and beef
    4. Potatoes and green vegetables

237. When a pregnant client with sickle cell anemia comes to the clinic each month, in addition to the routine observations, the nurse should also assess her for:
    1. Signs of hypothyroidism
    2. Hyperemesis gravidarum
    3. Symptoms of pyelonephritis
    4. Complaints related to hypoglycemia

238. On admission to the hospital, a primigravida, at 42 weeks' gestation, complaining of back pain and fluid leaking from the vagina, is assessed. The findings are: contractions every 3 to 4 minutes lasting 30 to 45 seconds; cervix 2 cm dilated and 70% effaced; presenting part floating; fetal heart rate of 140 beats per minute in the RLQ; streaks of blood from the vagina; and a positive nitrazine test. The nurse is aware that the finding that indicates that a problem may occur is that the:
    1. Nitrazine test is positive
    2. Presenting part is floating
    3. Streaks of blood from the vagina
    4. Fetal heart tones of 140 beats per minute are in the RLQ

239. When a breech presentation is suspected, the nurse should diligently observe the client for signs of:
    1. Precipitate labor
    2. Prolapse of the cord
    3. Primary uterine inertia
    4. Progression of normal labor

240. The membranes of a client whose fetus is in a breech position rupture spontaneously. The nurse then notes fresh meconium in the vaginal introitus and realizes that this:
    1. Indicates that the cord will prolapse
    2. Is evidence of fetal heart abnormalities
    3. Is a common occurrence in breech presentations
    4. Requires immediate notification of the physician

241. A laboring client is admitted and assessment reveals that the fetus is in a footling breech position. The nurse should be aware that:
    1. Meconium in the amniotic fluid is a sign of fetal hypoxia
    2. Severe back discomfort occurs with the fetus in this position
    3. The length of the labor often is shortened with the fetus in this position
    4. Because of the presentation, the client will probably deliver by cesarean birth

242. A client has a history of multiple preterm births followed by neonatal deaths. During the prenatal period, it is essential that the nurse teach this client that one of the most important danger signs to be aware of is:
    1. Leg cramps
    2. Pelvic pressure
    3. Early morning headaches
    4. Lack of fetal movement at 12 weeks

243. In her 30th week of gestation, a 16-year-old primigravida whose usual blood pressure is 120/70 mm Hg has a blood pressure of 130/88 mm Hg. She is admitted to the birthing room and says, "I don't know why the doctor is so worried about my blood pressure. According to a book I have, it's normal." The nurse should respond:
    1. "Your physician is just being very cautious."
    2. "Your blood pressure is high for your age group."
    3. "Your book is either for older women or outdated."
    4. "Your blood pressure is slightly elevated by pregnancy guidelines."

244. A pregnant client with a history of preterm labor is at home on bed rest. A teaching plan for this client should include the information that:
1. Blocks should be placed at the foot of the bed to raise it
2. She should sit upright with several pillows behind her back
3. She should lie on her side with her head raised on a small pillow
4. For 10 minutes every 2 hours she should assume the knee-chest position

245. The nurse explains to a client, who is 33 weeks pregnant with a history of treatment for preterm labor in this pregnancy, that coitus:
1. Is permitted if penile penetration is not deep
2. Is safe as long as she is in the side-lying position
3. Does not need to be modified in any way by either partner
4. Should be restricted because it may stimulate uterine activity

246. A client with type 1 diabetes is scheduled for an amniocentesis at 36 weeks' gestation. She asks the nurse why this is done so late in her pregnancy. The nurse explains that it is done to:
1. Ascertain the age of the fetus
2. Evaluate the fetal lung maturity
3. Schedule a cesarean birth early to avoid labor
4. Determine if the fetus is getting too large for a vaginal delivery

247. When caring for a client with type 1 diabetes on the first postpartum day, the nurse would expect her insulin requirements to:
1. Slowly decrease
2. Suddenly increase
3. Suddenly decrease
4. Remain unchanged

248. The assessment finding that the nurse would consider a cause for concern in a client at 35 weeks' gestation would be:
1. Frequent painless urination
2. Painful intermittent contractions
3. Increased fetal movement after eating
4. Difficulty sleeping because of lower back pain

249. A client who has had tocolytic therapy for preterm labor is being discharged. The nurse should include in the teaching plan that the client should:
1. Limit daily activities

2. Restrict her fluid intake
3. Monitor her urine for protein
4. Continue deep breathing exercises

250. A client who is at 34 weeks' gestation has been receiving terbutaline (Brethine) subcutaneously. Her contractions increase to every 5 minutes, and her cervix dilates to 4 cm. The tocolytic is discontinued. Priority nursing care during this time should be directed toward:
1. Promotion of maternal-fetal well-being during labor
2. Reduction of anxiety associated with preterm labor
3. Supportive communication with the client and her partner
4. Assisting the family to cope with the impending preterm birth

251. A woman at 39 weeks' gestation, whose membranes have ruptured at home, arrives at the clinic to be evaluated. Assessment reveals mild irregular contractions 10 to 15 minutes apart and a fetal heart rate of 186 beats per minute auscultated between contractions. This assessment indicates to the nurse that the fetus is:
1. Not at risk
2. Descending rapidly
3. Responding to an infection
4. In need of further assessment

252. A client is admitted to the hospital in labor 24 hours after her membranes have ruptured. It is important for the nurse to assess the client's amniotic fluid for signs of potential:
1. Cord prolapse
2. Placenta previa
3. Chorioamnionitis
4. Abruptio placentae

253. The husband of a client in labor asks what the indentation is on his wife's abdomen. The nurse immediately recognizes this as a retraction ring (Bandl's ring). The first action by the nurse should be to:
1. Inform him that this shows the baby's descent down the birth canal
2. Recognize that this is a danger sign and notify the physician immediately
3. Tell him that this indentation is expected and reflects the strength of the contractions
4. Explain that his wife is entering the second stage of labor and she should push at the next contraction

254. A client at 35 weeks' gestation is admitted to the hospital with a small amount of bright red

vaginal bleeding without contractions. After placing the client in bed, the nurse should:
1. Check fetal heart tones
2. Administer a Fleet enema
3. Obtain an amniotomy setup
4. Perform a vaginal examination

255. A client at 40 weeks' gestation is admitted to the birthing unit in early active labor. She tells the nurse that her membranes ruptured 26 hours ago. Several assessments of the fetal heart rate reveal rates between 168 and 174 beats per minute. When there is a history of prolonged ruptured membranes and a finding of fetal tachycardia, a priority nursing action would be to:
1. Prepare for an emergency birth
2. Administer oxygen via nasal cannula
3. Prepare for fetal scalp blood sampling
4. Assess the client's temperature, pulse, and respirations

256. A client's membranes rupture spontaneously during the latent phase of the first stage of labor, and the fluid is greenish-brown. The nurse understands that this indicates that:
1. Infection has already begun
2. A cesarean birth is necessary
3. Delivery should be immediate
4. The fetus may have been stressed in utero

257. While a multiparous client is in active labor, her membranes rupture spontaneously, and the nurse observes a loop of umbilical cord protruding from her vagina. The priority nursing action should be directed toward:
1. Monitoring the fetal heart rate
2. Covering the cord with a wet saline dressing
3. Holding the cord away from the presenting part
4. Keeping the presenting part away from the cord

258. A female client is being treated in a methadone maintenance program. On her next visit to the clinic she tells the counselor that she is three months pregnant and is receiving prenatal care. The client has been in the program for three months and has been taking 40 mg of methadone daily for treatment of an opiate addiction. The counselor calls the nurse, who should recommend that the client:
1. Continue with the methadone as prescribed to prevent withdrawal symptoms
2. Discontinue the methadone immediately to improve fetal and neonatal outcome
3. Discontinue the methadone slowly over the next two weeks to block drug cravings

4. Withdraw from the methadone maintenance program while she is pregnant and reenter when she has delivered

259. Aware of a client's history of opiate abuse, the nurse's initial plans for providing pain relief measures during labor should include:
1. Scheduling pain medication at regular intervals
2. Administering the medication only when the pain is severe
3. Avoiding the administration of medication unless it is requested
4. Recognizing that she will not need as much pain medication as others

260. When planning care for a client in labor who is a drug abuser and has tested positive for HIV, the nurse should know that the:
1. Client will need invasive fetal monitoring
2. Client has acquired immunodeficiency syndrome
3. HIV virus is transmitted primarily through body fluids
4. Incidence of HIV/AIDS is unaffected by the type of birth

261. The nurse should be aware that a postpartum client with a history of drug abuse may be experiencing drug withdrawal if she develops:
1. Paranoia and evasiveness
2. Extreme hunger and thirst
3. Depression and tearfulness
4. Irritability and muscle tremors

262. A client who is 4 cm dilated and in labor is admitted to the birthing room. An electronic fetal monitor is applied. The observation that would alert the nurse to notify the physician would be:
1. Beat-to-beat variability between contractions
2. Fetal heart accelerations at the beginning of a contraction
3. Contractions every minute, lasting 120 seconds each
4. Early fetal heart rate decelerations before the peak of a contraction

263. During early labor a client's membranes rupture, and her cervix is 3 cm dilated and 50% effaced. The fluid is clear and the fetal heart rate is stable. The nurse should anticipate that:
1. Birth of the fetus will occur within 24 hours
2. The second stage of labor will be prolonged
3. An oxytocin infusion will be required to stimulate labor
4. The delayed effacement will result in a difficult delivery

264. A client is admitted with the diagnosis of placenta previa. The nurse is aware that this diagnosis usually is confirmed by:
1. A laparoscopy
2. An ultrasound
3. A nonstress test
4. An amniocentesis

265. A client is admitted to the hospital with uterine tenderness and minimal, dark red vaginal bleeding. She is diagnosed as having abruptio placentae. Upon admission, the priority assessment would include vital signs, skin color, urine output, and:
1. Her past obstetric history
2. Fundal height or abdominal girth
3. The time and amount of last meal
4. Family history of bleeding disorders

266. A client at 36 weeks' gestation attends the prenatal clinic for a routine examination. The nurse identifies that the client's blood pressure has increased from 102/60 to 134/88 and is concerned she may be developing mild preeclampsia. The nurse should also assess the client for:
1. Proteinuria
2. Mild ankle edema
3. Episodes of faintness on arising
4. Weight gain of 2 pounds in 2 weeks

267. A client in the 38th week of gestation develops a slight increase in blood pressure. The physician advises her to remain in bed at home in a side-lying position. The client asks why this is important. The nurse's response would be based on the knowledge that this position:
1. Decreases intraabdominal pressure
2. Elevates the mean arterial pressure
3. Prevents the development of thromboses
4. Increases the circulation to the kidneys and uterus

268. An amniotomy is performed to stimulate labor in a client at 42 weeks' gestation. Immediately after this procedure, the nurse should observe for:
1. Prolapse of the umbilical cord
2. Increased fetal heart rate tracings
3. Lowered maternal blood pressure
4. Acceleration of the maternal heart rate

269. A nonstress test is scheduled for a client with preeclampsia. During the nonstress test the nurse should be aware that if nonperiodic accelerations of the fetal heart rate occur with fetal movement, it most likely indicates:

1. Fetal well-being
2. Head compression
3. Uteroplacental insufficiency
4. Umbilical cord compression

270. A nurse admits a client with preeclampsia to the hospital. After obtaining the vital signs, the nurse should:
1. Check the client's reflexes
2. Call the physician immediately
3. Determine the client's blood type
4. Administer intravenous normal saline

271. A client at 36 weeks' gestation is admitted because of a weight gain of 5 pounds in the previous week and a pronounced rise in blood pressure. Appropriate nursing care would include:
1. Preparing for an imminent cesarean birth
2. Providing a dark, quiet room with minimal stimuli
3. Instituting prescribed furosemide (Lasix) IV therapy
4. Administering prescribed calcium gluconate to lower blood pressure

272. Before administering IV magnesium sulfate therapy to a client with preeclampsia, the nurse should assess the client's:
1. Temperature, blood pressure, and respirations
2. Urinary glucose, acetone, and specific gravity
3. Urinary output, respirations, and patellar reflexes
4. Level of consciousness, funduscopic appearance, and knee reflex

273. A client is diagnosed as having mild preeclampsia. When instructing the client about diet before discharge, the nurse should advise her to:
1. Stay on a low-salt diet
2. Restrict her fluid intake
3. Continue on a regular pregnancy diet
4. Increase her carbohydrate consumption

274. A client with preeclampsia is admitted to the labor and birthing suite. Her blood pressure is 130/90, she has 2+ protein in her urine, and edema of the hands and face. As part of the admission history, the nurse should ask the client about:
1. Constipation, edema, visual problems, and headache
2. Visual disturbances, headache, constipation, and bleeding
3. Leakage of fluid, bleeding, edema, and abdominal pain

4. Headache, visual disturbances, edema, and abdominal pain

275. A client with severe preeclampsia is admitted to the hospital and given an IV infusion of magnesium sulfate (MgSO₄). The nurse recognizes that for this client magnesium sulfate is being given primarily because it is a:
   1. Hypotensive that relaxes smooth muscles
   2. Cholinergic that increases the release of acetylcholine
   3. Muscle relaxant that decreases the severity of uterine contractions
   4. Central nervous system depressant that blocks neuromuscular transmissions

276. An infusion of oxytocin (Pitocin) is administered to a client for induction of labor. After several minutes the fetal monitor indicates contractions lasting 100 seconds occurring every 95 seconds. The nurse should:
   1. Speed up the oxytocin flow
   2. Slow down the oxytocin flow
   3. Turn the client on her left side
   4. Discontinue the oxytocin flow

277. A client with a history of phenylketonuria, who was maintained on a low-phenylalanine diet until 9 years of age, is now pregnant. The nurse teaches this client that:
   1. The baby may be mentally retarded because of her history of PKU
   2. Reinstitution of the low-phenylalanine diet will protect her baby from PKU
   3. The fetus is at no risk prenatally but will require immediate care at birth to prevent PKU
   4. Phenylalanine should be avoided even when not pregnant so that her body is able to support a pregnancy

278. Diet counseling for a breastfeeding client with a history of phenylketonuria should include providing a list displaying foods containing:
   1. Lactose
   2. Glucose
   3. Fatty acids
   4. Amino acids

279. A client at 6 weeks' gestation who has type 1 diabetes is attending the prenatal clinic for the first time. The nurse explains that during the first trimester insulin requirements may decrease because:
   1. Body metabolism is sluggish during the first trimester
   2. Morning sickness may lead to decreased food intake

3. Fetal requirements of glucose in this period are minimal
4. The hormones of pregnancy decrease the body's need for insulin

280. The nurse teaching a prenatal class is asked why babies of mothers with diabetes are larger than those who are nondiabetic. The nurse should respond that these mothers:
   1. Take exogenous insulin, which stimulates fetal growth
   2. Have extra circulating glucose that causes fatty deposits in the fetus
   3. Consume extra calories to cover the insulin manufactured by the fetus
   4. Are usually overweight and some of the calories are utilized by the fetus

281. The nurse explains to a newly pregnant client with diabetes mellitus that to minimize fetal neonatal complications, the most important action for her to take would be to:
   1. Keep all the physician's appointments made for her
   2. Check her blood glucose level as ordered
   3. Adhere strictly to the prescribed diet to limit weight gain
   4. Comply with the management plan to maintain normal blood glucose levels

282. In the 35th week of gestation, a client with type 1 diabetes mellitus is scheduled for an amniocentesis. Nursing care for this client includes explaining that this test:
   1. Can reveal any structural defects of the placenta
   2. Is done to determine the approximate size of the fetus
   3. Will determine whether a cesarean birth is necessary
   4. Will provide information about the lung maturity of the fetus

283. A client with diabetes mellitus has an amniocentesis in the 37th week of gestation; the L/S ratio of the amniotic fluid indicates adequate lung maturity. Based on this information the nurse assesses that:
   1. A cesarean birth will be scheduled
   2. There will be no need for further fetal monitoring
   3. The baby will have to be delivered immediately
   4. The baby should be free from major respiratory problems

284. Aware of the signs of an impending postpartum hemorrhage secondary to laceration of the cervix, the nurse assesses a postpartum client for a firm uterus and:
    1. A decrease in pulse rate
    2. Persistent muscular twitching
    3. An increase in blood pressure
    4. Continuous trickling of blood

285. The nurse applies an electronic fetal monitor on the abdomen of a client in labor. When observing the relationship between the fetal heart rate and uterine contractions the nurse notes four late decelerations. The nurse recognizes that late decelerations are most frequently associated with:
    1. Head compression
    2. Maternal hypothyroidism
    3. Umbilical cord compression
    4. Uteroplacental insufficiency

286. A client who has undergone a cesarean birth because of the presence of active genital herpes is transferred to the postpartum unit. The nurse should plan to institute isolation precautions which include:
    1. Enteric
    2. Droplet
    3. Contact
    4. Airborne

287. A client with an abruptio placentae had an emergency cesarean birth. Subsequently the nurse observes that there is bloody urine in the indwelling catheter collection bag. The nurse recognizes that this is significant because the client may have:
    1. An incisional nick in the bladder
    2. A urinary infection from the catheter
    3. Uterine relaxation with increased lochia
    4. Disseminated intravascular coagulopathy

288. During an emergency birth the nurse should place the cord clamp
    1. 2 inches from the umbilicus
    2. 5 inches from the umbilicus
    3. 7 inches from the umbilicus
    4. 10 inches from the umbilicus

289. Two hours after giving birth, a client's physical assessment includes: BP, 86/40; TPR, 98/100/22; fundus firm, four finger-breadths above umbilicus; small spots of lochia rubra on perineal pad; bladder distended. After catheterization the client's fundus remains firm and four finger-breadths above the umbilicus. The nurse should:

1. Notify the client's physician immediately
2. Palpate the client's fundus every two hours
3. Recheck the client's vital signs again in 30 minutes
4. Catheterize the client again in one hour for residual urine

NORMAL NEONATE (NN)

290. In specific situations, gloves are being used when handling newborns whether they are HIV positive or not. The nurse understands that it is usually not necessary to wear gloves with infants when:
    1. Giving a feeding
    2. Changing the diaper
    3. Suctioning the infant
    4. Doing an admission bath

291. At one minute after birth the nurse notes that an infant is crying, has a heart rate of 140, has blue hands and feet, resists the suction catheter, and keeps the arms extended. What Apgar score should the nurse assign for this infant? Answer: _____.

292. The best place for the nurse to assess adequate tissue oxygenation in a neonate born of African-American parents would be the:
    1. Heels and buttocks
    2. Upper tips of the ears
    3. Nail beds on the hands and feet
    4. Mucous membranes of the mouth

293. Immediately after the birth of a neonate, the nurse's first action should be to:
    1. Dry and place the infant in a warm environment
    2. Perform an abbreviated systematic physical assessment
    3. Cut the umbilical cord and attach a clamp to the cord
    4. Administer oxygen by face mask until cyanosis clears

294. When checking a newborn's reflexes, the nurse is unable to elicit one reflex response that is often absent in babies born by vaginal breech delivery. The nurse attempts to elicit this response by:
    1. Moving the thumb along the sole of the baby's foot
    2. Stroking of the ulnar surface of the hand and fifth finger lightly
    3. Touching the skin fold of the mouth and cheek on the same side

4. Holding the baby upright and pressing the dorsal aspect of the feet on the crib mattress.

295. An assessment of a newborn includes the differentiation between cephalhematoma and caput succedaneum. When making this assessment, the nurse understands that with caput succedaneum the:
1. Edema crosses the suture line
2. Swelling increases within 24 hours
3. Scalp over the swelling becomes ecchymotic
4. Area surrounding the swelling will be tender

296. The nurse notes a right cephalhematoma on an otherwise healthy one-day-old newborn. A priority intervention at the time of discharge would be to instruct the parents:
1. How to observe for signs of jaundice
2. How to assess the fontanels for tenseness
3. To increase the infant's feeding to every three hours
4. To record the number of wet diapers the infant has in 24 hours

297. When assessing a newborn's grasp reflex, the nurse should elicit it by:
1. Putting direct pressure along the sole of the newborn's foot
2. Jarring the crib and watching the movement of the newborn's hands
3. Pressing the examining fingers against the palms of the newborn's hands
4. Holding the body upright and allowing the newborn's feet to touch a surface

298. Two hours after birth a newborn develops an area of soft swelling in the left parietal region. The nurse recognizes that the area of involvement would be:
1. Over the eyes
2. Behind the ears
3. Back of the head
4. Upper portion of the skull

299. During the physical assessment of a recently delivered newborn, the nurse palpates the infant's femoral pulses. This is done to detect the presence of:
1. Atrial septal defect
2. Coarctation of the aorta
3. Patent ductus arteriosus
4. Ventricular septal defect

300. Immediately after delivery a newborn is dried and then wrapped in warm blankets by the nurse. The drying of the newborn's skin helps to prevent body heat loss via:
1. Radiation
2. Convection
3. Conduction
4. Evaporation

301. When assessing a newborn's Moro reflex the nurse should elicit it by:
1. Turning the infant's head quickly to one side
2. Tapping briskly on the bridge of the infant's nose
3. Stroking the infant's back alongside the spine
4. Suddenly but gently jarring the infant's bassinet

302. The nurse informs the parents of a newborn that the petechiae on their infant's face and neck are a result of:
1. Excessive superficial capillaries
2. A rash called erythema toxicum
3. Increased intravascular pressure during birth
4. Decreased vitamin K level in the newborn infant

303. A newborn's total body response to noise or movement is often distressing to the parents. It is important for the nurse to teach the parents that this response is:
1. A reflex response that indicates normal development
2. An involuntary response that will remain for the first year of life
3. An automatic response that may indicate that the baby is hungry
4. A voluntary response that indicates insecurity in an unfamiliar environment

304. A baby weighing 5 pounds, 6 ounces is born via cesarean birth. The nurse expects the newborn's respiratory rate to range between:
1. 20 to 40 per minute
2. 30 to 60 per minute
3. 60 to 80 per minute
4. 70 to 90 per minute

305. The nurse recognizes that in the healthy, full-term neonate heat production is accomplished by:
1. Oxidizing fatty acids
2. Shivering vigorously
3. Breaking down brown fat
4. Increasing muscular activity

306. After the birth of her daughter, a mother states to the nurse, "I was told that my baby has to have an injection of vitamin K. She's so small to be getting a shot. Why does she have to have it?" The nurse's most appropriate response would be:
1. "Your baby needs the injection to help her develop red blood cells."
2. "An injection of vitamin K will help to prevent your baby from becoming jaundiced."
3. "Newborns are deficient in vitamin K. This treatment protects your baby from bleeding."
4. "A newborn's blood clots faster than it should. This injection helps decrease the clotting time."

307. When performing a discharge assessment on a 2-day-old newborn, a large amount of meconium is expelled. The nurse realizes that this would be:
1. A precursor of newborn diarrhea
2. Commonly found in a baby who is 2 days old
3. An abnormal finding, indicating a pathologic condition of the digestive system
4. Cause for concern because meconium is passed only on the first day of life

308. When assessing for developmental dysplasia of the hip (DDH) during the newborn assessment, the nurse should determine if the infant has extra skin folds in the:
1. Thigh
2. Abdomen
3. Calf muscles
4. Popliteal area

309. The nurse is performing the Ortolani test on a newborn. The finding that would indicate a positive result would be:
1. Dorsiflexion and fanning
2. Hypertonia and jitteriness
3. An arched back and crying
4. An audible click on abduction

310. To best assist new parents to understand the unique characteristics of a newborn, the nurse should discuss with them the:
1. Infant's response to a set feeding schedule
2. Newborn's behaviors and states of wakefulness
3. Testing of the normal newborn's auditory acuity
4. Importance of reading about parent-infant bonding

311. During the second reactive period a newborn becomes more alert and responsive. There is an increase in mucus production and gagging. The nurse should first:
1. Report this finding
2. Administer nasal oxygen
3. Lower the newborn's head
4. Remove secretions from the pharynx

312. When inspecting her newborn, a mother asks the nurse whether her newborn has flat feet. The nurse recalls that:
1. Flat feet are common in children and infants
2. This is difficult to assess because the feet are so small
3. Flat feet are associated with major deformities of the bones of the feet such as clubfoot
4. The arch of the newborn's foot is covered with a fat pad, giving the appearance of being flat

313. The nurse recognizes that survival in the neonatal period is largely related to:
1. Gestational age and birth weight
2. Reproductive history of the mother
3. Parental health habits and social class
4. Timing and adequacy of prenatal care

314. At one minute after birth a newborn's body is pink with blue extremities, the heart rate is 122, there is withdrawal when the soles are flicked, the respirations are easy with no evidence of distress, and the arms and legs are flexed and vigorously moving. The nurse assesses the Apgar score to be:
1. 7
2. 8
3. 9
4. 10

315. A newborn weighing 9 pounds, 14 ounces is delivered by cesarean birth because of cephalopelvic disproportion. The baby has an Apgar score of 9 at one minute and 10 at five minutes. Based on the assessment of this infant, an additional measure initiated by the nurse would be the:
1. Administration of 23% oxygen by hood
2. Determination of the blood glucose level
3. Passage of a gavage tube to give a formula feeding
4. Transfer of the infant to the neonatal intensive care unit

316. The nurse, observing a sleeping newborn, notes periods of irregular breathing and occasional twitching movements of the arms and legs.

The neonate's heart rate is 150 beats per minute; the respiratory rate is 50 breaths per minute; and the glucose strip reading is 60 mg/dl. The nurse's most appropriate assessment would be the:
1. Baby requires no intervention; all findings are normal
2. Twitching movements suggest the baby may be having seizures
3. Baby's blood glucose is low; twitching movements suggest hypoglycemia
4. Rapid respiratory rate and irregular breathing suggest respiratory distress

317. When assessing a newborn, the nurse notes several areas of raised white spots on the chin and nose. The nurse is aware that these are known as:
1. Milia
2. Lanugo
3. Vascular nevi
4. Erythema toxicum

318. A 1-day-old newborn has just had a thick, greenish-black stool. The nurse checks the chart and notes that this is the first stool. The nurse's first action would be to:
1. Document the stool in the infant's record
2. Assess the infant for an intestinal obstruction
3. Send the stool to the laboratory as per protocol
4. Notify the physician immediately, since this indicates bleeding

319. A client delivers a full-term male infant with an 8/9 Apgar score. The immediate nursing care of this newborn should include:
1. Assessing respirations, identifying the infant, and keeping him warm
2. Applying a prophylactic agent to the eyes, giving AquaMEPHYTON, and bathing him
3. Rushing him to the nursery while aspirating the oropharynx, and stimulating him often
4. Weighing him, placing him in a crib, and keeping him near until the mother is ready to hold him

320. The day after delivery a client asks the nurse if her baby had a test for PKU yet. The nurse answers, "We cannot:
1. Take any blood for the PKU test until your baby reaches 10 pounds."
2. Perform a heel stick for PKU today because newborns generally have sluggish pedal circulation."
3. Complete the PKU test because a newborn's liver does not produce measurable enzymes before seven days."
4. Perform the PKU test today because your baby has not had enough milk for the results to be accurate."

321. A newborn who has remained in the hospital because the mother had a cesarean birth is to be tested for phenylketonuria (PKU) on the morning of discharge. When educating the mother about PKU testing, the nurse should explain that it is done to:
1. Test for thyroid deficiency
2. Detect possible retardation
3. Measure protein metabolism
4. Identify chromosomal damage

322. Phenylketonuria (PKU) testing is performed on a newborn before discharge. The nurse plans to explain to the mother that the purpose of this screening test is to determine:
1. If the infant is positive for PKU
2. If the mother is a carrier for PKU
3. The incidence of the disease in the population
4. The risk for the infant's later development of PKU

323. On the second day of life, minutes after drinking $2\frac{1}{2}$ ounces of formula, a newborn regurgitates about half an ounce of milk. The mother states, "My baby spits up after every feeding." The nurse should:
1. Reassure the mother that all babies spit up some milk at first
2. Teach her to place the baby in a right-side-lying position after feedings
3. Take the baby back to the nursery and feed another $\frac{1}{2}$ ounce of fresh formula
4. Have her prop the baby at 20 degrees in an infant seat for an hour after feeding

324. A newborn male is circumcised. The nurse would recognize that the mother requires additional teaching regarding care of her son following the circumcision when she indicates that she plans to:
1. Change her son's diapers very frequently
2. Call the physician if there is excessive bleeding
3. Give the baby a tub bath the day after he is discharged
4. Place petrolatum gauze or A & D ointment on his penis with each diaper change

325. A newborn male is being discharged four hours after having had a circumcision. The nurse should teach the mother to:
1. Apply the diaper loosely for two to three days
2. Report a whitish exudate around the glans to the physician
3. Notify the physician if the baby fusses and cries with voiding
4. Check for bleeding every two hours during the first day home

326. A new mother asks the nurse why her baby seems to have a bowel movement after every feeding. When preparing a response to explain why this is an expected occurrence, the nurse should recall that it indicates an adequate:
1. Fluid intake
2. Cardiac sphincter
3. Gastrocolic reflex
4. Pancreatic amylase level

327. When changing her infant, a new mother notes a reddened area on the infant's buttock and reports it to the nurse. The nurse should:
1. Have the nursery staff change the infant's diaper
2. Use both lotion and powder to protect the involved area
3. Notify the pediatrician and request an order for a topical ointment
4. Encourage the new mother to cleanse and change the infant more often

328. A newborn develops jaundice 72 hours after birth. The nurse explains to the parents that the jaundice is probably a result of:
1. An allergic response to the feedings
2. Normal physiologic destruction of immature RBCs
3. An obstruction in the bile duct, which is common in newborns
4. Some Rh-negative blood that is still present in the baby's bloodstream

329. A community health nurse visits an infant who was born at home 24 hours ago. When assessing the infant, the nurse notes slight jaundice of the face and trunk. The first nursing action should be to:
1. Plan for immediate admission to the hospital
2. Arrange for the infant to have phototherapy in the home
3. Document this expected finding in the infant's record

4. Obtain a physician's order for a bilirubin determination

330. On a male newborn's first encounter with his mother the nurse encourages her to undress him. The mother strokes him with her whole hand and while looking at him intently says, "He feels so velvety, and he is going to be just as good looking as his daddy." The baby is alert and responsive while gazing at his mother. The nurse recognizes optimum:
1. Early parenting behavior
2. Attachment behavior in the newborn
3. Early maternal deprivation syndrome
4. Consummatory behavior in the newborn

331. To help the parents proceed with bonding behaviors immediately after birth, the nurse should:
1. Assess for proper parenting techniques
2. Demonstrate the desired behavior to the parents
3. Postpone footprinting the baby until late evening
4. Delay administering the antibiotic to the baby's eyes

332. After her baby's birth a client wishes to begin breastfeeding. The nurse assists the client by:
1. Positioning the infant to grasp the nipple to express milk
2. Giving the infant a bottle first to evaluate the baby's ability to suck
3. Leaving them alone and allowing the infant to nurse as long as desired
4. Touching the infant's cheek adjacent to the nipple to elicit the rooting reflex

333. The best indication that correct attachment to the breast has occurred is when the:
1. Baby's tongue is securely on top of the nipple
2. Baby's mouth covers most of the areolar surface
3. Baby makes frequent loud clucking sounds while nursing at each breast
4. Baby sucks each breast vigorously for five minutes before falling asleep

334. The nurse assures the breastfeeding mother that she will know that her infant is getting an adequate supply of breast milk if the infant gains weight and:
1. Rarely sucks on a pacifier
2. Has several hard stools daily
3. Voids six or more times a day
4. Awakens to feed every four hours

335. A mother is breastfeeding her newborn. She asks when she can switch the baby to a cup. The nurse would recognize that the mother understands the teaching about feeding when she says she will start to introduce a cup after the baby reaches:
    1. 4 months
    2. 6 months
    3. 12 months
    4. 16 months

336. The mother who is formula feeding her 1-month-old asks the nurse whether any vitamin or mineral supplements are required. The nurse bases the reply on the knowledge that babies who are fed with ready-to-use formula require:
    1. Iron
    2. Fluoride
    3. Vitamin K
    4. Vitamin B_{12}

337. A newborn is delivered vaginally in the breech presentation. When examining her baby the mother asks if the baby has been injured during birth because of the large black and blue areas on the buttocks and legs. The nurse should respond that:
    1. This is not a birth injury and probably just a birthmark
    2. These are caused by forceps used to aid in the delivery of the baby
    3. This is a temporary complication that will disappear in about a week
    4. These Mongolian spots, common in dark-skinned babies, disappear within a year

338. The nurse teaches a new mother that neonatal weight loss in the first three days of life is most often the result of:
    1. Allergy to formula
    2. A hypoglycemic response
    3. Inadequate breast- or formula feeding
    4. Excretion of fluid via lungs, urinary bladder, and bowels

339. When teaching a new mother care of the umbilical cord area, the nurse should recommend that:
    1. Neosporin ointment be placed around the cord after the sponge bath
    2. The area be cleansed daily with an alcohol swab and inspected for redness or drainage
    3. An elastic bandage be wrapped snugly around the body over the cord site to prevent umbilical hernia
    4. The clamp should remain on the cord until the umbilical cord stump separates about the seventh to tenth day of life

HIGH-RISK NEONATE (HN)

340. A male infant delivered at 28 weeks' gestation weighs 2 pounds, 12 ounces. When performing an assessment the nurse would probably observe:
    1. Wide, staring eyes
    2. Transparent, red skin
    3. An absence of lanugo
    4. A scrotum with descended testicles

341. On admission to the nursery a newborn is observed to be experiencing cold stress. The basis for the nursing intervention at this time would be to minimize:
    1. Shivering
    2. Hyperglycemia
    3. Oxygen consumption
    4. Metabolism of fat stores

342. A client with type 1 diabetes delivers a 9-pound, 10-ounce baby by cesarean birth in her 36th week of pregnancy. When monitoring the infant of a mother with diabetes, the nurse should monitor for signs of:
    1. Meconium ileus
    2. Respiratory distress
    3. Physiologic jaundice
    4. Increased intracranial pressure

343. A client at 24 weeks' gestation is admitted in early labor. Based on the nurse's knowledge of preterm births it is understood that:
    1. Birth at this gestational age may result in a severely compromised neonate
    2. If contractions are regular, labor cannot be effectively stopped and delivery will ensue
    3. Delivery after 34 weeks' gestation is usually safe because of advances in neonatal health care
    4. Attempts will be made to sustain the pregnancy for two more weeks to ensure neonatal survival

344. A nurse caring for a newborn of 33 weeks' gestation should observe the infant for:
    1. Flaring nares
    2. Acrocyanosis
    3. Abdominal breathing
    4. Respirations of 40 per minute

345. A client expresses a desire to breastfeed her preterm infant who is in the neonatal intensive care unit (NICU). The nurse should:
    1. Tell the client this is not possible because the infant is being fed by gavage
    2. Discourage the client because of the time and effort it will take to pump her breasts
    3. Support the client's decision and explain that even if her infant is able to nipple feed, the infant may be easily exhausted
    4. Instruct the client that breast milk is inadequate for a preterm infant because it does not contain all the necessary nutrients

346. The nurse assesses that a newborn is in respiratory distress when the infant exhibits:
    1. Apnea, grunting, wheezing, and crackles
    2. Wheezing, cyanosis, hiccups, and crackles
    3. Cyanosis, retraction, wheezing, and hiccups
    4. Tachypnea, retraction, grunting, and cyanosis

347. A neonate, born at 34 weeks' gestation and weighing 6 lbs, 10 oz (2750 g) is admitted to the nursery. The vital signs are: apical heart rate 130; respirations 58; blood pressure 60/20; temperature 98° F; Apgar scores of 4 and 8. The nurse should designate the highest priority health outcome to be:
    1. Oxygenation will remain adequate
    2. Body temperature will remain stable
    3. Weight will increase by 30 g per day
    4. Heart rate will recover to an acceptable range

348. Respiratory acidosis is confirmed in a neonate with respiratory distress syndrome when the nurse notes that the laboratory report of blood gases reveals:
    1. A pH of 7.35
    2. An elevated PCO_2
    3. A potassium level of 4.6 mEq/L
    4. An arterial O_2 level of 80 mm Hg

349. During the assessment of a newborn, it is most important for the nurse to report a:
    1. Temperature of 97.7° F
    2. Pale pink, rust-colored stain in the diaper
    3. Heart rate that drops to 120 beats/minute
    4. Breathing pattern that is diaphragmatic with sternal retractions

350. A preterm newborn is given oxygen via hood. The plan of care for a neonate receiving oxygen therapy should include:
    1. Assessing that the baby's skin remains bright pink at all times
    2. Ensuring that the oxygen is warmed and humidified at all times
    3. Monitoring and recording oxygen levels in the hood once per shift
    4. Informing the parents that blindness is not a risk if oxygen levels are kept low

351. A newborn with respiratory distress syndrome is receiving continuous positive airway pressure (CPAP) therapy via an endotracheal tube. The nurse notes that the infant's breath sounds on the right side are diminished, and the point of maximum impulse (PMI) of the heartbeat is in the left axillary line. Interpretation of this assessment data should lead the nurse to understand that:
    1. These are expected findings because infants with this disorder often have some degree of atelectasis
    2. The inspiratory pressure on the ventilator is probably too low and needs to be increased for adequate ventilation
    3. The endotracheal tube has probably slipped into the left main stem bronchus and needs to be pulled back to ventilate both lungs
    4. The infant may have a pneumothorax, and the physician should be contacted immediately so treatment can be instituted

352. When teaching the mother of a newborn with exstrophy of the bladder, the nurse should include how to:
    1. Measure intake and output daily
    2. Protect the skin surrounding the bladder
    3. Maintain sterility of the exposed bladder
    4. Apply a pressure dressing to the exposed bladder

353. A nursing intervention for a neonate with respiratory distress syndrome would be:
    1. Position to promote respiratory efforts
    2. Observe for possible congenital birth defects
    3. Set the incubator temperature at 85° F to prevent shivering
    4. Avoid handling to minimize overstimulation and conserve oxygen

354. When assessing a preterm infant, it is most important for the nurse to know the infant's gestational age and how it compares to the birth weight because:
    1. This information will help identify potential problems
    2. This information must be documented on the admission record

3. Evaluation and classification records are necessary for health insurance
4. The infant will lose 10% of birth weight during the first few days of life

355. After an emergency cesarean birth, a neonate born at 35 weeks' gestation is admitted to the neonatal intensive care unit (NICU). The neonate has a Silverman-Anderson score of 6, which reflects a need for:
   1. Continuous cardiac monitoring
   2. Assessment of neurologic reflexes
   3. Increased caloric intake and fluids
   4. Respiratory support and observation

356. A client delivers a baby girl by cesarean birth. The nurse monitors the baby's breathing because infants delivered by cesarean birth are more apt to have atelectasis because:
   1. The rib cage is not compressed and then released during birth
   2. Oxygen deprivation of the infant occurs following a cesarean birth
   3. The sudden change in temperature at birth causes the infant to aspirate
   4. There is no chance during the birth for gravity to drain the fluid from the lungs

357. The nurse is aware that in an infant born at 32 weeks' gestation the:
   1. Palms have clearly defined creases
   2. Ear pinnas spring back when folded
   3. Areolae and nipples are barely visible
   4. Square window sign shows a 0-degree angle

358. When assessing a newly delivered neonate, the nurse notes the following findings: arms and legs slightly flexed; skin smooth and transparent; abundant lanugo on the back; slow recoil of pinna; and few sole creases. In light of these findings, the care plan for this neonate should include nursing orders to monitor for:
   1. Polycythemia
   2. Hyperglycemia
   3. Postmaturity syndrome
   4. Respiratory distress syndrome

359. A client with chronic hypertension and superimposed preeclampsia gives birth to a 4-pound, 12-ounce infant at 39 weeks' gestation. The nurse would expect the neonate to have signs of:
   1. Prematurity
   2. Cardiac anomalies
   3. Respiratory infection
   4. Intrauterine growth restriction

360. The nurse would classify a newborn delivered at 39 weeks' gestation, weighing 2450 g (5.5 pounds), as being:
   1. Preterm and immature
   2. Small-for-gestational age
   3. Average-for-gestational age
   4. Average-for-gestational age but preterm

361. A neonate born at 39 weeks' gestation is determined to be small for gestational age. When planning care for this infant, the nurse must consider the most common immediate problem, which would be:
   1. Anemia
   2. Hypocalcemia
   3. Hypoglycemia
   4. Protein deficiency

362. A small-for-gestational age (SGA) newborn, who has just been admitted to the nursery, has a high-pitched cry, appears jittery, and has irregular respirations. The nurse is aware that these signs may be associated with:
   1. Hypovolemia
   2. Hypoglycemia
   3. Hypercalcemia
   4. Hypothyroidism

363. A finding in the nurse's physical assessment of a neonate that may indicate that the infant is preterm would be:
   1. Flexion of extremities
   2. Absent femoral pulses
   3. Many superficial veins
   4. A positive Babinski's reflex

364. The nurse suspects that a preterm neonate receiving gastric feedings may have necrotizing enterocolitis (NEC) when:
   1. An increased number of explosive stools are noted
   2. Circumoral pallor develops during gastric feeding
   3. Several severe bouts of projectile vomiting are observed
   4. Large amounts of residual formula are withdrawn before gavage

365. Nursing care for an infant with necrotizing enterocolitis (NEC) includes:
   1. Diluting the formula mixture as ordered
   2. Measuring abdominal girth every two hours
   3. Administering oxygen prior to gastric feeding
   4. Giving half-strength formula by gavage feeding

366. During the assessment of a preterm neonate, the nurse determines that the infant is experiencing hypothermia. The nurse should:
    1. Assess the infant for signs of hyperglycemia and begin temperature stabilization
    2. Rapidly rewarm the infant during the next hour until the temperature is stabilized
    3. Gradually rewarm the infant during the next several hours and monitor frequently
    4. Assess and record the infant's skin temperature every hour until the temperature is stable

367. A male infant, born at 35 weeks' gestation, is in the neonatal intensive care unit (NICU). When the mother is told that her infant's condition is now stable, she asks, "When will I be able to breastfeed my son?" The nurse's most appropriate response would be:
    1. "Even though he is preterm, he is stable. You may try now if you would like."
    2. "Preterm infants should not breastfeed. It takes more calories than bottle feeding."
    3. "He is preterm and sucks weakly so it will be several weeks before you may breastfeed."
    4. "Pump your breasts now and then feed him the milk by bottle to conserve his energy."

368. The nurse gives a nasogastric feeding to a male preterm infant. As the mother watches she asks, "Would it hurt my baby to suck on a pacifier during the feeding?" The nurse's most appropriate response would be:
    1. "It might tire him out because he's still so small. We don't want him to use up all his energy."
    2. "If he sucks on a pacifier a lot now, he may have problems learning how to suck from the breast or bottle later."
    3. "There's no real benefit in using a pacifier and there is a relationship between the use of a pacifier and buck teeth."
    4. "Sucking on a pacifier during tube feedings may help him associate sucking with food so that he'll adjust better to oral feedings."

369. When an apnea monitor sounds an alarm 10 seconds after cessation of respirations, the nurse should respond first by:
    1. Assessing skin color and respirations
    2. Using tactile stimuli on chest or extremities
    3. Resuscitating with face mask and Ambu bag
    4. Checking the device for signs of malfunction

370. The nurse is aware that a preterm neonate may have a potential nutritional problem because of:
    1. A poor sucking reflex

    2. A decreased metabolic rate
    3. Decreased caloric requirements
    4. Increased absorption of nutrients

371. To prevent the development of retinopathy of prematurity, it would be most beneficial for the nurse to:
    1. Place a shield over the neonate's eyes
    2. Assess the neonate every hour with a pulse oximeter
    3. Maintain a low concentration of oxygen in the blood
    4. Position the neonate in an elevated side-lying position

372. The nurse instills erythromycin ophthalmic ointment into a newborn's eyes. The nurse understands that this is done to prevent:
    1. Herpetic ophthalmia
    2. Retrolental fibroplasia
    3. Ophthalmia neonatorum
    4. Hemorrhagic conjunctivitis

373. The parents of a preterm infant are finally taking their baby home. To evaluate the parents' competency level in the care of their infant, it would be most effective to:
    1. Ask the parents what they plan to do at home
    2. Determine the rationale behind the parents' actions
    3. Give the parents a simple test concerning infant care practices
    4. Observe the parents in a return demonstration of care

374. The nurse would expect that the newborn of a woman with poorly controlled type 1 diabetes to be:
    1. Average for gestational age, term
    2. Small for gestational age, preterm
    3. Large for gestational age, postterm
    4. Large for gestational age, near term

375. The nurse, monitoring the blood glucose levels of an infant of a diabetic mother, identifies a blood glucose level of 48 mg/dl. The nurse should:
    1. Check the cord serum glucose level
    2. Secure an order for an intravenous of 50% glucose
    3. Continue to monitor the blood glucose for 24 hours
    4. Start the infant on oral feedings of 10% dextrose in water

376. A newborn's birth was prolonged because the shoulders were very wide. The nurse performing

the assessment would be particularly observant for a problem with the:
1. Moro reflex
2. Plantar grasp
3. Babinski reflex
4. Stepping reflex

377. The nurse should expect that the newborn of a mother with diabetes would be:
1. Red-faced
2. Long and thin
3. Hyperreflexive
4. Crying excessively

378. A newborn whose mother has type 1 diabetes mellitus has been receiving a continuous infusion of fluids with glucose. When discontinuing the IV infusion, the nurse should:
1. Slowly decrease the rate
2. Observe for metabolic alkalosis
3. Withhold oral feedings for four to six hours
4. Check for elevated blood glucose levels every hour

379. Three hours after birth, a newborn of a mother with diabetes becomes jittery, has a weak, high-pitched cry, and exhibits irregular respirations. The nurse recognizes that these signs are often associated with:
1. Hypovolemia
2. Hypocalcemia
3. Hypoglycemia
4. Hyperglycemia

380. A client developed a rubella infection during the fourth month of pregnancy. At the time of the infant's birth, the nurse should:
1. Use enteric precautions
2. Institute blood precautions
3. Use standard precautions at all times
4. Place the newborn in the isolation nursery

381. A preterm neonate develops physiologic jaundice and phototherapy is ordered. The nurse understands that this therapy:
1. Activates the liver to dispose of the bilirubin
2. Breaks down the bilirubin into a conjugated form
3. Activates vitamin K to facilitate excretion of bilirubin
4. Dissolves the bilirubin and allows it to be excreted from the skin

382. A newborn is being treated with phototherapy for hyperbilirubinemia. When providing phototherapy, the nurse should:
1. Dress the infant in just a diaper

2. Turn the infant every two hours
3. Maintain 24-hour continuous phototherapy
4. Place a sterile gauze pad on the infant's umbilical stump

383. When doing a newborn assessment of a male infant after a scheduled cesarean birth, the nurse notes that the infant's head circumference is 4 centimeters smaller than his chest. The nurse is aware that this finding:
1. Is indicative of anencephaly
2. Could indicate microcephaly
3. Commonly occurs in babies born by cesarean birth
4. Is expected in male newborns regardless of the mode of birth

384. The nurse is aware that an ABO incompatibility is most common when the mother is:
1. Type A
2. Type B
3. Type O
4. Type AB

385. The nurse understands that the effect PKU has on development will depend on:
1. Diagnosis within the first three days after birth
2. The level of phenylalanine in the blood at birth
3. Adherence to a corrective diet and how early it is instituted
4. The presence of excessive levels of epinephrine in the body

386. The nurse is aware that an infant with untreated PKU has a characteristic urinary odor best described as:
1. Fishy
2. Ammoniacal
3. Mousy or musty
4. Aromatic or pungent

387. A newborn's hands and feet appear cyanotic and there is circumoral pallor when crying or feeding. The best nursing action would be to:
1. Report the circumoral pallor to the physician because it could indicate cardiac problems
2. Take no specific action because both signs are expected in a newborn until two weeks of age
3. Take no specific action because circumoral pallor is an expected finding for the first 72 to 96 hours
4. Notify the physician because cyanosis and pallor can be indicative of increased intracranial pressure

388. The nurse assesses a newborn and observes central cyanosis. Central cyanosis is indicative of congenital heart defects that affect cardiac circulation by:
1. Shunting blood right to left
2. Shunting blood left to right
3. Obstructing flow of blood from the left side of the heart
4. Preventing shunting of blood between left and right sides of the heart

389. A mother's laboratory results indicate the presence of cocaine and alcohol. The characteristic in her newborn that would indicate to the nurse that the baby has been affected by fetal alcohol syndrome would be:
1. Cleft lip
2. Polydactyly
3. Umbilical hernia
4. Small upturned nose

390. Twelve hours after birth, the nurse observes that a newborn is hyperactive, jittery, sneezes frequently, has a high-pitched cry, and is having difficulty sucking. Further assessment reveals increased deep tendon reflexes and a decreased Moro reflex. The nurse should suspect:
1. Cerebral palsy
2. Neonatal syphilis
3. Fetal alcohol syndrome
4. Opioid drug dependence

391. A newborn has been exposed to HIV in utero. The finding that supports a diagnosis of HIV infection in the newborn would be:
1. A delay in temperature regulation
2. Continued bleeding after circumcision
3. Hypoglycemia within 12 hours after birth
4. Thrush that does not respond readily to treatment

392. After surgery for repair of a myelomeningocele the nurse should observe the baby for one of the first indications of impending hydrocephalus, which would be:
1. Frequent crying
2. Bulging fontanels
3. Change in vital signs
4. Difficulty with feeding

393. A newborn with a myelomeningocele is immediately transferred from the birthing room to the neonatal intensive care unit. The nurse in the unit should immediately:
1. Assess for paralysis
2. Start antibiotic prophylaxis

3. Apply a sterile saline dressing
4. Provide routine newborn care

394. A newborn is diagnosed as having a diaphragmatic hernia. An immediate nursing intervention after the neonate is admitted to the neonatal intensive care unit (NICU) should be:
1. Hydrating the infant with isotonic enemas
2. Limiting formula feedings to small amounts
3. Placing the infant in the Trendelenburg position
4. Providing gastric decompression via nasogastric tube

395. A client at term is admitted to the birthing room. Her membranes rupture spontaneously. The physician should be notified immediately if the nurse observes:
1. A bloody show
2. A greenish fluid
3. Clear fluid with specks of mucus
4. Shortened intervals between contractions

396. Twenty-four hours after birth, a newborn has not passed meconium. Hirschsprung disease is suspected. The nurse prepares for a diagnostic procedure that also may relieve the obstruction. This would be a:
1. Rectal tube
2. Rectal biopsy
3. Barium enema
4. Nasogastric tube

397. The mother of a newborn with exstrophy of the bladder tells the nurse that the doctor said her child may develop an unusual gait when learning to walk. The nurse explains that these children may develop a waddling gait because of:
1. Genu varum
2. Tibial torsion
3. Subluxation of the femur
4. Separation of the pubic bones

398. The nurse identifies that a newborn has not passed a meconium stool in the first 48 hours. The nurse should first assess the infant for:
1. Any episodes of vomiting
2. Presence of stool in the rectum
3. Intake and output during the last 12 hours
4. Fussiness during feedings in the next 24 hours

399. A newborn male is admitted to the nursery. He weighs 10 pounds, 2 ounces, which is 2 pounds more than the birth weight of any of his siblings. Because of the baby's weight, the nurse:
1. Places him in a heated crib

2. Performs serial glucose tests

3. Delays starting oral feedings

4. Calls the pediatrician immediately

400. A preterm newborn appears to have a strong sucking reflex. To prevent respiratory embarrassment, the nurse should plan to feed this infant:
1. Every four to six hours
2. Via a nasogastric feeding tube
3. Diluted formula more frequently
4. Small amounts of formula at each feeding

401. A client at 43 weeks' gestation has just delivered a typical postmature baby. The nurse would come to this conclusion because the newborn has:
1. Few creases on the soles of the feet
2. Vernix covering the back and buttocks
3. Dry peeling skin over the hands and feet
4. A red, puffy appearance of the face and neck

402. The nurse recognizes that the lungs of a preterm neonate at 28 weeks' gestation generally have alveoli that:
1. Have a tendency to collapse with each breath
2. Have a sufficient supply of pulmonary surfactant
3. Are fully mature in size, but cannot take in enough oxygen
4. Overinflate and trap oxygen because of excess surfactant

403. The mother of a neonate with Down syndrome visits the clinic one week after delivery. She explains that she is having problems feeding the baby. The nurse recognizes that these feeding difficulties probably are caused by:
1. Lack of teeth
2. Brain damage
3. Tongue thrust
4. Nasal congestion

404. The observations that would lead the nurse to suspect that a newborn with a spinal cord lesion has increased intracranial pressure is:
1. Irritability
2. Absence of crying
3. Depressed fontanels
4. Decreased urinary output

REPRODUCTIVE PROBLEMS (RP)

405. A client at 16 weeks' gestation is being treated for *Trichomonas vaginalis*. The statement that best indicates to the nurse that the client has learned measures to prevent recurrence is, "I will:
1. Void immediately after intercourse."

2. Persuade my sexual partner to be treated."
3. Insert a vaginal suppository after intercourse."
4. Douche immediately after having sexual intercourse."

406. While a client is being prepared for surgery because of a ruptured tubal pregnancy, the client complains of feeling light-headed. Her pulse is very rapid, and her color is pale. The nurse assesses that the client may be:
1. Hyperventilating
2. Going into shock
3. Extremely anxious
4. Developing an infection

407. A client, admitted to the hospital for surgery for a ruptured ectopic pregnancy, asks the nurse why she has shoulder pain. The nurse would base a response on the fact that the pain is caused by:
1. Anxiety about the diagnosis
2. Cardiac changes from hypovolemia
3. Blood accumulation under the diaphragm
4. Rebound tenderness from the ruptured tube

408. The most appropriate nursing diagnosis for a client with a ruptured ectopic pregnancy would be:
1. Risk for infection
2. Excess fluid volume
3. Decreased cardiac output
4. Ineffective health maintenance

409. A client calls the nurse midwife in the antepartum clinic complaining of sharp shooting pains in the lower abdomen and vaginal spotting. She is met at the emergency department of the hospital and a diagnosis of ruptured ectopic pregnancy is made. When obtaining information about the initial appearance of the symptoms, the nurse would expect that they started:
1. About the sixth week of pregnancy
2. At the beginning of the last trimester
3. Midway through the second trimester
4. Immediately after implantation occurred

410. A client has a child with Tay-Sachs disease and wants to become pregnant again. She tells the nurse, "I'm worried it will happen again." The nurse's best response would be:
1. "Did you discuss this with your physician?"
2. "Have you thought about genetic counseling."
3. "Can you remember if Tay-Sachs occurred before in your family?"
4. "It is a rare disease and statistically improbable that it will happen again."

411. A client who had a child with Tay-Sachs disease is pregnant and is to have an amniocentesis performed to determine if the fetus has the disease. The nurse counsels her to plan the procedure at the optimal time of:
1. 6 to 8 weeks' gestation
2. 14 to 16 weeks' gestation
3. 18 to 20 weeks' gestation
4. 22 to 24 weeks' gestation

412. After five years of unprotected intercourse, a childless couple comes to the fertility clinic. The husband tells the nurse that his parents have promised to make a down payment on a house for them if his wife gets pregnant this year. The nurse's best response to this comment would be:
1. "This must have been more difficult for you with this added pressure."
2. "You're lucky; I wish someone would give me a down payment for a house."
3. "Five years without a pregnancy is a long time. Do you think there is something wrong with both of you?"
4. "You know, you don't have to worry about satisfying your parents. Having a child should be a decision you make."

413. A couple is concerned about the risks associated with an in vitro fertilization embryo transfer (IVF-ET). The nurse's response should include the risk of:
1. Embryonic HIV
2. Ectopic pregnancy
3. Congenital anomalies
4. Hyperemesis gravidarum

414. A client comes to the fertility clinic for a hysterosalpingography using radioplaque contrast material to determine whether her fallopian tubes are patent. As part of the teaching before the test the nurse should tell the client:
1. "You will receive a local anesthetic to lessen the pain of the test."
2. "You will have to rest in bed for eight hours after the test is completed."
3. "You may become nauseated during the test, but the nausea will subside."
4. "You may have some persistent shoulder pain for 14 hours after the test."

415. Because an infertility workup involves both partners, a male client is to have a semen analysis. As part of his instructions the nurse should tell him to:
1. Use a condom to collect the semen specimen

2. Make sure that the specimen is collected as soon as he awakens
3. Ejaculate two to three days before collection to ensure a pure specimen
4. Deliver the specimen to the laboratory within two hours of obtaining it

416. On a return visit to the infertility clinic, a client whose temperature charts demonstrate an ovulatory pattern and a normal menstrual cycle despite an inability to become pregnant requests fertility drugs. The nurse should recognize that the client:
1. Has a right to receive this drug
2. Will require an endometrial biopsy
3. Must first be scheduled for a culdoscopy
4. Should have her husband's semen examined

417. A client at 12 weeks' gestation arrives in the prenatal clinic complaining of vaginal spotting and cramping. A pelvic examination reveals that the cervix is closed. The nurse plans care based on a probable diagnosis of:
1. Missed abortion
2. Inevitable abortion
3. Incomplete abortion
4. Threatened abortion

418. A client with a diagnosis of inevitable abortion is being monitored in the emergency department. The goal of nursing care would be to:
1. Explain all procedures
2. Sustain the pregnancy
3. Prevent or control hemorrhage
4. Follow the physician's orders carefully

419. A client at 10 weeks' gestation phones the prenatal clinic to report that she has been experiencing some vaginal bleeding and abdominal cramping. The nurse arranges for her to go to the local hospital. The vaginal examination reveals that her cervix is 2 cm dilated. The nurse concludes that the client is having:
1. A septic abortion
2. A threatened abortion
3. An inevitable abortion
4. An incomplete abortion

420. A client who is to have a vacuum and curettage abortion at 10 weeks' gestation should be told that:
1. General anesthesia will be used to insert the laminaria tent
2. A fever just above 100° F is common for the first 24 to 48 hours

3. The laminaria tent will have to be retained in the cervical canal for 4 to 24 hours

4. A heavy amount of bleeding will be present for three to five hours after the abortion

421. After a first-trimester aspiration abortion, the nurse knows that the instructions are understood when the client states:
1. "I will be able to resume intercourse in four to five days."
2. "After 24 hours I can substitute tampons for sanitary pads."
3. "I can expect my menstrual period to resume in two to three weeks."
4. "I will call the physician if I must change my sanitary pad more than once in four hours."

422. A client at 12 weeks' gestation expels the products of conception. Since the client's blood type is Rh negative, the nurse should:
1. Administer RhoGAM immediately after delivery
2. Administer RhoGAM within 72 hours after delivery
3. Not give RhoGAM because the gestation was only 12 weeks
4. Not give RhoGAM because it is not used when the fetus is dead

423. A client at 18 weeks' gestation visits the prenatal clinic stating she still is very nauseated and vomits frequently. She adds that now she has a brown vaginal discharge. When the blood pressure is found to be 148/90, the nurse should refer the client to the medical staff because these adaptations are suggestive of:
1. Dehydration
2. Choriocarcinoma
3. A hydatidiform mole
4. A spontaneous abortion

424. After the removal of a hydatidiform mole, the nurse monitors the client's laboratory data during a follow-up visit. The nurse recognizes that a prolonged elevation of the serum hCG level is frequently associated with:
1. Uterine rupture
2. Choriocarcinoma
3. Hyperemesis gravidarum
4. Disseminated intravascular coagulation

WOMEN'S HEALTH (WH)

425. When reviewing the role of hormones in the reproductive process, the nurse recalls that the corpus luteum secretes:
1. Cortisol

2. Prolactin
3. Oxytocin
4. Progesterone

426. A 13-year-old client whose menses began two years ago complains of having some lower abdominal pain between each period. The nurse explains that this:
1. Requires immediate medical attention
2. Usually occurs when menses first begin
3. Will disappear when ovulation is well established
4. Is a common occurrence known as mittelschmerz

427. A young client tells the nurse that her mother complains about having dysmenorrhea and asks the nurse what this means. The nurse can best describe dysmenorrhea as:
1. Cessation of menstruation
2. Abnormal vaginal bleeding
3. Uterine pain with menstruation
4. Spotting between menstrual periods

428. A 35-year-old woman presents to the Women's Health Care Center complaining of frequency and pain and burning when urinating. Her medical diagnosis is a urinary tract infection. When instructing this client it is important to:
1. Encourage her to void every two hours
2. Have her record her fluid intake and output
3. Pour warm water over her vulva when she voids
4. Teach her to wash her hands before and after voiding

429. A client is receiving antibiotics and antifungal medication to treat a recurring vaginal infection. To compensate for the effect of these medications, the nurse should encourage the client to:
1. Eat extra fruit
2. Eat yogurt daily
3. Avoid spicy foods
4. Take a daily enema

430. The nurse would determine that a woman with genital herpes (HSV-2) understands her self-care related to this infection when she states:
1. "When I get pregnant, I will have the baby normally."
2. "I can have sex when all the herpes sores have healed."
3. "When I finish the acyclovir prescription, I will be cured."
4. "I have to be careful when I have sex because herpes is a life-long problem."

431. A client, age 16, has a steady boyfriend and is having sexual relations with him. She is seeking advice as to how she can protect herself from contracting HIV. The nurse advises her to:
1. Have her partner withdraw before ejaculating
2. Seek counseling about various contraceptive methods
3. Make certain their relationship is monogamous
4. Have her partner use a condom during sexual activity

432. The nurse evaluates that a young female client who is being treated for a sexually transmitted infection understands instructions regarding future sexual contacts when she states:
1. "I need to ask my partners if they have a sexually transmitted infection before we have sex."
2. "If I have sex, nothing I do will really prevent me from getting another sexually transmitted infection."
3. "I am not allergic to any medicine so if I get a sexually transmitted infection I can take whatever you give me."
4. "I will not have unprotected sex again and I will tell my partners to be tested for sexually transmitted infections."

433. A 16-year-old female comes to the clinic complaining of increased vaginal discharge, intermittent vaginal bleeding, excessive bleeding during her periods, and pain in her lower abdomen. She relates an active sexual history with multiple partners. Based on this information, the nurse recognizes that the client probably has:
1. Herpes
2. Syphilis
3. Gonorrhea
4. Human papilloma virus

434. When assessing a female client who is suspected of having primary syphilis, the nurse should expect the client to exhibit the early sign of:
1. Flat wartlike plaques around the vagina and anus
2. An indurated painless nodule on the vulva that begins to drain
3. Glistening patches in the mouth covered with a yellow exudate
4. A maculopapular rash on the palms of the hands and soles of the feet

435. A client who has been diagnosed as having syphilis tells the nurse that it must have been contracted from a toilet seat. The nurse knows that this cannot be true because the causative agent of syphilis is:
1. Immobilized by body contact
2. Chelated by wood and plastic
3. Destroyed by warmth and moisture
4. Inactivated when exposed to a dry environment

436. The nurse recognizes that a 25-year-old client needs further teaching regarding breast self-examination when she states:
1. "I examine my breasts about a week after my period starts."
2. "I have been looking for dimpling as well as checking for lumps."
3. "I hate doing it. My breasts are so tender right before my period."
4. "My 65-year-old mother examines her breasts the first of each month."

437. To perform breast self-examination correctly, the nurse teaches a premenopausal female that she should be examining her breasts:
1. When she ovulates
2. The first of every month
3. The day her menses begins
4. About one week after her period

438. The nurse teaches a client that when performing breast self-examination she should be:
1. Squeezing the nipples to check for discharge
2. Using the right hand to examine the right breast
3. Placing a pillow under the shoulder opposite the side being examined
4. Pressing the palm of the hand against the breast to compress it to the chest wall

439. The factor in a woman's history that would have the nurse place her at increased risk for breast cancer would be:
1. Early menopause
2. Low-income background
3. Delayed onset of menarche
4. Late beginning of childbearing

440. A 26-year-old female, whose sister recently had a mastectomy, calls the local women's health center for an appointment for a mammogram. To prepare for the test, the nurse should teach the client that:

1. The room will be darkened throughout the procedure
2. Each breast will be firmly compressed between two plates
3. Food and fluid must be avoided for six hours before the test
4. She does not need a mammogram until she is 50 years old

441. A 38-year-old female client is admitted for a biopsy of a lump in her right breast. The nurse recognizes that the finding that could indicate a malignancy would be:
   1. A soft mass that is movable and nontender
   2. Hard, hot, reddened areas that are tender and painful
   3. Multiple bilateral lesions, well delineated and movable
   4. A single lesion in the upper, outer quadrant poorly delineated and nonmobile

442. A client who has had a lumpectomy is to have radiation therapy. At the client's first visit for this treatment the nurse should:
   1. Provide a protective skin lotion
   2. Assess the extent of wound healing
   3. Teach sterile technique for skin care
   4. Demonstrate how to dispose of her urine

443. After two weeks of radiation therapy for cancer of the breast, a client develops some erythema over the area being radiated. The area is sensitive but not painful. She states that she has been using tepid water and a soft washcloth when washing the area and applying an ice pack three times a day. The nurse concludes that:
   1. Further teaching on skin care is necessary
   2. No further intervention is needed at this time
   3. The radiation team should be notified of this occurrence
   4. Health teaching on the side effects of radiation is needed

444. A client is scheduled for a modified radical mastectomy for an adenocarcinoma of the right breast. It would be inappropriate for the nurse developing the client's preoperative teaching plan to include:
   1. Allowing the client time to vent her feelings
   2. Urging the client to have immediate reconstructive surgery
   3. Explaining the dressings and drains that the client will have after surgery

4. Teaching the client the postoperative pulmonary routines that will be followed

445. A client has just had a modified radical mastectomy. During the early postoperative period the nurse plans to teach the client to:
   1. Keep the arm in an elevated position
   2. Observe the incision site for redness and bleeding
   3. Maintain a high-Fowler's position with the affected arm on a pillow
   4. Do range-of-motion exercises including flexion, extension, and abduction of the affected arm.

446. A client who has had a mastectomy returns to her room on the unit. The primary nurse should anticipate that the:
   1. Drainage container will be kept level with the affected arm
   2. Hand and elbow of the affected arm will be elevated above the shoulder
   3. Affected arm will be abducted at the shoulder with the elbow extended
   4. Elbow and shoulder of the affected arm will be elevated with the hand resting on the abdomen

447. Before a client leaves the hospital after a mastectomy, it is most important that the nurse teach her to:
   1. Apply the breast prosthesis
   2. Curtail some of her usual activities
   3. Avoid household tasks that require stretching
   4. Regularly examine her remaining breast for abnormalities

448. When a client who had a mastectomy returns from surgery, a dressing and a portable wound drainage system to the axillary area are in place. The nurse observes an excessive amount of serosanguineous drainage on the mastectomy dressing. The nurse's next action should be to:
   1. Apply a pressure dressing
   2. Notify the physician immediately
   3. Check the function of the drainage system
   4. Elevate the affected arm on additional pillows

449. A client with breast cancer is scheduled for a lumpectomy. The physician tells the client that any affected lymph nodes will be removed and radiation therapy will be given postoperatively. The client blurts out, "My cancer has spread! That's why the doctor is doing more

surgery and giving me radiation." The nurse's most therapeutic initial response would be:

1. "Although the surgeon plans more extensive surgery and radiation therapy, you should not be upset at this time."
2. "Although more extensive surgery is planned along with radiation therapy, it means you will be disease free five years from now."
3. "Biopsies of the axillary lymph nodes are needed to determine whether the cancer has spread. Radiation therapy will not be needed if the lymph nodes are negative."
4. "Biopsies of the axillary lymph nodes are necessary to determine whether they are cancer free, and the radiation therapy is frequently used as follow-up care after a lumpectomy."

450. The nurse in the women's health clinic recognizes that a client who complains of swelling of the labia and throbbing pain in the labial area after sexual intercourse should be treated for:
1. Urethritis
2. Bartholinitis
3. Vaginal hematoma
4. Inflamed Skene's glands

451. A 62-year-old female client tells the nurse in the clinic that she has a cystocele, which was diagnosed a year ago. She has been having urinary frequency and burning. She asks, "The doctor wanted me to have surgery for the cystocele last year, but I can manage using peripads. It won't hurt not to have surgery, will it?" The best response by the nurse would be:
1. "Not really, but it should be done."
2. "Yes, you are risking kidney damage."
3. "Yes, you are risking bowel obstruction."
4. "No, but you would be more comfortable."

452. A 45-year-old client is admitted for an abdominal hysterectomy and bilateral salpingo-oophorectomy. The information from the admission interview that most likely reflects the reason the abdominal method was chosen over the vaginal method is that the:
1. Client has a prolapsed uterus
2. Client has large uterine fibroids
3. Client's cervical os has mild dysplasia
4. Client's bladder leaks urine when she coughs

453. During the discharge conference with a client who has had a hysterectomy, the nurse includes instructions for avoiding the thrombo-embolic phenomena that can occur as a complication. Specifically these instructions should include:
1. Regular blood coagulation studies
2. Limiting fluids to less than 2000 mL per day
3. Avoidance of sitting for long periods of time
4. Compliance with hormone replacement therapy

454. When providing preoperative teaching to a 60-year-old woman who is admitted for a vaginal hysterectomy and an anterior and posterior repair of the vaginal wall, the nurse should prepare the client for the immediate postoperative use of a:
1. Douche
2. Pessary
3. Rectal tube
4. Urinary catheter

455. Four days after a vaginal hysterectomy a client calls the telephone follow-up service and tells the nurse that she has a yellowish-green vaginal discharge. The nurse advises the client to return to the clinic because the nurse knows that there is a need to assess:
1. The blood pressure and pulse
2. The specific gravity of her urine
3. For the signs and symptoms of a urinary tract infection
4. For the presence of abdominal pain and a rising temperature

456. After a vaginal hysterectomy and an anterior and posterior repair of the vaginal wall, a client is returned to her room. The nurse should plan to:
1. Observe the dressing for bleeding
2. Check the client's vaginal packing
3. Elevate the client's lower extremities
4. Initiate sitz baths the following morning

457. During discharge teaching, a client who has had a radical hysterectomy states, "After this surgery, I don't expect to be interested in sex anymore." The nurse should base the response on the recognition that:
1. A surgically forced menopause usually will result in a decreased sex drive
2. Many women incorrectly equate hysterectomy with loss of libido
3. Body image changes occurring after this surgery prevent many women from resuming sexual activity

4. The loss of estrogen that results from this surgery will cause most women to experience a decrease in libido

458. A client is scheduled for a vaginal hysterectomy. She asks the nurse about the changes she should expect after surgery. The nurse should explain that she will:
1. No longer ovulate
2. Undergo a physiologic menopause eventually
3. Experience an immediate "surgical menopause"
4. Have some discomfort during sexual intercourse

459. When discussing future health management with a client who has had a radical hysterectomy, the nurse advises regular physical examinations. The client agrees and adds, "It won't be so hard to go now that I won't need the pelvic examination and Pap smear." The nurse should respond by:
1. Pointing out that pelvic examinations will be necessary until healing is complete
2. Suggesting that the client discuss the need for pelvic examinations with her physician
3. Explaining that regular pelvic examinations and Pap smears of vaginal secretions will still be necessary
4. Agreeing that other components of the physical examination will be more important in the future

460. A young sexually active client at the family planning clinic is advised to have a Pap smear. She has never had a Pap smear before. The nurse's explanation of the procedure should include:
1. A colposcope is used to magnify the cervix
2. A Pap smear can detect cancer of the cervix
3. Vaginal bleeding normally occurs after a Pap smear
4. Scraping the cervix usually is the most uncomfortable part

461. A client is admitted with a diagnosis of cervical cancer (carcinoma in situ, stage 0). When helping the client to understand her diagnosis and prognosis, the nurse should emphasize that:
1. The five-year survival rate for this cancer is nearly 100% if appropriate treatment is given
2. Radiation therapy has been as successful as surgery in the treatment of this type of cancer
3. The cancer has probably extended into the vaginal wall and may require a radical hysterectomy

4. This staging indicates that the cancer is invasive and may require surgery in addition to radiation therapy

462. Immediately after a rape, appropriate nursing care for a client should include:
1. Obtaining a gynecologic history from the client
2. Informing the police before the client is examined
3. Asking the client to collect a clean-catch urine specimen
4. Testing the client's urine for seminal alkaline phosphatase

463. A female client is tentatively diagnosed as having cystitis, pending laboratory results. The nurse recognizes that *Escherichia coli* is a common causative agent in cystitis because it is:
1. A particularly virulent bacteria
2. Commonly found in the kidneys
3. Usually found in the intestinal tract
4. A competitor with *Candida* for host sites

464. When performing a routine physical assessment on a client who is beyond her childbearing years, the nurse identifies that the client has enlarged breasts with galactorrhea. The nurse would expect the physician to order a test for:
1. Estrogen levels
2. Prolactin levels
3. Oxytocin levels
4. Progesterone levels

DRUG-RELATED RESPONSES (DR)

465. A 24-year-old, thin woman, who runs 10 miles weekly, asks the nurse for advice about preventing osteoporosis. The dietary supplement that the nurse should recommend is:
1. Ginseng tea and vitamin E
2. Ginkgo biloba and vitamin B
3. Calcium citrate and vitamin D
4. Glucosamine/chondroitin and vitamin C

466. While receiving betamimetic (tocolytic) therapy for preterm labor, the client begins to experience muscle tremors and nervousness and states, "My heart is racing." The nurse should:
1. Get an order to discontinue the medication
2. Recognize that these are the usual symptoms of preterm labor
3. Obtain the client's laboratory results for electrolyte and glucose levels
4. Reassure the client that these are expected side effects of the medication

467. The physician orders penicillin G benzathine suspension (Bicillin L-A) 2.45 million units for a client with a sexually transmitted disease. The drug is available in a multidose vial of 10 mL in which 1 mL = 300,000 units. The nurse should administer:
   1. 8.8 mL
   2. 8.2 mL
   3. 0.8 mL
   4. 0.008 mL

468. A client who is 33 weeks pregnant has contracted gonorrhea and is placed on probenecid (Benemid) and penicillin therapy. The nurse knows that the client understands the action of the drugs when she states that the probenecid will:
   1. "Minimize any allergy to penicillin."
   2. "Increase the penicillin in my blood."
   3. "Reduce the side effects of the disease."
   4. "Activate my immune defense mechanisms."

469. A pregnant client with an infection tells the nurse that she has taken tetracycline for infections on other occasions and would prefer to take it now. The nurse tells the client that tetracycline is avoided in the treatment of infection in pregnant women because it:
   1. Adversely affects breastfeeding
   2. Permanently stains the baby's teeth
   3. Produces allergies to the drug in the baby
   4. Increases the baby's tolerance to the drug

470. A client is placed on progesterone oral contraceptives (minipills) and is instructed by the nurse to take one pill daily:
   1. Throughout the menstrual cycle
   2. During the five days surrounding ovulation
   3. During the first five days of the menstrual cycle
   4. Throughout the first 21 days of the menstrual cycle

471. The nurse would know that a client taking oral contraceptives understood the teaching about estrogen when the client indicates that the most common side effect of estrogen would be:
   1. Amenorrhea
   2. Hypomenorrhea
   3. Nausea and vomiting
   4. Depression and lethargy

472. The nurse evaluates that a client understands the teaching about oral contraception when the client states that she will immediately cease taking the pill if she experiences:
   1. Chest pain
   2. Menorrhagia
   3. Mittelschmerz
   4. Increased leukorrhea

473. A pregnant client with iron-deficiency anemia is prescribed iron supplements daily. To increase iron absorption the nurse should suggest that the client eat foods high in:
   1. Vitamin C
   2. Fat content
   3. Water content
   4. Vitamin B complex

474. A pregnant client who has been receiving phenytoin (Dilantin) therapy now has developed megaloblastic anemia. It is most important for the nurse to:
   1. Offer counseling regarding termination of the pregnancy
   2. Refer her for nutritional counseling because of her increased protein needs
   3. Explain that this form of anemia will disappear in the second trimester
   4. Tell her why it is necessary to take her prescribed folic acid supplements

475. A 39-year-old woman who is Rh negative is seen by her primary care provider during the first trimester of pregnancy. The nurse's teaching is effective if the client understands that she will first receive Rho(D) immune globulin (RhIg) at:
   1. 12 weeks' gestation
   2. 28 weeks' gestation
   3. 36 weeks' gestation
   4. 40 weeks' gestation

476. A newly delivered client whose blood is Rh negative is to receive RhoGAM. The nurse understands that RhoGAM is given to mothers who are:
   1. Rh negative, have Rh negative infants, and positive antibody titers
   2. Rh negative, have Rh positive infants, and negative antibody titers
   3. Rh positive, have Rh negative infants, and positive antibody titers
   4. Rh positive, have Rh positive infants, and negative antibody titers

477. The nurse should be aware that an anticoagulant drug that a pregnant client with thrombophlebitis can safely receive is:
   1. Dicumarol
   2. Anisindione
   3. Heparin sodium
   4. Warfarin sodium

478. A pregnant client on anticoagulant therapy has blood drawn daily for activated partial

thromboplastin time (aPTT). One day her aPTT is 98 seconds. The nurse notifies the physician because the anticoagulant should be:
1. Increased for better clotting results
2. Discontinued because the aPTT is normal
3. Changed to one of the other effective anticoagulants
4. Omitted for today and the aPTT should be rechecked tomorrow

479. To halt preterm labor, a client is started on terbutaline (Brethine). The nurse is aware that a side effect of this drug is:
1. Bradycardia
2. Hyperkalemia
3. Widening pulse pressure
4. Hypertonic uterine contractions

480. Immediately after the third stage of labor, the nurse administers the prescribed oxytocin (Pitocin). This medication is administered to:
1. Lessen the uterine discomfort
2. Contract the uterus to minimize bleeding
3. Stimulate the breasts so that breastfeeding can be started
4. Aid in the separation of the placenta from the uterine wall

481. When a client is receiving oxytocin (Pitocin), the nurse, aware of the adverse effects of this oxytocic drug, should observe the client for:
1. Intrauterine pressure of 60 mm Hg
2. Contractions with a duration of 30 seconds
3. A fetal heart rate of 120 to 150 beats per minute
4. Contractions occurring more frequently than every two minutes

482. An adverse reaction from prolonged oxytocin (Pitocin) administration for which a client in labor must be monitored closely for is:
1. Hyperventilation
2. A change in affect
3. Water intoxication
4. An elevated temperature

483. A client with severe preeclampsia is receiving 2 g/hour of IV magnesium sulfate. To evaluate the effectiveness of this therapy, the nurse should assess for:
1. A decreased respiratory rate
2. An excessive urinary output
3. An increase in blood pressure
4. A diminished knee-jerk reflex

484. The nurse administers the prescribed dose of magnesium sulfate intravenously to a client with severe preeclampsia. When evaluating her response to the medication, it is important to observe for:
1. Visual blurring
2. Epigastric pain
3. Fetal tachycardia
4. Respiratory depression

485. A client with severe preeclampsia who has a BP of 170/110 mm Hg, a pulse of 108 beats per minute, and respirations of 24 per minute is placed on IV magnesium sulfate therapy. Eight hours later her BP is 150/110, the pulse is 98, and respirations are 10, and there is absence of the knee-jerk reflex. The nurse should:
1. Stop the infusion of magnesium sulfate and notify the physician
2. Administer calcium gluconate as an antidote for the magnesium sulfate
3. Continue the magnesium sulfate infusion because the blood pressure is still high
4. Wait one hour, monitor the vital signs and reflexes again, and then, if necessary, discontinue the infusion

486. When a client is receiving an intravenous infusion of magnesium sulfate the nurse should have its antidote readily available. The nurse knows that the antidote for magnesium sulfate is:
1. Protamine sulfate
2. Calcium gluconate
3. Sodium bicarbonate
4. Naloxone hydrochloride

487. Before giving medications to a client who is six hours postpartum, the nurse assesses the client and notes the following findings: BP 178/110 mm Hg; TPR 98/60/18; fundus firm, one finger below umbilicus; episiotomy edematous, red, and approximated; and one perineal pad saturated with lochia rubra in six hours. In light of these assessment findings, the nurse should contact the physician before administering:
1. Cephradine (Velosef)
2. Hydrocortisone acetate (Epifoam)
3. Methylergonovine maleate (Methergine)
4. Casanthranol and docusate sodium (Peri-Colace)

488. The nurse understands that a drug that is contraindicated for a woman who is breastfeeding would be:
1. Heparin
2. Propylthiouracil (PTU)
3. Gentamicin (Garamycin)
4. Diphenhydramine (Benadryl)

489. A client with severe preeclampsia is receiving magnesium sulfate. The nurse determines that the serum magnesium level may be elevated because the client has:
    1. An absent knee-jerk reflex
    2. A urine output of 100 mL/hour
    3. A blood pressure of 140/90 mm Hg
    4. An apical pulse of 80 beats per minute

490. When planning intervention for a newborn who is suspected of being addicted, the nurse should first:
    1. Examine the mother's arms for needle marks
    2. Observe the newborn closely for the first 48 hours
    3. Check the client's medication record since her hospitalization
    4. Apply a urine collection bag to the newborn to obtain a sample for testing

491. A preterm infant is started on digoxin (Lanoxin) and furosemide (Lasix) for persistent patent ductus arteriosus. The nursing assessment that would provide the best indication of the effectiveness of the Lasix would be that the:
    1. Pedal edema is reduced
    2. Fontanels appear depressed
    3. Urine output exceeds fluid intake
    4. Drug has not precipitated digitalis toxicity

492. A client at 32 weeks' gestation is admitted in active labor. Her cervix is effaced and 4 cm dilated. Betamethasone, 12 mg IM is ordered. The nurse should explain to the client that the medication primarily is given to:
    1. Increase cervical dilation
    2. Accelerate lung maturity in the fetus
    3. Reduce the possibility of a precipitous birth
    4. Minimize the potential of maternal hypertension

493. A client's preterm labor is to be treated with terbutaline (Brethine), a beta-adrenergic agent. The nurse understands that one of the maternal side effects of this drug is:
    1. Tachycardia
    2. Hyporeflexia
    3. Hyperkalemia
    4. Hypoglycemia

494. Based on knowledge of the side effects of terbutaline (Brethine), the nurse should expect that if antidote therapy is needed, the physician will order:
    1. Furosemide (Lasix)
    2. Ritodrine (Yutopar)
    3. Levodopa (L-Dopa)
    4. Propranolol (Inderal)

495. A woman in preterm labor at 32 weeks' gestation receives two serial IM injections of betamethasone (Celestone). The nurse is aware that this medication is given to:
    1. Stop the labor process
    2. Increase placental perfusion
    3. Help mature the fetus's lungs
    4. Reduce the intensity of contractions

496. A client with systemic lupus erythematosus (SLE) is at 39 weeks' gestation. The nurse should be aware that the client:
    1. Should discontinue her salicylate therapy
    2. May need temporary dialysis after delivery
    3. Would probably have a large-for-gestational age baby
    4. Will experience an increase in the butterfly-shaped rash during late pregnancy

497. A client with a large fetus is to have a pudendal block during the second stage of labor. The nurse plans to instruct the client that once the block is working she:
    1. May lose bladder sensation
    2. Will not feel an episiotomy
    3. May lose the ability to push
    4. Will no longer feel contractions

498. Before the administration of RhIg, the nurse reviews the laboratory data of a pregnant client. RhIg is given to pregnant women who are:
    1. Rh positive and Coombs' positive
    2. Rh negative and Coombs' positive
    3. Rh positive and Coombs' negative
    4. Rh negative and Coombs' negative

499. During a prenatal visit, the nurse explains to a client who is Rh negative that RhoGAM will be administered:
    1. To her infant immediately after birth if the Coombs' test is positive
    2. Within 72 hours after birth if the infant is found to be Rh positive
    3. Weekly during the ninth month, because this is her third pregnancy
    4. During the second trimester, if an amniocentesis indicates a problem

500. Vitamin K 0.5 mg is ordered for a newborn. The vial on hand is labeled 2 mg = 1 mL. How many mL should the nurse administer?
    Answer: _____.

Childbearing and Women's Health Nursing
Answers and Rationales

NURSING PRACTICE (NP)

1. 3 Legally, the person performing the surgery is responsible to inform the client adequately; the nurse may clarify information, witness the client's signature and cosign the consent form. (3) (SE; LE; EV)
   1 This is beyond the scope of nursing practice.
   2 The nurse could face criminal charges of assault and battery if proceeding when there is a lack of informed consent.
   4 This places blame on the client; it is the responsibility of the physician to impart the information and the nurse's role to clarify information and witness the client's written informed consent.

2. 2 This is the priority before anesthesia is administered. (2) (SE; LE; AS)
   1 This can be done later; it is not the priority.
   3 Same as answer 1.
   4 Same as answer 1.

3. 3 This response permits exploration of the parents' wishes and will lead to assisting them in making their own decision. (1) (SE; CJ; IM)
   1 This response blocks further discussion; the nurse can answer some of the questions and refer those that cannot be answered to the physician.
   2 This is a value judgment; it denies the parents' right to decide.
   4 This response might frighten the parents; it denies the parents their power of decision.

4. 2 This correctly done return demonstration can validate that desired learning has taken place from earlier teaching. (1) (PM; MR; EV)
   1 Teaching was already done and now must be evaluated.
   3 This is not necessary; a return demonstration provides feedback for evaluation.
   4 Same as answer 3.

5. 4 This is the required intervention when legally required eye treatment is refused. (2) (PM; LE; IM)
   1 This denies the parents' desires and implies wrongdoing on their part.
   2 The client has a right to refuse but must indicate refusal on an informed consent.
   3 This is shifting the responsibility to the physician.

6. 2 The client must be intellectually competent, that is, able to comprehend the outcome of the procedure to give informed consent. (3) (SE; LE; PL)
   1 This avenue may be pursued after the client is deemed unable to provide informed consent; the parent or guardian must be designated by the court to perform this function.
   3 This may be unrealistic with this client; it is more important for the client to understand the outcome of the procedure.
   4 The client should be free from the influence of others who might press to have the procedure performed; this is an individual decision by a mentally competent person.

EMOTIONAL NEEDS RELATED TO CHILDBEARING AND WOMEN'S HEALTH (EC)

7. 2 This is the most difficult part of labor, and the client needs encouragement and support to cope. (2) (PM; CJ; PL)
   1 Medication at this time is contraindicated because it can depress the newborn at birth.
   3 Fluids should be increased at this time because of the increase in metabolism; in addition, this is a dependent function of the nurse.
   4 Breathing patterns should be complex, not uniform, at this time because they require a high level of concentration to distract the client.

8. 1 During the taking-in phase, a woman is primarily concerned with being cared for and being cared about. (2) (PI; CJ; PL)
   2 This is best taught during the taking-hold phase of postpartum adjustment.
   3 Same as answer 2.
   4 This is not a primary concern during the immediate postpartum period.

9. 1 The mother needs to learn the realities of infant behavior and how to cope with them; holding and talking to the baby are consoling measures. (2) (PM; MR; PL)
   2 At this age a toy would not be meaningful and would be an inadequate substitute for parental attention.
   3 The infant is too young to be given cereal at this time.
   4 It is unhealthy to disrupt the baby's sleep pattern.

10. **2 This statement acknowledges the situation and suggests a possible solution to the problem. (3) (PI; CJ; IM)**
1 Postpartum blues occurs earlier; this may be postpartum depression and should not be dismissed lightly.
3 This is not true, and the response does not address the problem that is evident in the situation.
4 This is stereotyping and would not be therapeutic.

11. **1 The therapeutic regimen includes bed rest; peace of mind can best be achieved if the children are adequately cared for. (3) (PI; CJ; IM)**
2 This explores feelings without including a therapeutic regimen.
3 This is giving solutions rather than exploring the situation with the client.
4 Complete bed rest has been prescribed, and the suggested plan assumes that the client is able to afford it.

12. **3 Doing this will help the client relax and will lessen discomfort. (2) (PM; CJ; IM)**
1 The client may become more anxious if the procedure is hurried.
2 This may distract the client but will not produce relaxation.
4 This may make the client more anxious; holding the breath causes tightening of the perineum.

13. **3 This response is nonjudgmental; it permits the client to recognize her own feelings. (2) (PI; CJ; IM)**
1 This is judgmental; it leaves no room for the client's feelings.
2 This is judgmental; it gives the nurse's opinion on a moral question for the client.
4 This response leaves the burden of the decision to the client without offering assistance.

14. **1 This is a nonjudgmental response that encourages exploration of feelings. (2) (PI; CJ; IM)**
2 This response recognizes the client's feelings but cuts off communication because it ends the discussion.
3 This is a judgmental response that questions the mother's decision-making and deals only with the present.
4 Same as answer 3.

15. **3 The nurse's role modeling of the acceptance of the infant, even with the newborn's altered physical appearance, can help the parents to adjust. (2) (PI; CJ; IM)**
1 The parent's current major adjustment concern is the appearance of the child; odor is secondary.
2 This teaching would be appropriate later; the parents first need to deal with their feelings regarding the newborn's appearance.
4 This is false reassurance; there are no guarantees related to surgery.

16. **1 Before learning to care for her newborn emotionally and physically, the mother needs to begin to accept him. (2) (PI; CJ; PL)**
2 This concern is important but will be more easily dealt with after the mother accepts the child with the defect.
3 It is too soon to prepare the mother for surgery; this is a long-term goal.
4 The mother will be better able to meet her baby's emotional needs after she has accepted him.

17. **4 This reassures the client that her baby is all right at the moment and that the nurses are aware of and monitoring the baby's status. (1) (PI; CJ; IM)**
1 This response does not provide the mother with any reassurance of the baby's status or that anything is being done to monitor the baby.
2 This provides false reassurance; amniotic fluid makes the umbilical cord less vulnerable but does not protect against other causes of fetal distress.
3 This provides false reassurance; following instructions does not guarantee a healthy baby.

18. **4 Analgesia crosses the placental barrier; since birth of the fetus is imminent, it can cause respiratory depression in the newborn. (2) (PB; CJ; IM)**
1 The client is exhibiting fear and panic; a back rub at this time would not be effective and probably would be rejected.
2 This is incorrect information and provides false reassurance.
3 Although this is an empathetic response, an explanation as to why medication cannot be given is more appropriate.

19. **4 This intervention promotes bonding. (2) (SE; MR; PL)**
1 Although the infant's physical condition is a priority, the nurse must not overlook the psychosocial aspects of care.
2 Such planning may be unrealistic because the parents may have work and family responsibilities.
3 Postponing teaching until discharge limits its effectiveness; this action does not give the

parents time to demonstrate an understanding of and competence with skills that will be needed.

20. 2 **The mother should be reunited with the baby at the first opportunity and when the mother is emotionally prepared. (2) (PM; CJ; PL)**
   1 Grief work will go on for an extended period of time and has no relationship to when the baby is seen.
   3 There is no magic about the first 24 hours; some mothers are too ill or both parents may be too frightened to see the baby that soon.
   4 Some parents may be too frightened to think to ask to see the baby; the nurse can prepare the parents and then suggest a visit.

21. 3 **To cry in this situation is a normal response; it is also normal to be frightened about touching a small preterm infant; the nurse should provide support and encourage the mother to do so. (2) (PI; CJ; AN)**
   1 Bonding does not have a detachment behavior phase; the behavior indicates apprehension in a difficult situation.
   2 This is not incomplete bonding but fear in a difficult situation.
   4 The reaction to the baby is more complex than merely fear of the NICU.

22. 1 **Parent-infant bonding follows a natural progression involving touch; touching helps the parent overcome fear and initiates the bonding process. (2) (PI; CJ; IM)**
   2 The mother may not be ready for this step on her first contact and the newborn may not be well enough to be moved.
   3 In their state of anxiety the parents are not ready for detailed explanations.
   4 This may make the parents feel unwelcome and set a negative tone for future visits.

23. 4 **By participating in the infant's care, the client will gain confidence in her own ability to meet the infant's needs. (2) (PI; CJ; IM)**
   1 Watching the provision of care by others would only increase the client's sense of inadequacy.
   2 There is no need for a specialist to care for the infant after discharge.
   3 The mother should be involved with infant care as early as possible, not just a few days before discharge.

24. 4 **The client's response is appropriate to the situation; in addition, this is the time "postpartum blues" occur. (2) (PM; CJ; AN)**
   1 This may or may not occur; there is no indication that the feeling will pass or that bonding is involved.
   2 The client's statement is not indicative of depression.
   3 A woman's self-concept usually is not severely affected after a cesarean birth.

25. 3 **Giving the parents true information about what to expect during the procedure will help to allay their fears and encourage their cooperation. (2) (PM; CJ; IM)**
   1 The nurse should be able to provide information and interpretation of procedures for clients; delay in answering their questions may increase clients' concerns.
   2 Reassurance is nontherapeutic; an amniocentesis is a low-risk procedure, but some complications may occur.
   4 If the father is uninformed, viewing the procedure may increase his anxiety, even though his presence may be comforting to the mother.

26. 3 **During the second trimester the big event is palpation of movement. (2) (PM; CJ; EV)**
   1 This is true of the first trimester when the father's concern moves toward providing for financial needs.
   2 This is true of the first trimester when the father expresses excitement over confirmation of pregnancy and his virility.
   4 Childbirth classes are held during the third trimester; the father's response to childbirth cannot be predicted at this time.

27. 3 **This response encourages the client to verbalize concerns; verbalization is an outlet for discharging tension. (1) (PI; CJ; IM)**
   1 This response reinforces the client's fears; it conveys sympathy, not empathy.
   2 This response denies the client's feelings and gives false reassurance.
   4 Same as answer 2.

28. 4 **Anticipatory grief is to be expected with a potential loss; ventilation of feelings should be encouraged. (2) (PI; CJ; AN)**
   1 Gentle, not firm, handling is required to help the client cope with potential grieving; maintaining a positive attitude may provide false reassurance.
   2 This delays coping; it is more desirable to allow the client to ventilate feelings and work through the possible loss.
   3 The use of the word "it" relates to the fetus, not the birth; this is an expression of the grieving process.

29. 1 **The mother should see her infant as soon as possible so that she can acknowledge the reality of the birth and begin bonding. (1) (PM; CJ; PL)**
    2 A delay retards maternal-infant bonding.
    3 Same as answer 2.
    4 This is an independent nursing action.

30. 3 **An unplanned cesarean birth can result in guilt, disappointment, anger, and a sense of failure as a woman. (1) (PI; CJ; AN)**
    1 These are not usually common concerns.
    2 The hospital stay is not exceptionally prolonged; the client usually is discharged within two to four days.
    4 Mothers who deliver by cesarean birth can assume the mothering role.

31. 4 **This is important because deep breathing aids in fully expanding the alveoli and prevents stasis of pulmonary secretions. (3) (PM; CJ; IM)**
    1 This postpones needed pulmonary exercises which may result in atelectasis and retained respiratory secretions.
    2 This response does not deal directly with the problem; it states a fact and does not allow the client a sense of control.
    3 Although this response is empathetic, it postpones needed pulmonary exercises, which could compromise the client's respiratory status.

32. 2 **The nurse should assess the client to see if she is uncomfortable or needs assistance in proper breastfeeding technique. (1) (PM; CJ; AS)**
    1 Immediately providing the formula without assessing the situation does not meet the client's needs at this time.
    3 Pain may be a factor in the client's frustration with breastfeeding, but this would be determined as a result of the assessment process.
    4 It is the nurse's responsibility to assess the situation and arrive at a solution in collaboration with the client.

33. 3 **This opens communication and allows the client to verbalize thoughts and feelings. (2) (PI; CJ; IM)**
    1 This is judgmental; there are not enough data to make this assumption.
    2 This ignores the client's needs and cuts off communication.
    4 This does not give the client the opportunity to verbalize feelings and needs.

34. 3 **Because of the changes in body size, the adolescent may feel insecure as she struggles to establish her identity. (2) (PM; CJ; AN)**

1 There are no data to support this statement.
2 The optimum weight gain for an adolescent should be at the upper range for her body mass index (BMI) to prevent complications.
4 Although physiologic growth is rapid, the adolescent's gravid size falls within the expected parameters.

35. 3 **Vernix caseosa is a cheesy white substance that covers the fetus, which protects the fetus from the amniotic fluid while in utero; most of it disappears by 40 weeks' gestation. (2) (PM; CJ; IM)**
    1 Milia are white, pinpoint dots (sebaceous glands) on the newborn's nose, chin, and forehead that disappear within a few weeks.
    2 The nurse should explain only what vernix is; referring to the infant as preterm may unnecessarily alarm the mother.
    4 This is not answering the mother's question nor is it correct for neonates born at term or after.

36. 4 **Teenagers are capable of cognitively understanding the risk of unprotected sex but often believe themselves invulnerable, which leads to risk-taking behaviors. (1) (PM; CJ; IM)**
    1 This response would not help the mother to understand her daughter's behavior and may precipitate hostility toward the daughter.
    2 This may precipitate feelings of guilt and does not help the mother to understand her daughter's behavior.
    3 Sexual activity may be impulsive which is not conducive to a discussion; also, adolescents who are developing their sense of sexuality may feel too insecure to raise this discussion.

37. 4 **This statement allows parents an opportunity to obtain additional information and review their options to make an informed decision. (3) (PM; MR; IM)**
    1 Recent studies do not support any connection between circumcision and penile cancer.
    2 This information may have already been discussed with the physician; it may be more helpful for the nurse to review the information at this time.
    3 This is a partially true statement; however, the academy primarily emphasizes that there are no medical indications for this procedure.

38. 3 **This is an open-ended response that promotes ventilation of feelings and permits further assess-**

ment of the client's concerns. (2) (PB; CJ; IM)
1 This ignores the nurse's immediate responsibility to assess the client's needs; it cuts off communication and offers no support; ultimately the client may need to have a further discussion with the physician.
2 This not an accurate statement; there are alternatives for some people such as myomectomy, laser surgery, and vaginal hysterectomy; ultimately this discussion may take place with the physician; however, the nurse needs to meet the client's immediate emotional needs.
4 A vaginal hysterectomy can be done if the tumors are small and accessible; this client's tumors are large and multiple.

39. 2 Focusing on the mother's feelings permits her to express fears and concerns. (3) (PI; CJ; IM)
1 This is subjective and cuts off further communication.
3 This answer will frighten the client and cut off further communication.
4 Same as answer 3.

40. 2 This demonstrates understanding of grief work; the nurse first needs to help the individual resolve the current situation. (1) (PI; CJ; PL)
1 Although this is important, it focuses only on a part of the necessary interventions; the client needs to be helped to cope with her loss.
3 This does not demonstrate awareness of the process of grief work; the present loss must be dealt with.
4 Same as answer 3.

41. 1 This response utilizes empathy; the nurse is attempting to show understanding of the client's feelings. (3) (PI; CJ; IM)
2 This is nontherapeutic reassurance; the nurse has no way of knowing this.
3 This denies the client's feelings; it implies that the client should curb painful emotions.
4 This switches the focus away from the client, whose needs should be met at this time.

42. 1 Grieving is expected and necessary whenever a newborn is born less than healthy. (1) (PI; CJ; IM)
2 More data are needed to come to this conclusion; assessments every four hours may or may not be appropriate depending on the severity of the neurologic problem.
3 This may be done later, but it is not the priority at this time.
4 This may delay the client's ability to actively participate in dealing with feelings.

43. 2 Because of the critical home situation, this client probably has both positive and negative feelings about her pregnancy. (3) (PI; CJ; AN)
1 There are no data to indicate that the client has lost weight.
3 The client is attending the prenatal clinic which indicates that she is aware of reality and is not in denial.
4 These are caused by hormonal changes during the first trimester, not feelings.

44. 4 This is a reflective statement that opens the door for the client to express her feelings (3) (PI; CJ; IM)
1 There are insufficient data for this conclusion to be drawn.
2 This false reassurance does not address the client's concern; it may close the door for further discussion.
3 This is not true for all pregnant women.

45. 2 This response provides an opportunity for the client to discuss feelings. (2) (PI; CJ; IM)
1 This statement is contradictory and confrontational, which may cut off further communication.
3 This response dismisses the client's concern, can be answered with a yes or no response, and does not promote the client's further verbalization of feelings.
4 This response dismisses the client's concerns and cuts off further communication.

46. 2 This indicates recognition of expressed feelings; a nondirective response encourages verbalization. (2) (PI; CJ; IM)
1 This ignores the client's present emotional needs; direct questioning frequently does not elicit feelings and may cut off communication.
3 This is a judgmental response because it suggests that the client has been negligent.
4 Although this is a true statement, this response ignores the client's present emotional needs.

47. 2 This response denotes nonjudgmental interest in feelings and encourages open communication of thoughts. (1) (PI; CJ; IM)
1 Two healthy children do not influence the outcome of a third, especially in regard to Down syndrome related to advanced maternal age.
3 This is giving unwarranted information because no diagnosis has been made; this response would close communication.
4 The diagnosis has not yet been made, so information is inappropriate; also this response could close further communication.

48. **2 Anger is a coping strategy that allows a person to gain a sense of control over life; the husband feels a loss of control over the spontaneity of his intimate relationship with his wife; intercourse is based on administration of the medications. (2) (PI; CJ; AN)**
    1 There is no evidence that the client is feeling guilty; pregnancy is desired by both partners; anger is what is being expressed.
    3 The client is not withdrawing or expressing sadness, dejection, or lethargy.
    4 There is no evidence of the client feeling undeserving of an intimate relationship.

REPRODUCTIVE CHOICES (RC)

49. **1 Unless the condom is held, it can be displaced, allowing the sperm to enter the vagina. (2) (PM; MR; IM)**
    2 Spermicidal cream is needed because the diaphragm may be displaced in some positions.
    3 This is not true; sperm can be deposited at the beginning of intercourse without the man's knowledge.
    4 When the woman has a rise in her basal temperature, she is most fertile and should avoid intercourse.

50. **1 Studies have shown that women who smoke at least a pack of cigarettes a day are more prone to cardiovascular problems such as thrombophlebitis. (2) (SE; MR; IM)**
    2 There are no "safe" oral contraceptives for all women; women at risk should be informed of the potential consequences.
    3 Same as answer 2.
    4 This is not necessary if there are no contraindications; oral contraceptives are effective if used alone.

51. **4 Headaches, either sudden or persistent, may indicate hypertension or a cardiovascular event; visual disorders, such as partial or complete loss of vision or double vision, may indicate neuro-ocular lesions, which are associated with the use of oral contraceptives. (2) (SE; MR; EV)**
    1 These are expected side effects, and the client may need an adjustment in the dosage or have to change to another product.
    2 While there is controversy over the contribution of oral contraceptives to the development of breast cancer; the presence of breast pain, which may occur, is not a typical manifestation of a malignancy and is, therefore, not reportable; weight gain, not loss, occurs because of edema.
    3 Hypotension and amenorrhea do not occur; hypertension may occur with oral contraceptives and subsides when they are discontinued.

52. **4 Oral contraceptives may cause deficiencies of vitamins C, B$_6$, B$_{12}$, and B$_9$ (folic acid). (3) (PM; MR; IM)**
    1 It is unnecessary to increase the intake of calcium when taking oral contraceptives.
    2 There is no interrelationship between oral contraceptives and dietary intake of potassium.
    3 There is no clinical evidence that links oral contraceptives and a deficiency in this vitamin.

53. **4 This commonly occurs when women start using oral contraceptives; it is mid-cycle bleeding and if it persists, the dosage should be changed. (2) (PM; MR; PL)**
    1 There is no evidence that this is related to the use of oral contraceptives.
    2 Same as answer 1.
    3 Same as answer 1.

54. **3 This acts as a reminder that the oral contraceptive must be taken every day. (3) (PM; MR; EV)**
    1 A woman should wait two to three months after stopping the oral contraceptive pill before attempting pregnancy.
    2 If two consecutive menstrual cycles are missed, the client should stop the contraceptive pill and perform a pregnancy test.
    4 The client should use a barrier method of contraception for the first month of pill use and if a pill is missed to help prevent conception.

55. **3 This is the preferred method for clients with diabetes because it has no physiologic side effects. (1) (PM; MR; PL)**
    1 This requires a great deal of self-control and a strong desire to avoid pregnancy, and it is not as effective as a diaphragm.
    2 Because of the possibility of perforation, this method increases the risk of infection for diabetic women.
    4 Oral contraceptives have a diabetogenic effect; they alter carbohydrate metabolism, and insulin dosage must be adjusted.

56. **2 The diaphragm is used in conjunction with spermicidal jelly or cream, which remains active for only six to eight hours. (1) (PM; MR; EV)**
    1 Removal this soon would allow motile sperm to pass through the cervical os.
    3 The diaphragm may be left in place as a mechanical barrier, but the spermicidal jelly or cream becomes inactive after six to eight hours.

4 The diaphragm may be left in place for this period of time but it may cause an unpleasant odor.

57. 4 **The diaphragm should remain in place for at least six hours after intercourse; if coitus occurs within those six hours, additional spermicide should be added and the six-hour time frame begun again. (2) (PM; MR; IM)**
   1 The diaphragm must always be used with a spermicide to be effective.
   2 The diaphragm may be inserted with the dome facing either up or down and still be effective.
   3 Puckering, especially near the rim, could indicate thin spots that could rupture during intercourse; the diaphragm should not be used if puckering is noted.

58. 3 **In a normal, regular cycle, ovulation occurs two weeks (14 days) before the onset of the next menses. (1) (PM; MR; IM)**
   1 This would occur in a woman who menstruates every 28 days.
   2 This is too early in the cycle.
   4 Same as answer 2.

59. 2 **The ovum is viable for about 24 hours after ovulation and if not fertilized before this time it degenerates. (3) (SE; MR; IM)**
   1 The ovum is viable longer than 12 hours.
   3 The ovum is viable for a shorter length of time than this.
   4 Same as answer 3.

60. 2 **The fertile period is determined by subtracting 18 days from the length of the shortest cycle to determine the first unsafe day and subtracting 11 days from the length of the longest cycle to determine the last unsafe day. (2) (PM; CJ; EV)**
   1 This is how the last day, not the first day, of the unsafe period is determined.
   3 This is only true if the shortest cycle is 28 days; the date depends on a calculation based on the length of the woman's shortest and longest cycles.
   4 This is incorrect; the longest and shortest cycles are used, not the average length of a cycle.

61. 1 **The presence of the IUD thread should be verified before coitus; the IUD causes an inflammatory response of the myometrium; the inflammatory cells may be spermicidal or damage the ova, interfering with fertilization; also, increased local prostaglandins inhibit implantation. (2) (PM; CJ; IM)**

2 It is not common to have discomfort during coitus with an IUD in place; it is one of the warning signs that should be reported.
3 This is a rare, rather than a common, occurrence.
4 The incidence of vaginal infections is not increased with the use of an IUD; also, the risk of pelvic inflammatory disease is not increased if the couple's relationship is monogamous.

62. 4 **This is the most common side effect of the implantation of nonbiodegradable Silastic capsules containing progestin. (2) (PM; CJ; IM)**
   1 Although this is a side effect, it is less common than irregular menstrual bleeding.
   2 This may occur with some types of contraceptives that contain estrogen, not progestin.
   3 This is a side effect of estrogen excess; this product contains progestin, not estrogen.

63. 1 **Many couples in their thirties who are happy with their family and feel their family is complete choose sterilization as their method of contraception. (1) (PM; CJ; AS)**
   2 Sterilization via tubal ligation should have no effect on dysmenorrhea.
   3 The decision for sterilization should not be made by others, only by the woman herself.
   4 Decisions regarding sterilization should be made when the client is not pregnant and is not under stress.

64. 4 **This is true; some women find it emotionally unnerving to handle their genitals and discharges. (2) (PM; CJ; AN)**
   1 The data do not support this conclusion.
   2 Same as answer 1.
   3 Same as answer 1.

65. 1 **All of these, plus helping families to understand inheritance patterns and recurrence risks and then to select an appropriate course of action, are vital parts of genetic counseling. (2) (SE; MR; IM)**
   2 Laws of dominance, recessiveness, and probability, not predictability, govern which fetus will be defective; contraception may be recommended if risk for a defective fetus is calculated to be high.
   3 Abortion is one management option given to families; it is not specifically stressed for any condition.
   4 Genetic counseling offers all aspects of care, not just making the diagnosis; many family physicians are not well versed in the ramifications and management of genetic illness.

66. 4 According to Mendelian law, because both parents are carriers, this baby has a 50% chance of being a carrier, a 25% chance of having the disease, and a 25% chance of being unaffected. (3) (SE; CJ; IM)

1 This could occur with an X-linked inheritance, or in autosomal dominant inheritance patterns, but not in autosomal-recessive inheritance when both parents are carriers.
2 This would occur in an X-linked inheritance pattern.
3 Same as answer 2.

67. 3 This is important information; removing the diaphragm too early may allow for some still motile sperm to ascend into the uterus. (3) (PM; MR; IM)

1 Spermicidal jelly should be applied inside the dome so that it is directly over the cervical os.
2 Douching should not be done at all, especially while the diaphragm is in place, because it could wash away some of the spermicidal jelly and it interferes with the normal flora of the vagina.
4 Correct placement of the diaphragm affords a close fit from vaginal wall to vaginal wall while covering the cervix.

68. 2 Instructing the couple to have intercourse four times a week with at least 12 to 24 hours between ejaculations will increase the chance of conception and will correct the client's misconceptions in a nonthreatening manner. (3) (PM; MR; IM)

1 This is too vague; specific instructions should be given in a nonthreatening manner.
3 To openly discourage the mate without providing instruction could be harmful to the relationship between the couple itself or the couple and the nurse.
4 Twice daily intercourse is too frequent because it does not allow enough time between ejaculates for adequate spermatogenesis.

69. 3 Women in the childbearing years should be informed of all options available to preserve ovarian function. (3) (SE; MR; AN)

1 "Always" is too absolute.
2 This is an incorrect statement because radiation can influence or destroy ovarian functioning.
4 When ovarian function has been destroyed, it is permanent.

70. 1 Absence of sexual intercourse is the most effective form of birth control (100% effective),
because the egg and sperm do not come in contact with one another. (1) (PM; CJ; IM)

2 The birth control pill has a high, but not perfect (97% to 99%), effective rate when used correctly.
3 This is a fairly effective (82% to 98%) means of preventing pregnancy; effectiveness depends on correct, consistent use.
4 This is a fairly effective (94% to 99%) means of preventing pregnancy.

71. 4 The client should make up for the missed pill by taking two the next day; taking one in the morning and one in the evening lessens the chance of the client becoming nauseated. (3) (PM; CJ; IM)

1 This response does not tell the client what to do if a pill is missed; missing one pill can alter hormone levels and predispose the client to pregnancy.
2 It is unnecessary to call the physician unless other problems are noted.
3 This is wrong advice; missing one pill may alter hormone levels and predispose the client to pregnancy.

HEALTHY CHILDBEARING (HC)

72. 2 Nägele's rule for determining the estimated date of birth (EDB) is to subtract three months from the first day of the last menstrual period and add seven days. (2) (PM; CJ; AN)

1 This calculation is incorrect because it just subtracts seven days.
3 This calculation is incorrect because it subtracts two months and fails to add seven days.
4 This calculation is incorrect because it subtracts four months.

73. 2 Development proceeds in a cephalic to caudal progression. (1) (PM; MR; IM)

1 Both sides of the brain develop at the same time; which side of the brain becomes dominant develops later.
3 Development proceeds in a cephalic to caudal progression and from an internal to external direction.
4 Both sides of the brain develop and begin functioning at the same time.

74. 3 This response identifies the normalcy of Chadwick's sign and provides a simple explanation of the cause; women often need reassurance that the physical changes associated with pregnancy are expected. (2) (PM; CJ; IM)

1 This answers part of the question but fails to explain why it occurs.

2 There is no free blood circulating in the uterus during pregnancy.

4 This response is patronizing and does not really explain the finding.

75. 3 Clients experiencing nausea in early pregnancy often experience relief if they maintain something in their stomachs; it is best to avoid an empty or overloaded stomach. (1) (PM; MR; IM)

1 Low sodium antacids may be prescribed to be taken between meals to promote relief from heartburn, not nausea.

2 Carbonated beverages may or may not help, but women should be advised to take fluids between, not with meals.

4 This practice is more helpful for women who experience classic morning sickness during the immediate hours after awakening; it does not help control nausea late in the day.

76. 4 Although there are no limitations on sexual activity, the client and her partner may need some guidance in altering positions to make sexual activity more comfortable. (2) (PM; CJ; IM)

1 Intercourse may be continued throughout the entire pregnancy if no complications arise.

2 This is unnecessary if the cervical plug is still in place and the membranes are intact.

3 Sex information can be given by a professional nurse; it is not necessary to refer this to another care provider.

77. 1 Any regular activity that was typical before pregnancy can be continued in pregnancy if there are no complications such as bleeding, cramps, or pain. (2) (PM; CJ; IM)

2 It is not necessary to stop riding at six months unless the woman is uncomfortable or it is otherwise contraindicated.

3 A woman used to riding horses can continue; no exercise is too strenuous if it has been done consistently before pregnancy.

4 Both activities are acceptable as long as the woman is accustomed to doing them.

78. 4 Increased levels of hCG may cause nausea and vomiting, but the exact reason for this is unknown. (1) (PM; CJ; AN)

1 Some women do not experience nausea and vomiting.

2 Lightening occurs at the end of the third trimester; nausea and vomiting usually cease at the end of the first trimester.

3 Nausea and vomiting are unrelated to whether the pregnancy is desired or unwanted.

79. 1 There is reduced GI motility during pregnancy because of the high level of placental progesterone and displacement of the stomach superiorly and the intestines laterally and posteriorly; absorption of some drugs, vitamins, and minerals may be increased. (3) (PM; CJ; AN)

2 The glomerular filtration rate increases during pregnancy.

3 This is unrelated to the absorption of drugs.

4 This is unrelated to the absorption of drugs; the amount of gastric secretion is somewhat lower in the first and second trimesters but increases dramatically in the third trimester.

80. 1 The Salk vaccine (TOPV) may be given because it is a killed virus vaccine and will not have a teratogenic effect on the fetus. (3) (PM; CJ; IM)

2 This vaccine consists of an attenuated live virus that may be teratogenic to the fetus and is contraindicated during pregnancy.

3 Same as answer 2.

4 Same as answer 2.

81. 4 This amount is recommended by the Food and Nutrition Board of the National Academy of Sciences. (1) (PM; MR; IM)

1 This is less than the recommended requirement.

2 Same as answer 1.

3 Same as answer 1.

82. 4 Often there is a decrease in sexual desire in the first trimester, probably related to nausea and vomiting; if couples are informed about this, they are less likely to become distressed. (2) (PM; CJ; IM)

1 Calling the situation a problem may cause further anxiety in the client.

2 The client is asking the nurse for information; the client is unable to answer this question.

3 This does not tell the client why this feeling is occurring; this provides false reassurance.

83. 1 At 12 weeks' gestation the enlarging uterus begins to rise out of the pelvis and is palpable just above the symphysis pubis. (3) (PM; CJ; AS)

2 During the early weeks of gestation the uterus remains in the pelvic cavity.

3 Usually this occurs at about 16 weeks' gestation.

4 This occurs later than 12 weeks' gestation when the fundus has risen completely out of the pelvis.

84. 4 **Fasting results in hypoglycemia, which can cause nausea; in addition, the developing fetus should not be deprived of nutrients for any length of time. (2) (PM; MR; PL)**
1 Fluids need not be increased but should be consumed between meals.
2 This intake would not be sufficient to meet the normal nutritional needs of the mother and fetus.
3 Calcium intake will not change the nausea.

85. 4 **This is within the recommended weight gain for a woman who was of average weight for her height before pregnancy. (1) (PM; CJ; AN)**
1 This is less than the recommended weight gain for a woman who was of average weight for her height before pregnancy.
2 Same as answer 1.
3 Same as answer 1.

86. 3 **Most women feel movement by the 20th week of gestation. (2) (PM; CJ; IM)**
1 Twelve weeks is too early to feel movement.
2 Multiparas may feel movement this early, but for most primigravidas movement is felt between 18 to 20 weeks.
4 This is very late to feel initial movement; lack of movement by the 24th week might indicate a problem.

87. 1 **This avoids the possibility of ingesting cysts infected with the toxoplasma protozoa. (3) (PM; MR; IM)**
2 This disease, though more prevalent in foreign countries, is seen in the United States.
3 This is not related to toxoplasmosis.
4 Same as answer 3.

88. 4 **Increased estrogen and progesterone levels during pregnancy cause increased vascularization and resultant congestion of mucous membranes. (2) (PM; CJ; IM)**
1 Nasal decongestants are not advised during pregnancy; clients should consult a physician before using any medication.
2 The contrary is true; it is not common for women to develop allergies during pregnancy.
3 This is expected because of the higher estrogen and progesterone levels during pregnancy.

89. 4 **The fetal heartbeat can be heard with an electronic Doppler between 10 and 12 weeks' gestation. (1) (PM; CJ; IM)**
1 This is too early for the heartbeat to be heard with a fetoscope; a fetoscope cannot pick up the fetal heartbeat before the 17th week
2 Same as answer 1.

3 This is late; the fetal heart can be first heard with an electronic Doppler between 10 to 12 weeks.

90. 2 **The uterus remains in the pelvis until the second trimester, placing pressure on the bladder. (1) (PM; CJ; IM)**
1 The fetus is in the uterus; this is too early for the baby's head to descend, which occurs in the latter stages of pregnancy and can cause urinary frequency at that time.
3 Fetal waste products are very slight at this time.
4 Frequency is a physiologic, not a psychologic, symptom of pregnancy.

91. 3 **During pregnancy the need for water is increased; it is related to the increased metabolic rate and expanded blood volume; there is no indication of urinary infection. (1) (PM; CJ; PL)**
1 Fluids must be increased, not decreased.
2 This is unnecessary; there is no indication of urinary infection.
4 The bladder needs to be emptied often to prevent urinary stasis and potential ascending infection into the kidneys.

92. 2 **The issue of pregnancy is resolved by this time; awareness of the fetus as a person and the body changes of pregnancy lead the client to desire to learn about fetal growth, body changes, and nutrition. (2) (PM; MR; IM)**
1 This information would be appropriate for the last trimester.
3 This information would be appropriate for the first trimester.
4 Same as answer 1.

93. 3 **The funic souffle is blood rushing through the fetal umbilical cord and is therefore the same rate as the fetal heart rate. (3) (PM; CJ; AN)**
1 Twins would have different heart rates.
2 The maternal heart rate should be much slower than the fetal heart rate.
4 The uterine souffle is blood moving through the maternal side of the placenta and is the same as the mother's heart rate; the maternal heart rate should be less than 100.

94. 1 **The recommended weight gain averages 3 to 5 pounds during the first 12 weeks, then an additional pound per week until birth; the client could have gained 14 to 16 pounds and should be told she has gained the recommended amount. (2) (PM; CJ; IM)**
2 This response dismisses the client's concern, and the nurse's responsibility for teaching is

being abdicated by the referral to the physician.

3 This is inaccurate information.

4 Same as answer 3.

95. **4 Before the nurse can determine the adequacy of weight gain, it is necessary to determine the client's correct intake. (2) (PM; MR; AS)**

1 This may prevent further exploration of the diet because the client may answer yes or no.

2 Same as answer 1.

3 This assumes the client is not eating properly.

96. **2 Pelvic tilt exercises help relieve lower backaches, are easily learned, and can be done without any equipment. (2) (PM; MR; IM)**

1 A maternity girdle is not recommended routinely.

3 Sleeping in this position is not advised; it decreases venous return and impedes respirations.

4 Medication should be avoided during pregnancy; prescribing medications is beyond the scope of practice.

97. **2 This is an expected change during pregnancy; the gravid uterus is pressing upward against the diaphragm. (2) (PM; CJ; AN)**

1 It is not the presentation of the fetus but rather that the gravid uterus is pressing on the diaphragm thus impinging on respiratory expansion.

3 There are nursing interventions to relieve this type of shortness of breath; the client should be told to lie flat at times, with a lateral tilt, and keep her arms over her head.

4 There is no information given to suggest that the client's metabolic demands are exceeding O_2 consumption.

98. **3 This is the time when the fetus is laying down fat deposits and gaining the most weight. (2) (PM; CJ; IM)**

1 There is fetal weight gain throughout pregnancy, but it is most marked in the third trimester.

2 There is little fetal weight gain during this period of organ development.

4 Same as answer 1.

99. **3 This is the content of childbirth classes, to adequately prepare parents for childbirth. (2) (PM; MR; IM)**

1 This is only part of the class content.

2 This is not an absolute; most childbirth methods inform parents that analgesics are available if necessary.

4 Same as answer 1.

100. **2 There is much to be learned and practiced so that the client can vary the techniques through the stages of labor. (3) (PM; CJ; IM)**

1 The Read method can be quickly taught to an "unprepared" woman in labor.

3 Medication can be used if required.

4 The Read method focuses on naturalness and denial of pain.

101. **3 Effleurage is a gentle massage of the abdomen. (1) (SE; MR; EV)**

1 This is the pelvic rock; it is used during pregnancy to relieve backache.

2 This is a technique of breathing.

4 Same as answer 2.

102. **4 Kegel's exercises develop and strengthen the pubococcygeal muscle; they are done through repeated contractions of the vagina. (3) (SE; MR; EV)**

1 Tailor sitting aids in relaxing the muscles of the pelvic floor.

2 This is effective in relieving backaches.

3 Same as answer 2.

103. **2 The amniotic fluid is a protective environment; the fetus depends on the placenta, along with the umbilical blood vessels, for obtaining nutrients and oxygen. (2) (PM; CJ; EV)**

1 This is a true statement and would not require further teaching.

3 Same as answer 1.

4 Same as answer 1.

104. **4 Fatigue during labor decreases coping strategies which may result in increased discomfort; medication may be required. (1) (PM; MR; PL)**

1 Progesterone is decreased at this time.

2 Pushing is done during the second, not the first, stage of labor.

3 Energy will enhance the quality of contractions.

105. **2 To meet the metabolic demands of pregnancy during the second and third trimesters the average woman's daily caloric requirement increases by 300 calories. (2) (PM; MR; IM)**

1 This would not provide enough calories to meet the metabolic demands of pregnancy.

3 This is more than the recommended increase in calories for a pregnant woman.

4 Same as answer 3.

106. 3 This combination provides a complete protein for vegans because they do not eat foods from animal sources, which contain all the essential amino acids. (2) (PM; MR; IM)

1 This combination provides a complete protein and would be acceptable to ovolactovegetarians, who eat milk, eggs, and cheese, but not vegans.

2 Eggs are a complete protein but are not acceptable to vegans, only to ovolactovegetarians, who eat milk, eggs, and cheese.

4 These are both unrefined grains but together do not provide a complete protein.

107. 4 A conglomerate of incomplete proteins (vegetable proteins) can result in a combination that contains all the essential amino acids; the client must be taught which specific vegetables to include that would supply all the essential amino acids. (3) (PM; MR; IM)

1 Although important, the intake of optimum dietary nutrients is the priority.

2 The pregnant client should be consuming at least 60 g of protein daily.

3 Strict vegetarians do not drink milk.

108. 4 Folic acid supplements (0.4 mg/day) greatly reduce the incidence of fetal neural tube defects. (2) (PM; CJ; AN)

1 This is not the action of folic acid.

2 Same as answer 1.

3 This is related to the Rh factor and is not prevented by folic acid.

109. 4 Unless a lactose intolerance is present, the client should drink milk; eating dried fruits and high-fiber foods and increasing fluids and activity will aid in lessening constipation. (2) (PM; MR; IM)

1 These can cause constipation.

2 Megadoses of vitamins can be harmful; prenatal vitamins are not a substitute for milk.

3 Same as answer 1.

110. 4 Calcium supplements are available for people who do not tolerate milk or milk products. (1) (PM; CJ; PL)

1 Dental care and proper oral hygiene will be more beneficial for maintaining healthy teeth.

2 Calcium is essential to the pregnant woman's diet for the development of the fetal skeleton; it must be supplemented if the client dislikes milk and milk products.

3 If milk makes the client ill, this would be poor advice and compliance would be suspect.

111. 3 Broccoli is a good source of calcium because it contains approximately 150 mg of calcium per 6-ounce cup, compared with a 6-ounce cup of milk, which contains 216 mg. (2) (PM; CJ; PL)

1 Corn contains about 5 mg calcium per 6-ounce cup.

2 Liver contains about 18 mg calcium per 6-ounce serving.

4 Lean meat contains about 20 mg calcium per 6-ounce serving.

112. 1 Carrots provide the precursor pigment, carotene, which the body converts to vitamin A. (1) (PM; MR; AN)

2 These contain a very small amount of vitamin A precursor.

3 This contains only about half the needed vitamin A precursor.

4 These do not contain any vitamin A precursor.

113. 2 These animal proteins are complete proteins containing all nine indispensible (essential) amino acids. (2) (PM; CJ; EV)

1 Plant proteins are incomplete proteins.

3 Same as answer 1.

4 These are incomplete proteins; also, comparatively small amounts of protein are contained in these foods.

114. 2 A probable sign of pregnancy is a positive urine immunoassay pregnancy test because it is 95% accurate in detecting pregnancy; the basis for this test is the presence of hCG in the urine. (2) (PB; CJ; AS)

1 This is a presumptive sign of pregnancy; there are many other causes of amenorrhea.

3 This is a presumptive sign of pregnancy; there are other causes of frequency, such as urinary tract infection.

4 This is a presumptive sign of pregnancy; nausea can occur during the first trimester because of the secretion of hCG; there are many causes of nausea other than pregnancy.

115. 1 A reactive nonstress test is an expected finding because there are two or more increases in FHR greater than 15 beats per minute associated with fetal movement. (3) (PB; MR; EV)

2 A reactive nonstress test suggests fetal well-being.

3 Maternal movements have no bearing on nonstress test readings; fetal movements and fetal heart rate are monitored.

4 Same as answer 3.

116. 3 **This is a description of striae gravidarum; they occur from the stretching of the breast and abdominal skin. (1) (PM; CJ; AS)**

1 This is chloasma.

2 This is Chadwick's sign.

4 This is a linea nigra.

117. 1 **Measurement of the crown-rump length (CRL) is useful in approximating fetal age in the first trimester. (1) (PM; CJ; AS)**

2 This cannot be detected using ultrasonography.

3 Ultrasonography is used to detect structural defects in the second trimester.

4 It is too early to determine this.

118. 4 **Elevated levels of alpha-fetoprotein in pregnant women have been found to reflect open neural tube defects such as spina bifida and anencephaly. (1) (PB; CJ; AS)**

1 This is not associated with alpha-fetoprotein levels; there are, as yet, no maternal blood tests to determine if the fetus has cystic fibrosis.

2 A Guthrie test soon after ingestion of formula can determine if the infant has PKU.

3 This is associated with low alpha-fetoprotein levels.

119. 4 **A full bladder may improve resolution of the sonogram images in women at less than 20 weeks' gestation; a full bladder serves as an anatomic landmark and elevates the uterus out of the pelvis for better visualization. (1) (PB; CJ; IM)**

1 The procedure does not involve the colon.

2 This procedure does not affect the alimentary tract; fasting is contraindicated during pregnancy.

3 This is a noninvasive procedure that does not irritate the uterus or initiate labor.

120. 1 **A negative test implies that placental support is adequate; it is associated with a low fetal death rate within one week. (2) (PB; CJ; AN)**

2 Interpretable data did not show signs of hyperstimulation if a negative result was reported.

3 A positive test reveals that the fetus has late decelerations with contractions; it may indicate a fetus at risk

4 Fetal heart rate accelerations with movement are reassuring; an expeditious birth is not indicated.

121. 1 **Once the test is initiated the client will require continuous electronic monitoring and will be confined to bed; contractions are more uncomfortable with a full bladder. (1) (PB; CJ; IM)**

2 The client should be in the semi-Fowler's position to avoid supine hypotension.

3 The client should eat so that the fetus does not become hyperactive.

4 Only external monitoring is done.

122. 1 **The markers for true labor are cervical dilation and/or effacement. (1) (PM; CJ; AN)**

2 It is not uncommon for membranes to rupture before true labor begins.

3 The client's perception is not an indication of true labor; because of admission to the hospital and loss of diversionary activities, the client may perceive the contractions as becoming more intense.

4 A change in the fetal heart rate does not indicate true labor; the rate may be slowing because the fetus is resting or distress is occurring.

123. 2 **Walking may increase the frequency and intensity of the contractions. (2) (PM; CJ; IM)**

1 Although this may be a relaxing activity, it probably will not promote the progression of labor.

3 Activities such as walking are more likely to cause progress than bed rest; at this time there is no indication that she should assume the left-lateral position.

4 During early labor slow chest or abdominal breathing helps the client to relax; an accelerated-decelerated breathing pattern is more appropriate for active labor.

124. 4 **The priority is to evaluate the progress of labor so that the nurse can plan care. (2) (SE; CJ; PL)**

1 This question should be asked but it is not the priority.

2 Same as answer 1.

3 Same as answer 1.

125. 3 **Gravid means pregnant, so Gravida III indicates a third pregnancy. (1) (PM; CJ; AS)**

1 Para and Gravida do not refer to the gestational age.

2 Gravida does not indicate either an induced or a spontaneously aborted pregnancy.

4 Neither Para nor Gravida indicates a living child.

126. 1 **The nitrazine paper will turn dark blue if amniotic fluid is present; it remains the same color if urine is present. (1) (PM; CJ; AS)**
    2 Temperature assessment is not specific to ROM at this time; vital signs are part of the initial assessment.
    3 If ROM is suspected, a vaginal examination is done to confirm ROM and to assess cervical dilation and effacement and fetal presentation, position, and station.
    4 A urine test is unrelated to leaking amniotic fluid but this may be done as part of the initial assessment.

127. 4 **An over-distended urinary bladder prevents the uterus from contracting after birth, contraction of the uterus constricts blood vessels, preventing hemorrhage. (2) (PB; CJ; AN)**
    1 This does not interfere with the third stage of labor.
    2 A digital examination to assess vaginal dilation does not require an empty urinary bladder to be accurate.
    3 An over-distended urinary bladder may impede descent but does not interfere with the diagnosis.

128. 2 **This defines presentation; it may be cephalic, breech, or shoulder. (2) (PM; CJ; AS)**
    1 This defines fetal attitude; by palpating for their location, the fetal presentation and the position can be determined.
    3 This defines the position of the presenting part; it may be anterior or posterior.
    4 This defines fetal lie; it may be vertex or transverse.

129. 4 **Fetal heart sounds are heard through the fetus's back; when the position of the fetus is in the left occiput posterior (LOP) or left occiput anterior (LOA), the fetal heart sounds are located in the left lower quadrant of the mother. (2) (PM; CJ; AN)**
    1 The fetal position would be in the right sacrum anterior (RSA) for the fetal heart sounds to be located in the right upper quadrant of the mother.
    2 The fetal position would be in the left sacrum anterior (LSA) for the fetal heart sounds to be located in the left upper quadrant of the mother.
    3 The fetal position would be in the right occiput posterior (ROP) or right occiput anterior (ROA) for the fetal heart sounds to be in the mother's right lower quadrant

130. 1 **The fetus is in a left occiput anterior position because the buttock (firm mass) is in the fundus, the back is on the left, the small parts are on the right, and the head is flexed indicating an anterior occiput. (3) (PM; CJ; AN)**
    2 The right occiput anterior would reveal the back on the right side and the cephalic prominence on the left side; the occiput would be anterior.
    3 The left posterior would reveal cephalic prominence and the back on the same side, indicating an extended head and chin presentation.
    4 The mentum posterior would reveal the back and cephalic prominence on the same side (right), indicating an extended head and chin presentation.

131. 4 **Pressure on the sacral area during a contraction provides counterpressure to the gravitational force of the fetal head in the occiput posterior position. (2) (PM; CJ; IM)**
    1 This may promote relaxation but will not relieve the back pain caused by the force of the head during a contraction.
    2 This may aggravate the back pain because it increases the pressure of the fetal head on the sacral area.
    3 This will do nothing to alleviate the back pain caused by the force of the fetal head during a contraction.

132. 4 **A persistent occiput posterior position causes intense back pain because of fetal compression of the sacral nerves. (1) (PM; CJ; IM)**
    1 This position is not associated with back pain.
    2 Same as answer 1.
    3 This is the most common fetal position and generally it does not cause back pain.

133. 2 **Low back pain is aggravated when the mother is in the supine position because of increased fetal pressure on the sacral nerves. (2) (PM; MR; IM)**
    1 This position relieves back pain.
    3 Same as answer 1.
    4 Same as answer 1.

134. 3 **The major difference between true and false labor is that true labor can be confirmed by verifying dilation and effacement of the cervix. (2) (PM; CJ; AN)**
    1 Some women have a bloody show without cervical dilation.
    2 Fetal movements continue unchanged throughout labor.

4 The membranes may rupture before or after labor begins.

135. 2 **Identifying progress and providing encouragement motivate the client and promote positive feelings about the self. (1) (SE; MR; PL)**
1 A client in active labor should not be left alone.
3 Lying flat on her back may induce supine hypotension; side-lying should be encouraged to promote venous return.
4 There are no data to indicate which phase of labor the client is in; diversion is preferred during early labor.

136. 4 **The frequency of contractions is noted from the beginnings of contractions; these are the points of reference for one contraction cycle. (1) (PM; MR; IM)**
1 This may seem logical, but it is incorrect.
2 This is too long a time frame and would result in inaccurate information.
3 This is the duration of a contraction, not the frequency.

137. 2 **This is done to prevent pushing, because full dilation has not yet occurred. (1) (PM; CJ; EV)**
1 This is not done until full dilation; it may tire the mother and cause cervical edema.
3 This is done in the early part (preliminary phase) of the first stage of labor.
4 This is done in the middle part (accelerated phase) of the first stage of labor.

138. 2 **A full bladder can impede the forces of labor and is uncomfortable for the woman. (2) (PM; CJ; AS)**
1 The client's cervix has been dilating, and therefore it is in true, not false, labor.
3 Before this conclusion is considered, the client's bladder should be emptied to relieve the pressure of the presenting part on the uterus; the client can then be observed to see whether regular contractions resume.
4 This would have been established in the admission examination.

139. 2 **A full bladder encroaches on the uterine space and impedes the descent of the fetal head. (2) (PM; CJ; AN)**
1 The bladder can become atonic but is not physically damaged during the course of labor.
3 A full bladder may lead to prolonged labor but generally it does not jeopardize fetal status as long as placental perfusion continues.
4 A full bladder does not predispose the client to an infection.

140. 4 **This is a description of the contractions during the active portion of the first stage of labor. (2) (PM; CJ; AN)**
1 This adaptation occurs in the transition phase of the first stage of labor.
2 Same as answer 1.
3 Same as answer 1.

141. 3 **The client is experiencing supine hypotension, which is caused by the gravid uterus compressing the large vessels; side-lying will relieve the pressure, increase venous return, improve cardiac output, and raise blood pressure. (1) (PM; CJ; IM)**
1 This will not relieve uterine compression of large vessels; the client should be placed on her side.
2 Same as answer 1.
4 Same as answer 1.

142. 3 **Station −1 signifies that the fetal head is 1 cm above the ischial spines. (2) (PI; CJ; AS)**
1 When the fetal head is visible at the vaginal opening, it is at station +4.
2 When the fetal head is 1 cm below the ischial spines, it is at station +1.
4 When the fetal head is level with the ischial spines, it is at station 0.

143. 1 **The first stage of labor is from 0 cervical dilation to full cervical dilation (10 cm). (1) (PI; CJ; AS)**
2 This is the stage from full cervical dilation to delivery.
3 This is the stage before cervical dilation begins.
4 This is the phase of labor from 8 cm dilation to 10 cm dilation.

144. 4 **The cervix is 50% effaced and 6 cm dilated during the active phase of the first stage of labor. (2) (PM; CJ; AN)**
1 When the cervix is 6 cm dilated, the individual is beyond the early stage of labor.
2 The transition phase of the first stage of labor begins when the cervix is 8 cm dilated.
3 In the second stage of labor, the cervix is fully dilated and 100% effaced.

145. 4 **Meperidine is an opioid that can cause respiratory depression in the neonate if administered less than four hours before birth. (2) (PB; CJ; AN)**
1 Narcan is an opioid antagonist that reverses the effects of respiratory depression; it does not relieve pain.
2 This medication acts as a sedative and may be used to potentiate the effect of an opioid, but it does not relieve pain by itself.
3 Same as answer 2.

146. **4 The client is hyperventilating; these actions promote rebreathing of carbon dioxide, relieving respiratory alkalosis. (1) (SE; CJ; IM)**
 1 This may cause the client to hyperventilate further.
 2 Same as answer 1.
 3 This will not improve the client's respiratory alkalosis, the problem that is causing the client to hyperventilate.

147. **3 Inspection of the perineum is done to determine if rupture of the membranes has occurred; the fluid should be tested with a nitrazine strip. (2) (PM; CJ; AS)**
 1 The client probably does not have to void; rupture of the membranes should be documented.
 2 This can be done after testing the fluid to rule out rupture of the membranes; color, amount, and odor of fluid are assessed before change of linen.
 4 The fetal heart rate should be assessed after rupture of the membranes has been established.

148. **4 This provides accurate information about the labor pattern and fetal well-being; unless there are complications, a decision regarding intervention can be deferred. (3) (PM; CJ; PL)**
 1 There is no indication that the membranes have or have not ruptured.
 2 Labor would not be stimulated until other factors indicate the need to hasten the delivery.
 3 Fluoroscopy is contraindicated during pregnancy; cephalopelvic disproportion (CPD) is most frequently confirmed by assessing the size of the maternal pelvis via a bimanual examination and evaluating the progress of labor in the presence of adequate contractions.

149. **3 Piggybacking the oxytocin permits discontinuance of the drug if necessary while permitting the vein to remain open via the primary IV. (1) (PB; CJ; IM)**
 1 Cervical dilation is checked when there is believed to be a change, not on a regular basis.
 2 Unless specifically requested by the client, there is no reason to maintain this environment.
 4 Although this intervention is recommended, it is not the primary concern at this time; there are no signs of maternal hypotension.

150. **4 Internal monitoring requires the insertion of the probe into the fetal head inside the uterus,**
thus placing the mother and fetus at greater risk for infection. (2) (PM; CJ; AN)
 1 The monitor strips are the same.
 2 Each time the client with external monitoring moves, the baseline may need to be adjusted.
 3 Internal monitoring tends to be more accurate since the recording is not affected by the mother moving about.

151. **4 This is an expected occurrence caused by the interplay between the sympathetic and parasympathetic nervous systems. (3) (PM; CJ; PL)**
 1 There is no need for this intervention because this is an expected response.
 2 Same as answer 1.
 3 Same as answer 1.

152. **4 This fetal heart rate change is known as variable-type decelerations; this is indicative of umbilical cord compression that, if left uncorrected, may lead to fetal compromise; interventions are directed at improving umbilical circulation. (3) (PB; CJ; IM)**
 1 This is not an abnormal finding and therefore requires no action by the nurse.
 2 This is a normal variation of the fetal heart rate reflecting a well-oxygenated fetal nervous system.
 3 These are recurrent early decelerations, a result of fetal head compression during a contraction; they are a nonhypoxic reflex response requiring no immediate intervention.

153. **4 The infusion should be stopped because it is placing the fetus in danger. (1) (SE; CJ; IM)**
 1 This may not be necessary if late decelerations resolve with other interventions.
 2 This should be done after the oxytocin (Pitocin) has been discontinued.
 3 This can be done, but it is not the priority.

154. **2 Respiratory depression of the newborn will not occur if the medication is given at this time; it should not be given when birth is expected to occur within two hours. (2) (PB; CJ; AN)**
 1 The level of pain during this phase can usually be managed by other strategies such as breathing techniques or diversion; giving an opioid early in labor may slow the progress of labor.
 3 An opioid should be avoided within two hours of birth; giving it to a client in the transition phase could cause respiratory depression in the newborn.

4 Giving the medication when delivery is imminent (expulsion phase) is contra-indicated because it may cause respiratory depression in the newborn; the mother's level of consciousness would be altered as well, making it difficult to cooperate with pushing efforts.

155. 1 **If cord compression is allowed to occur, fetal hypoxia results in central nervous system damage or death; therefore, manual elevation of the presenting part is indicated. (2) (PB; CJ; IM)**

   2 This can be done after elevating the presenting part off the cord; this is necessary because with each contraction the umbilical cord becomes compressed between the maternal pelvis and the presenting part.

   3 This would be the next step; first, intervention is necessary to relieve pressure on the umbilical cord and prevent fetal hypoxia.

   4 Compression of the cord would continue in this position; the knee-chest or Trendelenburg's positions could be used to allow gravity to reduce pressure on the cord.

156. 2 **This prevents the cord from drying and the umbilical vessel, which supplies oxygen to the fetus, from collapsing. (2) (PB; CJ; IM)**

   1 The cord is never handled because it can cause the cord to spasm, shutting down the fetal blood supply.

   3 This is not the priority; the priority is to maintain cord integrity.

   4 Priority interventions are directed toward relieving compression on the cord and delivering the fetus promptly, not on monitoring.

157. 3 **This is the most difficult phase of labor; it is characterized by restlessness, irritability, nausea, and increased bloody show; this phase continues from 8 to 10 cm dilation. (1) (PM; CJ; AN)**

   1 The latent phase is early labor (1 to 4 cm dilation); it is relatively easy to tolerate and the client generally is in control and not too uncomfortable.

   2 The active phase lasts from about 6 to 8 cm dilation; it is difficult but is not accompanied by nausea, irritability, and increasing bloody show.

   4 The early active phase lasts from about 4 to 6 cm dilation; it is difficult but is not accompanied by nausea, irritability, and increasing bloody show.

158. 3 **These are some of the classic signs of the transition phase of the first stage of labor. (1) (PM; CJ; AS)**

   1 These are associated with the start of the second stage of labor.

   2 This signals that birth is imminent.

   4 This may signal uterine hypertonicity, which can occur throughout the first stage of labor.

159. 1 **This is the most difficult part of labor, and the client needs encouragement and support to cope. (2) (PM; CJ; PL)**

   2 Fluid management does not depend on the stage of labor.

   3 Breathing patterns should be complex and should require a high level of concentration to distract the client.

   4 An opioid at this time will depress the infant's respirations and is contraindicated.

160. 2 **All signs indicate impending birth; the perineum should be inspected for the appearance of caput. (2) (PM; CJ; AS)**

   1 Assessment of fetal status is important; however, the nurse must first determine if birth is imminent.

   3 This is important to know, but it does not assess the client's complaint.

   4 Same as answer 3.

161. 3 **A continuous blowing-breathing pattern overcomes the pressure urge to push; pushing before 10 cm may traumatize the cervix. (2) (PM; CJ; IM)**

   1 Expulsion breathing (pushing) should not be encouraged until the cervix is fully dilated; doing it too early may cause fatigue and cervical trauma.

   2 This type of breathing is used in early labor and the early active phase of labor for relief of discomfort; it is not used to overcome the desire to push.

   4 This breathing pattern is not effective in overcoming the urge to push.

162. 3 **Pushing when the cervix is not fully dilated and the head cannot emerge can cause cervical edema, predisposing the client to lacerations. (2) (PM; MR; AN)**

   1 This usually is associated with rupture of the membranes before the head is fully engaged; it occurs more frequently in multiparas.

   2 This may be caused by hypertonic uterine dysfunction or excessive oxytocic stimulation.

   4 This results from sudden, rapid labor and an uncontrolled birth

163. 4 The color of the amniotic fluid is indicative of meconium staining; the practitioner must therefore prepare for the potential fetal aspiration of meconium. (1) (PM; CJ; IM)
   1 The newborn should not be stimulated to cry until the airway is cleared of meconium.
   2 Oxygen would be administered only after a patent airway is established and if needed by the newborn.
   3 There is no indication that an umbilical transfusion will be necessary.

164. 1 Using a paper bag helps the client to rebreathe carbon dioxide which corrects respiratory alkalosis. (1) (PM; CJ; IM)
   2 The client needs to elevate the carbon dioxide, not the oxygen, level.
   3 Compressed air does not enhance the rebreathing of carbon dioxide.
   4 This is used to improve lung expansion, not to rebreathe carbon dioxide.

165. 4 Early decelerations are expected occurrences as the fetal head passes through the birth canal; the fetal heart rate returns to baseline quickly indicating fetal well-being. (2) (PM; CJ; AN)
   1 This would cause prolonged decelerations.
   2 Variable decelerations occur with umbilical cord compression.
   3 This would cause late decelerations because of fetal hypoxia.

166. 4 Mild toxic reactions occur because of vasodilation from direct action of these medications on maternal blood vessels; vertigo, dizziness, and hypotension may occur. (3) (PB; CJ; EV)
   1 Labor is not affected because there is no systemic effect.
   2 A local anesthetic does not affect the respiratory center in the central nervous system.
   3 A local anesthetic will not lower the level of consciousness, thus the loss of the swallowing reflex is avoided.

167. 4 The client should be pushing with each contraction; with the head at +3 station each push will bring the caput into view at the vaginal opening. (2) (PM; CJ; EV)
   1 It is too early for the perineum to be stretched to the point of tearing; if this should occur later, an episiotomy probably will be performed.
   2 This is an unexpected and unwanted finding that may indicate that the fetus is at risk.
   3 There are decreased, not increased, amounts of amniotic fluid at the end of labor.

168. 3 This will prevent rapid change in intracranial pressure after delivery of the head. (2) (PM; CJ; IM)
   1 This maneuver will not assist delivery of the head; it is used if shoulder dystocia occurs during delivery.
   2 This could interfere with the delivery and injure the baby.
   4 This could injure the baby; gentle pressure over the entire head is a safer action.

169. 3 The third stage of labor (from birth to expulsion of the placenta) may last as long as 30 minutes and still be within normal limits. (2) (PM; CJ; PL)
   1 Oxytocin is not administered before the delivery of the placenta.
   2 This is an outmoded procedure; it may cause eversion of the uterus.
   4 At the time of admission the client signed a consent form that covers all the stages of labor.

170. 2 As the placenta separates and drops down, the cord lengthens. (2) (PM; CJ; AS)
   1 The fundus contracts and becomes rounded and firmer.
   3 The client may feel a contraction, but it is not nearly as uncomfortable as the painful contractions at the end of the first stage of labor.
   4 Continual seepage occurs when there is hemorrhaging; a large sudden gush of blood heralds placental separation.

171. 4 Immediately after the birth of a neonate the uterus is 2 cm below the umbilicus; during the first several hours after the birth the uterus will rise slowly to slightly above the level of the umbilicus. (2) (PM; CJ; AS)
   1 This is unnecessary; if the bladder were full, the uterus would be higher and pushed to one side and also may be "boggy."
   2 These findings are expected and they should be recorded.
   3 Massage is used when the uterus is soft and "boggy;" when the uterus is firm and the expected size, it is not necessary to attempt to express clots.

172. 2 The third stage of labor is from the birth of the baby to the birth of the placenta; a firmly contracted uterus is desired to minimize blood loss. (1) (PM; CJ; AN)
   1 Providing comfort is a desirable goal but is secondary to the life-threatening possibility of hemorrhage associated with a boggy uterus.

3 This would be a concern in the first and second stages of labor; it is no longer applicable after the fetus is born.

4 The maternal respiratory rate may vary above or below this range.

173. 3 Red, distinctly blood-tinged vaginal flow (lochia rubra) is expected for two to four days after delivery; involution is progressing as it should. (1) (PM; CJ; EV)

1 Clots indicate uterine atony which prevents involution of the uterus.

2 The status of the episiotomy is unrelated to the status of the uterus.

4 Uterine cramps during breastfeeding are evidence that the uterus is involuting appropriately.

174. 2 Anesthesia blocks the sensory pathways so that the mother does not sense bladder distention and may be unable to void. (2) (PB; CJ; EV)

1 This is a side effect of spinal, not epidural, anesthesia.

3 An epidural anesthetic does not influence body temperature.

4 This occurs with general anesthesia, not epidural anesthesia; general anesthesia is used only in emergencies.

175. 2 Gentle massage stimulates muscle fibers and results in firming the tone of the fundus; it also helps expel any clots that may be interfering with the firming of the fundus. (1) (PM; CJ; IM)

1 Elevating the client's legs would increase return of blood from the extremities, but it would not firm the tone of the client's fundus.

3 This would be done only if massaging the uterus were ineffective; a physician's order is required.

4 This would not be the first action at this time; gentle massage to firm the fundus is the priority.

176. 4 This blood pressure is elevated; intervention may be necessary. (1) (PB; CJ; EV)

1 This is within expected limits.

2 Same as answer 1.

3 This is a slight elevation, which is consistent with the physiology of labor.

177. 2 A full bladder commonly elevates the uterus and displaces it to the right; even though the uterus feels firm, it may relax enough to foster bleeding; therefore, the bladder needs to be

emptied to increase uterine tone. (1) (PM; CJ; IM)

1 If part of the placenta, umbilical cord, or fetal membranes is not fully expelled during the third stage of labor, the retention limits uterine contraction and involution; a boggy uterus and bleeding would be evident.

3 Vigorous massage tires the uterus, and even with massage the uterus cannot contract over a full bladder.

4 This is not a sign of uterine stabilization; the uterus cannot remain contracted over a full bladder.

178. 3 Chances of postpartum hemorrhage are five times greater with large infants because uterine contractions may be impaired after the birth. (2) (PB; CJ; AN)

1 On the contrary, early breastfeeding will stimulate uterine contractions and lessen the chance of hemorrhage.

2 This does not contribute to postpartum hemorrhage because the anesthetic for a pudendal block does not affect uterine contractions.

4 This is a short third stage; a prolonged third stage of labor, 30 minutes or more, may lead to postpartum hemorrhage.

179. 4 There are several theories as to why this occurs; one theory is that it is caused by vasomotor instability resulting from fetus to mother transfusion that occurred during placental separation; comfort measures such as warm blankets or fluids are indicated. (2) (PM; CJ; IM)

1 Although the vital signs should be monitored during the fourth stage of labor, they are not being monitored because of the shivering, which is an expected response to the birth of a newborn.

2 Changes in blood pressure are unexpected.

3 Shivering is not a sign of dehydration.

180. 4 Pain becomes excruciating with hematoma development at the episiotomy site because of pressure on surrounding nerve endings; this pain is not relieved by the application of ice because ice only reduces edema formation around the incision. (3) (PM; CJ; AN)

1 There are no data to indicate the presence of hemorrhoids.

2 There are no data to indicate that the client has a low pain tolerance.

3 It is too early to assume that infection is present; pyrexia and local signs of infection would have to be present.

181. 2 **Voiding will be difficult because of periurethral edema and discomfort. (2) (PB; CJ; EV)**
1 This rarely occurs with primiparas, even when a lot of pushing occurs.
3 A second-degree laceration is unrelated to lactation.
4 A second-degree tear is unrelated to maladaptive bonding and attachment.

182. 4 **Prevention of infection is the priority. (2) (SE; CJ; EV)**
1 It is not necessary to stop sitz baths as long as they provide comfort.
2 Stair climbing may cause some discomfort but is not detrimental to healing.
3 This provides comfort but is not the priority.

183. 2 **A client's temperature may be elevated to 100.4° F during the first 24 hours postpartum as a result of dehydration from labor. (2) (PM; CJ; AN)**
1 Mastitis usually develops after breastfeeding has been established and mature milk is present.
3 This usually begins with a fever of 100.4° F or more on two successive days, excluding the first 24 hours postpartum.
4 Urinary tract infections usually become evident later in the postpartum period.

184. 2 **During the postpartum period a leukocytosis (WBC count of 15,000 to 20,000/mm^3) is normal and related to the physical exertion experienced during labor and birth, not infection. (2) (PM; CJ; EV)**
1 This is not a drop in the WBC count because the usual postpartum white blood cell count is between 15,000 and 20,000/mm^3.
3 The leukocytosis is normal and related to the physical exertion of labor and birth, not infection.
4 Same as answer 3.

185. 3 **This phase begins about the second or third day after delivery and involves concern about being a "good" mother; the new mother is most receptive to teaching at this time. (2) (PM; MR; AS)**
1 This is not related to bonding; the let-down reflex refers to the flow of milk in response to suckling and is caused by the release of oxytocin from the posterior pituitary.
2 This is the first period of adjustment to parenthood; it includes the first two days after birth; the mother is passive and dependent and preoccupied with her own needs.

4 The behavior described refers to the "taking-hold" phase of bonding; early parenting involves many behaviors, of which "taking hold" is only one.

186. 2 **Infection is most commonly transmitted through contaminated hands. (2) (SE; MR; IM)**
1 Tub baths are permitted.
3 Douching is contraindicated.
4 This is contraindicated in the postpartum period until the cervix is completely closed.

187. 2 **Ovulation can occur whether or not the client is breastfeeding; if not breastfeeding, prolactin diminishes, the ovaries again become active, and ovulation may occur before the first menstruation; if breastfeeding, ovulation also can occur before menstruation resumes. (3) (PM; MR; IM)**
1 There are general guidelines that the nurse should be able to share with the client; this response evades the question.
3 Ovulation precedes menstruation; the process of follicular maturation begins when prolactin levels decrease.
4 The nurse should answer the client's direct question; the response should not be postponed.

188. 4 **Varicose veins predispose the client to thrombophlebitis; warmth, redness, and pain in the calf are signs of thrombophlebitis. (1) (PB; CJ; AS)**
1 The clotting mechanism is not affected; clot formation results because of venous pooling and decreased venous return caused by the impaired vasculature.
2 These tests, while concerned with clotting factors, are not related to the development of thrombophlebitis.
3 These would be affected by the amount of bleeding that incurred during the birth, which usually is not severe enough to impair circulatory competency.

189. 4 **This indicates subinvolution and needs further assessment. (1) (SE; CJ; EV)**
1 This is an expected postpartal concern, especially with twins.
2 This is an expected postpartal diuresis.
3 This is the milk let-down reflex, which is expected.

190. 3 **Lochia serosa is the expected vaginal discharge around the third to tenth postpartum day; it is pinkish to brownish in color and consists of serous exudate, shreds of degenerating decidua, erythrocytes, leukocytes, cervical mucus, and numerous microorganisms. (1) (PM; MR; CJ)**

1 Lochia alba is the expected vaginal discharge that begins about 10 days after delivery and persists for one to two weeks; it is a creamy or yellowish color and consists of leukocytes, decidual cells, epithelial cells, fat, cervical mucus, cholesterol crystals, and bacteria.

2 Lochia rubra is the expected vaginal discharge on the first two to three days after delivery; it is dark red in color and consists of epithelial cells, erythrocytes, leukocytes, shreds of decidua, and occasionally fetal meconium, lanugo, and vernix caseosa.

4 There is no lochia known as purpura.

191. 2 Breastfeeding stimulates oxytocin release and uterine contractions, resulting in increased lochial flow. (2) (PM; MR; IM)

1 Weight loss may occur more slowly in the breastfeeding mother because of increased nutritional and caloric needs.

3 The increased levels of oxytocin and subsequent uterine contractions will enhance involution.

4 Heat is not contraindicated, and the client may take warm showers; heat is also used if the mother experiences problems such as engorgement or sore nipples.

192. 2 This measure will avert damage painlessly to the mother's nipple. (2) (PM; MR; IM)

1 This is somewhat cruel; breaking suction with a finger is less traumatic.

3 The mother may need to remove the baby from the breast before the baby is ready to let go, and the mother should be taught how to do this.

4 Pulling without first breaking the suction may traumatize the nipple.

193. 4 This dilates milk ducts, promotes emptying of the breasts, and stimulates further lactation. (1) (PM; MR; EV)

1 A large consumption of milk products is not required to stimulate the production of milk.

2 Breast binders may inhibit lactation; they fool the body into thinking that milk secretion is no longer needed.

3 This will contract the milk ducts and interfere with the milk let-down reflex.

194. 3 Exposure to air dries the nipples by evaporation; exposure also tends to harden the nipples, making them less tender. (2) (PM; CJ; IM)

1 Continuous ice packs are used to relieve the discomfort caused by engorged breasts, not sore nipples.

2 This may relieve discomfort but will do nothing to toughen the nipples.

4 If kept from the breast for a prolonged period, the baby may become accustomed to the bottle and not wish to breastfeed again; in addition, absence of suckling will inhibit lactation.

195. 2 If positions are changed for each feeding, the infant will exert pressure on different areas of the nipples while sucking, thus decreasing the possibility of soreness from constant pressure on one site. (2) (PM; MR; PL)

1 Persistent use of nipple shields does not foster effective breastfeeding; the rubber nipple of the shield may cause infant "nipple confusion."

3 The nipples should not be washed with soap because soap can cause further irritation.

4 The entire nipple and surrounding areolar tissue should be in the infant's mouth; pressure from the infant's jaw and mouth, combined with intraoral pressure, will bring milk into the mouth.

196. 4 Compared with the prenatal diet, the diet for lactation requires an increased intake of all food groups, vitamins, and minerals, plus increased fluid to replace that lost with milk secretion; calories should be increased by 500 calories daily over the prepregnant caloric intake. (2) (PB; CJ; IM)

1 Breastfeeding mothers need an additional 600 calories and 5 g of protein per day more than during pregnancy to maintain adequate milk production.

2 The client needs a well-balanced diet, not just additional milk.

3 This denies the client's concern; optimal nutrition is necessary to produce an adequate milk supply.

197. 2 Emptying the breasts limits engorgement, which causes pressure and tenderness in an already tender site. (3) (PM; CJ; PL)

1 Breastfeeding should be continued; it is not only unnecessary but also unwise to remove the infant from breastfeeding; sucking keeps the breasts empty, limits engorgement, and reduces pain.

3 Learning is difficult when in pain; this may be done eventually after the client has some relief from pain.

4 The milk culture may be negative because the infection may be limited to the connective tissue of the breast.

198. 1 **This is like binding the breasts; it reduces pain and prevents further engorgement. (1) (PM; MR; IM)**
2 Medication would reduce pain but would not prevent further engorgement.
3 Milk and fluids should not be restricted.
4 Cold compresses would prevent further engorgement in the non-breastfeeding mother.

199. 3 **If the client expresses milk from her breasts, she is stimulating milk production and this will not relieve engorgement; therefore additional teaching will be necessary. (2) (PM; MR; EV)**
1 This measure is used to give the body the message that milk production is not needed.
2 Non-breastfeeding mothers do not need extra fluids.
4 Warm water will promote vasodilation, lead to emptying of breasts, and support further milk production.

HIGH-RISK PREGNANCY (HP)

200. 4 **Fifteen percent of the women with gestational hypertension during the first trimester develop hydatidiform mole. (3) (PB; CJ; EV)**
1 This is an unlikely complication unless the hypertension becomes severe or there was preexisting hypertension.
2 This is not associated with hydatidiform mole, which is diagnosed before the third trimester; placenta previa is a hemorrhagic condition that creates problems in the third trimester.
3 Premature separation of the placenta is associated with uterine bleeding, uterine hypertonicity, abdominal pain, and a boardlike abdomen; usually it occurs in the last trimester.

201. 1 **Twins should be suspected with a more rapid increase in fundal height than normal; the nurse should assess for two distinct heartbeats. (3) (PB; CJ; AN)**
2 Fundal height, not the size of the fetus, should lead the nurse to suspect a multiple pregnancy.
3 This cannot be determined until an ultrasound is done.
4 Weight gain will not influence the height of the fundus.

202. 4 **Residual urine and catheterization increase the chance of introducing and promoting bacterial growth. (3) (PB; CJ; AN)**

1 A loss of 250 to 500 mL of blood is considered acceptable during delivery.
2 The size of the newborn does not predispose the mother to postpartum infection.
3 This does not reflect the highest risk for infection; a hemoglobin of 11 g is at the low end of the acceptable range.

203. 4 **The many risk factors attributed to this client place her at high risk in this pregnancy, and a high-risk specialist is the provider of choice. (1) (SE; MR; PL)**
1 A history of repeated early spontaneous abortions is not indicated, and it is not at all clear that a genetic evaluation is required.
2 A suggestion to quit or cut down on smoking is in order, but one cannot insist that an action be taken by the client.
3 There is no evidence that this client has an incompetent cervix, and a cerclage placement is a medical decision.

204. 4 **When there is a cephalopelvic disproportion, a cesarean birth is indicated; infusing oxytocin at this time could result in fetal distress and even uterine rupture. (1) (SE; MR; IM)**
1 The NPO status would be appropriate in anticipation of a cesarean birth.
2 A peripheral IV is needed not only for hydration but as a venous access if IV medications are required.
3 The client probably has an electronic monitor recording the FHR and uterine contractions; these assessments should be documented regularly according to hospital protocol.

205. 1 **Because of the client's multiple parity, postpartum uterine contractions may be ineffective. (1) (PM; CJ; AS)**
2 Primiparas would become more dehydrated because their labors are usually longer.
3 There is no evidence of an increased risk for a urinary tract infection; routine assessment of bladder tone should be performed.
4 Clients are encouraged to ambulate soon after delivery; it is too soon to be concerned about the effects of immobility.

206. 2 **Multiple parity contributes to an increased incidence of uterine atony because the uterine muscle may not contract effectively, thus leading to postpartal hemorrhage; a one-hour labor in a grand multipara is not uncommon. (3) (PB; CJ; AS)**

1 A primipara should maintain a well-contracted uterus because with only one pregnancy the uterus usually maintains its tone.

3 100 mg of Demerol is not considered excessive for a primipara and would not contribute to uterine atony.

4 The birth of the placenta 10 minutes after birth of the fetus is normal and would not affect tone of the uterus; multiparity contributes to uterine atony, so the woman who is a grand multipara is at a higher risk for hemorrhage.

207. 4 **An amniocentesis is commonly used to diagnose genetic problems, as well as fetal maturity and fetal hemolytic disease. (1) (PB; CJ; IM)**

1 This is not a reason for doing this invasive procedure.

2 Same as answer 1.

3 An amniocentesis is no longer done routinely if the mother is an older primipara; a sonogram is usually done.

208. 4 **The placement of the fetus and placenta is located by ultrasonography to avoid trauma from the needle during the amniocentesis. (2) (PB; CJ; PL)**

1 Although ultrasonography can be used to determine gestational age, this is not its purpose just before an amniocentesis.

2 The position of the placenta and fetus, not just the cord, is needed for safe introduction of the needle.

3 This is not the purpose of ultrasonography just before an amniocentesis.

209. 2 **Fetal size can be determined by ultrasonography, not by amniocentesis. (2) (PM; CJ; AN)**

1 At 16 weeks' gestation, sex of the fetus is established and can be identified by amniocentesis.

3 An assessment of fetal lung maturity can be made via amniocentesis; however, an amniocentesis is not done for this reason at 16 weeks' gestation.

4 Chromosomal abnormalities can be determined via amniocentesis.

210. 1 **This is done to determine whether any injury has occurred to the fetus or placenta during the procedure. (1) (PB; CJ; EV)**

2 This position enhances placental perfusion, but it serves no purpose in detecting complications.

3 This is unnecessary; the puncture site seals by itself immediately after removal of the needle.

4 There is no entry into the vaginal canal with this procedure; bleeding or discharge is not expected.

211. 3 **The lecithin concentration rises abruptly at 35 weeks, reaching a level that is twice the amount of sphingomyelin, which decreases concurrently. (1) (PB; CJ; AS)**

1 At about 30 to 32 weeks' gestation, the amounts of lecithin and sphingomyelin are equal; this result indicates lung immaturity.

2 The ratio is 2:1 when lung maturity is adequate; it is only early in pregnancy that the sphingomyelin concentration is higher than the lecithin concentration.

4 It is not until the L/S ratio is 2:1 that fetal lung maturity is attained.

212. 4 **It is possible that stimulation of the uterus resulting from the amniocentesis may cause uterine contractions. (1) (PB; CJ; EV)**

1 This is not necessary because an amniocentesis is not done via the vagina.

2 This is irrelevant because amniotic fluid is in no way influenced by the intake of fluid.

3 This should not be necessary because the pinprick opening seals immediately.

213. 3 **A nontender uterus and bright red bleeding are classic signs of placenta previa; as the cervix dilates the overlying placenta separates from the uterus and begins to bleed. (3) (PB; CJ; AN)**

1 There is no information to indicate that the client is in labor and no mention is made of any contractions.

2 Information does not indicate that the client had contractions, which have now ceased.

4 The classic adaptations of abruptio placentae are pain and a rigid boardlike abdomen; dark red blood may or may not be present.

214. 2 **In a healthy well-oxygenated fetus the heart rate increases with fetal movement; the test looks for accelerations of 15 beats with fetal movements. (2) (PB; CJ; AS)**

1 This is not a part of the evaluation of the fetus in the nonstress test.

3 Same as answer 1.

4 This is used in the contraction stress test (CST).

215. 4 During a CST uterine blood decreases, and, when there is too great a decrease, fetal hypoxia and late decelerations occur, reflecting diminished placental function. (2) (PB; CJ; AN)

  1 Although this may cause fetal problems, the CST cannot determine this.
  2 The CST cannot determine gestational age; this is accomplished through a sonogram.
  3 The CST cannot determine this because amniotic fluid is not obtained.

216. 2 Bleeding could indicate placenta previa or abruptio placentae, which would be aggravated by the contractions from the use of Pitocin. (1) (SE; CJ; AN)

  1 An oxytocin challenge test is not contraindicated; blurred vision may indicate preeclampsia; cardiac problems may diminish oxygen perfusion to the placenta and compromise the fetus during labor; fetal tolerance to the stress of contractions would be assessed.
  3 An oxytocin challenge test is not contraindicated; sickling may reduce oxygen perfusion to the placenta and compromise the fetus during labor.
  4 An oxytocin challenge test is not contraindicated; arteriolar spasms may diminish oxygen perfusion to the placenta and compromise the fetus during labor; fetal tolerance would be evaluated by this test.

217. 2 An ABO incompatibility may develop even in first-born infants since the mother has antibodies against the antigens of the A and B blood cells; these antibodies are transferred across the placenta and produce hemolysis of the fetal RBCs; if the infant were AB, an incompatibility may also occur. (3) (PB; CJ; AN)

  1 No problems will occur if the mother is Rh positive and the baby is Rh negative, only the other way around.
  3 A preterm birth will not produce an incompatibility; it may intensify problems if an incompatibility exists.
  4 If the baby is the same type and has the same Rh factor as the mother, no incompatibility occurs.

218. 3 This is premature placental separation; the classic signs are abdominal rigidity, a tetanic uterus, and dark red bleeding. (1) (PB; CJ; AS)

  1 Information on cervical effacement, dilation, and station would be required for this conclusion.

  2 This occurs with a low-lying placenta and is manifested by painless bright red bleeding.
  4 Fetal presentation is not related to the client's signs and symptoms.

219. 3 Early postoperative ambulation helps prevent many postpartal complications such as thrombophlebitis and constipation. (2) (PB; MR; PL)

  1 Clients are generally discharged by the third or fourth postpartum day.
  2 A bowel movement can occur spontaneously if early ambulation and adequate fluids are encouraged.
  4 Clients are permitted to shower within 48 hours.

220. 1 A tightly contracted uterus in the midline reflects normal physiologic functioning following birth of the fetuses and expulsion of the placenta; an atonic uterus is a common complication of a multiple birth. (1) (PM; CJ; EV)

  2 The woman may have complications but can still breastfeed her infants.
  3 When considering recovery following a multiple birth, physiologic stabilization takes precedence over psychologic concerns.
  4 Resting comfortably does not indicate an uncomplicated birth; a client can be resting quietly while hemorrhaging.

221. 4 Just as after any surgery, pain is a major postoperative problem during the first 24 hours after cesarean birth. (3) (PB; CJ; AN)

  1 Oral intake is not a priority concern.
  2 Promoting bowel function is not a priority concern.
  3 Gaseous distention is more likely to occur later.

222. 2 Palpation will indicate whether bladder distention is present; the increased intra-abdominal space available after birth can result in bladder distention without discomfort. (2) (PB; CJ; EV)

  1 A physician's order is needed for catheterization.
  3 Measurement alone is not sufficient for 24 to 48 hours postpartum.
  4 Trauma to the area makes surrounding organs atonic; the client may have a full bladder and not feel the urge to void.

223. 2 Because pregnant women with heart disease are more prone to anemia, there may be an additional need for iron and folic acid. (1) (PB; CJ; IM)

  1 If the pregnant client with heart disease is eating the recommended pregnancy diet

and taking prenatal vitamin and mineral supplements, there is no additional need for these nutrients.
3 Same as answer 1.
4 Same as answer 1.

224. 2 **Cardiac decompensation may occur because of the increased circulating blood volume after delivery which requires increased cardiac functioning. (1) (PB; CJ; EV)**
1 Although important, observation for cardiac decompensation is a higher priority.
3 Same as answer 1.
4 Instructions are an essential component of the care plan, but at this time it is not the highest priority.

225. 4 **Adequate analgesia and anesthesia are essential to reduce pain and anxiety which stress the heart; resting and limiting stress will conserve energy and reduce cardiac output. (3) (PM; CJ; PL)**
1 These interventions are appropriate for a client with advanced cardiac disease, not for a client with Class 1 heart disease.
2 Seizure precautions are not indicated at this time; however, other symptoms may indicate cardiac decompensation.
3 Clients with Class 1 cardiac disease should be advised to rest; protein monitoring and penicillin are inappropriate if preeclampsia and infection are not present.

226. 2 **This position is preferred for the cardiac client in labor since it promotes cardiac and respiratory function and prevents the gravid uterus from impinging on the diaphragm. (2) (PB; CJ; IM)**
1 If placed in this position, the client might develop supine hypotension syndrome because of the gravid uterus pressing on the inferior vena cava.
3 This position is uncomfortable for a client in labor; the gravid uterus would impinge on the diaphragm and impede respiratory excursion, which could lead to decreased cardiac output.
4 The gravid uterus would impinge on the diaphragm and respiratory and cardiac function would be compromised.

227. 4 **This is the accepted definition of placenta previa. (2) (PB; CJ; AN)**
1 This occurs in abruptio placentae.
2 Same as answer 1.
3 This may not lead to placenta previa but will place the fetus in jeopardy.

228. 4 **With a low-implanted placenta (placenta previa) the presenting part may have difficulty entering the pelvis. (3) (PB; CJ; AS)**
1 Engagement is difficult with a low-lying placenta.
2 Placenta previa does not make it difficult to palpate small fetal parts.
3 This occurs with abruptio placentae.

229. 1 **This position shunts blood to the upper body and vital organs. (3) (PB; CJ; AN)**
2 The bleeding will continue regardless of this position.
3 Pressure on the cervix is thought to have no bearing on bleeding episodes.
4 The placenta is implanted and positioning will not move it off the cervix.

230. 3 **A speculum examination may result in a sudden, severe hemorrhage because of the location of the placenta near the cervical os; blood should be ready for administration to prevent shock. (2) (PB; MR; PL)**
1 This is an incorrect response; fresh plasma may be used to restore coagulation factors when DIC occurs after severe blood loss.
2 Adults manufacture their own vitamin K, and an injection would not help to prevent bleeding from the placenta.
4 Giving heparin sodium is contraindicated in the presence of hemorrhage.

231. 1 **This will allow saliva to drain out of the mouth by gravity which will help to maintain a patent airway. (1) (PB; CJ; IM)**
2 This is contraindicated because it could cause an injury.
3 Although birth may be imminent, the priority is to maintain a patent airway.
4 During the seizure the priority is to protect the mother, not assess the fetus.

232. 1 **The symptoms indicate loss of blood; to compensate for the decreased cardiac output, oxygen is needed to maintain the well-being of both the mother and the fetus. (1) (PB; CJ; IM)**
2 This would decrease blood flow to the vital centers in the brain.
3 This would not be the first action; in view of the blood loss, providing oxygen is the priority.
4 This could mask abdominal pain and sedate an already compromised fetus.

233. 3 **A total placenta previa would necessitate a cesarean birth; early intervention helps ensure a healthy neonate and mother. (2) (PB; CJ; AN)**

1 This is a complication that may necessitate an early delivery to ensure a healthy neonate or mother.

2 Same as answer 1.

4 Induction of labor would be indicated if the fetus is at term, since prolonged rupture of membranes can lead to maternal and/or fetal sepsis.

234. 3 **As the cervix opens with labor, bleeding may ensue; blood loss is estimated and treatment is based on the maternal/fetal response. (2) (PB; CJ; AS)**

1 A fetal monitor would be indicated because it more accurately records fetal well-being.

2 This is done in the postpartum period, not while the client is in labor.

4 This is contraindicated; these examinations may stimulate greater bleeding if the placenta is accidentally dislodged.

235. 4 **Folic acid is needed to produce heme for hemoglobin. (3) (PB; MR; AN)**

1 Folic acid may reduce the risk of a sequestration crisis, but it will not prevent it.

2 There is no relationship between folic acid and the reduction of sickling.

3 There is no change in needs; sickling decreases the oxygen-carrying capacity of hemoglobin.

236. 2 **Raisins and dried figs have a greater iron content than other fruits. (2) (PM; MR; IM)**

1 These foods are poor sources of iron.

3 Same as answer 1.

4 Same as answer 1.

237. 3 **These clients are particularly vulnerable to infections, especially of the genitourinary tract; urine cultures should be performed frequently. (2) (PM; CJ; AS)**

1 Hypothyroidism affects 1 in 1500 women during pregnancy; women with sickle cell anemia are not at any higher risk for hypothyroidism than the general population.

2 Women with sickle cell anemia are not at an increased risk for this problem during pregnancy.

4 Same as answer 2.

238. 2 **A floating fetal head in a primigravida at 42 weeks' gestation who is in early labor is suggestive of disproportion because engagement usually occurs before labor in primigravidas. (3) (PM; CJ; AN)**

1 This test confirms the presence of ruptured membranes, which should not cause any problems.

3 This occurs during early labor when the presenting part bears down on the capillary structure of the cervix.

4 This falls within the normal range of 110 to 160 beats per minute.

239. 2 **The feet or buttocks are not effective in blocking the cervical opening, and the cord may slip through and be compressed. (2) (PB; CJ; AS)**

1 Rapid dilation and precipitate labor can occur with infants in cephalic positions as well.

3 Uterine inertia may result from fatigue or cephalopelvic disproportion and is not necessarily related to fetal position.

4 This is not specific to breech labors.

240. 3 **This occurs because pressure on the fetal abdomen from the contractions forces meconium from the bowel. (2) (PM; CJ; AN)**

1 Cord prolapse is not an absolute, but it may occur if the presenting part does not fill the pelvic cavity.

2 Fetal heart abnormalities are identified by auscultation or continuous electronic fetal monitoring, not by the presence of meconium.

4 This is unnecessary; this is a normal occurrence caused by pressure on the fetal abdomen during contractions when the fetus is in the breech position.

241. 4 **A cesarean birth may be performed when the fetus is in the breech presentation because there is an increased risk of morbidity and mortality. (2) (PB; CJ; AN)**

1 Meconium is a common finding in the amniotic fluid of a client whose fetus is in a breech presentation because contractions compress the fetal intestinal tract causing release of meconium.

2 Vertex presentations with occiput posterior cause back discomfort.

3 Labors are usually longer with a fetus in the breech presentation because the buttocks are not as effective as the head as a dilating wedge.

242. 2 **Pelvic pressure or a feeling that the baby is pushing down is one symptom of preterm labor and should be taught to the client so that she can present herself early for care. (3) (PM; CJ; IM)**

1 This is not a danger sign of preterm labor.

3 These are not danger signs of preterm labor.

4 Fetal movement is not normally felt until approximately 16 weeks.

243. 4 This provides accurate information; an increase of 30 mm Hg in the systolic reading or an increase of 15 mm Hg in the diastolic reading indicates hypertension during pregnancy. (2) (PM; CJ; IM)

1 This is false reassurance.
2 This could be frightening and elevate the blood pressure even more.
3 This response is demeaning.

244. 3 Bed rest keeps the pressure of the fetal head off the cervix; the side-lying position keeps the gravid uterus from impeding major vessels, thus enhancing uterine perfusion. (2) (PM; MR; PL)

1 These are used only when the cord is prolapsed or the client is in shock.
2 Sitting up in bed increases pressure on the cervix; this may lead to further dilation.
4 This may aid in relieving pressure of the fetus on the cervix, but it will not enhance uterine perfusion.

245. 4 Prostaglandins in semen may stimulate labor, and penile contact with the cervix may increase myometrial contractility. (1) (PM; MR; IM)

1 Sexual intercourse may cause labor to progress; birth is not desired in the 33rd week of pregnancy.
2 Same as answer 1.
3 Same as answer 1.

246. 2 A test of the amniotic fluid can determine the fetus's lung maturity; this determination can assist with the timing of a scheduled birth. (2) (PB; CJ; IM)

1 This can be done by a less invasive procedure such as an ultrasonography.
3 Cesarean births are not done routinely on women with diabetes unless a vaginal delivery has been ruled out.
4 The size of the fetus cannot be determined by amniocentesis; it may be approximated by palpation or sonographic measurements.

247. 3 Insulin requirements may fall suddenly during the first 24 to 48 hours postpartum because endocrine changes of pregnancy are reversed. (3) (PB; CJ; AN)

1 Insulin requirements suddenly, not slowly, decrease because of the rapid physiologic changes occurring after delivery.
2 Insulin requirements decrease, not increase, during the postpartum period.
4 Insulin requirements of women with diabetes fluctuate throughout pregnancy

and decrease suddenly during the postpartum period.

248. 2 Painful contractions at this time may indicate preterm labor; irregular intermittent contractions that move blood through the intervillous spaces aiding placental circulation may occur during pregnancy; these preparatory contractions (formerly called Braxton-Hicks contractions) may be painless or uncomfortable, but not painful. (2) (PM; CJ; AS)

1 Frequent urination is common during the last trimester because of the pressure of the enlarging fetus; painful urination may indicate a urinary tract infection.
3 Fetal movement usually increases after the mother eats.
4 Difficulty sleeping and lower back pain are both common adaptations during the third trimester.

249. 1 Although it has not been proven that bed rest prevents preterm labor, it is still often recommended; activities are restricted to bathroom privileges and movement to a daytime resting area. (2) (PB; CJ; PL)

2 Fluid intake should not be restricted; pregnancy nutrition should be maintained.
3 Monitoring the urinary protein level is included in the care of a client with preeclampsia, not preterm labor.
4 Deep breathing exercises do not prevent preterm labor.

250. 1 Labor is continuing, and the promotion of the well-being of the client and fetus is the priority for nursing care during this period. (2) (PM; CJ; PL)

2 This response addresses only one aspect of this client's needs; this problem must be dealt with in the context of her other needs.
3 Same as answer 1.
4 Same as answer 1.

251. 4 The normal fetal heart rate (FHR) is 110 to 160; an FHR of 186 is considered tachycardic and further evaluation is necessary. (1) (PB; CJ; AS)

1 The fetus may be at risk because an FHR of 186 is above the normal range of 110 to 160 beats per minute.
2 The speed of descent of the fetus is not related to the FHR except during a contraction.
3 Although fetal tachycardia is associated with infection, other causes must be ruled out as well; further assessment is needed.

252. 3 The risk of developing chorioamnionitis (intra-amniotic infection) is increased with prolonged rupture of the membranes; foul-smelling fluid is a sign of infection. (3) (SE; CJ; AS)

1 A prolapsed cord usually occurs shortly after the membranes rupture.

2 This is an abnormally implanted placenta; it is totally unrelated to ruptured membranes.

4 This is premature separation of a normally implanted placenta; it is totally unrelated to ruptured membranes.

253. 2 Bandl's ring is a pathologic retraction ring that is a ridge around the uterus at the junction of the upper and lower uterine segments; the upper segment is abnormally distended and thin and the lower segment is abnormally thick; Bandl's ring is a sign of impending uterine rupture. (3) (PB; MR; IM)

1 Bandl's ring does not reflect that the fetus is descending down the birth canal; it is associated with prolonged rupture of the membranes, dystocia, and prolonged labor.

3 Bandl's ring is pathologic, it is not expected.

4 Although Bandl's ring may occur during the second stage of labor, it is not a sign that the second stage of labor is beginning; pushing is contraindicated because uterine rupture may result.

254. 1 In light of the vaginal bleeding, the priority nursing action is ascertaining whether a viable fetus is present. (2) (PM; CJ; AS)

2 This is absolutely contraindicated; bright red bleeding is suggestive of placenta previa.

3 Same as answer 2.

4 Same as answer 2.

255. 4 Prolonged rupture of membranes and fetal tachycardia indicate a possibility for maternal infection; the maternal vital signs should be assessed for the presence of fever and increased pulse and respirations. (3) (SE; CJ; AS)

1 This is unnecessary unless the fetal status deteriorates and untrauterine resuscitation efforts fail.

2 Prolonged fetal decelerations would warrant oxygen administration; accelerations indicate increased cardiac activity, but sufficient oxygenation.

3 This may be done after additional data are collected and the cause of the tachycardia still cannot be determined.

256. 4 Greenish-brown amniotic fluid is a sign of meconium in utero, which may indicate that the fetus is stressed. (2) (PB; CJ; AN)

1 There is not enough information to come to this conclusion.

2 This may be necessary if the fetal heart rate becomes non-reassuring, then a cesarean birth would help ensure a viable newborn.

3 Meconium-stained fluid alone is not an indication for immediate delivery.

257. 4 This must be done immediately to maintain cord circulation and prevent the fetus from becoming anoxic. (3) (PB; CJ; IM)

1 The priority is maintaining cord circulation; although monitoring is important, it does not alter the emergency.

2 Keeping the cord moist is secondary; keeping the presenting part off it to maintain cord circulation is more important.

3 Holding the cord may increase pressure on the cord and further reduce oxygen to the fetus.

258. 1 Methadone is the only medication currently approved for the treatment of the pregnant woman with an opiate addiction; although the drug crosses the placenta, it is considered safer for the fetus than acute opiate detoxification if the methadone is not administered. (3) (SE; MR; PL)

2 This action would lead to withdrawal symptoms and place the client at risk for again using opiates.

3 Detoxification from methadone, a long-acting opioid, takes longer than two weeks.

4 This is not recommended; this will put the client and the fetus at risk once the opiate agonist is discontinued.

259. 1 This client will have lower tolerance for pain and greater need for pain relief. (2) (PB; CJ; PL)

2 Larger doses may be needed if this is done.

3 Delays increase anxiety and discomfort, and larger doses are needed.

4 Individuals who abuse drugs need more medication than do others because of tolerance.

260. 3 HIV is known to be transmitted through body fluids such as blood, semen, and vaginal secretions. (1) (SE; CJ; PL)

1 Invasive fetal monitoring is avoided to prevent vertical transmission.

2 HIV is the virus, not the disease; the diagnosis of AIDS is determined when the CD4T cell count drops below 200 per microliter.

4 Studies indicate that the type of delivery does not influence the transmission of HIV from mother to fetus; the fetus is exposed to the mother's body fluids in utero.

261. 4 The earliest sign of drug withdrawal is CNS overstimulation. (2) (PI; CJ; AS)
    1 These are related to drug use, not withdrawal.
    2 These have no relation to drug abuse; most postpartum women are hungry and thirsty.
    3 Same as answer 2.

262. 3 These contractions are too frequent and prolonged for a client who is only 4 cm dilated; the client could become exhausted, which would compromise the fetus. (2) (PB; CJ; AS)
    1 This is an expected finding and does not need medical intervention.
    2 Same as answer 1.
    4 Same as answer 1.

263. 1 Ruptured membranes of 24 hours or longer would predispose both the mother and fetus to sepsis; if the birth does not occur within this time frame, measures probably will be taken to stimulate labor. (1) (PM; CJ; PL)
    2 There is no relationship between ruptured membranes and the second stage of labor.
    3 Although this may be done eventually, it is too early to anticipate that labor would be stimulated.
    4 There are no data that indicate that effacement is delayed.

264. 2 This is a noninvasive, relatively harmless, way to visualize the location of the placenta. (2) (PB; CJ; AS)
    1 This is an invasive surgical procedure that is not used for this purpose.
    3 This provides information about the status of the fetus, not the placenta.
    4 This is used for removing amniotic fluid for fetal assessment.

265. 2 It is vital that a baseline measurement be obtained because increasing size is a sign of concealed hemorrhage; in abruptio placentae there is bleeding behind the placenta. (3) (PB; CJ; AS)
    1 This would be an appropriate assessment, but it is not a priority at this time.
    3 Same as answer 1.
    4 Same as answer 1.

266. 1 Preeclampsia is characterized by an elevated BP, proteinuria, and edema (as evidenced by excessive weight gain or edema of the hands and face). (2) (PM; CJ; AS)
    2 This is commonly seen in the third trimester; it is known as physiologic edema.
    3 This may occur in the third trimester because the enlarged uterus impedes venous return causing supine hypotension.

    4 Because it has been two weeks since the client's last visit, this weight gain is expected.

267. 4 This position moves the gravid uterus off the great vessels of the lower abdomen, which increases venous return, improves cardiac output, and promotes kidney and placental perfusion. (2) (PM; MR; AN)
    1 The side-lying position does not influence intraabdominal pressure.
    2 While on bed rest the blood pressure decreases and the interstitial fluid is mobilized into the intravascular space.
    3 The side-lying position does not prevent thromboses.

268. 1 As fluid gushes out of the amniotic sac, it may carry the umbilical cord out of the birth canal before the presenting part. (2) (PM; CJ; AS)
    2 There is a greater risk of decelerations because prolapse of the cord may occur; decelerations would indicate cord compression.
    3 Lowered maternal blood pressure occurs when the client is in the supine position, not when the membranes are ruptured.
    4 There is no change in the maternal heart rate after an amniotomy.

269. 1 Nonperiodic accelerations with fetal movement indicate fetal well-being. (3) (PB; CJ; AN)
    2 Early decelerations are associated with fetal head compression.
    3 Late decelerations are associated with uteroplacental insufficiency.
    4 Variable decelerations are associated with cord compression.

270. 1 The client is exhibiting signs of preeclampsia; the presence of hyperreflexia indicates central nervous system irritability, a sign of a worsening condition; this will help direct the physician to appropriate interventions while alerting the nurse to the possibility of seizures. (3) (PB; CJ; AS)
    2 The physician will need to be called, but a complete assessment should be done first to provide the physician with the most information.
    3 The client's blood type is not necessary at this time; assessment of the neurologic status is the priority.
    4 An IV may need to be started but should not precede a proper assessment; normal saline would not be preferred.

271. 2 Increasing cerebral edema may predispose the client to seizures; therefore stimuli of any kind should be minimized. (2) (PB; CJ; IM)

1 It is too early to plan for a cesarean birth; other therapies would be tried first.

3 The client probably would receive IV magnesium sulfate to prevent a seizure, not furosemide to promote diuresis.

4 Magnesium sulfate would be used; calcium gluconate is its antidote.

272. 3 An adequate urinary output, an indicator of adequate renal function, is necessary to prevent toxicity because magnesium sulfate is excreted by the kidneys; signs of magnesium sulfate toxicity are reduced respirations and absent patellar reflexes; therefore baseline assessments should be done. (2) (PB; CJ; PL)

1 Deviations in temperature are not relevant to magnesium sulfate.

2 These are urine tests; they are not relevant to magnesium sulfate.

4 These are assessments that may indicate worsening preeclampsia; they are not determinants of a baseline assessment.

273. 3 All pregnant women should increase their intake of all nutrients; if the client with mild preeclampsia has been following the recommended pregnancy diet, she should continue it. (2) (PM; MR; PL)

1 Salt restriction could activate an angiotensin response, which can elevate the blood pressure; a moderate salt intake is recommended.

2 Fluids should not be restricted during pregnancy.

4 There is no reason for the woman with mild preeclampsia to increase the intake of just carbohydrates.

274. 4 The presence of these clinical manifestations will determine the severity of the preeclampsia. (3) (PB; CJ; AS)

1 Constipation is not related to preeclampsia.

2 Constipation and bleeding are not related to preeclampsia.

3 Leakage of fluid and bleeding are not related to preeclampsia.

275. 4 Eclamptic seizures may be prevented by giving IV magnesium sulfate, which is a CNS depressant. (2) (PB; CJ; AN)

1 Although magnesium sulfate is a neuro-muscular sedative that relaxes smooth muscles and decreases BP, it is not considered an antihypertensive and is not given for that purpose.

2 Magnesium sulfate is considered a CNS depressant that decreases, not increases, the quantity of acetylcholine.

3 Increased uterine contractions are not associated with magnesium sulfate administration.

276. 4 Contractions lasting too long and occurring too frequently can lead to fetal hypoxia; stopping the oxytocin should stop the contractions, thus increasing the oxygen to the fetus. (1) (PB; CJ; IM)

1 Oxytocin will continue to promote uterine contractions; this is unsafe because the prolonged, frequent contractions decrease oxygen to the fetus.

2 Same as answer 1.

3 Same as answer 1.

277. 2 The fetus is at risk for retardation prenatally from a buildup of metabolites in the PKU-affected mother if a prescribed diet is not followed by the mother. (3) (PB; MR; IM)

1 This will not occur if the proper diet is maintained by the mother.

3 The fetus is at risk for mental retardation if the maternal diet contains phenylalanine; also, the infant can inherit phenylketonuria via an autosomal-recessive gene.

4 This is not true; the client should restart a phenylalanine-restricted diet when planning to become pregnant and continue it throughout pregnancy.

278. 4 PKU is an inborn error of metabolism involving an inability to properly metabolize phenylalanine, an essential amino acid. (2) (PB; MR; AN)

1 This is metabolized in those with PKU.

2 Same as answer 1.

3 Same as answer 1.

279. 2 Morning sickness, a common occurrence, contributes to decreased food intake; the insulin dosage must be reduced to prevent hypoglycemia. (2) (PB; CJ; IM)

1 The body's metabolism increases during pregnancy because the needs of the fetus as well as the mother must be met.

3 Rapid organogenesis requires large amounts of glucose.

4 If adequate intake is maintained, insulin requirements will be higher.

280. 2 It is difficult to maintain maternal normoglycemia throughout pregnancy; excess glucose passes into the fetus, where it is converted to fat. (2) (PB; MR; IM)

1 The problem is excess glucose, which is why exogenous insulin must be administered.

3 Although all pregnant women consume extra calories to meet the increased metabolism associated with pregnancy; fetal insulin does not pass from the fetus to the mother.

4 This is a stereotypical statement; not all clients with diabetes are overweight.

281. 4 The blood glucose level is important because hypoglycemia in early pregnancy can lead to congenital abnormalities; hyperglycemia in late pregnancy may lead to fetal hyperinsulinism and subsequent neonatal hypoglycemia. (2) (PM; CJ; PL)

1 Appointments should be made by the client; an authoritative approach takes control away from the client and may increase anxiety.

2 This is too limited a response; assessment without intervention is useless.

3 Dietary regulation is usually minimal, with a restriction on excessive carbohydrate ingestion; a limited diet to control weight gain could jeopardize both the fetus and the mother's nutritional status.

282. 4 Fetal lung maturation can be predicted by the presence of phosphatidylglycerol in amniotic fluid; if the results indicate fetal lung immaturity, birth is postponed provided the fetus and mother are not at risk. (2) (PB; CJ: IM)

1 Structural defects of the placenta cannot be identified by amniocentesis; however malposition of the placenta can be identified during pregnancy by a sonogram.

2 The approximate size of the fetus can be determined by a sonography, not an amniocentesis.

3 An amniocentesis will not be able to determine if a cesarean birth is necessary.

283. 4 An L/S ratio indicates adequacy of pulmonary function, and the baby should be free from major respiratory problems. (1) (PB; CJ; AN)

1 There is no indication of fetal distress; immediate birth is unnecessary.

2 The L/S ratio only determines fetal lung maturity; further fetal monitoring will be necessary in the future as with any pregnancy.

3 Same as answer 1.

284. 4 Blood pressure and pulse may not change significantly until large amounts of blood have been lost; the trickling of blood indicates continuous bleeding. (2) (SE; CJ; AS)

1 The pulse becomes very rapid, but not until a significant amount of blood is lost.

2 This is not a sign of impending hemorrhage.

3 Blood pressure is normotensive; it usually does not drop significantly until a large amount of blood is lost.

285. 4 Late decelerations are suggestive of fetal hypoxia and occur when there is uteroplacental insufficiency. (3) (PB; CJ; AN)

1 Head compression results in early decelerations; this is considered benign.

2 Hypothyroidism is unrelated to late decelerations.

3 Umbilical cord compression results in variable decelerations.

286. 3 Contact precautions include wearing a gown, mask, and gloves; these protect the nurse from the virus; the client should be in a private room. (1) (SE; MR; PL)

1 The CDC guidelines for isolation precautions do not include enteric precautions as a category.

2 These precautions are not necessary for a person with genital herpes.

4 Same as answer 2.

287. 1 During an emergency cesarean birth, the urinary bladder may be nicked while attempting to reach the uterus. (3) (PB; CJ; EV)

2 It is unlikely to develop bleeding associated with a urinary infection so soon after delivery.

3 This cannot occur; lochia is expelled from the vagina, not the urinary bladder.

4 With DIC there would be bleeding from other sites such as the incision and the IV, not just the bladder.

288. 2 The clamp should be placed four to six inches from the umbilicus to allow for use of the umbilical vein or artery if the newborn should need acute care. (2) (PM; CJ; PL)

1 The cord would be too short to allow for entering the umbilical vein or artery if required.

3 This is unnecessarily long.

4 Same as answer 3.

289. 1 **The physician should be notified because the increased height of the uterus may be due to accumulation of blood in the uterus from internal hemorrhaging; also, the blood pressure is low and the pulse is rapid, and this may be indicative of impending shock. (2) (PB; MR; EV)**
2 Further assessment to confirm hemorrhaging only delays immediate response to the problem; the physician should be notified immediately.
3 Same as answer 2.
4 The assessment points to possible hemorrhaging; with urinary distention the uterus is relaxed and lochia is heavy.

NORMAL NEONATE (NN)

290. 1 **Standard precautions do not include the use of gloves for feeding. (1) (SE; CJ; IM)**
2 Wearing clean gloves for diaper changes in all newborns is a standard protocol.
3 Clean gloves should be worn when suctioning an infant.
4 Clean gloves should be worn for all admission baths because the nurse will be exposed to blood and amniotic fluid.

291. Answer: **Apgar of 8.** A perfect score is 10; one point is deducted for lessened muscle tone (the baby's arms do not flex) and 1 point for acrocyanosis, which is manifested by bluish hands and feet. (2) (PM; CJ; AS)

292. 4 **Lack of skin pigmentation on the surfaces of the mucous membranes would give the best indication of this neonate's tissue oxygenation. (3) (PM; CJ; AS)**
1 These are usually highly pigmented areas and often contain mongolian spots.
2 The tips of the ears would indicate the skin color later in life.
3 Because of acrocyanosis of a neonate's hands and feet, a normal occurrence in the neonatal period, the nail beds may also be cyanotic.

293. 1 **Preventing heat loss conserves the infant's oxygen and glycogen reserves; this is a priority. (2) (SE; CJ; IM)**
2 Warming the infant will reduce cyanosis if no respiratory obstruction is present.
3 This is important but not a priority; assessment should be delayed until the infant is warm.
4 This can be done after provision has been made to prevent heat loss.

294. 3 **This action elicits the stepping response, which is absent when paresis is present or in babies born vaginally in the breech presentation. (2) (PM; CJ; IM)**
1 This should elicit the Babinski's reflex which is unrelated to a breech delivery.
2 This should elicit the rooting response reflex which is unrelated to a breech delivery.
4 This should elicit the digital response reflex which is unrelated to a breech delivery.

295. 1 **This is the sign that differentiates between these two conditions; with caput succedaneum the swelling crosses the suture line and it does not with cephalhematoma. (2) (PM; CJ; AN)**
2 The swelling decreases in size; if the swelling increases, the newborn would have to be observed for signs of increased intracranial pressure.
3 Bruising can occur with either condition.
4 Pain is not associated with either condition.

296. 1 **Bilirubin is a yellow pigment derived from the hemoglobin released with the breakdown of red blood cells as the hematoma resolves. (3) (PM; MR; PL)**
2 This action is not specific for a healthy infant with a cephalhematoma.
3 Same as answer 2.
4 Same as answer 2.

297. 3 **This action should elicit the grasp reflex of the newborn's hands. (1) (PM; CJ; IM)**
1 This action would cause the toes to hyperextend with dorsiflexion of the big toe (Babinski reflex).
2 This action would elicit symmetric abduction and extension of the arms with the thumb and forefingers forming a C, followed by adduction of the arms, and finally a return of the arms to a relaxed position (Moro reflex).
4 This action would elicit alternating flexion and extension of the feet that simulates walking (stepping reflex).

298. 4 **The upper portion of the skull is defined as the parietal area. (2) (PM; CJ; AN)**
1 The frontal area is the area over the eyes.
2 The temporal area is the area behind the ears.
3 The occipital area is the area at the back of the head.

299. 2 **Coarctation of the aorta results in diminished or absent femoral pulses. (3) (PM; CJ; AS)**

1 This has no effect on the volume of peripheral circulation (minimal shunting occurs in the newborn period).

3 This has minimal effect on the volume of peripheral circulation (left-to-right shunt).

4 Same as answer 3.

300. **2 Evaporative heat loss is a result of the conversion of moisture into vapor. (2) (PB; CJ; AN)**

1 Radiation is the loss of heat to colder solid surfaces not in direct contact.

3 Convective heat loss is a result of contact of the exposed skin with cooler surrounding air currents.

4 Conductive heat loss is a result of direct skin contact with a cold solid object.

301. **3 Sudden movement causes the startle response (Moro reflex) that begins with extension and abduction of the extremities with a C shape formed by the index finger and thumb, followed by flexion and adduction of extremities, and ending with return of the arms to a relaxed position. (1) (PM; CJ; IM)**

1 This action should elicit the asymmetric tonic neck reflex that simulates the fencing position.

2 Stroking elicits trunk incurvation or the Galant reflex.

4 This action causes the eyes to close tightly.

302. **3 Increased pressure during the birth process causes increased intravascular pressure, which may result in capillary rupture. (2) (PM; CJ; AN)**

1 These are intact capillaries; they may be distinguished from petechiae if they disappear when the area is blanched.

2 This is caused by the collection of eosinophils.

4 Bloody stools or oozing from the umbilicus is the most common sign of vitamin K deficiency.

303. **1 This is a Moro reflex, which indicates an intact nervous system. (2) (PM; CJ; IM)**

2 The Moro reflex is present up to the third month of life; if it persists, there may be a neurologic disturbance.

3 The Moro reflex has no relationship to hunger.

4 The Moro reflex is an involuntary response to environmental stimuli.

304. **2 After the respirations are established, the rate ranges from 30 to 60 breaths per minute with short periods of apnea. (1) (PM; CJ; AS)**

1 Twenty breaths per minute is too slow.

3 More than 60 breaths per minute is too rapid.

4 Same as answer 3.

305. **3 This metabolic process releases energy and increases heat production in the newborn. (3) (PM; CJ; AN)**

1 Fatty acids are byproducts of the breakdown of brown fat.

2 Shivering is the mechanism of heat production for the adult, not for the newborn.

4 This will not be successful unless plentiful brown fat is present.

306. **3 The absence of normal intestinal flora in the newborn results in low levels of vitamin K, causing a transient blood coagulation deficiency; an injection of vitamin K is given prophylactically to all infants on the day of birth. (1) (PM; CJ; IM)**

1 Vitamin K has no effect on erythropoiesis.

2 Vitamin K is important in the synthesis of clotting factor in the liver, but it will not prevent jaundice.

4 Newborns have a blood coagulation deficiency; the blood clots more slowly, not more quickly.

307. **2 Meconium usually is passed during the first several days of life. (1) (PM; CJ; AN)**

1 Meconium has no relationship to the pathologic state of diarrhea.

3 Passing meconium is desired in the newborn in that it indicates patency of the colon and a perforate anus, not pathology.

4 Although meconium usually is passed within the first 24 hours after birth, it can be passed for several days as it gradually mixes with milk waste products.

308. **1 With developmental dysplasia of the hip, there are extra folds in the affected thigh as a result of the shortening of the leg. (2) (PM; CJ; AS)**

2 There are no extra folds in this area in developmental hip dysplasia.

3 Same as answer 2.

4 Same as answer 2.

309. **4 As the head of the femur moves within the acetabulum, sometimes there is an audible click when there is developmental dysplasia of the hip. (1) (PM; CJ; AS)**

1 This is associated with the Babinski's test.

2 This is a neurologic finding.

3 This is opisthotonic posturing.

310. 2 This information assists parents to understand the unique features of their newborn and promotes interaction and care during periods of wakefulness. (3) (PM; MR; PL)

1 Infants should be on a demand feeding schedule, not a routine schedule; demand feeding provides for individuality.
3 This is too limited; the parents need a broader discussion of infant behaviors.
4 Printed instructions may be inadequate if unaccompanied by a discussion.

311. 4 An increase in mucus production is expected during the second reactive period; appropriate nursing intervention is to remove them either by swiping the oral cavity with a gloved finger or via aspiration. (2) (PM; CJ; IM)

1 This is unnecessary; identifying and treating human responses is within the scope of nursing practice.
2 Oxygen administration is useless if mucus is blocking the respiratory passages.
3 This may help the secretions to drain but the newborn cannot remove secretions that block respirations.

312. 4 The fat pad is present in newborns and infants; the arch develops when the child begins to walk. (2) (PM; CJ; AN)

1 Flat feet are no more common in children than in adults.
2 The size of the feet is not relevant; arch development is related to walking.
3 Flat feet are not associated with deformities of the bones.

313. 1 Adaptation to the extrauterine environment is largely dependent on the functional capacity of vital organ systems, which is established during intrauterine development; this is measurable in terms of gestational age and weight. (2) (PM; CJ; AN)

2 Although this factor may influence health, it is not critical to neonatal survival.
3 Although these factors may influence health, they are not critical to neonatal survival.
4 Same as answer 3.

314. 3 One point was removed from the Apgar score because the extremities were blue. (1) (PM; CJ; AS)

1 This score is too low and does not reflect the status of the newborn.
2 Same as answer 1.
4 This score is too high.

315. 2 This simple measure would detect hypoglycemia in this large for gestational age infant. (2) (PB; CJ; IM)

1 There are no data that indicate a need for oxygen.
3 Formula would not be given at this time, and there are no data that indicate a need for a gavage feeding.
4 The situation does not indicate such a need because the Apgar scores were excellent.

316. 1 During periods of active or irregular sleep it is normal for newborns to have some twitching movements and irregular respirations; the vital signs and blood glucose levels are within expected limits. (1) (PM; CJ; AN)

2 Twitching is a common finding in healthy neonates; it often occurs with crying or stimulation.
3 Hypoglycemia in newborns would be characterized by a blood glucose level less than 40 mg/dl.
4 The newborn respiratory rate ranges between 30 to 60 per minute; irregular breathing is expected.

317. 1 These are raised sebaceous cysts commonly found on the chin and nose of a newborn; they disappear spontaneously in a few days or weeks. (1) (PM; CJ; AS)

2 This is the fine downy hair covering the back and arms of the newborn.
3 These are elevated lesions of immature capillaries and endothelial cells that regress over a period of years; they are commonly called birthmarks.
4 This is an innocuous pink papular neonatal rash; it appears within 24 to 48 hours after birth and resolves spontaneously within a few days.

318. 1 The neonate's first stool is thick and greenish black and is called meconium; it is an expected occurrence and should be recorded. (1) (PM; CJ; IM)

2 This stool reflects an expected neonatal adaptation and there is no reason to suspect intestinal obstruction.
3 Meconium stool on the first day of life is expected and does not require further examination.
4 Meconium is not indicative of bleeding; meconium contains bile and other waste products produced by the fetus; it does not require notification of the physician.

319. 1 Establishing a patent airway, diminishing cold stress, and identification of the newborn are the priorities. (1) (SE; CJ; PL)

2 Application of eye prophylaxis and administration of vitamin K are often delayed to allow the parents to bond with the infant; a bath at this time would increase the risk of cold stress.

3 These measures would be appropriate in a compromised infant; an 8/9 Apgar is indicative of a healthy uncompromised newborn.

4 The newborn needs constant monitoring and should be placed in a warmer rather than a crib; the infant can be weighed later.

320. 4 **The test cannot be done until the infant has ingested high phenylalanine (formula or breast milk) diet for at least 48 hours. (2) (PM; CJ; IM)**

1 The test can be done at any weight; the important factor is ingestion of milk for at least 48 hours to obtain a reading.

2 This is not the reason for not testing for PKU.

3 Measurable enzymes are produced after the infant has ingested milk for at least 48 hours.

321. 3 **Phenylalanine, an essential amino acid necessary for growth and development, may be absent in infants with PKU; early diagnosis and treatment may prevent mental retardation. (1) (PM; MR; PL)**

1 This is done at the same time as PKU testing, but there is no relationship between thyroid deficiency and PKU.

2 This test will not detect mental retardation; recognition and treatment early in life can help prevent mental retardation.

4 Chromosomal damage cannot be detected with a PKU test.

322. 1 **The major purpose of this screening test is to determine if the infant has phenylketonuria (PKU); PKU can be detected after the infant has started ingesting milk. (1) (PM; MR; PL)**

2 Determination of the carrier state of the mother is not the objective of the testing of the infant.

3 Epidemiologic information is a purpose of genetic screening; in this instance the most important determination is whether or not the infant has PKU.

4 Risk for later development is not the purpose of PKU testing; it is to determine if the infant in fact has the disease.

323. 2 **Side-lying enables gravity to pull feeding through the pyloric sphincter; it lessens pressure of the cardiac sphincter and minimizes regurgitation. (2) (PM; CJ; IM)**

1 It is common for babies to regurgitate, but this response will not enhance mothering skills.

3 The baby has had enough formula and does not require more during this feeding.

4 A newborn should not be propped after eating, since this could worsen the condition because of pressure put on the esophagus.

324. 3 **The newborn should not be submerged in a tub; the penis should be gently cleaned with clear, warm water; in addition, sponge baths are given until the cord detaches. (1) (PM; CJ; EV)**

1 The diaper should be changed frequently to prevent irritation from the urine.

2 There should be only minimal bleeding; excessive bleeding requires immediate attention.

4 Petrolatum gauze or A & D ointment prevents the diaper from adhering to the operative site.

325. 1 **This is done to avoid pressure on the circumcision area because the glans remains tender for two to three days. (2) PM; MR; IM)**

2 This exudate is expected and does not indicate an infectious process.

3 The neonate may have pain with voiding for a few days, so this is to be expected.

4 The caregiver should check for bleeding every hour for the first 12 hours after the circumcision.

326. 3 **The gastrocolic reflex is stimulated when the newborn's stomach begins to fill with fluid; this causes an increase in peristalsis resulting in the passage of stool during or after a feeding. (3) (PM; CJ; IM)**

1 Six to 10 voidings a day of pale, straw-colored urine are indicative of adequate fluid intake, not the frequency of bowel movements.

2 The cardiac sphincter is unrelated to bowel movements; the cardiac sphincter, located between the esophagus and the stomach, is immature in the newborn and is the reason for the newborn's tendency to regurgitate feedings more easily.

4 Although this is a digestive enzyme, it is not the cause of bowel movements after a feeding.

327. 4 Proper cleansing and frequent changing will limit the presence of irritating substances. (1) (SE; CJ; IM)

1 Having the nurses change the diaper may lower the mother's self-esteem.

2 Powder and lotion will cake and retain moisture in the area.

3 This is a nursing, not a medical, problem.

328. 2 After birth, fetal erythrocytes hemolyze releasing bilirubin into the circulation which the immature liver cannot metabolize as rapidly as it is produced, resulting in physiologic jaundice. (2) (PM; CJ; AN)

1 Jaundice is not an allergic response.

3 This is not a common occurrence in newborns; also, symptoms would occur more quickly.

4 The infant and mother have independent blood supplies, and Rh-negative blood does not enter the baby's bloodstream.

329. 4 Jaundice that appears within 24 hours may be indicative of a pathologic process; if the bilirubin level is elevated, intervention is required. (2) (PM; CJ; IM)

1 Jaundice is not an indication for admission unless accompanied by a very high serum bilirubin level.

2 The infant may require phototherapy after further assessment factors have been carried out; this is not the first action.

3 Physiologic jaundice does not appear until 72 hours after birth; this observation indicates pathologic jaundice.

330. 1 This is typified by the touch that shows maternal bonding; attachment is manifested when the newborn is compared to the father. (2) (PM; CJ; EV)

2 Attachment behaviors in the newborn are defined as grasping and sucking the nipple.

3 There is no indication of maternal deprivation.

4 Consummatory behaviors in the newborn are coordinated sucking and swallowing.

331. 4 The parents need an opportunity for close, eye-to-eye contact in the first hour; any of the prophylactic eye medications may irritate the baby's eyes, preventing them from opening. (1) (PM; CJ; IM)

1 Assessment is appropriate but will not facilitate parent-child bonding; favorable conditions for bonding should be provided before assessment.

2 The nurse should assess, not demonstrate, behavior at this time.

3 Footprinting should be done immediately to ensure proper identification of the baby.

332. 4 Stimulating the rooting reflex is effective in making the infant grasp the nipple. (1) (PM; CJ; IM)

1 For milk to be expressed the infant must grasp the entire areola, which contains the secretory ducts.

2 Giving the neonate a bottle may interfere with the infant's learning to accept the breast.

3 The mother should be supervised for correct positioning of the infant's mouth on the nipple to avoid nipple soreness.

333. 2 This is the proper attachment and helps compress the milk glands. (1) (PM; CJ; EV)

1 The nipple must be on top of the tongue.

3 This indicates improper attachment.

4 This is not a good indication; the infant may be sucking on the nipple only.

334. 3 The presence of at least six to eight wet diapers each day indicates sufficient breast milk intake. (2) (PM; CJ; EV)

1 This is a poor indicator; not all babies need extra sucking stimulation.

2 This could indicate an inadequate amount of fluid ingestion.

4 This is not a reliable indicator; sleep patterns may vary.

335. 2 At about six months of age, infants are able to swallow independently of sucking and a cup can be introduced. (3) (PM; CJ; EV)

1 This would be inappropriate because the infant does not have the ability to swallow independently of sucking at this time.

3 Between 9 and 12 months of age, infants can swallow four to five times consecutively and hold and carry a cup to the mouth; introduction of a cup at 6 months of age makes the weaning easier at 9 to 12 months of age.

4 This is too late; by this time the child has teeth, and sucking on a bottle promotes the development of caries as well as a preference for milk over solid foods.

336. 2 Unless fluoridated water is used by the manufacturer, fluoride supplementation of 0.25 mg daily is required. (3) (PB; CJ; AN)

1 Commercial formulas are iron-fortified.

3 The supply of vitamin K is adequate after the first week of life.

4 This is unnecessary; vitamin B$_{12}$ may be needed if the mother is a vegetarian and is breastfeeding.

337. 4 **These areas of hyperpigmentation are commonly found in dark-skinned newborns; they are benign. (1) (PM; CJ; IM)**

1 Birthmarks are usually much smaller and red in color.

2 Marks from forceps are crescent shaped and are dark red.

3 This is not a complication.

338. 4 **The immediate weight loss is because of loss of excess fluid, not loss of body mass. (2) (PM; CJ; AN)**

1 Weight loss is expected; there are no data to support an allergic response.

2 Weight loss is not related to hypoglycemia.

3 Neither breast- nor formula feeding will prevent the 10% weight loss that is expected in the first few days of life.

339. 2 **The alcohol promotes drying of the skin; observation is necessary to detect signs of infection. (2) (PM; CJ; IM)**

1 Ointment would keep the cord moist; rapid drying of the cord is preferred.

3 This prevents the cord from drying and provides a dark, warm, moist medium for growth of organisms.

4 The cord clamp is removed when the cord stump is dry, usually at 24 hours.

HIGH-RISK NEONATE (HN)

340. 2 **This is expected because of the absence of subcutaneous fat tissue. (2) (PM; CJ; AS)**

1 This usually is observed in preterm infants born nearer to term.

3 Preterm infants generally are born with large amounts of lanugo that begins to thin just before term and by 40 weeks is found only on the shoulders, back, and upper arms.

4 The preterm infant's scrotum is small, and the testicles usually are high in the inguinal canal.

341. 4 **Increased brown fat metabolism (nonshivering thermogenesis) elevates fatty acids in the blood and may predispose the newborn to acidosis. (3) (PB; CJ; PL)**

1 Newborns do not shiver.

2 Hypoglycemia, not hyperglycemia, can occur because the newborn's glycogen reserves are depleted rapidly when under stress.

3 Although oxygen consumption increases during cold stress, it is not the priority; increased fat metabolism is more serious.

342. 2 **A 36-week, large-for-gestational-age infant of a mother with diabetes may have immature lung tissue that may predispose the infant to respiratory distress. (2) (PB; CJ; AS)**

1 Meconium ileus is highly suggestive of cystic fibrosis which is unrelated to diabetes.

3 This is manifested about 72 hours after birth when immature red blood cells begin to hemolyze; this is expected and unrelated to diabetes.

4 This may be associated with birth injury or hydrocephalus; it is unrelated to maternal diabetes.

343. 1 **Morbidity and mortality rates of preterm infants are highest between 24 and 26 weeks' gestation; these infants are prone to complications related to immature lung tissue, altered cardiac output, patent ductus arteriosus, and intraventricular hemorrhage; other complications are proneness to necrotizing enterocolitis and infections. (3) (PB; CJ; AN)**

2 Based on the status of cervical effacement and dilation a decision can be made to try to halt labor with the use of tocolytic medications and limited activity.

3 Although advances in neonatal health care have decreased infant mortality, neonates delivered at 34 weeks' gestation are still at high risk.

4 To prevent the complications of a preterm birth, the pregnancy should be maintained past 37 weeks' gestation.

344. 1 **Preterm neonates are prone to respiratory distress; flaring nares are a compensatory mechanism in a neonate with RDS that attempts to lessen resistance of narrow nasal passages and increase oxygen intake. (1) (PM; CJ; AS)**

2 Acrocyanosis is not related to respiratory distress but is caused by vasomotor instability; this is an expected occurrence in the newborn.

3 This is an expected finding in the newborn.

4 Same as answer 3.

345. 3 Exhaustion results from the extra sucking effort required to obtain milk flow from the breast. (2) (PB; CJ; IM)
1 If the infant is being fed by gavage, the mother's breasts can be pumped and the breast milk can be used for gavage feedings.
2 Time consumption and effort are insufficient reasons to discourage breastfeeding.
4 Breast milk provides adequate nutrition, protects the infant from necrotizing enterocolitis, and provides antibodies.

346. 4 These are the typical signs of respiratory distress in the newborn; immediate treatment is necessary. (3) (PB; CJ; AS)
1 Wheezing and crackles are not signs of respiratory distress in a newborn.
2 Hiccups, wheezing, and crackles are not signs of respiratory distress in a newborn.
3 Wheezing and hiccups are not signs of respiratory distress in a newborn.

347. 1 At 34 weeks' gestation the respiratory system is not fully developed; adequate oxygenation is a priority. (3) (PB; CJ; PL)
2 Although important, this is not as high a priority as oxygenation.
3 This is too rapid a weight increase; 20 to 25 g per day would be expected at this gestational age.
4 The heart rate of a newborn is 110 to 160 beats per minute; this heart rate is within the expected range.

348. 2 In respiratory acidosis, the pH falls and the carbon dioxide level rises. (2) (PB; CJ; AN)
1 This is a normal pH.
3 This is within the expected range of 3.5 to 5.0 mEq/L.
4 The arterial oxygen level may or may not change with acidosis.

349. 4 This breathing pattern is indicative of respiratory distress; the expected pattern is abdominal with synchronous chest movement. (1) (SE; CJ; IM)
1 This is within the expected range of 97.6° F to 99° F for a newborn.
2 This is caused by uric acid crystals from the immature kidneys; it is a common occurrence.
3 This is within the expected range of 110 to 160 beats per minute for a newborn.

350. 2 The oxygen must be warmed and humidified to avoid hypothermia and possible drying of the mucous membranes. (2) (SE; CJ; PL)
1 Bright pink skin may indicate an excessively high arterial oxygen level, which predisposes to retinopathy of prematurity.
3 Oxygen levels are monitored every one to two hours and are adjusted in response to the infant's condition.
4 Blindness develops with excessive arterial oxygen levels, which can occur at any percentage of oxygen.

351. 4 These are key signs of a pneumothorax, which can occur when an infant is receiving oxygen by positive pressure. (2) (PB; MR; AN)
1 These findings require immediate attention.
2 The findings do not indicate this occurrence.
3 Same as answer 2.

352. 2 Constant drainage of urine on the skin promotes excoriation and infection; it must be protected. (3) (PB; MR; IM)
1 Output would be difficult to measure because of constant leakage of urine.
3 Sterility is impossible to maintain because of the constant leakage of urine.
4 A pressure dressing is contraindicated because it would traumatize the bladder.

353. 1 Positioning with the head slightly hyperextended and changing the position every one to two hours helps to drain secretions which can increase oxygenation by enhancing respiratory efforts. (2) (PB; CJ; IM)
2 All newborns are assessed for the presence of congenital birth defects, not just those with RDS.
3 This is too low; preterm infants do not shiver.
4 Extensive handling is not desired, but infants do need to be touched.

354. 1 A preterm, small-for-gestational-age infant is at risk for problems not seen in the term small-for-gestational-age infant because of immaturity; this information will help the nurse to anticipate potential problems and aim interventions at prevention. (1) (PM; CJ; AN)
2 The information is documented in the infant's record, but this is not the overriding reason for obtaining the data.
3 Same as answer 2.
4 The infant will lose weight, but the comparison of weight and gestational age is important for the planning of appropriate nursing measures.

355. 4 The Silverman-Anderson score is an index of neonatal respiratory distress. (3) (PB; CJ; EV)

1 This score does not reflect cardiac function.
2 This score does not reflect neurologic status.
3 This score does not reflect caloric needs.

356. 1 **The release following compression of the chest during vaginal birth is the mechanism for expansion of the newborn's lungs; since this does not occur during a cesarean birth, lung expansion is incomplete and atelectasis may result. (1) (PB; CJ; AN)**
2 The infant is monitored closely to prevent this.
3 Temperature change is not implicated in aspiration.
4 Gravity could be used after a cesarean birth by holding the newborn upside down.

357. 3 **Breast tissue is not palpable in an infant of less than 33 weeks' gestation. (1) (PM; CJ; AS)**
1 Creases in the palms and on the soles of the feet are not clearly defined until after the 37th week of gestation.
2 The ear pinnas spring back in an infant at 36 weeks' gestation.
4 A 0-degree square window sign is present in an infant at 40 to 42 weeks' gestation.

358. 4 **The assessment findings are indicative of a preterm infant; therefore the nurse should closely monitor the infant for signs of respiratory distress syndrome; this occurs commonly in preterm infants because their lungs are immature. (2) (PB; CJ; AS)**
1 Preterm AGA infants do not develop polycythemia; preterm LGA infants may develop polycythemia, but there are no data to indicate the infant is LGA.
2 Preterm AGA infants may become hypoglycemic.
3 The neonate is preterm, not postterm.

359. 4 **The pathologic changes of chronic vascular disease cause uteroplacental insufficiency; vasospasms diminish fetal oxygenation and nutrition, which lead to slowed fetal growth. (2) (PB; CJ; AS)**
1 Prematurity is defined as gestational age of less than 37 weeks.
2 There is no greater incidence of cardiac anomalies in infants with intrauterine growth restriction.
3 There is no greater incidence of infection in infants with low birth weight; however, they may have lowered resistance to infection.

360. 2 **The infant would be classified as small-for-gestational age (SGA) because the weight is less than the 10th percentile on the growth curve for a term infant. (1) (PM; CJ; AN)**
1 An infant is considered to be preterm if born before the end of the 37th week of gestation; the wording "small-for-gestational age" rather than "immature" is used.
3 The infant's weight is less than the 10th percentile for a term infant; the infant is SGA.
4 Same as answer 3.

361. 3 **Hypoglycemia is common in newborns that are small for gestational age because of malnutrition in utero; the nurse can detect this with a blood glucose test and notify the medical staff. (2) (PB; MR; AS)**
1 Polycythemia, not anemia, occurs.
2 Although hypocalcemia may occur, it is not as common as hypoglycemia.
4 Although this may occur, it is not life-threatening at this time.

362. 2 **SGA infants may exhibit hypoglycemia, especially during the first two days of life, because of depleted glycogen stores and inhibited gluconeogenesis. (2) (PM; CJ; AN)**
1 Decreased BP, pallor with cyanosis, tachycardia, retractions, lethargy, and weak cry are present in hypovolemia.
3 Hypercalcemia is uncommon in newborns.
4 These signs are unrelated to hypothyroidism; signs of hypothyroidism are difficult to identify in the newborn.

363. 3 **Many superficial veins are common in the preterm infant because of the lack of subcutaneous fat deposits. (1) (PM; CJ; AS)**
1 Flexion of extremities is the posturing of normal term infants; preterm infants usually posture with extremities extended and flaccid.
2 Absent femoral pulses are indicative of coarctation of the aorta, a congenital heart defect.
4 A positive Babinski reflex is expected in the full-term, not preterm, newborn.

364. 4 **Primary manifestations of NEC are feeding intolerance, increased gastric residual of undigested formula, and bile-stained emesis. (3) (PB; CJ; AS)**
1 This occurs with diarrhea; stools in those with NEC are generally reduced in number and contain glucose and blood.
2 This may occur with a cardiac anomaly, not NEC.
3 This occurs with hypertrophic pyloric stenosis.

365. 2 Prolonged gastric emptying occurs with NEC; an increase in abdominal girth of greater than 1 cm in four hours is significant and needs immediate intervention. (2) (PB; CJ; IM)

1 Formula is stopped and the baby is placed on parenteral fluids.

3 This will have no therapeutic value for an infant with NEC.

4 Same as answer 1.

366. 3 Gradually rewarming an infant experiencing cold stress is essential to avoid compromising the infant's cardiopulmonary status. (3) (SE; CJ; IM)

1 An infant experiencing cold stress will become hypoglycemic; the infant uses up glycogen and glucose to maintain the core temperature.

2 Rapid rewarming of an infant may result in apnea and neonatal stress.

4 Skin temperatures should be taken at least every 15 minutes until stable.

367. 1 A preterm infant may have a weak suck but usually can be breastfed; the mother should attempt it if the infant is stable. (2) (PM; CJ; IM)

2 It does not necessarily take more calories to breastfeed; also, there are immunologic benefits to the preterm infant who receives antibodies through breast milk.

3 The suck may or may not be weak, but a supervised attempt to breastfeed should be encouraged.

4 Pumping the breasts may be necessary, but at 35 weeks if the infant is stable and the mother so desires, breastfeeding should be attempted.

368. 4 The pacifier may satisfy nonnutritive sucking needs and stimulate flow of saliva and digestive juices. (2) (PM; CJ; IM)

1 There is no evidence that nonnutritive sucking is harmful for a preterm infant.

2 Sucking on a pacifier promotes adaptation later to the breast or bottle.

3 Research has identified a benefit of nonnutritive sucking; buck teeth are associated with thumb sucking.

369. 2 The nurse applies tactile stimulation after validating that respirations are absent; this action may be sufficient to reestablish respirations in the high-risk neonate with frequent episodes of apnea. (2) (PB; CJ; IM)

1 Assessment will not interrupt the period of apnea; respirations must be immediately reestablished.

3 These measures are too invasive and aggressive for initial intervention; gentle stimulation should be attempted first.

4 The monitor should be assessed for proper functioning before use.

370. 1 The reflexes and muscles of sucking and swallowing are immature; this makes oral feeding ineffectual and exhausting. (3) (PM; CJ; AN)

2 The metabolic rate is increased because of fatigue and growth needs.

3 Caloric requirements are increased because of extra growth needs.

4 Absorption of nutrients is decreased because of immaturity of the intestines.

371. 2 Retinopathy of prematurity (ROP) is a complex disease of the preterm infant; hyperoxemia is one of the numerous causes implicated, and it can be monitored with pulse oximetry. (2) (PB; CJ; EV)

1 This will not prevent the development of ROP.

3 A low level of oxygen does not guarantee that ROP will be avoided.

4 Same as answer 1.

372. 4 This is caused by gonorrheal and/or chlamydial infections present in the vaginal tract; it is preventable by prophylactic use of erythromycin or tetracycline ophthalmic ointment after delivery. (2) (PB; CJ; IM)

1 Herpes affects the neonate systemically.

2 Retrolental fibroplasia (retinopathy of prematurity) occurs from prolonged exposure to a high oxygen concentration over long periods.

3 This usually is caused by rapid expulsion of the fetus's head from the vagina.

373. 3 Observing the care that the parents actually give the infant provides direct validation of their skill and comfort levels. (1) (SE; MR; EV)

1 This action is helpful in anticipatory guidance but is only a small part of competency evaluation.

2 Although this is helpful in identifying empirical knowledge, it does not test their skill or comfort level.

4 Same as answer 2.

374. 4 These newborns are large for gestational age because of macrosomia and usually are born at term. (1) (PB; CJ; AN)

1 Although these newborns generally are born at term, usually they are large, not average, for gestational age.

2 These newborns generally are large, not small, for gestational age; usually only

diabetic mothers with advanced vascular and renal disease may deliver infants that are small for gestational age.

3 Because of the risk for fetal death, women with diabetes are delivered before the 40th week of gestation.

375. **3 This is within the expected blood glucose level for the neonate (40 to 60 mg/dl) and requires no measures other than continued monitoring for the next 24 hours. (3) (PB; CJ; AS)**

1 Heel sticks are adequate for monitoring blood glucose levels in a neonate.

2 This would cause hyperglycemia in the neonate.

4 This would be done if the neonate's blood glucose level were low.

376. **1 A difficult birth because of broad fetal shoulders may result in a fractured clavicle, which can be assessed by the findings of a knot or lump, limited arm movement, and a unilateral Moro reflex. (2) (PM; CJ; AS)**

2 This is unrelated to a difficult birth of a baby with broad shoulders.

3 This reflex involves the feet; it is in no way related to a difficult birth because of broad shoulders.

4 Same as answer 3.

377. **1 Infants of diabetic mothers are polycythemic and therefore they appear flushed; the mechanism underlying this phenomenon is unknown. (3) (PM; CJ; AS)**

2 These infants generally are heavy due to macrosomia.

3 These infants are limp, not hyperreflexive.

4 These infants tend to lie quietly and not cry.

378. **1 Decreasing IV glucose slowly is necessary to prevent a hypoglycemic response. (3) (PB; CJ; IM)**

2 Metabolic alkalosis will not occur with discontinuation of the glucose; it occurs with excessive amounts of bicarbonate.

3 Withholding oral feedings while withdrawing IV glucose may result in hypoglycemia.

4 Hyperglycemia is unlikely to occur when decreasing the IV glucose because blood glucose levels will decrease.

379. **3 These signs are consistent with hypoglycemia; the newborn also may have difficulty feeding, lethargy, apnea, and cyanosis. (2) (PB; CJ; AN)**

1 The signs of hypovolemia include decreased blood pressure, pallor, tachycardia, tachypnea, weak pulses, and flaccid movements.

2 The signs of hypocalcemia are similar to the signs of hypoglycemia; however,

hypocalcemia occurs 24 to 36, not 3, hours after delivery.

4 Hyperglycemia rarely occurs because the newborn's pancreas continues to produce insulin.

380. **4 Because the virus is found in the respiratory tract and the urine, isolation is necessary; rubella is spread by droplets from the respiratory tract. (2) (SE; MR; PL)**

1 This is an outdated term that is no longer used; the techniques used with this precaution have been incorporated under contact precautions.

2 This is an outdated term that is no longer used; the techniques used with this precaution have been incorporated under standard precautions.

3 This would be unsafe; additional precautions must be taken to protect the nurse from droplet infection.

381. **2 Phototherapy changes unconjugated bilirubin in the skin to conjugated bilirubin bound to protein, permitting excretion. (1) (PM; CJ; EV)**

1 Phototherapy does not affect liver function; the liver does not dispose of bilirubin.

3 Vitamin K has no effect on bilirubin excretion; it is necessary for prothrombin formation.

4 The bilirubin is not excreted via the skin but in the urine and feces.

382. **2 The infant's position is changed every two hours to expose all skin surfaces to the phototherapy for maximum effect. (2) (PB; CJ; IM)**

1 The infant should be kept nude for maximum exposure to the lights.

3 The infant may be removed from the lights for feeding and the eye patches removed to assess the eyes for irritation.

4 The lights will dry the cord more quickly, which is a desired effect.

383. **2 The head circumference is usually 2 cm larger than the chest; a head circumference 4 cm smaller than the chest could indicate microcephaly. (3) (PM; CJ; AS)**

1 In anencephaly, the disparity between the head and chest circumference would be much larger than 4 cm.

3 No molding takes place in cesarean birth; therefore the head should be about 2.5 cm larger than the chest at birth.

4 According to growth charts, the range of head circumference for boys is just slightly (1.25 cm) larger than the chest.

384. 3 Mothers with type O blood have anti-A and anti-B antibodies that are transferred across the placenta; this is the most common incompatibility because the mother is type O in 20% of all pregnancies. (2) (PM; CJ; AN)
  1 This usually is not a problem.
  2 Same as answer 1.
  4 Same as answer 1.

385. 3 Adherence to the diet is necessary for optimal physical growth with little or no adverse effects on mental development; a diet that is instituted late will not reverse brain damage. (1) (PB; CJ; AN)
  1 Detection cannot occur until the infant has taken milk or formula that contains phenylalanine for 24 hours and metabolites accumulate in the blood; behaviors indicating mental retardation and CNS involvement usually are evident by about 6 months of age in the untreated infant.
  2 There is no phenylalanine at birth; it first becomes measurable after the infant ingests milk or formula.
  4 Epinephrine levels would be decreased, not increased; tyrosine, an amino acid produced by the metabolism of phenylalanine is absent in PKU; tyrosine is needed to form epinephrine.

386. 3 The term "phenylketonuria" is derived from phenylpyruvic acid, which gives urine a mousy, musty odor. (2) (PB; CJ; AS)
  1 This odor is not present with phenylketonuria.
  2 Same as answer 1.
  4 Same as answer 1.

387. 1 Cyanotic hands and feet (acrocyanosis) is common in the newborn; circumoral pallor is one sign of cardiac pathology and indicates a need for further investigation. (3) (PB; MR; IM)
  2 Circumoral pallor is not expected in the newborn; it may indicate cardiac pathology.
  3 Same as answer 2.
  4 These are not signs of increased intracranial pressure.

388. 1 Right-to-left shunts result in inadequate perfusion of blood; not enough blood flows to the lungs for oxygenation. (3) (PB; CJ; AN)
  2 Left-to-right shunts result in too much blood flowing to the lungs; blood is adequately perfused.
  3 Left-sided obstruction to the flow of blood results in decreased peripheral pulses, not cyanosis.

  4 There should be no shunting of blood between the right and left sides of the heart after the ductus arteriosus closes.

389. 4 The abnormal facies associated with fetal alcohol syndrome includes a small, upturned nose, which is distinctive in these infants. (3) (PB; CJ; AS)
  1 A cleft lip may occur without a precursor or with the trisomies.
  2 Multiple fingers are associated with the trisomies.
  3 An umbilical hernia can develop in early infancy and is not related to fetal alcohol syndrome.

390. 4 These signs are indicative of withdrawal from an opioid because of the changes occurring in the central nervous system; the newborn should be monitored during the first 24 to 48 hours. (2) (PB; CJ; AN)
  1 The signs of cerebral palsy are usually manifested later in infancy.
  2 The signs of syphilis are a low-grade fever with copious serosanguineous discharge from the nose.
  3 The signs of fetal alcohol syndrome are growth deficiencies in length, weight, and head circumference.

391. 4 Thrush, an oral infection caused by *Candida albicans*, is an opportunistic infection that may be indicative of HIV infection. (3) (SE; CJ; AS)
  1 This is more frequently associated with immaturity of the hypothalamus.
  2 Bleeding after a circumcision is associated with a bleeding disorder such as hemophilia.
  3 Hypoglycemia is usually associated with the infant born to a diabetic mother.

392. 2 After closure, spinal fluid may accumulate and back up into the brain, increasing intracranial pressure and causing the fontanels to bulge. (2) (PB; CJ; AS)
  1 This may be a typical pattern for the baby; it does not of itself indicate changes in intracranial pressure.
  3 Changes in vital signs are not among the early signs of increasing intracranial pressure in an infant.
  4 This can indicate changes in intracranial pressure but is not one of the first signs.

393. 3 This helps prevent infection while keeping the membranes moist. (1) (PB; CJ; IM)
  1 Although this should be done, it is not the priority.
  2 Antibiotics are not given prophylactically.

4 This newborn needs more than just routine care because of the outpouching of the meninges.

394. 4 **When a diaphragmatic hernia is present, the intra-abdominal pressure must be minimized; this is accomplished by the use of gastric decompression. (3) (PB; CJ; IM)**
1 This would not be a beneficial action; it might predispose the infant to diarrhea.
2 The infants are not fed orally; intravenous fluids are given with careful measurement of electrolytes and intake and output to guide replacement therapy.
3 This is contraindicated; the abdominal organs would increase pressure on the diaphragm.

395. 2 **This indicates the presence of meconium and is considered a sign that the fetus is compromised. (2) (SE; LE; IM)**
1 This is an expected occurrence and may increase at the end of the first stage of labor.
3 This describes normal amniotic fluid.
4 This should occur as labor progresses.

396. 3 **A barium enema can be both a diagnostic and therapeutic procedure; as barium is expelled, gas and meconium may be passed, temporarily relieving the obstruction. (2) (PB; CJ; PL)**
1 A rectal tube cannot relieve an intestinal obstruction; it promotes only the expulsion of gas.
2 A rectal biopsy is a diagnostic, not a therapeutic, procedure.
4 A nasogastric tube will relieve swallowed stomach contents; it will not help confirm the diagnosis.

397. 4 **The lack of completion of fetal bladder development may interfere with development of the pelvis. (2) (PB; MR; IM)**
1 Genu varum (bowlegs) can be congenital or caused by rickets; it is not related to exstrophy of the bladder.
2 This is a rotation of the tibia and is unrelated to exstrophy of the bladder.
3 This is a form of hip dislocation and is unrelated to exstrophy of the bladder.

398. 2 **If the rectum is empty of feces, this may indicate intestinal obstruction present at birth. (2) (PB; CJ; AS)**
1 Vomiting may occur, but vomiting may be related to any number of conditions.
3 Intake and output, while important, are not definitive information for making a diagnosis.

4 Fussiness during feeding is not definitive for making a diagnosis.

399. 2 **Large newborns may be the result of gestational diabetes; it is necessary to check the baby for hypoglycemia because maternal glucose is no longer available. (3) (PB; CJ; AS)**
1 This would be indicated if the temperature were low and the newborn needed additional warmth.
3 The infant may be hypoglycemic and would require the glucose in an oral feeding immediately.
4 Unless there is a low blood glucose or some other indication of a problem, the infant can be seen whenever the pediatrician arrives.

400. 4 **This prevents the neonate's stomach from becoming too distended and pressing upward against possibly compromised lungs. (2) (PM; CJ; PL)**
1 This is too long a period between feedings; preterm infants should be fed every two to three hours because it takes this amount of time for the preterm infant's stomach to empty.
2 This would not prevent respiratory embarrassment; more important, however, is the fact that the infant with a strong sucking reflex should be fed with a nipple, otherwise the sucking reflex will disappear.
3 Preterm infants need the full caloric value of formula; giving diluted formula has no bearing on preventing respiratory embarrassment.

401. 3 **Dry peeling skin is related to decreased vernix and prolonged immersion in amniotic fluid. (2) (PM; CJ; AS)**
1 Few sole creases are associated with preterm newborns.
2 Vernix would be found on a newborn at about 38 weeks' gestation.
4 Newborns of diabetic mothers usually have this appearance.

402. 1 **This occurs because of a lack of pulmonary surfactant to overcome surface tension in the alveoli. (2) (PB; CJ; AN)**
2 Surfactant is present in sufficient amounts when the birth is closer to term.
3 The alveoli tend to collapse and may stay collapsed resulting in atelectasis.
4 Fetal alveoli mature closer to term at about 35 to 36 weeks.

403. **2** Tongue extrusion, a reflex response to the tip of the tongue being touched, is characteristic of infants with Down syndrome and interferes with feeding; this reflex disappears approximately at 4 months of age. (1) (PB; CJ; AN)
   1 Newborns do not need teeth for sucking.
   3 Down syndrome is caused by a chromosomal defect, not brain damage; the feeding problem is related to the chromosomal defect.
   4 Nasal congestion is not a characteristic associated with newborns with Down syndrome.

404. **1** Pressure on the cerebral structures influences the central nervous system resulting in irritability. (2) (PB; CJ; AS)
   2 A high-pitched cry is common in neonates with increased intracranial pressure.
   3 The fontanels would be bulging, not depressed, with increased intracranial pressure.
   4 This is related to dehydration and kidney problems, not increased intracranial pressure.

REPRODUCTIVE PROBLEMS (RP)

405. **2** The male should be treated to prevent the infection from passing back and forth between him and his sexual partner. (1) (PM; CJ; EV)
   1 The organism is most likely present in the partner's urogenital tract; voiding will not prevent recurrence.
   3 This is an ineffective remedy and will not prevent recurrence.
   4 A douche is not recommended either during pregnancy or in the nonpregnant state.

406. **2** Hemorrhage can result from a ruptured tubal pregnancy and shock can ensue. (3) (PB; CJ; AS)
   1 The data do not include information related to respiratory patterns leading to hyperventilation and resulting respiratory alkalosis.
   3 Same as answer 1.
   4 There are no data, such as fever or rising white blood cell count, to support the conclusion that the client is experiencing an infection.

407. **3** Any blood from the rupture will accumulate, causing phrenic nerve irritation and pain. (3) (PB; CJ; AN)
   1 Anxiety can cause many things, but shoulder pain is an atypical symptom.
   2 The cardiac changes caused by hypovolemia do not cause shoulder pain.

4 A ruptured tube can cause rebound tenderness in the abdomen, not the shoulder.

408. **3** This is an appropriate nursing diagnosis; the bleeding is causing decreased circulating blood volume and therefore a decreased cardiac output. (3) (PB; CJ; AN)
   1 Infection could occur later but is not a problem at this time.
   2 There would be a fluid volume deficit, not excess.
   4 There are no data to justify this conclusion.

409. **1** At this time the fallopian tube is unable to expand to the size of the growing pregnancy. (1) (PB; CJ; AN)
   2 Tubal pregnancies are unable to advance to this stage because of the tube's inability to expand with the growing pregnancy.
   3 Same as answer 2.
   4 The size of the fertilized egg at this time is minuscule and would cause no problem.

410. **2** This response informs the client of the need for genetic counseling and gives her an option for decision making. (2) (SE; MR; IM)
   1 This shifts the responsibility to the physician; the nurse should be involved in teaching about resources.
   3 This response does not address the client's concern and changes the focus of the discussion.
   4 This is an autosomal recessive disorder; there is a 25% probability that it can occur again.

411. **2** An amniocentesis is done at this time because a therapeutic abortion can be legally and safely performed if desired by the parents. (2) (SE; CJ; IM)
   1 This is too early to perform an amniocentesis because the uterus has not ascended into the abdomen and there is little amniotic fluid present.
   3 Although an amniocentesis and therapeutic abortion can be performed at this time, it is preferred that they are done as early as possible.
   4 This is too late; the parents should not delay an amniocentesis if they are considering a therapeutic abortion.

412. **1** This response encourages the clients to verbalize their feelings. (1) (PI; MR; IM)
   2 The clients are not interested in the nurse's wishes; the focus should be on them.

3 This is a very insensitive and incorrect statement; there may be nothing wrong with either client.

4 The clients are not seeking advice about dealing with their parents.

413. 2 There is an increased risk of ectopic pregnancy with IVF-ET. (3) (PM; CJ; PL)

1 There is no increased risk for this complication with IVF-ET.

3 Same as answer 1.

4 Same as answer 1.

414. 4 This is referred pain from passage of contrast medium through the tubes; this is usually indicative of tubal patency. (2) (PB; MR; IM)

1 No anesthetic is given; the client's complaint of pain can be managed with position change and mild analgesis.

2 The client can resume usual activities as soon as the test is over.

3 The client does not usually experience nausea and/or vomiting.

415. 4 This is necessary to keep the sperm viable for determining sperm count and viability. (1) (PB; MR; IM)

1 Rubber solvents and preservatives may affect the semen specimen.

2 The specimen can be collected at any time.

3 This may lessen the amount of ejaculate needed for the specimen.

416. 4 Because the client is ovulating, the infertility may be a result of a seminal factor; the partner's semen should be examined before more extensive studies or treatments are begun with the woman. (2) (PM; CJ; AN)

1 All other potential problems should be ruled out first; the client does not have a right to receive the drug unless it is appropriate for the problem.

2 Before other potential problems are investigated, the husband's semen should be analyzed.

3 Same as answer 2.

417. 4 Since the cervix is closed, the abortion is threatened. (3) (PB; CJ; PL)

1 The lifeless products of conception are retained with a missed abortion.

3 Portions of the products of conception would have to be passed for a diagnosis of incomplete abortion.

2 Once the cervix is dilated, the abortion is inevitable.

418. 3 This is the most important goal for a client who is aborting the products of conception. (2) (PB; CJ; PL)

1 Although this is important, the primary concern at this time is to control the hemorrhage.

2 This is unrealistic.

4 Although the physician's orders should be followed, the nurse should monitor the client who is bleeding; observation for any change in maternal status is the nursing priority.

419. 3 Once cervical dilation has begun, the abortion is classified as inevitable. (2) (PB; CJ; AS)

1 In this type of abortion, the cervix is dilated and bleeding; it is also malodorous.

2 Bleeding and cramping may be present, but the cervix is still closed in a threatened abortion.

4 The products of conception have been partially expelled with an incomplete abortion.

420. 3 Since the laminaria tent is left in place for this length of time, it increases in size from absorption of moisture and dilates the cervix two to three times its original diameter before the suction procedure is done. (2) (PM; CJ; IM)

1 A local anesthetic agent is usually injected into the cervix (paracervical block) and may cause mild cramping or light spotting.

2 A temperature over 100° F is a danger sign and the client should be alerted to call her health care provider if this occurs.

4 Cervical bleeding is reduced by the use of the laminaria tent and is usually equivalent to a heavy menstrual period; the client is usually observed for one to three hours following the procedure.

421. 4 This indicates that the bleeding is excessive and the physician should be notified. (1) (SE; MR; EV)

1 Although instructions vary among health care providers, sexual intercourse usually may be resumed in one to three weeks.

2 Although instructions vary among health care providers, tampons usually are denied for three days to three weeks.

3 The menstrual period will usually resume in four to six weeks.

422. 2 RhoGAM should be given within 72 hours after delivery to have an impact on future pregnancies. (2) (PM; CJ; PL)

1 It is not necessary to administer RhoGAM at this time.

3 RhoGAM is always indicated at the termination of a pregnancy, whether it is at term or before term and whether the fetus is alive or dead.

4 Same as answer 3.

423. 3 A hydatidiform mole, in which chorionic villi degenerate into grapelike vesicles, causes these signs and symptoms. (3) (SE; MR; AS)

1 While vomiting could cause dehydration, this ignores the vaginal discharge and hypertension.

2 Choriocarcinoma is a sequela of hydatidiform mole; the hCG blood levels are monitored for one year after removal of the mole; if they decrease to normal limits and remain there for one year the client can plan for another pregnancy.

4 Although a vaginal discharge is related to a spontaneous abortion, an elevated blood pressure and severe nausea and vomiting are not.

424. 2 Human chorionic gonadotropin (hCG) increases shortly after the onset of pregnancy, peaks at the end of the second month, then falls and is sustained at a lower level until the end of pregnancy; a continued elevation indicates retained trophoblastic tissue and possible choriocarcinoma. (3) (PB; CJ; EV)

1 This is characterized by persistent, localized abdominal pain; it does not have a higher incidence in women with hydatidiform mole.

3 Hyperemesis gravidarum cannot occur after termination of a pregnancy.

4 This is manifested by shock, bleeding, a low platelet count, and elevated PT and PTT levels; it does not have a higher incidence in women with hydatidiform mole.

WOMEN'S HEALTH (WH)

425. 4 This is known as the hormone of pregnancy; together with estrogen it helps prepare the endometrium for the fertilized ovum, helps maintain pregnancy, and prepares the mammary glands for milk secretion. (1) (PM; CJ; AN)

1 This is secreted by the adrenal cortex, and affects carbohydrate metabolism.

2 This is secreted by the anterior lobe of the pituitary gland; it starts and maintains milk secretion by the mammary glands.

3 This is secreted by the posterior pituitary gland; it stimulates labor contractions and

contractile tissue around the nipple during breastfeeding.

426. 4 Mittelschmerz is pain that sometimes occurs at ovulation when the ovum erupts from the follicle. (1) (PM; CJ; IM)

1 The pain is mild, cyclic, and characteristic of mittelschmerz; it requires no medical intervention.

2 When menses first begin, the client is usually anovulatory and would not experience the pain known as mittelschmerz.

3 The pain probably will occur most often when ovulation is well established.

427. 3 This is the correct definition of dysmenorrhea. (1) (PM; CJ; IM)

1 This occurs with menopause and during pregnancy.

2 This is any bleeding that occurs at any time other than during the menstrual period; there may or may not be any pain.

4 This is known as menometrorrhagia.

428. 4 This medical aseptic technique should limit the spread of microorganisms and help prevent future urinary tract infections if incorporated into her health practices. (1) (SE; MR; IM)

1 This is unnecessary, but the client should be encouraged to void when the urge occurs.

2 Intake and output do not need to be measured.

3 This is unnecessary with cystitis; it may be employed as a part of perineal care for other problems.

429. 2 Yogurt contains *Lactobacillus acidophilus* bacteria, which will replace those destroyed by antibiotics. (2) (PB; CJ; IM)

1 This is not relevant to antibiotics or intestinal flora.

3 Same as answer 1.

4 Same as answer 1.

430. 4 Genital herpes (HSV-2) is characterized by remissions and exacerbations; it cannot be cured. (1)(SE; CJ; EV)

1 Most pregnant women with HSV-2 have children by cesarean birth to prevent the newborns from contracting the disease while passing through the vagina.

2 Clients should abstain from sex until 10 days after the lesions heal.

3 Herpes can be controlled, not cured.

431. 4 A condom covers the penis and contains the semen when it is ejaculated; semen contains a

high percentage of HIV in infected individuals. (1) (SE; MR; IM)

1 Preejaculatory fluid carries the HIV in an infected individual.

2 This is not what the client is asking; most contraceptives do not provide protection from the HIV.

3 Although a monogamous relationship is less risky than having multiple sexual partners, if the one partner is HIV positive, the other person is at risk for acquiring the HIV.

432. 4 **The most effective strategies for preventing sexually transmitted infections in one's self and sex partners is through the use of condoms and having sex partners tested to identify their status and be treated if necessary. (1) (SE; MR; EV)**

1 Asking does not always elicit truthful answers; protection is necessary to help prevent sexually transmitted infections.

2 There are protective measures that can be used to help prevent sexually transmitted infections.

3 The emphasis should be on prevention, not treatment; some sexually transmitted infections have no cure.

433. 3 **The client has signs and symptoms indicative of pelvic inflammatory disease (PID), which is a complication of gonorrhea. (2) (PM; MR; AN)**

1 Herpes is noted for its painful lesions on the genitals; there are no data to indicate the presence of these lesions.

2 The client does not have the signs and symptoms associated with this disease.

4 Same as answer 2.

434. 2 **This is a description of a chancre, which is the initial sign of syphilis. (3) (SE; CJ; AS)**

1 These are condylomata lata, which are typical of the secondary stage.

3 This is typical of the secondary stage of systemic involvement, which occurs from two to four years after the disappearance of the chancre.

4 This is typical of the secondary stage.

435. 4 **A dry environment inactivates the *Treponema pallidum*, making it incapable of causing disease. (1) (SE; CJ; AN)**

1 The organism is transferred by sexual contact; warm, moist body contact supports growth of the organism.

2 Nothing chelates the organism.

3 These support the growth of the organism.

436. 3 **Breast self-examination should be done about a week after menstruation when the**

breasts are less engorged and tender. (2) (PM; MR; EV)

1 This is when menstruating women should examine their breasts.

2 Dimpling may occur when a tumor attaches to the skin or underlying tissues and therefore should be reported.

4 After menopause, selection of a specific time each month for breast self-examination reduces the possibility of forgetting.

437. 4 **Breast engorgement has abated at this time, limiting lumps that may occur because of fluid accumulation. (1) (PM; MR; AS)**

1 Breast engorgement begins before ovulation and does not subside until several days after menses ends; engorgement interferes with accurate palpation.

2 Inaccurate assessment could result because examination would occur at different times of the menstrual cycle; accurate comparisons could not be made from month to month; this is appropriate for post-menopausal women.

3 Same as answer 1.

438. 1 **Serous or bloody discharge from the nipple is pathologic. (2) (PM; MR; AS)**

2 The right hand should examine the left breast because this allows the flattened fingers to palpate the entire breast including the tail (upper, outer quadrant toward the axilla) and axillary area.

3 A small pillow or rolled towel should be placed under the scapula of the side being examined.

4 The flat part of the fingers, not the palm or fingertips, should be used for palpation.

439. 4 **Advanced age at birth of a first child is one of the risk factors for malignancy of the breast because of prolonged exposure to unopposed estrogen. (1) (PM CJ; AN)**

1 This is not considered a risk factor.

2 Same as answer 1.

3 Same as answer 1.

440. 2 **Compression of the breast flattens mammary tissue and maximizes the penetration of the breast by x-rays; this is especially important for the dense breast tissue of adolescents, young nulliparous women, and women with large breasts. (1) (PB; MR; IM)**

1 This usually is done with sonography.

3 This is not necessary.

4 The American Cancer Society recommends that women at risk for breast cancer should have routine mammographies regardless of age or relationship to menopause.

441. 4 Most breast malignancies are painless, fixed, and in the upper outer quadrant; painful, mobile lesions are usually benign. (2) (PB; CJ; AN)
1 These findings are suggestive of a lipoma.
2 These findings are suggestive of a lactation breast abscesses.
3 These findings are suggestive of fibrocystic benign tumors.

442. 2 Radiation will interfere with wound healing if initiated too soon; inadequate healing should be reported. (2) (PB; CJ; AS)
1 Topical preparations should not be used unless prescribed.
3 Sterile technique is not necessary unless there is a break in the skin.
4 Urine or other excreta of a client receiving radiation to the breast area are not affected by this form of therapy.

443. 1 Further teaching is needed because extremes of temperature should be avoided; ice constricts blood vessels, interfering with circulation. (3) (SE; CJ; EV)
2 Continued application of cold is contraindicated because it may cause tissue damage.
3 Erythema is an expected reaction; however, pain, vesicle formation, or sloughing of tissue requires medical intervention.
4 The knowledge deficit relates to skin care, not the side effects of radiation therapy.

444. 2 Pressure to follow a course of therapy is never appropriate, especially at such a stressful time. (1) (PI; CJ; PL)
1 This would be therapeutic.
3 Knowledge of procedures decreases anxiety and would be therapeutic.
4 This would help decrease postoperative complications and would be therapeutic.

445. 1 Elevation promotes drainage by gravity and reduces the risk of developing lymphedema. (2) (SE; MR; PL)
2 This is not the responsibility of the client at this time.
3 A high-Fowler's position would keep the arm in a dependent position thus limiting venous return and promoting lymphedema.
4 Abduction, moving the arm away from the body, increases tension on the suture line and is contraindicated at this time.

446. 2 This position supports venous return by gravity and promotes mobility of the arm. (2) (PB; CJ; PL)

1 The container should be lower, not level, with the affected arm; although portable wound drainage systems work by negative pressure, gravity assists the flow of drainage.
3 Abduction could put unnecessary stress on the suture line at this time; slight flexion of the elbow promotes functional alignment.
4 When the hand is held lower than the elbow and shoulder, venous stasis and edema of the hand can occur.

447. 4 Clients who have cancer of one breast are at risk for development of cancer in the other breast. (2) (SE; MR; PL)
1 A breast prosthesis is not used until healing has occurred.
2 Most clients can resume full activity as strength returns.
3 Stretching activities are considered helpful in regaining full movement.

448. 3 If the tubing is patent and negative pressure is present, the wound should practically be free of exudate. (2) (PB; CJ; IM)
1 Pressure dressings are not used with portable wound drainage systems because the latter are effective in removing interstitial fluid.
2 Drainage is expected; it is the nurse's responsibility to maintain the drainage system.
4 Although elevating the arm may facilitate drainage, it is not the priority in relation to the data presented.

449. 4 This is an honest response; surgery that removes less than all of the breast tissue is combined with irradiation and removal of affected axillary lymph nodes. (1) (PB; CJ; IM)
1 This is an unfeeling response that denies the woman's feelings.
2 This gives false hope; it is not possible to state that the client will be disease free in five years.
3 This gives inaccurate information regarding the radiation therapy and false hope that radiation will not be needed.

450. 2 The Bartholin glands are located beneath the vaginal vestibule; if cysts form and they become infected they cause labial, vaginal, or pelvic pain particularly during or after intercourse (dyspareunia). (3) (SE; CJ; AN)
1 Urethritis, not bartholinitis, would cause painful urination.

3 A vaginal hematoma causes swelling in the vaginal wall, not the labia.

4 Skene's glands are located in the urethra, not the labia.

451. **2 A cystocele is a herniation of the bladder through the vaginal wall because of weakened pelvic structures; the herniated bladder does not empty properly and urinary stasis, chronic infection, and renal failure can develop. (3) (PB; CJ; IM)**

1 The surgery improves bladder function and prevents renal failure; it is needed.

3 Bowel obstruction is a complication of a rectocele, not cystocele.

4 Although corrective surgery will reduce perineal pressure, its primary purpose is to improve bladder function and prevent complications.

452. **2 Attempting to remove a uterus with large uterine fibroids vaginally could cause trauma, resulting in hemorrhage. (2) (PB; CJ; AN)**

1 Vaginal hysterectomy is indicated for prolapsed uterus because the uterus is usually collapsed into the vagina.

3 A hysterectomy is not the treatment of choice for mild cervical dysplasia; when a hysterectomy is necessary, the vaginal route is usually preferred.

4 When a cystocele also needs to be repaired, a vaginal hysterectomy, rather than an abdominal one, is indicated.

453. **3 This leads to pooling of blood in the pelvic area, predisposing the client to thrombus formation. (1) (PB; MR; PL)**

1 This is not done routinely because clotting elements usually are not disturbed by a hysterectomy.

2 Fluids should be increased to 3000 mL daily to decrease blood viscosity, which can lead to thrombus formation.

4 Hormone replacement therapy is not considered unless an oophorectomy was performed; hormone replacement therapy continues to be controversial.

454. **4 After surgery the urethral orifice may be distorted and edematous; a catheter keeps the bladder completely empty, limiting pressure on the operative site. (2) (PB; MR; PL)**

1 A cleansing douche may be ordered before, not after, surgery.

2 A pessary placed in the vagina is used for a displaced uterus; following an anterior/posterior repair (colporrhaphy), vaginal packing is used to support the surgical repair.

3 A rectal tube is used for abdominal distention caused by flatulence; it rarely is necessary.

455. **4 A yellowish-green vaginal discharge indicates the presence of an infection; further assessment for adaptations related to an infection is necessary. (2) (SE; CJ; EV)**

1 Although all the vital signs should be taken, changes in the blood pressure and pulse are not as specific for infection as pain and temperature.

2 This is unrelated to a vaginal infection; this reflects the concentrating ability of the kidneys and fluid balance.

3 Cystitis is characterized by frequency and burning on urination, not a vaginal discharge.

456. **2 Vaginal packing supports the repair and provides slight pressure to prevent bleeding; the packing needs to be checked for possible bleeding. (2) (PB; CJ; PL)**

1 There is no dressing, only vaginal packing and a sanitary pad.

3 Elevation of the legs is unnecessary; leg exercises and a gradual increase in ambulation are encouraged to prevent pulmonary emboli.

4 Sitz baths are not instituted until the packing is removed; an ice pack and/or a heat lamp may be used to promote comfort.

457. **2 The uterus is often erroneously believed necessary for a satisfying sexual life. (2) (PI; CJ; AN)**

1 Sexuality should not be diminished, particularly because the fear of pregnancy no longer exists.

3 Although body image changes can interfere with sexuality, this is not an expectation for most women.

4 Although estrogen levels are reduced, libido is influenced by psychologic as well as hormonal factors.

458. **2 As the term "hysterectomy" implies, only the uterus is removed; therefore, the client will eventually have a physiologic menopause. (2) (PM; CJ; IM)**

1 The client will ovulate; the ovaries are not removed with a hysterectomy

3 When the ovaries are removed along with the uterus, the client will have a surgical menopause.

4 There should be no discomfort if an appropriate period of healing has occurred before resuming sexual intercourse.

459. 3 These will be necessary to screen for atypical changes in vaginal tissue. (3) (PB; CJ; IM)

1 Pelvic examinations and Pap smears will always remain a priority for this client.

2 This suggestion transfers the nurse's responsibility for client teaching to the physician.

4 Same as answer 1.

460. 2 Pap smears can detect cancer of the cervix by screening for atypical as well as cancerous cells. (1) (PM; MR; IM)

1 A colposcopy is not part of a routine Pap smear.

3 Scraping the cells can cause a few drops of blood to come to the surface; vaginal bleeding does not occur.

4 Insertion of the speculum usually is the most uncomfortable part of the test.

461. 1 With carcinoma in situ the epithelium is eroded and replaced by rapidly dividing neoplastic cells; there is no distinct tumor; prognosis with treatment is excellent. (1) (PB; CJ; IM)

2 Preinvasive lesions of the cervix are treated with cryotherapy, laser therapy or loop electrosurgical excision procedure (LEEP); radiation therapy is used for invasive cervical cancer.

3 Stage II would involve the vaginal wall; stage 0 is preinvasive.

4 Stages I to IV are considered invasive by increasing degrees; stage 0 is preinvasive; treatment is based on the staging.

462. 1 This routine screening for information provides a basis for assessing trauma; in a younger client it also assesses risk for pregnancy. (3) (PM; CJ; AS)

2 Examination may precede reporting; the decision to report is mandated by law, not the client.

3 Using water or antiseptic solution would wash away spermatic or bloody evidence.

4 A test specifically for seminal acid phosphate, not alkaline phosphatase, is performed.

463. 3 It is a fact that *E. coli* is commonly found in the bowel and, because of close anatomic proximity and improper hygiene after bowel movements, may spread to the urethra. (1) (PM; CJ; AN)

1 *E. coli* is no more virulent than other infective agents.

2 *E. coli* is not commonly found in the kidneys.

4 *E. coli* does not compete with *Candida* organisms for host sites.

464. 2 Prolactin is a hormone that is produced and secreted by the anterior pituitary; a pituitary tumor is the most probable cause of elevated prolactin levels that result in lactation not associated with childbirth or nursing (galactorrhea). (3) (PB; CJ; AN)

1 If the client were taking oral contraceptives, estrogen levels would increase, causing galactorrhea in some women; in this situation the client is postmenopausal and would not be receiving oral contraceptives.

3 The production of this hormone is not related to the occurrence of galactorrhea.

4 Same as answer 3.

DRUG-RELATED RESPONSES (DR)

465. 3 Premenopausal women should ingest over 1000 mg of calcium daily; if the client is unable to ingest enough calcium in food, then supplements of calcium and vitamin D are recommended; calcium is essential for the formation of bone as well as other vital metabolic processes; vitamin D promotes the absorption of calcium and phosphorus from the gastrointestinal tract. (1) (PB; CJ; IM)

1 These supplements do not help prevent osteoporosis; ginseng is noted by some as a tonic for the heart, an aphrodisiac, and a stimulant; vitamin E functions as an antioxidant to prevent tissue damage from other unstable molecules.

2 These supplements do not help prevent osteoporosis; ginkgo biloba is used to inhibit platelet aggregation, repair damage to nerve cells, and act as an antioxidant to limit cell damage from free radicals; the B complex vitamins are water-soluble vitamins that are different structurally and function in a variety of ways as coenzymes in the body.

4 These supplements maintain cartilage and connective tissue integrity but they do not help prevent osteoporosis.

466. 4 Betamimetics have the unpleasant side effects of nervousness, tremors, and palpitations; clients should be informed that these side effects are expected. (3) (PB; CJ; EV)

1 If contractions are lessened and the heart rate is less than 120 and regular, the medication is performing as expected and does not need to be discontinued.

2 These are not the usual symptoms of preterm labor.

3 Although glucose levels can increase, electrolyte levels are unrelated to these symptoms.

467. 2 Use ratio and proportion:

2,450,000 units : 300,000 units = X mL : 1 mL
300,000 X = 2,450,000
X = 8.2 mL

(2) (PB; CJ; AN)

1 This would deliver more than the ordered amount.

3 This would deliver less than the ordered amount.

4 Same as answer 3.

468. 2 **Probenecid reduces renal tubular excretion of penicillin. (2) (PB; CJ; EV)**

1 This is unrelated to the concomitant administration of penicillin and probenecid.

3 Same as answer 1.

4 Same as answer 1.

469. 2 **Tetracycline has an affinity for calcium; if used during tooth bud development, it may cause discoloration of teeth. (2) (PM; CJ; IM)**

1 This is untrue; it is associated only with the discoloration of teeth.

3 Same as answer 1.

4 Same as answer 1.

470. 1 **Maintenance of serum progesterone levels keeps cervical mucus thick and hostile to sperm at all times. (1) (PM; CJ; IM)**

2 This is insufficient information; the pill must be taken throughout the menstrual cycle.

3 Fertility drugs are often taken during the first part of the cycle to encourage ovulation, not for contraception.

4 Combined estrogen and progesterone oral contraceptives are taken during the second, third, and fourth weeks of the cycle.

471. 3 **Nausea and vomiting are related to excessive amounts of estrogen; these symptoms usually can be controlled by reducing the dosage. (1) (PB; CJ; EV)**

1 Amenorrhea is associated with pregnancy; with estrogen, breakthrough bleeding is more common than amenorrhea.

2 Hypomenorrhea is caused by estrogen deficiency.

4 Depression and lethargy can be related to both excessive estrogen and excessive progesterone but are not common side effects.

472. 1 **Oral contraceptives should be discontinued with any symptom that could be related to a pulmonary embolus. (1) (PB; CJ; EV)**

2 Menorrhagia is a side effect related to excessive amounts of estrogen; immediate discontinuance of contraceptives is unnecessary.

3 Mittelschmerz is pain midway in the menstrual cycle, usually at ovulation.

4 This may be a sign of infection, not a side effect of oral contraceptives.

473. 1 **Iron absorption is pH dependent; therefore, iron should be taken with a source of ascorbic acid to enhance duodenal absorption. (2) (PB; CJ; PL)**

2 This is unrelated to the absorption of iron.

3 Same as answer 2.

4 Same as answer 2.

474. 4 **Phenytoin therapy interferes with folate absorption causing megaloblastic anemia; it is a priority that this client take folic acid supplements. (3) (PB; CJ; IM)**

1 Termination of pregnancy is not necessary because of this anemia.

2 This is not a physiologic anemia associated with pregnancy; this anemia can occur in any client receiving phenytoin therapy.

3 Although all pregnant clients have increased protein needs, the need for even more protein is not necessary because of phenytoin therapy.

475. 2 **RhIg administration during the 28th week of gestation reduces an active antibody response in an Rh-negative individual exposed to the positive blood of the fetus; this drug is used during pregnancy. (3) (PB; MR; EV)**

1 An unsensitized pregnant woman receives RhIg at 28 weeks' gestation as prophylaxis.

3 RhIg is given earlier in the pregnancy; it is a preventive measure.

4 Same as answer 1.

476. 2 **Unsensitized women who are Rh negative with Rh positive infants should receive RhoGAM within 72 hours after delivery to prevent sensitization. (1) (PM; CJ; AN)**

1 RhoGAM is not indicated for Rh negative women with Rh negative infants because these women have not been exposed to Rh positive blood from their newborns.

3 RhoGAM is not indicated for Rh positive women.

4 Same as answer 3.

477. 3 **Heparin can be used during pregnancy because it does not cross the placental barrier and will not cause hemorrhage in the fetus. (3) (PB; CJ; AN)**
1 This drug can cross the placental barrier and cause hemorrhage in the fetus.
2 Same as answer 1.
4 Same as answer 1.

478. 4 **Heparin should not be given because 98 seconds is almost 3 times the normal time it takes a fibrin clot to form (25 to 36 seconds) and prolonged bleeding may result; the therapeutic range with heparin is 1½ to 2 times the normal range. (3) (PB; MR; EV)**
1 Heparin must not be increased; the client already has received too much.
2 The aPTT is not normal but prolonged; it is almost 3 times the normal rate.
3 The medication does not need to be changed; it needs to be stopped.

479. 3 **This is one commonly occurring side effect of this drug. (2) (PB; CJ; EV)**
1 Tachycardia, not bradycardia, commonly occurs.
2 Hypokalemia, not hyperkalemia, is a potential side effect.
4 These do not occur with terbutaline.

480. 2 **Oxytocin given after delivery will stimulate the uterus to contract and remain contracted. (1) (PB; CJ; PL)**
1 Oxytocin has no analgesic effect.
3 Prolactin, not oxytocin, stimulates milk production.
4 Oxytocin usually is administered after the placenta has been expelled.

481. 4 **Frequent contractions with short relaxation periods may lead to fetal hypoxia. (2) (PB; CJ; EV)**
1 This intensity is within the normal limits of 50 to 75 mm Hg.
2 An adverse response to Pitocin is a contraction lasting more than 90 seconds; contractions lasting 30 seconds usually occur in early labor.
3 This is within the expected fetal heart rate range of 110 to 160 during labor.

482. 3 **Oxytocin (Pitocin) has an antidiuretic effect, acting to reabsorb water from the glomerular filtrate. (3) (PB; CJ; EV)**
1 Hyperventilation is caused by inappropriate breathing patterns, not by prolonged use of Pitocin.
2 Affect is not altered by the use of Pitocin.

4 Fever occurs with infection or dehydration, not with prolonged use of Pitocin.

483. 4 **Magnesium sulfate is used to depress CNS irritability; diminished reflexes would indicate the medication's effectiveness. (1) (PB; CJ; EV)**
1 This is a sign of toxicity.
2 Magnesium sulfate is not a diuretic; it acts as an anticonvulsant.
3 A transient lowering of blood pressure after a loading dose may occur, but within an hour the blood pressure should rise.

484. 4 **This is a late indicator of toxicity; if the respiratory rate falls below 12 per minute the infusion should be discontinued. (2) (PB; CJ; EV)**
1 This is associated with worsening of preeclampsia which may lead to a seizure; it is not a toxic effect of the magnesium sulfate.
2 Same as answer 1.
3 The fetal heart rate is not affected by the infusion of magnesium sulfate.

485. 1 **Near-toxic levels of magnesium sulfate are suggested by the disappearance of the knee-jerk reflex and by depressed respirations (less than 12 per minute). (3) (PB; CJ; EV)**
2 This is given as an antidote only when ordered by the primary care provider.
3 Magnesium sulfate is not an antihypertensive.
4 Waiting could put the client in jeopardy of respiratory arrest; signs of toxicity require immediate intervention.

486. 2 **Calcium gluconate will reverse the central nervous system depressant action of magnesium sulfate. (2) (PB; CJ; PL)**
1 Protamine sulfate is the antidote for heparin toxicity.
3 Sodium bicarbonate counteracts acidosis.
4 Naloxone hydrochloride is an opiate antagonist.

487. 3 **Methergine, an oxytocic, is used to promote uterine contractions; its vasoconstrictive action can also lead to hypertension, and it should not be used when hypertension is already present. (2) (SE; MR; EV)**
1 This medication generally is not given to a postpartum client unless an infection is present; there are no data to support the presence of an infection.
2 There is no contraindication to using this medication to relieve the discomfort of an episiotomy.

4 There is no contraindication for use of this drug; there are no data to support the fact that the client is constipated.

488. 2 **The concentration of propylthiouracil excreted in breast milk is 3 to 12 times higher than its level in maternal serum; this may cause agranulocytosis or goiter in the infant. (3) (PB; CJ; AN)**
1 Heparin is not excreted in breast milk.
3 The amount of breast milk excretion of gentamicin is unknown, but it can be given to infants directly without adverse effects.
4 Diphenhydramine is excreted in breast milk, but it does not adversely affect the infant when therapeutic doses are given to the mother.

489. 1 **This is a manifestation of hyporeflexia; it is one indication of magnesium sulfate toxicity. (1) (PB; CJ; EV)**
2 This is an adequate urinary output; a urinary output of less than 30 mL/hr indicates inadequate excretion of magnesium sulfate and the potential for toxicity.
3 The maternal blood pressure is not related to magnesium sulfate administration or toxicity.
4 This is a typical pulse rate; it is not indicative of toxicity.

490. 4 **This is the most reliable method to confirm newborn addiction. (3) (PB; CJ; PL)**
1 This will not determine the amount of drugs the mother used or the last time the drug was taken.
2 The priority is to determine if the newborn is addicted before clinical signs of withdrawal occur.
3 It is the mother's drug habit before hospitalization that is important, not the medications she has received since she has been hospitalized.

491. 3 **This is the expected outcome; if output exceeds intake, it indicates that the infant is diuresing from the effect of the Lasix. (1) (PB; CJ; EV)**
1 Although important to assess, this is subjective; intake and output would be an objective assessment.
2 This is not the desired outcome; this would indicate dehydration, which could occur with excessive administration of Lasix.
4 Although Lasix can cause hypokalemia, which can precipitate digitalis toxicity, this is not the desired effect of Lasix administration.

492. 2 **Steroids such as betamethasone (Betacort) and dexamethasone (Decadron) administered to the mother cross the placenta and promote lung maturity in the fetus; they have other beneficial effects including reducing the incidence and severity of intraventricular hemorrhage. (1) (PB; CJ; AN)**
1 Steroids will not have this effect.
3 Same as answer 1.
4 Same as answer 1.

493. 1 **Terbutaline stimulates beta receptors in the heart, which cause excitation resulting in tachycardia; pulse rates over 120 beats per minute should be reported to the physician, and the dosage will be decreased. (1) (PB; CJ; EV)**
2 It is more likely that the client will experience tremors.
3 Hypokalemia is a maternal side effect.
4 Maternal hyperglycemia is a side effect; hypoglycemia can occur in the neonate.

494. 4 **This is a beta-blocking agent that reverses the uterine inhibitory responses and cardiovascular effects of terbutaline. (3) (PB; MR; PL)**
1 This is a diuretic; it will not reverse the cardiovascular effects indicated.
2 This may cause symptoms similar to those of terbutaline; it is sometimes used to halt premature labor because it inhibits beta 2 receptors.
3 This is not an antidote for terbutaline; it is used for Parkinson's disease.

495. 3 **Corticosteroids stimulate surfactant production; they also have been shown to reduce the incidence of intraventricular hemorrhage. (2) (PB; CJ; AN)**
1 Betamethasone does not affect the labor process.
2 Betamethasone does not increase placental perfusion.
4 Betamethasone does not affect the intensity of contractions.

496. 1 **Salicylate therapy is used because clients with SLE have an increased risk for thrombus formation; as the time of birth approaches, salicylate therapy should be discontinued to reduce the possibility of bleeding in the newborn. (3) (PB; CJ; AN)**
2 There would be no need for dialysis during the postpartum period.
3 There is a greater probability that the infant would be small for gestational age.
4 The butterfly-shaped rash that can occur with SLE does not worsen late in pregnancy.

497. 2 A pudendal block provides anesthesia to the perineum. (1) (PB; CJ; IM)

1 This affects only the perineum, not the bladder.
3 This does not affect muscle control.
4 This anesthetizes only the perineum, not the cervix or the body of the uterus.

498. 4 RhIg is given to prevent active formation of antibodies when an Rh-negative individual is at risk for sensitization; if given to an Rh-positive person, an injection of RhIg would cause hemolysis of RBCs. (3) (PB; CJ; AN)

1 RhIg is never given to an individual with Rh antibodies.
2 A positive Coombs' test indicates that the woman has Rh antibodies; RhIg is never given to an individual with Rh antibodies.
3 Administration of RhIg to an Rh-positive woman causes hemolysis of RBCs.

499. 2 RhoGAM will be given to the mother only if the infant is Rh positive and the Coombs' test is negative. (3) (PB; MR; PL)

1 RhoGAM is never given to the baby; it is given only to Rh-negative mothers to prevent antibody formation and protect future pregnancies.
3 This is not done; however, a minimal dose of RhoGAM may be given prophylactically in the 28th week of gestation to decrease antibody response in the presence of transplacental bleeding.
4 RhoGAM might be given after the 28th week if the amniocentesis procedure resulted in the escape of some fetal blood into the maternal circulation.

500. Answer: 0.25 mL. Solve for X by using ratio and proportion.

$$\frac{\text{Desired 0.5 mg}}{\text{Have 2 mg}} = \frac{\text{X mL}}{\text{1 mL}}$$

$$2X = 0.5$$

$$X = 0.5 \div 2$$

$$X = 0.25 \text{ mL}$$

(2) (PB; CJ; IM)

Childbearing and Women's Health Nursing Quiz 1

1. A client at 38 weeks' gestation, who is having periods of bright red, painless bleeding, is in the high-risk unit because of a placenta previa. The nurse is aware that the client's labor has started when assessment demonstrates:
   1. Decreased fetal heart rate
   2. Lessened vaginal spotting
   3. Increased vaginal bleeding
   4. Rhythmic uterine contractions

2. During the first two hours after a cesarean birth, the priority nursing intervention would be to:
   1. Evaluate fluid needs and provide fluid as ordered
   2. Encourage bonding to promote parent-child interaction
   3. Assess lochia to prevent hemorrhagic complications
   4. Monitor the incision to prevent complications from infection

3. When planning nursing care for a client who delivered a preterm male infant, the nurse should understand that the mother will:
   1. Suffer from feelings of guilt and withdrawal
   2. Experience feelings of helplessness, failure, and loss of control
   3. Be unable to form a healthy relationship with the baby until he is out of danger
   4. Have increased feelings of attachment resulting from greater concern over the baby

4. The nurse understands that true labor is characterized by:
   1. Contractions 10 minutes apart with no change in frequency over two hours; cervix closed
   2. No contractions; cervix 3 cm dilated and 50% effaced; no change after four hours of walking and sitting
   3. Contractions every 5 to 10 minutes; cervix dilated 2 cm and 75% effaced; dilation increased to 3 cm in two hours
   4. Contractions irregular, every 10 to 15 minutes; cervix dilated a fingertip and 50% effaced; no change with four hours of bed rest

5. If involution is progressing as expected, one hour after birth the nurse should expect the fundus to be located:
   1. At the level of the umbilicus
   2. 2 cm below the umbilicus
   3. 3 cm above the umbilicus
   4. 2 cm above the symphysis pubis

6. During the first 24 hours after birth of an infant at 36 weeks' gestation, the nurse must monitor the infant for:
   1. Duration of cry
   2. Respiratory distress
   3. Frequency of voiding
   4. An increase in body temperature

7. The nurse is aware that a common adaptation during pregnancy would be:
   1. Increased ovarian activity
   2. Increased pulmonary capacity
   3. Decreased gastrointestinal motility
   4. Decreased glomerular filtration rate

8. A client attending the prenatal clinic for the first time tells the nurse that her last menstrual cycle began on January 11. The client also states that she had one day of light spotting on February 7. The expected date of birth (EDB) is calculated to be:
   1. October 14
   2. October 18
   3. November 14
   4. November 18

9. A client with preeclampsia is placed on intravenous magnesium sulfate therapy. The nurse caring for this client should immediately notify the physician if the client's:
   1. Blood level is 5 mEq/L
   2. Respirations are 18 per minute
   3. Patellar reflexes can be elicited
   4. Output is less than 100 mL in four hours

10. A public health campaign is planned to immunize children and women in the childbearing age group. The nurse knows that the immunization that can be safely administered to a pregnant woman would be:
    1. Polio
    2. Mumps
    3. Rubella
    4. Rubeola

11. A client who is at four months' gestation is scheduled for a sonogram followed by an amniocentesis. The nurse should instruct the client to drink 8 oz of fluid before the test. This is done to:
    1. Hydrate the mother and increase circulation
    2. Improve ultrasonic visualization of the fetus
    3. Hydrate the fetus and decrease fetal movement
    4. Replace fluid that may be lost during the procedure

12. When a new mother sees her newborn son assume a fencing position as she turns his head, she becomes concerned. The nurse should explain to the mother that this:
    1. Is an expected response
    2. Reflex disappears around 2 months of age
    3. Reflex may indicate neurologic damage in the newborn
    4. Is a suspicious response and the physician has been notified

13. A woman in the family planning clinic asks the nurse why contraceptives are necessary since she is still breastfeeding her baby. The nurse's most appropriate response would be:
    1. "It is best to delay any sexual relations until you have your first menstrual period."
    2. "It is best to use contraceptive measures since ovulation may occur without a menstrual period."
    3. "Since lactation suppresses ovulation, you probably don't have to worry about becoming pregnant."
    4. "As long as you have no menstrual period, you won't have to worry about using contraceptives."

14. The nursing care for a drug-dependent newborn should include:
    1. Administering methadone
    2. Offering small, frequent feedings
    3. Increasing environmental stimuli
    4. Reducing elevated body temperature

15. While being prepared for her first prenatal examination, a pregnant woman complains to the nurse of feeling very tired and being sick to her stomach, particularly in the morning. The best response by the nurse would be:
    1. "These symptoms should be discussed with your doctor."
    2. "This is expected considering all the changes going on in your body."
    3. "This occurs frequently during the early part of pregnancy. You need not worry."
    4. "These are common occurrences. You say your sick feelings bother you most often in the morning?"

16. When assessing a client with an abruptio placentae, the nurse would expect to observe:
    1. A flaccid uterus
    2. Painless bleeding
    3. Bright red bleeding
    4. A boardlike abdomen

17. The nurse is aware that diabetes mellitus can affect pregnancy by:
    1. Promoting abnormal placental implantation
    2. Predisposing the client to hypertensive states
    3. Increasing the appetite and causing excessive weight gain
    4. Decreasing the amount of amniotic fluid present at term

18. When discovering the presence of a prolapsed cord, the nurse anticipates that the client's delivery will be:
    1. Via a cesarean birth
    2. Induced with oxytocin
    3. A low forceps vaginal birth
    4. Postponed as long as possible

19. In the eighth month of pregnancy, a client tells the nurse that she is experiencing dyspareunia. The nurse should plan to teach the client to:
    1. Avoid intercourse
    2. Try alternative positions
    3. Douche to lubricate the vaginal mucosa
    4. Consult a therapist for sexual counseling

20. After a cesarean birth, a client is receiving IV fluids and has an indwelling catheter. The client's fluid intake should be increased via the physician's order when the nurse notes:
    1. Dark amber urine
    2. Urinary suppression
    3. Tinges of blood in the urine
    4. Blood pressure of 100/60 mm Hg

21. The physician prescribes and the nurse administers vitamin K intramuscularly to a newborn immediately after birth to:
    1. Promote the synthesis of prothrombin
    2. Limit elevated levels of serum bilirubin
    3. Facilitate the growth of normal intestinal flora
    4. Decrease calciferol until renal clearance can take over

22. The nurse should plan the postpartum care for a new mother with a history of rheumatic heart disease based on the knowledge that:
    1. The client should increase her fluid intake, particularly if she is breastfeeding
    2. Clients with cardiac problems should be kept on bed rest for a minimum of four days

3. The first 48 hours postpartum are the most stressful on the cardiopulmonary system

4. The client is out of immediate danger because the stress associated with pregnancy is over

23. A client is receiving subcutaneous terbutaline (Brethine) tocolytic therapy. During the initial administration of Brethine, the nurse should:
   1. Check the client's reflexes every two hours
   2. Monitor the client's pulse every 15 minutes
   3. Institute safety measures because of altered consciousness
   4. Insert an indwelling catheter to monitor the urinary output

24. The nurse prepares a client with a ruptured tubal pregnancy for immediate surgery. The nurse understands that an informed consent will have to include permission for a:
   1. Myomectomy
   2. Hysterectomy
   3. Salpingectomy
   4. Dilation and curettage

25. A strict vegetarian (vegan) becomes pregnant and asks the nurse whether there is anything special she should do in relation to her diet during pregnancy. The nurse should teach the client the importance of:
   1. Eating at least 40 g of protein a day
   2. Drinking at least 1 quart of milk per day
   3. Taking a vitamin supplement and iron tablet daily
   4. Including a variety of vegetable proteins in her diet

26. A client with a possible ovarian tumor undergoes laparoscopic surgery. Following this surgery, the nurse should instruct the client that:
   1. Betadine douches should be used daily
   2. Her usual activities may be resumed in 12 hours
   3. Shoulder pain may be present for 12 to 24 hours
   4. Vaginal bleeding may be present for one to three days

27. One hour postpartum the nurse identifies that a client's uterus has become relaxed and boggy. The initial nursing response should be to:
   1. Notify the physician
   2. Massage it until firm
   3. Check the blood pressure
   4. Observe the amount of bleeding

28. At 40 weeks' gestation a client is scheduled for a contraction stress test, and the nurse explains the procedure. The nurse is satisfied that the mother understands the teaching when she says:
   1. "I hope the baby doesn't get too restless after this procedure."
   2. "If this test causes my labor to begin early, it may affect my baby."
   3. "I hate having needles in my arm, but now I understand why it's necessary."
   4. "If my baby's heart reacts normally during the test I will not need to have my labor induced today."

29. To support the body's natural defense mechanisms, a client who has had recurrent infections prior to and during pregnancy should be instructed to eat a nutrient-rich diet that emphasizes:
   1. The fat-soluble vitamins
   2. Dietary fiber and oat bran
   3. Low fat with essential fatty acids
   4. Vitamins A, C, and E and selenium

30. A newborn has sustained an intracranial hemorrhage because of a tear in the tentorial membrane sustained during birth. The nurse should expect this infant to display:
   1. Extreme lethargy
   2. Weak, timorous cry
   3. Generalized purpura
   4. Abnormal respirations

31. Before a client signs the informed consent for a modified radical mastectomy, the nurse should be certain that the client knows the surgery includes the removal of:
   1. Pectoral muscles
   2. Skin overlying the breast tissue
   3. The involved half of the breast and nodes
   4. Axillary lymph nodes on the affected side

32. An 18-year-old primigravida in the 36th week of gestation is admitted to the hospital with a diagnosis of mild preeclampsia. The nurse admitting this client is aware that nursing care measures will be directed chiefly toward reducing:
   1. Anxiety
   2. Bleeding
   3. Blood pressure
   4. Circulating blood volume

33. A client, wishing to postpone having children until she and her husband are financially sound, has been on oral contraceptive pills for several years. The nurse is aware that an assessment finding that would indicate a potential risk with continuing use of birth control pills would be:
   1. Dysmenorrhea
   2. Midcycle bleeding
   3. The lack of ovulation
   4. A blood pressure of 140/90 mm Hg

34. A client finds a lump in her breast and is hospitalized for a biopsy and possible surgery. As the nurse is preparing her for surgery, the client says, "I'm really scared. My mother and sister went through this. It was awful." The nurse's most appropriate response would be:
    1. "Breast cancer has an excellent cure rate."
    2. "You know, most breast lumps are benign."
    3. "What happened with your mother and sister?"
    4. "You are worried about the results tomorrow?"

35. Immediately after a client has completed the third stage of labor, the nurse administers 10 units of oxytocin (Pitocin) as ordered. The desired response from this medication will:
    1. Lessen the discomfort of the episiotomy
    2. Relax the uterus so that it can be emptied
    3. Prevent profuse bleeding following separation of the placenta
    4. Stimulate the client's breasts so that breast-feeding can be started

36. A woman who is admitted to the hospital for poorly controlled gestational diabetes during her third pregnancy has two other children at home. An applicable nursing diagnosis is interrupted family processes related to hospitalization. Nursing care for this client should include:
    1. Suggesting that she be allowed to leave the hospital every few days to visit with her other children
    2. Suggesting that a social worker visit the family weekly to perform a home and child-care evaluation
    3. Providing family members the opportunity to discuss their feelings regarding the hospitalization
    4. Supporting her efforts to be discharged from the hospital as soon as she learns to administer insulin

37. A primigravida in her first trimester visits her obstetrician for the first time. The statement that illustrates a psychologic reaction to pregnancy that commonly occurs in the first trimester would be:
    1. "I know I'm going to be a terrible mother. I'll forget the baby somewhere the first time I go shopping."
    2. "I know I'm having a little girl. I dreamed she would be a doctor or a lawyer and be very successful."
    3. "I want to be pregnant, and I'm excited about the baby, but I'm not sure I'm ready to become a mother."

    4. "I'm so excited about this baby, but I'm so afraid of losing control during labor. I know I'll be a terrible patient."

38. In a preparation for childbirth class, the nurse would teach that labor:
    1. Should be painless and uneventful
    2. Can be painful, but clients will be taught how to tolerate it
    3. Will cause discomfort; however, medication will not be needed
    4. May be uncomfortable, but medication is available when needed

39. The nurse realizes that the greatest influence on the perception of pain for a woman in labor is the:
    1. Parity of the client
    2. Length of the labor
    3. Tension of the client
    4. Difficulty of the labor

40. At 42 weeks' gestation a client delivers an 8-pound, 5-ounce infant. The nurse is aware that the characteristics that would be indicative of a postterm infant are:
    1. Abundant lanugo, abundant vernix, and fine woolly hair
    2. Smooth, edematous skin, with many blood vessels visible
    3. Breast buds 5 mm, veins barely visible, and superficial peeling of skin
    4. Thick, wrinkled and parchment-like skin with generalized peeling of epidermis

41. A client seeking family planning information asks the nurse during which phase of the menstrual cycle an IUD should be inserted. The nurse responds that the insertion is usually done on the:
    1. 1st to 4th day
    2. 5th to 11th day
    3. 14th to 16th day
    4. 25th to 28th day

42. When assessing a newborn, the nurse identifies that the baby's skin is mottled. The nurse should first:
    1. Administer oxygen
    2. Notify the physician
    3. Encourage an oral feeding
    4. Place the baby under the radiant warmer

43. The nurse assesses the hips of a newborn for dislocation and is aware that dislocation would be indicated by:
    1. Legs of equal length

2. Resistance to flexion of the hips
3. Limitation in abduction of either hip
4. Ability to abduct each hip 90 degrees

44. About six hours after birth the nurse notes that a client's fundus is two finger-breadths above the umbilicus and is deviated to the right of the midline. The nurse suspects that the client has:
   1. Begun involution
   2. Bladder distention
   3. Second-degree uterine atony
   4. Retained placental fragments

45. A client with endometriosis asks the nurse what side effects to expect from leuprolide (Lupron). The nurse's response would be:
   1. Weight gain
   2. Increased libido
   3. Frequent urination
   4. Heavy menstrual bleeding

46. A client with a history of rheumatic heart disease is admitted in early labor. The nurse should encourage this client to assume the:
   1. Supine position
   2. Semi-Fowler's position
   3. Trendelenburg position
   4. Left lateral recumbent position

47. A 60-year-old woman is admitted for a vaginal hysterectomy and an anterior and posterior repair of the vaginal wall. A current adaptation the nurse would expect the client to divulge during the nursing history would be:
   1. Hematuria
   2. Dysmenorrhea
   3. Pain on urination
   4. Stress incontinence

48. During preconceptual counseling, a couple with a history of congenital defects in the family has been advised to have an amniocentesis when the woman becomes pregnant. They ask when the test will be performed. The nurse should tell them that the test will be scheduled sometime during the:
   1. 8th to 10th week
   2. 14th to 16th week
   3. 20th to 24th week
   4. 28th to 32nd week

49. The day after a client has a cesarean birth, the indwelling catheter is removed. The nurse can best evaluate that the client's urinary function has returned to normal when the:
   1. Client's urinalysis indicates no bacteria present
   2. Client has a residual urine of 90 mL after voiding
   3. Client's daily urinary output is at least 1500 mL
   4. Client voids at least 300 mL four hours after catheter removal

50. A client who has just begun breastfeeding her newborn complains that her nipples feel very sore. The mother should be encouraged to:
   1. Apply continuous ice packs to her nipples to reduce the pain
   2. Take the analgesic medication prescribed to limit the discomfort
   3. Remove the baby from the breast for a few days to rest the nipples
   4. Assume a different position when breastfeeding to adjust the infant's sucking

1. 4 **Rhythmic uterine contractions are positive signs of beginning labor. (2) (PM; CJ; AS; HP)**
   1 This is not a sign of labor but may be indicative of fetal compromise that would demand medical attention.
   2 This is not a sign of labor; it may indicate that placental separation has lessened.
   3 This may or may not be related to contractions or the onset of labor.

2. 3 **The amount and character of the lochia must be checked after a cesarean birth just as it is after a vaginal birth. (2) (PB; CJ; EV; HP)**
   1 Although it is important to maintain hydration, the priority is to prevent hemorrhage.
   2 Bonding is an important consideration after the mother and infant have stabilized.
   4 The incisional area is observed for signs of hemorrhage; it is too early for evidence of infection.

3. 2 **Attachment theory states that the experience of the birth of a preterm infant carries with it feelings of loss of control for the mother. (3) (PI; CJ; PL; EC)**
   1 Withdrawal from the situation is maladaptive and requires special help.
   3 A healthy relationship can occur regardless of the baby's state of health.
   4 There is no basis to believe that increased attachment occurs, especially if the infant must remain in the hospital.

4. 3 **Progressive cervical dilation and regular contractions that get progressively closer and increase in intensity are indications of true labor. (2) (PM; CJ; AS; HC)**
   1 These are not indications of true labor.
   2 Same as answer 1.
   4 Same as answer 1.

5. 1 **The first hour after birth is called the fourth stage of labor; during this time the uterus is at the level of the umbilicus and each succeeding day it descends one finger-breadth. (3) (PM; CJ; AS; HC)**
   2 This should happen on the second postpartum day because the uterus descends one finger-breadth each day.
   3 The uterus descends below the umbilicus, rising above it if the bladder is full.
   4 This occurs on the fourth or fifth postpartum day because the uterus descends one finger-breadth per day.

6. 2 **Respiratory distress is a common response indicative of possible immaturity of the infant's respiratory tract, such as small lumen, weakness of the respiratory musculature, paucity of functional alveoli, or insufficient calcification of the bony thorax. (2) (PB; CJ; EV; HN)**
   1 Tone (i.e., high, shrill) would be more pertinent than duration of the cry.
   3 This would not yet be important, since the infant's intake is limited during the first 24 hours.
   4 The temperature of the preterm infant would decrease because of immature thermoregulation.

7. 3 **The influence of progesterone and the pressure of the gravid uterus slows GI motility. (1) (PM; CJ; AN; HC)**
   1 There is a decrease in ovarian activity.
   2 The pulmonary capacity stays relatively stable as the thoracic cage widens to accommodate lung volume.
   4 There is an increase in the glomerular filtration rate because of the increased fluid volume.

8. 2 **Using Nägele's rule to calculate, the estimated date of birth (EDB) is the date of the last menstrual period (LMP) plus seven days, minus three months; spotting is fairly common at the time of the expected menstrual period. (1) (PM; CJ; IM; HC)**
   1 This is too early.
   3 This is too late.
   4 Same as answer 3.

9. 4 **A decreased urinary output of less than 25 mL/hour may be indicative of kidney damage, secondary to the preeclampsia, and impending renal failure; magnesium sulfate is excreted by the kidneys and magnesium toxicity can occur. (2) (SE; MR; EV; DR)**
   1 This is within the therapeutic magnesium blood levels of 2.5 to 7.5 mEq/L.
   2 Respirations at this rate are within the expected range; a rate of at least 16 breaths per minute should be present before each dose of magnesium sulfate.
   3 Loss of the patellar reflex is suggestive of magnesium sulfate toxicity.

10. 1 Salk vaccine (IPV) may be given because it is a killed virus vaccine and will not have a teratogenic effect on the fetus. (2) (SE; CJ; PL; HC)

2 This vaccine is not administered during pregnancy because it is an attenuated live virus vaccine and may be teratogenic to the fetus.

3 Same as answer 2.

4 Same as answer 2.

11. 2 A full bladder helps support the uterus in proper position for the imaging during the scan. (2) (PB; CJ; AN; HP)

1 Increased circulation is not required before an ultrasound and amniocentesis; 8 ounces of fluid will not increase fluid volume significantly.

3 The purpose of increasing maternal fluid intake is not to hydrate the fetus or to decrease fetal movement.

4 After the procedure hydration is encouraged to decrease uterine activity caused by the amniocentesis and support fluid volume.

12. 1 The tonic neck reflex is expected in the healthy newborn and disappears within three to four months. (2) (PM; MR; IM; NN)

2 This response disappears between three and four months.

3 Lack of this reflex may indicate neurologic impairment.

4 This is an expected newborn response and does not need medical attention.

13. 2 Anovulation occurs in nursing mothers for varying periods; generally it is not a reliable method of birth control. (2) (PM; CJ; IM; RC)

1 Menstrual periods may not occur for several months; sexual relations need not be delayed this long.

3 Lactation may delay menses but does not reliably suppress ovulation.

4 Ovulation can occur without menstruation.

14. 2 Drug-dependent newborns are poor feeders because of hyperactivity, vomiting, respiratory distress, excessive mucus, and pyrexia; small, frequent feedings are given to prevent dehydration. (3) (PB; CJ; PL; HN)

1 These infants need supportive care during the time the drug is leaving their systems; methadone only modifies withdrawal, it does not prevent it.

3 To minimize extraneous stimulation, environmental stimuli should be decreased.

4 Infants of drug-addicted mothers are prone to hypothermia, not hyperthermia.

15. 4 Knowing that others share the same problems may be comforting; the second part of the nurse's statement is open-ended and allows the client to describe her physical and emotional feelings. (2) (PM; CJ; IM; HC)

1 This discussion is within the purview of the nurse; the discussion should take place at this time.

2 This is too factual; it closes off communication; the client should explore with the nurse the means for feeling better.

3 Telling the client not to worry closes off communication; this does not allow exploration of avenues for further discussion.

16. 4 Extravasation of blood at the separation site into the myometrium causes a tetanic, boardlike uterus. (2) (PB; CJ; AS; HP)

1 The uterus is rigid because it is filled with blood and clots.

2 This is associated with placenta previa; abdominal pain and uterine tenderness occur in abruptio placentae.

3 Bleeding with abdominal pain can be concealed or apparent; the color is usually port wine.

17. 2 The likelihood of gestational hypertension increases fourfold in clients with diabetes mellitus, probably because of a preexisting vascular disorder. (1) (PB; CJ; AN; HP)

1 Abnormal implantation may occur because of scarring or uterine abnormalities, not because of diabetes.

3 Most pregnant women have increased appetites; excessive weight gain may be caused by a macrosomic infant and hydramnios.

4 Decreased fluid volume may occur secondary to underlying vascular disease which affects placental perfusion; there is no direct cause and effect.

18. 1 Immediate delivery is necessary to prevent fetal hypoxia and death. (1) (SE; CJ; PL; HP)

2 Contractions would increase pressure on the cord, causing fetal hypoxia.

3 This would increase pressure on the cord.

4 The fetus may be compromised, and immediate delivery is necessary.

19. 2 Pain caused by deep penetration by the male partner is common in late pregnancy and can be

reduced by using alternative positions such as rear entry. (1) (PM; MR; PL; HC)

1 This should not be suggested until other alternatives have been tried.

3 Douching is not recommended and does not lubricate the vagina; a water-soluble lubricant is more effective.

4 This is unnecessary because this is common during the third trimester.

20. 1 **Dark amber or tea-colored urine indicates highly concentrated urine and requires additional hydration of the client. (1) (SE; MR; IM; HP)**

2 Increasing the IV rate in the presence of urinary suppression would be unsafe because it could cause hypervolemia.

3 Tinges of blood in the urine may indicate bladder injury and are not related to the client's fluid status.

4 This reading is meaningless unless a comparison with other readings indicates a decrease and the possibility of shock.

21. 1 **Vitamin K stores are almost absent in the newborn because the intestinal flora that produce this vitamin are not present; vitamin K is an essential precursor of prothrombin, which is part of the clotting mechanism. (2) (PB; CJ; IM; NN)**

2 Elevated bilirubin levels in the blood occur in newborns because of the rapid breakdown of RBCs and the immature liver's difficulty in conjugating such large amounts; it is not influenced by vitamin K.

3 The normal intestinal flora develop as the newborn is exposed to extrauterine living conditions.

4 The young kidneys operate at a functional level appropriate to the needs of a healthy infant; this is not influenced by vitamin K.

22. 3 **The blood volume was increased during pregnancy. The rapid fluid shift after the placenta is delivered causes an increase in cardiac output, making the first 48 hours postpartum crucial. (2) (PB; CJ; PL; HP)**

1 This is not recommended because it will further increase the circulating blood volume and necessitate an increased cardiac output.

2 Progressive ambulation as tolerated is recommended.

4 The first 48 hours are crucial because of the rapid fluid shift and the increased cardiac output.

23. 2 **Tachycardia is an expected side effect of terbutaline, a beta-mimetic agent; the pulse rate should be no greater than 120 beats per minute;**

pulmonary edema is a rare side effect that can occur with tocolysis. (3) (PB; CJ; EV; DR)

1 The reflexes are not affected by this drug, which relaxes uterine musculature.

3 This drug does not affect the client's level of consciousness.

4 Although intake and output are assessed, an indwelling catheter is not indicated.

24. 3 **The ruptured fallopian tube may be removed rather than repaired; repair of the tube may result in scarring, predisposing the client to another tubal pregnancy. (1) (SE; LE; PL; NP)**

1 This is a procedure for removing leiomyomas (fibroids) from the uterus.

2 The uterus is usually uninvolved in a tubal pregnancy and does not need to be removed.

4 A D&C would be effective in cleaning out the uterine cavity; there are no products of conception in the uterus with a tubal pregnancy.

25. 4 **A variety of incomplete proteins (vegetable proteins) can be combined to provide all the essential amino acids. (3) (PB; MR; PL; HC)**

1 The pregnant client should receive at least 60 g of protein in her diet.

2 Strict vegetarians do not drink milk.

3 These are not the most important factors in diet planning; other nutrients also must be provided.

26. 4 **The postoperative teaching should include instructing the client to expect shoulder pain, secondary to the insufflated carbon dioxide, for 12 to 24 hours. (2) (PB; MR; PL; WH)**

1 There is no need to douche postoperatively.

2 Vaginal spotting may occur, not frank bleeding.

3 Usual activities should not be resumed until two to three days postoperatively and no heavy lifting or strenuous exercise for four to seven days.

27. 2 **Immediate action to prevent excessive bleeding is to massage the fundus until it is firm; this stimulates uterine muscle contraction. (1) (SE; CJ; IM; HC)**

1 This would not be necessary unless bleeding persists after massaging of the uterus.

3 The immediate action is to promote uterine contraction; obtaining the BP would be indicated if a large amount of bleeding occurred or bleeding persisted.

4 If the uterus does not contract after massage, the nurse should notify the physician, not just observe the bleeding.

28. 4 **This indicates that the mother understands that the well-being of the infant will be established by the testing. (2) (PB; MR; EV; HP)**
1 The baby is not affected by the use of external monitoring.
2 This procedure should not precipitate labor.
3 This test does not always require an intravenous infusion; nipple stimulation can be used to initiate uterine activity.

29. 4 **Vitamins A, C, and E and selenium are immune-stimulating nutrients. (2) (PM; MR; IM; HC)**
1 Too much emphasis on the fat-soluble vitamins could result in an inadequate intake of important water-soluble vitamins and minerals.
2 These have no known effect on natural defenses.
3 Same as answer 2.

30. 4 **Tears in the tentorial membrane cause bleeding into the cerebellum, pons, or medulla oblongata; the respiratory regulation centers are located in the medulla and pons. (3) (PB; CJ; AN; HN)**
1 Lethargy would be more indicative of cerebellar injury.
2 A weak, timorous cry would be more indicative of cardiac or respiratory difficulty; a high-pitched, shrill cry is usually present with CNS problems.
3 Purpura is unrelated to tentorial or other CNS injuries.

31. 4 **Axillary lymph nodes are an early site of metastasis and thus are removed and examined to determine if or how much of the cancer has metastasized. (1) (PB; LE; EV; NP)**
1 Pectoral muscles are not removed in a modified radical mastectomy.
2 This is not removed in this type surgery; leaving the skin intact improves healing and enhances breast reconstruction.
3 The entire breast is removed in this type surgery.

32. 3 **Treatment is directed primarily toward reducing the blood pressure and preventing seizures. (1) (PB; CJ; PL; HP)**
1 Anxiety may be present, but the blood pressure is the priority problem.
2 Bleeding is not generally a problem with preeclampsia unless abruptio placentae occurs.
4 In preeclampsia there is already a decrease in circulating blood volume, which causes hemoconcentration and decreased organ perfusion.

33. 4 **The estrogen and progesterone in birth control pills increase the amount of renin produced in** the kidney, which in turn increases production of angiotensin, a potent pressor substance. (1) (SE; CJ; EV; RC)
1 Dysmenorrhea does not occur.
2 This is not usually serious; it often indicates a low hormone level; it is corrected by changes in the type of medication prescribed.
3 Anovulation is the desired effect of oral contraceptives.

34. 4 **Reflecting these feelings gives the client the opportunity to express fears and provides a chance to explore the family history. (2) (PI; CJ; IM; EC)**
1 This supports the client's fears of cancer and blocks communication.
2 Although true, this provides false reassurance.
3 This statement is probing and does not address the client's fears.

35. 3 **Pitocin will cause the uterus to contract after the placenta has been expelled, preventing hemorrhage. (2) (PB; CJ; EV; DR)**
1 Pitocin has no analgesic effect.
2 Relaxation of the uterus is undesirable because it promotes bleeding.
4 Prolactin, not Pitocin, stimulates milk production; Pitocin stimulates the let-down reflex.

36. 3 **The appropriate nursing action is to assist the family in discussing their feelings about hospitalization and loss of the mother's presence. (3) (PI; CJ; IM; EC)**
1 Leaving the hospital while attempts are being made to stabilize her diabetes would be counterproductive.
2 A social worker is necessary only if ineffective coping is identified; it is not indicated in this situation.
4 This is not related to the stated nursing diagnosis; the client also needs to understand the interaction between diet, medication, and exercise.

37. 3 **This response reflects the ambivalence about the pregnancy that is typical during the first trimester. (1) (PM; CJ; EV; EC)**
1 This is a typical response during the third trimester when the client begins to doubt her ability to be a good parent.
2 Fantasizing about the infant, its sex, and its future is common during the second trimester.
4 Expressing fears about the labor and delivery experience and parenting is common during the third trimester.

38. 4 **Preparation for parenthood classes should help couples develop realistic expectations of the laboring process, including associated discomfort and ways of dealing with it. (2) (SE; MR; IM; HC)**
1 Contractions are uncomfortable, but childbirth preparation helps the client cope with discomfort.
2 Clients are taught what to expect and the proper exercises to expedite labor; the focus should not be on pain.
3 There is no way of predicting whether medication will be needed; however, the client should be assured of its availability.

39. 3 **Tension in the woman prevents relaxation and has the greatest influence on how she will progress through labor and on her perception of pain; tension is related to the expectation of pain, which is based on cultural norms and past experiences. (1) (PI; CJ; AN; EC)**
1 Parity does not play a major role in the woman's perception of pain.
2 Although the woman often becomes more uncomfortable and tired near the end of labor, the length of labor does not play a major role in her perception of pain.
4 Although the difficulty of labor affects the amount of pain, it does not play a major role in the woman's perception of pain.

40. 4 **This describes the skin of a postterm infant who has been exposed to amniotic fluid too long. (3) (PM; CJ; AS; HN)**
1 These are characteristics of a preterm infant.
2 Same as answer 1.
3 These are characteristics of a term infant.

41. 1 **Intrauterine devices should be inserted during menses because the cervical os is slightly dilated and there is little chance of pregnancy. (3) (PM; CJ; IM; RC)**
2 An IUD should not be inserted at this time; this is the proliferative phase of the menstrual cycle.
3 An IUD should not be inserted at this time because pregnancy may have occurred.
4 Same as answer 3.

42. 4 **Mottling of the newborn's skin results from hypothermia. (1) (PB; CJ; IM; NN)**
1 This is not necessary; this is a phenomenon that usually indicates falling temperature; the infant requires warming.
2 Same as answer 1.
3 Feeding will not increase temperature.

43. 3 **Dislocation of the hip limits abduction to less than 90 degrees. (2) (PB; CJ; AS; HN)**
1 The legs should be of equal length.
2 Flexion of the hips is not affected by dislocation.
4 This is an expected finding in the newborn; maternal hormones cause loosening of ligaments, which allows abduction to 90 degrees.

44. 2 **Bladder distention causes uterine displacement, which interferes with uterine contractions and may lead to postpartum hemorrhage. (1) (PB; CJ; AS; HC)**
1 During involution the uterus is not deviated to the right.
3 There is no such thing as second-degree uterine atony.
4 Retained placental fragments often cause bright red bleeding and a boggy uterus; there are no data to support this.

45. 1 **The nurse should teach the client that the side effects of leuprolide include edema, which causes an increase in weight. (3) (PB; CJ; EV; DR)**
2 This medication causes decreased libido.
3 Frequent urination is not a side effect of leuprolide.
4 Clients who take leuprolide do not experience menstrual periods because both FSH and LH are suppressed.

46. 2 **The head of the bed should be elevated 45 degrees; this allows for maximum chest expansion for ventilation. (1) (PB; CJ; IM; HP)**
1 The laboring woman should not assume the supine position because she may develop hypotension because of impeded venous return.
3 Trendelenburg position would interfere with optimum cardiac function during labor.
4 The head of the bed should be elevated, not flat.

47. 4 **Increased intraabdominal pressure associated with lifting, coughing, or laughing, in conjunction with a relaxed pelvic musculature and a bladder displaced into the vagina, results in an inability to control the urinary stream. (1) (PB; CJ; AS; WH)**
1 Usually this is associated with a urinary tract infection, bladder tumor, or renal calculi, not with a cystocele or rectocele.
2 Usually this is associated with pelvic inflammatory disease, endometriosis, or cervical stenosis, not with cystocele or rectocele; the client is probably postmenopausal.
3 Usually this is associated with a urinary infection, not with a cystocele or rectocele.

48. 2 **This timing allows for decision making and intervention before viability; the uterus has risen into the abdomen and there is enough amniotic fluid to be withdrawn and tested. (3) (PB; MR; IM; HP)**

1 An amniocentesis before 14 weeks is associated with an increase in complications such as fetal loss and fetal talipes.

3 This timing is late; the results can take two weeks and may limit options if pathology is identified.

4 Same as answer 3.

49. 4 **This would indicate that the urinary sphincter tone has not been affected by the catheter and urinary retention with overflow is not present. (2) (PB; CJ; EV; HP)**

1 The absence of bacteria indicates the absence of infection but does not portend the return of urinary function.

2 This indicates retention with overflow; the client urinates small amounts but does not completely empty the bladder.

3 Although the total amount of urine indicates adequacy of kidney function, it does not reflect sphincter control or the possibility of retention.

50. 4 **Altering the breastfeeding position may ensure that the entire nipple and as much of the areola as possible is in the infant's mouth; when the infant is latched on the nipple correctly and a finger is used to release suction at the end of a feeding, trauma to the nipple is reduced. (2) (PB; CJ; PL; HC)**

1 This is contraindicated because it suppresses lactation; also, ice applications of any kind should never be continuous because they can result in tissue damage.

2 Analgesics should not be necessary; soreness is common; it usually occurs only at the beginning of a feeding and is temporary until the nipples become accustomed to the infant's sucking.

3 Removing the infant from the breast will result in engorgement, which will increase the discomfort.

Childbearing and Women's Health Nursing Quiz 2

1. A client with severe preeclampsia is receiving magnesium sulfate therapy. When monitoring this client's response to therapy, the priority assessment would be:
   1. Urinary output
   2. Respiratory rate
   3. Deep tendon reflexes
   4. Level of consciousness

2. During a pelvic examination of a 24-year-old woman, the nurse suspects a vaginal infection because of the presence of a white, curd-like vaginal discharge. Additional assessments that the nurse should make at this time include the presence of:
   1. A foul odor
   2. Perineal itching
   3. An ischemic cervix
   4. A forgotten tampon

3. The nurse midwife should assist a mother to deliver a baby's anterior shoulder by:
   1. Guiding the head upward
   2. Guiding the head downward
   3. Flexing the head toward the thigh
   4. Extending the head above the pubic symphysis

4. The nurse assesses a newborn using the Apgar score. At one minute after birth, the baby has a heart rate of 120, slow and irregular respirations, weak cry, some flexion of extremities, and a pink body with blue extremities. The one-minute Apgar score should be recorded as:
   1. 5
   2. 6
   3. 7
   4. 8

5. During the initial newborn assessment the nurse finds several dark round spots on the buttocks of a newborn. The nurse's next action would be to:
   1. Report that there are forceps marks on the newborn
   2. Note in the chart that the newborn has several stork bites
   3. Notify the physician that there are bruises on the buttocks
   4. Describe the Mongolian spots on the nursing assessment form

6. Pregnant women with cardiac problems must be assessed routinely. The nurse should suspect early decompensation if the client exhibits:
   1. Hemoptysis
   2. Tachycardia
   3. Increasing fatigue
   4. Generalized edema

7. The breathing technique that the nurse instructs a mother to use as the head crowns on the perineum would be:
   1. Blowing
   2. Slow chest
   3. Shallow breathing
   4. Accelerated-decelerated

8. During a newborn neurological assessment, the nurse should expect to find an:
   1. Absent Babinski's reflex and intact grasp reflex
   2. Absent Babinski's reflex and intact startle reflex
   3. Intact Babinski's reflex and intact tonic neck reflex
   4. Intact Babinski's reflex and absent tonic neck reflex

9. The nurse teaches a postpartum client with type 1 diabetes that the safest and most reliable method of birth control would be:
   1. The vaginal sponge
   2. The rhythm method
   3. An oral contraceptive
   4. A diaphragm with spermicidal gel

10. A couple seeking genetic counseling are heterozygous carriers of Tay-Sachs disease. They ask the nurse what the chances are for their child inheriting the disease. The nurse responds that the probability would be:
    1. 0%
    2. 25%
    3. 50%
    4. 100%

11. A 20-year-old developmentally disabled woman is a resident in a group home. She has had four abortions in the last two years, and the agency supervisor recommends that she be sterilized. The client is brought to the gynecological clinic for evaluation. It is obvious that the client is unable

to exercise informed consent for sterilization. The nurse should be aware that the procedure cannot be performed without legal consent from the:
1. Next of kin
2. Court appointed individual or group
3. Agency designated to perform the abortion
4. Organization licensed to administer the group home

12. During the discharge evaluation of a two-day-old newborn, the nurse observes a swelling confined to the right side of the scalp. The nurse would recognize that this is:
1. Molding
2. Hydrocephalus
3. Cephalhematoma
4. Caput succedaneum

13. A client with a fourth-degree perineal laceration is being assessed six hours after delivery. The most important nursing intervention at this time would be to:
1. Encourage fluid intake and a high-fiber diet
2. Offer sitz baths at least three times each day
3. Apply a premoistened anesthetic pad to the area
4. Administer a Fleet enema to prevent straining at stool

14. A 24-year-old client complains to the nurse in the women's health clinic that her breasts become tender before her menstrual period. The nurse should recommend that the client:
1. Take salt tablets daily
2. Increase dietary protein by 40%
3. Reduce daily exercise to three times weekly
4. Decrease caffeine intake a week before menstruation

15. A client, who is a mother for the first time, appears anxious about her new parenting role. With encouragement, she has joined the new mothers support group at the local YWCA. This is an example of:
1. Tertiary prevention
2. Primary prevention
3. Therapeutic alliance
4. Secondary prevention

16. A client who suspects that she is six weeks pregnant appears mildly anxious as she is waiting for her first obstetrical appointment. A symptom the nurse would expect this client to exhibit is:
1. Dizziness
2. Breathlessness
3. Increased alertness
4. Abdominal cramps

17. To ensure proper nutrition during pregnancy for a client who is a vegetarian, the nurse should:
1. Advise the client to include meat in her diet at least once daily
2. Encourage the client to join a diet group to teach her good nutrition
3. Help the client plan nutritious meals that use foods that she is willing to eat
4. Tell the client to discontinue the vegetarian practice entirely until she delivers

18. A client in her 30th week of gestation is in preterm labor and the physician orders betamethasone. The client asks the nurse why she is receiving the drug. The nurse explains that it is used to:
1. Prevent chorioamnionitis
2. Increase uteroplacental exchange
3. Promote neonatal pulmonary maturity
4. Treat fetal respiratory distress syndrome

19. After a client's membranes rupture spontaneously, the nurse observes the umbilical cord protruding from the vagina. The nursing action that should receive the highest priority in this situation is:
1. Raising the foot of the bed
2. Preparing for a cesarean birth
3. Administering oxygen by mask
4. Auscultating the fetal heartbeats

20. A woman who is breastfeeding her newborn is taught breastfeeding techniques. The nurse explains how to relieve breast engorgement. The nurse would recognize that further teaching is necessary when the woman states she will:
1. Manually express breast milk
2. Breastfeed the infant more frequently
3. Take a warm shower to increase the milk flow
4. Apply ice packs immediately before breastfeeding

21. A 16-year-old primipara, at 32 weeks' gestation, is admitted to the hospital. Her blood pressure is 170/110 mm Hg and she has 4+ proteinuria. She has gained 50 pounds during the pregnancy and her face and extremities are edematous. The nurse assesses that the client probably has:
1. Eclampsia
2. Mild preeclampsia
3. Severe preeclampsia
4. Chronic hypertensive disease

22. A client at 36 weeks' gestation, with severe preeclampsia, is admitted to the high-risk labor unit and placed on a fetal monitor as well as on an automated machine for blood pressure monitoring.

Frequent monitoring of the blood pressure is essential to reduce the potential for:
1. Brain attack
2. Hemorrhage
3. Precipitous labor
4. Disseminated intravascular coagulation

23. As part of a high school sex education program, the school nurse discusses herpes genitalis. The nurse should tell the students that:
    1. Herpes genitalis is curable with penicillin
    2. The disease generally is painless in women
    3. The disease is transmitted via fomites such as toilet seats
    4. Herpes genitalis causes both local and systemic reactions

24. Postoperatively, the nursing care plan for a client who has had pelvic surgery should include:
    1. Encouraging the client to ambulate in the hallway
    2. Assisting the client to dangle her legs over the side of the bed
    3. Elevating the client's lower extremities by gatching the bed
    4. Maintaining the client on bed rest until the bandages are removed

25. The nurse understands that gonorrhea is difficult to control because:
    1. The blood test is expensive and time consuming
    2. The causative organism has become resistant to treatment
    3. There is no specific diagnostic test for the causative organism
    4. The symptoms are vague and the incubation period is relatively short

26. When teaching cord care, the nurse should explain to the parents about the care of the cord. The teaching should include:
    1. Swabbing the base of the cord daily with alcohol at each diaper change
    2. Taping a pressure dressing over the umbilicus to protect it until the cord dries and falls off
    3. Applying an antibiotic ointment to the base of the cord with each diaper change until the cord falls off
    4. Placing the diaper over the umbilical cord to prevent infection and to protect the umbilicus from injury until the cord falls off

27. When preparing a client to breastfeed, the nurse is aware that:
    1. High levels of progesterone stimulate the secretion of oxytocin
    2. High levels of estrogen stimulate secretions of lactogenic hormones

3. Milk secretion is under the control of hormones and starts immediately after the birth
4. Suckling stimulates the posterior pituitary gland to release oxytocin, which initiates the let-down reflex

28. A client arrives in the birthing room with the fetal head crowning. The nurse recognizes that birth is imminent and tells the client to:
    1. Push with all her power
    2. Use the pant-breathing pattern
    3. Assume the Trendelenburg position
    4. Hold her breath and turn to the left side

29. A new mother is inspecting her baby girl for the first time. The baby's breasts are swollen, and there is a red vaginal discharge. When the mother asks what is wrong the nurse should respond:
    1. "Your baby appears to have a problem. I will notify the pediatrician."
    2. "I do not see anything unusual. What exactly do you see on the baby?"
    3. "It is nothing to worry about. The swelling and discharge will go away."
    4. "The swelling and discharge are expected and are due to hormonal stimulation."

30. Examination of a client in active labor reveals fetal heart sounds in the right lower quadrant. The head is in the anterior position, is well flexed, and cannot be dislodged from the pelvic outlet. The nurse should chart:
    1. ROA, station 0
    2. LOP, station –2
    3. ROP, station –3
    4. LOA, station +1

31. A client has had a dilation and curettage (D&C) after a spontaneous abortion. Later in the day, the nurse finds her crying quietly. The most appropriate statement for the nurse to make would be:
    1. "This must be a very hard experience for you to deal with."
    2. "You will have other children to take the place of the one you lost."
    3. "I know you are sad now, but at least you know you can get pregnant."
    4. "I know how you feel, but when a woman miscarries it is usually for the best."

32. A woman in labor with her third child is 4 cm dilated. The fetal head is not engaged. Suddenly her membranes rupture. The nurse should first:
    1. Notify the physician
    2. Check the fetal heart rate
    3. Assess the color of the fluid
    4. Place a sterile towel under the buttocks

33. A postpartum client is being prepared for discharge. Her blood laboratory report indicates a white blood cell count of 16,000/dL. The nurse should:
    1. Check with the nurse manager to see if the client can go home
    2. Reassess the client for signs of infection by checking her vital signs
    3. Place the report in the client's chart because this is an expected postpartum finding
    4. Delay the client's discharge until the physician performs a complete examination

34. When preparing a client for an amniocentesis, the nurse should:
    1. Instruct her to empty her bladder before the test is started
    2. Encourage her to drink three glasses of water before the test
    3. Advise her to take nothing by mouth for four hours before the test
    4. Administer the ordered sedative to prevent fetal movement during the test

35. An infant is admitted to the hospital nursery and is classified as being small for gestational age (SGA). A priority intervention for this infant would be to:
    1. Test the infant's stools for occult blood
    2. Monitor the infant's blood glucose levels
    3. Place the infant in the Trendelenburg position
    4. Measure the infant's head circumference every shift

36. A newborn's discharge is being delayed because of a rising reticulocyte count. The infant's mother, who is being discharged, asks the nurse why the baby must stay. The nurse's response is based on an understanding that the infant needs to be observed for:
    1. Bleeding tendencies
    2. Significant jaundice
    3. A bacterial infection
    4. Adequate oxygenation

37. A 17-year-old client tells the nurse that her sister had an ectopic pregnancy about three months ago and had to have her tube removed. The nurse knows that this young woman needs further explanation when she states:
    1. "I guess I'll have to wait awhile to become an aunt."
    2. "This kind of thing can happen to my sister again."

    3. "This kind of thing can happen after a pelvic infection."
    4. "My sister is lucky because she'll never have a period again."

38. The nurse instructs and encourages a client admitted to the hospital with placenta previa about the importance of:
    1. Breathing deeply to ensure that the fetus gets oxygen
    2. Remaining on her back to minimize pressure on the cervix
    3. Lying on her side to avoid putting pressure on the vena cava
    4. Keeping all movement to a minimum to diminish bleeding

39. The nurse understands that a positive contraction stress test (CST) may be indicative of potential fetal compromise. The test demonstrates that during contractions the fetal heart rate shows:
    1. Late decelerations
    2. Early decelerations
    3. A normal baseline
    4. Variable decelerations

40. A 24-year-old client is admitted at 40 weeks' gestation. The cervix is 5 cm dilated and is 100% effaced, and the presenting part is at station 0. The nurse assesses that the fetal heart tones are just above the umbilicus. The presentation that the fetus probably is in would be:
    1. Face
    2. Brow
    3. Breech
    4. Shoulder

41. Epidural anesthesia is administered to a client. A primary responsibility of the nurse is to assess for:
    1. Tachycardia
    2. Hypotension
    3. Decreased urinary output
    4. Precipitous second stage of labor

42. A large-for-gestational age (LGA) infant of a diabetic mother (IDM) should be assessed for:
    1. The presence of mongolian spots
    2. A blood glucose level less than 40
    3. A body temperature less than 98° F
    4. Elevated bilirubin levels in the first 24 hours

43. While a client is receiving IV magnesium sulfate for preeclampsia, a primary nursing intervention would be:
    1. Limiting her fluid intake to 1000 mL/24 hours

2. Preparing for the possibility of a precipitate birth
3. Restricting visitors and keeping the room darkened and quiet
4. Obtaining magnesium gluconate for use as an antagonist if necessary

44. A few weeks after discharge, a postpartum client develops mastitis and telephones for advice concerning breastfeeding. The nurse should tell the client to:
1. Start to wean the baby from the breast to reduce the pain
2. Get an antibiotic from the physician and start formula feedings
3. Pump her breasts and wear a tight-fitting bra to suppress milk production
4. Breastfeed often because this will keep the breasts empty and reduce pain

45. A 40-year-old client arrives at the women's health clinic stating she has missed two menstrual periods. When preparing the client for a gynecological examination, the nurse places her in the:
1. Supine position with knees and hips flexed and the feet flat on the table
2. Sims' position with the uppermost thigh and knee fully flexed and the other leg partly flexed
3. Knee-chest position with the knees separated, head turned to the side, and chest and face on a pillow
4. Dorsal recumbent position with the knees and hips flexed and the heels resting on the footrests

46. The nurse assesses that a one-day-old newborn has a heart rate of 138 beats per minute. The best nursing action at this time would be to:
1. Rewrap the baby quickly
2. Continue the assessment

3. Place the baby in a heated crib
4. Take the heart rate again in one hour

47. A high-risk preterm infant is placed in the neonatal intensive care unit. A common concern that the nurse can anticipate for this mother would be:
1. Failure to bond with the infant
2. Fear of touching and handling the infant
3. Inability to provide breast milk for the infant
4. Anxiety that the father may not accept the infant

48. When assessing a newborn with exstrophy of the bladder, the nurse should be aware that a defect associated with exstrophy of the bladder is:
1. Absence of one kidney
2. Congenital heart disease
3. Pubic bone malformation
4. Tracheoesophageal fistula

49. A 60-year-old woman who is to have a total abdominal hysterectomy for a noninvasive endometrial cancer may have difficulty in emotionally adjusting to this type of surgery. The nurse recognizes that the reason for this would be because she:
1. Will have diminished sexual desire
2. May be concerned about her femininity
3. Needs to cope with body image changes
4. Will recover more slowly because of her age

50. A client had a blood pressure of 90/50 during her first visit to the prenatal clinic. At 34 weeks' gestation her blood pressure is now 120/76. The nurse recognizes that this can occur because of:
1. The possible development of preeclampsia
2. The development of essential hypertension
3. An increased stroke volume during the third trimester
4. An expected rise in blood pressure as pregnancy progresses

1. 2 **Respiratory depression occurs with toxic levels of this medication; calcium gluconate should be readily available to counteract toxicity. (2) (PB; CJ; EV; DR)**
   1 Although this is an important observation, assessment of respiratory status is more critical.
   3 Same as answer 1.
   4 Same as answer 1.

2. 2 **This type of vaginal discharge usually occurs with candidiasis, a fungal infection; pruritus is the most common symptom. (3) (SE; CJ; AS; WH)**
   1 An odorous, frothy, greenish discharge occurs with trichomoniasis, a protozoal infestation.
   3 Ischemia of the cervix is not associated with candidiasis; the vagina and cervix usually are inflamed with candidiasis.
   4 This may cause a bacterial, not fungal, vaginitis.

3. 2 **After the newborn's head has externally rotated, the nurse guides the head gently downward to deliver the anterior shoulder. (2) (PM; CJ; IM; HC)**
   1 This will deliver the posterior shoulder.
   3 This will not assist with the delivery of the anterior shoulder.
   4 Same as answer 3.

4. 2 **According to the Apgar scoring scale: heart rate above 120 = 2, respirations below 30 = 1, some flexion of extremities = 1, weak cry = 1, color-blue extremities = 1; the total Apgar is 6. (2) (PB; CJ; AS; HN)**
   1 Based on the data, this score is too low.
   3 Based on the data, this score is too high.
   4 Same as answer 3.

5. 4 **Mongolian spots are bluish-black areas of pigmentation commonly near the back and buttocks of dark-skinned newborns; they fade gradually over time. (1) (PM; CJ; AS; NN)**
   1 Forceps marks are red and have a distinctive imprint matching the configuration of the instrument.
   2 Stork bites are short red marks commonly near the base of the neck of newborns.
   3 These are not bruises and should not be reported as such.

6. 3 **This is one of the early signs of decompensation resulting from an increased cardiac workload. (2) (PB; CJ; AS; HP)**
   1 This is a late sign of cardiac decompensation that is associated with pulmonary edema.
   2 This is a later sign of cardiac decompensation and may be accompanied by other signs of heart failure.
   4 Same as answer 2.

7. 1 **Blowing forcefully through the mouth controls the strong urge to push and allows for a more controlled delivery of the head. (2) (PM; MR; IM; HC)**
   2 This is not helpful in overcoming the urge to push; this is used during the latent phase of the first stage of labor.
   3 This breathing pattern does not help to control the expulsion of the fetus.
   4 This is not helpful in overcoming the urge to push; this is used during active labor when the cervix is 3 to 7 cm dilated.

8. 3 **Both reflexes are intact in the healthy newborn. (2) (PM; CJ; AS; NN)**
   1 The Babinski reflex is intact in the healthy newborn.
   2 Same as answer 1.
   4 The tonic neck reflex is intact in the healthy newborn.

9. 4 **This mechanical device, if used correctly, offers the lowest risk with a high degree of reliability for a person with type 1 diabetes. (3) (PM; MR; IM; RC)**
   1 This can be used by people with diabetes mellitus but it is less reliable than the diaphragm with spermicidal gel.
   2 This is not reliable because the menses during the postpartum and lactation periods are often irregular; partner cooperation is also required.
   3 Even a low-dose contraceptive increases the risk for vascular complications; people with type 1 diabetes mellitus are already at risk for vascular complications.

10. 2 **Since Tay-Sachs disease is an autosomal recessive disorder, there is the probability that 25% of the offspring of two unaffected heterozygous parents will inherit it. (2) (SE; CJ; IM; RP)**
   1 This occurs if one parent is a Tay-Sachs carrier and the other does not have the gene.
   3 This occurs if one parent is heterozygous and the other is homozygous; however, this does

not occur because children with Tay-Sachs disease do not live long enough to reproduce.

4 This does not occur because children with Tay-Sachs disease do not live long enough to reproduce.

11. 2 **In the United States individual states each have their own restrictions; the approval of a court-appointed individual or group is required to give legal consent. (1) (SE; LE; AN; NP)**

1 This would not meet the legal requirements for granting consent; the states have an obligation to oversee the best interests of the mentally disabled and the court must be involved.

3 Same as answer 1.

4 Same as answer 1.

12. 3 **This is a collection of blood beneath the periosteum of the skull bone; the blood mass does not cross the suture line and is confined to one side of the head; it reabsorbs spontaneously in three to six weeks. (2) (PM; CJ; EV; NN)**

1 This is overlapping of the cranial bones or shaping of the fetal head to accommodate and conform to the bony and soft parts of the mother's birth canal during labor; it disappears spontaneously.

2 This is an enlargement of the entire head (macrocephaly) caused by an abnormal enlargement of the cerebral ventricles and skull which results from an obstruction in the flow of cerebral spinal fluid.

4 This is an edematous swelling of the scalp that extends across the suture line; it disappears spontaneously in three to four days.

13. 1 **Fluid intake and fiber help promote soft stools and defecation; promoting defecation is a priority because a fourth-degree laceration impinges on the rectal sphincter. (3) (PM; CJ; IM; HP)**

2 Although comfort measures should be employed to relieve pain, managing bowel elimination is the priority to prevent further trauma to the rectum.

3 Same as answer 2.

4 This would cause additional unnecessary trauma to the rectum; administering a Fleet enema is contraindicated when there is damage to the rectum.

14. 4 **The client is exhibiting one symptom of premenstrual syndrome (PMS); deleting food and beverages containing caffeine can limit breast swelling. (1) (PB; CJ; IM; WH)**

1 Salt intake should be reduced premenstrually to limit the development of edema.

2 This is an excessive intake of protein; whole grains, vegetables, and fruits should be increased in the diet.

3 Exercise should be increased premenstrually to help reduce the symptoms of PMS.

15. 2 **Primary prevention is directed toward health promotion and illness prevention. (2) (SE; MR; PL; NP)**

1 Tertiary prevention is focused on rehabilitation and the reduction of residual effects.

3 Therapeutic alliance relates to the relationship between the client and a professional provider of care.

4 Secondary prevention is related to early detection and treatment.

16. 3 **Increased alertness is an expected common behavior that occurs in new or different situations when a person is mildly anxious. (2)(PI; CJ; AS; EC)**

1 This is a common sign of moderate to severe anxiety.

2 Same as answer 1.

4 Same as answer 1.

17. 3 **Various foods, such as nuts and soy products, can be substituted for meat or animal-related products when planning nutritious meals for the pregnant woman who is a vegetarian. (1) (PB; MR; PL; HC)**

1 This would ignore the client's beliefs and lifestyle.

2 The client may know healthy nutrition; this client needs help to adapt the vegetarian diet to meet pregnancy needs.

4 Same as answer 1.

18. 3 **Betamethasone accelerates lung maturity and reduces intravascular hemorrhage and necrotizing enterocolitis in the preterm neonate if given 24 hours before birth. (1) (PB; CJ; IM; DR)**

1 Chorioamnionitis will be treated with antibiotic therapy; this problem may occur if the membranes are ruptured prematurely and birth does not occur within 24 hours.

2 The drug has no effect on uteroplacental exchange.

4 The neonate, not the fetus, develops respiratory distress syndrome (RDS); if given to the mother 24 hours before the preterm birth, the drug will decrease the severity and incidence of RDS in the neonate.

19. 1 **This eases the pressure of the presenting part on the umbilical cord and receives the highest priority. (2) (PB; CJ; IM; HC)**

2 A cesarean birth may be necessary; however, the priority is to ease the pressure on the cord to prevent fetal hypoxia.

3 Oxygen can be given, but this is not the priority.

4 Time should not be wasted trying to locate the fetal heart when the fetus is at risk for hypoxia because of cord compression.

20. **4 Applying ice packs will cause constriction of vessels, inhibit lactation, and interfere with successful breastfeeding. (2) (PM; MR; EV; HC)**

1 Manual expression initiates milk flow, empties the ducts, and relieves engorgement.

2 Frequent nursing empties the milk ducts, thus relieving engorgement.

3 This exhibits adequate understanding by the client; warmth will dilate ducts and facilitate flow of milk, thus relieving engorgement.

21. **3 Arteriolar spasms cause hypertension; decreased arterial perfusion of the kidneys causes an alteration in the glomeruli resulting in oliguria and proteinuria; sodium and water are retained resulting in edema. (2) (PB; CJ; AS; HP)**

1 This is characterized by seizures; there are no data to indicate that the client is having or has had seizures.

2 The symptoms are less severe in mild preeclampsia, especially the BP, which usually is not higher than 150/110 mm Hg.

4 The client would have been hypertensive before the pregnancy.

22. **1 The likelihood of a brain attack increases with rising blood pressure readings. (1) (PB; CJ; EV; HP)**

2 The degree of hypertension is not associated with hemorrhage.

3 The course of labor is not affected by blood pressure changes except in the presence of abruptio placentae.

4 Fluctuations in blood pressure do not affect the status of the clotting factors.

23. **4 Fever, malaise, and headache may accompany local reactions. (2) (SE; MR; AS; WH)**

1 Herpes is of viral origin; there is no cure, and antibiotics are ineffective.

2 Vesicles on genitalia rupture, causing painful ulcerations.

3 Most transmissions occur through intimate sexual contact with acute or healing lesions.

24. **1 Muscle contraction during ambulation improves venous return, which prevents venous stasis and thrombus formation. (2) (PB; CJ; PL; WH)**

2 Dangling the legs places pressure on the popliteal spaces, limiting venous return and increasing the risk of thrombus formation.

3 Gatching the bed places pressure on the popliteal spaces, limiting venous return and increasing the risk of thrombus formation.

4 Bed rest is associated with venous stasis, which increases the risk of thrombus formation.

25. **4 Many clients are asymptomatic; the incubation period is three to five days. (3) (SE; CJ; AN; WH)**

1 There is no effective readily available blood test for gonorrhea.

2 Gonorrhea responds well to treatment; however, at times back-up secondary medications have to be utilized.

3 Urethral/vaginal smears or cultures are specific for the identification of the gonococcal organism.

26. **1 The alcohol will dry the cord and facilitate its falling off. (2) (SE; CJ; PL; NN)**

2 Although this is practiced in some cultures, using a pressure dressing is ineffective and could promote infection because the air circulation needed to promote drying is decreased.

3 If no infection is present, antibiotic ointment is not used.

4 The warm, moist environment inside a diaper is a good medium for bacterial growth; the diaper should be turned down below the umbilicus.

27. **4 If suckling or nipple stimulation is discontinued, acinic cells degenerate, regressive changes occur, and lactation ends. (2) (PM; CJ; AN; HC)**

1 Other than suckling, the stimulant for oxytocin secretion is unknown.

2 High levels of estrogen inhibit anterior pituitary gland secretion of lactogenic hormones.

3 Milk secretion starts on the third or fourth postpartum day.

28. **2 Panting will slow the process so the nurse can support the head as it is delivered. (1) (SE; MR; IM; HC)**

1 Pushing will speed up the birth and could injure the mother and the baby.

3 This will have no effect on the progress of the second stage of labor.

4 Usually holding the breath causes involuntary pushing, and it also depletes the mother and baby of oxygen.

29. **4 This response emphasizes that these findings are expected and explains why they occur; this should relieve the client's anxiety. (2) (PM; CJ; IM; EC)**
   1 Calling the physician is not necessary; these findings are expected.
   2 This response denies that there is anything to explain to the mother; this comment is somewhat belittling.
   3 This tells the mother that the findings are expected, but offers no explanation; this comment is somewhat belittling.

30. **1 The fetal heart is in the right quadrant, therefore the fetus' head and back are on the right side; the head is engaged and is at 0 station. (3) (PM; CJ; AS; HC)**
   2 In this position the fetal heart would be on the left side; at station −2 the head would be mobile.
   3 The information presented stated that the head is anterior and flexed; at −3 station the head would be mobile.
   4 In this position the fetal heart would be heard on the left side; at +1 station the head would be below the ischial spines.

31. **1 This acknowledges the validity of the grief and provides the client with an opportunity to talk if she wishes. (2) (PI; CJ; IM; EC)**
   2 Children cannot and should not be substituted for a lost fetus.
   3 Getting pregnant is not the issue; this statement belittles the lost fetus.
   4 The nurse can not know how the client feels; this comment is patronizing and diminishes the significance of the lost fetus.

32. **2 Assessment of the fetal heart rate is necessary because a prolapsed cord can occur when the membranes rupture and the fetus can become compromised if the cord is compressed. (2) (PB; CJ; IM; HP)**
   1 After careful observation for any change in the fetal heart rate because of the possibility of a prolapsed cord, the physician should be notified.
   3 Although important because meconium staining may indicate fetal distress, checking the fetal heart rate is the priority.
   4 A sterile pad is not needed and should not be the first action.

33. **3 Leukocytosis (15,000 to 20,000 WBC) typically occurs during the postpartum period as a** compensatory defense mechanism. (3) (PM; CJ; PL; HC)
   1 There is no need for further intervention because the client is exhibiting an expected postpartum leukocytosis.
   2 Same as answer 1.
   4 Same as answer 1.

34. **1 This is done to prevent injury to the bladder as the needle is being introduced into the amniotic sac. (2) (PB; CJ; PL; HP)**
   2 This would fill the bladder and make it vulnerable to injury as the needle is inserted into the amniotic sac.
   3 There is no reason to withhold food or fluid because the test does not involve the gastrointestinal tract.
   4 A preprocedure sedative is unnecessary.

35. **2 SGA infants have little subcutaneous fat or glycogen stores. (2) (PB; CJ; AS; HN)**
   1 Intestinal bleeding is not common in SGA infants.
   3 This would provide no therapeutic value for this SGA infant.
   4 Changes in head circumference are not characteristic of SGA infants.

36. **2 A rising reticulocyte count indicates accelerated erythropoietic activity that may reflect increased RBC destruction; increased RBC destruction raises the bilirubin level, causing jaundice. (3) (PB; CJ; AN; HN)**
   1 Although the reticulocyte count may be elevated with chronic blood loss, there are no data to indicate the baby is bleeding.
   3 In this instance the sedimentation rate or WBCs, not the reticulocytes, would be elevated.
   4 This test does not reflect respiratory functioning; however, ultimately with hemorrhage the respiratory rate will be elevated.

37. **4 Removing the tube does not bring a halt to menses; endometrial proliferation and shedding will occur as long as the ovaries and uterus are present. (1) (PM; CJ; EV; RP)**
   1 Pregnancy should be delayed 6 to 12 months after a tubal pregnancy.
   2 There is evidence that clients who have one tubal pregnancy are highly susceptible to having another.
   3 Pelvic infections can lead to constriction of tubes, and a fertilized ovum may become trapped.

38. **3 The side-lying position decreases pressure on the vena cava from the gravid uterus, ensuring**

adequate oxygenation of the fetus. (1) (PM; CJ; IM; HP)

1 Without proper positioning, breathing techniques will be less effective.

2 Lying on the back will increase pressure on the vena cava, further compromising the fetus.

4 Although the client would probably have an order for bed rest, all movement would not be restricted.

39. 1 **The fetus with a borderline cardiac reserve will demonstrate hypoxia by a decreased heart rate when there is minimal stress, making the test positive. (2) (PB; CJ; AN; HP)**

2 These decelerations are a response to head compression.

3 A baseline fetal heart rate characteristically occurs between contractions and between accelerations and/or decelerations of the heart rate.

4 These are nonuniform drops in FHR before, during, or after a contraction; variable decelerations during an CCT do not make the test positive.

40. 3 **In the breech presentation the fetal head is in the fundal portion of the uterus; the chest or back is at or above the umbilicus, where fetal heart tones can be heard. (2) (PM; CJ; AS; HC)**

1 In the vertex presentation, the head is the presenting part; the chest and back are in lower quadrants, where the fetal heart is heard.

2 The brow presentation is a type of cephalic presentation, where the fetal head is partially extended; the fetal heart would be heard in the lower abdomen, not above the umbilicus.

4 In the shoulder presentation the fetal heart usually is heard in the midabdominal region.

41. 2 **Regional anesthesia lowers the blood pressure. (2) (PB; CJ; EV; DR)**

1 The blood pressure, not the heart rate, will be affected first.

3 The client may not have the sensation to void but the amount of urine in the bladder does not decrease because a regional block does not affect the kidneys.

4 An epidural does not shorten the second stage of labor.

42. 2 **At birth, circulating maternal glucose is removed; however, the infant still has a high level of insulin and may develop rebound hypoglycemia. (2) (PB; CJ; AS; HN)**

1 These are not related to diabetes mellitus in the mother; mongolian spots are pigmented nevi found primarily on the skin of the sacrum and buttocks of Asian and African-American babies.

3 The temperature-regulating ability of a neonate born to a mother with diabetes mellitus is similar to that of a normal neonate unless the infant is preterm.

4 Pathologic jaundice is associated with hemolytic diseases such as Rh and ABO incompatibility and sepsis, not diabetes mellitus.

43. 3 **A quiet room helps to reduce stimuli, which is essential for limiting or preventing seizures. (2) (PB; CJ; PL; HP)**

1 All infusions are closely monitored and are usually maintained at a volume of 125 mL/hr.

2 Precipitous birth is not a usual side effect of magnesium therapy.

4 Calcium gluconate, not magnesium gluconate, is the antagonist for magnesium sulfate and should be on hand if symptoms of toxicity appear.

44. 4 **This keeps the breasts as empty as possible, limiting pressure within the ducts, thereby reducing pain. (1) (PB; CJ; IM; HC)**

1 Weaning will cause stasis of milk ducts and increase the fullness of the breasts at this time, thereby increasing pain.

2 The causative organism is probably already in the baby's nose and mouth; weaning is not always necessary with mastitis.

3 A tight-fitting bra will increase pain and suppress milk production; this will impede breastfeeding.

45. 4 **This is a description of the lithotomy position; it allows for visualization and direct access to the genital organs. (2) (PM; CJ; IM; WH)**

1 This is the dorsal recumbent position; it is difficult to separate the knees when the feet are kept flat on the examining table.

2 This position is appropriate for the administration of an enema.

3 This is the desired position for a sigmoidoscopy.

46. 2 **This is within the expected range of a heart rate for a newborn; the assessment can continue. (2) (PM; CJ; AS; NN)**

1 This is not necessary.

3 Same as answer 1.

4 Same as answer 1.

47. 2 The fear stems from the size and frailty of the newborn and the overwhelming environment of the intensive care area; parents should be encouraged to touch and handle their infant when possible. (3) (PI; CJ; PL; EC)

1 Bonding is possible and can be enhanced when the fear of touching has been overcome.
3 The breasts can be pumped and the milk administered via gavage feedings.
4 Although this may be a concern, it is not the most common initial concern.

48. 3 Incomplete formation of the pubic bone is associated with exstrophy of the bladder. (2) (PB; CJ; AS; HN)

1 This is not associated with exstrophy of the bladder.
2 Same as answer 1.
4 Same as answer 1.

49. 2 Removal of the uterus may produce changes in how some women view themselves sexually because it is a reproductive organ. (3) PI; CJ; AN; EC)

1 The libido of a postmenopausal woman probably would not be altered unless there are concerns about sexuality.
3 Although this could occur, it is less likely than surgery that has obvious external changes.
4 A 60-year-old otherwise healthy woman should have an uneventful recovery.

50. 1 During the second trimester the blood pressure usually decreases; an increase in systolic pressure of 30 mm Hg and diastolic pressure of 15 mm Hg warrants close observation for a preeclampsia that may develop. (3) (PB; CJ; AN; DR)

2 The client's baseline blood pressure was low normal suggesting that the increase in blood pressure is pregnancy related.
3 This physiologic change does not cause a rise in blood pressure.
4 An increase in blood pressure of this amount at 34 weeks' gestation is not expected.

Chapter 3

Pediatric Nursing

NURSING PRACTICE (NP)

1. An infant is admitted to the hospital with gastroenteritis. The infant vomits shortly after admission. When cleaning the infant after the vomiting episode, the nurse following standard precautions should wear:
   1. Gloves
   2. A mask
   3. A gown
   4. Goggles

2. A 16-year-old, her 1-month-old baby, and the baby's grandmother come to the emergency room saying that the infant accidentally fell down the stairs. Legally, consent for the baby's medical care:
   1. Must be decided by family court because the baby's mother is a minor
   2. Is not necessary because this is an emergency and no consent is needed
   3. Should be obtained from the grandmother, who must sign the consent
   4. Is the responsibility of the baby's mother, and she should sign the consent

3. An 8-year-old girl visits the school nurse several times a week with vague ailments. The nurse spends time listening to the girl, takes her temperature, and always sends her back to class. One Thursday, the girl tells the nurse that she no longer wants to visit her grandfather in his home, as he "hugs me too tight and touches me down there" (pointing to her genitals). She told her mother that she does not want to spend the weekend there, but her mother stated that she has no choice. The nurse should:
   1. Advise the child to tell her mother exactly why she does not want to go to her grandfather's house
   2. Plan a home visit to assess the home situation and tell the mother what her daughter has shared with her
   3. Call a meeting with the teacher, principal and the child's mother to discuss her concerns of child molestation

   4. Call the local child protective agency to report the alleged abuse and encourage an investigation before the coming week-end visit

4. An infant is scheduled for emergency surgery. The nurse notes that the baby's mother is 13 years old and the father is 16 years old. The baby's father and the paternal grandmother, who cares for the baby, are at the bedside. The nurse should obtain the informed consent from the:
   1. Paternal grandmother
   2. Hospital administrator
   3. Sixteen-year-old father
   4. Thirteen-year-old mother

5. When a nurse suspects that a child has been abused, the nurse's primary responsibility must be to:
   1. Treat the child's traumatic injuries
   2. Confirm the suspected child abuse
   3. Protect the child from any future abuse
   4. Have the child examined by the physician

GROWTH AND DEVELOPMENT (GD)

6. The nurse manager of a home health care agency is teaching a group of nursing assistants about pica practice. The nurse explains why this practice is more common among:
   1. Toddlers
   2. Older adults
   3. Preschoolers
   4. Pregnant women

7. When asked about spanking as a disciplinary technique, the nurse's best response would be:
   1. "It really depends on the child's age."
   2. "It is strongly suggestive of negative role modeling."
   3. "This may be the only option when no other technique works."
   4. "Research studies have shown it to be an effective disciplinary technique."

8. A 1-month-old infant grasps a rattle placed in the hand. The mother is impressed with this skill. The nurse should explain that this is:
   1. The palmar grasp reflex, which is expected at this age
   2. Atypical behavior and further evaluation is required
   3. Voluntary behavior usually observed in an older infant
   4. The pincer grasp, which should disappear in 3 to 4 months of age

9. An appropriate toy that the nurse should offer to a 3-month-old infant would be a:
   1. Push-pull toy
   2. Stuffed animal
   3. Metallic mirror
   4. Large plastic ball

10. The nurse is aware that the play of a 5-month-old infant would probably consist of:
    1. Picking up a rattle or toy and putting it into the mouth
    2. Exploratory searching when a cuddly toy is hidden from view
    3. Simultaneously kicking the legs and batting the hands in the air
    4. Waving and clenching fists and dropping toys placed in the hands

11. A mother tells the nurse that her 7-month-old child has just started sitting without support. The nurse should inform the mother that this:
    1. Is an expected developmental behavior at this age
    2. Activity signifies the upper 10% of physical development
    3. Could be a developmental delay that requires further evaluation
    4. Behavior is early and indicates that the baby will be walking soon

12. The nurse counsels a mother of an 8-month-old infant to make sure the floors are free of small objects when her child is crawling on the floor. The major rationale for this instruction would be that:
    1. An 8-month-old infant can easily pick up small objects
    2. Sharp objects can injure the fragile skin of an 8-month-old
    3. It is a health hazard for babies to pick things up off the floor
    4. The infant could hide small objects, making them difficult to locate

13. After teaching a mother about the appropriate play for an 8-month-old infant, the nurse is aware that the mother needs additional teaching when the mother states that she will buy a:
    1. Stuffed animal
    2. Play telephone
    3. Hanging mobile
    4. Book with textures

14. The nurse's developmental assessment of a 9-month-old child would be expected to reveal:
    1. A two- to three-word vocabulary
    2. An ability to feed self with a spoon
    3. The ability to sit steadily without support
    4. Closure of both anterior and posterior fontanels

15. A mother brings her 9-month-old infant to the clinic. The nurse is familiar with the mother's culture and knows that "belly binding" is a common practice. While accepting the mother's cultural practices and still promoting safety for the infant, the nurse should discourage the use of:
    1. A binder that encircles the waist
    2. Adhesive tape across the umbilicus
    3. A coin to prevent extrusion of the umbilicus
    4. Any binders because they do not prevent umbilical hernias

16. While caring for a 6-month-old infant, it is likely that the nurse will observe the presence of the reflex called:
    1. Startle
    2. Babinski
    3. Extrusion
    4. Tonic neck

17. The nurse recognizes that behaviors frequently first exhibited in an 8-month-old infant include:
    1. Smiling spontaneously, clasping hands, and keeping the head steady when sitting
    2. Removing some clothing, building a tower of two cubes, and stooping to pick up toys
    3. Drinking from a cup, using the words "mama" and "dada," and standing alone
    4. Being shy with strangers, playing peek-a-boo, and standing by holding onto furniture

18. An infant who weighed 7.5 pounds at birth now weighs 15 pounds at 1 year. The nurse at the pediatric clinic recognizes that this infant:
    1. Has probably been neglected
    2. Is the expected weight for this age
    3. Is not receiving the proper nourishment
    4. Should be 3 times the birth weight at one year

19. When planning nursing care for a 1-year-old infant, the nurse should assess the infant's abilities in relation to the developmental level. The nurse should expect a 1-year-old to be able to:

1. Jump with both feet
2. Attempt climbing stairs
3. Communicate in simple sentences
4. Build a tower of four to five blocks

20. A 15-month-old girl is brought to the clinic for her well-baby examination. During an interview with the mother, the nurse becomes aware that teaching regarding toddler development is needed when the mother states:
    1. "She's always trying to get out of her car seat."
    2. "I just can't seem to get her to sit on the potty chair."
    3. "Lately, she's been crying when I leave her with the sitter."
    4. "At home she gets into everything. Toys are scattered everywhere."

21. When teaching a parents' class, the nurse explains that medication and household cleaning products should be kept out of the reach of toddlers because:
    1. They have a high level of oral activity
    2. Their sense of taste is developing at this time
    3. Their appetite is greater to support rapid growth
    4. They rebel against parental authority during this phase

22. A mother indicates to the nurse in the pediatric clinic that she is concerned that her 20-month-old baby's bedtime thumb-sucking will cause the teeth to protrude. The nurse's most appropriate response would be:
    1. "You should seek counseling; the thumb-sucking may indicate an emotional problem."
    2. "You should switch the baby to a pacifier in the next two months to prevent protrusion of the teeth."
    3. "You need to restrain the baby from sucking the thumb because it prematurely loosens the first teeth."
    4. "You need not be concerned about the teeth protruding unless thumb-sucking persists after permanent teeth appear."

23. The nurse notes that a 22-month-old uses two- or three-word phrases (telegraphic speech), has a vocabulary of about 200 words, and often uses the word "me." The nurse would interpret the child's language development as being:
    1. A developmental lag
    2. Slow for the child's age
    3. Normal for the child's age
    4. Advanced for the child's age

24. A mother expresses concern that her 2-year-old daughter has become a "finicky eater and is eating less." The nurse's best response would be:
    1. "She has become manipulative"
    2. "She is probably experiencing the stress of the "terrible 2s""
    3. "I can refer you to have her evaluated for an eating disorder"
    4. "This is expected behavior because her growth has slowed"

25. Several 3-year-old girls in the day care center are having a tea party with their dolls. The center's nurse would assess this behavior to be:
    1. Evidence of abstract thought
    2. Appropriate make-believe play
    3. Inappropriate exclusion of boys
    4. Maladaptive use of magical thinking

26. A mother in the postpartum unit expresses concern that her 3-year-old daughter will be jealous of her newborn brother. The nurse should suggest neutralizing the jealousy by:
    1. Allowing the daughter to watch her baby brother when the mother naps
    2. Explaining in simple terms that the mother must spend more time with the baby
    3. Ignoring any negative comments or actions that her daughter makes toward the baby
    4. Bringing home a new baby doll for her daughter when her baby brother is brought home

27. A 3-year-old child is a "picky" eater. The mother expresses concern about her child's nutritional status. The nurse can assist the mother in meeting the child's nutritional requirements by suggesting that she:
    1. Include some of the foods the child will eat in every meal plan
    2. Cook nutritious meals and stay with the child until the food is eaten
    3. Serve a regular diet to the family and a special meal that the child will eat
    4. Explain that there will be no dessert until the child eats the food on the plate

28. A mother tells the office nurse that her 3-year-old child is afraid to sleep alone because of the "monsters under the bed." The mother asks for suggestions on how to handle this problem. The nurse should suggest:
    1. Telling the child that monsters do not exist
    2. Allowing the child to sleep with the parents temporarily
    3. Looking under the bed and saying, "I don't see any monsters."
    4. Stating that monsters aren't allowed in the house and leaving a small light on at night

29. When caring for a 4-year-old, the nurse bases the nursing-care plan on the knowledge that the child is in Erikson's psychosocial stage of:
    1. Trust vs. mistrust
    2. Initiative vs. guilt
    3. Industry vs. inferiority
    4. Autonomy vs. shame and doubt

30. When planning self-care that would foster independence, the nurse would expect a 4-year-old child to be able to:
    1. Tie shoelaces
    2. Button a shirt
    3. Part and comb hair
    4. Cut the meat at dinner

31. When assessing a 4-year-old, the nurse would expect the child to:
    1. Ask the definitions of new words
    2. Have a vocabulary of 1500 words
    3. Name two or three different colors
    4. Use just three- or four-word sentences

32. During a clinic visit, a 4-year-old girl suddenly screams, "Don't sit on Erin!" The parent whispers that Erin is an imaginary friend. The nurse's health teaching plans for this family should include:
    1. Special instructions for discipline
    2. Referral for counseling regarding "Erin"
    3. Investigation by child protective services
    4. Increasing social interaction between their daughter and her peers

33. When talking with a 4-year-old, the nurse observes that the child is shy and stutters. The nurse is aware that stuttering in a 4-year-old child would be considered:
    1. A sign of a delay in neural development
    2. A common characteristic of a preschooler
    3. The result of a serious emotional problem
    4. An indication of a serious permanent impairment

34. A 4-year-old child's concept of death is based on a sense of causality. The nurse plans care for a terminally ill child of this age based on the stage of cognitive thought that is characterized by:
    1. Formal operations
    2. Preoperational thought
    3. Sensorimotor operations
    4. Concrete operational thought

35. A 5-year-old is brought to the pediatric clinic for a routine visit. When assessing the child's relationship with other children, the nurse would expect to observe:
    1. Team play
    2. Parallel play
    3. Initiative play
    4. Cooperative play

36. The nurse knows that a child is performing the expected developmental tasks for a 5-year-old when the child:
    1. Is ritualistic when playing
    2. Makes up rules for a new game
    3. Asks for a pacifier when uncomfortable
    4. Plays near others quietly, but not with them

37. A Girl Scout leader arrives in the emergency department with a 7-year-old child who may have a broken leg. The nurse obtains a history of the accident and finds out that the child fell about one mile from the camp while on a hike with the scout leader and four other 7-year-old girls. Assuming that the scout leader intervened safely, the nurse would expect her to say she:
    1. Left the girls and went for help
    2. Sent 2 of the girls back to camp for help
    3. Carried the injured girl and led the rest of the girls back to camp
    4. Stayed with the injured girl and sent all the other girls back to camp for help

38. A 12-year-old is to be hospitalized for several weeks. The most appropriate activity for the nurse to include when planning diversionary activities would be:
    1. Offering to play card games
    2. Permitting television watching
    3. Providing supplies for drawing pictures
    4. Encouraging continuation of school work

39. A 15-year-old girl is grounded for two weeks by her parents for smoking in school. The adolescent tells the school nurse, "It's not fair that I get punished when my friends get away with doing the same thing." The nurse's most appropriate response would be:
    1. "The others will pay someday for lying to school authorities."
    2. "I intend to report your friends to the principal so they can also be punished."
    3. "When errors in judgment are made, people must be prepared to take the consequences of their actions."
    4. "It is difficult enough to get teenagers to obey the rules. If the parents don't act, it reinforces the behavior."

40. The nurse working in an adolescent clinic in a large city should be aware that the best avenue for communication with an adolescent would be:
    1. Relating on a peer level
    2. Dealing in concrete terms

3. Using typical teenage language
4. Establishing a relationship over time

41. The nurse is aware that corrective surgery for an infant with hypospadias probably will be done:
1. Shortly after birth
2. At approximately 4 years of age
3. Within a few months after birth
4. After 6 months and before 18 months of age

42. The primary nurse, assigned to a 4-month-old girl being admitted to the hospital, understands that the infant's emotional development should make the infant:
1. Cry when the nurse approaches her for the first time
2. Smile socially in recognition of the primary nurse's face
3. Welcome the attention that the primary nurse gives her
4. Cling furiously to her mother when the nurse tries to take her away

43. The mother of a 7-month-old infant, who is to be catheterized to obtain a sterile urine specimen, expresses fear that this procedure may traumatize the child psychologically. The nurse should reassure the mother that:
1. Her fear is justified and the nurse will obtain a "clean catch" specimen
2. She has every right to refuse catheterization since her concerns are realistic
3. Her concern is appropriate but the need for a sterile specimen is a higher priority
4. The procedure, though slightly uncomfortable, should not have any damaging effect

44. A 6-month-old infant is admitted with a diagnosis of failure to thrive. The birth weight was 7 pounds. Based on growth and development charts, the nurse should expect an infant at 6 months to weigh approximately:
1. 10 pounds
2. 14 pounds
3. 18 pounds
4. 21 pounds

45. A 1-year-old infant is brought to the pediatric clinic for the first time. While assessing the infant's physical and social skills, the nurse suspects there is a developmental problem because of an inability to:
1. Say six words
2. Stand without support
3. Respond to "peek-a-boo"
4. Build a tower of two cubes

46. The parents of an 18-month-old child are anxious to know why their child has experienced several episodes of suppurative otitis. The nurse should explain the:
1. Immunologic difference between the young child and the adult
2. Structural difference between the eustachian tube of younger and older children
3. Difference between the size of the middle ear cavity in infants and older children
4. Functional difference between an infant's eustachian tube and that of an older child

47. When teaching parents to instill eardrops in an 18-month-old child, the nurse shows them how to:
1. Cleanse the ear canal by pulling the pinna up and down
2. Straighten the auditory canal by pulling the earlobe up and back
3. Straighten the auditory canal by pulling the pinna down and back
4. Apply medicated ear wicks tightly before instilling the eardrops

48. A 2½-year-old male child who has fallen from a tree tells his parents, "Bad, bad tree." The nurse recognizes that the child is within the cognitive developmental norm of Piaget's:
1. Concrete operations
2. Concept of reversibility
3. Preconceptual operations
4. Sensorimotor development

49. A 2½-year-old girl whose older sibling has recently died has started hitting her mother and refusing to go to bed at night. The nurse in the pediatric well-child clinic tells the mother that the toddler is probably:
1. Fearful of dying in her sleep
2. Trying to get more of her mother's attention
3. Just going through the "terrible twos" developmental stage
4. Reacting appropriately to anxiety generated by the family upheaval

50. A 3-year-old girl has been hospitalized with nephrotic syndrome. The child is oliguric and has generalized edema. The nurse recognizes that the factor that will have the greatest effect on the child's adjustment to hospitalization would be the:
1. Inability to select a variety of foods for meals
2. Ability to participate in cooperative play activities
3. Response of peers to her appearance while edematous
4. Hospital policy restricting visitors to four hours daily

51. An IV catheter is to be inserted into a 3-year-old toddler's peripheral vein. As local topical anesthetic is applied, the toddler starts to cry and asks if it is going to hurt. The nurse's best response would be:
    1. "Yes, it may hurt, but not for very long."
    2. "A little, but remember big children don't cry."
    3. "If you hold still, I'll hurry and then it won't hurt as much."
    4. "Only a little, because I'm very good at getting the needle into your arm."

52. Based on an understanding of typical preschool behavior, during hospitalization the nurse is aware that a 4-year-old will probably:
    1. Refuse to cooperate with nurses during the parents' absence
    2. Demonstrate despair if parents do not visit at least once a week
    3. Cry when the parents leave and return but not during their absence
    4. Be unable to relate to peers in the playroom if there are parents present

53. The nurse would assess a 4-year-old child's abdominal pain by:
    1. Asking the child to point to where it hurts
    2. Asking the parents about the child's bowel habits
    3. Auscultating the abdomen for bowel sounds
    4. Observing the position and behavior while the child is moving

54. The nurse plans care of 4-year-old hospitalized children based on their developmental level. The nurse recognizes that children in this age group are vulnerable to:
    1. Separation anxiety
    2. Altered family roles
    3. Intrusive procedures
    4. Enforced dependency

55. The nurse is planning recreational activities for a 4-year-old with nephrotic syndrome. The most appropriate activities based on the child's developmental level and physical status would be:
    1. Riding a tricycle and playing with large blocks
    2. Reading animal stories and playing video games
    3. Leading a pull toy and playing with a map puzzle
    4. Watching cartoon videos and listening to stories

56. The most appropriate play activity that the nurse should provide for a 4-year-old whose arm is immobilized during intravenous therapy would be:
    1. Watching television
    2. Cutting out paper dolls
    3. Looking at comic books
    4. Playing with jigsaw puzzles

57. The nurse is aware that the most therapeutic play activity for a 4-year-old child on bed rest would be:
    1. Finger-painting on blank sheets of paper
    2. Using crayons to color in a coloring book
    3. Engaging in a checker game with the father
    4. Playing dominos with an 8-year-old roommate

58. After surgery, a 5-year-old is experiencing intense pain, and an analgesic is prescribed. When administering the analgesic, the nurse should consider that:
    1. Even though children do not like medicines, analgesics will make them more comfortable
    2. Pain is not as strongly felt by children as by adults, so analgesics are not needed frequently
    3. Children do not need analgesics because they are easily distracted and quickly return to playing or sleeping
    4. Children should rarely receive analgesics because this may result in addiction or respiratory depression

59. The nurse knows that an appropriate toy for a 6-year-old child on complete bed rest would be a:
    1. Game of checkers
    2. Set of building blocks
    3. Game of ball and jacks
    4. Coloring book and crayons

60. The mother of a 6-year-old child in the acute phase of nephrotic syndrome asks the nurse about play activities for her child. The nurse should suggest:
    1. Action toys such as a hula hoop
    2. Stuffed animals, large puzzles, and large blocks
    3. CD player, computer games, and children's magazines
    4. Table games, checkers, simple card games, and crayons

61. A 7-year-old child, admitted to the hospital for intrathecal methotrexate chemotherapy, is prescribed allopurinol (Zyloprim) and asks the nurse why this medication has to be taken.

The nurse's best response would be:
1. "Because this pill helps the other medicines get rid of the things that are making you sick."
2. "To protect your body from developing other problems after your treatment has been stopped."
3. "To stop your sick white cells from going to other parts of your body where they can cause problems."
4. "Because your doctor ordered it. Your doctor would not order anything for you unless it was very important."

62. An 8-year-old child is being prepared for surgery the next day. Preoperative teaching should:
1. Be repeated often
2. Provide time for needle play
3. Utilize several abstract examples
4. Focus on simple anatomical diagrams

63. An 11-year-old is diagnosed with acute lympho-cytic leukemia (ALL), and the physician discusses the diagnosis and treatment with the family. The nurse is aware that age-appropriate behavior for an 11-year-old regarding a diagnosis implying death and dying would be that the child:
1. Is rude, impolite, and insolent
2. Says that an uncle died and went to heaven
3. Is afraid to go to sleep for fear of not awakening
4. Tells the nurse that death is punishment for not being good

64. The mother of a 15-year-old girl with a history of allergies that have resulted in chronic sinusitis tells the nurse in the clinic that she thinks her daughter is becoming a hypochondriac. The nurse can be most therapeutic by:
1. Discussing the developmental behavior of adolescents
2. Discussing the underlying causes of hypochondriasis
3. Explaining the potentially serious complications of sinusitis
4. Explaining that the mother may be transferring her own fears to her daughter

65. When caring for a 15-year-old client receiving chemotherapy for leukemia, the nurse should keep in mind that an adolescent of this age will:
1. Feel dependent and enjoy the "sick role"
2. Be most bothered by having to limit activities
3. Feel different because of an altered body image

4. Be preoccupied by concerns about missed schoolwork

66. Once the crisis has passed, when listing all the problems of a teenage client who has sickle-cell anemia, the nurse recognizes that priority must be given to the client's:
1. Restriction of movement during periods of arthralgia
2. Altered body image resulting from skeletal deformities
3. Separation from family during periods of hospitalization
4. Interruption of learning as a result of multiple hospitalizations

67. An adolescent who has had type 1 diabetes for five years becomes noncompliant with therapy. The nurse is aware that the noncompliance is developmentally related to:
1. The need for attention
2. A denial of the diabetes
3. The struggle for identity
4. A regression associated with illness

EMOTIONAL NEEDS RELATED TO HEALTH PROBLEMS (EH)

68. When working with a family as the unit of service, the public health nurse should consider that:
1. Certain members of the family may be capable of providing more support than the nurse can
2. Separating health problems from other aspects of this family's life is essential to help them
3. Assessing each member of this family is not necessary to plan the care for the family as a whole
4. Values, beliefs, and attitudes held by the family have limited influence on how they will perceive assistance

69. The parents of a sick child constantly blame each other for their child's illness. The response by the parents that would indicate that the nurse's attempts to point out reality had been successful would be:
1. The father bringing the child many expensive gifts
2. The parents promising the child a trip to Disney World
3. The parents making an appointment with a family counselor
4. The mother assuming the blame for not paying attention to the child's complaints

70. The parents of an infant with a congenital heart anomaly have just been told the diagnosis. They appear overwhelmed and anxious. The nurse's action that will best help the parents would be:
    1. Explaining the diagnosis in a variety of ways
    2. Allowing the parents to express their feelings
    3. Encouraging the parents to talk with other parents
    4. Assuring the parents that surgery will probably correct the problem

71. When the adolescent mother of an infant admitted to the hospital with multiple trauma sees her infant in the intensive care unit for the first time, she cries out, "I didn't mean to hurt her." The nurse should:
    1. Encourage the young mother's family to come and comfort her
    2. Respond by saying, "You caused your baby's injury and feel guilty."
    3. Notify the Child Abuse Hotline of this probable instance of abuse
    4. Put an arm around the young mother and say, "This must be difficult for you."

72. The mother of an infant with meningitis is concerned that if she stays at the hospital, her toddler at home will feel neglected. The nurse's most appropriate response would be:
    1. "What has made you feel this way?"
    2. "It's best to divide your time evenly between the two children."
    3. "The baby will benefit greatly by your constant presence."
    4. "Have you talked with anyone about staying with the baby while you are at home?"

73. A mother of three children who was abandoned by her husband shortly after the birth of her youngest daughter brings the child, now 9 months old, to the hospital with a diagnosis of failure to thrive. As the mother leaves, the nurse is not surprised to see the daughter react by:
    1. Clinging to the mother and expressing fear of the nurse
    2. Crying at first but then letting the nurse hold and comfort her
    3. Sustaining eye contact with the mother and refusing the nurse's arms
    4. Readily allowing the nurse to take her but remaining stiff while being held

74. When assessing the family dynamics of a suspected abusing family, the nurse would be surprised to observe that the:
    1. Parents provide little emotional support to the child
    2. Parents offer consistent, detailed stories about the injuries
    3. Child cringes and appears unduly afraid when approached
    4. Child has many unexplained old injuries, scars, and bruises

75. A 9-year-old male child, who has been newly diagnosed with type 1 diabetes, is being discharged. The nurse suspects that there may be a problem with family dynamics when the child's mother states:
    1. "We want to encourage our son to do as much as he can for himself."
    2. "We know our child is special, and we'll have to go easy on the discipline for him."
    3. "We know our child and the rest of the family are in for a lot of ups and downs over the years."
    4. "We really hope our son can still be in the Boy Scouts and participate with his Little League baseball team."

76. A child who has barely survived a near-drowning episode is in critical condition in an intensive care unit. At one point the child opens the eyes and smiles, prompting the mother to say to the nurse, "Look, I think my child will get better now." The nurse's best response would be:
    1. "Yes, you are right; this is a very good sign."
    2. "See if you can get your child to hold your hand, too."
    3. "God must have certainly been watching over your child."
    4. "We are doing everything we can to help your child to recover."

77. A toddler who has been physically abused is admitted to the pediatric unit. When approaching this child, the nurse should expect the child to:
    1. Smile readily when anyone enters the room
    2. Be wary of physical contact initiated by anyone
    3. Pay little attention to anyone standing at the bedside
    4. Begin to cry and scream when anyone approaches the bedside

78. When caring for children in a family that is economically deprived, the nurse should understand that the characteristic most common to those living in poverty would be:
    1. Long-term feelings of powerlessness

2. Open and direct expressions of anger
3. A willingness to postpone gratification
4. Compliance with health recommendations

79. A female client who has been abusing her son is undergoing treatment to control her behavior. A statement by the client that indicates the development of some insight into her behavior as a parent would be:
1. "I promise that I won't get so angry when my son causes trouble again."
2. "Once my son gets straightened out, we should not have these problems."
3. "I think the root of the problem is when my husband comes home after drinking."
4. "If I feel angry at my son again, I'm going to go into the bedroom and punch a pillow."

80. A 16-month-old male infant has been in the hospital for two weeks and has become increasingly withdrawn and mute. It would be most appropriate for the nurse to:
1. Move him in with other children
2. Provide him with distracting toys
3. Encourage the parents to stay with him as much as possible
4. Assign different nurses to be with him to provide sensory stimuli

81. During the course of treatment, a toddler is to receive an intramuscular injection. The most supportive intervention at this time would be:
1. Distracting the toddler's attention with a toy car
2. Explaining to the parents in detail what is being done
3. Giving the toddler the choice of having the injection now or later
4. Involving the parents in comforting the toddler after the injection

82. The primary nursing objective for a child newly diagnosed with celiac disease would be to:
1. Prevent celiac crisis and resulting complications
2. Minimize complications from respiratory involvement
3. Teach the parents to control the diet to promote normal growth
4. Help the parents and child adjust to the long-term dietary restrictions

83. To be most therapeutic when giving a 3-year-old toddler an intramuscular injection, the nurse should approach the child and say:
1. "You are afraid of having a shot because of the pain."

2. "Act like a big child and we can be done quickly."
3. "I know this might hurt, but it's important that you hold still."
4. "I brought another nurse along to help me give your medicine."

84. Before a 4-year-old child with a new colostomy is discharged, the nurse prepares a teaching plan for the parents that includes telling them that:
1. An enterostomal therapist is available to assist with home care
2. They should try correcting the child's poor eating habits at mealtime
3. Fluids should be limited between meals, although permitted at meals
4. The child should not take part in physical education when attending school

85. A 4-year-old boy with Reye syndrome is beginning to show signs of recovery. The intracranial pressure has receded, the vital signs are stable, the fever has subsided, and urinary output is as expected for weight and fluid intake. The nurse's statement to the parents should be:
1. "His illness has resolved."
2. "He is out of danger now."
3. "He seems free of any complications."
4. "We are hopeful that he is recovering."

86. A 5-year-old child is admitted for an appendectomy. The question that is most effective in eliciting information about what the child thinks is the reason for the hospitalization would be:
1. "Do you know what this place is?"
2. "Why did you come to the hospital?"
3. "Do you know what is going to happen to you?"
4. "You know why you are in the hospital, don't you?"

87. A 5-year-old girl is receiving a course of chemotherapy. One day the nurse observes the child crying. The child tells the nurse, "All my hair is gone and everyone stares at me." The nurse's most appropriate response would be:
1. "I will help you take the hair off your doll so you two will look alike."
2. "I'm going to take this terrible mirror out of your room and then we'll play a game."
3. "No, they're not. You just think they are because you feel funny without your hair."
4. "Why don't we ask mother to bring in a hat for you to wear until your hair grows back?"

88. A 5-year-old, newly arrived from Latin America, attends a nursery school where everyone speaks English. The child's mother tells the nurse in the well-child clinic that her child is no longer outgoing and is very passive in the classroom. The nurse suspects that the child:
    1. May be experiencing discrimination
    2. Lacks adequate motivation for school
    3. Is undergoing a state of cultural shock
    4. Is not mature enough for kindergarten

89. After treatment for Lyme disease, a child expresses fear of going camping again because of the ticks. The nurse's best response would be:
    1. "You are afraid to go camping just because of a tick?"
    2. "Frequent checks for ticks are a defense against infection."
    3. "Tell me more about your fears about camping."
    4. "Oh, camping is fun. Just think of what you will be missing."

90. A 6-year-old boy is receiving chemotherapy for a neuroblastoma, stage IV. He had his first chemotherapy session last week and has arrived with his mother for this week's session. The nurse should approach the child and his mother by asking:
    1. "Did you vomit after the last dose?"
    2. "How did you feel after your last medicine?"
    3. "Aren't you happy that two sessions will be finished?"
    4. "How are you feeling this week? Ready for another dose?"

91. The nursing plan for an 8-year-old boy with celiac disease should include helping the child to:
    1. Express his feelings, while focusing on ways in which he can still be normal like his friends
    2. Select meals from those high-residue, high-carbohydrate foods that are gluten-free and permitted
    3. Understand the relationship of diet to disease so that he will be more willing to adhere to his diet and refrain from eating snack foods
    4. Learn which foods can be eaten that are low in gluten, such as frankfurters and hamburgers that have wheat fillers, because occasional noncompliance is permitted

92. Three days after being admitted to the hospital with meningococcal meningitis, a 12-year-old child is afebrile and asymptomatic but appears very sad and cries frequently. To assist the child to verbalize thoughts and feelings, the nurse should:
    1. Encourage the parents to speak with their child
    2. Ask the child directly what seems to be the trouble
    3. Show the child some photos of hospitalized children and have the child tell stories about them
    4. Have the child watch videotapes about sick children and answer any questions that the child may have

93. After assessing that an adolescent with type 1 diabetes has sufficient knowledge of the disorder, the nurse should:
    1. Set goals with the client
    2. Develop a rapport with the client
    3. Teach how to give insulin injections
    4. Explain how to monitor blood glucose

94. An adolescent with a diagnosis of osteogenic sarcoma is to have the affected leg amputated followed by chemotherapy. The parents are concerned about what to tell their child and ask the nurse for advice. The nurse responds that the best approach would be:
    1. A detailed explanation of amputation and chemotherapy
    2. Straightforward honesty about the amputation with brief information about chemotherapy
    3. A discussion of choices of treatment, indicating that the final one cannot be made until the time of surgery
    4. Provision of information about chemotherapy and the suggestion that amputation may be a possibility

95. A 16-year-old with full-thickness burns of the entire right arm states, "I'll never be able to use my arm again. I'll be scarred forever." The nurse's best initial response would be:
    1. "The staff will take steps to minimize scarring."
    2. "Think about how lucky you are. You are alive."
    3. "I know you are worried, but it is still too early to tell."
    4. "Try not to worry; concentrate on doing your range-of-motion exercises."

BLOOD AND IMMUNITY (BI)

96. The nurse in the pediatric clinic has been asked to write a brochure explaining the governmental requirements for the receipt of the hepatitis B vaccine series in children. The statement that accurately explains hepatitis B or its vaccine to parents would be:

1. Only children of immunosuppressed families require it
2. This hepatitis vaccine protects against all types of hepatitis
3. Hepatitis B is transmitted through contaminated food or water
4. There are three injections in the hepatitis B series which are given during infancy

97. The nurse is aware that, with the exception of hepatitis B, immunization of infants does not begin until 2 months of age because:
    1. Younger infants rarely are exposed to infectious diseases
    2. The neonatal spleen is unable to produce efficient antibodies
    3. Maternal antibodies interfere with the development of active antibodies by the infant
    4. The immunization would attack the immature infant's body and produce the disease

98. A 2-month-old is to receive the first DTaP immunization. The infant's response to this immunization would be influenced by a history of:
    1. Allergy to eggs
    2. Febrile seizures
    3. Lactose intolerance
    4. Infectious dermatitis

99. Before giving a 2-month-old infant the first series of immunizations, the nurse should discuss with the mother the possible reactions that may occur because these reactions are:
    1. Often serious and may require hospitalization
    2. Usually responsible for permanent neurologic damage
    3. Quite common and may be either local or systemic
    4. Sometimes responsible for deep ulceration at the site of injection

100. The nurse administers the first series of immunizations to a 2-month-old. The nurse instructs the mother that, if the site becomes inflamed, she should give the prescribed acetaminophen and:
    1. Place a warm compress on the area
    2. Put a witch hazel compress on the site
    3. Give a cool sponge bath for 15 minutes
    4. Apply an ice pack to the inflamed area for 20 minutes

101. When teaching a mother about the immunization schedule for her baby, the nurse explains that the measles vaccine should be given between:
    1. 2 to 5 months
    2. 6 to 8 months
    3. 9 to 11 months
    4. 12 to 15 months

102. A 13-month-old child is having a lumbar puncture to confirm a diagnosis of bacterial meningitis. During the procedure the nurse notices that the spinal fluid is cloudy. This finding is indicative of:
    1. A normal spinal fluid
    2. An increased glucose level
    3. A rising number of red blood cells
    4. An elevated white blood cell count

103. A mother tells the nurse that her 8-month-old will eat only mashed potatoes and drink only milk, and she is concerned about the baby's diet, even though the baby is receiving Poly-Vi-Sol daily. The nurse recognizes that the child's diet could lead to:
    1. A potassium deficit
    2. A vitamin deficiency
    3. An amino acid deficiency
    4. An iron-deficiency anemia

104. A 1-year-old is diagnosed as having iron deficiency anemia. The nursing intervention that would be unnecessary is:
    1. Conserving the infant's energy
    2. Protecting the infant from infection
    3. Teaching the parents about nutrition
    4. Giving the infant small, frequent feedings

105. The nurse should suggest to the mother of an 18-month-old with anemia that the child be fed:
    1. Pieces of pumpkin pie
    2. Slices of a whole apple
    3. A cup of seedless grapes
    4. Bread pudding with raisins

106. When an infant receives the first immunizations at 2 months, the nurse should instruct the parent to:
    1. Apply heat to the injection site for the first day; afterward apply ice if the arm is sore
    2. Apply ice to the injection site if soreness is present; call the physician if a fever develops
    3. Give the baby aspirin for pain; if swelling at the injection site develops, call the physician
    4. Give acetaminophen for fever; call the physician if marked drowsiness or seizures occur

107. A 2-year-old child has been admitted to the pediatric unit with a diagnosis of thalassemia (Cooley's anemia). The parents are told that there is no cure, but the anemia can be treated with frequent transfusions. The father tells the nurse he is glad that there is a treatment that "fixes" his child's problem. The nurse should respond:
    1. "Blood transfusions correct the anemia but also present a risk of hepatitis."
    2. "While blood transfusions temporarily correct the anemia, this treatment may cause other problems."
    3. "Blood transfusions are a supportive treatment, and as your child grows older fewer of them will be needed."
    4. "Yes, a blood transfusion replaces the defective red blood cells. It's like giving insulin to a person with diabetes."

108. A child with leukemia is to continue taking prednisone at home after discharge. The nurse discovers that the child's sibling is home with chickenpox. The nurse plans the discharge teaching based on the knowledge that:
    1. The child must be immunized before going home
    2. Chickenpox can be fatal to individuals with leukemia
    3. Clients receiving prednisone are immune to chickenpox
    4. If direct contact between the two siblings is prevented, the child can go home

109. A 4-year-old child has been admitted for a tonsillectomy. When reviewing the child's preoperative laboratory work the nurse should pay particular attention to the:
    1. Potassium level
    2. Coagulation studies
    3. Red blood cell level
    4. Erythrocyte sedimentation rate

110. Upon return to the pediatric unit after a tonsillectomy, the admitting nurse notes that a 4-year-old is swallowing frequently. The nurse is aware that this response is indicative of:
    1. Pharyngeal edema
    2. Postoperative bleeding
    3. Tenacious oral secretions
    4. Increased salivary response

111. A 4-year-old child is admitted with a tentative diagnosis of acute lymphocytic leukemia (ALL). When obtaining a health history from the parents, the nurse would expect that the child has:
    1. Alopecia and petechiae
    2. Anorexia and insomnia
    3. Anorexia and petechiae
    4. Alopecia and bleeding gums

112. When obtaining a health history from the parents of a toddler who is admitted to the hospital with acute lymphocytic leukemia (ALL), the nurse would be surprised if the parents report that the first sign they observed was:
    1. A loss of appetite
    2. Sores in the mouth
    3. A paleness of the skin
    4. Purplish spots on the skin

113. To confirm a tentative diagnosis of leukemia a bone-marrow aspiration is to be performed on a 4-year-old child. In addition to providing an age-appropriate explanation of the procedure the nurse should:
    1. Tell the child that there will be pressure, but no pain
    2. Administer the prescribed sedation before the procedure
    3. Place the child in the semi-Fowler's position supported by pillows
    4. Have the child help by holding some of the nonsterile equipment

114. A 4-year-old child is admitted with a tentative diagnosis of acute lymphoid leukemia (ALL). The mother states that the changes in behavior and the "black and blue" marks were noticed several days ago. She blames herself for not bringing the child to the clinic when the child first appeared ill. The nurse's response to the mother is based on the knowledge that:
    1. If leukemia is diagnosed, the child's prognosis is probably poor
    2. Diagnosis can be certain only after a blood smear is taken and analyzed
    3. Symptoms of leukemia are initially similar to many mild illnesses of childhood
    4. With such severe symptoms, the child has probably been ill longer than one week

115. A 3-year-old child with sickle-cell anemia is admitted to the hospital with a pain episode. Splenomegaly is identified. The nurse understands that splenomegaly usually is:
    1. Common in infancy
    2. Not easily palpable in children
    3. Initiated by a vaso-occlusive crisis
    4. Most evident during late childhood

116. A 10-year-old child who has sickle-cell anemia is admitted to the hospital with vaso-occlusive

crisis. When assigning a room, it is most appropriate for the nurse to place the child with a roommate who has:
1. Pneumonia
2. Thalassemia
3. Osteomyelitis
4. Acute pharyngitis

117. A child with sickle-cell anemia is admitted to the hospital with a vaso-occlusive pain episode. The nurse is aware that this is a result of:
1. Diminished red blood cell production by the bone marrow
2. Pooling of blood in the spleen with resultant splenomegaly
3. Blockage of small blood vessels with clumped red blood cells
4. Severe depression in circulating thrombocytes (blood platelets)

118. Included in discharge planning for a child who was hospitalized for a vaso-occlusive pain episode would be instruction to the child and parents to:
1. Keep ice packs on painful joints
2. Participate in active indoor sports
3. Drink large amounts of fluids daily
4. Get plenty of fresh air and sunshine

119. After being bitten by a rabid dog, a child is to receive a series of anti-rabies inoculations. The nurse understands that rabies is:
1. An acute bacterial infection characterized by encephalopathy and opisthotonos
2. An acute bacterial septicemia that results in seizures and a morbid fear of water
3. A viral infection, characterized by seizures and difficult swallowing, that affects the nervous system
4. A nonspecific immune response to organisms deposited under the skin by a rabid animal bite

120. The nurse in the clinic must give a booster immunization for polio to a child. The recommended vaccine would be the:
1. Hib
2. IPV
3. OPV
4. DTaP

121. The mother of a child who has been recently diagnosed as having hemophilia is pregnant with her second child. She asks the nurse what the chances are that this baby will also have hemophilia. The nurse's best response would be:

1. "There is no chance the baby will be affected."
2. "There is a 25% chance the baby will be affected."
3. "There is a 50% chance the baby will be affected."
4. "There is a 75% chance the baby will be affected."

122. The nurse is aware that the most common area for bleeding to develop in a child with hemophilia would be the:
1. Brain
2. Joints
3. Abdomen
4. Pericardium

123. When giving nursing care to a child with leukemia, the nurse notes blood on the pillow case and several bloody tissues. The nurse should check the child's laboratory report for the:
1. Platelet count
2. Uric acid level
3. Prothrombin time
4. Red blood cell count

124. The nurse should recognize that the parents of a child with leukemia need further teaching regarding oral care for their child when they indicate that they should use:
1. A plastic straw
2. Mild toothpaste
3. Saline mouthwash
4. An electric toothbrush

125. There are many nursing interventions that are important for a child with leukemia who is receiving chemotherapy. The priority should be:
1. Employing techniques to prevent infection
2. Promoting normal growth and development
3. Using measures to improve nutritional status
4. Providing emotional support for the child and family

126. A child with leukemia who is receiving chemotherapy is susceptible to rectal ulcerations. To lessen the severity of this problem nursing care should be directed toward:
1. Keeping the child positioned on the abdomen
2. Having the child wear cotton pants while in bed
3. Applying rectal ointments liberally four times a day
4. Cleaning and washing the perianal area after each bowel movement

127. A child with leukemia is to be sent home on a protocol that includes several antineoplastics after an intrathecal administration of methotrexate. Before discharge the nurse should instruct the child's parents to:
1. Limit contact with peers because they tend to have communicable diseases
2. Return weekly for bone marrow aspiration to determine effectiveness of therapy
3. Schedule routine laboratory appointments for evaluation of response to medication
4. Withhold medications when nausea occurs to prevent additional episodes of vomiting

128. When discharging a 5-year-old girl who is to continue chemotherapy at home, the nurse would know that the parents understood the discharge instructions when they say, "We should:
1. Isolate her from other children her age."
2. Allow her to eat her food at her own pace."
3. Provide her with structured activities each day."
4. Have her rinse her mouth with mouthwash."

129. The most important discharge teaching for the parents of a child who has just completed a chemotherapy protocol should include:
1. Purchasing a wig or hat
2. Providing adequate rest
3. Offering sufficient fluid intake
4. Exercising proper handwashing

130. The nurse is aware that children with AIDS are more prone to infection than adults with AIDS because:
1. Even the immune system of a healthy child is incapable of producing antibodies
2. The AIDS virus attacks children's immune systems through different mechanisms
3. Children with AIDS are exposed to many more pathogens than are adults with AIDS
4. Children have fewer circulating antibodies resulting from a lack of previous exposure to pathogens

131. When a child with AIDS is awaiting adoption, to protect the staff, the nurse should immediately institute:
1. Droplet precautions
2. Contact precautions
3. Airborne precautions
4. Standard precautions

132. A child with partial-thickness burns on 21% of the total body surface area (TBSA) has progressed from the acute phase of burn care to the management phase. The most important nursing intervention at this time would be:
1. Recording intake and output
2. Monitoring for signs of infection
3. Instituting a pain management plan
4. Maintaining a high nutritional intake

133. A child with Cooley's anemia is being discharged from the hospital. The nurse should plan to instruct the parents regarding the need to:
1. Restrict activity
2. Encourage fluids
3. Prevent infection
4. Provide small, frequent meals

134. A child with a puncture wound of the sole of the foot is brought to the emergency department. Because of a language barrier, a caregiver cannot provide a clear history of previous tetanus immunizations. The physician orders tetanus immune globulin. The nurse understands that this drug is given because it:
1. Produces lifelong passive immunity
2. Induces longer-lasting active protection
3. Confers immediate passive protection of short duration
4. Stimulates increased production of antibodies immediately

135. One of the aims of therapy for sickle-cell anemia is the prevention of the sickling phenomenon, which is responsible for the pathologic sequelae. A plan of care directed toward prevention of a crisis should consist of:
1. Promotion of adequate oxygenation and hemodilution
2. Administration of an iron-fortified formula as nourishment
3. Measures to decrease tissue oxygen requirements and maintain hemoconcentration
4. Enforced periods of bed rest to minimize energy expenditure and oxygen utilization

136. The mother of a 13-year-old who has sickle-cell anemia tells the nurse that the family is going camping this summer. She asks what activities would be appropriate for the child. The nurse should suggest:
1. Softball games with the family
2. Collecting logs for the campfire
3. Motorboat rides around the lake
4. Walking along the mountain trails

137. The nurse recognizes that the teaching about sickle-cell anemia was understood when a

16-year-old with the disease states, "I know that symptoms will appear when I have:
1. A low iron intake."
2. A decreased amount of fluids."
3. A breakdown of thrombocytes."
4. An increased WBC production."

138. The nurse, preparing a 12-year-old child for a bone marrow aspiration, would know that the child does not understand the teaching about the procedure when the child states:
1. "I can get out of bed when I stop feeling sleepy."
2. "I will have a tight dressing to put pressure on the area."
3. "The doctor is going to inject a needle into the center of one of my hip bones."
4. "The only pain I should feel is when the doctor puts in the shot so it won't hurt."

139. An adolescent visits the allergy clinic because of seasonal environmental allergies. Blood is drawn for evaluation. The nurse would expect that the blood will indicate an allergic response with:
1. A decreased platelet count
2. An elevated eosinophil level
3. An elevated lymphocyte count
4. A decreased immunoglobulin level

140. A 16-year-old student, who was injured while skateboarding, arrives in the emergency department with a deep gash on his leg. He does not remember when he received his last tetanus immunization. The nurse explains that he will receive tetanus immune globulin instead of tetanus antitoxin because it:
1. Is more convenient to administer
2. Is not likely to cause anaphylaxis
3. Can be as effective as the antitoxin
4. Can be safely given to anyone who needs it

141. If a 9-month-old's immunization schedule is up-to-date, the nurse should inform the parent that the next immunization the infant will receive at 15 months of age is:
1. Hepatitis A
2. Polio vaccine
3. Tetanus toxoid
4. Measles, mumps, and rubella vaccine

CARDIOVASCULAR (CV)

142. The nurse is aware that in infants with heart failure:
1. The illness is an acquired congenital anomaly

2. The treatment differs vastly from adult treatment
3. Treatment is experimental because infants rarely develop heart failure
4. Digoxin (Lanoxin) and furosemide (Lasix) are the most commonly used medications

143. A parent asks the nurse, "The doctor said my baby has pulmonic stenosis. What does that mean?" The nurse's best response would be:
1. "What else did your doctor say?"
2. "Your baby has a heart problem."
3. "Are you concerned about your baby?"
4. "I'll page your physician so that you can discuss this again."

144. A 3-month-old infant is admitted with a diagnosis of tetralogy of Fallot. Assessment reveals that the infant's weight is in the 5th percentile. The nurse is aware that the reason for this poor weight gain would be:
1. Cyanosis leading to cerebral changes
2. Decreased arterial PO_2 resulting in polycythemia
3. Exercise intolerance resulting in deficient caloric intake
4. Pulmonary hypertension resulting in recurrent respiratory infections

145. The parents of an infant with tetralogy of Fallot ask the nurse to explain what is wrong with their baby's heart. Before explaining the problem in words they will understand, the nurse recalls that in tetralogy of Fallot there is:
1. Overriding of the aorta, aortic stenosis, patent ductus, and mitral insufficiency
2. Tricuspid atresia, ventricular septal defect, atrioventricular canal, and coarctation of the aorta
3. Atrial septal defect, right ventricular hypertrophy, patent ductus, and mitral insufficiency
4. Right ventricular hypertrophy, ventricular septal defect, pulmonic stenosis, and overriding of the aorta

146. When attempting to identify the presence of tetralogy of Fallot in an infant, the nurse should understand that:
1. In the absence of cyanosis, poor sucking is insignificant
2. Many infants retain mucus that may interfere with feeding
3. Poor sucking and swallowing may be early indications of heart defects
4. Feeding problems are fairly common in infants during the first year

147. The nurse is aware that a common adaptation of children with tetralogy of Fallot is:
    1. Clubbing of fingers
    2. Slow, irregular respirations
    3. Subcutaneous hemorrhages
    4. Decreased red blood cell count

148. An infant with tetralogy of Fallot becomes cyanotic and dyspneic after a crying episode. To relieve the cyanosis and dyspnea, the nurse should place the infant in the:
    1. Knee-chest position
    2. Orthopneic position
    3. Lateral Sims' position
    4. Semi-Fowler's position

149. The nurse teaches the parents of an infant with a cardiac defect how to detect impending heart failure. An early sign would be:
    1. Increased urinary output
    2. Tachycardia and dyspnea
    3. Gasping and grunting respirations
    4. Distended neck and peripheral veins

150. The physician orders a complete blood workup for a 5-month-old infant with tetralogy of Fallot. Because of the infant's heart disease, the nurse would expect the report to show:
    1. Polycythemia
    2. Agranulocytosis
    3. Thrombocytopenia
    4. A decreased hematocrit level

151. An appropriate nursing action to include in the care of an infant with congenital heart disease who has been admitted with heart failure would be:
    1. Positioning flat on the back
    2. Encouraging nutritional fluids
    3. Providing small frequent feedings
    4. Measuring the head circumference

152. An infant with a cardiac defect is fed in the semi-Fowler's position. After the nurse feeds and burps the infant and changes the infant's position, the infant has a bowel movement and almost immediately becomes cyanotic, diaphoretic, and limp. These symptoms are most likely caused by the:
    1. Burping
    2. Formula
    3. Position change
    4. Bowel movement

153. A newborn is diagnosed with coarctation of the aorta. The baby is discharged with a prescription for digoxin (Lanoxin) 0.01 mg po q12h. The bottle of digoxin is labeled 0.01 mg in $^{1}/_{2}$ teaspoon. The nurse should teach the mother to administer the medication by using:
    1. A nipple
    2. A plastic baby spoon
    3. The calibrated dropper in the bottle
    4. The small size baby bottle with 1 oz of water

154. A 1-month-old infant is admitted for confirmation of the diagnosis of ventricular septal defect. During the initial admission assessment, the nurse would expect to find:
    1. Bradycardia at rest
    2. Bounding peripheral pulses
    3. Cyanosis on increased activity
    4. A murmur at the left lower sternal border

155. The mother of a child with a congenital cardiac defect asks the nurse why her child squats after exertion. The nurse should reply that this position:
    1. Reduces muscle aches
    2. Increases cardiac efficiency
    3. Enhances the pull of gravity
    4. Decreases blood volume in the extremities

156. The nurse explains to the parents that a cardiac catheterization is scheduled for their 5-year-old with a ventricular septal defect to:
    1. Identify the degree of cardiomegaly present
    2. Demonstrate the exact location of the defect
    3. Confirm the presence of a pansystolic murmur
    4. Establish the presence of ventricular hypertrophy

157. A 3$^{1}/_{2}$-year-old child returns to the room after a cardiac catheterization. Post-procedure nursing care for the child should include:
    1. Encouraging early ambulation
    2. Monitoring the insertion site for bleeding
    3. Restricting fluids until blood pressure is stabilized
    4. Comparing blood pressure in affected and unaffected extremities

158. An infant with a congenital heart defect has just returned to the unit after a cardiac catheterization. The nurse manager immediately intervenes when the infant's nurse:
    1. Performs range-of-motion exercises
    2. Administers fluids and foods as tolerated
    3. Assesses pulses distal to catheterization site
    4. Monitors the apical pulse for rate and rhythm

159. When planning to give discharge instructions to the parents of a child who has had a cardiac catheterization, the nurse should include:
    1. Giving a sponge bath for the first three days at home
    2. Using ice compresses to relieve swelling at the entry site
    3. Limiting fluid intake for the next three days to prevent nausea
    4. Returning to the clinic in five days for removal of the pressure dressing

160. A 4-month-old who has a congenital heart defect develops heart failure and is exhibiting marked dyspnea at rest. The nurse is aware this finding can be attributed to:
    1. Anemia
    2. Hypovolemia
    3. Pulmonary edema
    4. Metabolic acidosis

161. The mother of a 5-month-old infant with heart failure questions the necessity of weighing the infant every morning. The nurse's response should be based on the fact that this daily information is important in determining:
    1. Renal failure
    2. Fluid retention
    3. Nutritional status
    4. Medication dosage

162. When examining the laboratory work of a child with the diagnosis of rheumatic fever, the nurse would expect the findings to demonstrate:
    1. A negative C-reactive protein
    2. An elevated reticulocyte count
    3. A positive antistreptolysin titer
    4. A decreased erythrocyte sedimentation rate

163. A 5-year-old returns to the pediatric intensive care unit after cardiac surgery. The child has a left chest tube attached to water-seal drainage, an IV of D5 ½NS at 40 mL/hr, and a nasogastric tube to gravity. The child is attached to a cardiac monitor and has a left chest dressing. Upon admission to the unit, the nurse should first:
    1. Take the vital signs
    2. Check the identification bracelet
    3. Measure the chest and gastric drainage
    4. Check the suction pressure of the water-seal drainage

164. As part of the discharge teaching for the parents of a child who has had cardiac surgery, the nurse should inform them of the need for antibiotic prophylaxis to prevent:
    1. Pericarditis
    2. Myocarditis
    3. Upper respiratory infections
    4. Subacute bacterial endocarditis

ENDOCRINE (EN)

165. The nurse should anticipate that an infant of a mother with diabetes will have a precipitous drop in the blood glucose level about:
    1. ½ hour after birth
    2. 1 to 3 hours after birth
    3. 5 to 12 hours after birth
    4. 24 to 36 hours after birth

166. When reviewing the plan of care for a child with diabetes, the nurse is aware that the most accurate method to evaluate the effectiveness of diet and insulin therapy over time is the laboratory test that measures:
    1. Urine ketones
    2. Serum protein levels
    3. Serum glucose levels
    4. Glycosylated hemoglobin

167. A child with type 1 diabetes, whose diabetes has been under control for several years, is admitted with the diagnosis of ketoacidosis. Based on this history, the nurse should suspect that this episode of ketoacidosis may have been precipitated by:
    1. A recent weight loss
    2. An increase in exercise
    3. The presence of an infection
    4. The administration of too much insulin

168. A child with type 1 diabetes has been admitted in ketoacidosis. The nurse would expect the child to exhibit:
    1. Pyrexia
    2. Hyperpnea
    3. Bradycardia
    4. Hypertension

169. A 9-year-old child, who has had type 1 diabetes mellitus for several years, is brought to the emergency department of a community hospital. The child is displaying deep, rapid respirations, flushed, dry cheeks, abdominal pain with nausea, and increased thirst. The nurse would expect laboratory tests to reveal a blood pH of:
    1. 7.20 and blood glucose of 60 mg/dl
    2. 7.50 and blood glucose of 60 mg/dl
    3. 7.50 and blood glucose of 460 mg/dl
    4. 7.20 and blood glucose of 460 mg/dl

170. A 9-year-old child with diabetes is hospitalized for dosage regulation of insulin. The child appears to be very manipulative and has been observed sneaking food and trying to talk the mother into providing sweets. Based on this behavior, when the child complains of hypoglycemia, the most appropriate nursing action would be to:
1. Test the urine for glucose
2. Obtain a blood glucose level
3. Administer orange juice with sugar
4. Ask the child the last time food was eaten

171. A child with diabetes who is also learning disabled has trouble correctly measuring the required insulin dose. The child frequently draws up 42 units of insulin instead of the prescribed 24 units. The most appropriate intervention to ensure dosage safety would be to:
1. Teach the child to use a magnifying glass to read the numbers on the syringe
2. Provide the child with preset syringe guides that were developed for the blind
3. Exchange the insulin syringe the child has been using for a tuberculin syringe
4. Allow the child to have the number written down on paper when filling the syringe

172. The nurse teaches an adolescent who has just been diagnosed with type 1 diabetes that regulation of the disorder can be accomplished with dietary control, exercise and:
1. Insulin therapy
2. Prophylactic antibiotics
3. Blood glucose monitoring
4. Oral hypoglycemic agents

173. An adolescent, newly diagnosed as having type 1 diabetes, asks what will happen when the blood glucose declines. Before answering, the nurse recalls that a hormone secreted by the islets of Langerhans causes liver glycogenolysis. This hormone is:
1. ACTH
2. Insulin
3. Glucagon
4. Epinephrine

174. After assessing what a newly diagnosed child knows about diabetes, the nurse should:
1. Develop a rapport with the client
2. Set goals with the client and the client's family
3. Teach the client how to do blood glucose testing
4. Teach the client how to administer the insulin injections required daily

175. The nurse is caring for a child with diabetes and suspects that the child is experiencing an episode of hyperglycemia. Which assessments of the child led the nurse to this conclusion? Select all that apply:
1. _____ Headache
2. _____ Irritability
3. _____ Diaphoresis
4. _____ Increased thirst
5. _____ Redness of the face
6. _____ Deep, rapid breathing

176. A 16-year-old type 1 diabetic adolescent is brought to the emergency room unconscious. The adolescent's blood glucose level is 742 mg/dl. During the initial assessment the nurse would expect to note:
1. Pyrexia
2. Hyperpnea
3. Bradycardia
4. Hypertension

177. A 15-year-old adolescent, who has type 1 diabetes mellitus, is admitted to the pediatric intensive care unit (PICU) in ketoacidosis with a blood glucose level of 700 mg/dl. The teenager has a history of fluctuating blood glucose levels and difficulty adhering to the therapeutic regimen. A continuous insulin infusion is started. When developing a plan of care, the nurse should be alert for the evidence of:
1. Hypokalemia
2. Hypovolemia
3. Hypernatremia
4. Hypercalcemia

178. When teaching about insulin self-administration to a 10-year-old child newly diagnosed with diabetes, the nurse should teach the child to:
1. Always wash the hands prior to preparing the insulin injection
2. Shake the bottle of insulin thoroughly before drawing the dose
3. Briskly rub the injection site for a minute after giving the injection
4. Give the insulin injections alternately in both the upper and lower extremities

179. The nurse plans to teach a child with diabetes, who is receiving both Humulin N and Humulin R insulin daily, how to self-administer the insulin before discharge. When learning to give the injections, the child should:
1. Alternate the sites until the best one to use is found
2. Learn to use the needle and syringe by practicing on an orange first

3. Administer the injections immediately after being taught the technique

4. Draw up the Humulin N insulin first and then draw up the Humulin R insulin

180. An 8-year-old child is receiving 45 units of Humulin N (NPH) insulin at 7 AM and 7 PM. The most appropriate information for the nurse to give the parents concerning a bedtime snack would be:

1. Provide a snack at bedtime to prevent hypoglycemia during the night

2. Give the child a snack at bedtime if any signs of hyperglycemia are displayed

3. Keep the snack at the bedside in case the child becomes hungry during the night

4. Bedtime snacks are not recommended for diabetic children treated with long-acting insulin

181. The nurse is able to determine that an adolescent with type 2 diabetes understands the nutritional teaching when the adolescent states:

1. "I can eat pizza at a party."

2. "I can eat low fat, low calorie candy bars."

3. "Regular soft drinks are better than diet ones."

4. "My fasting blood sugar should be no higher than 150."

182. Since prevention of infection is of utmost importance in children with diabetes, the nurse should emphasize to the child and parents the importance of:

1. Inspecting both feet frequently and carefully

2. Soaking the feet at least once daily for 30 minutes in hot water

3. Drying the feet thoroughly after a bath by rubbing vigorously with a towel

4. Treating minor cuts on the feet immediately with a strong antiseptic such as iodine

183. An adolescent, who had been admitted to the hospital with ketoacidosis, has been stabilized and is now receiving Humulin R subcutaneously. One hour after its administration, the nurse enters the room and identifies that the client is diaphoretic and irritable. The nurse should first:

1. Delay the client's lunch tray

2. Obtain a blood glucose reading

3. Administer a glass of orange juice

4. Cover the client with a light blanket

184. If surgery is to be performed on a child with diabetes, the nurse should be cognizant that:

1. Urine test results provide the best gauge of diabetic control after the surgery

2. The greatest danger during the surgical procedure is from diabetic ketoacidosis

3. The stress of surgery causes a rise in blood glucose levels during the postoperative period

4. If insulin was not required before surgery, it generally will not be required in the postoperative period

185. A 14-year-old with diabetes wants to go for a pizza after a volleyball game. The teenager asks the school nurse whether this would be permissible on the insulin-diet-exercise regimen prescribed. The most appropriate response by the nurse would be:

1. "Fast foods are unhealthy, especially for teenagers with diabetes."

2. "It would be best if you ate at home where your diet can be controlled."

3. "Go with your friends but make an effort to eat something other than pizza."

4. "I will teach you how to use a fast food exchange list for individuals with diabetes."

186. The statement that reflects why the nurse teaches the mother of a young child with diabetes how to test the child's urine at home even though blood glucose testing is being done four times a day is:

1. Blood glucose testing before meals and at bedtime may be stopped once the child is stabilized on insulin

2. The urine should be tested for acetone during illness and when the blood glucose level is more than 250

3. Urine testing remains the most accurate way to check for high glucose levels if double-voided specimens are used

4. It is now thought that voided urine specimens reflect short-term glucose levels more accurately than blood glucose, especially in children

187. A young girl with diabetes has just joined the school's soccer team, and her mother is unsure whether to tell the coach of her child's condition. The mother asks the nurse in the pediatric clinic for guidance. The nurse's response to the mother's concern should be based on the fact that:

1. The coach might discuss the child's condition with other faculty members

2. Hyperglycemia can be treated by the school nurse if symptoms are recognized early

3. The child would be dropped from the team if school authorities learn she has a chronic disease

4. Episodes of hypoglycemia are associated with children with diabetes who participate in sports activities

FLUIDS AND ELECTROLYTES (FE)

188. A severely dehydrated infant has been admitted to the hospital, too lethargic to be started on oral rehydration therapy (ORT). An intravenous infusion is begun. The nurse's priority responsibility regarding the intravenous infusion would be to:
    1. Limit cuddling during the infusion
    2. Monitor the prescribed rate of flow
    3. Record changes in the baby's behavior
    4. Explain the purpose of the infusion to the parent

189. To best ascertain the magnitude of fluid loss in an infant with gastroenteritis and diarrhea, the nurse should:
    1. Evaluate the infant's skin turgor carefully
    2. Note the elevation of the infant's hematocrit value
    3. Assess the moistness of the infant's mucous membranes
    4. Compare the infant's pre-illness weight with the current weight

190. A dehydrated 2-month-old infant with a history of diarrhea is admitted to pediatrics. Oral rehydration therapy is instituted. The most accurate method for monitoring the infant's hydration status would be:
    1. Counting wet diapers
    2. Obtaining daily weights
    3. Measuring the intake and output
    4. Checking skin turgor of the abdomen

191. A 4-month-old infant is brought to the emergency department with a 2-day history of diarrhea. The baby is listless, with sunken eyeballs, depressed fontanelle and minimal tissue turgor. Breathing is deep, rapid, and unlabored. The mother states that there have been 10 liquid stools and no voiding. Based on the history and observations, the nurse concludes that the infant is in a state of:
    1. Mild dehydration
    2. Metabolic acidosis
    3. Respiratory alkalosis
    4. Compensated acid-base balance

192. A 5½-month-old infant is admitted to the hospital with a fever and a history of vomiting for 48 hours. In view of this infant's responses, the assessment by the nurse that initially influences the child's care would be:
    1. Inspecting the baby's skin for poor turgor
    2. Determining the baby's vital signs and weight
    3. Checking the baby's neurologic status and urinary output
    4. Asking the mother whether the baby is breastfed or bottle fed

193. A mother arrives in the emergency department with her severely dehydrated infant. After being treated aggressively, the infant is rehydrated and ready to be discharged. A priority concern that the nurse includes in the teaching plan for the mother would be the:
    1. Effects of antibiotics on viral gastroenteritis
    2. Importance of a well-balanced diet for her baby
    3. Need for cleanliness of foods and feeding utensils
    4. Potential hazards of fluid loss in young children

194. A 3-week-old infant, who has been vomiting for three days, is admitted to the pediatric unit with the diagnosis of hypertrophic pyloric stenosis (HPS). During the admission procedure it would be most important for the nurse to determine the:
    1. The size and shape of the abdominal mass
    2. Character, amount, and times when the infant vomited
    3. Time of the last feeding, type of formula, and amount taken
    4. Skin turgor, respiratory status, amount and color of the last voiding

195. An infant is diagnosed with hypertrophic pyloric stenosis (HPS). The physician schedules a pyloromyotomy to relieve the pyloric obstruction. The nurse understands that this procedure has a high success rate when preoperatively:
    1. Fluid and electrolyte imbalances have been vigorously treated
    2. Decreased serum chloride levels have been restored to normal
    3. Replacement intravenous infusions have been carefully monitored
    4. General malnutrition and respiratory problems have been corrected

196. The best indicator of fluid balance in children with nephrotic syndrome is the daily measurement of:
    1. Body weight
    2. Urinary output
    3. Abdominal girth
    4. Urine osmolality

197. A child's adaptation associated with nephrotic syndrome that requires the nurse to assess the child's vital signs, especially the blood pressure and pulse quality and rate, would be:

1. Hypovolemia
2. Hyperkalemia
3. Pulmonary emboli
4. Chronic heart failure

198. A 6-month-old infant, weighing 15 pounds, is admitted with a diagnosis of diarrhea and dehydration. An order for oral rehydration therapy (ORT) reads: 40 to 50 mL/kg of Pedialyte over 4 hours. The amount the baby should ingest during the four hours would be approximately:
1. 260 mL
2. 320 mL
3. 360 mL
4. 420 mL

199. The physician orders that potassium chloride be added to the IV fluids of a 6-month-old infant with diarrhea. The assessment by the nurse that should be brought to the physician's attention is that the:
1. Child is crying
2. Child has poor skin turgor
3. Child's intake is 120 mL for 8 hours
4. Child's urinary output is 50 mL for 8 hours

200. A 2-year-old is brought into the emergency department having ingested a half-full bottle of aspirin. The nurse recognizes that initially, respiratory alkalosis is seen in aspirin toxicity. This is the result of the:
1. Lowered renal excretion
2. Rapid absorption of aspirin
3. Presence of hyperventilation
4. Change in pH of the gastric contents

201. A priority in planning care for a toddler who has ingested aspirin is the frequent monitoring of the child's:
1. Blood pressure
2. Abdominal girth
3. Body temperature
4. Blood glucose level

202. The nurse notes that an infant with a diagnosis of failure to thrive, who has been on tube feedings for three days, has very dry skin and mucous membranes. The nurse verifies that all feedings have been retained, but the daily urinary output is consistently 250 mL and the infant has lost weight. The nurse should:
1. Realize this is probably normal for babies and infants with failure to thrive
2. Increase the intravenous flow of half-normal saline and call the physician
3. Recognize undernutrition and call the physician to increase the caloric intake

4. Identify underhydration and call the physician to increase the infant's fluid intake

203. When assessing a 4-month-old infant with gastroenteritis and dehydration, the nurse would expect to find a:
1. Specific gravity of 1.014
2. Urinary output of 50 mL/hr
3. Depressed anterior fontanel
4. History of allergies to various foods

204. After surgery for the repair of a meningomyelocele, an infant develops diarrhea and metabolic acidosis with a decreased urinary output. Because of the infant's status, the nurse would anticipate an order for:
1. Albumin
2. Isotonic saline
3. Sodium lactate
4. Potassium chloride

205. When a 3-month-old infant is receiving IV fluids via a scalp vein, the nurse should:
1. Check the baby's pupils for reaction every hour
2. Restrain the baby's arms when no one is with the child
3. Observe behind the baby's ear and occiput for infiltration
4. Explain to the parents why they can't hold the baby during IV therapy

206. An 8-month-old infant who weighs 18 lb, 12 oz is receiving 8 oz of full-strength formula every four hours. Based on the recommended caloric intake of 108 kcal/kg, the nurse determines that this amount:
1. Meets the recommended requirements for growth
2. Exceeds the recommended requirements for growth
3. Is less than the recommended requirements for growth
4. Is difficult to evaluate without more information

207. The mother of an infant with a congenital heart defect, who was admitted with heart failure, questions why her baby must be weighed each morning. The nurse's response should be based on the fact that this daily information is important in determining:
1. Renal failure
2. Fluid retention
3. Nutritional status
4. Medication dosage

208. The nurse teaches the parents of a 4-year-old child, weighing 33 pounds, who has sickle-cell anemia about their child's fluid needs. The nurse identifies the understanding of the teaching when one of the parents states, "Every day I should give my child:
    1. Two to 3 quarts of fluid."
    2. Four 6-ounce glasses of fluid."
    3. About 10 small glasses of fluid."
    4. Approximately 2 quarts of fluid."

209. A child with Reye's syndrome is receiving an intravenous solution of 10% glucose and mannitol to reduce cerebral edema. The child's vital signs should be monitored for changes to prevent the occurrence of:
    1. Seizures
    2. Over-hydration
    3. Acute heart failure
    4. Hypovolemic shock

210. An IV of D5W is infusing when a child returns to the pediatric unit from surgery. The postoperative orders do not indicate the desired rate of infusion. The most appropriate action for the nurse to take would be to:
    1. Reduce the flow rate to keep the vein open and obtain an order
    2. Adjust the flow to the rate the child was receiving before surgery
    3. Regulate the flow rate to 25 mL per hour until the physician makes rounds
    4. Maintain the present flow rate and call the operating room to verify the correct rate

211. After abdominal surgery, a priority nursing intervention for a young infant with an IV would be:
    1. Administering oral fluids
    2. Limiting handling by the parents
    3. Weighing the diapers after voiding
    4. Stabilizing the intravenous site with tape

212. The nurse would expect a child with acute glomerulonephritis to be placed on a diet low in:
    1. Fat
    2. Protein
    3. Glucose
    4. Potassium

213. A 6-year-old child with acute glomerulonephritis is restricted to 600 mL of fluid for 24 hours. The nursing intervention that would be most appropriate to assist the child to cope with this limitation is:
    1. Dividing fluid intake equally among each shift (200 mL each shift)
    2. Allowing the child to drink fluids as desired until the 600 mL limit is reached
    3. Withholding fluids from 7 PM to 7 AM and giving the entire 600 mL from 7 AM to 7 PM
    4. Providing the child a minimum of one ounce of fluid in small, 1-ounce cups each waking hour

214. A critically ill child develops Cheyne-Stokes respirations, and the nurse suspects an increasing acid-base imbalance related to:
    1. Respiratory alkalosis from overbreathing and excess carbon dioxide output
    2. Respiratory acidosis from impeded breathing and the retention of carbon dioxide
    3. Metabolic acidosis from the concentration of cations in body fluids, which displace bicarbonate
    4. Metabolic alkalosis from an increase in base bicarbonate resulting from the primary health problem

215. In the immediate period after admission to the hospital for severe burns, a 5-year-old child requests a drink of water. The nurse's reply is based on the knowledge that most burn clients will be:
    1. Given ice chips when desired
    2. Limited to 15 mL of oral fluid q4h
    3. Permitted water unless unconscious
    4. NPO for approximately 24 to 48 hours

216. When caring for a child with partial and full-thickness burns of the extremities, the nursing action that should have the highest priority would be:
    1. Administering oxygen
    2. Inserting a urinary catheter
    3. Giving the prescribed pain medication
    4. Starting and maintaining an IV infusion

217. An adolescent is hospitalized with multiple internal injuries after an automobile accident. The adolescent is being kept NPO and is receiving an intravenous solution at 125 mL/hour and an antibiotic reconstituted in 100 mL of normal saline q6h (10 AM, 4 PM, 10 PM, 4 AM). When computing the intake and output for this adolescent, what is the intake for the 7 AM

to 3 PM shift?

Answer: _____.

218. The physician orders multielectrolyte solution (MES) 150 mL per kg of body weight every 24 hours for a child weighing 13 pounds. The nurse calculates that the intake of MES for this child should be:
    1. 500 mL/24 hr
    2. 750 mL/24 hr
    3. 885 mL/24 hr
    4. 965 mL/24 hr

219. The nurse should recognize that the sequence of events that occurs in a child's respiratory response to acidosis is:
    1. Hypoventilation; increased CO_2 elimination; decreased blood H ions; increased pH
    2. Hyperventilation; increased CO_2 elimination; decreased blood H ions; increased pH
    3. Hyperventilation; decreased CO_2 elimination; decreased blood H ions; decreased pH
    4. Hypoventilation; decreased blood H ions; increased CO_2 elimination; decreased pH

220. The nurse recognizes that the physiologic compensatory mechanism that is activated to counteract the effects of acid-base imbalance in a child with severe dehydration is:
    1. Profuse diaphoresis
    2. Elevated temperature
    3. Renal retention of H^+
    4. Increased respirations

221. The nurse manager of an infection control unit presents an educational class for nurses regarding the care of young children with viral-related diarrhea. The nurse manager emphasizes that the most important intervention would be administering the prescribed:
    1. Kaopectate after each stool
    2. Antibiotics every four hours
    3. Antiviral agent at 6-hour intervals
    4. Oral rehydration therapy until diarrhea subsides

222. The blood gas report that would most likely reflect the acid-base balance found in a child admitted to the hospital with severe dehydration is:
    1. A pH of 7.50 and a PCO_2 of 34 mm Hg
    2. A pH of 7.20 and a PCO_2 of 20 mm Hg
    3. A pH of 7.23 and a PCO_2 of 70 mm Hg
    4. A pH of 7.56 and a PCO_2 of 20 mm Hg

223. A child with acute glomerulonephritis (AGN) has fluid intake restricted to the previous day's output plus 400 mL. The child's output in the last 24 hours was 140 mL. If the child were to receive one third of the total fluid permitted from 3 to 11, the nurse should limit the evening intake to:
    1. 60 mL
    2. 90 mL
    3. 180 mL
    4. 270 mL

GASTROINTESTINAL (GI)

224. The mother of an infant diagnosed with hypertrophic pyloric stenosis (HPS) states she has never heard of this disorder and asks many questions. When responding, the nurse should emphasize that:
    1. It is unlikely that surgery will be necessary
    2. This is a disorder with an excellent prognosis
    3. This disorder results from an inborn error of metabolism
    4. Her baby will need special feedings and handling for several months

225. A 4-week-old infant is admitted with a tentative diagnosis of hypertrophic pyloric stenosis (HPS). During the admission assessment, the nurse bicycles the infant's legs before palpating the abdomen. This enables the nurse to:
    1. Assess abdominal rebound
    2. Palpate abdominal contour
    3. Relax the abdominal muscles
    4. Detect weak abdominal muscles

226. A 6-week-old infant is brought to the clinic by the parents. They state that their baby has been vomiting with increasing frequency and force after feeding. Hypertrophic pyloric stenosis (HPS) is diagnosed. The nurse is aware that the manifestations of pyloric stenosis are:
    1. Avid hunger and non-bile-stained vomitus
    2. Severe abdominal pain and visible peristaltic waves
    3. Vomiting several hours after a feeding and tarry stools
    4. Bile-stained vomitus and generalized abdominal distention

227. The nurse is assessing a 1-month-old infant suspected of having hypertrophic pyloric stenosis. Using the Figure below, select the area where the nurse would expect to palpate an olive-shaped mass:

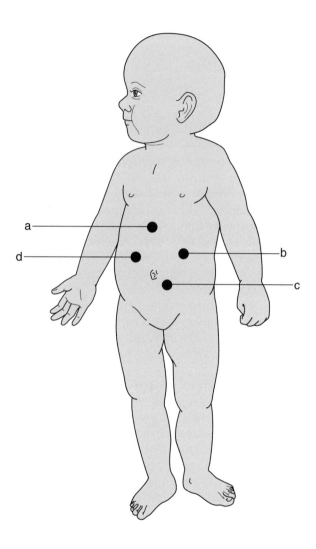

1. a
2. b
3. c
4. d

228. The nurse explains to the parents of an infant with pyloric stenosis that the type of surgery scheduled for this problem has a high success rate when:
1. The fluid and electrolyte imbalances are corrected preoperatively
2. Gastric decompression is monitored for amount and type of drainage
3. It is performed before the infant's vomiting becomes severe and projectile
4. The infant receives small, frequent feedings of thickened formula preoperatively

229. The mother of an infant with hypertrophic pyloric stenosis (HPS) asks the nurse many questions about the problem. When answering these questions the nurse should convey the idea that:
1. Surgery will be necessary
2. Chromosomal mutation is the cause of HPS
3. Slow feeding will be necessary for a few months
4. Dietary restrictions will be required throughout childhood

230. A 10-week-old is diagnosed as having pyloric stenosis and is scheduled for surgery. Oral feedings are usually initiated a few hours after surgery. The nurse expects that initially the baby will receive:
1. Clear liquids
2. Full-strength formula
3. Half-strength formula
4. Thickened formula with cereal

231. An infant who has had surgery for hypertrophic pyloric stenosis (HPS) is being fed by the mother. To decrease the chance of vomiting after feedings, the nurse teaches her that after a feeding the baby should be:
1. Rocked for 20 minutes
2. Placed in an infant seat
3. Positioned flat on the right side
4. Kept awake with sensory stimulation

232. An infant is to be discharged following surgery for pyloric stenosis. The mother should be instructed to:
1. Give the baby creamy cereal at each feeding followed by the regular formula
2. Continue the regular formula, hold the baby during all feedings, feed the baby slowly, and burp frequently
3. Give the baby about 1 ounce of regular formula per hour for the next two weeks; progressing slowly, as tolerated, to larger amounts
4. Feed the regular formula while the baby is in the crib positioned on the right side; handle the baby as little as possible for two hours after each feeding

233. A newborn with a cleft lip is fed with a special nipple. To minimize regurgitation of the feedings the nurse instructs the mother to:
1. Hold and burp the baby frequently while feeding
2. Give the baby the thickened formula as ordered
3. Feed the baby while sitting the baby up in an infant seat

4. Lay the baby on the side with the bottle firmly propped

234. Immediate nursing care for a neonate born with a cleft lip is directed primarily toward:
1. Modifying feeding methods
2. Keeping the baby from crying
3. Minimizing handling by parents
4. Preventing the occurrence of infection

235. During the initial postoperative period after a one-month-old infant has had a cleft lip repair, the nurse should feed the infant using a:
1. Spoon
2. Soft nipple
3. Ten mL syringe
4. Nasogastric tube

236. The first action by the nurse after each feeding of an infant with a recent surgical repair of a cleft lip should be to:
1. Burp the infant several times
2. Place the infant on the abdomen
3. Cuddle the infant for a few minutes
4. Clean and rinse the suture line of the lip

237. A priority nursing measure for an infant during the immediate postoperative period following a surgical repair of a cleft lip is to:
1. Minimize the infant's crying
2. Restrain the infant at all times
3. Oxygenate the infant frequently
4. Handle the infant as little as possible

238. Several days after a baby girl's birth she begins to vomit and lose weight. Galactosemia is diagnosed. The nurse explains to the parents that galactosemia is an inherited autosomal recessive disorder which is the result of:
1. An intolerance to wheat and rye
2. An inborn error of carbohydrate metabolism
3. The inability to metabolize an essential amino acid
4. The absence of parasympathetic ganglion cells in the colon

239. To provide appropriate instructions for parents caring for an infant with galactosemia, the nurse should include teaching them to:
1. Eliminate milk from the diet
2. Avoid soybean-based formulas
3. Substitute cheese for meat in the diet
4. Keep penicillin on hand for respiratory infections

240. When performing a physical assessment on a 15-month-old toddler, the nurse suspects evidence of a disorder when the child's:
1. Anterior fontanelle is still palpable
2. Liver is palpated 3 cm below the costal margin
3. Respiratory movements are observed as abdominal
4. Apical pulse rate of 104 beats/minute is auscultated

241. A 2-month-old infant is to have a nasogastric tube inserted. The nurse should expect that:
1. A pacifier may be used to lessen gagging and allow easier insertion of the tube
2. Gastric contents would not appear in the tube because the baby has been NPO
3. The tube will be passed about four inches, the distance from the chin to the tip of the sternum
4. Coughing, irregular breathing, and even slight cyanosis are expected during the initial introduction of the tube.

242. Before an infant is to receive a tube feeding, the nurse inserts a nasogastric tube. When the infant begins to cough and gag, the nurse's initial action should be to:
1. Validate tube placement
2. Remove and reinsert the tube
3. Administer the tube feeding slowly
4. Auscultate the chest for breath sounds

243. To help a child retain tube feedings and avoid aspiration, the nurse should place the child in the:
1. Prone position
2. Semi-Fowler's position
3. Left side-lying position
4. Supine position with head turned

244. A 6-week-old infant is admitted to the pediatric unit with a diagnosis of gastroesophageal reflux. When discussing care with this child's mother, the nurse plans to include:
1. Giving formula thickened with cereal with frequent burping
2. Ways of handling the child after surgery to repair the esophageal defect
3. Discontinuing breast-feeding and placing the child in an infant seat after feedings
4. Feeding cereal with a spoon and administering a drug to help the stomach to empty

245. Because of the relaxation of the lower esophageal sphincter and the frequent return of stomach contents into the upper GI tract, the nurse should monitor an infant with gastroesophageal reflux for:
1. Increased hematocrit
2. Abdominal distention
3. Respiratory symptoms
4. Lower bowel obstruction

246. A mother asks why her 1½-year-old toddler's cleft palate was not repaired at the time the cleft lip was repaired at 3 months of age. The nurse's best response would be:
   1. "Waiting leaves time for other birth defects to be detected and corrected."
   2. "The cleft lip was so disfiguring that plastic surgery was done as quickly as possible."
   3. "Your surgeon prefers to separate the operations to minimize and prevent complications."
   4. "The palate is corrected after teething and before your child talks so that correct speech may be learned."

247. The physician orders arm restraints for a 1½-year-old who just had surgery for a cleft palate. The nurse is aware that the reason for the restraints is to prevent the child from:
   1. Playing with unsterile toys
   2. Rolling to a supine position
   3. Putting fingers into the mouth
   4. Pulling out the nasogastric tube

248. When a toddler with a cleft palate repair is able to tolerate fluids, the nurse should administer the fluids with a:
   1. Small cup
   2. Bulb syringe
   3. Lamb's nipple
   4. Teflon-coated spoon

249. An infant with persistent diarrhea is placed on NPO. The nurse understands that this is done to:
   1. Allow the intestinal tract to rest
   2. Correct the electrolyte imbalance
   3. Determine the cause of the diarrhea
   4. Prevent irritation of the perineum from diarrhea

250. The parents of an infant admitted to the hospital with gastroenteritis and dehydration want to be involved with the baby's care. The nurse recognizes that they understand the teaching about the maintenance of standard precautions when they state, "We should:
   1. Wear a mask when we are holding the baby."
   2. Weigh the diaper each time we change the baby."
   3. Wear gloves each time we change the baby's diaper."
   4. Keep the door to the baby's room closed most of the time."

251. A mother whose 20-month-old toddler has just developed diarrhea calls the pediatric clinic and asks what she should do. The nurse practitioner tells the mother to:
   1. Allow the child to continue normal activities, hold all feedings for 24 hours, and call back tomorrow
   2. Limit the child's activities, hold all oral feedings, observe carefully, and call back in four hours
   3. Wrap the child snugly, give child sugar water, and bring the child in to see the physician immediately
   4. Continue to feed the child as usual, make an appointment with the receptionist, and bring the child to the clinic tomorrow

252. After receiving and tolerating an oral rehydration solution (Pedialyte) because of dehydration from diarrhea, a 20-month-old toddler improves, and the diet is advanced to soft foods. The nurse understands that a food that would be contraindicated is:
   1. Creamed soup
   2. Strained carrots
   3. Animal crackers
   4. Mashed bananas

253. The mother of a 2-month-old bottle-fed infant asks the nurse how much formula is required per day. The nurse ascertains that the formula contains 20 calories per ounce. After determining that the baby weighs 11 pounds, the nurse tells the mother that her baby's total daily requirement would be about:
   1. 12 oz.
   2. 28 oz.
   3. 54 oz.
   4. 89 oz.

254. The nurse teaches the mother of a young child that thiamine, which helps to produce more energy for both children and adults, is found in foods such as:
   1. Eggs
   2. Fruits
   3. Green vegetables
   4. Whole or enriched grains

255. After an emergency appendectomy, the nurse should place the child in a semi-Fowler's or right Sims' position because:
   1. The lungs can aerate fully in both of these positions
   2. Drainage is facilitated, preventing subdiaphragmatic abscesses
   3. Movement is easier, thus reducing complications from immobility
   4. Splinting of the wound is accomplished by pressure on the operative site

256. The nurse's charting for a child who has had an appendectomy should include, in addition to coughing and deep breathing, documentation of:
   1. Intake and output and bowel sounds
   2. Mouth care and frequency of dressing changes
   3. Bowel sounds and teaching about the low-residue diet
   4. Teaching to prevent dumping syndrome and early ambulation

257. The nurse is aware that the food choice that would ensure maintenance of nitrogen balance after surgery in a 5-year-old child would be:
   1. Chicken soup
   2. A bacon sandwich
   3. Cut-up orange slices
   4. A hamburger on a bun

258. The nurse epidemiologist of a large urban hospital is called to the pediatric unit to investigate an outbreak of diarrhea. Suspecting a *Salmonella* infection, the nurse would be particularly concerned if the children had eaten:
   1. Raw carrots and apples
   2. Grapefruit juice and ice cream
   3. Hamburgers and soft-boiled eggs
   4. Ham and cheese sandwiches and milk

259. When caring for a child with diarrhea caused by a *Salmonella* infection, the physician's order that the nurse should question would be:
   1. Oral rehydration fluids
   2. Kaopectate 2 teaspoons after each stool
   3. Notify physician if blood is present in stool
   4. Tylenol liquid 3 mL for temperature above 101° F

260. A 1-day-old neonate with an imperforate anus undergoes a pull-through procedure with an anoplasty. The nurse knows that it is most appropriate postoperatively to place the infant:
   1. In Buck's traction
   2. In Trendelenburg position
   3. Prone with the head of the crib elevated
   4. Supine with the head of the crib elevated

261. The nurse working with infants who are preterm should be alert to the fact that these infants may later develop intestinal obstruction because of:
   1. Meconium ileus
   2. Imperforate anus
   3. Duodenal atresia
   4. Necrotizing enterocolitis

262. After several episodes of abdominal pain and vomiting, a 5-month-old child is taken to the hospital. A diagnosis of intussusception is made. To assist in confirming the diagnosis, the priority nursing assessment should be:
   1. Noting frequency of crying
   2. Listening for bowel sounds
   3. Observing characteristics of stools
   4. Measuring fluid intake and output

263. When obtaining a health history from the mother of a 2-month-old with a diagnosis of pyloric stenosis, the nurse should record the significant finding that the infant's:
   1. Birth was preterm and the weight was four pounds
   2. Older brother had idiopathic vomiting during infancy
   3. First cousin had surgery for hypertrophic pyloric stenosis
   4. Older sister had an episode of intestinal obstruction in early infancy

264. A child who has successfully completed the emergent (resuscitative) phase of treatment for a severe burn injury is started on a high-protein, high-calorie diet. As a snack between meals the nurse should encourage:
   1. Crackers and cheese
   2. White bread and honey
   3. Orange juice and cookies
   4. Jell-O and whipped cream

265. The nurse bases the care plan for an infant with celiac disease on the pathophysiology believed to cause this disorder, which would be an inborn error of metabolism characterized by:
   1. Excessive salt in the sweat glands
   2. An absence of the enzyme peptidase
   3. Excessive viscosity of the mucous glands
   4. An absence of the enzyme phenylalanine

266. When obtaining a health history from the mother of an infant with celiac disease, the nurse would expect the mother to say that her baby:
   1. Is irritable all the time
   2. Has bulky, foul, frothy stools
   3. Drinks large amounts of fluid
   4. Voids strong, concentrated urine

267. The nurse recognizes that the diagnosis of celiac disease can be confirmed when a jejunal biopsy reveals:
   1. Small areas of fatty plaques
   2. Atrophic changes in the mucosal wall
   3. Irregular areas of superficial ulcerations
   4. Diffuse degenerative fibrosis of the acini

268. The nurse recognizes that anemia in a child with celiac disease is caused by:
    1. The poor absorption of iron and folic acid
    2. The small amount of iron included in the diet
    3. An inadequate amount of the intrinsic factor
    4. A low food intake and the child's minimal appetite

269. Discharge planning for a toddler newly diagnosed with celiac disease includes instructions related to dietary restrictions. The nurse recognizes that the mother understands the instructions when she states that the foods she will withhold from the diet include:
    1. Beef, pork, chicken
    2. Eggs, milk, Rice Krispies
    3. Corn crisps, spinach, cheese
    4. Chocolate milk, whole-wheat toast, fruit

270. After being on a dietary regimen for celiac disease for six months, the child's compliance to the diet can be evaluated by assessing the:
    1. Physical and emotional progress
    2. Ability to handle stressful situations
    3. Understanding of the disease process
    4. Knowledge of foods allowed on the diet

271. In addition to teaching the mother of a toddler with celiac disease the specific foods allowed on the gluten-restricted diet, the nurse should help the mother understand that:
    1. This diet will be discontinued in three to five years
    2. She must read the labels of all prepared foods carefully
    3. All grains contain gluten; therefore none can be included in the diet
    4. The caloric intake will be adjusted to compensate for the deficient protein intake

272. The nurse teaches a mother to collect a specimen from her child who is suspected of having a pinworm infestation. It is recommended that she collect the cellophane tape specimen:
    1. At night after the child has had a bath
    2. At night before the child has a bowel movement
    3. In the late morning after the child has had a bowel movement
    4. In the morning before the child has had a bowel movement or bath

273. A child who has been diagnosed with congenital aganglionic megacolon (Hirschsprung's disease) is to be managed at home on isotonic enemas. The nurse should teach the parents that they should use:
    1. Tap water
    2. Fleet enemas
    3. Soapsuds and water
    4. Diluted saline solution

274. The nurse evaluates that teaching has been effective when the mother of a child on a low–residue diet states that she will serve:
    1. Frankfurter on a roll
    2. Ripe peaches with ice cream
    3. Peanut butter and jam on white bread
    4. Poached eggs and toasted white bread

275. The mother of an 11-month-old child who just had surgery to create a temporary colostomy is concerned about care at home. The nurse's teaching plan about colostomy care would include instructions to:
    1. Limit the intake of milk
    2. Change the bag frequently
    3. Irrigate the colostomy with as much water as possible
    4. Report slight bleeding from the stoma site to the physician immediately

276. The nurse is aware that enterobiasis (pinworm infestation) is most commonly diagnosed by:
    1. Anal itching
    2. Scaly skin patches
    3. Maculopapular rash
    4. A bald spot on the head

277. When advising the mother of a child who may have a pinworm infestation, the nurse's first responsibility would be to teach the mother:
    1. Strategies to avoid reinfestation
    2. How to identify a pinworm egg
    3. When to obtain a pinworm specimen
    4. Why hands should be washed before eating

278. The mother of a toddler who has been treated for pinworm infestation is taught how to prevent a recurrence. The nurse evaluates that the teaching has been effective when the mother states, "I'll:
    1. Need to be sure that the cat stays off my child's bed."
    2. Be sure to disinfect the bathroom and kitchen for the next few days."
    3. Have to reinforce my child's handwashing before eating or handling food."
    4. Report my child's infestation to the school nurse because it was probably contracted from the school's dirty toilets."

279. The mother of a 3-year-old tells the nurse that her child frequently has constipation. The nurse asks how the mother handles the child's toileting. The nurse plans further teaching when the mother says:
1. "I give my child a lot of those high-fiber foods at meals and as snacks."
2. "I encourage my child to drink a lot of fluids, including prune juice, every day."
3. "I notice that my child always has just one bowel movement a day except when ill."
4. "I schedule my child's toileting time first thing in the morning so we are done before breakfast."

INTEGUMENTARY (IT)

280. As a mother leaves the hospital with her newborn, the nurse notes that the mother covers the infant with a blanket. The nurse understands that the mother is preventing heat loss by the principle of:
1. Radiation
2. Conduction
3. Active transport
4. Fluid vaporization

281. During an infant's routine visit to the pediatric clinic, the nurse observes white patches adhering to the mucosa of the infant's mouth. The nurse should:
1. Obtain a swab culture of the patches
2. Scrape off the patches with a tongue blade
3. Instruct the mother to apply neomycin ointment
4. Note the finding and continue with the examination

282. A 3-month-old with severe dehydration has an excoriated diaper area. The infant's mother is quite upset when she finds the nurse has left her infant without a diaper. The nurse should explain that:
1. Increasing the exposed areas helps to reduce the infant's fever
2. Air drying of the skin prevents the diaper from sticking to it
3. Cleansing of the skin followed by air drying reduces excoriation
4. This action allows the nurse to observe more quickly when the infant stools

283. To preserve suture line integrity after a cleft lip repair, the nurse should position the infant on the:
1. Side
2. Back
3. Abdomen
4. Mother's shoulder

284. The mother of a male infant who just had a cleft lip repair tells the nurse, "My baby seems restless. Can I hold him?" The nurse's response would be influenced by the knowledge that:
1. The baby should be sedated to decrease activity before being held
2. Handling may increase irritability and place tension on the suture line
3. Holding may meet the needs of the infant and reduce tension on the suture line
4. The mother will be unable to control the infant's arm movements, thereby endangering the suture line

285. The most important nursing care for infants with eczema is:
1. Promotion of physical growth
2. Provision of sufficient hydration
3. Identification of causative factors
4. Prevention of secondary infections

286. The nurse evaluates that the mother of a 6-month-old with eczema needs more teaching regarding her baby's care when the mother states:
1. "I will be careful not to cut the baby's nails short."
2. "I will make sure not to give the baby any whole milk products."
3. "I have given all of the baby's woolen blankets to my nephew."
4. "I am going to buy my baby a whole new wardrobe of cotton clothing."

287. The nurse in the pediatric clinic is taking a health history of a toddler with an exacerbation of eczema. The nurse should assess if the toddler has been:
1. Eating well and drinking sufficient milk
2. Wearing new clothes or eating new foods
3. Near anyone with a streptococcus infection
4. In close contact with anyone with eczema recently

288. The nurse learns that a 12-month-old infant recently had a fever, runny nose, cough, and white spots in the mouth for three days. A rash developed that started on the face and spread to the whole body. The nurse should suspect that the child has:
1. Rubella
2. Rubeola
3. Varicella
4. Scarlet fever

289. A child with rubella should be isolated from an unimmunized:
1. 20-year-old brother living at home
2. 3-year-old girl friend who lives next door
3. 12-year-old sister who had rubeola as a child
4. 18-year-old female cousin who has recently married

290. The nurse is aware that rubeola often causes children to have:
1. A macular rash
2. A paroxysmal cough
3. Enlarged parotid glands
4. Generalized vesicular lesions

291. To hasten the drying of the lesions and relieve the itch in a child with chickenpox, the nurse suggests that the mother should try:
1. Patting the lesions gently with calamine lotion
2. Rubbing bacitracin ointment into the open lesions
3. Using wet to dry saline dressings over the oozing vesicles
4. Having the child wear mittens and cutting the fingernails short

292. When teaching a mother about communicable diseases, the nurse informs her that chickenpox is:
1. Communicable until all the vesicles have dried
2. Still communicable even when just dry scabs remain
3. No longer communicable after a high fever has subsided
4. Not communicable as long as the vesicles are intact and surrounded by a red areola

293. A 10-year-old child has sustained partial-thickness burns on the anterior surfaces of both arms and hands and the upper half of the chest. Based on the grading system of the American Burn Association, the nurse estimates that the total body surface area (TBSA) involved would be approximately:
1. 12%
2. 15%
3. 17%
4. 20%

294. A child is admitted with partial thickness burns of both arms and the chest. The nursing care plan is based on the knowledge that:
1. Some grafting of the burned area will be required
2. The burns are extremely painful and disfiguring

3. Pressure dressings and prolonged hydrotherapy will be required
4. Spontaneous epithelial regeneration should occur within two to six weeks

295. When extensive eschar formation is present on the arms of a child admitted to the hospital with severe burns, the priority nursing action would be to:
1. Remove blisters
2. Check radial pulses
3. Perform range of motion
4. Enforce respiratory isolation

296. A child who had full-thickness burns is to have skin grafts. The nurse explains to the child's parents that for permanent grafts the child must have:
1. Steroids
2. Autografts
3. Homografts
4. Immunosuppressives

297. When performing a dressing change for a child with severe burns, the nurse understands that a basic principle of surgical asepsis is that:
1. The entire sterile field is considered sterile
2. Sterile items held below the waist are considered sterile
3. Sterile objects in contact with clean objects are considered clean
4. Wounds with exudates are contaminated, and dry wounds are sterile

298. When fever is suspected in preschool children with leukemia who are receiving chemotherapy, the nurse recognizes that:
1. Rectal temperatures are too upsetting for this age group
2. Oral temperatures alone are inaccurate in children with leukemia
3. Rectal temperatures are avoided to reduce the risk of rectal trauma
4. Tympanic temperatures are not accurate when a fever is suspected

299. A child is receiving radiation therapy for a brain tumor. When planning skin care for this child, the nurse should:
1. Rinse the child's head with plain water
2. Wash the child's head with mild soap every day
3. Apply baby oil to the child's head and neck daily
4. Have the child shower rather than bathe in a bathtub

300. The nurse teaches a teenager about the need for special mouth care because of the potential

for lesions from the chemotherapy being administered. The nurse evaluates that the instructions were understood when the teenager says, "I should:
1. Brush my teeth with baking soda."
2. Swish my mouth with hydrogen peroxide."
3. Rinse my mouth with undiluted mouthwash."
4. Brush my teeth with a soft-bristled toothbrush."

301. The mother of a kindergartner tells the nurse that her daughter is constantly scratching behind her ears. The nurse, suspecting pediculosis capitis (head lice), would expect to observe:
1. Small grayish-brown threadlike lines
2. Scaly patches within areas of alopecia
3. Streaked blisters surrounding a larger one
4. White spots attached to the base of hair shafts

302. The nurse is aware that the most common secondary infection from head lice (pediculosis capitis) is:
1. Eczema
2. Cellulitis
3. Impetigo
4. Tinea capitis

303. The instructions that the nurse gives to a parent of a 5-year-old regarding the application of Permethrin 5% cream (Elimite) for scabies should be to apply the medication:
1. Sparingly and rinse it off in four hours
2. At bedtime and wash it off in the morning
3. After bathing and rinse it off in 15 minutes
4. Each morning for three days and wash it off on the last day

304. A child, recently returned from a camping trip, complains of a rash, chills, fever, and a headache and is taken to the clinic by the parents. The nurse in the clinic recognizes that this child's history and physical assessment should include:
1. A history of allergies and duration of symptoms
2. A developmental screening and history of exposure to chickenpox
3. Sports played on the trip and when the child has to return to school
4. The date the child received a flu vaccination and a history of any sunburn

305. When a 12-year-old boy who received several tick bites on a camping trip becomes ill, he is told that he may have Lyme disease. He asks the nurse, "What is Lyme disease?" The nurse's best response would be:

1. "It's a spirochetal infection that penicillin will treat."
2. "You are concerned. Why don't you ask me what you want to know."
3. "You sound upset, but we have medicine that will make you better."
4. "The tick bites gave you an infection, but there is medication that will stop it."

306. The mother of an adolescent asks the nurse what the best way is to remove a tick from the skin. The nurse should reply:
1. "Touch the tick with a lighted cigarette."
2. "Remove the tick carefully with tweezers."
3. "Pour ammonia over the tick and it will shrivel up."
4. "Spray the tick with insect repellent and it will fall off."

307. A 10-year-old boy arrives with his mother at the emergency department after being bitten by a stray dog. There is a bleeding soft tissue injury on the inner aspect of the left forearm. The first nursing action would be to:
1. Notify the police department to capture the dog
2. Ask the mother if her son is allergic to horse serum
3. Assess the injury, vital signs, and past health history
4. Inoculate the child with human rabies immune globulin

NEUROMUSCULAR (NM)

308. The nurse understands that the genetic etiologic factor of Down syndrome is an:
1. Extra chromosome
2. Intrauterine infection
3. X-linked chromosome
4. Autosomal recessive gene

309. The nurse should recognize that the most common serious anomaly associated with Down syndrome is:
1. Renal disease
2. Hepatic defects
3. Congenital heart disease
4. Endocrine gland malfunction

310. The nurse is aware that infants with a myelomeningocele, not just a meningocele, usually have:
1. Hydrocephalus
2. Lower extremity paralysis
3. A sac over the lumbar area
4. Infections of the spinal fluid

311. The nursing assessment that would supply data about a major complication in an infant with a myelomeningocele is:
1. Obtaining the infant's weight daily
2. Monitoring the infant's output every shift
3. Measuring the infant's head circumference daily
4. Assessing the infant's blood pressure every 12 hours

312. The abnormal finding that a nurse would expect to observe during an assessment of a 1-month-old infant admitted to the hospital with hydrocephalus would be that the:
1. Infant's anterior fontanelle is tense on palpation
2. Infant demonstrates poor eye/muscle coordination
3. Infant is unable to support the head and shoulders while prone
4. Infant's head circumference is larger than the chest circumference

313. An infant with a myelomeningocele is scheduled for surgery to close the defect. The nursing action that would best facilitate parent-child relationships in the preoperative period would be:
1. Allowing the parents to cuddle the child in their arms
2. Demonstrating feeding techniques in the prone position
3. Encouraging the parents to stroke and comfort the child
4. Referring the parents to the Spina Bifida Association of America

314. A 3-month-old infant has a ventriculoper toneal (VP) shunt inserted. The nurse should plan to:
1. Keep the infant in the prone position
2. Apply sterile moist dressings to the incision
3. Observe for signs of leakage of cerebrospinal fluid
4. Teach the parents the signs of increased intracranial pressure

315. Preoperatively, the parents of a child undergoing an insertion of a right ventriculoperitoneal (VP) shunt for hydrocephalus are taught about postoperative positioning. The nurse can evaluate their understanding of the teaching when they state, "We will avoid putting pressure on the shunt site by positioning our baby:
1. In the position that provides the most comfort."
2. On the back with a small support beneath the neck."
3. On the abdomen with a small support against the left side of the head."
4. Flat and side-lying on the unoperated side with a small support against the head and back."

316. The nurse assesses a 5-year-old child after a shunt procedure to correct increased intracranial pressure. The observation that is of most concern would be:
1. Marked irritability
2. Complaints of pain
3. A temperature of 99.4° F
4. A pulse of 100 beats per minutes

317. On the day after surgery for insertion of a ventriculoperitoneal shunt for hydrocephalus, an infant's temperature rises to 103° F. The nurse should first notify the physician and then:
1. Sponge the infant with tepid alcohol
2. Recheck the temperature in two hours
3. Remove any excess clothing from the infant
4. Record the temperature on the infant's chart

318. The nurse should teach the parents of an infant with cerebral palsy to:
1. Focus on cognitive rather than motor skills
2. Maintain prolonged immobility of limbs with splints
3. Preserve muscle tone to prevent contractures
4. Encourage strenuous exercise to build the infant's muscle tone

319. The mother of a 1-year-old, earlier diagnosed with cerebral palsy, brings the baby to the clinic because she has noticed the development of slow writhing movements. The nurse explains that these movements characterize a specific type of cerebral palsy known as:
1. Atonic
2. Ataxic
3. Spastic
4. Athetoid

320. The nurse is concerned about helping the parents of an infant with cerebral palsy to set long-term goals for the family. These goals will be set with the understanding that:
1. Special education will be needed because of the related cognitive impairments
2. Continual adjustments will be necessary until the full extent of the disability is known
3. This disorder causes progressive deterioration and future institutionalization will be necessary

4. The baby will have to be protected from infections because of lowered immune responses

321. A 9-month-old infant is admitted to the pediatric unit with a tentative diagnosis of meningitis. A lumbar puncture is performed. The nurse recognizes that the primary reason for this procedure is to:
1. Reduce intracranial pressure
2. Identify the presence of bleeding
3. Measure spinal fluid glucose level
4. Determine the causative organism

322. When holding an infant for a lumbar puncture, the nurse should position the baby in a:
1. Prone position with the head extended and the extremities mummified
2. Sitting position with the buttocks at the edge of the table and the head flexed
3. Lateral recumbent position with the back at the edge of the table and the head and legs extended
4. Side-lying position with the back at the edge of the table, head flexed, and knees brought up to the chin

323. When the nurse caring for an infant with meningitis extends the baby's leg, the hamstring muscles go into spasm. The nurse recognizes that the baby is exhibiting a positive:
1. Kernig's sign
2. Babinski reflex
3. Chvostek's sign
4. Cremasteric reflex

324. A child is admitted to the hospital with a diagnosis of meningococcal meningitis. The nurse is aware that isolation:
1. Of any kind is not required
2. Will be required for seven days
3. Must be maintained during the incubation period
4. Is required for 24 to 72 hours after onset of antibiotic therapy

325. The purpose of placing a child with an infectious disease in isolation with airborne precautions would be to:
1. Separate the infected child from noninfected persons
2. Interrupt the infectious process as quickly as possible
3. Protect the child with a decreased resistance to infection
4. Prevent nosocomial infection during the hospitalized period

326. While in the playroom, a 7-year-old child has a twitching of the right arm and leg that almost immediately progresses to a generalized tonic-clonic seizure with clenched jaws. The nurse's best initial action would be to:
1. Take the other children to their rooms
2. Place a large pillow under the child's head
3. Put a plastic airway into the child's mouth
4. Move the toys and furniture away from the child

327. When reviewing nursing care of the child with seizures, the nurse charts a clonic episode as:
1. Generalized rigidity
2. A loss of consciousness
3. Tremors of the upper extremities
4. A spasmodic jerking of the entire body

328. A 4-year-old is admitted to the pediatric neurological service with a seizure disorder. Shortly after admission, while in bed, the child experiences a generalized seizure. The nurse should respond by raising the padded side rails and:
1. Holding the child gently and speaking softly
2. Taking the child's vital signs and calling for help
3. Placing the child on the side and assessing the seizure
4. Loosening the child's clothing and administering oxygen

329. The mother of a 2-year-old child tells the nurse that she is concerned about her child's vision. The nurse suspects that the child has strabismus when the mother states that, when her child is tired, she has noticed:
1. One eyelid droops
2. Both eyes look cloudy
3. One eye moves inward
4. Both eyes blink excessively

330. A major goal for the surgical correction of strabismus in a child would be to:
1. Improve appearance
2. Prevent legal blindness
3. Restore peripheral vision
4. Avoid the need for glasses

331. A 2-year-old child is admitted with a tentative diagnosis of lead poisoning. To aid in confirming the diagnosis, the nurse should observe the toddler for:
1. Epistaxis
2. Clumsiness
3. Excessive salivation
4. Decreased pulse rate

332. The nurse, teaching dietary management to the parents of a child with lead poisoning, explains that they should offer a diet that is:
    1. Low in salt content
    2. Free of refined sugar
    3. High in calcium and phosphorus
    4. High in calories and low in protein

333. After oral surgery, the physician writes an order for pain medication for an 18-month-old child. The nurse should question an order for:
    1. Aspirin
    2. Codeine
    3. Percodan
    4. Acetaminophen

334. An 8-year-old child is admitted to the emergency department with signs and symptoms of Reye syndrome. When obtaining information, the nurse should place emphasis on a:
    1. Recent rash
    2. History of tonsillitis
    3. Recent viral infection
    4. History of high fevers

335. The parents of a child with Reye syndrome ask the nurse to define this disorder. The nurse's response would be based on the knowledge that it is:
    1. A newly identified genetic disorder requiring genetic counseling if more children are desired
    2. A bacterial infection affecting the brain and nervous system, resulting in slowly advancing paralysis
    3. An encephalopathy of unknown etiology that results in permanent disability depending on the severity of the illness
    4. An acute illness primarily of the brain and liver, with problems in maintaining normal blood glucose levels, fluid balance, and intracranial pressure

336. A 15-year-old arrives at the emergency department with vague symptoms of acute, crampy abdominal pain, anorexia, fever, and deficits in sensory perception. While assessing the adolescent, the nurse notes the presence of black lines between the gums and teeth. Further assessment is needed because this finding is characteristic of:
    1. Perthes' disease
    2. Lead poisoning
    3. Salicylate toxicity
    4. Neonatal exposure to tetracycline

337. The nurse suspects that a 7-month-old infant, who is brought to the well-baby clinic for the first time, may have a hearing deficit when the:
    1. Mother says the infant is unable to learn the word "Mama"
    2. Infant does not always turn the head when the name is called
    3. Infant fails to demonstrate a Moro reflex in response to hand clapping
    4. Mother says the infant stopped making verbal sounds about a month ago

338. When obtaining the health history of an infant who has had repeated episodes of otitis media the nurse asks the mother:
    1. "How many times has your son had otitis media?"
    2. "Does your son go to bed with a bottle in his mouth?"
    3. "Did any of your other children have this problem?"
    4. "What do you give your son when he has otitis media?"

339. The mother of a 10-month-old infant with otitis media tells the nurse in the pediatric clinic that this is her baby's third episode in three months. The nurse is aware that with otitis media:
    1. The labyrinth and cochlea both become severely inflamed
    2. Young children are most susceptible to otitis media because their eustachian tubes are shorter and more horizontal
    3. After a myringotomy, the child should be positioned on the unaffected side to facilitate drainage from the ear
    4. When pressure-equalizer or tympanostomy tubes are used for a myringotomy, the ear should be irrigated with saline twice a day

340. When explaining a myringotomy procedure, the nurse should emphasize that the incision:
    1. Takes several days to heal and often leaves a scar
    2. Provides immediate relief of pressure in the middle ear
    3. Widens the perforation in the eardrum to allow for drainage
    4. Often results in permanent perforation of the tympanic membrane

341. To help the parents promote the effectiveness of their child's myringotomy procedure, the nurse suggests that they should:

1. Maintain the child in the supine position
2. Position the child with the affected ear down
3. Keep the child with the affected ear uppermost
4. Observe the child for bleeding from the operative site

342. Before discharge after a myringotomy, a potential complication the nurse should teach the child's parents to report is:
    1. Mild or moderate hearing loss
    2. Bleeding and diminished pain
    3. Lack of drainage and increased pain
    4. Low-grade temperature and headache

343. When a child visits the clinic after an adenoidectomy, the nurse should include an assessment of hearing, as well as:
    1. Smell and taste
    2. Speech and taste
    3. Swallowing and smell
    4. Swallowing and speech

344. The nurse is aware that discharge planning related to care of a child with Duchenne's muscular dystrophy should include teaching the parents about:
    1. Range-of-motion exercises
    2. Instituting seizure precautions
    3. Maintaining a high-calorie diet
    4. Restricting the use of larger muscles

345. The nurse should teach the parents that when a child with Duchenne's muscular dystrophy reaches adolescence, additional problems will probably develop with the:
    1. Neurologic system
    2. Gastrointestinal system
    3. Musculoskeletal system
    4. Cardiopulmonary system

346. A 4-year-old girl, with a brain tumor diagnosed as an astrocytoma, is admitted accompanied by her parents for treatment. During the physical assessment while she is lying supine, she states that her "head hurts" and begins to cry. The nurse recognizes that the headache is probably attributable to:
    1. Blood pooled by gravity, which increases intracranial pressure
    2. Separation anxiety, which often manifests in physical symptoms
    3. Mutilation anxiety, which is common in children in this age group
    4. Tension from hospitalization, which may result in symptoms of headache

347. The morning after admission, the nurse is feeding breakfast to a child who has a brain tumor. Because of increasing intracranial pressure the child then vomits. The nurse should:
    1. Increase the drop rate on the IV
    2. Administer the prescribed antiemetic
    3. Clean the child, and refeed the breakfast
    4. Keep the child NPO, call the physician and request new orders

348. After a child has a craniotomy, the nurse performs an assessment of the child's neurologic status by observing the level of consciousness, pupillary activity, reflex activity, and:
    1. Blood pressure
    2. Motor function
    3. Rectal temperature
    4. Head circumference

349. A child is about to be admitted to the pediatric intensive care unit after surgery for removal of a brain tumor. The nurse manager should immediately intervene when the child's nurse:
    1. Places a hypothermic blanket on the bed
    2. Raises the foot of the bed on shock blocks
    3. Secures an IV pump to closely monitor IV fluid intake
    4. Obtains a cardiorespiratory monitor and sphygmomanometer

350. The day after brain surgery, a 9-year-old child with diabetes mellitus develops a temperature of 103° F. The nurse understands that:
    1. A slight fever is to be expected following any surgery
    2. Anyone with diabetes will develop an infection following surgery
    3. Edema following the surgery often causes pressure on the hypothalamus
    4. An excess of viscid secretions has caused inadequate respiratory ventilation

351. The nurse in the emergency department is caring for a 9-year-old child suspected of having a spinal cord injury after a bicycle accident. The most appropriate nursing intervention would be to:
    1. Place a pillow under the child's head for support
    2. Log roll the child to check for lacerations on the back
    3. Move the child to a stretcher that does not have a mattress
    4. Immobilize the child's spine to minimize additional injury

352. The mother of an 8-year-old boy who has a mild concussion is instructed to check her child for responsiveness every two hours, even when sleeping. She telephones the nurse that she is afraid to allow him to go to sleep. The nurse should respond:
1. "Would you prefer your son be admitted to the hospital?"
2. "There is no need to worry. Your son is past the critical period."
3. "If your son becomes difficult to waken, bring him to the hospital."
4. "Awakening your son throughout the night will alert you to any change."

353. A child is brought to the emergency department with a head injury. When assessing a child with an acute head trauma, the nurse initially should check:
1. Ocular signs
2. Muscular strength
3. Level of consciousness
4. Superficial injuries to the head

354. The mother of a 7-year-old boy arrives at the clinic with her son. The history reveals that he fell from his tree house. He continued playing until lunch, at which time he told his mother he fell and "saw stars" after hitting his head. Soon after, he complained of a headache and feeling sick to his stomach. His mother telephoned the pediatric nurse who suggested the child be brought to the clinic. The child's motor responses would best be assessed by his ability to:
1. Draw a picture
2. Walk around the room
3. Squeeze the nurse's hand
4. Perform the Romberg test

355. A 12-year-old child was admitted to the neurosurgical unit for observation after receiving a head injury. The details of how the injury occurred are unknown. It is now 12 hours after the injury and the child has demonstrated no signs or symptoms of a head injury. The priority intervention for the nurse would be to:
1. Promote rest by creating a quiet environment
2. Administer opioids for complaints of a headache
3. Monitor the level of consciousness every hour as ordered
4. Question the child about the circumstances leading to the injury

356. The nurse suspects that the concept that a developmentally disabled child could probably learn the fastest would be:
1. Love vs hate
2. Life vs death
3. Large vs small
4. Right vs wrong

357. When parents ask the nurse what to do about their preschooler's stuttering, the nurse should suggest that they:
1. Identify situations that increase stuttering and avoid or ignore the hesitancy
2. Avoid looking at the child when the child has difficulty forming or expressing words
3. Help the child by supplying the correct word when the child is experiencing a block
4. Stop the conversation and tell the child to speak slowly and think before starting again

RESPIRATORY (RE)

358. The nurse understands that in the child, as in the adult, respiratory patterns are controlled by the:
1. Medulla
2. Cerebellum
3. Hypothalamus
4. Cerebral cortex

359. A nursing diagnosis of impaired gas exchange is made for an infant with a diaphragmatic hernia. The causative factor for this diagnosis is the:
1. Diaphragmatic hernia
2. Decrease in oxygen intake
3. Presence of excessive secretions
4. Increase in the basal metabolic rate

360. In addition to raising the head of the bed of an infant who has had a surgical repair of a diaphragmatic hernia, the nurse should place the infant in the:
1. Contour position in an infant seat
2. Supine position with the knees flexed
3. Prone position with the head to the side
4. Side-lying position on the operative side

361. After the repair of a diaphragmatic hernia, the nursing assessment indicating that the infant's respiratory condition is improving would be that:
1. The infant stops crying
2. The blood pH decreases to 7.31
3. Breath sounds are heard bilaterally
4. 1 oz of formula is ingested and retained

362. A young baby has an open repair of a fractured

sternum and has a chest tube. The nurse explains to the baby's mother that the chest tube:
1. Will be removed once the baby is feeding well and is afebrile
2. Does not cause discomfort and is put in place for emergency use
3. Is left in to drain the air from the chest cavity that entered during surgery
4. Drains the extra air in the baby's chest that accumulated following the punctured lung

363. After returning from surgery, an infant suddenly becomes cyanotic. The nurse's priority should be to:
1. Administer oxygen
2. Suction the nasopharynx
3. Turn the baby on the side
4. Check the baby's vital signs

364. A child in the pediatric intensive care unit (PICU) is on a ventilator. One of the nurses asks what should be done when condensation, due to humidity, collects in the ventilator tubing. The nurse manager should respond:
1. "Notify the physician's assistant."
2. "Decrease the amount of humidity."
3. "Empty the fluid and reconnect the tubing."
4. "Measure the fluid and mark it on the tubing."

365. When making an assessment of a 6-month-old infant with bronchiolitis, the nurse would expect:
1. A decreased heart rate
2. Increased breath sounds
3. A prolonged expiratory phase
4. Intercostal and subcostal retractions

366. The nurse organizes care for an infant with bronchiolitis to allow for uninterrupted periods of rest. This plan would be:
1. Appropriate because the cool mist helps to maintain hydration status
2. Inappropriate because frequent assessment by auscultation is required
3. Appropriate because this action promotes decreased oxygen demands
4. Inappropriate because constant care is necessary in the acute stage

367. An important nursing measure for a 6-month-old infant with bronchiolitis would be:
1. Promoting stimulating activities that meet the infant's developmental needs
2. Making frequent observations of the infant's skin color, anterior fontanelle, and vital signs
3. Discouraging visits from the parents during the acute phase to conserve the infant's energy
4. Keeping the infant on airborne precautions and using a gown, cap, mask, and gloves when giving care

368. A 2-year-old is admitted with croup and 1/4 liter humidified oxygen via cannula is started because it:
1. Congeals the mucous secretions and relieves the dyspnea
2. Triggers the cough reflex and facilitates the expectoration of mucus
3. Dilates the blood vessels in the bronchi and alleviates the congestion
4. Liquefies the mucous secretions making them easier to expectorate

369. A child is brought to the emergency department because of a barking cough, a loud inspiratory stridor and sternal retractions. A diagnosis of croup is made. The signs and symptoms subside after treatment with nebulized epinephrine. Discharge instructions should include recommending that when a croup episode starts, the parents:
1. Use a cool mist vaporizer
2. Perform postural drainage
3. Return to the emergency department
4. Have the child expel all the air after inspiration

370. The parents of a 3-year-old child, who has recurrent attacks of croup, asks the nurse why this happens to their child. The best rationale to explain why croup is a disorder of young children is that they:
1. Have small airways
2. Are mouth breathers
3. Have difficulty resisting infection
4. Are prone to communicable diseases

371. An 8-year-old child with asthma is being assessed by the nurse. An assessment that requires immediate intervention would be:
1. A round face
2. Persistent wheezing
3. Regular use of inhalers
4. A respiratory rate of 30 per minute

372. The nurse should caution parents of a child who has been newly diagnosed with asthma that the symptoms usually worsen:
1. At night
2. At mid-morning
3. In the afternoon
4. Soon after dinner

373. The nurse instructs the mother of a child with asthma how to make the bedroom "allergy proof." Further teaching would be needed when the mother states that she will:
1. Remove the stuffed animal collection
2. Put plastic slipcovers over the mattress and box spring
3. Store her child's off-season clothes in another room
4. Cover the hardwood floors with flat indoor-outdoor carpeting

374. A child who had been admitted for status asthmaticus appears to be improving. The best way for the nurse to evaluate the child's response to therapy would be to:
1. Auscultate the child's breath sounds
2. Observe the client's respiratory pattern
3. Ask the client if breathing is getting easier
4. Assess the client for a decrease in cyanosis

375. A child who was rescued from a burning building is brought to the hospital via emergency medical services. Smoke inhalation has caused the child's condition to deteriorate within 24 hours. The nurse should be particularly alert for signs of:
1. Infection
2. Tracheobronchial edema
3. Posttraumatic stress disorder
4. Generalized adaptations to stress

376. A 10-year-old child who has been rescued from a house fire has been brought to the emergency department with burns of the extremities. When assessing the child, the nurse would be most concerned with an observation of:
1. Burns around the mouth
2. A blood pressure of 115/80
3. An increasing activity level
4. Edema distal to the burns on the extremities

377. The nurse understands that the pathophysiologic factor primarily responsible for respiratory manifestations of cystic fibrosis is that:
1. Endocrine glands secrete abnormal levels of hormones
2. Increased irritability of airways causes obstruction
3. There is acute inflammation of lung parenchyma
4. Abnormally thick mucus leads to obstruction of the airways

378. The nurse provides clapping, percussion, and postural drainage every four hours for a 3-month-old infant with cystic fibrosis.

The nurse is aware that the best time for scheduling this chest physiotherapy is:
1. After every feeding
2. Before every feeding
3. During every feeding
4. Midway between every feeding

379. The nurse recognizes that a male teenager who has a sibling with cystic fibrosis understands genetic counseling when he states, "To determine whether I am a carrier, I will have to undergo:
1. A chest x-ray."
2. Enzyme assays."
3. DNA probe testing."
4. Sweat chloride tests."

380. The respiratory assessment of an 8-year-old admitted with viral pneumonia demonstrates bronchial breath sounds over areas of consolidation, mild substernal retractions, profuse mucus production, pallor, and temperature of 102° F. The nursing action with the highest priority would be to:
1. Contact the respiratory therapist to set up oxygen
2. Start an intravenous line to provide fluids and electrolytes
3. Notify the physician of the fever so an antipyretic can be given
4. Place the child in a semi-Fowler's position and suction the nasopharynx

381. The nurse is aware that when administering oxygen therapy to a child the oxygen:
1. Should be labeled as flammable
2. Is warmed before administration
3. Must be humidified before administration
4. May be administered without a prescription

382. A 15-year-old high school student with hay fever has been taking a prescribed long-acting antihistamine/decongestant q8h for the past 3 days. The adolescent tells the nurse, "This medication is making me sleepy. Can you change it to something else?" The nurse's best response would be:
1. "Take only half a tablet before school."
2. "I think you should omit the early morning dose."
3. "The drowsiness will usually diminish after a few days."
4. "I'll ask the physician to change you to a medication containing ephedrine."

383. A 14-year-old develops sinusitis and is placed on a broad-spectrum oral antibiotic to be taken four times a day. To maintain the blood level,

the nurse should recommend that the medication be taken at:
1. 8 AM, 12 PM, 4 PM, and 8 PM
2. 8 AM, 4 PM, 12 AM, and 4 AM
3. 6 AM, 12 PM, 6 PM, and 12 AM
4. 10 AM, 2 PM, 10 PM, and 2 AM

384. A child who has just returned to the unit after surgery is drowsy and not alert to commands. To maintain an airway the nurse should:
1. Have a tongue blade available
2. Keep the child in a supine position
3. Use nasotracheal suction as needed
4. Place the child in a lateral Sims' position

385. An adolescent has an order for placement of a pulse oximeter. To ensure accuracy of the pulse oximeter reading, the nurse should:
1. Place the probe on a finger or earlobe
2. Calibrate the oximeter at least every eight hours
3. Place the probe on the abdomen or upper leg
4. After application wait 30 minutes before obtaining a reading

386. A child who was found face down in a water-filled ditch is brought to the emergency room. The child, who has a pulse of 50 beats per minute but no spontaneous respirations, is intubated and bagged with 100% oxygen. The most important nursing measure at this time would be to:
1. Assist the physician in delivering intracardiac medications
2. Suction the endotracheal tube, mouth, and nasal passages
3. Start an intravenous line to provide fluid and electrolytes
4. Call the pediatric ICU to inform them of the child's admission

387. A child survives a near-drowning episode in a cold pond but still has many problems to overcome. The nurse is aware that the ultimate prognosis will depend mainly on the extent of damage resulting from the:
1. Hypoxia
2. Hyperthermia
3. Emotional trauma
4. Aspiration pneumonia

388. A 10-year-old child who is developmentally delayed and blind must be fed all meals. The child has problems swallowing and frequently chokes and coughs during the feeding. When feeding this child, the nurse should:

1. Liquefy the feedings and use a soft-tip bulb syringe
2. Place the child in the supine position with the head turned to the right
3. Prop the child in a semi-sitting position, chop up the food, and place it into the child's mouth with plastic tableware
4. Seat the child in the wheelchair and give small bites of food with metal tableware, encouraging the child's participation

389. When examining the throat of a 5-year-old child, the nurse should position a tongue blade to the side of the child's tongue primarily to avoid:
1. Eliciting the gag reflex
2. Obstructing the airway
3. Hurting any of the teeth
4. Interfering with the visual examination

REPRODUCTIVE AND GENITOURINARY (RG)

390. A nursing diagnosis that should have priority for an infant born with exstrophy of the bladder is:
1. Risk for infection
2. Urinary retention
3. Sexual dysfunction
4. Deficient fluid volume

391. An infant has exstrophy of the bladder. To protect the exposed bladder area, the nurse should expect the physician to order:
1. Antibacterial ointments
2. Warm moist compresses
3. Pediatric urine collectors
4. Sterile non-adherent dressings

392. A child is admitted for urinary diversion surgery. The ureters are transplanted to a section of the colon, with one end attached to the abdominal wall as an ileostomy. The nurse explains to the parents that the procedure is known as:
1. A cystostomy
2. An ileal conduit
3. An ureterosigmoidostomy
4. A cutaneous ureterostomy

393. After surgical repair of a urinary tract malformation, a child is to be discharged with an indwelling catheter. The nurse should teach the parents that if no urine appears in the urinary drainage bag for a period of an hour or longer, they should first:
1. Call the physician
2. Give the child extra fluids to drink
3. Check for blockage of the drainage tubing
4. Place firm pressure on the abdominal wall just above the bladder

394. The nurse explains to parents whose infant son has hypospadias that this defect occurred in the:
1. First trimester
2. Third trimester
3. Second trimester
4. Implantation phase

395. The plan of care for an infant with hypospadias should include:
1. Keeping the penis wrapped with petrolatum gauze
2. Preparing the infant for the insertion of a cystostomy tube
3. Explaining to the parents why a circumcision will not be done
4. Carefully explaining the genetic basis for the defect to the parents

396. After a child has a surgical correction for hypospadias, during the postoperative period it is important for the nurse to:
1. Ensure that the child's privacy is maintained
2. Maintain the surgically implanted tension device
3. Keep the child properly immobilized with restraints
4. Gradually increase the time that the catheter is clamped

397. The nurse is aware that if a child with chordee does not have corrective surgery, when he becomes an adult, he will be at increased risk for:
1. Renal failure
2. Testicular cancer
3. Testicular torsion
4. Reproductive dysfunction

398. When admitting a 4-year-old child with nephrotic syndrome to the hospital, the nurse should assess for:
1. Severe lethargy
2. Chronic hypertension
3. Dark, frothy urine output
4. Flushed, ruddy complexion

399. A 3-year-old is admitted to the hospital with a diagnosis of nephrotic syndrome. The child has ascites, oliguria, respirations of 40 per minute, and a recent weight gain of 10 pounds. The nurse plans to relieve the child's respiratory difficulty by:
1. Feeding the child small amounts frequently
2. Assigning the child to a well-ventilated room
3. Placing the child on bed rest in a semi-Fowler's position

4. Administering oxygen to the child at 2 L/minute by mask

400. A 6-year-old child is admitted with a diagnosis of nephrotic syndrome. Nursing care for this child in the acute phase should include:
1. Encouraging fluids every hour
2. Providing time for active play periods
3. Encouraging frequent changes of position
4. Offering low protein, high carbohydrate, and low salt foods

401. The nurse should assign a 4-year-old boy admitted to the hospital with nephrotic syndrome to a room with a:
1. 2-year-old boy with croup
2. 3-year-old boy with impetigo
3. 4-year-old girl with conjunctivitis
4. 5-year-old girl with a fractured femur

402. When planning nursing care for a child with nephrotic syndrome, the nurse should include:
1. Provision of meticulous skin care
2. A diet low in carbohydrates and protein
3. Restriction of fluids to 500 mL each shift
4. A laboratory test for blood type and crossmatch

403. The nurse realizes that the parents of a child with nephrotic syndrome need further discharge instructions when they state, "We will:
1. Ignore any weight gain since it's normal."
2. Look at our child's eyelids every morning."
3. Need to test our child's urine for albumin."
4. Give our child the prednisone with meals or milk."

404. A boy with nephrotic syndrome has been in remission for several months. One day the mother calls the clinic nurse to report that for the past week her child's skin has had a muddy, pale appearance, his appetite has been poor, and he has been unusually tired after school. The nurse suspects that the child:
1. Is not taking his medication
2. Is developing a viral infection
3. May be in impending renal failure
4. May be extending himself at school

405. The mother of a 6-year-old brings the child to the pediatric clinic and complains that the child has malaise, weakness, lethargy, anorexia, headaches, and smoky urine. When taking the nursing history, the nurse asks the mother whether the child has had a:
1. Pain in the shoulders and knees
2. Recent weight loss of at least 2 pounds

3. Streptococcal infection within the last two weeks
4. Rash on the palms and feet within the last three weeks

406. A child is admitted to the hospital with a tentative diagnosis of acute glomerulonephritis. When the laboratory results are reported, the nurse would expect to see:
   1. An increased hematocrit value
   2. A low urine specific gravity result
   3. A decreased blood urea nitrogen level
   4. An elevated antistreptolysin O (ASO) titer

407. When assessing a child with acute glomerulonephritis the morning after admission to the hospital, the nurse should expect a:
   1. Normal blood pressure, anorexia, proteinuria of 1+, and glycosuria
   2. Proteinuria of 1+, anorexia, hematuria, and decreased blood pressure
   3. Decreased blood pressure, periorbital edema, proteinuria of 1+ and decreased urine specific gravity
   4. Moderately elevated blood pressure, periorbital edema, proteinuria of 4+, and increased specific gravity

408. The mother of an 8-year-old child with the diagnosis of acute glomerulonephritis is concerned that a 4-year-old sibling might be developing the disorder. When preparing to explain the cause of the disease, the nurse is aware that it is:
   1. Caused by some unknown factor and therefore is difficult to prevent
   2. Caused by a clot in the small renal tubules secondary to a systemic infection
   3. An antigen-antibody response secondary to a group A beta-hemolytic streptococcus infection
   4. Inherited by an autosomal recessive trait, and there is a 25 percent chance that the sibling will develop it

409. A 10-year-old child with acute glomerulonephritis is marking the dietary menu for dinner. The nurse encourages the child to choose the most appropriate combination of food, which would include:
   1. Baked ham, bread and butter, peaches, and milk
   2. Corn on the cob, baked chicken, rice, apple, and milk
   3. Baked potato, ground beef, banana, and buttermilk
   4. Hot dog on a bun, potato chips, dill pickle slices, and brownie

410. The nurse, caring for a child with acute glomerulonephritis, observes the child for signs of possible cerebral stem involvement. This would be indicated by the development of:
   1. Headache, drowsiness, and vomiting
   2. Cardiac decompensation, slow pulse, and vomiting
   3. Anuria, temperature above 103° F, and confusion
   4. Generalized edema, anorexia, and restlessness

411. A child who has been treated for acute glomerulonephritis is to be discharged. The nurse should plan to provide the parents with:
   1. Suggestions about activities to keep the child active for long periods of time
   2. The nurse's phone number so that the parents can call if they have any questions
   3. Instructions as to when the child should return for a workup for a kidney transplant
   4. A sample of a sodium-restricted diet because the child will continue on this diet at home

412. The adaptation that indicates that a child may have nephrotic syndrome rather than glomerulonephritis is the presence of:
   1. Edema
   2. Lethargy
   3. Protein in the urine
   4. A slightly decreased blood pressure

413. The nurse understands that surgery is needed for a 2-year-old child with undescended testes because:
   1. Future malignancy may be prevented
   2. Maturation of the testes starts at about age 7
   3. The puboscrotal ring is more elastic at this age
   4. Early surgery produces less psychologic damage

414. When assessing a child with vesicoureteral reflux, the nurse should be especially alert for:
   1. Dysuria
   2. Oliguria
   3. Glycosuria
   4. Proteinuria

415. A 4-year-old child has a nephrectomy because of a Wilms' tumor. After a nephrectomy, it is essential that the nurse teach the parents to:
   1. Prepare for a kidney transplant
   2. Restrict the child's intake of sodium
   3. Maintain the child's fluid restrictions
   4. Recognize the signs of a urinary tract infection

416. The urinary output of a child with acute glomerulonephritis decreases to less than 100 mL/24 hours and the creatinine clearance is 60 mL/min. The physician determines that the child has acute renal failure. The nurse notes that the child has an irregular apical pulse. The most significant laboratory finding would be:
    1. Serum sodium 126 mEq/L
    2. Serum creatinine 1.3 mg/dl
    3. Serum potassium 6.1 mEq/L
    4. Blood urea nitrogen 40 mg/dl

417. A child in renal failure, who has had the creation of an arteriovenous fistula access, begins hemodialysis three times a week. The nurse would know the child's mother needs further teaching when the mother states, "I will:
    1. Check the pulse at the wrist of the arm with the fistula daily."
    2. Take a blood pressure in the arm with the fistula twice a day."
    3. Call the doctor if my child develops vomiting or diarrhea."
    4. Ensure that my child drinks the appropriate amount of fluid in warm weather."

418. A child with chronic kidney disease is receiving peritoneal dialysis. To monitor for complications associated with this procedure, the nurse should assess the:
    1. Blood glucose levels
    2. Abdomen for a bruit
    3. Clarity of return dialysate solution
    4. Skin and mucous membrane for petechiae

419. A 7-year-old child must remain quietly in bed while having peritoneal dialysis. The most appropriate activity the nurse should plan for this child would be:
    1. Learning to play chess with one parent
    2. Gluing together a model airplane without help
    3. Working a 100-piece puzzle with another child
    4. Using a sponge ball to play catch with a roommate

420. To confirm a suspected diagnosis of gonorrhea in a 16-year-old male who has come to the clinic with a complaint of a thick urethral discharge, the nurse should:
    1. Get a sexual history
    2. Draw blood for a VDRL
    3. Collect a urine specimen
    4. Obtain a urethral culture

421. The nurse in an adolescent clinic is aware that an early diagnosis of syphilis is important, and its presence is often determined by:
    1. Evidence of a rash
    2. A lesion on the genitals
    3. Multiple gummatous lesions
    4. A discharge from the genitals

422. A 16-year-old male client is inquiring about the use of condoms. The client states, "I have used condoms in the past but I'm not sure I'm using them properly." As part of the teaching plan about condoms, the nurse should tell the client that:
    1. Vaseline should be used as a lubricant when using condoms
    2. Condoms must be positioned after an erection has occurred
    3. The condom should be fitted against the tip of the penis, leaving no space
    4. Withdrawal after ejaculation should be delayed until the penis becomes flaccid

SKELETAL (SK)

423. The nurse is aware that the finding that would differentiate talipes equinovarus as a true clubfoot from a pseudoclubbed foot is that the affected foot:
    1. Exhibits little movement
    2. Cannot be rotated past the midline
    3. Is cooler to the touch than the other foot
    4. Rotates past the midline but returns quickly when released

424. After a boot cast is applied to an infant with a clubfoot, a nursing diagnosis of "Ineffective tissue perfusion related to casting" is considered. The vascular assessment that could not be determined while the cast is in place would be:
    1. Color
    2. Warmth
    3. Blanching
    4. Pedal pulse

425. Teaching for parents whose baby is undergoing frequent casting to correct a foot deformity should include information on cast care, such as:
    1. Covering damp cast edges with adhesive petals
    2. Applying lotion to the skin at cast edges to keep it soft
    3. Checking the skin at the edges of the cast daily for redness
    4. Immersing the cast briefly during the tub bath and wiping it lightly

426. The statement by the mother of a 6-week-old female infant that would lead the nurse to assess the child for the presence of an abnormality would be:
1. "Her feet look very flat when I put both of her booties on her."
2. "She wants to sleep curled up on her stomach all the time."
3. "I seem to have a hard time getting her diaper between her legs."
4. "I can't get her to straighten out her legs when I try to stand her up."

427. When assessing a child suspected of having developmental dysplasia of the hip, the nurse would expect that an assessment of the child's orthopedic status would reveal:
1. An apparent shortening of one leg
2. A limited ability to adduct the affected leg
3. A narrowing of the perineum with an anal stricture
4. An inability to palpate movement of the femoral head

428. An 18-month-old child is admitted with a diagnosis of developmental dysplasia of the left hip. During the assessment the nurse should elicit the Trendelenburg sign by positioning the toddler:
1. Sitting
2. Supine
3. Standing
4. Side-lying

429. Six weeks after birth, an infant is diagnosed with developmental dysplasia of the hip. The nurse is aware that corrective measures will be instituted immediately because:
1. Infants are easier to manage in spica casts than toddlers
2. Mobility will be delayed if correction is postponed until later
3. Traction is effective if it is used before the child reaches 2 years of age
4. The infant's hip joint is still cartilaginous, and molding of the acetabulum is possible

430. A 2-year-old has a hip spica cast applied for developmental dysplasia of the hip. The mother asks the nurse how to keep the cast clean. The nurse's best response would be:
1. "Place plastic wrap around the perineal edges."
2. "Tuck a folded diaper above the perineal opening."
3. "Do the best you can; it will get soiled no matter what you do."

4. "Wash the cast with a wet cloth and sprinkle it with baby powder."

431. Three days following the application of a spica cast, a child has a temperature of 101.4° F. Suspecting an infection, the nurse should first assess the child for:
1. Rapid irregular respirations
2. A foul smell coming from the cast
3. Any complaints of tingling in the toes
4. The presence of itching around the top of the cast

432. When preparing to teach a 10-year-old about crutch walking, the nurse should include in the teaching plan to:
1. Use only one crutch at a time
2. Explore the child's fear of falling
3. Demonstrate the use of the 4-point gait
4. Ensure that there are plastic tips on the ends of the crutches

433. A 16-year-old has sustained an ankle injury while playing soccer. The physician prescribes no weight bearing and crutches. When adjusting the crutches, the nurse must ensure that they:
1. Provide a snug fit under the axillae when walking
2. Keep the elbows extended when the crutches are held by the crossbars
3. Allow the shoulders to be slightly stooped when the crutches are bearing body weight
4. Are 2 inches below the axillae when the crutch tips are 6 inches to the side of the feet

434. The nurse determines that an adolescent with a sprained ankle needs no further teaching regarding the use of a crutch for ambulation when the teen states:
1. "The crutch should not be used on the stairs."
2. "I will place the crutch in front of my bad ankle."
3. "I will use the crutch on the side of my good ankle."
4. "After one month I can stop using the crutch."

435. A child hospitalized with rheumatoid arthritis complains of pain in the knees. The intervention that would most likely relieve some of the discomfort is:
1. Immobilizing the affected joints
2. Supporting the knees with pillows
3. Massaging the swollen areas gently
4. Applying moist heat to the affected areas

436. The main objective of care for a child with juvenile rheumatoid arthritis would be preventing and correcting:
1. Infection
2. Hemarthrosis
3. Contracture deformities
4. Delayed intellectual development

437. The nurse is helping a child with juvenile rheumatoid arthritis perform range-of-motion exercises. The nurse knows that the exercises have been effective when the:
1. Child states that there is less pain
2. Knees can be flexed and extended
3. Child's pedal pulses become stronger
4. Subcutaneous nodules at the joints recede

438. When teaching a school-age child with rheumatoid arthritis activities to prevent the loss of joint function, the nurse should caution the child to avoid:
1. Riding a bicycle
2. Walking to school
3. Isometric exercises
4. Sitting for prolonged periods

439. When doing an assessment of a child who has just had a cast applied to the right arm, the nurse finds that the fingers of the child's hand are cool. The nurse should first:
1. Clip the edge of the cast to reduce pressure
2. Elevate the right arm to reduce the swelling
3. Compare the temperature of the right and left hands
4. Call the physician to report the circulatory impairment

440. During the initial assessment of a 7-year-old child with a compound fracture of the wrist, the nurse notices a dark, wet area on the cast. The nurse's next action would be to:
1. Notify the physician about the stain
2. Wash off the stain with soap and water
3. Check if the child was playing with a "magic marker"
4. Circle the area with a pen noting the date and time

441. A child sustains a fractured femur in a bicycle accident. However, the admission x-ray films reveal evidence of fractures of other long bones in various stages of healing. The nurse determines that this child should be assessed for:
1. Child abuse
2. Vitamin D deficiency
3. Osteogenesis imperfecta
4. Inadequate calcium intake

442. A child is placed in traction to align a fractured bone in a lower extremity. The nurse observes the traction weights touching the floor. The nurse should:
1. Raise the foot of the bed
2. Lengthen the traction rope
3. Notify the physician to reapply the traction
4. Move the child up toward the head of the bed

443. The nurse understands that the correct way to turn a 10-year-old child in a spica cast is to:
1. Logroll the body as one unit
2. Use the crossbar between the legs
3. Have the child assist by using the overhead trapeze
4. Teach the child to sit up and help when changing position

444. After an above-the-knee amputation for bone cancer, an adolescent male is returned to his room. To temporarily control hemorrhaging from the residual limb the nurse should plan to keep at the bedside a:
1. Hemostat
2. Tourniquet
3. Pressure dressing
4. Protamine sulfate

445. A child has had a leg amputated for bone cancer. To prevent contractures, the position that the nurse would plan to encourage the child to assume would be:
1. Lying on the abdomen
2. Sitting in high Fowler's
3. Supine with pillows between the thighs
4. Recumbent with a pillow under the residual limb

446. The nurse is aware that scoliosis usually is most notable when the child is:
1. 3 to 5 years of age
2. 6 to 9 years of age
3. 10 to 13 years of age
4. 14 to 18 years of age

447. During a routine physical examination, a 9-year-old is discovered to have scoliosis. The curve is diagnosed as mild and functional. A daily exercise program is established for the child. During a follow up visit in one month, the nurse recognizes acceptance of the program when the child states:
1. "I like doing my exercises with my brother, so he can get stronger."
2. "I think my exercises will help me improve in baseball and basketball."

3. "I do my exercises every day; my mother stays with me and watches."
4. "I do my exercises and count out loud, so my mother can be sure I'm doing them all."

448. The mother of a 10-year-old boy with mild scoliosis asks the nurse, "How long will my son have to continue his exercises before he is better?" The nurse responds:
   1. "Wearing a brace daily would probably lead to a quicker improvement."
   2. "At your son's age the exercise program is only done for a few months."
   3. "Surgery is a likely eventuality, but it will be less involved if the exercises are done."
   4. "Even though he continues the exercises, we won't know until his growth is complete if the curvature has improved."

449. A spinal fusion is performed on an adolescent with scoliosis. Postoperative care that is specific for this client would include:
   1. Log-rolling every 2 hours
   2. Checking the dressing frequently
   3. Supervising coughing and deep breathing
   4. Lying in the supine position for several days

DRUG-RELATED RESPONSES (DR)

450. Digoxin (Lanoxin) has been prescribed for a 1-month-old infant. At the next clinic visit the nurse observes that the apical pulse is 88. The nurse should:
   1. Notify the physician immediately
   2. Tell the mother to continue the digoxin
   3. Suggest that the physician lower the dose
   4. Ask the mother if this is the baby's usual heart rate

451. When reviewing medication instructions with the parents of an infant who is receiving digoxin (Lanoxin) and spironolactone (Aldactone), the nurse would know that the parents understood the instructions when they indicate:
   1. Their infant must have orange juice daily
   2. Their infant's activity should be carefully restricted
   3. Any vomiting should be reported to the physician
   4. Aspirin should be avoided while the infant is taking Aldactone

452. The nurse is teaching the parents of an infant with a cardiac defect how to administer digoxin (Lanoxin). The mother asks what she should do if she forgets whether she has given the dose of digoxin. The best response by the

nurse would be:
   1. "Wait two hours and then give the medication."
   2. "Give the dose since this is an essential medication."
   3. "Omit the dose and give it at the next prescribed time."
   4. "Take the baby's pulse and give the medication if the pulse is over 90."

453. An infant with congenital heart disease who had been admitted to the hospital in heart failure is to be discharged with digoxin and furosemide (Lasix). The nurse instructs the mother to notify the physician if:
   1. Her baby's pulse rate goes above 100
   2. Feeding difficulties and vomiting occur
   3. Her baby requires several naps each day
   4. Cyanosis occurs during periods of crying

454. An infant with a seizure disorder is prescribed phenobarbital. The mother brings the baby to the clinic a week later because of lethargy and prolonged sleep periods. The nurse may reduce the mother's anxiety by telling her:
   1. "The doctor will probably order another drug to counteract this side effect."
   2. "These signs probably mean your baby's dose of medication needs to be adjusted."
   3. "This is probably a temporary response to the drug and usually stops after a couple of weeks."
   4. "Many children experience the same problem, but your baby needs the medication and should continue to receive it."

455. The nurse teaches the parents of a child on long-term phenytoin (Dilantin) therapy about care pertinent to this medication. The nurse recognizes that the teaching is effective when the parents say, "We should:
   1. Provide oral hygiene, especially gum massage and flossing of teeth."
   2. Supplement the diet with high-calorie foods and encourage fluids."
   3. Give our child the medication two hours after breakfast and dinner."
   4. Observe our child's urine for the complication of a reddish-brown discoloration."

456. Ferrous fumarate (Feostat) 30 mg is ordered for an infant. The Feostat solution contains 45 mg/0.6 mL. The nurse should administer:
   1. 0.2 mL
   2. 0.4 mL
   3. 0.6 mL
   4. 0.9 mL

457. An adolescent who is receiving prednisone and vincristine for leukemia complains of constipation. The nurse is aware that the constipation is most probably:
1. A side effect of the vincristine
2. A toxic effect of the prednisone
3. Caused by the spleen compressing the bowel
4. Caused by the leukemic mass obstructing the bowel

458. A 2-year-old is admitted with a tentative diagnosis of cystic fibrosis. As part of the diagnostic process, pilocarpine is used. The nurse should explain to the parents that this medication stimulates:
1. Secretion of mucin
2. Activity of the sweat glands
3. The excretion of pancreatic enzymes
4. The release of bile from the gall bladder

459. A 12-year-old with cystic fibrosis is to receive three Pancrease capsules five times a day. The nurse is aware that this medication is given to:
1. Promote excretion of fats
2. Promote adequate oxygenation
3. Prevent iron-deficiency anemia
4. Facilitate utilization of nutrients

460. A child with cystic fibrosis is ready for discharge and the nurse is reviewing the discharge instructions with the mother. The statement by the mother that would indicate that she knows how to administer the pancreatic enzyme replacement would be:
1. "I will give the medication with feedings."
2. "I will give the pills in applesauce every morning."
3. "I must dissolve the enteric-coated pills in the formula."
4. "I must give the medication every six hours including during the night."

461. A child who had a craniotomy for the removal of a brain tumor complains of incisional pain. The nurse administers the prescribed ibuprofen. The mother asks the nurse why her child isn't receiving stronger pain medication such as codeine. The nurse's answer should be based on the fact that opioids:
1. May suppress the cough reflex
2. Are contraindicated in the young child
3. Are addicting when given for long periods of time
4. May interfere with the assessment of the level of consciousness

462. The nurse explains to the parents of a child who is receiving mannitol (Osmitrol) after a craniotomy that the medication is being given to:
1. Increase the filtration rate of the bladder
2. Decrease the peripheral retention of fluid
3. Reduce the amount of glucose in the urine
4. Relieve cerebral pressure following surgery

463. When a 5-year-old child is receiving dactinomycin (Cosmegen) and doxorubicin (Adriamycin) therapy following a nephrectomy for a Wilms' tumor, nursing care should include:
1. Administering aspirin for pain
2. Serving citrus juices with meals
3. Using an anesthetic mouthwash
4. Providing age-appropriate books

464. When caring for a child receiving prednisone, it is important for the nurse to know that adrenocorticosteroid therapy:
1. Accelerates wound healing
2. May produce hyperkalemia
3. Increases production of antibodies by the blood
4. Suppresses the inflammatory symptoms of infection

465. An important nursing intervention for a child who has been receiving long-term prednisone therapy for nephrotic syndrome would be:
1. Daily checking of pulse for irregularities
2. Regular checking of urine for mucous threads
3. Frequent checking of stools for occult blood
4. Daily checking of the oral mucous membrane for ulcers

466. The nurse, caring for a child with acute glomerulonephritis would expect the physician to order:
1. Penicillin and digoxin
2. Morphine and cortisone
3. Furosemide and hydralazine
4. Phenytoin and phenobarbital

467. When formulating a plan of care for a child receiving chemotherapy, the most important nursing consideration should be:
1. Increasing caloric intake
2. Limiting nausea and vomiting
3. Preventing formation of hematomas
4. Compensating for decreased immune response

468. A child newly-diagnosed with acute lymphoid leukemia (ALL) is to receive induction therapy with prednisone, vincristine and L-asparaginase. After several days it is noted that the child is constipated. The nurse recognizes that this has occurred because of:

1. The child's relative inactivity
2. The child's diet, which lacks bulk
3. The prednisone, which reduces intestinal tract motility
4. The neurotoxicity of vincristine, which decreases peristalsis

469. When assessing the status of a child with leukemia who is receiving vincristine (Oncovin), the nurse would know that the fluid intake should be increased when the child's:
1. Temperature is 99.8° F
2. Uric acid level is elevated
3. Urine's specific gravity is 1.026
4. Output for the last 24 hours totaled 1700 mL

470. For a child receiving chemotherapy, an important nursing intervention based on managing problems of drug toxicity would be:
1. Restricting fluid intake
2. Instituting contact precautions
3. Keeping the hair shortly cropped
4. Giving special mouth care several times a day

471. An 8-year-old girl in the hospital who is receiving methotrexate and cranial radiation is very weak, and her mother asks the nurse whether her daughter could receive some vitamin therapy to give her strength. The nurse's best response would be:
1. "Some vitamins contain folic acid, which interferes with methotrexate."
2. "That is an excellent idea; I'll ask the physician to order some for her."
3. "Unfortunately, vitamin supplements won't make her feel any better now."
4. "Your daughter will benefit from vitamins and will be receiving them soon."

472. When considering the side effects of dactinomycin (Cosmegen) and doxorubicin (Adriamycin) therapy, the nurse can suggest to the parents of a child receiving these drugs that the child:
1. Wear a baseball cap
2. Avoid dairy products
3. Dress in light clothing
4. Eat three large meals daily

473. An adolescent with acute lymphocytic leukemia (ALL) completes parenteral chemotherapy and is discharged home with a prescription for mercaptopurine (6-MP) one tablet daily by mouth. The statement by the adolescent that indicates an understanding of the reason for this therapy would be:
1. "These pills prepare me for additional IV drugs."

2. "These pills will be better than having brain radiation."
3. "This medication should help prevent another relapse of my disease."
4. "This medication should prevent the cancer from spreading to my stomach."

474. A 5-year-old-child is receiving chemotherapy. The mother is concerned that the child has not completed the required immunizations for school. The nurse's best response would be:
1. "By this time your child has developed sufficient antibodies to provide the needed immunity."
2. "Maintaining current immunizations is critical for all children, so your child should complete the series."
3. "It is important to complete the immunizations to provide protection from childhood diseases that could be fatal."
4. "This is not the best time to finish the immunizations because your child's immune system is suppressed."

475. After taking levothyroxine (Synthroid) for three months for congenital hypothyroidism, an infant is brought to the clinic for a checkup. The nurse evaluates that the drug is effective when the mother states that the infant's:
1. Activity level has decreased
2. Fine tremors have decreased
3. Skin is cool and dry to the touch
4. Bowel movements have increased to two soft stools daily

476. A 1-year-old is in the pediatric unit for management of AIDS. The child is receiving zidovudine (AZT) every six hours. The nurse evaluates that the child is in life-threatening AZT toxicity when the child manifests:
1. Fatigue and lethargy
2. A progressive weight loss
3. An increased urine output
4. Multiple bruises on the limbs and trunk

477. A 10-year-old child is newly diagnosed with type 1 diabetes, and insulin therapy is instituted. The child and the family are taught how to give the injections. The child dislikes the injections and asks the nurse why the insulin cannot be taken by mouth. The nurse explains that insulin:
1. Is a protein and would be inactivated by digestion
2. Would irritate the stomach lining and lose its potency
3. Has a carbohydrate portion that would add to the blood glucose
4. Is alkaline and would be neutralized by gastric hydrochloric acid

478. The mother of a child with type 1 diabetes asks why her child needs an insulin pump rather than insulin injections. The nurse explains that the major advantage of the pump would be that it:
1. Minimizes dietary restrictions
2. Allays fears of daily injections
3. Offers more freedom for the child
4. Eliminates blood glucose monitoring

479. When the nurse teaches a child about the use of the insulin pump, it is most important that the child understands that the:
1. Needle must be changed every 24 hours
2. Glucose monitoring will be necessary only once daily
3. Pump is an attempt to mimic the way a healthy pancreas works
4. Pump will be implanted in a subcutaneous pocket near the abdomen

480. The physician orders succimer (Chemet), an oral chelating agent, for a child with lead poisoning. The nurse recognizes that chelating agents cause:
1. Lead to be removed from the bone
2. Free lead to be secreted in the feces
3. Free lead to combine with hemoglobin
4. Lead to bind and be excreted in the urine

481. The nurse is supervising an adolescent who is self-administering 3 units of Humulin N insulin. The nurse should plan to instruct the adolescent to administer the insulin:
1. When lunch is eaten
2. One hour after lunch
3. One hour before lunch
4. In the middle of the afternoon

482. A chelating agent is prescribed for a child with lead poisoning. Because the chelating agent may cause hypocalcemia, the child should be encouraged to choose a menu consisting of:
1. Beef broth soup, glazed ham, potato salad, and green beans with almonds
2. Vegetable soup, roast beef with meat gravy, mashed potatoes, peas, and fruit
3. Cream of pea soup, fried shrimp, and broccoli covered with cheese sauce
4. Chicken vegetable soup, liver and onions, creamed carrots, white bread and butter, and fruit

483. Priority nursing care for children on chelation therapy for lead poisoning should include:
1. Scrupulous care of the skin
2. Providing a high-protein diet
3. Careful monitoring of intake and output
4. Drawing blood daily for liver function tests

484. The pediatrician has ordered ampicillin 160 mg IV every four hours. A vial containing 250 mg/5 mL is available. The nurse should administer:
1. 2.2 mL
2. 3.0 mL
3. 3.2 mL
4. 4.0 mL

485. A broad-spectrum oral antibiotic is prescribed for an adolescent with a bacterial infection. The prescription reads, "Take 4 times a day." To maintain the blood level, the nurse should recommend that the medication be taken at:
1. 8 AM, 12 PM, 4 PM, and 8 PM
2. 8 AM, 4 PM, 12 AM, and 4 AM
3. 10 AM, 2 PM, 10 PM, and 2 AM
4. 6 AM, 12 PM, 6 PM, and 12 AM

486. The nurse would determine that the teaching about the side effects of tetracycline was understood when the client says that the medication could cause:
1. Vertigo
2. Tinnitus
3. Diarrhea
4. Constipation

487. The nurse would know that the teaching about administration of tetracycline was effective when a teenage client says that the drug should be taken:
1. Just before meals
2. With meals or milk
3. At least one hour before meals
4. Approximately 30 minutes after meals

488. Screening for hearing loss should be planned for the child who is receiving:
1. Penicillin
2. Gentamicin
3. Tetracycline
4. Chloramphenicol

489. The nurse explains to a teenager who is receiving penicillin G and probenecid for syphilis that the rationale for both drugs being used is:
1. Each drug attacks the organism during different stages of cell multiplication
2. The penicillin treats the syphilis whereas the probenecid relieves the severe urethritis

3. Probenecid delays excretion of penicillin by the kidneys to maintain effective blood levels for longer periods
4. Probenecid decreases the potential for an allergic reaction developing to the penicillin, which treats the syphilis

490. A 7-year-old boy has been diagnosed with attention deficit hyperactivity disorder (ADHD). Methylphenidate (Ritalin) has been prescribed. The child's mother expresses concern that he will be "doped up." The nurse should explain that:
1. The medication usually causes an increase in appetite
2. Your child must continue to take the medication until adulthood
3. This is a short-acting medication that must be administered four times a day
4. Stimulants often have a calming effect when given to children who are hyperactive

491. After the severe effects of dehydration are under control in a 3-month-old infant, the physician orders lactobacilli granules (Lactinex) to:
1. Diminish inflammatory mucosal edema
2. Relieve the pain of gas in the gastrointestinal tract
3. Recolonize the normal flora of the gastrointestinal tract
4. Relieve the pain caused by gastric hyperacidity

492. Mebendazole (Vermox) is prescribed for a child with pinworms. When teaching about the medication, the nurse tells the mother and child that:
1. The drug may precipitate transient diarrhea
2. Rectal itching will be relieved rapidly once the drug is started
3. Only the child and no other family member will need treatment
4. A single course of treatment is all that is needed to control the problem

493. Cough syrup ½ tsp is ordered for a 4-year-old. Each teaspoonful contains dextromethorphan hydrobromide 7.5 mg. When administering the cough syrup, the nurse should provide:
1. 0.5 mL
2. 2.5 mL
3. 7.5 mL
4. 3.75 mL

494. The nurse tells a 13-year-old child with hay fever that the ordered phenylephrine nasal spray must be used exactly as directed to prevent the development of:
1. Nasal polyps
2. Bleeding tendencies
3. Tinnitus and diplopia
4. Increased nasal congestion

495. The physician prescribes astemizole (Hismanal) for a 15-year-old student with hay fever. The student tells the school nurse that she took her first dose early in the morning and she is concerned that she will be sleepy for a quiz that the teacher just scheduled for the next day. The nurse's best response would be to:
1. Explain that this medication rarely causes drowsiness
2. Advise her to take only half a tablet tomorrow before school
3. Suggest that she skip tomorrow's dose if she can tolerate the hay fever
4. Recommend that she call the allergist for a prescription containing a stimulant

496. The nurse evaluates that pancreatic enzyme replacement being taken by a child with cystic fibrosis is inadequate when the child complains of:
1. Anorexia
2. Constipation
3. Sudden weight gain
4. Abdominal cramping

497. A nurse is planning discharge teaching for a 10-year-old male who is taking prednisone for asthma. A critical medication instruction for the child and his parents would be:
1. "Observe for a moon-shaped face."
2. "Do not stop taking prednisone abruptly."
3. "Prednisone may cause an earlier growth spurt."
4. "This drug will protect you from infection."

498. A 15-year-old adolescent is admitted in status asthmaticus. An IV with theophylline is started. During the administration of this drug, immediate intervention is required if the nurse identifies the occurrence of:
1. Tinnitus
2. Drowsiness
3. Tachycardia
4. Blurred vision

499. A 14-year-old female has a spinal fusion. On the first postoperative day, her face is red and she is rigid and crying that she hurts. She has orders for both morphine and an acetaminophen-codeine compound. When considering analgesia for this client, the nurse should remember that:

1. One dose of morphine can be given, but she should be restricted thereafter because morphine is highly addictive

2. Adolescents often tend to exaggerate their discomfort, particularly when they are hospitalized and immobilized by surgery or injury

3. Spinal fusion results in considerable pain during the first few postoperative days, and morphine would be the most effective analgesic medication

4. It would be better to give her the acetaminophen-codeine compound, because morphine can cause respiratory depression, addiction, and respiratory arrest

500. The nurse is caring for a 15-year-old adolescent with an acetaminophen overdose after a suicide attempt. The diagnostic study that is most important for the nurse to monitor closely should be the:

1. Blood gas levels
2. Liver function tests
3. Complete blood counts
4. Glycosylated hemoglobin findings

Pediatric Nursing Answers and Rationales

NURSING PRACTICE (NP)

1. 1 Gloves should be worn when the nurse is exposed to blood and body fluids; this provides a barrier and protects the nurse. (1) (SE; LE; IM)
2 This personal protective equipment is not required unless the vomiting is projectile.
3 The use of a gown may be necessary if there is a risk of contamination of the nurse's clothing; however, in this situation, gloves are of greater importance.
4 Same as answer 2.

2. 4 In most states, the age of majority is 18 years; however, mothers younger than 18 years are considered emancipated minors and can sign consents for themselves and their children. (2) (SE; LE; AN)
1 The client is an emancipated minor; this confers adult status.
2 Consent is always needed; the 16-year-old mother is present and can legally give consent.
3 The grandmother has no legal right to give consent; the 16-year-old mother is present and can legally give consent.

3. 4 When alleged child abuse (neglect, sexual, or physical) is brought to the attention of a nurse, by law it must be reported to the proper state agency for further investigation. (1) (PI; LE; IM)
1 This is inappropriate because the student has already talked with her mother who is not hearing her concerns; the child expects the nurse, an adult she trusts, to help her.
2 This action circumvents the law.
3 Same as answer 2.

4. 3 Regardless of age, parenthood confers the rights of an adult on the teenager. (2) (SE; LE; PL)
1. It is unnecessary and not legal for the grandmother to sign the consent; the father is present.
2 This would be done only if neither parent were available to give consent in an emergency.
4 The mother has a legal right to give consent but is not available.

5. 3 Most injuries to abused children are not life-threatening; protection takes priority over immediate treatment. (3) (SE; LE; PL)

1 Treatment of medical injuries is the physician's primary responsibility.
2 An accurate diagnosis of child abuse may take time and must be fully investigated.
4 The nurse is often the first individual to see the abused child and must establish protection even before the physician arrives.

GROWTH AND DEVELOPMENT (GD)

6. 1 Mouthing is a typical activity of young children from 18 to 36 months, thus toddlers are at the highest risk for lead ingestion and other problems related to poisoning. (1) (PM; MR; IM)
2 There is no evidence of this in the older population.
3 Children from 3- to 6-years of age may mouth objects, but not as frequently as toddlers.
4 Pica occasionally occurs in pregnant women; but pica is most often associated with toddlerhood.

7. 2 Children who are spanked tend to use aggressive behavior as they get older; they learn their own behavior through their parents' behavior. (2) (PM; CJ; IM)
1 Age is not significant in the effectiveness of spanking.
3 This response is not appropriate; spanking is a form of child abuse.
4 Research studies dispute this as an effective disciplinary technique.

8. 1 The palmar grasp reflex, an involuntary behavior, is strong at one month of age and disappears by 3-4 months of age. (1) (PM; CJ; IM)
2 The palmar grasp reflex is expected at one month of age, begins to fade at 2 months of age and disappears by 4 months of age.
3 It is an involuntary, not voluntary behavior; it is a reflex that occurs in infants up to 4 months of age, not older infants.
4 The pincer grasp is a fine motor voluntary behavior that begins to be used at 8 months of age.

9. 3 The 3-month-old infant is interested in self-recognition and playing with the baby in the mirror. (3) (PM; CJ; IM)
1 This is not appropriate for a 3-month-old.
2 Same as answer 1.
4 Same as answer 1.

10. 1 During the oral stage, infants tend to complete the exploration of all objects by putting the objects in the mouth as a final step. (2) (PM; CJ; AS)

2 Infants 9 to 10 months old play this way as they learn that objects continue to exist even though they are not visible.

3 These are the random reflexive movements of 1- to 2-month-olds, whose voluntary control of distal extremities has not developed.

4 This is the momentary grasp reflex of neonates before the development of eye-hand-mouth coordination.

11. 1 This behavior is within the expected range; a 7-month-old child can sit without assistance by extending the legs to the side and leaning forward on the hands; by 8 months a child should sit steadily unsupported. (1) (PM; CJ; IM)

2 Most children can sit without assistance by 7-8 months of age.

3 Same as answer 2.

4 Sitting alone is not a predictor of when the infant will walk.

12. 1 Eight-month-old infants have the ability to use their fingers and thumbs in opposition (pincer grasp); this enables them to pick up small objects and put them in their mouths and aspirate them. (1) (SE; MR; AN)

2 Although this is true, the major concern is preventing infants from putting foreign objects in their mouths where they can be aspirated.

3 It is not a health hazard if the floor is clean and the object is large enough so that there is no danger of the child aspirating it.

4 The danger is not that the items would be hidden but that they would be put into the mouth and aspirated.

13. 2 This is inappropriate for an 8-month-old; this is appropriate for a toddler to promote imitative play. (3) (PM; CJ; EV)

1 A stuffed animal promotes manipulative play.

3 A hanging mobile promotes visual stimulation.

4 A textured book promotes tactile stimulation and touch discrimination.

14. 3 This usually occurs by age 8 months. (1) (PM; CJ; AS)

1 Two- to three-word vocabulary is an expectation of a 12-month-old child

2 This is accomplished by the 2-year-old, not the 9-month-old.

4 The posterior fontanelle is closed by age 2 months and the anterior fontanelle closes between ages 18 to 24 months.

15. 3 A coin can become dislodged and the infant could put it in the mouth creating a safety issue. (3) (SE; MR; IM)

1 This will not endanger the child; cultural beliefs that do not place the infant at risk need not be discouraged.

2 Same as answer 1.

4 Same as answer 1.

16. 2 The Babinski reflex, present at birth, should remain positive throughout the first 12 months of life. (2) (PM; CJ; AS)

1 This reflex, present at birth, disappears by 4 months of age.

3 Same as answer 1.

4 Same as answer 1.

17. 4 These are typical behaviors of an 8-month-old. (2) (PM; CJ; AS)

1 These are typical behaviors of a 3-month-old.

2 These are typical behaviors of an 18-month-old.

3 These are typical behaviors of a 12-month-old.

18. 4 This is an accurate, nonjudgmental conclusion based on the weight charts of the National Center for Health Statistics. (2) (PM; CJ; AN)

1 This is a judgmental reaction; more evidence is needed to come to this conclusion.

2 This is the expected weight for a 6-month-old infant weighing 7.5 lb at birth.

3 Same as answer 1.

19. 2 A 1-year-old child has the physical ability to attempt to climb stairs; this skill will not be accomplished before 15 months of age. (2) (PM; CJ; AN)

1 This is beyond the ability of a 1-year-old; a 15-month-old child can jump with both feet but may still fall.

3 A 1-year-old infant's vocabulary is limited.

4 This is beyond the ability of a 1-year-old; a 15-month-old child can do this.

20. 2 The toddler develops voluntary sphincter control between 18 and 24 months of age; at this age the child should be developmentally ready for potty training. (2) (PM; MR; EV)

1 This demonstrates autonomous behavior and the need to explore the environment; this is typical of a 15-month-old toddler.

3 This demonstrates separation anxiety, which is common in a 15-month-old toddler.

4 This is typical behavior of a 15-month-old child exploring the environment.

21. 1 One way toddlers explore their environment is by putting objects in their mouths. (1) (PM; MR; IM)

2 The sense of taste is well developed at birth.

3 An expected decline in appetite occurs during this period; it is called physiologic anorexia.

4 Toddlers assert themselves but are not rebellious of adult authority; adolescents rebel against adult authority.

22. **4 Lips and teeth closed around the finger create suction and can move permanent teeth forward, causing malocclusions. (1) (PM; CJ; IM)**

1 If thumb-sucking is practiced only in relation to sleep, no treatment is necessary because it involves only a short period of time.

2 The pacifier can cause malocclusions when permanent teeth appear.

3 There is no indication that the first teeth are loosened by thumb-sucking.

23. **3 Brief messages, with only essential words included (telegraphic speech), are a normal pattern for a child 18 months to 2½ years of age. (2) (PM; CJ; AN)**

1 A child with a severe developmental lag would have no obvious recognizable speech pattern and would only make a few sounds.

2 A child slow for this age would have a smaller vocabulary and would use only single words to identify familiar objects.

4 A child advanced for this age would have a larger vocabulary and would use three- to four-word sentences rather than telegraphic speech.

24. **4 Growth slows during toddlerhood and children generally do not eat as much as during infancy; this is called physiologic anorexia, which is typical of this age group. (1) (PM; CJ; IM)**

1 Toddlers may try to manipulate as they assert their autonomy, but usually not through eating behaviors unless the parents express anxiety and concern over their food intake.

2 Although toddlers have difficulty withstanding frustration and are prone to temper tantrums, these eating behaviors are within the norm for toddlers.

3 Eating disorders usually do not occur in children this young; these behaviors are typical of healthy toddlers.

25. **2 Preschool children use imitation of adult situations to help learn social skills, they enjoy make-believe play. (1) (PM; CJ; AN)**

1 Abstract thinking does not develop until adolescence.

3 Same gender play is common among preschoolers.

4 Magical thinking is expected in toddlers and early school-age children.

26. **4 Being brought a gift will minimize feelings of being ignored; the child can role-play with the new doll, which is an age-appropriate activity. (2) (PM; CJ; IM)**

1 The child is too young to be responsible for the baby.

2 This may increase the child's feelings of jealousy if told that the mother must stay with the baby rather than with her.

3 Ignoring the child will reinforce insecurity and may promote acting-out behavior.

27. **1 The mother should ignore the picky eater's food intake and not let it become a major point of contention; by including some of the foods the child will eat in every meal plan, the mother can ensure that the child eats without giving in to the child's demands. (1) (PM; CJ; IM)**

2 This would produce a battle for control between the toddler and the parent, which is nontherapeutic.

3 Fixing two meals is not appropriate because it draws attention to the toddler's eating habits.

4 Dessert should not be used for disciplinary control; as the child gets older, desert-like food may take on too much significance.

28. **4 This response may reduce the toddler's level of stress without loss of self esteem; toddlers see their parents as capable of all things and would be accepting of this "house rule"; light allows the toddler to see familiar objects in the room and reduces fears associated with a dark environment. (3) (PM; CJ; PL)**

1 This denies the toddler's concerns and is beyond the concrete thinking of a toddler.

2 This may interfere with the parents' ability to get a restful night's sleep; with additional emotional support, the child should be encouraged to remain in his or her own bed.

3 A toddler thinks in concrete terms and this may not relieve the fear of monsters; it also denies the toddler's concerns.

29. **2 This is Erikson's early childhood or preschool stage, which includes children from 3 to 6 years of age. (1) (PM; CJ; PL)**

1 This is Erikson's infancy stage, which includes children from birth to 1 year of age.

3 This is Erikson's middle childhood or school-age stage which includes children from 6 to 12 years of age.

4 This is Erikson's toddler stage which includes children 1 to 3 years of age.

30. **2 A 4-year-old can manage large buttons on a shirt. (1) (PM; CJ; AS)**

1 A child of 4 years can put on shoes but is usually unable to tie them until age 5.
3 A child of 4 years will be able to comb, but not part the hair.
4 A child of 4 years can handle a fork and spoon but cannot hold the meat with the fork to cut it with the knife; the child is usually 7 years old before this can be managed.

31. **2 Because of expanded experiences and developing cognitive ability, the 4-year-old should have a vocabulary of approximately 1500 words. (2) (PM; CJ; AS)**

1 By 5 years of age, children ask the definitions of new words.
3 By 2½ to 3 years of age, children can name colors.
4 By 3 years of age, children use three- or four-word sentences.

32. **4 Imaginary friends are typical of children of this age; children who have few social contacts with peers are more likely to be involved with imaginary friends. (1) (PM; MR; PL)**

1 This is an inappropriate intervention for this situation; the child was protecting an imaginary friend, and having imaginary friends is typical of a 4-year-old child.
2 Counseling is unnecessary; this is typical behavior for a 4-year-old child.
3 There is no evidence of child abuse or neglect.

33. **2 Stuttering occurs because the child's advancing mental ability and level of comprehension exceed the vocabulary acquisitions in the preschool years. (2) (PM; CJ; AN)**

1 Stuttering is common in the preschool years; it is not a problem at this age.
3 Same as answer 1.
4 Same as answer 1.

34. **2 According to Piaget, this describes the thought processes associated with the preschool-age child. (3) (PM; CJ; PL)**

1 According to Piaget, this describes adolescent thought processes.
3 According to Piaget, this describes the infant's thought processes.
4 According to Piaget, this describes the school-age child's thought processes.

35. **4 This form of organized play is typical of 5-year-olds as they learn to share and take turns without becoming frustrated. (2) (PM; CJ; AN)**

1 This kind of play is typical of older, school-age children who play games with other children and learn to abide by the rules.
2 This play is typical of the toddler-age group; they have not yet learned to interact with other toddlers in a social situation.
3 This term does not identify any age group; it is not a recognized term for social play.

36. **2 A 5-year-old is able to negotiate and use make-believe to play. (3) (PM; CJ; AS)**

1 Older children in the middle-childhood years need conformity and rituals, whether they play games or amass collections; rules to games are fixed, unvarying, and rigid; knowing the rules means belonging.
3 The use of a pacifier for oral satisfaction is typical of infants.
4 Parallel play occurs in children ages 2 to 3 years.

37. **3 This action provides adult supervision for all the children. (1) (SE; MR; AN)**

1 This is unsafe; 7-year-olds should not be without supervision.
2 This puts too much responsibility on children who are too young and who may get lost or hurt.
4 Same as answer 2.

38. **4 This activity provides the child with a familiar routine; it encompasses the age-appropriate developmental tasks of Industry vs. Inferiority. (2) (PM; CJ; PL)**

1 Although social interaction and mental stimulation are important at this age, continuing with schooling is the priority.
2 This is satisfactory but should not replace active participation.
3 This activity is best for the preschooler.

39. **4 As part of the maturation process, adolescents should be taught to accept the consequences of their actions. (1) (SE; CJ; IM)**

1 There is no way to predict what will be the outcome of friends' behavior in the future.
2 The focus should be on pointing out that the adolescent should be accountable for self-behavior, not that friends should also be punished.
3 The focus should be on the adolescent's actions and not those of friends' parents.

40. **4 Several meetings with an adolescent provide an opportunity to develop trust and establish a relationship. (1) (PM; CJ; AN)**

1 This is unrealistic because the nurse is not an adolescent's peer.

2 It is not necessary to deal in concrete terms because the adolescent is capable of abstract thought; this would be necessary with a young child.

3 Using teenage language is not necessary and may even impede the establishment of a relationship.

41. **4 This is the preferred age before the development of body image and fear of castration; if necessary, testosterone may be administered to increase the size of the penis. (3) (PM; CJ; PL)**

1 The phallus is not developed enough for surgery to be done at this age.

2 The child is in the oedipal stage of development, which is accompanied by fear of mutilation.

3 Same as answer 1.

42. **3 The infant has not yet recognized boundaries between self and mother and is not particular about who meets and resolves needs. (1) (PM; CJ; EV)**

1 The infant does not yet differentiate familiar faces from those of strangers.

2 This behavior does not indicate recognition of a specific person but only a human face.

4 Because the concept of self-boundaries has not yet developed, the infant does not really know or fear separation from the mother.

43. **4 A 7-month-old infant is used to having the perineal area exposed and cared for and is not in a developmental stage where fears related to sexuality are present. (1) (PM; CJ; IM)**

1 A "clean catch" at this age is often contaminated; the physician ordered a catheterization.

2 The mother does have the right to refuse, but these concerns are not realistic for an infant at this age.

3 Although the mother may be concerned, a catheterization is not a problem for an infant and the mother needs to be educated.

44. **2 The average infant doubles the birth weight at 6 months. (1) (PM; CJ; AN)**

1 This is below the expected weight gain.

3 This is above the expected weight gain.

4 This is expected at one year of age when the birth weight usually triples.

45. **3 Typically, infants respond to social play by 10 months. (3) (PM; CJ; AS)**

1 This behavior is typical of a 15-month-old.

2 Same as answer 1.

4 Same as answer 1.

46. **2 The eustachian tube in young children is shorter and wider, allowing a reflux of nasopharyngeal secretions. (3) (PM; CJ; IM)**

1 Immunologic differences are not a factor in the development of otitis media.

3 The size of the middle ear does not play a role in the common occurrence of otitis media in very young children.

4 There is no difference in the functioning of the eustachian tube among age groups.

47. **3 The canal curves upward in children under 3 years of age; this straightens the canal so that medication will reach the eardrum. (3) (PM; CJ; IM)**

1 The auditory canal must be pulled down and back to straighten it.

4 This is not advised; it can only add more pressure within the ear and prevent the drops from reaching the middle ear.

2 This is an incorrect technique for children younger than 3 years because it will not straighten the ear canal.

48. **3 Attributing lifelike qualities to inanimate objects (animism) is associated with preconceptual thought. (3) (PM; CJ; AN)**

1 This is related to school-age children.

2 This is a phase of concrete operations seen in school-age children.

4 This is related to infants.

49. **4 Changes in the daily routines in the home and anxiety expressed by family members lead to anxiety in toddlers. (2) (PI; CJ; IM)**

1 The toddler has no reality-based concept of death.

2 Although this may be true, the primary motivation for the behavior is a response to the upheaval in the family.

3 This is false reassurance; it fails to acknowledge the family upheaval.

50. **4 Hospitalization is traumatic to the preschooler because of separation from significant family members; it is rare to find a pediatric unit that restricts a significant caregiver's visitation. (2) (PM; CJ; AN)**

1 Preschoolers are not interested in food, and appetite tends to vary with the menu; children with nephrotic syndrome have notoriously poor appetites.

2 Massive edema results in easy fatigability and a lack of interest in play.

3 Preschoolers are not concerned about attitudes and opinions of peers; it is too early in their social development to have this concern.

51. 1 **Although the local anesthetic will help minimize the discomfort, this is an honest, simple answer that is appropriate for a 3-year-old child. (2) (PM; CJ; IM)**
    2 This is a judgmental response that is inappropriate for a 3-year-old child; children sometimes need to cry to express their feelings; if the child does not move, crying is acceptable.
    3 Although the child should hold still, there is no guarantee that it will not hurt.
    4 This gives false reassurance; there is no guarantee of success.

52. 3 **Preschoolers can tolerate brief periods of separation from their parents; however, emotions associated with separation and perhaps anger at being left are difficult to hide when parents arrive or leave. (2) (PM; CJ; AN)**
    1 Preschoolers usually are quite docile and cooperative because they are afraid of being totally abandoned.
    2 The child would demonstrate despair long before the week was over.
    4 The presence of other children's parents would be unrelated to their relationship with peers.

53. 4 **The child with abdominal pain may assume the side-lying position with the knees flexed to the abdomen and/or may self-splint when moving. (1) (PM; CJ; AS)**
    1 A 4-year-old may be unable to define the exact location of the pain; in addition, the pain may be generalized rather than localized.
    2 This might be included in the health history, but it is not specific to the assessment of pain.
    3 This might be included in the physical assessment, but it is not specific to the assessment of pain.

54. 3 **According to Freud, preschool-age children are in the Oedipal phase of development; they fear procedures that intrude on their body integrity. (2) (PM; CJ; PL)**
    1 This is a fear that toddlers experience.
    2 This is a fear that adults experience.
    4 This is a fear that school-age and adolescent children experience.

55. 4 **Enjoyment of fantasy is a pleasurable pastime for a 4-year-old; this also provides for rest. (2) (PM; CJ; PL)**
    1 These activities are below a 4-year-old child's ability; they also do not provide for rest.
    2 Although a 4-year-old may enjoy video games, he is not expected to be able to read for enjoyment.

3 The pull toy is below a 4-year-old child's developmental level, and the puzzle is too advanced.

56. 4 **Playing with age-appropriate puzzles is intellectually stimulating and can be done with an intravenous infusion in place. (2) (PM; CJ; IM)**
    1 This is a passive activity and not especially stimulating.
    2 The child needs both hands for this activity.
    3 Same as answer 1.

57. 1 **This is appropriate for this age child; it would give the child the opportunity for free expression and its free-form nature can give the child a sense of mobility. (3) (PM; CJ; PL)**
    2 This is less than optimal because coloring within lines of pictures in a coloring book requires more skill than most 4-year-olds possess; also this does not allow freedom of expression or movement.
    3 Checkers is a game with too many rules for a 4-year-old to comprehend.
    4 Playing dominos requires the ability to count and conserve numbers, which most 4-year-olds do not possess.

58. 1 **Children feel pain and should receive analgesics when needed. (3) (PB; CJ; AN)**
    2 This is a myth; it may be difficult for children to communicate pain.
    3 Some sources suggest this may be a child's way of coping with unrelieved pain; however, it is no reason to withhold medication.
    4 This is a common, but unsound belief; addiction and respiratory depression are rare.

59. 4 **This is appropriate for the child's age and suited to the child's limited mobility. (1) (PM; CJ; AN)**
    1 The child is too young for this activity; children of 7 years or older are able to play checkers.
    2 Building blocks would be difficult to play with while on bed rest.
    3 The child will not have enough mobility to engage in this type of play and is too young for this activity.

60. 4 **School-aged children enjoy competition, have manipulative skills, and are creative. (2) (PM; CJ; IM)**
    1 This activity is inappropriate during the acute phase of nephrotic syndrome; it requires too much energy.

2 These toys are appropriate for the toddler who is developing fine motor skills.

3 Magazines would interest an older child; a 6-year-old child is just beginning to learn to read; listening to a CD is not mentally stimulating; computer games may be too stimulating.

61. 1 This is the most accurate and age-appropriate response to the question. (3) (PM; CJ; IM)

2 This is inaccurate; not being truthful interferes with the development of trust.

3 This is inaccurate and may instill more fear.

4 This response is insensitive to the child's concern and does not provide an explanation.

62. 4 According to Piaget, an 8-year-old child's level of development is in the stage of concrete operations; the child will benefit from simple concrete examples. (2) (PM; MR; IM)

1 The preschooler and younger child require repetition, not the school-age child.

2 This might be done if the child were to receive an injection; there is no indication of this.

3 The child who is in the period of concrete operations can not abstract; the ability to abstract occurs during adolescence.

63. 1 This is appropriate for an 11-year-old, who sees dying as loss of control over every aspect of living; the child may convey this meaning by physically attempting to run away or by pushing others away by rude behavior; it is a plea for some self-control and power. (3) (PI; CJ; AS)

2 This is characteristic of the toddler, who is egocentric and has a vague separation of fact and fantasy, which makes it impossible to understand the absence of life.

3 This is characteristic of the preschooler, who does not have logical thinking.

4 This is more typical of the adolescent, who sees deviation from accepted behavior as the reason for becoming ill.

64. 1 Adolescents are very aware of their changing bodies and become especially concerned with any alteration. (2) (PM; CJ; IM)

2 This does not educate the mother about concepts concerning the developing adolescent; a discussion about hypochondriasis may reinforce the mother's concern.

3 This does not address concepts related to growth and development of the adolescent and could cause unnecessary concern about the daughter's physical condition.

4 This could reinforce the mother's concern as well as promote feelings of guilt.

65. 3 The 15-year-old is normally preoccupied with appearance; the side effects of the antineoplastics and prednisone could result in the adolescent feeling different, which can cause an impaired body image. (1) (PM; CJ; AN)

1 A 15-year-old enjoys and strives for independence; the sick role would force the client to be dependent.

2 This may be a concern but is not likely to be the outstanding concern or feeling.

4 Same as answer 2.

66. 2 The teenage child is concerned with body image and fears change or mutilation of body parts; in sickle-cell anemia, bone weakened because of hyperplasia and congestion of the marrow can cause lordosis and kyphosis. (1) (PM; CJ; AN)

1 Restriction of movement is not a major problem because when the pain is relieved and the crisis is over, activity can be resumed; for the teenager, the change in body image produces greater anxiety.

3 Teenagers can easily tolerate extended periods of separation from the family.

4 Although this could be a concern at this time for a teenager, altered body image is a more fearful threat.

67. 3 Striving to attain identity and independence is a task of the adolescent, and rebellion against established norms may be exhibited. (3) (PM; CJ; AN)

1 This behavior is not a bid for attention; rather it is an attempt to establish an identity, which is a developmental task of the adolescent.

2 Although the adolescent may be using denial, denial is not developmentally related to adolescence.

4 This behavior is not regression; it is an attempt to attain identity by rebellion against established norms.

EMOTIONAL NEEDS RELATED TO HEALTH PROBLEMS (EH)

68. 1 Family strengths must be identified and utilized by the nurse. (3) (SE; MR; AN)

2 The family members and their problems must be viewed as a whole.

3 The opposite is true.

4 Values, beliefs, and attitudes greatly influence perceptions.

69. 3 **The parents need assistance in exploring their feelings and their family relationships with a professional. (1) (SE; MR; EV)**
    1 The gifts are attempts to relieve guilt feelings; the parent still feels responsible.
    2 This is a gift to the child that helps the parents relieve their guilt feelings.
    4 The parent is assuming the martyr role and accepting responsibility for the child's illness.

70. 2 **The parents need to express and deal with their feelings before they can move forward with other coping strategies. (1) (PI; CJ; IM)**
    1 This does not focus on the needs of the parents at this time.
    3 Although important, this is not the priority at this time.
    4 This is premature reassurance and does not meet the parent's present needs.

71. 4 **This response is accepting of the individual and communicates concern. (3) (PI; CJ; IM)**
    1 This is the nurse's responsibility and should not be transferred immediately to the client's family.
    2 This response interprets the client's statement as guilt, which may or may not be the true interpretation.
    3 There is no indication that the injuries were deliberate abuse.

72. 4 **This response accepts the mother's concern and offers an option. (2) (PM; CJ; IM)**
    1 This response evades the mother's concern and may cause the mother to become defensive.
    2 This is a judgmental response and does not explore the feasibility of this advice.
    3 This response offers no options; it may increase the mother's guilt if she cannot stay.

73. 4 **Going to a stranger without protest usually indicates the lack of a meaningful relationship with the mother. (1) (PI; CJ; AS)**
    1 This is a healthy reaction to strangers that is uncommon in children with nonorganic failure to thrive syndrome.
    2 Same as answer 1.
    3 Children with nonorganic failure to thrive avoid eye contact with their mothers and do not prefer them over others.

74. 2 **Because parents are trying to hide the fact of abuse, the explanations are fabricated and vague. (2) (PI; CJ; AS)**
    1 This is expected; the parents are unable to provide emotional support.

3 The child behaves in this manner because in past experiences adults have inflicted pain rather than provided comfort.
    4 This is no surprise; parents do not discuss them because this would be an admission of child abuse.

75. 2 **Children with diabetes should be treated normally; they need discipline and should have limits set for their behavior. (1) (PI; MR; EV)**
    1 Parents should foster independence in the child with diabetes mellitus.
    3 It is realistic to think that the family will have ups and downs.
    4 The child with diabetes should be encouraged to maintain previous interests and activities.

76. 4 **The nurse must emphasize that everything possible is being done because the outcome cannot be predicted. (3) (PI; CJ; IM)**
    1 The outcome is still in doubt; encouraging the parent's positive interpretation of the child's reflexive behavior raises false hope.
    2 Same as answer 1.
    3 The outcome is still in doubt; this response by the nurse may raise false hope; the parent's statement did not ask for the nurse's religious viewpoint.

77. 2 **Abused children distrust anyone who touches them because it may be a precursor to abuse. (2) (PI; CJ; AS)**
    1 Abused children are fearful of others and do not smile when approached.
    3 Abused children would be acutely aware of anyone at the bedside; they would be alert to the possibility of attack.
    4 Abused children usually do not cry because they have learned not to expect comforting or soothing from others.

78. 1 **People living in poverty have long-term feelings of powerlessness because they do not have buying power or social status to influence change. (1) (PI; CJ; AN)**
    2 Their anger is covert and not direct; in addition, the anger rarely resolves their situation, resulting in feelings of powerlessness and hopelessness.
    3 The opposite is true; they are focused on the present, not the future.
    4 People in poverty tend to focus on today; health recommendations may be delivered in less than optimal circumstances or may be misunderstood, confusing, or of little value.

79. 4 **This plan for behavior shows the potential for increased impulse control, which is important for the prevention of further abuse. (2) (PI; CJ; EV)**
   1 This is unrealistic because all parents become angry with their children at some time or another.
   2 This places the blame on the child, rather than on the parent's own behavior.
   3 This places the blame on the spouse, rather than the self.

80. 3 **These behaviors are associated with separation anxiety; parental contact should be encouraged. (1) (PM; CJ; PL)**
   1 Separation anxiety can be minimized by increasing contact with parents, not peers.
   2 Separation anxiety can be minimized by increasing contact with parents, not by distraction with toys.
   4 This would increase feelings of anxiety; the same nurse should care for the child to promote consistency, continuity, and the development of trust.

81. 4 **Parental involvement in comforting the child is the most supportive intervention for the toddler. (3) (PB; CJ; PL)**
   1 Distraction does not provide an outlet for the toddler's feelings.
   2 An explanation is required and expected; the depth of the explanation depends on the needs of the parents.
   3 The toddler will probably refuse both times; a choice is not an option.

82. 4 **Adherence to dietary restrictions can prevent future complications and celiac crisis. (2) (PB; CJ; PL)**
   1 Celiac crisis usually develops as a result of non-adherence to the diet, so adherence would be a primary objective.
   2 Respiratory involvement is not a primary problem in celiac disease.
   3 Regardless of adherence to the diet, there may be an interference with normal growth.

83. 3 **This is an honest statement; the nurse recognizes the fact that this might hurt and requests expected behavior. (2) (PB; CJ; IM)**
   1 This puts a thought in the mind of the child.
   2 This puts unrealistic expectations on the child.
   4 This might be too threatening for the child.

84. 1 **Colostomy care may seem overwhelming to the parents, and it may reassure them to know that a therapist is available. (1) (SE; MR; PL)**
   2 Mealtime should be a pleasant time; also, this assumes that eating habits are poor.

   3 Increased fluids are often needed to compensate for fecal fluid loss.
   4 Physical activity will probably not be limited.

85. 4 **This is a realistic and optimistic appraisal of the child's status. (2) (PI; CJ; IM)**
   1 This conclusion is premature, since the acute phase of the illness may not have passed.
   2 Same as answer 1.
   3 Same as answer 1.

86. 2 **This is an open-ended question that should elicit the desired information. (2) (PM; CJ; IM)**
   1 This question can be answered with a yes or a no and does not elicit what the child knows or feels about the situation.
   3 Same as answer 1.
   4 Same as answer 1.

87. 4 **This meets her present need while assuring her this is a temporary condition. (3) (PI; CJ; IM)**
   1 This response denies and demeans the child's feelings.
   2 Same as answer 1.
   3 Same as answer 1.

88. 3 **The child learned to think and solve problems in a very different culture and language and may feel helpless in the new classroom. (1) (PI; CJ; AN)**
   1 There are not enough data to substantiate this.
   2 This is untrue; 5-year-olds are inquisitive and adapt well to school.
   4 Most 5-year-olds adapt well to kindergarten.

89. 2 **This response identifies concern and presents an appropriate protective intervention; regular and prompt removal of ticks decreases the chances of the spread of Lyme disease to humans. (2) (SE; CJ; IM)**
   1 This response belittles the child's feelings.
   3 This response centers on camping, not on the fear of ticks.
   4 This is an inappropriate response because it focuses on the wrong fear.

90. 2 **This allows the child to volunteer information first and thus feel in control; the nurse can ask validating questions later. (1) (PB; CJ; AS)**
   1 This focuses the assessment on vomiting, thus predisposing the child to vomiting during this treatment.
   3 This is an unfeeling response; it reminds the child and mother of the many sessions remaining and brings little consolation to the child for the discomfort or to the mother for her worry about the prognosis.
   4 This statement is flippant and insensitive.

91. 1 **This child needs help adjusting; focusing on feelings and abilities promotes effective coping and raises self-esteem. (2) (PI; CJ; PL)**

2 In general, the diet is limited to simple carbohydrates; bowel inflammation necessitates avoidance of high-roughage foods.

3 Teaching the relationship of diet to the disease process does not ensure compliance with the diet.

4 Occasional non-adherence to the regimen is not permitted; it can cause a relapse.

92. 2 **The child is old enough to respond when asked a direct question. (2) (PI; MR; IM)**

1 The parents are too emotionally involved with the child and may not be trained in principles of mental health and therapeutic communication.

3 A younger child would benefit from this projective technique.

4 This may be productive with a younger child.

93. 1 **Negotiation of goals is essential to successful learning; mutual goal-setting provides a focus for learning. (1) (SE; CJ; PL)**

2 A rapport should already be developed before beginning the teaching-learning process.

3 If the client does not identify this need or set a goal, motivation could be minimal.

4 Same as answer 3.

94. 2 **Honesty is essential to help the client accept the loss of the leg; only a brief discussion of chemotherapy is needed to avoid overwhelming the client. (2) (PI; CJ; IM)**

1 A detailed explanation of surgery and chemotherapy would only overwhelm the client at this time.

3 This would only serve to avoid the issue and would destroy the client's trust in parents and staff.

4 Same as answer 3.

95. 3 **This is a truthful answer that offers some hope without false reassurance. (2) (PI; CJ; IM)**

1 This response shuts off communication and discourages further ventilation of feelings.

2 This response produces guilt and denies the adolescent's realistic fears.

4 This response denies the adolescent's feelings.

BLOOD AND IMMUNITY (BI)

96. 4 **The first dose is given at birth; the second dose is given 4 to 6 weeks after the birth dose; the last dose should be administered at 6 months of age. (1) (SE; MR; PL)**

1 All children should receive the hepatitis B vaccine.

2 The hepatitis B vaccine protects against hepatitis B, not hepatitis A or hepatitis C.

3 Hepatitis B is a blood-borne disease; hepatitis A is transmitted through contaminated food or water.

97. 3 **The passive antibodies to DTaP received from the mother would be diminished by age 8 weeks and would not interfere with the development of active immunity after this time. (2) (PM; CJ; AN)**

1 Infants are often exposed to infectious diseases; passive immunity from the mother offers some protection.

2 The spleen does not produce antibodies.

4 These immunizations are attenuated; they may cause irritability and fever, but they will not cause the related disease.

98. 2 **Recurrent seizures can cause brain damage; therefore, if the immunization causes another febrile seizure, future immunization with DTaP may be contraindicated. (3) (PM; CJ; EV)**

1 This is not a contraindication for the administration of DTaP; it may be a contraindication to the measles vaccination.

3 This is not a contraindication for DTaP.

4 This is not a contraindication for the administration of DTaP; it may be a contraindication to the smallpox vaccination.

99. 3 **Mild reactions are redness and induration at the injection site, slight fever, and irritability. (2) (PM; MR; EV)**

1 Serious reactions are not common.

2 Occasionally a DTaP injection may precipitate a febrile seizure, but it does not cause permanent brain damage.

4 Induration at the site of injection may occur, but deep ulceration does not.

100. 1 **This will promote circulation, reduce swelling and relax muscles, thus lessening the inflammation. (1) (PM; MR; IM)**

2 This will not lessen inflammation or promote relaxation.

3 Fever is not a response; therefore, the cooling effect of a sponge bath is not necessary.

4 Cool applications will not provide relief because they reduce circulation to the area.

101. 4 **This is the optimum age because maternal antibodies to measles are no longer present to block the formation of the child's own antibodies. (2) (SE; MR; IM)**
   1 It is not given at this time because of the questionable efficacy of the vaccination due to the presence of maternal antibodies.
   2 Same as answer 1.
   3 Same as answer 1.

102. 4 **A high white blood cell count makes the spinal fluid appear cloudy and possibly milky white; it is a sign of infection. (2) (SE; CJ; AS)**
   1 Normal spinal fluid is clear.
   2 Elevated glucose levels do not affect the color of the spinal fluid.
   3 Red blood cells would make the spinal fluid appear sanguineous; they do not appear in normal spinal fluid.

103. 4 **Potatoes and whole milk are not adequate sources of iron; at age 8 months, fetal iron stores are depleted. (2) (PB; CJ; AN)**
   1 Potatoes are a rich source of potassium.
   2 The infant is receiving Poly-Vi-Sol, which contains vitamins but no iron; Poly-Vi-Sol with iron exists, but the data indicate that plain Poly Vi-Sol is being used.
   3 There are some amino acids in the foods that are being eaten.

104. 4 **The time and amount of feedings do not require special consideration when caring for an infant with iron deficiency anemia. (2) (PM; CJ; EV)**
   1 Conservation of energy preserves the infant's energy level because these babies are usually fatigued.
   2 A malnourished anemic state frequently leads to decreased resistance to infections.
   3 Teaching the parents that inclusion of foods or formula high in iron content is essential.

105. 4 **This supplies iron and some protein; it can be eaten with a spoon, encouraging mastery of fine motor muscles. (1) (PB; CJ; PL)**
   1 This provides some protein and iron but has a spicy taste that is not generally a favorite of this age group.
   2 This is low in protein and iron.
   3 Although grapes contain iron, a cup portion would be difficult to finish for an 18-month-old child.

106. 4 **Fever is a common reaction to the immunizations; acetaminophen helps to reduce fever;**

both loss of consciousness and seizures are rare but serious complications of the pertussis vaccine. (2) (PM; MR; IM)
   1 These data do not indicate that an inflammatory response has occurred.
   2 Infants do not respond well to the application of ice; fever is expected and requires no intervention other than administration of acetaminophen.
   3 Aspirin should not be given to children because it is associated with Reye syndrome.

107. 2 **Excess iron from hemolysis of the replaced red blood cells is deposited in the organs and body tissue causing hemosiderosis; chelation therapy is then required. (2) (PB; CJ; IM)**
   1 With proper asepsis and screening of donated blood, this should not occur.
   3 Red blood cell replacement depends on the child's hematological picture; the number of transfusions is not related to age.
   4 Although red blood cells are replaced, this treatment cannot be compared to insulin therapy.

108. 2 **Children with leukemia are immunosuppressed; the chickenpox virus can cause death in the individual without an intact immune system. (2) (SE; MR; PL)**
   1 The vaccine against chickenpox is a live virus and should not be given to an immunosuppressed child.
   3 Prednisone does not confer immunity to the chickenpox virus.
   4 This would be unsafe; chickenpox can be spread by airborne droplets in the prodromal stage and by fomites that have come in contact with pox that are oozing.

109. 2 **Tonsillectomy may result in hemorrhage because of the vascularity of the oropharynx; adequate clotting function must be present. (2) (PB; CJ; AS)**
   1 This is not significant for this type of surgery if the child is otherwise healthy.
   3 Same as answer 1.
   4 Same as answer 1.

110. 2 **Increased swallowing occurs with bleeding in the oropharynx. (2) (PB; CJ; EV)**
   1 Signs of respiratory distress, not increased swallowing, would be noticed with pharyngeal edema.
   3 Tenacious secretions may cause gagging, not increased swallowing.
   4 There is a decreased, not increased, salivary response after a tonsillectomy.

111. 3 These are indicative of catabolism and bone marrow depression that are expected in a child with ALL. (2) (PB; CJ; AS)

1 There would be no change in hair growth until chemotherapy is instituted.

2 Because of the bone marrow depression, the child will be lethargic and sleep excessively.

4 Same as answer 1.

112. 2 Sores in the mouth are not a presenting sign but often result from chemotherapy. (3) (PB; CJ; AS)

1 Anorexia is a presenting symptom of leukemia and may be the result of enlarged lymph nodes and areas of inflammation in the intestinal tract.

3 Pallor is a presenting sign of leukemia and reflects the anemia present because of decreased erythrocytes.

4 Decreased platelet production with petechiae and bleeding is a presenting sign of leukemia.

113. 2 Before the procedure sedation is administered to minimize discomfort. (3) (PB; CJ; IM)

1 This is a painful procedure requiring sedation.

3 The child should be placed prone with a towel roll under the hips for aspiration of marrow from the posterior iliac crest.

4 The child can handle some of the equipment as part of the explanation of the procedure; during the procedure, the child will be sedated.

114. 3 To allay parental guilt and anxiety, it is important to acknowledge how difficult it is to recognize severe illness based on changes in the child's behavior and ecchymoses that could have been caused by banging into objects—which young children often do. (2) (PB; CJ; AN)

1 Between ages 2 and 10 the prognosis is favorable based on such factors as the child's age when diagnosed, the WBC, the type of cell involved. etc.

2 The only certain diagnosis that can be made is with a bone aspiration or biopsy.

4 Even if the mother missed the fact that her child was so ill, mentioning this would raise even more anxiety and guilt and interfere with rapport.

115. 3 Vaso-occlusive crisis (pain episode) often precipitates a pooling of blood in the liver and in the spleen resulting in its enlargement (splenomegaly). (3) (PB; CJ; AN)

1 Splenomegaly is not common during infancy.

2 An enlarged spleen is easily palpable in a child.

4 Splenomegaly is not common during late childhood; the spleen of a child with sickle-cell anemia may be smaller by adolescence because of chronic repeated infarcts.

116. 2 Thalassemia is a hemolytic anemia that is not communicable; roommates with infectious diseases should be avoided because a child with sickle-cell anemia is susceptible to infections. (2) (SE; MR; PL)

1 The child with sickle-cell anemia is susceptible to infection; pneumonia is an infection of the lung.

3 The child with sickle-cell anemia is susceptible to infection; osteomyelitis is an infection of the bone.

4 The child with sickle-cell anemia is susceptible to infection; pharyngitis is an upper respiratory infection.

117. 3 The crescent shape of sickle cells makes them fragile; they then clump together to occlude blood vessels. (2) (PB; CJ; AN)

1 This is called an aplastic crisis resulting in severe anemia.

2 This is known as a sequestration crisis.

4 The platelet count is not severely depressed in vaso-occlusive crisis.

118. 3 Adequate hydration promotes hemodilution, which helps prevent sickling and thrombus formation. (2) (PB; MR; PL)

1 This would cause vasoconstriction and enhance sickling.

2 Muscle contraction increases oxygen demands, which would decrease oxygen tension resulting in increased sickling.

4 Sunshine may cause dehydration and hemoconcentration resulting in increased sickling.

119. 3 This is the definition of the characteristics of a rabies infection; it is usually fatal if allowed to go untreated. (3) (PB; CJ; AN)

1 Rabies is not a bacterial infection.

2 Same as answer 1.

4 The virus specifically attacks the nervous system and is carried in the saliva of infected animals.

120. 2 The current polio vaccine is the inactivated polio vaccine (IPV) (Salk vaccine) that is injectable. (2) (PB; CJ; IM)

1 This is the *Haemophilus influenzae* type b (Hib) vaccine.
3 The oral polio vaccine (OPV) (Sabin vaccine) is no longer administered because it is related to vaccine-associated polio paralysis (VAPP)
4 This is the diphtheria, tetanus, and pertussis (DTaP) vaccine.

121. **2 Before the sex of the unborn child is known, the odds are 25%; 50% of pregnancies will result in boys, and each has a 50% chance of having hemophilia. (3) (PM; CJ; IM)**
1 Because the disease is genetically transmitted, this is not likely.
3 This is too high; there is only a 25% chance that the baby will be affected.
4 Same as answer 3.

122. **2 Joints are the most commonly involved areas, probably because of weight bearing and constant movement of joints. (3) (PB; CJ; AS)**
1 This is not the most common site; however, bleeding can occur here.
3 Same as answer 1.
4 Same as answer 1.

123. **1 The platelet count is reduced as a result of the bone marrow depression associated with leukemia. (3) (PB; CJ; IM)**
2 The uric acid level reflects urinary function, not blood clotting.
3 Prothrombin time is influenced by vitamin K factors, not lack of platelets.
4 The red blood cell count will indicate the hematocrit and hemoglobin levels, which would neither provide the reason for nor cause the bleeding.

124. **4 An electric toothbrush vigorously massages the gums; this may be irritating, causing the gums to hemorrhage. (1) (SE; CJ; IM)**
1 This can be used because it will not injure the mucous membranes.
2 Same as answer 1.
3 A saline mouthwash is isotonic and will not injure the mucous membranes.

125. **1 Overwhelming infection is the leading cause of death because of the depressed immune system resulting from chemotherapy. (2) (PB; CJ; PL)**
2 Although this is important, prevention of infection is the priority.
3 Same as answer 2.
4 Same as answer 2.

126. **4 Meticulous toilet hygiene is essential to prevent infection and promote comfort. (3) (PB; CJ; IM)**

1 Changing positions is preferable to maintenance of one position.
2 This may keep the area moist and promote bacterial growth; it is preferable to leave the area exposed to air even if under bed linens.
3 Ointments tend to occlude and trap organisms, thus promoting infection.

127. **3 Blood tests indicate response to therapy; if the WBC count drops severely, therapy may be temporarily halted. (2) (PB; MR; PL)**
1 These children receive therapy for extended periods, and prolonged isolation from their peers may lead to destructive social isolation.
2 This is a very painful procedure and is not done weekly.
4 Nausea commonly occurs with this therapy; although antiemetic measures are instituted, the drug is not withdrawn.

128. **2 Adequate nutrition is extremely important to the child's overall health; best results are attained when a child receiving chemotherapy is allowed to eat as desired. (2) (PB; MR; EV)**
1 The child should be isolated only from other children with known or possible infections.
3 Although activities are important to the child's health, these should be provided according to the child's interest and should not always be structured.
4 Mouthwashes can irritate the fragile mucosa, so saline should be used; nutrition is the priority.

129. **4 Effective handwashing helps prevent infection; this is the most important intervention when caring for a child with a suppressed immune system. (1) (SE; CJ; PL)**
1 Although this is important, it is not the priority.
2 Same as answer 1.
3 Same as answer 1.

130. **4 Previously formed antibodies, acquired through active immunity, offer some resistance to infection; adults have higher levels of antibodies than children because over time they have been exposed to more pathogens. (1) (PM; CJ; AN)**
1 The immune systems of children are as capable of producing antibodies as are those of adults.
2 The pathophysiologic mechanism of AIDS is the same in both children and adults.
3 Exposure to pathogens in the environment does not differ significantly between children and adults.

131. 4 **The Centers for Disease Control and Prevention recommends standard precautions when caring for those who have HIV infection and/or AIDS without opportunistic infections. (1) (SE; LE; IM)**
   1 Droplet precautions are not necessary because HIV is not transmitted by large particle respiratory droplets.
   2 Contact precautions would not be necessary unless the HIV or AIDS were complicated by the presence of disease or infection, necessitating the addition of these precautions to standard precautions.
   3 Airborne precautions are unnecessary because HIV is not spread by airborne droplet nuclei; these precautions would be used in addition to standard precautions if an opportunistic infection such as Mycobacterium tuberculosis were present.

132. 2 **The major complication of a partial-thickness burn injury is wound infection; once it occurs it is difficult to treat and can be life-threatening. (2) (PB; CJ; EV)**
   1 Although this is important, it is not the priority.
   3 Same as answer 1.
   4 Same as answer 1.

133. 3 **Children with a chronic illness should not be exposed to the additional stress of an infection. (2) (SE; MR; PL)**
   1 The child should be encouraged to lead an active, ordinary life during periods of well being.
   2 Fluid intake can be according to the child's wishes.
   4 The child should be encouraged to lead as regular a life as possible and eat meals with the family.

134. 3 **Tetanus immune globulin contains antibodies and only confers short-term passive immunity. (2) (PM; CJ; AN)**
   1 The passive immunity is temporary.
   2 Passive, not active, protection is provided.
   4 Immune globulins are antibodies and therefore may block the formation of natural antibodies if given with the tetanus toxoid.

135. 1 **Low oxygen tension may precipitate sickling; therefore adequate oxygenation is desirable; hemodilution prevents increased viscosity, which can cause sickling and thrombus formation. (2) (PB; CJ; PL)**
   2 The intake of oral iron may aggravate the condition by causing hemoconcentration.
   3 Hemoconcentration results in increased viscosity, which would promote thrombus formation and sickling.
   4 This would be desirable during a pain episode, but it is not employed routinely to prevent a crisis.

136. 3 **This is a relatively passive, innocuous activity that would not increase oxygen demands of the body, which could precipitate sickling. (2) (PB; CJ; IM)**
   1 This may lead to increased cellular metabolism and increased tissue hypoxia, which could precipitate sickling.
   2 Same as answer 1.
   4 High altitudes should be avoided because of the lower oxygen concentration of the air, which might trigger a crisis.

137. 2 **Dehydration is a major causative factor for a sickle-cell episode. (2) (PB; MR; EV)**
   1 It is not the iron intake but ineffective hemoglobin that causes the anemia.
   3 A breakdown of platelets (thrombocytes) is unrelated to sickle-cell episodes.
   4 The WBCs are not increased unless infection is present.

138. 4 **The physician probably will use conscious sedation as well as a local anesthetic; the child should not feel any discomfort, pain, or pressure when the bone marrow is withdrawn. (3) (PB; CJ; EV)**
   1 The child will need to recover from the conscious sedation and then may prefer to remain quiet; activity usually is not restricted.
   2 This is done to prevent bleeding from the puncture site.
   3 The anterior or posterior iliac crest is the site most often used for a bone marrow aspiration in children.

139. 2 **The eosinophil count increases to inhibit the acute inflammatory response to histamine, which is released in allergic reactions. (2) (PB; CJ; AN)**
   1 Platelets are unrelated to an allergic reaction.
   3 Lymphocytes are unrelated to an allergic reaction.
   4 Immunoglobulins would increase, not decrease, in response to an allergic reaction.

140. 2 **Tetanus immune globulin should not cause anaphylaxis because it is derived from human serum. (3) (PM; CJ; IM)**

1 Both drugs are equally convenient to administer.

3 Tetanus immune globulin is not as effective as the antitoxin.

4 These medications always carry a risk of hypersensitivity; it cannot be assumed that they can be given safely to everyone

141. 4 **The American Academy of Pediatrics (AAP) recommends that infants be given the MMR combination vaccine at 12 to 15 months of age. (1) (SE; MR; PL)**

1 The AAP recommends that the vaccine be given at 24 months.

2 The infant should have received this immunization at 2 months, 4 months, and 6 months of age; the next booster will be at 18 months.

3 Same as answer 2.

CARDIOVASCULAR (CV)

142. 4 **Because the mechanism of heart failure is the same in all children, the same basic treatment of a cardiac glycoside and a loop diuretic (Lasix) is used, although the dosage may vary. (1) (PB; CJ; AN)**

1 Heart failure in infants is not in itself a congenital defect but results from a congenital defect of the heart.

2 The treatment of heart failure is basically the same whether the client is an infant or a senior citizen.

3 Children can develop heart failure just as adults can; if there is cardiac decompensation, the treatment is the well-established combination of Lanoxin and Lasix.

143. 1 **The nurse needs to know how much information the parent has before responding; pulmonic stenosis is a narrowing at the entrance to the pulmonary artery and may vary in severity; treatment may vary from balloon angioplasty to valvotomy. (3) (PB; CJ; IM)**

2 This response is too blunt; the nurse needs to know how much the parent knows and understands first.

3 The parent is concerned or the question would not have been asked.

4 This response abdicates the nurse's role.

144. 3 **Because the infant tires so easily, it is impossible to ingest sufficient calories to meet nutritional needs. (3) (PB; CJ; AN)**

1 Although this occurs, it does not directly relate to growth.

2 Although decreased PO_2 does lead to polycythemia, it would not affect growth.

4 Same as answer 1.

145. 4 **This is an accurate description of tetralogy of Fallot. (3) (PB; CJ; AN)**

1 Only the overriding aorta is associated with tetralogy of Fallot.

2 Only the ventricular septal defect is found in tetralogy of Fallot.

3 Only right ventricular hypertrophy is found in tetralogy of Fallot.

146. 3 **Compromised heart function and inadequate oxygen reserves in the infant often result in feeding problems such as cyanosis and fatigue while sucking and swallowing. (2) (PB; CJ; AN)**

1 Poor sucking is always significant.

2 This may be true in the first days of life but is not true as the infant grows, unless there is a major health problem.

4 Same as answer 2.

147. 1 **Hypoxia leads to poor peripheral circulation; clubbing occurs as a result of additional capillary development and tissue hypertrophy of the fingertips. (2) (PB; CJ; AS)**

2 Respirations will be increased.

3 The child's problems are related to decreased oxygenation, not to a clotting deficit.

4 The body attempts to compensate for the hypoxemia by increased erythropoiesis.

148. 1 **Flexing the hips and knees decreases venous return to the heart from the legs; when venous return to the heart is decreased, the cardiac workload is decreased. (1) (PB; CJ; IM)**

2 Although this would reduce pressure of abdominal organs on the diaphragm, it does not put enough pressure on the femoral veins and vena cava to sufficiently reduce venous return to the heart.

3 This position does not reduce venous return to the heart.

4 Same as answer 2.

149. 2 **These occur in infants when there is impaired myocardial function; they are the direct result of sympathetic stimulation; the pulse is elevated even when the infant is at rest. (3) (PB; MR; IM)**

1 Urinary output is decreased as a result of sodium and water retention.

3 This is a late sign of heart failure; it occurs when pulmonary congestion develops.

4 This only occurs in adults when heart failure has progressed to systemic congestion.

150. 1 The body responds to the chronic hypoxia caused by the heart defect by increasing the production of red blood cells in an attempt to increase the oxygen-carrying capacity of the blood. (3) (PB; CJ; AS)

2 This does not result from hypoxia; it occurs in disease processes in which the WBCs drop to very low levels and neutropenia becomes pronounced.

3 Thrombocytopenia (low platelet production) does not result from hypoxia; it occurs in disease processes in which platelet production is suppressed, as in leukemia.

4 The hematocrit level would be elevated because the body increases the production of red blood cells in an attempt to make more cells available to carry oxygen.

151. 3 Small frequent feedings with adequate rest periods will improve the infant's total intake; these infants become extremely fatigued while sucking. (2) (PB; CJ; IM)

1 Lying flat restricts lung expansion and should be avoided; positioning with the head elevated facilitates respiration.

2 Fluids are often restricted in infants with heart failure because it reduces the cardiac workload.

4 The head circumference is not a parameter that must be monitored with congenital heart disease; head measurement would be done for infants with hydrocephaly.

152. 4 During a bowel movement the Valsalva maneuver can occasionally initiate a hypercyanotic spell (tet spell, blue spell); the Valsalva maneuver causes increased intrathoracic pressure, slowing of the pulse, decreased return of blood to the heart, and increased venous pressure. (3) (PB; CJ; AN)

1 This would not influence cardiovascular functioning.

2 Same as answer 1.

3 Same as answer 1.

153. 3 A calibrated dropper is the most accurate way to measure the medication. (1) (PB; CJ; IM)

1 This is not an accurate way to measure medication.

2 Same as answer 1.

4 If the dose of medication is diluted in 1 oz of water and the infant does not drink the entire ounce, the resulting dose will be insufficient.

154. 4 This murmur is the most characteristic finding in children with a ventricular septal defect (VSD). (3) (PB; CJ; AS)

1 These children generally have tachycardia.

2 This is not a finding in VSD.

3 Children with VSD usually are acyanotic.

155. 2 When the child squats, blood pools in the lower extremities because of flexion of the hips and knees; less blood returns to the heart enabling the heart to beat more effectively. (2) (PB; CJ; IM)

1 Flexion of the hips and knees decreases blood flow to the extremities; muscle aches will not improve.

3 Squatting position is not related to the pull of gravity.

4 Squatting increases blood volume in the extremities.

156. 2 A cardiac catheterization will identify the exact location of the ventricular septal defect as well as assess pulmonary pressures. (1) (PB; CJ; AN)

1 This is demonstrated by electrocardiographic and echocardiographic examinations.

3 Murmurs can be heard with a stethoscope placed at the left lower sternal border.

4 Same as answer 1.

157. 2 Postprocedure hemorrhage is a major life-threatening complication following cardiac catheterization because arterial blood is under pressure and the catheter has entered an artery. (2) (PB; CJ; PL)

1 The child has an oxygen deficit; rest should be encouraged; flexion of the insertion site should be avoided to prevent disturbance of the clot.

3 The blood pressure should not be unstable unless a problem developed; fluids should be administered as ordered.

4 This is unnecessary; the distal pulses would be monitored.

158. 1 A range-of-motion exercise to the limb that has the catheterization site might cause hemorrhage or the dislodging of a clot. (2) (PB; MR; EV)

2 Intake should start with fluids and progress as tolerated.

3 This should be done because formation of thrombi is a complication of catheterization.

4 This should be done because a common complication after catheterization involves disturbances of cardiac rate and rhythm.

159. 1 The catheter insertion site should not be submerged in water; sponge baths limit trauma and infection at the insertion site. (1) (PB; MR; IM)

2 This is contraindicated; ice will cause vasoconstriction and could compromise circulation.

3 Fluids should be encouraged to enhance excretion of the contrast media used during the procedure.

4 The child is not sent home with a pressure dressing.

160. 3 **The increased blood volume and pressure in the lungs resulting from left ventricular failure cause pulmonary edema; dyspnea, an early sign of failure, is probably caused by the decreased distensibility of the lungs. (3) (PB; CJ; AN)**

1 Anemia is fairly well tolerated in infants and does not cause dyspnea.

2 Dyspnea, not hypovolemia, is an early sign of pulmonary edema; hypovolemia would cause signs of shock.

4 Respiratory, not metabolic, acidosis could develop; this occurs because of the pulmonary insufficiency resulting in retention of carbon dioxide.

161. 2 **Fluid retention is reflected by an excessive weight gain in a short period of time in a child with heart failure; inadequate cardiac output decreases blood flow to the kidneys, thus leading to increased intracellular fluid and hypervolemia. (1) (PB; CJ; IM)**

1 This would be an appropriate answer if a renal condition or hypovolemia were present; however, other assessments such as hourly output and BUN values would then also be indicated.

3 Weight gain resulting from nutritional intake is gradual and would not vary greatly on a day-to-day basis.

4 Weight is helpful in determining drug dosages, but the drug dosage would not need to be recalculated daily according to weight changes.

162. 3 **A positive antistreptolysin titer is present with rheumatic fever because of previous infection with streptococci. (3) (PB; CJ; AS)**

1 A positive, not a negative, C-reactive protein would be present; this is indicative of an inflammatory process.

2 This is usually related to a decrease in mature RBCs caused by hemorrhage or other blood diseases; it is unrelated to an infectious or inflammatory process.

4 The ESR would be elevated, not decreased, indicating the presence of an inflammatory process.

163. 1 **The vital signs must be taken first to determine the child's postoperative status and to compare them with the previously recorded vital signs. (3) (PB; CJ; AS)**

2 Although this is important, obtaining the vital signs is the priority.

3 Same as answer 2.

4 Same as answer 2.

164. 4 **Prophylaxis before an invasive procedure can prevent endocarditis, which occurs often in children and adults with heart abnormalities. (2) (PB; MR; IM)**

1 The endocardium is more susceptible to infection than the pericardium.

2 This is an infection of the myocardium, which is not found in children with congenital heart anomalies.

3 Avoidance of crowds, not the administration of antibiotics, is recommended to prevent upper respiratory infections.

ENDOCRINE (EN)

165. 2 **Although the maternal glucose supply is interrupted, the newborn's pancreas continues to produce large amounts of insulin for one to three hours after birth. (3) (PB; CJ; PL)**

1 This is too soon; hypoglycemia occurs later.

3 This is too late for hypoglycemia to occur.

4 Same as answer 3.

166. 4 **The glycosylated hemoglobin (GHb) test provides an accurate long-term index of the client's average blood glucose level for the 100- to 120-day period before the test; the more glucose the RBC was exposed to, the greater the GHb percentage; the test result is not affected by short-term variations. (3) (PB; CJ; AS)**

1 The presence of ketones in the urine may indicate only short-term variations and extreme hyperglycemia.

2 Serum protein levels do not reflect the effectiveness of glucose management in diabetes mellitus.

3 Serum glucose levels reflect short-term (hours) variations.

167. 3 **The stress of an infection increases the body's metabolism, and the presence of glucocorticoids results in hyperglycemia and an increased need for insulin. (2) (PB; CJ; AS)**

1 This causes a decrease in insulin demands resulting in hypoglycemia, not hyperglycemia and ketoacidosis.

2 This would decrease insulin demands and cause an episode of hypoglycemia, not hyperglycemia and ketoacidosis.

4 Excessive insulin would result in hypoglycemia, not hyperglycemia and ketoacidosis.

168. 2 Deep, rapid breathing (hyperpnea) is an attempt by the respiratory system to eliminate excess carbon dioxide; it is a characteristic compensatory mechanism of metabolic acidosis. (2) (PB; CJ; AS)

1 Increased body temperature (pyrexia) occurs when an infection is present.

3 Tachycardia, not bradycardia, results from the hypovolemia caused by the polyuria associated with ketoacidosis.

4 Hypotension, not hypertension, may result from the decreased vascular volume caused by the polyuria associated with ketoacidosis.

169. 4 These are both expected values; the pH indicates acidosis (metabolic) and the blood glucose is elevated above the normal range of 90 to 110 mg/dl. (2) (PB; CJ; AN)

1 Although the blood pH indicates acidosis, the blood glucose is below the normal range of 90 to 110 mg/dl; with ketoacidosis the client would be hyperglycemic.

2 Both values are not expected with ketoacidosis; with ketoacidosis the pH would be lowered and the blood glucose elevated.

3 Although the blood glucose would be elevated in ketoacidosis, the pH would be lowered, not elevated; a pH of 7.50 indicates alkalosis.

170. 2 A quick check of the blood glucose level will confirm whether the client is hypoglycemic. (2) (PB; CJ; AS)

1 This is inaccurate and does not reflect the present status.

3 Although this might be appropriate to counter hypoglycemia, it does not determine whether the client is hypoglycemic or is being manipulative.

4 Same as answer 3.

171. 2 The client's trouble stems from perceptual difficulties; the preset syringe removes the need to differentiate between 24 and 42 units. (2) (SE; CJ; PL)

1 This would not solve the transposition of the numbers; the problem is not caused by the inability to see the numbers but by the child's perception of them.

3 This would not solve the transposition of the numbers.

4 Same as answer 3.

172. 1 Because clients with type 1 diabetes have little or no endogenous insulin, they must take insulin; dietary control and exercise reduce the amount of exogenous insulin needed. (2) (SE; MR; IM)

2 Although infection increases insulin requirements, the administration of prophylactic antibiotics is not required.

3 While this is an important aspect of therapy for clients with diabetes, it is used to evaluate the effectiveness of diabetic control.

4 Oral hypoglycemics are ineffective in stimulating insulin secretion in clients with type 1 diabetes.

173. 3 Glucagon promotes liver glycogenolysis, resulting in the release of glucose into the blood. (3) (PB; CJ; AN)

1 ACTH is not directly related to glycogenolysis; it is released from the anterior pituitary.

2 The level of insulin will decrease as the glucose level declines; it is not directly related to glycogenesis.

4 Epinephrine is not directly related to glycogenolysis; it is released from the adrenal medulla and sympathetic nerve endings.

174. 2 Negotiation of goals precedes and is essential to successful learning; mutual goal-setting provides a focus for learning. (3) (SE; MR; AN)

1 A rapport should already be developed before beginning the teaching-learning process.

3 If the client does not identify this need or set this as a goal, there will probably be little motivation to learn this task.

4 Same as answer 3.

175.

1 _____ Headache—Headache is an adaptation associated with hypoglycemia, not hyperglycemia, that is caused by impaired cerebral function.

2 _____ Irritability—Irritability is an autonomic nervous system response to hypoglycemia, not hyperglycemia.

3 _____ Diaphoresis—Sweating with pale, cool skin is an autonomic nervous system response associated with hypoglycemia, not hyperglycemia.

4 **_x_ Increased thirst—Hyperglycemia acts as an osmotic diuretic resulting in an increased urine output (polyuria) and dehydration; as a result, thirst as a compensatory mechanism causes the**

person to drink increased amounts of fluid (polydipsia). (2) (PB; CJ; AS)

5 __x__ Redness of the face—Warm, dry, flushed skin is related to the dehydration associated with ketoacidosis.

6 __x__ Deep, rapid breathing—Kussmaul breathing is the body's attempt to blow off carbon dioxide in an attempt to correct the metabolic acidosis associated with hyperglycemia.

176. **2 This is an attempt by the respiratory system to eliminate the excess carbon dioxide; it is a characteristic compensatory mechanism to correct metabolic acidosis. (1) (PB; CJ; AS)**
1 An increased temperature will only occur if an infection is present.
3 Tachycardia, not bradycardia, results from the hypovolemia of dehydration.
4 Hypotension, not hypertension, may result from decreased vascular volume.

177. **1 Insulin mobilizes potassium to move into the cells along with glucose, thus lowering serum potassium levels. (3) (PB; CJ; EV)**
2 Insulin does not lead to reduced blood volume.
3 Insulin does not directly alter sodium levels.
4 Insulin does not affect calcium mobilization.

178. **1 Proper handwashing is the best infection-prevention technique and should always precede preparation of an injection. (1) (SE; CJ; PL)**
2 Shaking causes air bubbles, which can interfere with preparing the dosage accurately; the bottle should be gently rotated.
3 The injection site should not be rubbed because this affects absorption of the insulin and also causes reactions at the site.
4 The abdomen, not the extremities, is the preferred site for self-administration of insulin; sites should be rotated.

179. **2 The child's confidence, readiness, and skill for giving self-injections is essential for long-term management of diabetes. (3) (PB; CJ; PL)**
1 The sites must be rotated at all times.
3 Learning responsibility for injections should be a gradual process with continuous support and guidance.
4 The recommended procedure is to draw up the Humulin R first and then the Humulin N to prevent contamination of the multidose vial of Humulin R by the intermediate-acting Humulin N.

180. **1 Humulin N peaks in 8 to 12 hours; a bedtime snack will prevent hypoglycemia during the night. (1) (PB; MR; PL)**
2 This is unsafe because it would intensify the hyperglycemia; if hyperglycemia is present, the child needs insulin.
3 When hypoglycemia develops the child will be asleep; the snack should be eaten before going to bed.
4 Humulin N is an intermediate, not a long-acting insulin for which bedtime snacks are recommended.

181. **1 Pizza contains complex carbohydrates and protein; children can include a slice in their diets on special occasions. (3) (PB; CJ; EV)**
2 Although candy bars can be low in fat, they may still have a high simple sugar content, which would be contraindicated.
3 Diet, not regular, soft drinks are preferred for a client with diabetes; regular soft drinks are high in simple sugars.
4 A euglycemic fasting blood glucose should be 70-105 mg/dl.

182. **1 Adequate inspection of the feet should become a habit; it is the quickest and easiest measure to identify pressure sites and prevent infection. (1) (PB; MR; IM)**
2 Hot water should never be used because it can cause injury by burning the skin.
3 The feet should be patted dry, not rubbed vigorously; rubbing can cause abrasion and injure the skin.
4 Strong antiseptics are too harsh and should not be used because they can cause injury to the skin.

183. **2 The client is exhibiting signs of hypoglycemia; the blood glucose level should be identified to document the client's status so that appropriate treatment can be determined and implemented; a carbohydrate and protein may be administered to restore a normal blood glucose level. (2) (PB; CJ; EV)**
1 It may be necessary to administer food rather than withhold food if the client is having a hypoglycemic reaction.
3 This may be done if the blood glucose level indicates hypoglycemia is present.
4 This will delay appropriate intervention and is unsafe.

184. 3 The stress of surgery causes the release of epinephrine and glucocorticoids, which raise blood glucose levels. (2) (PB; CJ; AN)

1 Urine test results are affected by many variables, such as renal threshold, so they are not accurate enough when control is precarious; serum glucose levels are preferred.

2 Hypoglycemia can result because the client has taken nothing by mouth and body fluids are being lost.

4 Most clients with diabetes who are diet-controlled require insulin for a short period after surgery, especially when receiving IV glucose; most children have type 1 diabetes.

185. 4 A fast food exchange list allows participation in postgame activities without feeling different from peers, which is important to the adolescent. (1) (PB; CJ; IM)

1 The nutritional benefits of fast foods are not the issue.

2 The adolescent needs to learn how to select appropriate foods when away from the home environment; this promotes social interaction with peers.

3 This would make the adolescent feel different from peers.

186. 2 Urine testing is primarily helpful in detecting ketones, which are most likely to be present during illness and hyperglycemia. (3) (PB; CJ; AN)

1 Because of the complexity of the medical regimen and the variety of factors that influence serum glucose levels, such as food ingested, exercise, medications, and the stresses of growth and development, serum glucose levels in children can fluctuate and should therefore be measured by monitoring the serum glucose levels before meals and at bedtime.

3 Blood, not urine, is the best specimen to be tested for determining glucose levels.

4 The opposite is true.

187. 4 The coach needs to know because there is difficulty in balancing food, exercise, and insulin in active children. (1) (SE; MR; AN)

1 The people associated with the school who are interacting with the child need to know about the child's condition, but should be asked to keep the information confidential.

2 With increased activity, the child will experience episodes of hypoglycemia, not hyperglycemia.

3 This would be a form of discrimination; the child with diabetes mellitus should be allowed to engage in activities as long as the diabetes remains under control.

FLUIDS AND ELECTROLYTES (FE)

188. 2 It is critical to infuse the prescribed fluid over the prescribed time to gradually restore fluid and electrolyte balance. (2) (PB; CJ; IM)

1 Cuddling should be offered, preferably by the significant caregiver.

3 Although this is important, the priority at this time is related to the infusion itself; an improvement in behavior would indicate a probable institution of ORT.

4 The infant's caregiver should understand the purpose of the infusion, but this is secondary to the physiologic safety of the baby.

189. 4 Loss of weight is the most accurate measurement to evaluate the magnitude of fluid loss in an infant; 1 liter of fluid weighs 2.2 pounds. (2) (PB; CJ; AS)

1 This is a subjective assessment; measurement of weight is an objective assessment.

2 Although this would indicate dehydration, it is not an effective monitoring method for assessing fluid loss.

3 This is a subjective assessment.

190. 2 This provides an objective measurement because a weight loss indicates a loss of fluid; approximately 1 kg is equal to l liter of fluid. (2) (PB; CJ; EV)

1 Although the number of diapers counted is an objective measure, the extent of fluid contained in the diaper is not an accurate measure.

3 Although intake can be measured accurately, output—especially with diarrhea—is difficult to measure.

4 This is too subjective and open to a variety of interpretations.

191. 2 Metabolic acidosis occurs with loss of alkaline fluid through diarrhea and is manifested by lethargy and Kussmaul breathing; all of the observations indicate severe dehydration. (2) (PB; CJ; AS)

1 All data indicate that there is a severe fluid-volume deficit.

3 Respiratory alkalosis is not caused by diarrhea; it is caused by hyperventilation.

4 Acid-base compensation may occur, but the history and observations give no supporting evidence for this.

192. 2 **The degree of dehydration is correlated with weight loss; 1 liter of fluid is equivalent to 2.2 pounds; continued fever aggravates fluid losses through evaporation. (2) (PB; CJ; AS)**
1 Decreased skin turgor is not an initial sign of dehydration.
3 This is not relevant; the neurologic status is not altered; the urinary output may show signs of decreasing.
4 This is not relevant because the child has been vomiting and may be NPO until the vomiting subsides.

193. 4 **A priority concern is that immediate treatment is necessary for severe diarrhea; because infants and toddlers have a greater proportion of body fluid to tissue, they cannot maintain fluid balance when there is a large loss of fluid via diarrhea and vomiting. (2) (PB; MR; PL)**
1 The data do not indicate administration of antibiotics.
2 Although this is important, the priority at this time is to assure that the mother understands how serious a problem diarrhea can be.
3 This is important but not the priority; diarrhea can be contracted despite cleanliness.

194. 4 **"Tenting" when assessing skin turgor, increased depth of respirations, and scanty urine—in conjunction with prolonged vomiting—reflect dehydration and metabolic alkalosis; metabolic alkalosis results from hydrochloric acid and potassium depletion. (3) (PB; CJ; AS)**
1 Although these assessments would eventually be made, they are not the immediate priority.
2 Although this information should eventually be obtained, it is not the priority.
3 Same as answer 2.

195. 1 **The outcome of surgery can be altered by uncorrected metabolic alkalosis caused by prolonged vomiting preoperatively. (3) (PB; CJ; AN)**
2 This is only partly correct; there is a concurrent fluid deficit.
3 This is only partly correct; electrolyte imbalance also exists.
4 Respiratory problems are not associated with pyloric stenosis.

196. 1 **In nephrotic syndrome a large proportion of the child's body weight is composed of retained fluid; the loss of fluid would be readily reflected by a loss of weight. (3) (PB; CJ; AS)**
2 It is very difficult to get an accurate recording of output in a young child.
3 With nephrotic syndrome it would be difficult to evaluate return to fluid balance in this way because the edema is generalized, not concentrated in the abdomen.
4 Osmolality reflects kidney activity, not the reduction of edema.

197. 1 **The shift of fluid from the intravascular to the interstitial compartment predisposes to hypovolemia; a weak thready pulse and hypotension are signs of impending shock. (3) (PB; CJ; EV)**
2 Tubular reabsorption of sodium is increased to replenish the vascular volume; therefore, potassium is excreted.
3 This is not a complication of nephrotic syndrome, although pulmonary effusion may occur.
4 This does not usually occur as an early complication; it is a major complication of glomerulonephritis.

198. 2 **At 15 pounds the infant weighs about 7 kg; 40 mL/kg in four hours would be 280 mL; 50 mL/kg in four hours would be 350 mL; 320 mL falls within these parameters. (3) (PB; CJ; AN)**
1 This amount is not enough.
3 This amount is too much.
4 Same as answer 3.

199. 4 **A decreased urinary output will result in retention of potassium, causing hyperkalemia. (3) (PB; CJ; AS)**
1 This is a normal response of a 6-month-old infant to illness; there is no need to notify the physician.
2 This is an indication of dehydration, which is the reason for the fluids being ordered by the physician.
3 The IV fluids ordered will provide appropriate hydration.

200. 3 **Hyperventilation occurs with aspirin toxicity; there is a loss of carbon dioxide resulting in respiratory alkalosis. (3) (PB; CJ; AN)**
1 Decreased renal excretion may lead to metabolic acidosis.
2 The stomach contents would be made more acidic leading to metabolic acidosis.
4 Same as answer 2.

201. 3 **The temperature is altered by aspirin because of increased metabolism, which leads to increased oxygen consumption and heat loss. (2) (PB; CJ; PL)**

   1 This is not directly affected by aspirin ingestion.

   2 Ascites does not occur as a result of aspirin ingestion; it may occur if the child develops liver failure

   4 Aspirin ingestion does not affect the blood glucose level.

202. 4 **These are classic signs of dehydration; an order to increase fluids is needed. (2) (PB; MR; EV)**

   1 It is not common for the condition of these infants to continue to deteriorate once therapy is implemented.

   2 The nurse must have an order for this; also, the data do not indicate that the infant is receiving an IV.

   3 The symptoms indicate dehydration, not undernutrition.

203. 3 **This is a classic sign of fluid volume deficit in infants. (1) (PB; CJ; AS)**

   1 This is within the normal limits of 1.010 to 1.030 for a urine specific gravity.

   2 This indicates adequate hydration; the urinary output would be decreased in dehydration.

   4 Dehydration is unrelated to allergies.

204. 3 **Sodium lactate is converted to sodium bicarbonate; it helps correct the sodium deficit and the metabolic acidosis. (3) (PB; CJ; PL)**

   1 Albumin is a colloid used as a substitute when plasma is needed; it is not used in the treatment of metabolic acidosis.

   2 Saline results in the chloride combining with the hydrogen ion, intensifying the acidosis.

   4 Potassium is not administered until urinary function is restored.

205. 2 **The extremities need to be restrained because the child will use all extremities in an attempt to dislodge the needle. (2) (PM; CJ; IM)**

   1 Pupillary responses are unrelated to dehydration and fluid replacement.

   3 Scalp veins used for IVs are not located in these areas.

   4 The parents can be taught how to hold a child with an IV infusing via a scalp vein.

206. 2 **The present caloric intake for a 24-hour period is 8 oz × 20 calories × 6 feedings = 960 calories; the recommended intake is 108 calories × 8.52 kg = 920.16 calories. (3) (PB; CJ; EV)**

   1 The present caloric intake exceeds the daily recommended requirements by 40 calories.

   3 Same as answer 1.

   4 The data can be used to calculate the child's daily caloric intake (oz × calories × number of feedings), which can be compared with the recommended caloric intake (108 calories × kg of body weight).

207. 2 **Fluid retention is reflected by an excessive weight gain in a short period of time; inadequate cardiac output decreases blood flow to the kidneys, thus leading to increased intracellular fluid and hypervolemia. (1) (PB; CJ; AN)**

   1 This would be appropriate if renal disease or hypovolemia were present; however, other assessments, such as hourly output and BUN values, also would be indicated.

   3 Weight gain resulting from nutritional intake is gradual and weight would not vary on a day-to-day basis.

   4 Weight is helpful in determining medication dosages, but dosages need not be recalculated daily according to weight changes.

208. 4 **Hydration requirements are calculated by the formula 125 mL/kg/day; 33 pounds is equal to 15 kg; 15 kg multiplied by 125 mL equals 1875 mL, which is slightly less than 2 quarts of fluid. (3) (PB; MR; EV)**

   1 This would provide an excessive amount of fluid.

   2 This would provide an insufficient amount of fluid to prevent dehydration and acidosis.

   3 Depending on the size of the glass, the fluid intake could be either inadequate or acceptable.

209. 4 **These therapies cause diuresis; the child should be monitored for excessive fluid loss. (3) (PB; CJ; EV)**

   1 Changes in vital signs are not indicative of impending seizures.

   2 These therapies will cause a fluid loss, not gain.

   3 An increased fluid volume can lead to heart failure; these therapies will cause a fluid loss, not gain.

210. 1 **To prevent fluid overload, the IV infusion should be maintained at the slowest rate possible to keep the circulatory access patent until the physician can be reached to verify the correct rate. (2) (SE; LE; IM)**

   2 After surgery all previous orders are canceled and new orders must be written.

3 This is unsafe; the administration of intravenous fluids requires a physician's order.

4 Same as answer 3.

211. 4 **Safety is a priority; the infant may inadvertently dislodge the circulatory access. (2) (SE; CJ; IM)**

1 This is contraindicated; oral fluids are not administered until peristalsis returns.

2 Parent-infant contact should be encouraged.

3 This is unnecessary; the number of voidings should be assessed.

212. 4 **Potassium is always restricted in the presence of oliguria to prevent cardiac dysrhythmias associated with hyperkalemia. (3) (PB; CJ; PL)**

1 Fat is not restricted; usually it is the prime source of calories.

2 Protein restriction is used only when severe azotemia with prolonged oliguria is present.

3 Glucose is not restricted; it is a prime source of calories.

213. 4 **This allows the child to get a full cup (1 oz medicine cup) without long waits; a full cup, even if it is a small cup, creates the illusion of receiving more. (3) (PB; CJ; PL)**

1 When fluid is limited, a smaller amount should be apportioned to sleeping hours.

2 If the child were allowed to drink as much as desired until the limit is reached, 15 to 20 hours might elapse before any fluid would be permitted again.

3 Although fluids can be limited more easily during sleeping hours, 12 hours is too long for a young child to tolerate.

214. 3 **Metabolic acidosis results from an excess concentration of hydrogen cations; potassium increases; the kidneys cannot convert ammonium (NH_3) to ammonia (NH_4); there is inadequate base bicarbonate to maintain an appropriate acid-base balance. (3) (PB; CJ; AN)**

1 The child has an excess of hydrogen ions, resulting in metabolic acidosis; carbonic acid blown off as carbon dioxide results in respiratory alkalosis.

2 The child has an excess of hydrogen ions from a metabolic problem rather than an excess of carbonic acid resulting from retained carbon dioxide.

4 The child has an excess of hydrogen ions, the opposite of an excess of base bicarbonate.

215. 4 **NPO is maintained during the early emergent/resuscitative phase to monitor and control fluid and electrolyte balance. (2) (PB; CJ; AN)**

1 This is unsafe and interferes with monitoring and controlling the client's fluid and electrolyte status.

2 Same as answer 1.

3 Same as answer 1.

216. 4 **Because of the location and degree of burns, an IV line for fluid restoration is the priority. (2) (PB; CJ; PL)**

1 No airway involvement or oxygen deprivation has been identified in this situation.

2 Until fluids are administered, this is a secondary action.

3 Although this is important, an IV line for fluid restoration to prevent hypovolemic shock is the priority.

217. Answer: 1100 mL; 125 mL × 8 hours = 1000 mL; one dose of the reconstituted antibiotic is administered at 10 AM = 100 mL; 1000 mL + 100 mL = 1100 mL. (1) (PB; CJ; EV)

218. 3 **2.2 lb = 1 kg; 13 lb = 5.9 kg; 150 × 5.9 = 885 mL. (2) (PB; CJ; PL)**

1 This is less than the ordered amount of fluid.

2 Same as answer 1.

4 This exceeds the ordered amount of fluid.

219. 2 **Respiratory compensation to acidosis involves increased CO_2 elimination through hyperventilation, with a resulting increase in pH to normal limits. (2) (PB; CJ; AN)**

1 Hypoventilation would not increase expiration of CO_2 with the ultimate increase in pH.

3 With hyperventilation, there would be an increase in CO_2 elimination, not a decrease; the pH would increase, not decrease.

4 If the child is hypoventilating, blood H ions would increase, not decrease, because of CO_2 retention, not elimination; pH would decrease.

220. 4 **In metabolic acidosis the lungs try to compensate by blowing off excess carbonic acid in the form of carbon dioxide. (3) (PB; CJ; AN)**

1 This is a compensatory mechanism to reduce fever by evaporation.

2 This is not an adaptation to metabolic acidosis; fever with dehydration results from inadequate fluid for perspiring and cooling.

3 This indicates renal compensation for respiratory alkalosis.

221. 4 **The percentage of fluid to body mass is higher in young children than adults, and fluid and electrolyte imbalance with shock can occur more rapidly. (1) (SE; MR; PL)**
    1 Kaopectate may be harmful because it slows the course of the disease by retaining stool containing the virus in the intestine.
    2 Antibiotics are not effective against a virus and may do harm by eliminating normal flora.
    3 There are no antiviral agents for treating viral-related diarrhea.

222. 2 **A low blood pH and bicarbonate level indicate metabolic acidosis. (3) (PB; CJ; AS)**
    1 These findings indicate metabolic alkalosis.
    3 These findings indicate respiratory acidosis.
    4 Same as answer 1.

223. 3 **The child should receive 400 mL plus 140 mL = 540 mL per day. There are three 8-hour segments in a day. 540 divided by 3 equals 180 mL per 8-hour segment. (2) (PB; CJ; IM)**
    1 This amount is too little.
    2 Same as answer 1.
    4 This amount is too much.

GASTROINTESTINAL (GI)

224. 2 **If the infant is dehydrated and rehydration therapy is successful, followed by surgery, the outcome results in full recovery. (2) (PB; MR; IM)**
    1 Medical treatment is not widely used because the success rate with surgery is greater and more rapid.
    3 There is no known metabolic deficiency; hypertrophy of the circular muscle of the pylorus causes obstruction at the pyloric sphincter.
    4 After surgery, the infant should be feeding normally within a week.

225. 3 **Bicycling increases abdominal relaxation enabling the examiner to palpate the abdomen easily. (3) (PB; CJ; PL)**
    1 Abdominal rebound is assessed by palpation, which is done after bicycling the legs.
    2 Abdominal contour is assessed by inspection, not palpation.
    4 Muscular anomalies of the abdomen are detected by palpation, which is done after bicycling the legs.

226. 1 **The vomitus is white (color of milk) because the obstruction is above the ampulla of Vater;**

because the feedings are expelled before digestion and absorption take place, there is avid hunger as evidenced by irritability. (2) (PB; CJ; AN)
    2 The infant is usually not in pain, but cries from hunger; peristaltic waves are common because of hypermotility.
    3 Vomiting usually occurs immediately after feeding; tarry stools are caused by intestinal bleeding, which does not occur with HPS.
    4 Because the obstruction is above the ampulla of Vater, the vomitus is not bile-stained; there is an insignificant amount of distention.

227. 4 **Hypertrophic pyloric stenosis (HPS) occurs when the circumferential muscle of the pyloric sphincter of the stomach becomes thickened; this thickening may be palpated as an olive-like mass in the upper right quadrant just to the right of the umbilicus. (2) (PB; CJ; AS)**
    1 This area is over the cardiac sphincter, where the esophagus and stomach are connected, which is unrelated to HPS.
    2 This area is over the spleen, which is unrelated to HPS.
    3 The olive-like mass associated with HPS is on the right, not left, side of the umbilicus.

228. 1 **This corrects the metabolic alkalosis; fluid and electrolytes should be in balance when the child is undergoing the stress of anesthesia and surgery. (2) (PB; CJ; IM)**
    2 This does not include the necessary fluid replacement.
    3 Conservative treatment rather than surgery would be used if vomiting were not severe and projectile.
    4 This may help restore protein, but it will not balance fluids and electrolytes.

229. 1 **The success rate with surgery is extremely high and produces a rapid recovery; surgery is usually necessary. (1) (PB; CJ; IM)**
    2 Pyloric stenosis is a structural defect; hypertrophy of the circular muscle of the pylorus causes obstruction at the pyloric sphincter; it is not caused by a mutation.
    3 The infant will be feeding normally within a week following surgery.
    4 Once fluids are tolerated, a special diet is not required.

230. 1 **Initial feedings postoperatively consist of clear fluids until tolerance for feeding is determined. (2) (PB; CJ; PL)**

2 An increase in feeding osmolarity is attempted after the tolerance for clear liquids is assessed.

3 Same as answer 2.

4 Thickened formula with cereal is used when an infant experiences gastroesophageal reflux.

231. 2 An elevated position allows gravity to aid in emptying the stomach's contents, thereby limiting vomiting. (2) (PB; MR; IM)

1 This would increase the chance of vomiting.

3 Same as answer 1.

4 Same as answer 1.

232. 2 When there are no complications, the infant is usually feeding normally within a few days of the surgery. (2) (SE; MR; IM)

1 Within a few days of the surgery, the infant will be feeding normally and needs no special dietary modification.

3 Same as answer 1.

4 Holding the infant should be encouraged because it is an important part of the parent-child relationship at this age.

233. 1 Because of the cleft (opening) in the lip, the infant tends to suck in more air than usual; burping will prevent frequent regurgitation of formula. (1) (PB; CJ; PL)

2 Thickened formula is given to an infant with reflux problems, such as vomiting after each feeding.

3 The baby should be held while being fed.

4 The infant's bottle should never be propped; the infant can aspirate.

234. 1 Because of the anomalous structure of the upper lip, the neonate may have difficulty sucking on a nipple; duckbill nipples and other modified devices may have to be used. (1) (PB; CJ; PL)

2 This is not an immediate concern; it is necessary after surgery to prevent tension on the suture line.

3 The infant should be cuddled like any newborn.

4 The cleft lip does not predispose the neonate to infection; difficulty in feeding is the main problem.

235. 3 Feeding with a syringe provides nutrition without placing stress on the suture line. (2) (PB; CJ; IM)

1 A spoon may injure the suture line.

2 Sucking stresses the suture line.

4 This is unnecessary; fluid can be taken orally.

236. 4 Meticulous care of the suture line is necessary because inflammation and sloughing of tissue disrupt healing. (1) (PB; CJ; IM)

1 This would be done throughout the feeding; the priority care after a feeding is cleansing the suture line.

2 This is contraindicated; the infant may rub the face on the sheet and irritate the suture line.

3 The infant can be cuddled at all times; priority care after feeding is cleansing the suture line.

237. 1 This is important; crying would put tension on the suture line. (2) (SE; CJ; PL)

2 The infant should be out of restraints periodically.

3 This is unnecessary; the infant should have no respiratory difficulty.

4 The infant needs to be cuddled frequently; parents are encouraged to pick the baby up as much as possible.

238. 2 Galactosemia results from an absence of the hepatic enzyme that converts galactose to glucose. (2) (PB; MR; IM)

1 This is found in celiac disease.

3 Inability to metabolize an essential amino acid (phenylalanine) describes phenylketonuria.

4 When parasympathetic ganglion cells are absent from the colon, megacolon develops.

239. 1 Milk and dairy products have a high lactose content and should therefore be avoided. (1) (PB; MR; IM)

2 Soybean-based formulas are permissible because they do not contain lactose.

3 Cheese and other dairy products should be avoided, since they contain lactose; meat is permissible.

4 Penicillin may contain lactose as a filler; antibiotics should be prescribed, not kept in the home.

240. 2 A 15-month-old child's liver should be palpable 1 to 2 cm below the right costal margin. (3) (PB; CJ; AS)

1 The anterior fontanelle closes at about 18 months of age.

3 Abdominal or diaphragmatic breathing is expected in children younger than 7 years of age.

4 This is within normal range (100 to 110 beats/min) for a 15-month-old child.

241. 1 **Sucking and swallowing (the infant's response to a pacifier) reduce gagging and facilitate the insertion of the nasogastric tube. (3) (PB; CJ; PL)**
2 A small amount of gastric juice is always present and will appear in the tube.
3 The tube is passed 9 to 10 inches, the distance from the tip of the nose to the distal end of the sternum.
4 These signs indicate that the tube has passed into the larynx, not the stomach.

242. 2 **This indicates that the tube may be in the trachea rather than the stomach; the tube should be removed, reinserted, and verified for its placement before beginning the feeding. (3) (PB; LE; IM)**
1 This is unsafe and would result in aspiration if the tube were not in the stomach.
3 The feeding should not begin until the tube definitely is in the stomach.
4 This is unnecessary because this assessment would provide no information about the placement of the nasogastric tube.

243. 2 **This position limits the potential for aspiration; the infant will be partially upright, and fluid is held in the stomach by gravity. (2) (SE; CJ; IM)**
1 This position allows gastric reflux and may lead to aspiration.
3 Same as answer 1.
4 Same as answer 1.

244. 1 **This is the most currently accepted form of therapy: the thickened formula and gravity limit reflux. (2) (PB; CJ; PL)**
2 Surgery would be done only if complications, such as respiratory distress, esophagitis, or esophageal stricture, occur.
3 Breast milk can be placed in a bottle and cereal can be added to thicken it; for infants with GERD this method of positioning has been replaced by the prone position with the head of the mattress elevated.
4 A 6-week-old baby cannot take food from a spoon and swallow it.

245. 3 **Reflux of gastric contents to the pharynx predisposes the infant to aspiration and the development of respiratory problems. (2) (PB; CJ; AS)**
1 This would occur with excessive vomiting that produces dehydration, not just reflux.
2 This does not occur because gastric contents are forcefully vomited.

4 There is no obstruction in the lower bowel; the problem is a relaxed or incompetent lower esophageal sphincter.

246. 4 **This surgical repair is done after the teeth appear to prevent damage to the tooth buds and before the child talks, so that the child can speak with the proper anatomic structures in place in the mouth. (2) (PB; CJ; IM)**
1 While both cleft lip and palate may occur with other birth defects, it is not always so; most birth defects are diagnosed early, not at 1½ years of age.
2 Focusing on the disfigurement may raise anxiety and precipitate feelings of guilt, which can delay acceptance.
3 This response may raise anxiety; the statement implies that the surgical decision is based on the whim of the surgeon.

247. 3 **The suture lines in the mouth must be protected from accidental harm; because an infant explores the world through the mouth, elbow restraints must be used to prevent the placement of fingers or objects in the mouth. (2) (SE; CJ; PL)**
1 The child should have time to play with toys, but with supervision to prevent mouthing activities that would disrupt the suture line.
2 This is an acceptable position; the prone position is contraindicated because friction from the bed linen could harm the suture line.
4 A nasogastric tube is not used.

248. 1 **Feeding with a small cup is best because liquids can be given slowly without stress on the suture lines; also, using a cup is age-appropriate for a toddler. (2) (SE; CJ; IM)**
2 Feeding with a syringe increases the chance of aspiration.
3 Sucking on a nipple may cause pressure on the suture line; also, a cup is more age-appropriate.
4 Feeding with a spoon increases the risk of damage to the suture line.

249. 1 **Withholding food decreases intestinal activity, thus minimizing the diarrhea and loss of fluid. (1) (PB; CJ; AN)**
2 An electrolyte imbalance is corrected by IV therapy.
3 Stool cultures are used to determine the cause of the diarrhea.
4 Irritation of the perineum is prevented by meticulous skin care, not by withholding food.

250. 3 The organisms causing gastroenteritis are eliminated along with the feces; gloves provide a protective barrier and are used for medical asepsis. (2) (SE; MR; EV)
  1 This is required with airborne, not standard, precautions.
  2 This is not necessary with standard precautions; this is necessary for an accurate measure of intake and output.
  4 Same as answer 1.

251. 2 This reduces activities, allows the intestines to rest, and provides for early follow-up. (1) (SE; MR; IM)
  1 This provides neither for rest nor for more immediate contact with a health professional.
  3 Wrapping elevates temperature; sugar water does not include electrolytes and may cause further gastric irritation; there is no emergency.
  4 Food may increase the diarrhea; the immediate intervention does not support the mother's attempt to manage the situation at home; there is no emergency.

252. 1 This contains milk, which may irritate the gastrointestinal tract in some children. (2) (PB; CJ; PL)
  2 These are an appropriate soft food; they also replace the sodium lost in diarrhea.
  3 These are an appropriate bland food; they are not irritating to the GI tract.
  4 This is an appropriate soft food; it also replaces the potassium lost in diarrhea.

253. 2 The infant weighs 11 lb = 5 kg (2.2 lb/kg); the daily caloric needs are 550 cal (5 kg × 110 cal/kg = 550 cal); at 20/cal/oz this equals 27.5 oz. (3) (PB; CJ; IM)
  1 This intake is inadequate.
  3 This intake is excessive.
  4 Same as answer 3.

254. 4 Whole grains, legumes, and meat are excellent sources of thiamine, an essential coenzyme factor in energy metabolism, with an RDA standard of 0.5 mg/1000 kcal intake. (3) (PB; CJ; IM)
  1 Eggs are only a fair source of thiamine.
  2 Fruits do not contain thiamine.
  3 Vegetables are only a fair source of thiamine.

255. 2 Drainage is promoted by the principle of gravity, preventing fluid accumulation and possible subdiaphragmatic abscess formation. (2) (PB; CJ; PL)
  1 The lungs aerate well in any position if a subdiaphragmatic abscess does not form;

with an abscess, the child will splint when breathing.
  3 Deep breathing and coughing, leg exercises, and ambulation must be employed to prevent problems with immobility; maintaining a constant position does not provide mobility.
  4 Splinting of an abdominal wound is best accomplished by direct external pressure to the site, not by positional changes.

256. 1 Assessment of fluid balance and possible paralytic ileus are important aspects of care after surgery. (1) (PB; CJ; PL)
  2 Mouth care is not specific, and following an appendectomy there is little drainage.
  3 A low-residue diet is considered to be one of the factors leading to appendicitis because it tends to decrease peristalsis.
  4 Dumping syndrome is a phenomenon associated with a gastrectomy.

257. 4 This is the best source of the complete protein that is needed to maintain nitrogen balance. (2) (PB; CJ; PL)
  1 This is a source of protein, but not the best source.
  2 Same as answer 1.
  3 This is high in vitamin C, which is needed for healing but not for nitrogen balance.

258. 3 *Salmonella* is present in animal sources such as meat, poultry and eggs but is destroyed when cooked adequately. (2) (SE; MR; AS)
  1 *Salmonella* infection is not associated with fruits and vegetables.
  2 Juices and ice cream are not associated with *Salmonella* infections.
  4 Cheese and milk carry many organisms, but not specifically *Salmonella*; ham is cooked thoroughly.

259. 2 Kaopectate has adsorbent and demulcent effects; it will keep stool in the intestine longer, which could allow the organism to infect the intestinal mucosa. (3) (SE; LE; EV)
  1 This is an appropriate intervention because it will replace fluid and electrolyte losses.
  3 This is an acceptable physician's order; observation of the client and communication of findings are important functions of the nurse.
  4 This is an appropriate order that provides comfort for a child with a fever.

260. 4 **This is one of the preferred positions to prevent pressure on the perineal sutures following this surgery, which is done to correct intermediate anorectal malformations. (3) (PB; CJ; IM)**

1 Buck's traction is usually applied in the supine position, and this would put pressure on the perineal sutures; it would also contribute to prolonged contamination of the operative site by feces.

2 This would not promote healing of the anal area and could impede respiratory excursion.

3 This would increase pressure in the perineal area; the child may be placed in the side-lying prone (Sims') position with the hips elevated, not with the head of the bed elevated.

261. 4 **Necrotizing enterocolitis (NEC) is an inflammatory disease of the gastrointestinal mucosa related to several factors including prematurity, hypoxemia, and high-solute feedings; it includes shunting of blood from the GI tract, decreased secretion of mucus, greater permeability of the mucosa, and increased gas-forming bacteria, eventually causing obstruction. (3) (PM; CJ; AS)**

1 Meconium ileus is not related to the development of NEC; it is a common complication of cystic fibrosis.

2 Imperforate anus is the failure of fetal tissue to connect early in gestation and is present at birth.

3 Duodenal atresia may be a genetic or environmental defect that occurs early in gestation and is present at birth.

262. 3 **Because intussusception creates intestinal obstruction where the intestine "telescopes" and becomes trapped, passage of intestinal contents is lessened; stools are red and currant jelly–like from the mixing of stool with blood and mucus. (2) (PB; CJ; AS)**

1 This is not as important to assessment as is observable behavior associated with crying.

2 Bowel sounds would not be significantly affected.

4 Accurate fluid intake and output records are important, but they are not essential to confirming this diagnosis.

263. 3 **The higher incidence of HPS among first-degree relatives seems to indicate a hereditary cause. (2) (SE; CJ; AN)**

1 Full-term infants are more likely to be affected than preterm infants.

2 This is not related to other gastrointestinal disorders, even among close relatives.

4 This condition is not related to other intestinal-obstructive disorders.

264. 1 **The cheese increases protein intake, which is needed for tissue repair, and the crackers provide carbohydrates that provide calories for anabolism. (2) (PB; CJ; PL)**

2 Although this snack increases caloric and vitamin intake, it furnishes little protein needed for tissue repair.

3 Although this snack increases vitamin and fluid intake, it supplies no protein, which is needed for tissue repair.

4 Although this snack increases caloric intake, it supplies little protein, which is most important.

265. 2 **Although the exact cause of celiac disease is not yet known, it is believed to be an inborn error of metabolism, specifically an absence of peptidase; this absence results in an inability to digest gluten. (3) (PB; CJ; AN)**

1 This is related to cystic fibrosis, not celiac disease.

3 Same as answer 1.

4 This is related to phenylketonuria, not celiac disease

266. 2 **Steatorrhea (fat, foul, frothy, bulky stools) occurs with celiac disease because of an intolerance to gluten; as a result toxic substances, which damage the intestinal mucosal cells, accumulate causing diarrhea. (2) (PB; CJ; AS)**

1 This is symptomatic of many problems ranging from cutting teeth to leukemia; although these infants are irritable, this is too vague to evaluate accurately.

3 Some thirst could occur but it would not be continuous; this is more a sign of dehydration or diabetes mellitus.

4 This is associated with a urinary tract infection or dehydration; it is too vague to evaluate accurately.

267. 2 **Celiac disease is a primary defect in which the intestinal mucosal transport system is impaired; the inability to digest gliadin results in an accumulation of glutamine, which is toxic to mucosal cells and causes atrophy of the villi. (3) (PB; CJ; AS)**

1 This does not occur in celiac disease.

3 Same as answer 1.

4 The pancreatic acini degenerate in cystic fibrosis.

268. 1 **Because mucosal lesions limit nutrient absorption, there are inadequate nutrients (iron and folic acid) for hemoglobin synthesis causing anemia. (1) (PB; CJ; AN)**
   2 This child's anemia is caused by poor absorption rather than the quantity consumed.
   3 This causes pernicious anemia.
   4 Same as answer 2.

269. 4 **Primary sources of gluten are wheat, rye, barley, and oats; whole wheat bread contains wheat flour or wheat by-products. (2) (PB; MR; EV)**
   1 Meats, in small to average portions, are allowed on a gluten-free diet because their protein is digestible.
   2 Eggs and milk are gluten free; rice is a grain that can be tolerated.
   3 Spinach and cheese are gluten free; corn is a grain that can be tolerated.

270. 1 **Weight gain, improved appetite, improved behavior, and the disappearance of steatorrhea should have occurred. (1) (PB; CJ; EV)**
   2 This is not a stress-related disease; it is caused by a basic defect in metabolism or an immunologic response.
   3 Even when the child understands the disease process, adherence to the diet may be relaxed; in time, symptoms may recur.
   4 It is important to assess this, but it does not guarantee the child will select the foods on the diet.

271. 2 **The labels of foods such as gravy, sauces, and other prepared foods must be checked for hidden gluten. (2) (PB; MR; IM)**
   1 The diet will be continued at least through adolescence if not for one's entire life.
   3 Rice and corn are grains that are virtually gluten free and can be used.
   4 The diet should be high in calories and protein; it should be low in fat and residue as well as gluten free.

272. 4 **Pinworms emerge from the rectum when the child is asleep and lay eggs; these can be collected in the morning on cellophane tape placed against the perianal area. (1) (PB; MR; IM)**
   1 Any eggs on the perianal area would have been removed by the bath.
   2 The eggs would not have been deposited yet because the adult pinworm would still be in the bowel.

3 Any eggs that were present in the morning would probably have been wiped away.

273. 4 **This is an isotonic solution approximating the salinity of body fluids that can easily be made at home. (2) (PB; MR; IM)**
   1 This is a hypotonic solution that should not be used because it can cause fluid and electrolyte imbalance.
   2 This is a hypertonic solution that should not be used because it can cause fluid and electrolyte imbalance.
   3 Soap can be irritating to the intestinal mucosa.

274. 4 **A low-residue diet should have minimal roughage; eggs prepared any way but fried are permitted; refined bread and toast also are permitted. (2) (PB; MR; EV)**
   1 Although meat is permitted, spicy, fried or tough meats are not.
   2 Raw fruits are not permitted because they are high in roughage.
   3 Nuts and jams are not permitted because they are high in roughage.

275. 2 **This limits odor and promotes cleanliness. (2) (SE; MR; PL)**
   1 Milk does not have to be limited.
   3 Only 50 to 100 mL of saline solution should be used for irrigation to prevent fluid reabsorption and retention.
   4 This is expected in the immediate postoperative period; it should be reported on the next routine visit.

276. 1 **With enterobiasis, the adult worm lays her eggs around the anal opening, producing an irritation and thus an itch. (2) (SE; CJ; AS)**
   2 This is commonly seen with eczema or dermatitis.
   3 This may be seen with hookworm infestations but is more commonly associated with a localized allergen
   4 This is produced by a ringworm fungus, tinea capitis.

277. 3 **A specimen must be obtained in the morning because pinworms move to the anus at night to lay eggs. (2) (SE; MR; IM)**
   1 Although important, the infestation must be confirmed first.
   2 A pinworm, not the eggs, is visible to the naked eye.
   4 Although important, toddlers touch dirt that may be infested and then put their hands in their mouths.

278. 3 This infestation is transferred by the oral-anal route; handwashing is the most effective method to prevent transmission. (2) (SE; CJ; EV)

1 Cats do not transmit pinworms.

2 Disinfecting surfaces does not help prevent transmission; washing clothing and bed linens daily will help limit transmission.

4 This is not the usual mode of transmission; the rectal/oral cycle must be completed.

279. 4 Evacuation time should be unhurried and with-out time limits; evenings are often less hurried. (2) (SE; CJ; EV)

1 High-fiber foods aid treatment of constipa-tion; no additional teaching is needed.

2 Increasing fluid intake may help to relieve or allay constipation; no additional teaching is needed.

3 One bowel movement per day makes scheduling easier; no additional intervention is needed.

INTEGUMENTARY (IT)

280. 1 Radiation, or the transferring of heat from a warm object to the atmosphere, is prevented by reducing the surface and covering the child with a blanket. (2) (PB; CJ; AN)

2 Conduction is the transfer of heat from one molecule to another with contact between the two; very little body heat is lost by conduction.

3 Active transport is not related to loss of heat; this is a process that moves ions or molecules across a cell membrane against a concentration gradient.

4 Vaporization is the conversion of liquid or solid into a vapor; it would occur if a person were perspiring.

281. 1 The microorganism causing the patches should be determined; commonly they are caused by candidiasis (thrush), a fungal infection. (2) (SE; CJ; IM)

2 The patches should never be forcibly removed because it could further injure the delicate oral mucosa.

3 Prescribing antibiotics is not within the legal role of the nurse; also, the micro-organism causing the problem should be identified first because it may require treatment other than an antibiotic.

4 A further assessment of the oral cavity should be conducted immediately.

282. 3 Air drying promotes healing; moisture macerates the skin and provides a medium

for the growth of microorganisms. (1) (PB; CJ; IM)

1 This is not the reason for leaving the baby exposed; body heat effectively leaves the body through the head; also, the situation does not convey that the baby has a fever.

2 Although this statement is true, it is not the reason for leaving the baby without a diaper.

4 Same as answer 1.

283. 2 Lying supine prevents incisional contact with the bed and is the preferred position for infants who are not able to turn. (1) (SE; CJ; IM)

1 This could cause stress on the suture line.

3 Lying prone allows frictional contact with the bed and can cause stress on the suture line; it is not recommended for any infant because of its relationship to sudden infant death syndrome (SIDS).

4 Same as answer 1.

284. 3 Touching and cuddling would provide a sense of well-being and relieve strain resulting from restlessness and crying. (2) (PM; CJ; AN)

1 It is inappropriate to sedate an infant to calm or decrease activity.

2 Careful handling will not damage the suture line.

4 Elbow restraints usually are applied to prevent the infant's hand from touching the suture line.

285. 4 The skin integrity of these children is highly compromised because of their constant scratch-ing; they are prone to streptococcal and staphy-lococcal infections. (1) (SE; CJ; PL)

1 This is always important for infants, but the priority is prevention of secondary infections.

2 Same as answer 1.

3 This is the physician's, not the nurse's, responsibility.

286. 1 The baby's nails should be cut very short to minimize injury from scratching. (1) (SE; MR; EV)

2 This is a correct statement; infants with eczema should avoid milk.

3 This statement is correct; woolens tend to further irritate the eczematous rash.

4 This is a correct statement; this kind of clothing seems to be less irritating.

287. 2 Eczema is a common manifestation of allergies in the young child and is often related to foods and clothing. (2) (SE; CJ; AS)

1 Appetite plays no role in the occurrence of eczema.

3 Eczema is an allergic manifestation, not an infectious process.

4 Eczema is not contracted by contact with someone else who has eczema.

288. **2 White spots (Koplik's spots) and the rash with coryza are very indicative of rubeola (measles). (3) (SE; CJ; AN)**

1 Rubella (German measles) does not cause Koplik's spots.

3 Varicella (chickenpox) causes skin lesions rather than a rash and lesions in the mouth.

4 Scarlet fever does not cause Koplik's spots but a strawberry-red tongue.

289. **4 An unimmunized woman who is exposed to the rubella virus may contract the disease and transmit it to the fetus; there is a potential for pregnancy in this cousin. (1) (SE; CJ; PL)**

1 There is less risk if a young male adult contracts rubella than if a young adult female, who may be pregnant, does.

2 If the playmate should contract the rubella from the child, the disease would probably be mild and confer immunity.

3 Rubeola has no relationship to rubella; the sister would be at risk only if she were pregnant.

290. **1 Measles starts with a discrete maculopapular rash on the face and spreads downward, eventually becoming confluent. (2) (SE; CJ; AS)**

2 This occurs with whooping cough.

3 This occurs with mumps.

4 This occurs with chickenpox.

291. **1 Patting the lesions will not disturb them, and calamine lotion is an effective drying agent. (1) (PB; CJ; IM)**

2 This may prevent secondary infection but has no drying effect.

3 This may tear off the vesicles and lead to scar formation.

4 This may minimize scratching but will not relieve pruritus.

292. **1 When all vesicles are dried, chickenpox is no longer transmissible; dried vesicles do not harbor the varicella virus. (2) (SE; CJ; IM)**

2 This is not true; dry scabs do not transmit the virus.

3 Chickenpox is not associated with a high fever unless a bacterial complication such as pneumonia is present.

4 These vesicles are mature vesicles that occur in successive crops; these vesicles contain the varicella virus.

293. **3 The estimation of the TBSA that has been burned is 5.25% for each anterior portion of the arm and hand (10.5% total) and 6.5% for the upper half of the chest; 17% is the TBSA burned. (3) (PB; CJ; AS)**

1 This percentage is too low for the TBSA of the burns.

2 Same as answer 1.

4 This percentage is too high for the TBSA of the burns.

294. **4 If there is no subsequent infection of the burned areas, wound healing should be uneventful. (3) (PB; CJ; PL)**

1 Regeneration will occur unless there is further insult to the burn injury such as infection; grafting should not be necessary.

2 Although partial thickness burns are painful, they usually heal with little or no scarring.

3 Occlusive dressings may be applied to minimize the discomfort of frequent dressing changes; hydrotherapy or grafting is usually not required in partial-thickness burns.

295. **2 Eschar is rigid and may restrict circulation and lead to loss of limb perfusion. (3) (PB; CJ; AS)**

1 This is not the role of the nurse; blisters are a protective adaptation.

3 Although this would be done, adequate arterial perfusion is the priority.

4 This is unnecessary.

296. **2 These grafts use tissue from the client's own body; there is a minimal chance of rejection. (2) (PB; CJ; IM)**

1 This is not part of the therapy related to skin grafts.

3 These grafts use tissue from genetically different members of the same species, usually a cadaver; they are used as a temporary graft.

4 Same as answer 1.

297. **3 Once a sterile object comes into contact with any object that is not sterile, it is no longer considered sterile. (1) (SE; CJ; AN)**

1 This is untrue; a 1-inch border around the sterile field is considered contaminated.

2 This is untrue; the object is considered contaminated.

4 This is untrue; dry wounds are considered clean.

298. 3 Chemotherapy causes severe alteration in mucous membranes; a rectal thermometer may damage delicate rectal tissue. (2) (SE; CJ; AN)

1 Although this may be true, it is not the primary reason to avoid taking rectal temperatures in children receiving chemotherapy for leukemia.

2 Oral temperatures are accurate, provided the child can hold the thermometer in the mouth correctly.

4 Tympanic temperatures are accurate.

299. 1 A child receiving radiation therapy usually has dry, sensitive skin; the nurse should use plain water to remove perspiration and cellular debris on the skin. (1) (PB; CJ; PL)

2 This could remove the marks on the skin which are essential for accurate directions for the radiation therapist.

3 Oil-based products are contraindicated because they may cause the radiation beam to scatter resulting in excessive tissue damage and inadequate radiation to the tumor site.

4 Same as answer 2.

300. 4 Soft bristles will not damage the oral mucosa. (1) (PB; CJ; EV)

1 This would not be effective oral hygiene.

2 Hydrogen peroxide will irritate the mucosa and has an offensive taste.

3 Mouthwash may irritate the oral mucosa and should always be diluted.

301. 4 Head lice are common among enclosed groups of children in nursery and primary schools; the eggs (nits) adhere to the hair shafts, about $\frac{1}{4}$ inch from the scalp; they commonly are found behind the ears and at the nape of the neck. (1) (SE; CJ; AS)

1 This is typical of scabies, which is a mite infestation.

2 This is typical of dermatitis caused by poison ivy and is found on exposed areas of the body such as the extremities.

3 This is typical of tinea capitis (ringworm), which is caused by a fungal infection.

302. 3 Impetigo may develop as a secondary bacterial infection because of breaks in the skin from scratching. (3) (SE; CJ; AN)

1 Eczema is an allergic response, not an infection.

2 This is an extended inflammation that is not commonly found in children with pediculosis.

4 This is a fungal infection of the scalp; it usually occurs by itself, not as a secondary infection to pediculosis.

303. 2 Permethrin 5% cream (Elimite) is rubbed on all skin surfaces and left in place from 8 to 14 hours before it is washed off. (3) (PB; MR; IM)

1 This would not provide an adequate dose to promote eradication of the scabies; the medication must be applied liberally, not sparingly, and washed off in 8 to 14, not 4, hours.

3 This would not provide an adequate dose to promote eradication of the scabies; the medication must be left in place for 8 to 14 hours, not 15 minutes.

4 Three days of treatment is not necessary; one liberal application usually is sufficient to be curative.

304. 1 The nurse needs to gather information regarding the symptoms because they can be related to many factors. (2) (PM; CJ; AS)

2 A developmental screening is not necessary in an acute situation.

3 This is unnecessary; this information is not related to the situation.

4 A child in good health would not be in a high-risk group and receive an influenza vaccination; a rash is unusual after a sunburn.

305. 4 This is a straightforward, truthful answer at a level that a 12-year-old would comprehend. (2) (PM; CJ; IM)

1 This answer is full of medical jargon that the child might not understand.

2 This identifies a feeling but disregards the fact that the child has already asked a question.

3 This identifies a feeling but avoids answering the question.

306. 2 The tick must be carefully removed with tweezers or forceps so that the tick does not further inoculate the individual. (1) (SE; MR; IM)

1 This is an unsafe method of removing a tick; the tick may further inoculate the individual, and the method may hurt the child.

3 Same as answer 1.

4 Same as answer 1.

307. 3 To make effective decisions, baseline information on the child's condition, extent of the injury, and significant past health history are required. (3) (PB; CJ; AS)

1 Authorities should be notified after the injured client has received care.

2 Hyperimmune anti-rabies serum is not a preferred treatment; it is not necessary to obtain this information.

4 Inoculation for establishment of short-term, passive immunity to rabies follows initial

care of injuries; the priority is assessment and treatment of the injury.

NEUROMUSCULAR (NM)

308. 1 Down syndrome (trisomy 21) results from an extra chromosome 21. (1) (PM; CJ; AN)
2 Down syndrome is not infectious in origin.
3 Down syndrome is not related to an X-linked or Y-linked gene.
4 This is not a cause of Down syndrome, although translocation of chromosomes 15 and 21 or 22 is a genetic aberration found in 4% to 6% of the children with Down syndrome.

309. 3 Forty percent of children with Down syndrome have cardiac anomalies. (2) (PM; CJ; AN)
1 This is not a characteristic finding in children with Down syndrome.
2 Same as answer 1.
4 Same as answer 1.

310. 2 A defective development of the spinal cord resulting in lower extremity paralysis is found only in myelomeningocele. (3) (PB; CJ; AN)
1 Hydrocephalus results from associated ventricular abnormalities and can occur with either defect.
3 A saclike cyst containing meninges and spinal fluid may be present in either defect.
4 Infection is possible with either defect because of the exposure of the meninges.

311. 3 Hydrocephalus is a major complication of myelomeningocele, typically after surgical correction. (3) (PB; CJ; EV)
1 Although important, it is not specific to developing hydrocephalus.
2 An infant's output is unrelated to hydrocephalus.
4 Vital signs should be taken every 2 to 4 hours.

312. 1 This sign is indicative of increased intracranial pressure, which is caused by the fluid accumulation associated with hydrocephalus. (1) (PB; CJ; AS)
2 This is a normal finding; conjugate gaze does not occur until 3 to 4 months of age when eye muscles are mature.
3 This is a normal finding; a baby does not do this before 1 to 1½ months of age.
4 This is a normal finding; the head is the largest part of the body at this age.

313. 3 Because the infant cannot be readily held, tactile stimulation meets the infant's needs and fosters bonding with the parents. (1) (PI; CJ; IM)
1 An infant with an unrepaired myelomeningocele cannot be held in the arms.
2 Demonstration of feeding techniques is helpful but may not improve parent-child relationships.
4 This intervention will be more beneficial at a later time.

314. 4 The parents must be taught to identify increased intracranial pressure, since this can develop if shunt malfunction occurs. (3) (SE; MR; IM)
1 The prone position places too much pressure on the shunt; the infant should be flat and turned on the unoperative side.
2 Dry, sterile dressings are applied postoperatively to prevent infection.
3 Cerebrospinal fluid would not drain from the incision.

315. 4 The side-lying position on the unoperated side and use of supports avoids pressure on the shunt; the flat position prevents too rapid drainage of cerebrospinal fluid. (3) (PB; CJ; EV)
1 This is inappropriate in the immediate postoperative period; the infant should be kept flat.
2 Neck supports should not be used with infants; they may cause airway occlusion.
3 The prone position is contraindicated; in the prone position the head would have to be turned to one side or the other which would put pressure on the shunt.

316. 1 Marked irritability could be a sign of malfunction or infection and should be reported immediately. (2) (PB; CJ; EV)
2 Complaints of pain are expected after surgery.
3 A low-grade fever is expected after the stress of surgery.
4 A pulse rate of 100 beats per minute is within the expected range (70 to 110) for children between the ages of 2 to 10 years.

317. 3 This may help to reduce the infant's temperature; chilling should be avoided. (2) (PB; CJ; IM)
1 Alcohol should never be used with infants or children; it causes severe chilling, which can lead to increased metabolic activity and a higher temperature.
2 This fever requires more frequent readings than every two hours.
4 This is not a priority; temperature reduction should be done first; recording can be done later.

318. 3 Children with cerebral palsy are especially prone to muscle tone disorders, including spasticity, which can lead to contractures. (1) (SE; MR; PL)

1 The therapy program must be balanced to promote progress in all areas of growth and development.

2 This is contraindicated because prolonged immobility promotes the development of contractures.

4 In a therapeutic regimen there must be a balance between exercise and rest.

319. 4 The athetoid type consists of slow, wormlike, writhing movements. (3) (SE; MR; IM)

1 The atonic type is characterized by rigidity and lack of active movements.

2 The ataxic type is characterized by rapid, repetitive movements.

3 The spastic type is characterized by hypertonicity of muscles.

320. 2 This infant is too young for long-term plans; different problems manifest as the child grows older. (2) (PB; CJ; PL)

1 Children with cerebral palsy may or may not have cognitive impairments.

3 Cerebral palsy does not get progressively worse; placement of the child depends on the child's needs and the parent's abilities and desires.

4 There is no relationship between cerebral palsy and a lowered immune response.

321. 4 Organisms that cause meningitis are often harbored in the spinal fluid; the lumbar puncture helps determine if meningitis is bacterial or viral. (2) (PB; CJ; AN)

1 More conservative measures, such as medications or positioning, would be used to reduce intracranial pressure.

2 Although some RBCs may be present, bleeding is not a usual diagnostic confirmation of meningitis.

3 This finding would not be relative to confirming a diagnosis of meningitis; more important is the determination of the causative organism.

322. 4 This position separates the vertebrae so that the needle insertion is easier; it provides for better restraint by the nurse. (2) (PB; MR; IM)

1 This position prevents the head from being flexed and the spine curved outward for the correct insertion of the needle.

2 This position is used at times for adults; it is not recommended for children because of difficulty keeping the child still.

3 This position is unacceptable; it does not curve the spine.

323. 2 A positive Kernig's sign, demonstrated by a spasm of the hamstring muscles, occurs when the legs are extended. (3) (PB; CJ; AS)

1 A positive Babinski sign is a dorsiflexion and fanning of the toes resulting from stroking the sole of the foot.

3 Chvostek's sign is elicited by tapping on the facial nerve in the region of the parotid gland; spasm indicates tetany.

4 In a male, the cremasteric reflex is elicited by stroking on the inner thigh; retraction of the scrotal sac occurs.

324. 4 The meningococcal organism is rendered inactive after 24 to 72 hours of antibiotic therapy; therefore isolation is required at least for this time. (2) (SE; CJ; PL)

1 Treatment with antibiotic therapy for 24 to 72 hours will render the microorganism inactive; after that, isolation is usually not required.

2 Meningococcal meningitis is a serious contagious disease; isolation is required for at least 24 to 72 hours after beginning antibiotics.

3 The disease is not evident in the incubation period; because the disease is undiagnosed, isolation would not have been instituted.

325. 1 This precaution reduces the transmission of infection from client to client (cross-infection). (1) (SE; CJ; AN)

2 The enacting of precautions has no effect on the infectious process.

3 This is protective (reverse) isolation; it is not used for infectious clients but rather to protect clients with lowered resistance; for example, clients receiving chemotherapy.

4 Thorough handwashing and careful aseptic technique limit nosocomial infections.

326. 4 Safety is the priority during the seizure. (2) (SE; CJ; IM)

1 It would be unsafe to leave the child having the seizure.

2 This may cause airway occlusion by forcing the chin onto the neck; a small, flat blanket is more effective.

3 Attempting to open clenched jaws could result in injury to the child's teeth and jaw.

327. 4 Clonus is the rapid rhythmic extension and relaxation of muscle groups during seizure. (2) (PB; CJ; AN)

1 This occurs during a tonic seizure.

2 This is not synonymous with clonus; however, a client can lose consciousness during a clonic seizure.

3 Clonus generally occurs throughout the entire body; the movements during a clonic seizure are more marked than the movements of a tremor.

328. 3 **Preventing trauma is the priority; placing the child on the side allows for drainage of secretions that cannot be swallowed during the seizure; therapeutic management is based on an accurate description of the seizure. (3) (SE; CJ; IM)**

1 The child may be injured if held during a seizure; the child is not conscious during a seizure; there can be no verbal communication.

2 Although calling for help is advisable, during the clonic phase of the seizure it would be impossible to take vital signs.

4 Although, if possible, the clothes should be loosened, administering oxygen is useless because the child does not breathe during a seizure.

329. 3 **This is one form (tropia) of strabismus, also known as squint. (2) (PB; CJ; AS)**

1 This is ptosis; it may be congenital or traumatic.

2 This is associated with congenital cataract.

4 This is not related to strabismus; it may be a tic.

330. 1 **Cosmetic improvement is a major goal for children because with crossed eyes they may be teased by their peers. (3) (PM; CJ; AS)**

2 Strabismus does not affect vision to the extent of blindness.

3 Peripheral vision is intact with strabismus.

4 The child may still need glasses because surgery does not always correct the defect and there may be other visual problems.

331. 2 **Behavioral disturbances such as clumsiness are important clues to early identification of lead poisoning. (3) (SE; MR; AS)**

1 This is not a clinical sign of lead poisoning.

3 Same as answer 1.

4 Same as answer 1.

332. 3 **Calcium and phosphorus enhance the deposition of lead in bones, thus lowering blood levels. (3) (PB; MR; IM)**

1 There is no basis for such a restriction in children with lead poisoning.

2 Same as answer 1.

4 Protein should not be restricted because it may be lost through the urine in children with lead poisoning.

333. 1 **Aspirin should not be given to infants and small children because it is associated with the occurrence of Reye syndrome. (2) (SE; CJ; EV)**

2 This drug is not contraindicated for a child who has had oral surgery.

3 Same as answer 2.

4 Same as answer 2.

334. 3 **There is a strong relationship between Reye syndrome and an antecedent viral infection, especially if treated with aspirin. (3) (PB; CJ; AS)**

1 This is not specifically related to Reye syndrome.

2 Same as answer 1.

4 Same as answer 1.

335. 4 **This is a comprehensive description; stating it in laymen's terms prepares the parents for an explanation of therapeutic goals. (2) (SE; CJ; IM)**

1 Reye syndrome is not genetic; the nurse is giving misinformation.

2 Reye syndrome is not infectious, and most children recover.

3 Although the etiology is obscure, it is known that there is a relationship between a febrile viral illness and the ingestion of aspirin as an antipyretic; there may be some residual impairment.

336. 2 **This is a common finding in lead poisoning (plumbism) attributable to the deposition of lead on the teeth at the gum line. (2) (PB; CJ; AS)**

1 Perthes' disease is characterized by pain and hip dysfunction.

3 ASA toxicity affects the eighth cranial nerve, causing tinnitus.

4 This would manifest itself in yellow discoloration of the teeth.

337. 4 **Deaf infants commonly babble until they are 6 months old; if they cannot hear, their vocalizations are not reinforced and often stop at this time. (2) (PM; CJ; AS)**

1 This skill is learned by the infant at about 11 to 12 months of age.

2 Infants with no hearing impairment do not respond to a name all of the time.

3 This is an inappropriate test at 7 months; the Moro reflex usually disappears when the infant is 3 to 4 months old.

338. 2 **Drinking milk from a bottle in a recumbent position may lead to pooling of fluid in the pharyngeal cavity, which hinders normal eustachian tube drainage. (2) (PM; CJ; AS)**

1 Although this is important information, the factor that precipitated the otitis media is more significant.

3 This question is irrelevant because otitis media is an inflammatory response, not a hereditary-related disease.

4 Although it is important to ascertain what medication is taken for otitis media, it is more important to determine if the infant feeds in the recumbent position.

339. 2 **These anatomical differences in young children permit easier migration of microorganisms from the oral cavity into the middle ear, which predisposes them to otitis media. (2) (PB; CJ; AN)**

1 The labyrinth and cochlea are part of the inner ear and are not affected in otitis media.

3 A myringotomy is a surgical opening into the middle ear; placing the child on the affected, not unaffected, side puts the ear in a dependent position, which promotes drainage.

4 A major requirement of this surgical intervention is to keep water out of the ears; therefore irrigation of the ears is contraindicated because it would increase pressure in an already congested area.

340. 2 **The incision allows for drainage, which produces relief of pressure and results in immediate relief of pain. (2) (PB; CJ; IM)**

1 This incision does not leave any scar because healing by primary intention occurs within 24 hours.

3 A myringotomy is performed to prevent the trauma of perforation.

4 This incision is very small and heals spontaneously within 24 hours.

341. 2 **This position facilitates drainage by gravity. (1) (PB; MR; IM)**

1 This position will not allow for proper drainage.

3 This position will promote pooling of drainage in the operative site and may lead to reinfection.

4 This is rare and should not occur from this tiny incision.

342. 3 **These may indicate the need for a repeat myringotomy because of ineffective drainage. (2) (PB; CJ; EV)**

1 This is characteristic of otitis media and does not indicate an infection.

2 Bleeding is not seen in otitis media or after a myringotomy.

4 These are not expected complications of a myringotomy.

343. 1 **Adenoids can obstruct nasal breathing, interfering with the senses of taste and smell; these senses should have improved. (3) (PM; CJ; EV)**

2 Speech should not be affected because the vocal cords are not within the operative area.

3 Swallowing should not be affected because this ability is not related to the operative area.

4 Speech and swallowing should not be affected because these abilities are not related to the operative area.

344. 1 **Range-of-motion exercises are essential to help achieve the primary objectives of maintaining optimal muscle function as long as possible and preventing the development of contractures. (1) (PM; MR; PL)**

2 Seizures usually are not associated with Duchenne's muscular dystrophy.

3 A high-calorie diet may result in obesity, which may accelerate the time when a wheelchair will be necessary.

4 Restricting the use of large muscles may result in disuse atrophy and contractures.

345. 4 **Muscular degeneration is advanced in the adolescent; the disease process involves the diaphragm, auxiliary muscles of respiration, and the heart, resulting in life-threatening respiratory infections and heart failure. (3) (PB; MR; IM)**

1 Central nervous system functioning is not affected by Duchenne's muscular dystrophy.

2 Nutritional problems related to the gastrointestinal system are less significant than cardiopulmonary problems.

3 Although the musculoskeletal system will exhibit marked degeneration, it is secondary to the cardiopulmonary changes.

346. 1 **A headache is a sign of increased intracranial pressure; lying supine increases the blood flow to the brain adding to the brain and tumor mass. (3) (PB; CJ; AN)**

2 Both parents are present; therefore, separation anxiety is not likely.

3 Although this is true for children in this age group, it is not appropriate for this behavior.

4 Although tension can result in a headache, there is no indication that the child is tense.

347. 3 **Refeeding breakfast is appropriate because the vomiting was caused by increased intracranial pressure, not nausea. (3) (PB; CJ; IM)**
1 There is no indication that an IV is in place; if it were, increasing the drop rate would require a physician's order.
2 Since nausea is not associated with this diagnosis, antiemetics would not be effective.
4 This action may contribute to dehydration and nutritional deficiency; vomiting is expected and nutrition should be maintained.

348. 2 **These activities are part of a neurologic assessment and provide information about cerebral functioning. (2) (PB; CJ; AS)**
1 This is not a direct measure of neurologic status.
3 Same answer as 1.
4 This provides information as to skeletal development and brain growth, not neurologic data; a change in head circumference as a result of increased intracranial pressure is not expected in a 4-year-old whose cranial bones have already fused.

349. 2 **Raising the foot of the bed would increase blood flow to the brain, thereby increasing intracranial pressure, and is contraindicated. (2) (PB; MR; EV)**
1 Extreme temperature elevations are likely to occur after a craniotomy because of stimulation of the hypothalamus.
3 IV fluids should be monitored closely to reduce the possibility of cerebral edema.
4 Monitoring vital signs is a major component of postoperative care.

350. 3 **Pressure on the hypothalamus, the temperature-regulating mechanism of the brain, causes temperature imbalances. (2) (PB; CJ; EV)**
1 After an operation, a temperature from the inflammatory response rarely exceeds 101° F; this temperature is not slight.
2 This is not true when aseptic technique is observed.
4 These would not cause such a high temperature unless infection were present.

351. 4 **Immobilization of the spine is most important to minimize additional injury during a further assessment of the child. (1) (PB; CJ; IM)**
1 This is contraindicated because it could move the vertebral column and spinal cord causing additional damage to the spinal cord.
2 This would not be a safe intervention without first immobilizing the spine.

3 Same as answer 2.

352. 4 **This reassures the parent that there is no danger in allowing the child to sleep as long as responsiveness is periodically evaluated. (3) (PB; CJ; IM)**
1 Since there is no change warranting care by health professionals, there is no reason for hospitalization.
2 This is false reassurance; a change in the child's condition is possible.
3 This does not answer the mother's concern about sleep.

353. 3 **A declining level of consciousness (LOC) reflects cerebral edema related to head trauma because after infancy the cranium does not allow for expansion, resulting in increased intracranial pressure. (1) (PB; CJ; AS)**
1 Ocular signs are less definitive for increased intracranial pressure than a lowered LOC.
2 Muscular strength is less definitive for increased intracranial pressure than a lowered LOC.
4 Superficial injuries of the scalp do not cause increased intracranial pressure because the injuries are outside the cranium.

354. 3 **Motor responses are tested by strength of hand grasps, movement, and strength of upper and lower extremities. (3) (PB; CJ; AS)**
1 Drawing is utilized for assessing hand-to-eye coordination.
2 Gait and balance are indications of cerebellar integrity.
4 The Romberg test is utilized to evaluate cerebellar integrity.

355. 3 **Evidence of a subdural hemorrhage may take hours or even days to develop; early recognition is important to reduce neurologic damage. (1) (PB; CJ; AS)**
1 Although important, preventing further damage is the priority.
2 This is contraindicated because it may mask the signs and symptoms of increasing neurologic injury.
4 This is not the priority; the child needs rest at this time.

356. 3 **Children who are mentally challenged can learn concrete concepts faster than they can learn abstract concepts. (1) (PM; CJ; AN)**
1 This is an abstract concept that a child begins to learn between the ages of 7 and 11 years.
2 Same as answer 1.
4 Same as answer 1.

357. 1 This prevents placing undue emphasis on the speech pattern, thus preventing inadvertent reinforcement of the pattern. (3) (SE; CJ; IM)

2 Same as answer 3.

3 This is demeaning; it may decrease self-esteem and increase stuttering.

4 Same as answer 3.

RESPIRATORY (RE)

358. 1 The medulla oblongata contains the respiratory center, and the neurons that supply the respiratory muscles originate here; they produce the rhythmic pattern of inspiration and expiration. (2) (PB; CJ; AN)

2 This is concerned with the control of skeletal muscles.

3 This links the nervous system to the endocrine system and functions as a relay station between the cerebral cortex and the lower autonomic centers.

4 This is unrelated to respirations; this is the thin surface layer of the cerebrum.

359. 2 The presence of abdominal viscera in the thoracic cavity impinges on the lung, limiting the amount of air that can enter. (3) (PB; CJ; AN)

1 A medical diagnosis cannot be used as part of a nursing diagnosis.

3 There are no excessive secretions with a diaphragmatic hernia.

4 The basal metabolic rate is not increased with a diaphragmatic hernia.

360. 4 Placing the infant on the operative side promotes gas exchange in the unimpaired lung. (3) (PB; CJ; IM)

1 This would not maximally promote aeration of the unaffected lung.

2 Same as answer 1.

3 This would not maximally promote aeration of the unaffected lung; the prone position increases the effort of breathing because respiratory excursion is impeded by the weight of the body.

361. 3 Bilateral lung sounds indicate that the hypoplastic lung has begun functioning. (3) (PB; CJ; EV)

1 This is not a reliable indicator that the respiratory status is improving; it could actually indicate that the infant is hypoxic and too fatigued to cry.

2 A normal pH is 7.35 to 7.45; a decreasing pH indicates respiratory acidosis, which can be attributed to decreased gas exchange.

4 Retention of formula is unrelated to gas exchange.

362. 3 The chest was opened during surgery for the sternal repair, and air was allowed into the thorax; the air must be removed for the lungs to expand properly. (2) (PB; CJ; IM)

1 The chest tube is unrelated to the baby's ability to retain feedings.

2 Chest tubes are uncomfortable; also, this response discounts the importance of the chest tube to the baby's respiratory status.

4 The baby did not have a punctured lung.

363. 2 The airway must be cleared of secretions for effective air exchange. (1) (PB; CJ; IM)

1 This would be ineffective if secretions were not first cleared from the airway.

3 This may assist in promoting drainage of secretions only after the airway has been cleared.

4 Valuable time would be lost while the infant's brain is being deprived of oxygen.

364. 3 The course of action is to empty the fluid from the tubing and reconnect it because accumulated fluid may flood the trachea. (3) (SE; MR; EV)

1 This problem does not require assistance from a physician's assistant; the nurse or respiratory therapist, depending on hospital protocol, is responsible for this remedial action.

2 Humidity is necessary to preserve moistness of the respiratory tract.

4 The amount of condensation is irrelevant in terms of recording fluid level.

365. 3 The infectious and mechanical changes narrow the bronchial passages and make it difficult for air to leave the lungs. (2) (PB; CJ; AS)

1 As a result of increased respiratory effort and decreased oxygen exchange, tachycardia may develop.

2 Breath sounds may be diminished because of the swelling of the bronchiolar mucosa and filling of the lumina with mucus and exudate.

4 Costal retractions are unlikely because of the overinflation of the chest with air and the shallow, rapid breathing.

366. 3 The infant is having difficulty with breathing; disturbing the infant frequently causes an excessive expenditure of energy and increases oxygen demands. (2) (PB; CJ; PL)

1 Cool mist helps to liquefy secretions and keeps the temperature down; cool mist does not maintain hydration.

2 Too frequent auscultation will disturb the infant's rest, causing an excessive expenditure of energy and increased oxygen demands.

4 Constant observation, not constant physical disturbance, is important; the infant needs to rest to minimize oxygen demands.

367. 2 **These observations are vital to assess the child's hydration status. (2) (PB; CJ; AS)**
1 The child is too ill to be involved in stimulating activities; energy should be conserved and oxygen demands kept at a minimum.
3 The child needs the parents to limit separation anxiety.
4 Contact precautions are recommended for bronchiolitis; airborne precautions are recommended for diseases such as measles, varicella, and tuberculosis.

368. 4 **Respiratory distress will be reduced when excess mucus is mobilized and removed from the respiratory system. (3) (PB; CJ; AN)**
1 Congealed mucus would obstruct air passageways and increase respiratory distress.
2 Cool moist air will not stimulate this reflex.
3 Cool moist air constricts the blood vessels in the bronchi; if dilation of the blood vessels occurred, airway diameters would be narrowed and respiratory distress increased.

369. 1 **The cool mist provides relief for most children. (2) (PB; MR; IM)**
2 This is not necessary and would probably increase the child's anxiety.
3 This would be necessary only if respiratory distress increased despite the introduction of cool moist air.
4 It would be useless to attempt this maneuver with a child fighting to inhale air.

370. 1 **Swelling and edema in airways with small diameters lead to the signs and symptoms of croup. (2) (PB; MR; IM)**
2 It is the small airway becoming edematous that causes the problem, not mouth breathing.
3 This is too general a statement; it depends upon the specific resistance of the individual child.
4 This causative factor does not explain why only small children get croup.

371. 2 **Wheezing is indicative of bronchopulmonary constriction or obstruction. (3) (PB; CJ; AS)**
1 Clients with asthma often receive corticosteroids, which could cause a round face; however, this does not require nursing intervention.

3 The use of inhalant medications is expected.
4 This is the normal respiratory rate for an 8-year-old child.

372. 1 **Asthma symptoms worsen in the middle of the night because of low epinephrine and cortisol levels in the blood. (2) (PB; MR; IM)**
2 This is not the time that most children with asthma experience exacerbations.
3 Children with asthma tend to feel better in the afternoon.
4 Same as answer 2.

373. 4 **Hardwood floors can be mopped daily and are more hypoallergenic than indoor-outdoor carpeting. (1) (SE; MR; EV)**
1 Stuffed toys are frequent sources of dust and mold.
2 This action tends to reduce the child's exposure to dust and mold generated by the mattress and box spring.
3 Out-of-season clothing harbors dust and should not be stored in the allergic child's room.

374. 1 **Auscultating the lungs for the absence of wheezing that is caused by bronchial constriction is the most accurate assessment to determine the effectiveness of bronchodilators, the therapy for asthma. (3) (PB; CJ; EV)**
2 Respirations are under both voluntary and involuntary control; when being observed, the client may consciously or unconsciously alter respirations.
3 This elicits a subjective response; it is not as accurate as objective data.
4 Common manifestations of asthma are labored breathing, bilateral wheezing, prolonged expirations, and a tight cough; cyanosis usually is not present.

375. 2 **Heat and inhaled smoke-product antigens may cause fluid to shift from the intravascular compartment into the interstitial compartment resulting in an obstructed airway. (1) (PB; CJ; AS)**
1 Although important, a patent airway is the priority.
3 Same as answer 1.
4 Same as answer 1.

376. 1 **The child may have inhalation burns; respiratory tract injury may result in edema causing an airway obstruction. (1) (PB; CJ; AS)**
2 This is an expected blood pressure for a 10-year-old child.
3 This would be desirable, indicating that the burns were not severe.
4 This is expected with burns of the extremities.

377. 4 **Dysfunction of the exocrine glands leads to an abnormal accumulation of thick mucus, a slower flow rate of mucus, and incomplete expectoration of mucus, all of which contribute to airway obstruction. (1) (PB; CJ; AN)**
    1 The endocrine glands are not affected in cystic fibrosis.
    2 This is associated with hyperactive airway disease.
    3 This is associated with pneumonia.

378. 4 **Chest physiotherapy is done midway between feedings to lessen vomiting and increase drainage for suctioning. (3) (PB; CJ; IM)**
    1 This is inadvisable; the infant may vomit and nutritional intake will be impaired.
    2 Doing chest physiotherapy at this time will tire the infant and possibly lead to an impaired nutritional intake.
    3 Same as answer 1.

379. 3 **This test establishes genotype with the lowest margin of error. (3) (PB; CJ; EV)**
    1 The results of this test will not determine whether the individual is a carrier of CF; this may be part of the testing that is conducted when a client is suspected of having CF.
    2 The results of these tests will not determine whether the individual is a carrier of CF; these may be part of the testing that is conducted when a client is suspected of having CF.
    4 Same as answer 2.

380. 4 **Maintenance of a patent airway is always the priority. (2) (PB; CJ; PL)**
    1 An order is needed to begin routine oxygen.
    2 An IV will probably be started but this is not essential immediately; establishing a patent airway takes priority.
    3 This delays attention to the immediate problem of respiratory distress.

381. 3 **Because of the drying nature of oxygen, most oxygen is humidified before it is administered. (2) (PB; CJ; PL)**
    1 Oxygen is combustible and supports fire; it does not ignite; it is not flammable.
    2 Oxygen is not usually warmed before administration; it is cool on routine administration.
    4 Oxygen is considered a drug and therefore must be prescribed.

382. 3 **This reply addresses the client's concern; CNS depressant effects may diminish or sponta-** neously disappear after several days. (2) (PB; CJ; IM)
    1 Administration of medication is a dependent function of the nurse, and the nurse has no legal authority to tell the client to alter the dose.
    2 Administration of medication is a dependent function of the nurse, and the nurse has no legal authority to tell the client to omit a dose.
    4 This is unnecessary because the side effect of drowsiness should diminish in several days; the client needs teaching about the drug.

383. 3 **Antibiotics should be administered with doses equally spaced over 24 hours so that a constant blood level of the drug is maintained. (2) (PB; CJ; IM)**
    1 The 12 hours between the 8 PM and 8 AM doses is too long; the blood level of the drug will drop and the therapy will not be as effective.
    2 Doses are not equally spaced over 24 hours, and the blood level of the drug will not remain constant.
    4 Same as answer 2.

384. 4 **The lateral Sims' position will prevent aspiration of emesis or other obstructive fluid, which could lead to an obstructed airway. (2) (PB; CJ; IM)**
    1 Tongue blade insertion will not prevent aspiration.
    2 The supine position predisposes to aspiration of blood, mucus, or vomitus.
    3 Nasotracheal suction might be used in the postanesthesia care unit; by the time the child is returned to the pediatric unit, it should not be needed.

385. 1 **Capillary beds are closest to the surface in a finger or earlobe; this proximity allows for more accurate measurement of the arterial oxygen saturation. (1) (SE; CJ; IM)**
    2 The pulse oximeter requires no routine calibration.
    3 Capillary beds are closest to the surface in a finger, toe, or earlobe and not on the abdomen or upper thigh.
    4 An almost instantaneous accurate readout can be obtained with the pulse oximeter.

386. 2 **Maintenance of a patent airway is always the priority. (2) (PB; CJ; IM)**
    1 The primary focus now is to establish breathing; the child has a pulse of 50, which can be addressed later.

3 An IV can be started later; suctioning to ensure airway patency is the priority.

4 The ICU can be called once the child's vital signs are stabilized and a patent airway is ensured.

387. 1 The degree of the hypoxia and asphyxia the child had will determine the extent of the neurologic, liver, and renal damage. (3) (PB; CJ; AN)

2 The child is hypothermic, not hyperthermic.

3 Although emotional trauma can be all encompassing, it usually does not influence the ultimate physical prognosis as does hypoxia.

4 Although initially severe, aspiration pneumonia does not result in long-term sequelae as does hypoxia.

388. 4 An upright position helps prevent aspiration; metal tableware is safer than plastic because it is unbreakable; encouraging participation attempts to socialize and treat the client with dignity. (3) (PB; CJ; IM)

1 Using a syringe is essentially a form of forced feedings; in addition, the client should be encouraged to eat solids.

2 Feeding the client in the supine position puts the client at risk for aspiration and choking.

3 A mentally challenged client can easily bite down on plastic tableware and break it.

389. 1 The gag reflex is elicited by pressing on the posterior pharynx, resulting in glossopharyngeal stimulation; inserting the tongue blade on the side of the mouth limits this stimulation. (1) (PB; CJ; IM)

2 Although this is important, it is not the reason for inserting the tongue blade on the side of the tongue.

3 Same as answer 2.

4 Same as answer 2.

REPRODUCTIVE AND GENITOURINARY (RG)

390. 1 The constant seepage of urine from the exposed ureteral orifices makes the area very susceptible to infection; infection must be prevented or controlled because an infection could ultimately lead to renal failure. (1) (SE; CJ; AN)

2 This will not occur because of the constant seepage of urine.

3 Although this could be a problem when the child reaches puberty or later, it is not the primary nursing diagnosis at this time.

4 Although this could occur if the infant is not well hydrated, risk for infection is the priority nursing diagnosis for the infant at this time.

391. 4 These help prevent infection and ulceration of the surrounding skin and prevent the diaper from adhering to the mucosa. (3) (SE; MR; PL)

1 Seepage of urine would prevent ointments from remaining on the exposed mucosa for more than a few moments; also, ointments may irritate the mucosa and result in bleeding.

2 These are contraindicated because they would increase the moisture and temperature in the area, which would enhance the growth of microorganisms and the potential for infection.

3 Pediatric urine collectors would not adhere because of the moist environment; also, the adhesive backing would be irritating to the skin.

392. 2 This is the transplantation of the ureters to a section of the colon with one end attached to the abdominal wall. (2) (PB; MR; IM)

1 This is the opening into the bladder through the abdominal wall that allows urine to flow out.

3 This procedure involves transplanting the ureter into the colon so that the urine is excreted through the rectum.

4 This procedure involves the surgical creation of an opening from the ureter to the skin surface of the abdomen.

393. 3 Kinking or twisting of the tubing, which can result in an obstruction of urine flow, can be easily resolved by the parents. (1) (PB; MR; IM)

1 This is not the first action; the parents should not call the physician until they have attempted to resolve the problem.

2 Although it is important to keep the child adequately hydrated, the patency of the tubing should be assessed first.

4 Although this eventually may be done to assess for distention, the first action should be to determine patency of the tubing.

394. 1 This is the critical period of organogenesis, during which fetal development is most likely to be adversely affected. (1) (PM; CJ; IM)

2 The fetus is less vulnerable during this period because development is almost complete.

3 The fetus is less vulnerable to major anomalies during this period because all major organ systems are already formed.

4 At the time of implantation, cellular differentiation has not occurred; the genital bud appears in the seventh week.

395. 3 Circumcisions are never done because the foreskin may be needed for repair and reconstruction of the penis. (2) (PB; CJ; PL)
1 The penis does not need to be wrapped in petrolatum gauze because no surgery has been done.
2 A cystotomy tube is not inserted because there is no interference with voiding.
4 Hypospadias is not a genetic disorder, although there appears to be some evidence that it may be familial.

396. 3 Immobilization and sedation are necessary to maintain the position of the urethral stent to ensure optimum healing of the newly formed urethra. (3) (SE; CJ; PL)
1 Although this is important, the site must be assessed frequently and safety is the priority.
2 There is no tension device.
4 The indwelling catheter is never clamped because backup pressure may disturb the suture line.

397. 4 The presence of an uncorrected chordee can affect a child's future reproductive capabilities because of the inability to inseminate directly. (3) (PM; CJ; AN)
1 Kidney function is not affected.
2 The incidence of testicular cancer is not increased.
3 The risk of testicular torsion is not increased.

398. 3 This is characteristic of a child with nephrotic syndrome; large amounts of protein in the urine cause it to have a dark, frothy appearance. (2) (PB; CJ; AS)
1 The child may be somewhat lethargic but usually not severely.
2 Blood pressure is normal or decreased; hypertension is associated with glomerulonephritis.
4 These children are usually pale.

399. 3 The semi-Fowler's position decreases pressure on the diaphragm from the abdominal organs and the ascites thereby increasing respiratory excursion. (3) (PB; CJ; PL)
1 Frequent feedings may lead to fatigue and increased respirations, which would further distress the child.
2 This action will not alleviate the cause of the respiratory problems, which is pressure on the diaphragm from the ascites.
4 Oxygen therapy is not necessary; the dyspnea results from pressure on the diaphragm, not lack of oxygen.

400. 3 Severe edema is usually present and changes of positions are necessary to prevent the breakdown of tissue. (2) (PB; CJ; IM)
1 Fluids are not encouraged and may even be curtailed during periods of edema.
2 Active play periods would be permitted during remission but not during the acute phase to limit energy expenditure.
4 A low-protein diet is used for renal failure with azotemia; a high protein diet should be offered.

401. 4 In children with nephrotic syndrome, infection is always a threat because of lowered resistance; the child with a fractured femur is noninfectious and therefore is appropriate as a roommate; in addition, the closeness of age will provide for preschool socialization. (3) (SE; CJ; IM)
1 This disorder is caused by a pathogen; it exposes the client to infection.
2 Same as answer 1.
3 Same as answer 1.

402. 1 The massive edema predisposes to skin breakdown. (3) (PB; CJ; PL)
2 Carbohydrates and proteins are not restricted.
3 This is far too much fluid; the damaged kidneys would not be able to handle this amount.
4 These children usually do not receive blood transfusions.

403. 1 This is incorrect; weight gain must be monitored carefully because it could be indicative of an accumulation of fluid. (1) (SE; MR; EV)
2 The child should be monitored for edema.
3 This is to determine whether kidney functioning is impaired.
4 Steroids are given with milk or food to prevent gastric irritation.

404. 3 The associated anemia with renal failure accounts for the pallor and decreased energy; the decreased appetite and decreased energy are related to the accumulation of toxic wastes. (3) (PB; CJ; AN)
1 Discontinuing the corticosteroids and diuretics, if prescribed, might result in a recurrence of edema in the steroid-dependent child; it is not a sign of renal failure.
2 An elevated temperature probably would be present; an infection would not cause a muddy pallor.

4 Once remission has occurred, usual activities can be resumed with discretion.

405. 3 In view of the smoky urine and the other symptoms, the nurse may suspect glomerulonephritis, which usually occurs after a recent streptococcal infection. (2) (PB; CJ; AS)

1 This kind of pain is found in rheumatic fever, which never results in smoky-colored urine.
2 Weight loss generally occurs with children who have developed diabetes mellitus, not glomerulonephritis.
4 This rash would be related to scarlet fever, with which there is no smoky-colored urine.

406. 4 An elevated ASO titer indicates the presence of a previous streptococcal infection; levels are highest with acute glomerulonephritis, bacterial endocarditis and scarlet fever. (3) (PB; CJ; AS)

1 The hematocrit would be decreased, not increased, because of blood lost in the form of hematuria.
2 The specific gravity would probably be high because of hematuria and oliguria.
3 The blood urea nitrogen level is elevated, not decreased, because of impaired glomerular functioning resulting in azotemia.

407. 4 The glomerular filtration rate is reduced, resulting in sodium retention, protein loss, and fluid accumulation producing these adaptations. (3) (PB; CJ; AS)

1 The blood pressure would be elevated; proteinuria would be greater than 1+; glycosuria is unrelated; anorexia would be present.
2 The blood pressure would be elevated; proteinuria would be greater than 1+; anorexia and hematuria would be present.
3 The blood pressure and urine specific gravity would be elevated; proteinuria would be greater than 1+; and periorbital edema would be present.

408. 3 The beta hemolytic streptococcus immune complex becomes trapped in the glomerular capillary loop, causing glomerulonephritis; it usually is precipitated by a localized pharyngitis. (3) (PB; CJ; AN)

1 The cause is known; prevention depends on treating infected individuals with antibiotics to eliminate the organism before there is an immune response.
2 Clots do not form in the small renal tubules.
4 This is an acquired, not inherited, disorder.

409. 2 All these foods are permitted on a low-sodium, low-potassium diet that the child should be following. (3) (PB; CJ; IM)

1 All but the peaches are high in sodium and all but the butter are fairly high in potassium.
3 A banana is high in potassium and buttermilk is high in both sodium and potassium.
4 All of these foods are fairly high in sodium and/or potassium.

410. 1 These adaptations can occur if the blood pressure remains elevated leading to cerebral edema. (3) (PB; CJ; AS)

2 Although the pulse may be altered and vomiting can occur, cardiac decompensation is not related to cerebral involvement.
3 Although a fever and confusion could occur, anuria is not specific to cerebral edema.
4 Drowsiness, not restlessness, would occur; generalized edema and anorexia are not specific to cerebral edema.

411. 4 Sodium is usually limited to control or prevent edema and/or hypertension until the child is asymptomatic. (2) (PB; MR; PL)

1 The child should not be kept active for long periods because rest is needed; the child will not usually need a long convalescence.
2 The nurse would not give a home phone number; the mother should contact the physician for follow-up care.
3 Glomerulonephritis does not cause such severe kidney damage that a kidney transplant would be necessary.

412. 4 With nephrotic syndrome, the child's blood pressure will be normal or slightly decreased; with glomerulonephritis, the child's blood pressure will be elevated. (3) (PB; CJ; AS)

1 This occurs in both nephrotic syndrome and glomerulonephritis.
2 Same as answer 1.
3 Same as answer 1.

413. 4 Surgery at this age reduces concerns about body image that would occur at an older age. (2) (PM; CJ; AN)

1 Malignancy may develop with or without surgical correction.
2 Maturation of testes starts about age 5; surgery should be done before maturation to prevent sterility.
3 The puboscrotal ring has nothing to do with the outcome of this surgical procedure.

414. 1 Discomfort when urinating (dysuria) is a symptom of a urinary tract infection that is common with vesicoureteral reflux; when voiding, urine is swept up the ureters and then ultimately flows back to the bladder resulting in a residual that provides a medium for a urinary tract infection. (3) (PB; CJ; AS)

2 This commonly does not occur with vesicoureteral reflux.

3 Same as answer 2.

4 Same as answer 2.

415. 4 Because the child has only one kidney, efforts to prevent urinary tract infections, which can compromise kidney function, must be ongoing. (3) (SE; CJ; AN)

1 With a unilateral tumor, a kidney transplant is not necessary because the child still has one kidney.

2 After surgery, sodium is usually not restricted.

3 Fluids are not restricted; adequate fluid is encouraged to prevent urinary tract infections.

416. 3 High potassium levels can cause cardiac dysrhythmias; the normal range for serum potassium in the child is 3.4 to 4.7 mEq/L. (1) (PB; CJ; AS)

1 Hyponatremia is expected with acute renal failure.

2 An increase is expected with acute renal failure.

4 Same as answer 2.

417. 2 This is contraindicated because the pressure of the inflated cuff could disrupt the integrity of the arteriovenous fistula. (1) (SE; MR; EV)

1 Not only should this be done to assess vascular functioning distal to the arteriovenous fistula, but this assessment should be done bilaterally and the results compared.

3 This would be desirable because vomiting or diarrhea could lead to dehydration and an acid-base imbalance.

4 This would be desirable because an inadequate fluid intake could result in dehydration and an acid-base imbalance.

418. 3 A return of cloudy dialysate solution is indicative of infection. (2) (SE; CJ; EV)

1 Dialysis does not affect blood glucose level.

2 There is no danger of an abdominal bruit developing during dialysis.

4 Petechiae do not occur during dialysis treatments.

419. 3 This provides quiet activity that will not jeopardize placement of the peritoneal cathether; also, it is appropriate for the child's cognitive level and allows for social interaction with a peer. (2) (SE; CJ; PL)

1 Chess requires cognitive abilities beyond the scope of a 7-year-old.

2 Although this is a quiet activity, it would probably be too difficult for a 7-year-old to do without help from an adult.

4 This activity could result in displacement of the peritoneal catheter.

420. 4 If the gonococcus organism is present in the genitourinary tract of males, it is easy to identify with a culture. (1) (PM; CJ; IM)

1 This does not confirm the diagnosis; it may identify sexual activity and partners.

2 The gonococcus organism is in the genitourinary tract, not the blood; VDRL is a test for syphilis, not for gonorrhea.

3 Although urine may contain gonococcus organisms, the urine would dilute the concentration; the organisms are more concentrated in the urethral discharge.

421. 2 A chancre is the earliest sign of syphilis; a dark-field examination of the scraping will reveal the Treponema organism. (3) (SE; CJ; AS)

1 A rash is found in the secondary stage of syphilis; if a rash is found, it is too late for early diagnosis.

3 These are late manifestations of syphilis.

4 This is associated with gonorrhea.

422. 2 Proper positioning and fitting of the condom will occur after the penis is erect and should be applied at this time. (1) (PM; MR; PL)

1 Vaseline may break down the material used for the condom; a water-based lubricant can be used.

3 A space should be left at the tip of the penis to provide room for the ejaculate and prevent breakage of the condom.

4 The penis should be withdrawn immediately after ejaculation while the penis is still erect; if the penis is allowed to become flaccid, semen may leak from the loose fitting condom.

SKELETAL (SK)

423. 2 This finding indicates that tendons, ligaments, and bone changes are involved. (2) (PM; CJ; AS)

1 Club foot is not associated with neurologic damage; there is no paralysis.

3 This finding could indicate vascular damage; it is not related to club foot.

4 This finding indicates a positional (pseudo) club foot.

424. 4 **This would not be measurable under a boot cast. (2) (PB; CJ; EV)**

1 This is an appropriate neurovascular check and it is measurable.

2 Same as answer 1.

3 Same as answer 1.

425. 3 **Rough cast edges can cause skin irritation and breakdown; the skin at the edges of the cast should be assessed for edema, signs of pressure, and evidence of skin breakdown. (1) (PB; CJ; EV)**

1 Adhesive petals will not adhere to a damp cast; even if the cast is composed of fiberglass, it takes about a half-hour for it to dry.

2 Lotions applied to the skin at the edges of a cast can promote skin breakdown.

4 The skin under the cast may become macerated from inadequate drying after water immersion.

426. 3 **Difficulty with abduction may indicate developmental dysplasia of the hip. (1) (PB; CJ; AS)**

1 This is a normal finding in a young infant.

2 Flexion of extremities is the normal position for a young infant.

4 Same as answer 2.

427. 1 **The affected leg appears to be shorter because the femoral head is displaced upward. (2) (PM; CJ; AS)**

2 There is a limited ability to abduct, not adduct, the affected leg.

3 This does not occur with developmental hip dysplasia.

4 When the femoral head slips out of the acetabulum, it is easily palpable.

428. 3 **When standing and bearing weight, the pelvis tilts downward instead of upward, indicating a positive Trendelenburg's sign. (3) (PM; CJ; AS)**

1 This position would not accomplish the desired effect because weight bearing is needed to tilt the pelvis.

2 Same as answer 1.

4 Same as answer 1.

429. 4 **This is the basis for abduction devices (e.g., Pavlik harness) and spica casts when the infant is very young. (1) (PM; MR; AN)**

1 This may be true, but the easy moldability of the bones at this age favors corrective devices.

2 Congenital hip dysplasia usually is not painful and does not limit ambulation for the young child.

3 Traction is not used to correct developmental dysplasia of the hip.

430. 1 **This suggestion is supportive, constructive, practical, and factual. (2) (PB; CJ; IM)**

2 This may keep the area above the opening clean; there will be no protection beneath the area.

3 This response gives neither a suggestion nor support to the mother.

4 Although water may or may not cause dissolution of cast material, the baby may inhale baby powder dust, which may cause respiratory difficulties and should be avoided.

431. 2 **This may be indicative of an infection under the cast and would probably cause a fever. (1) (SE; CJ; AS)**

1 Respirations may increase but do not become irregular with a fever.

3 This would not cause a fever; it may indicate neurovascular impairment.

4 This would not cause a fever.

432. 2 **This is a common, realistic fear; the child should be encouraged to ventilate concerns. (2) (PM; MR; PL)**

1 The gait depends on the needs and abilities of the child; the gait used would be the one with the widest base of support.

3 Same as answer 1.

4 Plastic tips would be too slippery; crutch tips should be made of rubber.

433. 4 **This provides the maximum base of support when the adolescent ambulates and does not put pressure on the brachial plexus. (2) (SE; CJ; IM)**

1 This is unsafe because it would cause trauma to the brachial plexus.

2 The elbows should be flexed, not extended, when holding the crossbars.

3 This is unsafe because it would cause trauma to the brachial plexus; the crutches would be too short.

434. 3 The crutch is positioned on the unaffected side and advanced with the affected leg; the crutch supports the body's weight while the client is walking on the affected leg. (3) (PB; CJ; EV)
    1 The crutch should be used on the stairs to provide a wide base and extra support when going up or down the stairs.
    2 This would place the affected foot in a weight bearing position without support, defeating the purpose of using the crutch.
    4 A sprained ankle should heal in less than one week and the crutch would no longer be needed.

435. 4 Moist heat increases circulation to the involved areas, thereby reducing the swelling and relieving joint pain and stiffness. (2) (PB; CJ; IM)
    1 Immobilization until pain is completely gone would contribute to contracture deformity.
    2 This is contraindicated because it will promote flexion contractures.
    3 This will aggravate the inflammation and cause more pain.

436. 3 Severe joint pain and swelling cause the child to immobilize the affected parts for prolonged periods, causing joint deformities. (2) (PB; CJ; PL)
    1 The rheumatoid process is inflammatory but usually non-infectious.
    2 Bleeding into the joints is not part of the rheumatoid process, but this may occur if the client is on prolonged salicylate therapy.
    4 Rheumatoid arthritis bears no relationship to the mental development of the child but it may contribute to a physical developmental delay.

437. 2 The exercises are done to preserve function by mobilizing restricted joint motion. (2) (PB; CJ; EV)
    1 Exercises are done to restore joint function; they do not necessarily relieve pain.
    3 Circulation is not affected by the arthritic process.
    4 Exercising does not affect the subcutaneous nodules in the joints

438. 4 Prolonged sitting or lying in one position can lead to stiffness and flexion contractures and should be avoided. (1) (PB; MR; IM)
    1 This helps to maintain joint mobility, which is advantageous.
    2 This promotes functional movement and would be advantageous.
    3 This helps maintain muscle tone and is advantageous.

439. 3 Cool fingers are a sign of circulatory impairment caused by the pressure of the cast; however, if both hands feel cool, it indicates some factor other than circulatory impairment is responsible. (1) (PB; CJ; EV)
    1 This should not be done without a physician's order.
    2 Further assessment to determine the cause of temperature change is indicated before taking immediate remedial action.
    4 Further assessment should be done before informing the physician.

440. 4 The dark stain indicates that there is bleeding; by circling the area the nurse could determine that more bleeding has occurred when the stained area spreads beyond the circle. (2) (PB; CJ; IM)
    1 This is a premature action; a compound fracture may bleed initially and the site should continue to be monitored; if the stain extends beyond the initial stain, then the physician should be notified.
    2 This is contraindicated because it would remove the evidence that there was bleeding; there would be no baseline for future assessments.
    3 The professional nurse should recognize that the stain is blood, not coloring matter.

441. 1 Injuries in various stages of healing are the classic sign of child abuse. (1) (PI; CJ; AS)
    2 This can be evaluated after child abuse has been ruled out.
    3 Same as answer 2.
    4 Same as answer 2.

442. 4 This is an independent nursing intervention that will produce sufficient countertraction to keep the weights off the floor. (2) (PB; CJ; IM)
    1 This would decrease countertraction and keep the weights on the floor.
    2 Same as answer 1.
    3 This is unnecessary; intervening to maintain correct traction is within the scope of nursing practice.

443. 1 The child should be rolled as one unit, with shoulders and hips turned at the same time to prevent injury. (1) (PB; CJ; IM)
    2 The crossbar is not used to turn because it may dislodge and weaken the cast.
    3 This would be used for lifting, not turning.
    4 The child will not be able to sit up because the cast immobilizes the hips.

444. 3 A pressure dressing will control hemorrhage until surgical intervention can be instituted. (3) (PB; CJ; PL)

1 A hemostat is not practical since bleeding can be internal.

2 While a tourniquet can readily be applied, the residual limb may be damaged.

4 This is the antidote for an excessive amount of heparin; the client is not receiving heparin.

445. 1 **The prone position will prevent flexion contractures of the affected limb. (2) (PB; CJ; PL)**

2 Sitting would contribute to flexion contractures, especially when prolonged, and should be avoided.

3 Supine with pillows between the thighs would promote external rotation and hip abduction contributing to contractures.

4 Elevating the residual limb after the first 24 hours would cause flexion contractures.

446. 3 **Preadolescence is the time when scoliosis is most likely to become evident. (2) (PM; CJ; AN)**

1 Although scoliosis may occur at any time, idiopathic scoliosis, the most common type, tends to become evident during the preadolescent growth spurt.

2 Same as answer 1.

4 Same as answer 1.

447. 2 **This reflects positive internal motivation, which would probably maintain the child's interest and willingness to continue with the program. (2) (PM; CJ; EV)**

1 This focuses on the brother rather than the child's need to do them.

3 This reflects that the exercises are done to please others; this is external motivation, which is not as desirable as internal motivation.

4 Same as answer 2.

448. 4 **As the child grows, the curvature may progress despite the exercise program; the child should be checked often because a brace may become necessary. (3) (PM; CJ; IM)**

1 A brace may or may not be necessary; specific daily exercises may be all that are necessary for functional scoliosis.

2 The younger the child is, the longer the need to exercise; the program should be continued until growth is complete.

3 Surgery may not be necessary if the exercises are done regularly.

449. 1 **Logrolling is necessary to prevent damage to the newly positioned vertebrae and spinal nerves. (2) (PB; CJ; PL)**

2 Checking the dressing is done for all postoperative clients; this action is nonspecific.

3 Coughing and deep breathing are done on all postoperative clients; this action is nonspecific.

4 The client who had a spinal fusion can be turned and still protected from injury by logrolling.

DRUG-RELATED RESPONSES (DR)

450. 1 **Bradycardia (pulse rate less than 90 to 110 beats/minute in infants) is an early sign of digitalis toxicity. (3) (SE; MR; IM)**

2 Additional dosages of digoxin would add to the toxicity.

3 The medication should be stopped; when bradycardia is no longer present, the physician may modify the dosage.

4 This is not a reliable source; the nurse should rely on previous pulse readings before the digoxin was prescribed.

451. 3 **Vomiting is a classic sign of digoxin toxicity, and the physician must be notified. (3) (PB; MR; EV)**

1 This is rarely needed because Aldactone spares potassium.

2 This is rarely necessary except when the heart condition is severe; infants are usually not overactive.

4 There is no restriction on taking aspirin with Aldactone; however, infants and children are generally not given aspirin because of its association with Reye syndrome.

452. 3 **An additional dose may cause overdosage leading to digitalis toxicity; it is better to omit. (3) (SE; MR; IM)**

1 This may cause overdosage leading to digitalis toxicity.

2 Same answer as 1.

4 This is not a reliable method for determining a missed dose; 90 to 110 bpm is within the expected range for this age.

453. 2 **Vomiting and feeding difficulties are early signs of digoxin toxicity. (2) (PB; MR; IM)**

1 The pulse rate of an infant receiving digoxin should remain above 100 beats per minute.

3 This is expected; infants routinely require several naps, and a child with heart disease requires even more rest periods daily.

4 Cyanosis will be pronounced in a crying infant with heart disease because the energy expenditure exceeds the body's ability to meet the oxygen demand.

454. 3 Drowsiness frequently is a side effect of barbi-turate therapy because it depresses the central nervous system; the child will adapt to this over time. (3) (PB; MR; IM)
1 Stimulants are not routinely administered because they would counteract the desired effect of seizure reduction.
2 This response demonstrates little understanding of barbiturate therapy.
4 This negates the mother's concerns about the drug's side effects.

455. 1 This may reduce the risk of gingival hyperplasia, a common side effect of Dilantin. (2) (PB; MR; EV)
2 Avoidance of overeating and of overhydration may result in better seizure control.
3 The drug is strongly alkaline and should be administered with meals to avoid gastric irritation.
4 A pink, not reddish-brown, color may occur during drug excretion; it is not a complication.

456. 2 This is the correct amount; no conversion is necessary because desired and available dosages are both in milligrams. (2) (PB; CJ; AN)
1 This is too little.
3 This is too much.
4 Same as answer 3.

457. 1 Constipation is a common side effect of vin-cristine because gastrointestinal motility is slowed. (3) (PB; CJ; EV)
2 This is not a toxic effect of prednisone.
3 An enlarged spleen would put pressure on the stomach and diaphragm, not on the large bowel.
4 This is not likely.

458. 2 Pilocarpine is a cholinergic that is applied to the skin to stimulate sweat production. (3) (PB; CJ; IM)
1 This is not the action of pilocarpine.
3 Same as answer 1.
4 Same as answer 1.

459. 4 Pancreatic enzyme replacement (Pancrease) is needed because pancreatic enzymes are absent in children with cystic fibrosis. (1) (PB; CJ; AN)
1 Pancrease promotes the body's ability to metabolize and absorb fat rather than excrete it.
2 This is not the effect of Pancrease; Pancrease contains enzymes to break down fats, proteins, and carbohydrates.

3 Same as answer 2.

460. 1 Pancreatic enzyme replacements are given just before or with every meal to help aid digestion. (2) (PB; MR; EV)
2 The medication must be given just before or with every meal to aid digestion.
3 Breaking up and dissolving the medication will enhance its degradation by gastric secretions and interfere with its efficiency.
4 Same as answer 2.

461. 4 Assessing the level of consciousness is primary in the postoperative period; opioids may depress responses and interfere with an accurate assessment. (2) (PB; CJ; AN)
1 This is an inadequate justification for withholding opioids.
2 Opioids are used judiciously for children who require them.
3 Although opioids are addicting, long-term therapy is not expected.

462. 4 Mannitol is an osmotic diuretic used to relieve cerebral edema. (2) (PB; CJ; AN)
1 The bladder is a storage basin and is not involved with filtration; mannitol acts in the kidneys.
2 Mannitol is an osmotic diuretic that does not reduce peripheral edema.
3 Mannitol is an osmotic diuretic that has no effect on the body's glucose.

463. 3 This would minimize oral discomfort; ulceration of the oral mucosa occurs as a result of the antineoplastic effect on the rapidly dividing GI epithelium. (2) (PB; CJ; PL)
1 Although pain may be present, aspirin would be avoided because doxorubicin is also being used, and a side effect of this medication is thrombocytopenia.
2 These would aggravate the stomatitis that is a common side effect of Cosmegen.
4 This is not related to the administration of medications.

464. 4 Because of the suppression of the inflammatory symptoms of infection, such as an increase in body temperature, the nurse must be alert to the subtle signs of infection such as changes in appetite, sleep patterns, and behavior. (1) (PB; CJ; AS)
1 Adrenocorticosteroid therapy delays, not accelerates, wound healing.

2 Adrenocorticosteroid therapy may cause hypokalemia, not hyperkalemia, because of the retention of sodium and fluid.

3 Adrenocorticosteroid therapy decreases, not increases, the production of antibodies.

465. 3 **Because steroids are irritating to the gastric mucosa, a peptic ulcer with bleeding may occur; stools should be checked for occult blood. (3) (PB; CJ; EV)**

1 Steroids do not cause this to occur.

2 Same as answer 1.

4 Same as answer 1.

466. 3 **The child with acute glomerulonephritis (AGN) is hypertensive and oliguric; diuretics (such as furosemide) are used to increase urinary output and antihypertensives (such as hydralazine) are used to reduce the blood pressure. (3) (PB; CJ; AN)**

1 Penicillin is administered only if there is still evidence of a streptococcal infection; heart failure does not occur and therefore digoxin is not necessary.

2 Children with AGN do not have pain and therefore morphine is not necessary; corticosteroids are administered for nephrotic syndrome, not AGN.

4 Seizures do not occur with AGN if the hypertension is controlled and, therefore, these medications are not necessary.

467. 4 **Chemotherapy suppresses the immune system; the child is in danger of contracting an overwhelming infection. (2) (PB; CJ; PL)**

1 Although this is important, it is not the priority.

2 This is a side effect of chemotherapy that is expected and can be limited somewhat with pharmacologic therapy; it is not the priority.

3 Gentle handling is important to prevent hematomas but not as important as preventing infection.

468. 4 **Constipation is a sign of neurotoxicity from vincristine which can result in paralytic ileus. (2) (PB; CJ; AN)**

1 Inactivity can contribute to but is not the prime cause of constipation in this case.

2 Lack of bulk can contribute to constipation, but it is not the prime cause of constipation in this case.

3 Prednisone may cause nausea and vomiting, but it does not cause constipation

469. 2 **Elevated uric acid levels from destroyed cells may lead to renal problems; increased fluid intake helps dilute urine. (3) (PB; CJ; AS)**

1 This will have to be monitored, but it is not of primary importance at this time.

3 Same as answer 1.

4 Same as answer 1.

470. 4 **Children receiving chemotherapy are prone to mucosal cell damage that can produce ulcers throughout the GI tract; oral ulcers are a frequent side effect and cause extreme discomfort. (2) (PB; CJ; IM)**

1 Increased fluid intake is encouraged to enhance the excretion of uric acid crystals.

2 Chemotherapy causes the child to be prone to infection; contact precautions protect the care provider from contracting an infection from the child; it is the child who needs to be protected.

3 This will not prevent the hair from falling out, which is expected; it is not a sign of toxicity.

471. 1 **Many vitamins contain folic acid, which is contraindicated with methotrexate, a folic acid antagonist. (1) (PB; MR; IM)**

2 Vitamins would be contraindicated because folic acid interferes with the action of methotrexate.

3 This is true but does not answer the question; it permits vitamin use in the near future, which long-term chemotherapy contraindicates.

4 This is inaccurate; vitamin use is contraindicated.

472. 1 **Antineoplastic drugs exert their effect on rapidly dividing tissues such as hair follicles, resulting in alopecia. (2) (PB; CJ; IM)**

2 This is not related to any of the side effects of the antineoplastics that are being used.

3 Same as answer 1.

4 Same as answer 1.

473. 3 **The objective of the oral chemotherapy is to achieve a remission and prevent further relapses. (1) (PB; CJ; EV)**

1 If the oral chemotherapy is effective, additional IV drugs will be unnecessary.

2 Oral chemotherapy is an adjunct to other therapies, not an alternative of other therapies.

4 The prime site of metastasis of ALL is to the central nervous system.

474. 4 **Introduction of an attenuated vaccine at this time may be fatal because of the child's suppressed immune system. (3) (PB; MR; IM)**
    1 The child has not developed sufficient antibodies; the child needs booster immunizations but giving them at this time could be fatal.
    2 Administering immunizations at this time could be fatal.
    3 Same as answer 2.

475. 4 **Because Synthroid speeds up the basal metabolic rate, an absence of constipation is a therapeutic response to the medication. (3) (PB; CJ; EV)**
    1 This is a clinical sign of hypothyroidism and is related to a slow basal metabolic rate.
    2 Fine hand tremors are related to hyperthyroidism and would not have been present in an infant with hypothyroidism.
    3 Same as answer 1.

476. 4 **AZT can cause life-threatening blood dyscrasias including thrombocytopenia. (3) (PB; CJ; EV)**
    1 With AZT toxicity, the child would demonstrate agitation, restlessness, and insomnia, not fatigue and lethargy.
    2 This is usually a response to the disease rather than the therapy.
    3 Urinary output is unrelated to AZT toxicity; a decreased urinary output can be related to a decreased fluid intake, vomiting, and diaphoresis associated with fever.

477. 1 **Insulin is a hormone containing protein; when taken orally it is destroyed by the digestive enzymes, particularly pepsin. (2) (PB; CJ; IM)**
    2 The potency of insulin is not just reduced, it is totally inactivated.
    3 This is untrue; insulin does not contain a carbohydrate that would raise the blood glucose.
    4 Insulin is not neutralized, it is inactivated by digestive enzymes.

478. 3 **Continuous insulin therapy allows the child and family freedom to monitor blood glucose levels at convenient times. (2) (PB; CJ; IM)**
    1 The child must still adhere to an ADA diet; dietary control minimizes the amount of exogenous insulin needed.
    2 The pump still requires a subcutaneous injection site; increased flexibility is the major advantage.
    4 Blood glucose monitoring is required regardless of the method of insulin administration.

479. 3 **The basal infusion rate mimics the low rate of insulin secretion during fasting, and the bolus**
before meals mimics the high output after meals. (3) (PB; MR; EV)
    1 The subcutaneous needle may be left in place for as long as three days.
    2 Blood glucose monitoring is done a minimum of four or more times a day.
    4 Most insulin pumps are battery-driven syringes external to the body.

480. 4 **Chelating agents mobilize lead from blood and soft tissues into the urine. (2) (PB; CJ; AN)**
    1 Chelating agents act to deposit lead in the bone.
    2 Free lead is excreted primarily through the urine, not feces; secretions are substances produced by glandular organs.
    3 Chelating agents do not deposit iron in hemoglobin or displace appreciable quantities of iron from hemoglobin.

481. 1 **Humulin N insulin is a long-acting insulin and should be given at lunch time. (3) (PB; CJ; PL)**
    2 This is too late.
    3 This is too early.
    4 Same as answer 2.

482. 3 **This menu is the highest in calcium, which is important because chelating agents pull calcium from the body along with the lead. (3) (PB; CJ; IM)**
    1 This menu does not have enough calcium to counteract the calcium lost through chelation.
    2 Same as answer 1.
    4 Same as answer 1.

483. 3 **Kidney function must be adequate to handle the lead being excreted; if kidney function is not adequate, nephrotoxicity or kidney damage may result. (2) (PB; CJ; PL)**
    1 There is no skin breakdown with chelation therapy.
    2 A normal protein intake is adequate; excessive protein is not lost unless kidney damage is present.
    4 This would not be a nursing function; liver damage does not occur with chelation therapy.

484. 3 **Use ratio and proportion to solve this problem.**

$$\frac{\text{Desired 160 mg}}{\text{Have 250 mg}} = \frac{\text{x mL}}{\text{5 mL}}$$
$$250x = 800$$
$$x = 3.2 \text{ mL of solution contains 160 mg of ampicillin}$$

(2) (PB; CJ; AN)

1 This would deliver less than the ordered dose.

2 Same as answer 1.

4 This would deliver more than the ordered dose.

485. 4 **Antibiotics should be administered with doses equally spaced so that constant blood levels of the medication are maintained. (1) (PB; CJ; IM)**

1 Twelve hours between the 8 PM and 8 AM doses is too long; the blood level of the drug will drop.

2 If doses are not equally spaced over 24 hours, blood levels of the drug will not remain constant.

3 Same as answer 2.

486. 3 **Diarrhea is initially related to GI irritation; later, overgrowth of drug-resistant microbes can result in superinfection, which also causes diarrhea. (2) (PB; CJ; EV)**

1 Vertigo is unrelated to tetracycline.

2 Tinnitus is unrelated to tetracycline; this is associated with ASA toxicity.

4 The opposite occurs because GI irritation increases motility.

487. 3 **Absorption of tetracycline is enhanced when the stomach is empty. (3) (PB; MR; EV)**

1 Food interferes with absorption.

2 Same as answer 1.

4 Same as answer 1.

488. 2 **Gentamicin is potentially ototoxic and nephrotoxic. (3) (PB; MR; PL)**

1 Penicillin reactions are usually allergic reactions.

3 Tetracycline causes discoloration of forming teeth.

4 Chloramphenicol may cause blood dyscrasias.

489. 3 **Probenecid results in better utilization of the penicillin by delaying the excretion of the penicillin through the kidneys. (3) (PB; MR; IM)**

1 This is untrue; the penicillin destroys the Treponema during all stages of its development; the probenecid delays the excretion of penicillin.

2 The probenecid does not treat the urethritis; it delays excretion of the penicillin.

4 Probenecid does not prevent allergic reactions.

490. 4 **Although the exact mechanism is not known, clinical improvement of the signs and symptoms of ADHD have been reported with sympathomimetic amines such as Ritalin. (2) (PB; CJ; IM)**

1 The child's appetite usually diminishes.

2 The child should be medicated for as short a time as possible; the medication should be used as part of a total treatment plan.

3 Ritalin may be given twice a day before breakfast and lunch; it is never given before bedtime because of the side effect of insomnia; Ritalin SR (sustained time-release) is given once a day.

491. 3 **The purpose of administering lactobacilli, normally found in the GI tract, is to help recolonize the normal flora excreted with the diarrheal stools. (1) (PB; MR; AN)**

1 This is not the action of this medication.

2 Same as answer 1.

4 Same as answer 1.

492. 1 **This is expected; parents should be advised so that they do not become alarmed and can protect clothing and bedding. (1) (PB; MR; IM)**

2 The drug will not affect rectal itching; it will eliminate the pinworms, and this takes some time to accomplish.

3 All family members should be treated.

4 Reinfestation is common; the drug may be needed again.

493. 2 **5 mL = 1 teaspoon; therefore 2.5 mL = ½ (0.5) teaspoon. (2) (PB; CJ; AN)**

1 This is too little; 0.5 mL = 0.10 teaspoon.

3 This is too much; 7.5 mL = 1½ teaspoons.

4 This is too much; 3.75 mL = 0.75 teaspoon.

494. 4 **Phenylephrine, with frequent and continued use, can cause rebound congestion of mucous membranes. (2) (PB; CJ; IM)**

1 Nasal polyps may be associated with allergies but are unrelated to phenylephrine.

2 Bleeding tendencies are related to inadequate clotting mechanisms; nasal bleeding may be associated with dry mucous membranes, but with rebound congestion the tissues are full of fluid.

3 These symptoms are unrelated to this drug; phenylephrine may cause hypotension, tachycardia, and tingling of the extremities.

495. 1 **This response provides accurate information; astemizole causes little or no drowsiness or anticholinergic side effects. (2) (PB; CJ; IM)**

2 The administration of medication is a dependent function of the nurse, and the nurse has no legal authority to alter the prescribed dose.

3 Same as answer 2.

4 This is not necessary because astemizole rarely causes drowsiness.

496. 4 Abdominal cramping and distention are associated with inadequate pancreatic enzyme replacement because foods are inadequately digested. (2) (PB; CJ; EV)
  1 The opposite is true; they would have a voracious appetite.
  2 Diarrhea, not constipation, would result.
  3 There would be a weight loss because of decreased digestion and absorption, not a weight gain.

497. 2 Gradual weaning from prednisone is necessary to prevent adrenal insufficiency or adrenal crisis. (2) (PB; MR; IM)
  1 This may occur, but it is not life threatening.
  3 Prednisone may cause a suppression of growth.
  4 Because of its depressing effect on the immune system, prednisone may increase susceptibility to infection.

498. 3 Children are sensitive to the central–nervous-system-stimulating effects of the xanthines, such as theophylline; toxicity is evidenced by nausea, vomiting, tachycardia, palpitations, headache, and nervousness. (3) (PB; CJ; EV)
  1 Tinnitus is associated with aspirin toxicity.
  2 Drowsiness is associated with sedatives or anticonvulsive medications.
  4 This is not related to xanthines.

499. 3 True; this type of surgery results in considerable pain for several days afterward and requires a strong analgesic. (2) (PB; CJ; PL)
  1 The first postoperative day is too early to begin weaning the client from opioids.
  2 Adolescents are no more prone to exaggerate discomfort than any other age group.
  4 A more potent analgesic, such as morphine, is necessary because the pain from this type of surgery is considerable.

500. 2 Acetaminophen is metabolized by the liver and an excess may result in an elevated aspartate aminotransferase (AST), bilirubin, and prothrombin time; hepatic involvement may last up to seven days and liver damage may be permanent. (1) (PB; CJ; EV)
  1 Blood gas results are not the priority at this time; they will become important if the child develops hepatic failure or respiratory distress.
  3 The hematologic components measured in a complete blood count are not profoundly affected by an acetaminophen overdose.
  4 Glycosylated hemoglobin is a measure of diabetic control, not a measure of response to an acetaminophen overdose.

Pediatric Nursing Quiz 1

1. The nurse understands that a child with asthma is receiving albuterol (Proventil) to:
   1. Relax smooth muscle
   2. Thin pulmonary secretions
   3. Enhance intercostal contractility
   4. Stimulate respirations at the CNS level

2. The nurse knows that the treatment of choice for a 1-year-old child who has a risk of a hearing loss because severe otitis media has not responded to antibiotic therapy will probably be:
   1. Myringotomy
   2. Mastoidectomy
   3. Steroid therapy
   4. Lubricating ear drops

3. When teaching a 12-year-old to use crutches, the nurse should teach the child to avoid:
   1. Taking short steps of equal length
   2. Looking forward to maintain balance
   3. Maintaining an erect posture when walking
   4. Looking down to watch where the crutches should be placed

4. A child is admitted to the hospital with acute lymphocytic leukemia (ALL). When performing the admission history and physical assessment, the nurse should assess the child for the common early signs of ALL including:
   1. Nosebleeds and papilledema
   2. Fever and areas of ecchymosis
   3. Enlargement of the liver and spleen
   4. Abdominal pain and reddened complexion

5. The physician orders a gavage feeding for an infant. To determine the length of tube needed to reach the stomach, the nurse should:
   1. Advance the tube until resistance is met
   2. Advance the tube as far as necessary to aspirate gastric contents
   3. Measure from the mouth to the umbilicus and add half the distance
   4. Measure the distance from the nose to the earlobe to the epigastric area of the abdomen

6. A pyloromyotomy is performed on an infant who has hypertrophic pyloric stenosis. Postoperatively the nurse should instruct the mother to feed the infant in:

   1. The supine position to reduce pressure on the sutures
   2. A comfortable position and then rock after feedings to reduce crying
   3. The semi-Fowler's position and then afterward place the infant prone
   4. An upright position and then place the infant on the right side with the head slightly elevated

7. A 5-year-old is admitted to the hospital with a diagnosis of acute glomerulonephritis. A nursing diagnosis of excess fluid volume would be correct if the assessment data included:
   1. Dysuria, pruritus, weight loss
   2. Diarrhea, polyuria, weight gain
   3. Hypotension, tachycardia, hematuria
   4. Periorbital edema, smoky urine, headaches

8. An 8-year-old who is experiencing a sickle-cell pain episode is admitted to the hospital. Appropriate nursing care during this period should include:
   1. Administering analgesics
   2. Restricting fluids until the crisis is over
   3. Applying cold compresses to painful joints
   4. Performing active range-of-motion exercises to all joints

9. The mother of a school-age child asks the school nurse how her child could have gotten head lice. When replying, the nurse should remember that:
   1. Transmission occurs through household pets
   2. Infestation is most common where crowded conditions exist
   3. Transmission just occurs through direct personal contact
   4. Infestation is more widespread among lower socioeconomic groups

10. A client brings her 3-week-old infant to the well-baby clinic for a checkup. The client is upset and states, "The baby cries all the time, and I don't know what to do." The nurse's initial response should be:
    1. "When did the baby eat last?"
    2. "What is the baby's daily schedule like?"
    3. "Did you sleep last night? You look exhausted."
    4. "Why don't you tell the pediatrician that the baby is colicky?"

11. Despite the physical distress and discomfort caused by the activity of weighing, the nurse must accurately weigh a young child with burns because the weight provides a:
    1. Baseline for future growth
    2. Measure of the burned surface area
    3. Basis for fluid replacement and medications
    4. Guideline for dietary and fluid management

12. When teaching a child with the diagnosis of acute glomerulonephritis about the ordered diet, the nurse should explain that appropriate food choices include:
    1. Corn on the cob, baked chicken, rice, apple, and milk
    2. Canned green beans, baked ham, bread and butter, peach, and milk
    3. Baked potato, ground beef, canned carrots, banana, and buttermilk
    4. Hot dog on a bun, potato chips, dill pickle slices, brownie, and buttermilk

13. The most appropriate play activity for a 4-year-old whose arm is immobilized during IV therapy would be:
    1. Watching TV
    2. Reading comic books
    3. Cutting out paper dolls
    4. Manipulating jigsaw puzzles

14. A 1-year-old child with a distended abdomen is admitted to the hospital with the diagnosis of Hirschsprung's disease. When planning nursing care, the most appropriate position for the child would be:
    1. Prone
    2. Sitting
    3. Supine
    4. Side-lying

15. When teaching an adolescent client about diabetes and self-administration of insulin, the nurse should first:
    1. Set specific and realistic short- and long-term goals
    2. Find out what the client knows about the health problem
    3. Begin the teaching program at the client's level of understanding
    4. Collect all the equipment needed to demonstrate giving an injection

16. When planning a menu for an adolescent with type 1 diabetes whose height and weight are average, the nurse should consider a meal pattern that:
    1. Limits calories to prevent weight gain
    2. Avoids using potatoes, bread, and cereal
    3. Discourages substitutions on the menu pattern
    4. Allows for adequate growth and developmental needs

17. An infant is born with talipes equinovarus (clubfoot) and the physician applies a cast to the lower extremity. The nurse knows that the mother will have to bring the baby back to the physician's office for a cast change:
    1. Each week
    2. Once a month
    3. Every other day
    4. When the cast is soiled

18. A 3-month-old with acute spasmodic bronchitis (spasmodic croup) is admitted to the hospital with severe dyspnea and a temperature of 104° F. The infant is receiving cool mist via a face mask. The nurse is aware that the main reason cold mist is preferred to steam is that it:
    1. Dries up the mucosal secretions
    2. Aids in reducing mucosal edema
    3. Is more readily absorbed by the mucosa
    4. Produces a more comfortable environment

19. A platelet transfusion is ordered for a child with acute lymphocytic leukemia (ALL), and an IV is started. The nurse should:
    1. Administer the platelets rapidly
    2. Have the platelets infuse for two hours
    3. Flush the line with 5% dextrose and normal saline
    4. Check vital signs three hours after the transfusion

20. An 18-month-old child is admitted to the hospital with an immunodeficiency syndrome. The toddler has never been hospitalized or separated from the mother prior to admission. Given this information, the nurse, during the initial admission, would expect the toddler to:
    1. Withdraw, sit quietly, and not be interested in playing
    2. Cry relentlessly and be consoled by no one except the mother or father
    3. Initially be unhappy and cry but become contented after meeting roommates
    4. Cry when people enter the room but respond with a smile after a few minutes

21. To evaluate kidney function, the nurse must accurately measure the hourly urinary output

for a 1½-year-old child with severe, extensive burns. The minimum safe output per hour for this child would be:
1. 10 to 20 mL
2. 21 to 40 mL
3. 41 to 60 mL
4. 61 to 80 mL

22. A child with a fractured leg is to have no weight bearing on the affected leg. When measuring the child for crutches, the nurse knows that:
1. The elbows should be in extension when the crutches are held at the crossbar
2. There should be a snug fit under the axillae when walking to provide support
3. There should be a slight stoop of the shoulders when the crutches are used
4. The tips of the crutches should be resting 6 inches from the feet when crutches are 2 inches below axillae

23. The parents of a newborn discuss with the nurse their child's need for immunizations. The nurse should explain the entire immunization schedule, including the fact that after 12 months of age their child will receive the first immunization against:
1. Polio
2. Tetanus
3. Measles
4. Pertussis

24. The nurse can help a child with cystic fibrosis achieve optimum growth and development by planning to teach the parents about the importance of a diet high in calories and:
1. Low in protein
2. Moderate in fat
3. High in calcium
4. High in potassium

25. An 8-year-old has a tonsillectomy. During the immediate postoperative period it would be most important for the nurse to ensure that the child maintains:
1. Hydration by providing cool liquids frequently
2. Aeration by assisting with coughing and deep breathing
3. Airway patency by placing the child in a side-lying position
4. Consciousness by encouraging the mother to interact with the child

26. The nurse in a pediatric health clinic would be especially observant for signs of cerebral palsy in a 6-month-old infant who:
1. Weighed less than 1500 g at birth
2. Had a positive Moro reflex at birth
3. Was born by elective cesarean birth
4. Was born to a mother older than 35 years

27. A preadolescent brings home a note from the school nurse informing the parents that the child should be evaluated for scoliosis. The mother calls the school nurse to ask what scoliosis is. To answer the question the nurse must understand that it is a:
1. Pathologic process involving the vertebrae
2. Concave lumbar curvature that is exaggerated
3. Lateral curvature of the spine with a rotary deformity
4. Curvature of the thoracic spine that has an increased convex angulation

28. After a successful craniotomy for the removal of a brain tumor in a 9-year-old, the nurse notes an area of serosanguineous drainage on the child's dressing about the size of a quarter. The nurse should:
1. Notify the physician immediately
2. Mark the area with nonabsorbable ink
3. Reinforce the dressing with gauze pads
4. Remove the dressing and check the sutures

29. An intravenous line is started in the scalp vein of an infant, and the mother asks why the IV is not placed in the hand as for an adult. The nurse responds:
1. "Putting the IV in the scalp improves the absorption rate of the IV."
2. "Inserting the IV in the scalp decreases the need to restrain the baby."
3. "Veins are closer to the surface of the scalp, making it easier to insert the IV."
4. "The IV solution is too irritating to be introduced through a vein in the hand."

30. A mother brings her 6-month-old infant to the emergency room with signs of gastroenteritis. The nurse should immediately prepare for
1. Insertion of an IV line
2. Placement in an incubator
3. Blood type and crossmatch
4. Intestinal intubation with continuous suction

31. The most important clinical indication of the degree of dehydration in a young infant that the nurse should assess for would be:
1. Dry skin
2. Weight loss
3. Sunken fontanelle
4. Decreased urine output

32. To facilitate optimum growth and development in a 10-week-old infant, the nurse should encourage the parents to provide age-appropriate activities such as:
1. Giving the baby push-pull toys
2. Playing pat-a-cake with the baby
3. Placing the baby in an infant seat
4. Keeping the baby in a carriage in the living room

33. To promote growth and development, the nurse should instruct the mother of a 4-month-old to provide the infant with:
1. Push-pull type toys
2. Snap beads and strings
3. Nesting blocks and cups
4. Soft squeeze toys with squeakers

34. A child with AIDS is admitted to the hospital, and bed rest and oxygen via nasal cannula are ordered. The mother, having just been informed that her child has AIDS, is visibly upset at the child's bedside. The nurse's most therapeutic statement would be:
1. "You must really feel like screaming."
2. "Let me give you a referral for social service."
3. "Your child will get excellent care at this hospital."
4. "It is a shame that your child has become ill so suddenly."

35. The nurse must assess the child who had a bone marrow transplant for infection, as evidenced by:
1. Fever and lethargy
2. Blood antibody titers
3. Delayed bone growth
4. The presence of leukopenia

36. A male toddler is scheduled to receive methotrexate for treatment of leukemia. The mother asks the nurse whether the child can be started on vitamin supplements because he seems so weak. The nurse's best response would be:
1. "Vitamin supplements won't help him feel any better right now."
2. "That's a fine suggestion; I'll ask the physician to order some for him."
3. "Yes, he will benefit from a vitamin supplement and will be receiving it soon."
4. "Some vitamin preparations contain folic acid, which interferes with the drug's effectiveness."

37. The nurse should understand when an adolescent with epilepsy who is taking Dilantin develops status epilepticus that the most common reason for its development is that the prescribed dosage of Dilantin was:
1. Ineffective for the seizures
2. Insufficient to cover activities
3. Probably not taken consistently
4. Maintained at a therapeutic level

38. A 3-week-old infant has just had surgery for esophageal atresia. An immediate postoperative nursing care priority for this infant would be:
1. Giving the oral feedings very slowly
2. Reporting any vomiting to the physician
3. Checking the patency of the nasogastric tube
4. Observing for signs of infection at the incisional site

39. An 8-year-old is admitted to orthopedics after falling out of a tree and suffering a supracondylar fracture of the right humerus. With this type of fracture, the nurse should immediately report the presence of:
1. Bruising near the right elbow
2. Restlessness and apprehension
3. A weak radial pulse in the right wrist
4. Complaints of aching pain near the right elbow

40. The nurse teaches the mother of a 1-year-old who has frequent ear infections that the major cause of otitis media in young children is:
1. Sinusitis
2. Recurrent tonsillitis
3. An inflamed mastoid process
4. A malfunctioning eustachian tube

41. Phenobarbital is prescribed for an infant who experiences repeated seizures. One week later the child becomes lethargic and sleeps excessively. The nurse knows that:
1. Another drug will be ordered to counteract this side effect
2. Everyone has these responses, but the drug must be continued for life
3. The child is getting too much medication and the dosage will be reduced
4. This is probably a temporary response to the drug that will subside eventually

42. The nurse should be alert to identify the early signs of chronic lead poisoning (plumbism) in children such as:
1. Anemia
2. Oliguria
3. Seizures
4. Mental retardation

43. When assessing a child after the administration of epinephrine, a side effect the nurse should be aware of is:
1. Tachycardia
2. Hypoglycemia
3. Constricted pupils
4. Decreased blood pressure

44. A 4-year-old is admitted to the hospital for a diagnostic workup for pulmonic stenosis. The nurse understands that pulmonic stenosis is:
1. Narrowing of the valve between the left atrium and left ventricle
2. Hardening of the valve between the right atrium and right ventricle
3. Hardening of the lining of the pulmonary artery at a point close to the lungs
4. Narrowing of the valve between the right ventricle and the pulmonary artery

45. Three siblings are termed accident prone because of frequent incidents. The community health nurse involves the parents in a teaching program and instructs them to lower the risk of accidents by using discipline that emphasizes:
1. Realistic rigidity
2. Rational consistency
3. Guarded indifference
4. Serious overprotection

46. An infant is born with a cleft lip. The nursing care of this infant, unlike that of other infants, would include:
1. Changing the infant's position frequently
2. Using modified techniques to feed the infant
3. Keeping the infant's head elevated at all times
4. Maintaining the infant on strict intake and output

47. An 18-month-old with celiac disease is placed on a gluten-free diet. A teaching program about the diet is instituted with the child's parents. The nurse knows that the parents understand the teaching about food substances that must be avoided when they state that their child cannot have:
1. Steamed rice
2. Mashed corn
3. Fresh applesauce
4. Grilled frankfurter

48. While informing the parents about the significance and the causes of cleft lip and palate, the nurse should:
1. Emphasize that the two defects follow laws of mendelian genetics
2. Assess the family history for presence of the defect in other siblings or relatives
3. Stress that the defect is rare and will probably never happen twice in the same family
4. Prepare the parents for the likelihood of mental and psychologic problems in the child

49. A 2-year-old requires an intramuscular injection. As the nurse enters the room with the medication, the child begins to scream and flail about the bed. The father is sitting at the child's bedside and gets up to leave. The nurse could best handle this situation by:
1. Allowing the child to say good-bye to the father before giving the injection
2. Asking the father to stay to comfort and hold the child while the injection is given
3. Telling the father that he can return to comfort the child after the injection is given
4. Leaving the room and asking another nurse to come in to hold the child during the injection

50. The nurse generally does not use the gluteal muscle when administering IM injections to young children because they:
1. Fear intrusive procedures
2. Associate this area with punishment
3. Have an undeveloped muscle mass in this area
4. Are able to wiggle and change position when placed on their abdomen

1. 1 **Albuterol is an adrenergic drug that stimulates beta receptors and leads to relaxation of the smooth muscles of the airway. (2) (PB; CJ; AN; DR)**
   2 Albuterol does not affect the consistency of pulmonary secretions.
   3 Albuterol will not affect intercostal contractility.
   4 Albuterol provides no CNS stimulation.

2. 1 **This is an opening into the eardrum to allow for drainage. (2) (SE; CJ; PL; NM)**
   2 Removal of the mastoid will in no way relieve the pressure within inflamed ears.
   3 Antibiotics, not steroids, are used for an infectious process.
   4 These are not used because they obscure the view of the tympanic membrane.

3. 4 **The child should maintain proper walking posture and not look down to ensure equilibrium and avoid losing balance. (2) (SE; MR; PL; SK)**
   1 This is a proper technique for safe ambulation while crutch walking.
   2 Same as answer 1.
   3 Same as answer 1.

4. 2 **These signs of early ALL are caused by unrestricted white blood cell proliferation and resultant decreased platelet production. (1) (PB; CJ; AS; BI)**
   1 Papilledema is not a common presenting sign because the blood-brain barrier is an initial deterrent.
   3 These are not the presenting signs; these occur through infiltration of the vascular organs of the reticuloendothelial system by immature WBCs.
   4 Pain is not an early symptom; the skin will be pale.

5. 4 **Prior to inserting the gastric tube, the nurse measures the anatomic pathway the tube will follow— i.e., from the nose to the earlobe (corresponding to the nasopharynx) to the epigastric area of the abdomen (lower end of stomach); it is then marked and inserted to this point. (2) (PM; CJ; IM; GI)**
   1 Resistance to the passage of a gastric tube may be felt, and rotation of the tube often changes placement enough to continue insertion to the point marked by measurement.
   2 This distance might not place the tube well into the stomach and would increase the risk of aspiration.
   3 This distance would be much too long.

6. 4 **During and after feeding, the position most favoring gravity is employed to promote retention of fluid and prevent vomiting. (3) (PB; MR; IM; GI)**
   1 Feeding any child in the supine position greatly increases the risk of aspiration.
   2 Vomiting may continue postoperatively so limited movement after feedings is suggested.
   3 Postoperative positioning with the head elevated helps to assist food passage; the prone position is avoided to prevent SIDS.

7. 4 **Periorbital edema is indicative of fluid retention; the kidneys are inflamed and the output of urine is lessened; hematuria can occur. (2) (PB; CJ; AS; RG)**
   1 These signs do not indicate excess fluid.
   2 Diarrhea and polyuria would lead to fluid deficit and, perhaps, weight loss.
   3 Same as answer 1.

8. 1 **The first priority is pain management; severe pain requires analgesics. (1) (PB; CJ; IM; BI)**
   2 Increased hydration is necessary to promote hemodilution, improve circulation, and prevent more sickling.
   3 Cold will constrict blood vessels, further depleting oxygenation to affected parts; warmth is preferable.
   4 There are too much swelling and pain in the joints during a crisis for this intervention.

9. 2 **Transmission occurs through direct contact with infected individuals and indirect contact with contaminated articles; crowded conditions aid transmission. (1) (SE; CJ; IM; IT)**
   1 Head lice are not carried or transmitted by household pets.
   3 Pediculosis also can be transmitted by contact with infested clothing, personal articles, or bedding.
   4 All socioeconomic groups are equally affected.

10. 2 **This provides the client with the opportunity to express feelings and gives the nurse more data. (3) (PM; MR; AS; EH)**
1 This could put blame for the crying on the mother by inferring that the baby is not being fed on time.
3 This is empathetic but gives the mother no opportunity to respond.
4 This is making a diagnosis without sufficient data collection.

11. 3 **Body weight is used in the calculation of body surface area; it is the main criterion for determining drug dosage and fluid requirements. (3) (PB; CJ; AN; IT)**
1 It is inappropriate to be concerned about growth in the face of an acute situation.
2 Measurement of the burned surface is determined by the parts of the body involved.
4 Dietary management is a later consideration.

12. 1 **All these foods are permitted on low-sodium, low-potassium diets. (3) (PB; MR; IM; RG)**
2 Canned beans and ham are both very high in sodium.
3 Canned carrots are high in sodium, banana is high in potassium, and buttermilk is high in both.
4 All are high in sodium and/or potassium.

13. 4 **This is intellectually stimulating and can be done with an IV in place. (2) (PM; CJ; PL; GD)**
1 This is a passive activity, which is neither the most appropriate nor especially stimulating.
2 The child is not old enough to read.
3 The child needs both hands to do this activity.

14. 4 **In this position the distended abdomen does not press against the diaphragm and lung expansion is facilitated. (3) (PB; CJ; PL; GI)**
1 This position is not conducive to easier breathing, and it is difficult to assume because of abdominal distention.
2 The distended abdomen may press against the diaphragm and hinder full lung expansion.
3 The supine position will interfere with respiration because of the pressure of the abdominal distention.

15. 2 **Before planning and instituting a teaching plan, the nurse must assess the client's attitudes, experience, knowledge, and understanding of the health problem. (2) (PM; MR; AS; EN)**
1 Before goals can be set, assessment must be carried out.
3 Before teaching can begin, assessment of the present level of knowledge is necessary.

4 Before teaching begins, assessment and planning must occur.

16. 4 **As a result of hormones involved in growth and development, adolescents with type 1 diabetes have different and changing needs regarding nutrition and exogenous insulin. (1) (PM; CJ; PL; GD)**
1 Adequate caloric intake is needed by the average-size adolescent because adolescence is a time of growth.
2 Potatoes, bread, and cereal contain necessary fiber and nutrients.
3 Some flexibility is needed to promote adherence to any dietary regimen.

17. 1 **Casts are changed weekly to accommodate the rapid growth in early infancy. (2) (SE; CJ; PL; SK)**
2 This is not frequent enough in early infancy; the cast could become too tight because of rapid growth of the infant.
3 This is too frequent; muscles and tendons would not be stretched and relaxed enough between cast changes to affect foot position.
4 Soiling is not usually a problem because casts for clubfoot do not extend to the perineal area.

18. 2 **Cool mist causes vasoconstriction and reduces edema; it may also help to reduce fever. (2) (PB; CJ; AN; RE)**
1 Heat, not cold, dries secretions.
3 Absorption via the mucosa is insignificant.
4 Cool mist is less comfortable because the environment is cold and damp.

19. 1 **Platelets are rapidly administered after hanging the IV to prevent their destruction. (2) (SE; CJ; IM; BI)**
2 Platelets should not remain in the IV bag for a long time because of their fragility.
3 Dextrose solution is not appropriate for flushing a blood derivative line because the line may become clogged.
4 This is too long an interval; during infusion of blood derivatives, vital signs are monitored more frequently.

20. 2 **The first stage of separation anxiety is protest, which is characterized by loud crying, rejection of all strangers, and inconsolable grief. (2) (PM; CJ; AS; EH)**
1 This would be indicative of despair, the second stage of separation anxiety.
3 Toddlers do not socialize well with peers.
4 An 18-month-old is not so easily consoled when separated from parents.

21. 1 **The minimum safe urine volume is 10 to 20 mL per hour in children younger than 2 years. (2) (PB; CJ; EV; RG)**
  2 This is the minimum safe output for children older than 2 years.
  3 This volume is more than the minimum for any age group.
  4 Same as answer 3.

22. 4 **This provides a maximum base of support when the child ambulates and there is no pressure on the brachial plexus. (2) (SE; CJ; AN; SK)**
  1 When holding the crossbar, the elbows should be flexed and the shoulders straight.
  2 This could cause a brachial plexus injury.
  3 This would indicate that the crutches are too short.

23. 3 **This vaccine is not usually given before 12 months of age because of passive natural immunity from the mother. (2) (PM; MR; IM; GD)**
  1 This is given in the first 6 months of life.
  2 Same as answer 1.
  4 Same as answer 1.

24. 2 **Moderate fat is recommended because of increased caloric needs related to growth and development. (2) (PB; MR; PL; GD)**
  1 High protein is recommended to overcome protein maldigestion
  3 High calcium is not recommended.
  4 Unless potassium levels are low, this would be contraindicated.

25. 3 **Positioning on the side permits flow of oral secretions that could block the child's airway; a patent airway takes precedence; if the child is not able to take air in, all other measures are futile. (1) (PB; CJ; AN; RE)**
  1 This becomes important after a patent airway is established; the child can receive tepid or cool liquids.
  2 After airway patency is established, deep breathing can be encouraged; coughing is contraindicated because it could dislodge a clot.
  4 Airway patency is of primary importance.

26. 1 **Studies indicate that a large percentage of children with cerebral palsy had birth weights less than 1500 g. (2) (PM; CJ; AS; NM)**
  2 The Moro reflex is normally present at birth.
  3 There is no greater incidence of cerebral palsy in children born by a cesarean delivery that is not done because of fetal distress.
  4 Studies do not indicate any greater incidence of cerebral palsy in children born to women older than 35 years.

27. 3 **This is the correct definition of scoliosis. (1) (PM; CJ; AN; SK)**
  1 There are no pathologic changes in the vertebrae.
  2 This is a description of lordosis.
  4 This is a description of kyphosis.

28. 2 **If the drainage progresses beyond the markings, it would enable the nurse to determine that there is an increasing amount of drainage occurring. (1) (PB; CJ; EV; NM)**
  1 This is not an emergency; some drainage is expected.
  3 This would not enable the nurse to monitor progression of the drainage.
  4 In the immediate postoperative period, the dressing is to be removed only by the neurosurgeon.

29. 3 **This provides an accurate statement of why scalp veins are used in infants. (2) (PB; CJ; IM; CV)**
  1 The absorption rate through a peripheral vein is the same regardless of placement.
  2 The infant will still need to be restrained to prevent pulling out the IV or rolling over on it.
  4 Placement of the needle is not related to whether the solution is irritating.

30. 1 **Gastroenteritis causes a disturbance in intestinal motility and absorption, accelerating excretion so that IV fluids are necessary; severe dehydration and fluid and electrolyte imbalance occur rapidly and can lead to death because of the infant's large fluid content. (2) (PB; CJ; IM; FE)**
  2 Incubators serve to isolate, warm, and, if necessary, oxygenate small infants and newborns; a 6-month-old infant does not need the protection an incubator offers.
  3 This test is used to determine blood type when a transfusion is indicated.
  4 Intestinal intubation with suction is utilized to remove intestinal contents when there is an obstruction or when it is necessary to have the GI tract clear of contents.

31. 2 **Loss of fluid as a result of dehydration is most objectively assessed by measuring the infant's weight because total body water (TBW) accounts for approximately 75% of an infant's body weight. (3) (PB; CJ; AS; FE)**
  1 Dry skin may be indicative of conditions other than dehydration.
  3 This is a clinical sign of dehydration but is not an accurate way to measure hydration.
  4 Decreased urine output cannot always be measured accurately in infants and children who are not toilet trained.

32. 3 This is a suggested activity for a 2- to 3-month-old so that the infant can more readily observe the environment. (2) (PM; MR; IM; GD)

　1 This is a suggested activity for a 12- to 24-month-old.

　2 This is a suggested activity for a 6- to 9-month-old.

　4 This is a suggested activity for a 4- to 6-month-old.

33. 4 This is appropriate for a 4-month-old; the child enjoys squeezing and hearing the sound of the squeaker. (1) (PM; MR; IM; GD)

　1 This is appropriate for a child 12 to 24 months of age.

　2 This is appropriate for a child 10 to 12 months of age.

　3 This is appropriate for a child 16 months of age.

34. 1 This statement acknowledges the mother's feelings. (3) (PI; CJ; IM; EH)

　2 This statement does not address the mother's feelings.

　3 Although this statement may be true, it gives false hope for recovery.

　4 Same as answer 2.

35. 1 A fever occurs with an infection because pyrogens affect the temperature-regulating center in the hypothalamus; lethargy occurs with an infection because of the related increased basal metabolic rate. (1) (SE; CJ; EV; BI)

　2 Antibody titers only indicate exposure to the microorganisms, not the presence of disease.

　3 This is not an indication of infection.

　4 Infection usually causes an increase, not a decrease, in white blood cells.

36. 4 Many vitamins contain folic acid and are contraindicated with methotrexate, a folic acid antagonist. (2) (PB; CJ; IM; DR)

　1 This does not answer the question and leaves open vitamin use in the near future, which long-term chemotherapy contraindicates.

　2 Folic acid, which vitamin supplements contain, interferes with the action of methotrexate.

　3 Same as answer 2.

37. 3 This behavior is a form of denial that may occur once the seizures are controlled; also, adolescents have a need to be like their peers, and they avoid anything that makes them seem different. (2) (PM; CJ; EV; GD)

　1 Drugs are prescribed according to the type of seizure and are effective if taken consistently.

　2 The dosage is not based on activity but on the type of seizure.

　4 This is desired and indicates that the drug is effective.

38. 3 A nasogastric tube is used postoperatively to decompress the stomach and limit tension on the suture line. (2) (PB; CJ; IM; GI)

　1 To limit pressure on the suture line, oral feedings should not be used in the immediate postoperative period when the nasogastric tube is in place.

　2 Vomiting indicates obstruction of the nasogastric tube; the initial action should be to check the patency of the tube.

　4 This is too soon for signs of infection to occur.

39. 3 Edema at the fracture site may increase pressure on the radial artery, interrupting the blood supply to the hand of the affected extremity. (2) (PB; CJ; EV; SK)

　1 This is an expected occurrence caused by tissue trauma.

　2 By themselves these do not relate to the specific complication of radial artery pressure associated with a supracondylar fracture; with these findings further assessments regarding pain, bleeding, and respiratory distress should be made.

　4 Same as answer 1.

40. 4 A blocked eustachian tube impairs drainage and creates negative pressure; when the tube opens, bacteria are pulled into the middle ear. (2) (PM; CJ; AN; NM)

　1 This is usually not related to otitis media.

　2 Usually, this is caused by adenoiditis.

　3 This is a complication, not a cause, of otitis media.

41. 4 Drowsiness is a common side effect of barbiturate therapy because of its sedative properties. (2) (PB; CJ; EV; DR)

　1 Stimulants are not routinely administered because they would counteract the desired effect of seizure reduction.

　2 Although these are common responses, they are not expressed by everyone; the length of therapy depends on the client's status.

　3 This demonstrates little understanding of this drug therapy; this is a usual response to barbiturates.

42. 1 The bone marrow is most susceptible to lead toxicity; interference with hemoglobin biosynthesis leads to early signs of anemia. (3) (PB; CJ; AS; NM)

2 This is a late response indicating kidney shutdown; loss of protein and other substances occurs first.

3 This is a serious late response.

4 This is a late response indicating CNS involvement.

43. 1 **Epinephrine is a sympathetic nervous system stimulant that causes tachycardia. (1) (PB; CJ; EV; NM)**

2 Hyperglycemia, not hypoglycemia, may result.

3 The pupils will be dilated, not constricted.

4 Epinephrine is more likely to cause hypertension.

44. 4 **The cusps of the valves may be fused or the infundibulum below may be hypertrophied, thus restricting blood flow to the lungs. (3) (PB; CJ; AN; CV)**

1 The mitral valve is not involved in pulmonic stenosis.

2 The tricuspid valve is not involved in pulmonic stenosis.

3 Pulmonic stenosis is a congenital condition that results from the failure of tissues to develop normally in utero.

45. 2 **Unwavering adherence to the same principles and regulations promotes safe, firm limits. (1) (PM; MR; PL; GD)**

1 This stifles the child's natural development in learning to explore.

3 Injuries are promoted when there is lack of attention.

4 This hinders the child's freedom to explore and enjoy the surroundings.

46. 2 **With a cleft in the lip, the baby will be unable to suck like other newborns. (1) (PM: CJ; PL; GI)**

1 This is common for all infants, not just a baby with a cleft lip.

3 This is contraindicated because the normal alignment of the spine will be interfered with if the head is elevated at all times.

4 This is not necessary because intake and output will be normal once a feeding method is established.

47. 4 **Many frankfurters have grain filler; parents should read labels and, unless they are sure of ingredients, should not feed the food to the child. (2) (PB; MR; EV; GI)**

1 This does not contain gluten; this is a substitute for grain foods.

2 Same as answer 1.

3 This does not contain gluten.

48. 2 **Cleft lip and palate demonstrate a familial pattern of inheritance that is significantly increased when a close relative is similarly affected. (2) (PM; CJ; AS; GI)**

1 Mendelian laws of inheritance do not apply to these defects.

3 The defects are familial; however, no exact pathogenesis has been found.

4 The way the young child responds to these defects depends on the parental response.

49. 2 **The 2-year-old child is extremely fearful of separation as well as intrusive procedures; if parents are present, they should be encouraged to stay and give comfort. (2) (PI; CJ; IM; EH)**

1 Two-year-olds still depend on their parents for comfort and control.

3 The father may provide comfort to the child during the procedure as well.

4 Two-year-olds are still dependent on their parents; the parent should be encouraged to participate in care.

50. 3 **Infants and small children have small buttocks with a very proximal sciatic nerve. (2) (PM; CJ; AN; GD)**

1 Children of this age fear the procedure no matter what site is chosen.

2 Preschoolers tend to associate many treatments, and illness itself, with punishment.

4 Children properly restrained can be held still in this position.

Pediatric Nursing Quiz 2

1. A 13-month-old child is admitted to the hospital with a tentative diagnosis of bacterial meningitis. A lumbar puncture has been ordered. When preparing the baby for the lumbar puncture, the nurse should first:
   1. Use a doll to demonstrate the procedure to the baby
   2. Shave and prep the child's lumbar region for the procedure
   3. Ask the parents if the procedure has been explained to them
   4. Obtain a pacifier for the child to suck on during the procedure

2. The nurse initiates preparation of a 9-year-old girl for an infratentorial craniotomy. The nurse plans to:
   1. Encourage doll play with blunt tools and dressings
   2. Schedule role-playing with others having similar surgery
   3. Have the child draw her concept of a brain and briefly clarify any misconceptions
   4. Provide a minutely detailed explanation of anatomy and the surgery to be performed

3. Based on the problems associated with bronchiolitis caused by the respiratory syncytial virus, the nurse recognizes the treatment of choice for an infant with this illness should consist of:
   1. Postural drainage and corticosteroids
   2. Humidified air and adequate hydration
   3. Adequate hydration and bronchodilators
   4. Oxygen by hood and broad-spectrum antibiotics

4. An 8-year-old is being discharged after recovery from a sickle-cell pain episode. The nurse teaches the parents all the "do's and don'ts" concerning the child's care. The nurse is satisfied that the parents understand the principles of care when they state that they are:
   1. Keeping the child's fluid intake restricted at night
   2. Not permitting the child to play soccer or football
   3. Not allowing the child to play with other children
   4. Getting the child a private tutor to help with school work

5. The nurse plans with the parents of an infant with a cardiac defect how to decrease their baby's cardiac demands. The nurse should teach them:
   1. Why the infant cannot be picked up and cuddled
   2. Why care should be organized to allow for uninterrupted sleep
   3. To feed the infant at two-hour intervals throughout the day
   4. To stimulate the infant periodically to promote respiratory excursion

6. A client brings her 4-week-old son to the clinic. She states, "He cries all the time and always acts hungry, but he throws up everything. He looks like a skinny old man." Based on this information, the nurse should concentrate the physical assessment on:
   1. A rectal observation that would confirm rectal prolapse
   2. An abdominal assessment that would confirm pyloric stenosis
   3. The color of vomitus that would confirm a bile duct obstruction
   4. An elimination history that would confirm an imperforate anus

7. A 6-year-old is admitted to the hospital with a tentative diagnosis of leukemia. On admission the most important nursing assessment would be to determine:
   1. What the child has been told about the diagnosis
   2. The parents' ability to cope in stressful situations
   3. The growth percentile and developmental abilities of the child
   4. What the child's previous experience with illness and hospitalization has been

8. With persistent diarrhea an infant is subject to significant fluid and electrolyte alterations. Because of this the nurse should be aware that an infant with diarrhea may develop:
   1. Hypovolemia, hypercalcemia
   2. Hypernatremia, hypervolemia
   3. Metabolic acidosis, hypovolemia
   4. Decreased hematocrit, hyponatremia

9. The nurse is caring for an 11-year-old child with type 1 diabetes. Two hours after breakfast, the child becomes pale, diaphoretic, and shaky. The nurse should:
1. Notify the physician
2. Administer the supplemental order of insulin
3. Compare these findings with those in the child's chart
4. Give the child 4 ounces of orange juice and a slice of bread

10. When obtaining a health history of a 7-year-old admitted to the hospital with acute glomerulonephritis, the nurse would expect the child's mother to report that the:
1. Child had just gotten over the measles
2. Child had a sore throat three weeks ago
3. Child's father has a history of urinary infections
4. Child's immunizations for camp were completed last week

11. At a routine visit to the pediatric clinic, the mother of a 6-week-old infant states that her baby has the "cutest little folds on her legs, two on one side, three on the other." The nurse recognizes that this may indicate the presence of:
1. Neonatal obesity
2. A slipped epiphysis
3. Talipes equinovarus
4. Dysplasia of the hip

12. An adolescent male is admitted with a tentative diagnosis of a bone tumor of the left femur. During the admission procedure he casually asks, "Do they ever have to cut off a leg if someone has bone cancer?" The nurse should respond:
1. "Why are you asking? Do you think this may happen to you?"
2. "Most times the leg can be saved, although sometimes it is necessary."
3. "Sometimes it is necessary. What do you think about such a treatment?"
4. "Such a decision can only be made when the kind of bone cancer is determined."

13. An order for an infant with a severely reddened diaper rash that the nurse should question is:
1. Use cloth diapers only
2. Expose the buttocks to air
3. Direct a heat lamp to the buttocks prn
4. Apply A&D ointment to the diaper area

14. While in the hospital's playroom, a child suddenly has a nosebleed spreading blood on the play table. The nurse's first response in this situation should be:
1. Taking the child back to the room for care
2. Calling the housekeeping staff to clean up the room
3. Providing nursing care to stop the child's nosebleed
4. Notifying the supervisor so that all those in the playroom be tested for HIV

15. The nurse is aware that uncorrected bilateral cryptorchidism can cause:
1. Sterility
2. Hydrocele
3. Varicocele
4. Epididymitis

16. When discussing feeding techniques with the mother of a toddler in a spica cast, the nurse should suggest that she use a:
1. Padded, adjustable tilt board
2. Football hold, facing the mother
3. Supine position with the head on a pillow
4. Position that is upright on the mother's lap

17. Postoperatively a 2-month-old returns to the pediatric unit with an intravenous infusion and a nasogastric tube in place. The initial nursing action should be to:
1. Assess the infant's status
2. Administer a mild sedative
3. Connect the IV to an infusion pump
4. Attach the nasogastric tube to wall suction

18. A 4-year-old is admitted to the hospital with a diagnosis of Wilms' tumor. The nurse should place a sign on the child's bed that states:
1. Strain all urine
2. No IV medications
3. Use cloth diapers only
4. Do not palpate abdomen

19. An 8-year-old with a history of severe asthma is admitted to the hospital after an asthma attack at home. The child is extremely short of breath. To facilitate breathing and to promote respiratory drainage, the nurse should place the child in a:
1. Supine position
2. Left lateral position
3. High-Fowler's position
4. Trendelenburg position

20. After reduction with traction for developmental dysplasia of the hip (DDH), a toddler is placed in a bilateral hip spica cast. The nurse should teach

the parents to monitor their child and report to the physician the occurrence of:
1. Warmth
2. Numbness
3. Skin desquamation
4. Generalized discomfort

21. The signs that would most probably lead the nurse to suspect that a 1-year-old child has rubella are:
1. Conjunctivitis and sensitivity to light
2. Buldging fontanelle and nuchal rigidity
3. Koplik's spots on the soft palate and buccal mucosa
4. Enlargement of the posterior cervical and postauricular nodes

22. A 4-year-old child is diagnosed with acute lymphoid leukemia (ALL) and induction therapy includes vincristine (Oncovin). The nurse recognizes that a side effect unique to this drug would be:
1. Diarrhea
2. Alopecia
3. Anorexia
4. Paresthesia

23. An abused child, after being hospitalized for severe injuries, is being placed in temporary foster care. The foster family is coming into the hospital to meet the child. The nurse should plan to facilitate this meeting by:
1. Decorating the child's room with "welcome" signs
2. Providing a private room for the foster family and the child
3. Encouraging the child to draw a picture for the new mother
4. Answering all the child's questions about the foster family ahead of time

24. After the insertion of a shunt to treat hydrocephalus, the nurse should evaluate the function of the shunt by:
1. Assessing for periorbital edema
2. Noting the frequency of voiding
3. Palpating the child's anterior fontanel
4. Observing for symmetric Moro reflexes

25. The nurse explains to a newly diagnosed child that regulation of diabetes is best accomplished by:
1. Insulin, dietary control, and exercise
2. Dietary control, exercise, and urine testing
3. Exercise, dietary control, and blood glucose monitoring
4. Oral hypoglycemic agents, dietary control, and exercise

26. The nurse confers with the nutritionist about the diet of a child with decreased mobility because of a fracture. In addition to being non-constipating, the diet should be:
1. Low in calories and purine
2. High in calories and phosphorus
3. Moderate in calories and high in protein
4. Adequate in calories and high in calcium

27. Abdominal surgery will be performed on a 2-month-old. Recognizing the developmental level, on the day of surgery the nurse should provide the infant with a:
1. Rattle to shake
2. Pacifier to suck
3. Mobile to watch
4. Music box for listening

28. A 15-year-old adolescent with newly diagnosed type 1 diabetes is admitted for evaluation and the institution of protocol for insulin therapy. The primary long-term goal would be that the adolescent:
1. Comply with the diabetic diet
2. Develop a non-stressful lifestyle
3. Adhere to a routine exercise program
4. Maintain normoglycemia with few episodes of hypo- or hyperglycemia

29. A four-year-old is admitted with burns over the entire right arm and the anterior and posterior aspects of both legs. Using the percentages of total body surface area (TBSA) that was burned, the nurse estimates that the TBSA affected would be approximately:
1. 36%
2. 41%
3. 47%
4. 52%

30. The alkylating agent cyclophosphamide (Cytoxan) is ordered for a child with cancer. When the child is receiving this drug the nurse should assess for:
1. Unexpected nausea
2. Extent of hydration
3. Increased irritability
4. Hyperplasia of gums

31. The nurse should plan to place a child admitted with meningitis in:
1. A semiprivate room in the middle of the unit
2. A corner of a four-bed room next to the nurses' station
3. A private room two doors away from the nurses' station
4. An isolation room away from activity at the far end of the unit

32. A child returns to the unit after a cardiac catheterization. The statement on the child's progress made during the change-of-shift report two hours after the catheterization that should be questioned by the incoming nurse would be that the child:
    1. Is on bed rest with bathroom privileges
    2. Has a pressure dressing over the entry site
    3. Has voided only 100 mL since the procedure
    4. Is to have the blood pressure checked every two hours

33. After a pyloromyotomy, the mother is asked to offer her baby son his first feeding. He sucks it eagerly and vomits immediately. The nurse should explain to the mother that:
    1. He is ridding himself of postoperative mucus
    2. Her feeding technique may need to be changed
    3. His feeding will have to be stopped until peristalsis improves
    4. His postoperative vomiting is a common response and will decrease

34. A 3-year-old is admitted to the hospital for chelation therapy for lead poisoning. The child's mother asks the nurse how the child got lead poisoning. The nurse should base the response on the knowledge that this problem in children is:
    1. Clearly related to the child's ingestion of nonfood substances
    2. Attributed to an indigent and passive mother who fails to supervise them
    3. Considered to be environmental, with lead available for oral exploration by children who are unsupervised
    4. Associated with high-risk groups including those with pica and those exposed to hazards present in the environment

35. A child with asthma is being discharged from the hospital on oral theophylline. The nurse recognizes that the parents understand the discharge teaching when they tell the nurse that they will monitor the child for the side effect of:
    1. Apneic episodes
    2. Frequent urination
    3. Nausea and vomiting
    4. Spasmodic hiccoughs

36. From the nurse's knowledge of preschoolers, the nurse should predict a 4-year-old's reaction to illness and hospitalization will be characterized by:
    1. Feeling lonely, bored, depressed over separation from family, and fearing death
    2. Being out of control, regressing to overdependency and fearing bodily mutilation

    3. Anger, frustration, and resentment over depersonalization and loss of peer support
    4. Experiencing intense panic and loss of security over separation from parents and having a low frustration tolerance

37. To meet the nutritional needs of a 5-month-old with congenital heart disease, the nurse would instruct the mother to:
    1. Use 1½ strength formula
    2. Feed the infant slowly, allowing for rest
    3. Administer an iron supplement with meals
    4. Avoid giving solid food until the infant is 1 year old

38. A 4-week-old infant with hypertrophic pyloric stenosis is admitted for corrective surgery. The nurse recognizes that the primary objective of the preoperative period would be to:
    1. Stabilize vital signs
    2. Improve nutritional status
    3. Correct fluid and electrolyte imbalances
    4. Document the number of times and character of vomitus

39. When the nurse assesses the renal function of a child with acute glomerulonephritis (AGN), the expected findings would be:
    1. Dysuria and azotemia
    2. Oliguria and hematuria
    3. Glycosuria and polyuria
    4. Nocturia and proteinuria

40. When planning teaching for the parents of a child with tetralogy of Fallot, who are both employed full time, the nurse should:
    1. Schedule a whole evening for teaching
    2. Insist both parents attend the teaching sessions
    3. Provide written and oral information in short sessions
    4. Point things out to them when they are visiting their child

41. For a few days after the repair of a cleft lip, the nurse should feed the infant via:
    1. A nasogastric tube
    2. A rubber-tipped syringe
    3. An intravenous infusion
    4. A bottle with a preemie nipple

42. The nurse is planning the discharge of a child who has had a tonsillectomy. The mother is told that the child may have a mouth odor, slight ear pain, and a low-grade fever for a few days. The nurse should recommend that the mother:
    1. Apply an ice collar for pain

2. Give aspirin for pain as necessary
3. Let the child suck on peppermint candies as desired
4. Have the child gargle with a warm saline solution

43. A 16-month-old has had large, frothy, foul-smelling stools since the introduction of table food and cow's milk into the diet. The child's mother also notes that the child has changed from pleasant and outgoing to irritable and apathetic. The child is diagnosed as having celiac disease and is placed on a gluten-free diet. When evaluating the child's response to the diet after two days, the nurse anticipates the first change will be:
1. A return of appetite
2. An increase in weight
3. A cessation of diarrhea
4. An improved personality

44. Chelation therapy with Ca EDTA is started on a child with chronic lead poisoning. The nurse can evaluate the success of this therapy by monitoring for:
1. Fecal excretion of lead
2. Elevated blood-lead levels
3. Increased urinary excretion of lead
4. Decreased deposition of lead in the bones

45. The nurse understands that dialysis will be necessary when a child with chronic kidney disease exhibits:
1. Hypotension
2. Hypokalemia
3. Hypervolemia
4. Hypercalcemia

46. A child with leukemia is receiving vincristine. Nursing care for this child includes checking and recording bowel sounds bid. This action is necessary because a side effect of this drug is:
1. Decreased innervation of the GI tract

2. Hyperactivity of the bowel with diarrhea
3. Nausea that decreases fluid intake and produces constipation
4. Increased antigen/antibody reactions, which cause edematous bowels

47. The best method for assessing an infant's response to rehydration therapy would be for the nurse to:
1. Measure the infant's abdominal girth
2. Observe the color of the infant's stools
3. Weigh the infant at the same time daily
4. Monitor the infant's skin turgor frequently

48. The nurse is aware that developmentally, 2-year-old children are at risk for lead poisoning primarily because:
1. Lead is easily available to them
2. Their vascular system is very fragile
3. They have a high level of oral activity
4. Motor vehicle use and pollution have increased

49. A 4-year-old boy with acute lymphocytic leukemia is to have a bone marrow aspiration. While involving the child in therapeutic play prior to the procedure, the nurse should help him understand that:
1. He needs to have a positive attitude
2. His parents are concerned about him
3. He did nothing to cause his present illness
4. His problem was caused by an environmental factor

50. The nurse is aware that 18-month-old children with normal hearing have usually acquired a vocabulary sufficient to enable them to communicate by:
1. Pointing and grunting
2. Using at least six words
3. Making babbling sounds
4. Using complete sentences

Pediatric Nursing Quiz 2 Answers and Rationales

1. 3 An informed consent is required; the procedure should be explained to the parents by the physician; the nurse should confirm their comprehension and have them sign the consent form. (2) (SE; LE; AS; NP)

1 A signed consent form is the priority; the child is too young to comprehend a demonstration of the procedure.

2 A signed consent form is the priority.

4 Same as answer 2.

2. 3 This indicates the child's level of understanding to the nurse, and an explanation can then proceed at this level. (3) (SE; MR; PL; GD)

1 Doll play is more appropriate for younger children; it is inappropriate in this instance.

2 Role-playing is inappropriate and nontherapeutic at this time.

4 Although the school-age child appreciates some detail, extensive detail is inappropriate.

3. 2 Adequate hydration and high humidity are essential to loosen tenacious secretions and minimize fluid loss. (1) (PB; CJ; PL; RE)

1 Corticosteroids are not used because they have not proved effective.

3 Bronchodilators are not used because the bronchial tree is not in spasm.

4 Oxygen is used only if the infant has severe dyspnea and hypoxia; antibiotics are ineffectual because the etiologic agent is viral.

4. 2 Strenuous exercise leads to increased cellular metabolism, causing tissue hypoxia, which can precipitate sickling. (2) (SE; MR; EV; BI)

1 Fluid should never be restricted; keeping the child well hydrated helps to prevent sickling.

3 This is unnecessary unless the other children have an infectious disease; peer relationships should be encouraged.

4 This is detrimental to the child's developmental needs and may result in social isolation.

5. 2 Long periods of rest must be promoted; activities should be organized to minimize interruptions. (2) (PB; MR; PL; CV)

1 Parents should be encouraged to provide cuddling to help the infant sleep more soundly.

3 The feeding plan should be flexible to accommodate the infant's sleep and wake needs and patterns.

4 Crying should be minimized to decrease the work load of the heart.

6. 2 With a history that strongly suggests hypertrophic pyloric stenosis, the nurse should assess the abdomen for an olive-shaped mass and visible peristalsis. (2) (PB; CJ; AS; GI)

1 The data presented are not consistent with rectal prolapse.

3 Although the color of vomitus is important for a diagnosis of pyloric stenosis, bile duct obstruction is not indicated by the history.

4 The data presented are not consistent with imperforate anus; because the infant is 4 weeks old, this condition should have been discovered already.

7. 4 Positive and negative experiences connected with previous illness or hospitalization will influence the child's response and adaptation to this and subsequent hospitalization. (3) (PM; CJ; AS; EH)

1 This will not be too meaningful because a 6-year-old may not have too great an understanding of the illness.

2 Although this is an influence, the priority care at this time should be directed to the child's coping abilities.

3 This is not a priority; the child's present acute illness must be attended to first.

8. 3 Loss of bicarbonate and sodium in the stools causes metabolic acidosis; fluid loss in liquid stools causes hypovolemia. (2) (PB; CJ; AN; FE)

1 Fluid loss does cause hypovolemia, but hypercalcemia does not occur.

2 Hypovolemia, not hypervolemia, would result from diarrhea; there may or may not be an increase in sodium.

4 The hematocrit would be elevated because of fluid loss (hemoconcentration); sodium may be increased, decreased, or normal.

9. 4 **The client is demonstrating signs and symptoms of hypoglycemia and needs glucose. The orange juice is a simple carbohydrate, and the bread is a complex carbohydrate. (1) (PB; CJ; IM; EN)**

 1 This may be done after the child receives glucose.

 2 Administering insulin will exacerbate the hypoglycemia and endanger the client.

 3 Same as answer 1.

10. 2 **Glomerulonephritis is associated with a history of prior streptococcal infection of the throat. (1) (SE; CJ; AS; RG)**

 1 A streptococcal infection, not the measles virus, is associated with the development of glomerulonephritis.

 3 Glomerulonephritis is not an inherited disease; it usually follows a streptococcal infection.

 4 There are no immunizations that would cause glomerulonephritis.

11. 4 **Asymmetric hip and thigh folds are indicative of developmental dysplasia of the hip. (2) (PM; CJ; AN; SK)**

 1 Extra folds would be bilateral if the infant were obese.

 2 This is found in the school-age child; it is characterized by a lump and pain in the leg.

 3 This is clubbed feet; there are no extra folds, only deformities of the feet.

12. 3 **This response honestly answers the question and encourages further discussion about the client's feelings. (1) (PI; CJ; IM; EH)**

 1 This response is too direct; not only does it not deal with feelings, but it attacks the basis for these feelings.

 2 This response is evasive and does not deal with feelings.

 4 Same as answer 2.

13. 3 **The order should include intervals and frequency of lamp application to prevent overexposure to heat. (2) (SE; CJ; IM; IT)**

 1 Plastic-lined disposable diapers hold heat and stool close to the skin, thereby increasing irritation.

 2 This will promote drying and healing of the diaper area.

 4 Ointment protects the buttocks from the irritating contents of stool.

14. 3 **The nurse's priority is to care for the child; once the child's problem has been resolved, the nurse can address the problem of the blood on the play table. (1) (PB; CJ; IM; BI)**

 1 The child's needs must be met immediately, even if the intervention must be performed in the play room.

 2 Cleaning up the blood in the play room would be done after the child's immediate needs are met; the hospital protocol for the removal of the blood should be followed.

 4 This is not necessary unless others in the play room have been contaminated; the hospital's protocol should be followed.

15. 1 **In cryptorchidism, sperm-producing abilities of the testes are destroyed, resulting in sterility. (1) (PM; CJ; AN; RG)**

 2 This is enlargement of the scrotum with fluid; it is not related to cryptorchidism.

 3 This is an abnormal dilation and tortuosity of the scrotal veins; it is not caused by undescended testicles.

 4 Inflammation of the epididymis may occur whether or not cryptorchidism is corrected.

16. 1 **Because of the child's age, this is the best position; it permits upright feeding while fostering growth and development needs. (1) (PB; CJ; IM; GD)**

 2 This is a more appropriate position for an infant.

 3 This position makes feeding and digestion difficult.

 4 This position is difficult for the mother because the combination of child and cast would be too cumbersome; it would be difficult for the toddler as well.

17. 1 **Assessment is the first step of the nursing process and is the priority because it influences all future interventions. (2) (SE; CJ; IM; NP)**

 2 Although important, this can be done later.

 3 Same as answer 2.

 4 Same as answer 2.

18. 4 **Palpation would create a risk of rupturing the tumor mass. (2) (SE; MR; IM; RG)**

 1 This is unnecessary; no calculi are present.

 2 There is no contraindication for IV medication.

 3 Cloth or disposable diapers can be worn as long as there is no palpation.

19. 3 **This position allows the lungs more room to expand, thus affording more comfort. (1) (PB; CJ; IM; RE)**

 1 This position would increase dyspnea; it does not allow for chest expansion.

 2 Same as answer 1.

 4 Same as answer 1.

20. 2 **Numbness is a neurologic symptom that should be reported immediately because it indicates**

pressure on the nerves and blood vessels. (2) (PB; MR; IM; SK)

1 Warmth is an expected reaction to a new plaster cast; the cast may be plastic and warmth would occur only if there were an infection, which would be unusual.

3 This is the result of inadequate skin care, but can be managed easily with lotion or oil.

4 Some degree of discomfort is expected after cast application.

21. 4 **Lymphadenopathy and the development of a rash after a day of fever, sneezing, and coughing characterize rubella. (2) (SE; CJ; AS; IT)**

1 These are symptoms of rubeola, not rubella.

2 These are symptoms associated with meningitis and encephalitis, not rubella.

3 Koplik's spots are present with measles (rubeola) not rubella (German measles).

22. 4 **Paresthesia is a major, unique side effect because of the medication's neurotoxic effects on the cranial and peripheral nerves. (2) (PB; CJ; AN; DR)**

1 This is a common side effect of chemotherapy; it is not unique to vincristine (Oncovin).

2 Same as answer 1.

3 Same as answer 1.

23. 2 **A private room will provide a secure environment for the child and the family to get to know one another. (2) (SE; MR; PL; EH)**

1 This is not therapeutic because it may make the child feel guilty about leaving the biologic family.

3 Same as answer 1.

4 Although some information may be given, too much information about the family may promote preconceived ideas that may be inaccurate.

24. 3 **A bulging fontanel is the most significant sign of increased intracranial pressure in an infant. (3) (PB; CJ; EV; NM)**

1 This is not a significant indicator of increased intracranial pressure.

2 Same as answer 1.

4 Same as answer 1.

25. 1 **Most juveniles are type 1 diabetics and have little or no endogenous insulin; diet control and exercise reduce the amount of exogenous insulin needed. (2) (PB; MR; PL; EN)**

2 Those having type 1 diabetes have little or no endogenous insulin and need exogenous insulin; this regimen is for type 2 diabetics; blood glucose monitoring is usually used.

3 Those having type 1 diabetes need insulin for control because of a lack of endogenous insulin.

4 Oral hypoglycemics are ineffective in stimulating insulin secretion in clients having type 1 diabetes because they have no endogenous insulin.

26. 4 **Calcium promotes osteoblastic activity, and calories support the growth and energy needs of the child. (1) (PB; CJ; PL; SK)**

1 The level of purine does not affect bone repair; a decrease in calories would not support growth and development.

2 Extra calories are converted to adipose tissue; if calcium needs are met, sufficient phosphorus will be ingested.

3 Bone tissue responds to sufficient calcium in the diet; if injury had occurred to the soft tissues, a high-protein diet would be necessary.

27. 2 **The infant is NPO and satisfying the sucking need is the priority at this age. (1) (PM; CJ; IM; GD)**

1 Although this is age appropriate, the sucking need is the priority.

3 Same as answer 1.

4 Same as answer 1.

28. 4 **This is a realistic goal; maintaining normoglycemia decreases the risk of developing complications such as neuropathy, retinopathy, and atherosclerosis. (1) (PM; MR; PL; EN)**

1 This is an unrealistic goal; adolescents are notoriously noncompliant.

2 This is an unrealistic goal.

3 Same as answer 2.

29. 2 **Using the TBSA percentage for a child between 1 and 5 years of age, the total arm is 8.5% and each total leg is 16.25%; thus, 32.5% for both legs and 8.5% for the arm equals a total of 41% of TBSA burned. (3) (PB; CJ; AS; IT)**

1 This percentage is too small.

3 This percentage is too large.

4 Same as answer 3.

30. 2 **Cystitis is a potentially serious adverse reaction to Cytoxan, which can sometimes be prevented by increased hydration because the fluid flushes the bladder. (3) (PB; CJ; PL; DR)**

1 This is an expected but not serious side effect of Cytoxan.

3 Irritability may be present but is not necessarily a result of Cytoxan administration.

4 This is unrelated to Cytoxan administration; it occurs with Dilantin therapy.

31. 3 A private room will provide isolation; also, being close to the nurses' station will facilitate frequent neurologic monitoring. (2) (SI; PL; PE; NM)

 1 This would permit cross-infection; a private room is necessary to prevent transmission of airborne droplets.
 2 Same as answer 1.
 4 This interferes with frequent monitoring of the child.

32. 1 Children are kept on complete bed rest after a cardiac catheterization to reduce the risk of bleeding or trauma to the insertion site; the order for bathroom privileges should be questioned. (3) (PB; MR; EV; CV)

 2 This is an expected part of postcatheterization care; a pressure dressing is placed over the insertion site to reduce the possibility of bleeding.
 3 This urinary output is within acceptable limits; the child was kept NPO before and during the procedure; after the procedure oral fluids need to be encouraged to promote hydration and voiding.
 4 Frequent blood pressure checks are part of routine postcatheterization care.

33. 4 This provides correct information while supporting the anxious parent. (2) (PB; CJ; IM; GI)

 1 This is not a result of mucus accumulation.
 2 This places guilt on the parent for the child's physical condition; although feeding techniques may need to be changed eventually, discussing this at this time is inappropriate.
 3 Feedings are continued and vomiting subsides on its own.

34. 4 Three factors appear to be related to lead poisoning: lead in the environment; toxins in the environment; and characteristics of the child and the parents. (3) (SE; MR; AN; NM)

 1 This is only one of the three etiologic factors.
 2 Same as answer 1.
 3 Same as answer 1.

35. 3 Theophylline is a local irritant to the GI tract. (3) (SE; MR; EV; DR)

 1 This is not a side effect; theophylline is given to improve respirations.
 2 Frequent urination is expected because this drug often produces diuresis.
 4 This is not a side effect.

36. 2 Piaget's preoperational stage focuses on egocentricity and concrete thoughts and Freud's phallic stage supports this response. (3) (PM; CJ; AN; GD)

 1 These feelings are typical of the school-aged child.
 3 These feelings are typical of the adolescent.
 4 These feelings are typical of the toddler.

37. 2 Because of poor exercise tolerance and fatigue, these children become too tired to eat; allowing for rest, and feeding slowly limit the fatigue associated with eating. (2) (PB; CJ; IM; CV)

 1 The child should be fed the same type of diet and foods as other infants.
 3 This will impede absorption; it should be given with orange juice between meals.
 4 Same as answer 1

38. 3 Preoperative restoration of fluid and electrolyte balance improves the likelihood of a successful outcome after surgery. (2) (PB; CJ; AN; FE)

 1 Vital signs can be stabilized only after fluid and electrolyte balances have been corrected.
 2 Fluid and electrolyte balance is of priority importance; nutritional status should improve after surgery.
 4 The number of episodes and character of vomitus are important, but not the primary objective of preoperative nursing care.

39. 2 Urinary output is decreased (oliguria) because of reduced glomerular filtration; red blood cells are in the urine (hematuria) because of local or diffuse nephron damage. (2) (PB; CJ; AS; RG)

 1 Although azotemia does occur resulting in proteinuria, there is no pain on urination (dysuria).
 3 These occur with uncontrolled diabetes mellitus, not AGN.
 4 Although there is proteinuria, nocturia would not be expected.

40. 3 The parents will probably be anxious and will benefit most from short teaching sessions and written material to review at their leisure. (1) (SE; MR; PL; EH)

 1 This would be overwhelming, and the parents would not be able to retain everything presented.
 2 The nurse could recommend, but not insist, that both parents attend the teaching sessions.
 4 The most effective teaching and learning sessions occur in an area with minimal distractions; being in the room with their child at this time would present a major distraction to the parents.

41. 2 **This would minimize sucking and yet not be irritating to the suture line. (2) (PM; CJ; PL; GI)**
1 This is not used because it would be irritating to the nostrils and is unnecessary.
3 Intravenous infusions do not supply the necessary caloric intake.
4 No nipple should be used because the baby should not suck.

42. 1 **This produces vasoconstriction, limits edema, and prevents hemorrhage; also, it anesthetizes the area, thus reducing pain. (2) (PB; MR; PL; BI)**
2 Aspirin has anticoagulant properties that could increase the risk of bleeding; also, it should not be given to children because it can cause Reye syndrome.
3 Hard candies can traumatize the operative site and cause bleeding.
4 This could traumatize the operative site and cause bleeding.

43. 4 **Favorable personality change within one to two days attests to the effectiveness of the diet; other improvements take longer. (3) (PB; CJ; EV; GI)**
1 Usually anorexia is not a problem; if it does occur, it does so during bouts of diarrhea.
2 This occurs after the personality change.
3 Same as answer 2.

44. 3 **The desired outcome is the increased excretion of lead in the urine. (2) (PB; CJ; EV; DR)**
1 The elimination of lead via the GI tract is less than via the urinary tract and would be an unsatisfactory measure of the success of the chelation therapy.
2 This is expected when lead initially equilibrates to the blood; until the lead is excreted in the urine, the treatment is not considered a success.
4 This is a desirable effect, but it does not determine the success of therapy; also, the amount is difficult to determine.

45. 3 **This will result when kidneys have failed and are no longer excreting urine, the blood pressure is high, and cardiac overload is imminent. (2) (PB; CJ; AN; RG)**
1 Hypertension is present when there is kidney failure.
2 Hyperkalemia occurs in kidney failure and is relieved by dialysis.
4 Hypocalcemia is present when kidney failure occurs.

46. 1 **Constipation and paralytic ileus are common problems because of decreased nerve innervation**

of the GI tract; they are symptomatic of neurotoxicity. (2) (PB; CJ; EV; DR)
2 This is not a toxic effect of vincristine.
3 This is not a factor in the development of constipation; fluids can be given intravenously if nausea is present.
4 Vincristine causes leukopenia, which increases susceptibility to infection; it does not cause antigen/antibody reactions.

47. 3 **This is the most objective and accurate way to assess fluid loss or gain; weights measured at the same time each day provide for daily comparisons. (2) (PB; CJ; EV; FE)**
1 This would be appropriate for assessing the progression of ascites, not for assessing rehydration.
2 The color of stools is unrelated to fluid balance; noting consistency would be more important, although subjective.
4 Although this would be done, it is subjective.

48. 3 **Young children have an increased propensity for putting things in their mouths; this age group uses this as a means of exploring the environment. (1) (PM; CJ; AN; GD)**
1 Although this may be true in older homes or in the inner city, it is the activity of putting things into the mouth that is the primary cause.
2 This is untrue; toddlers do not have a fragile vascular system; children with a fragile vascular system are severely compromised.
4 This is not true; although gas fumes in areas of heavy traffic have increased pollution, most gasoline used today does not contain lead.

49. 3 **This will help to elicit any fantasy the child may have; it helps the child understand that treatment is not a punishment. (3) (PI; CJ; IM; EH)**
1 This is inappropriate for a 4-year-old and does not elicit feelings.
2 This is inappropriate; it may be frightening.
4 This is not currently supported as a cause; this is an inappropriate discussion for a 4-year-old.

50. 2 **A vocabulary consisting of a minimum of six words with telegraphic-type speech is normal for a child this age. (2) (PM; CJ; AS; GD)**
1 The child with a hearing impairment communicates in this way because the child has not acquired the rudiments of language.
3 Babbling is the expected communication for an 8-month-old infant, even one with a moderate hearing loss.
4 This language skill is seen in the 5-year-old child.

Chapter 4

Mental Health Nursing

NURSING PRACTICE (NP)

1. A male lawyer has been committed to a psychiatric facility after being diagnosed with schizophrenia. One morning while walking outside with the nurse, the client runs away. The immediate responsibility of the nurse would be to notify the:
1. Client's psychiatrist of the elopement
2. Probate judge who committed the client
3. Client's family that the client has left the hospital
4. Local law enforcement officers of the client's escape

2. After caring for a terminally ill client for several weeks, the nurse becomes increasingly aware of a need to get away from this assignment. The best initial action by the nurse would be to:
1. Request vacation time for a few days
2. Seek support from colleagues on the unit
3. Withdraw emotional involvement with the client
4. Stay with the client and try to work through feelings

3. A female nurse, who works in the intensive care unit of a large city hospital, has been working double shifts to pay for a new car. These are stopped when frequent headaches and fatigue ensue. The nurse manager notices that the care the nurse is providing is barely adequate, that she is working harder, and accomplishing less even staying an extra hour every day. The nurse manager should handle this situation by stating:
1. "I think you are trying to do too much."
2. "What can I do to help you to get finished on time?"
3. "I've noticed you've been staying late almost every night."

4. "I'll help you get more organized so you can leave on time."

4. A client with dementia often assaults the nursing staff, and the staff decides to develop a plan that will make this client's personal care less of a problem. The plan should include:
1. Limiting staff time with the client
2. An outline of the consequences for uncooperative behavior
3. Identification of nursing staff members whom the client prefers
4. The client's likes and dislikes for use as a reward or punishment

5. The nurse should first discuss terminating the nurse-client relationship with a client during the:
1. Working phase when the client brings it up
2. Orientation phase when a contract is established
3. Working phase when the client shows some progress
4. Termination phase when discharge plans are being made

6. On a home visit to an older adult who has chronic heart failure, the nurse observes that a 6-month-old grandchild lies quietly in a crib, rarely smiles or babbles, and barely has basic needs attended. The client is the primary caregiver for the infant. The nurse should:
1. Advise purchasing appropriate toys designed for this age level
2. Inform the client that the child will be retarded if not stimulated
3. Explain the need for the family to hire a mother's helper for the home
4. Initiate a referral to an appropriate agency to assess the need for a home health aide

7. When planning nursing care for a client with severe agoraphobia, the nurse should first:
   1. Determine the client's degree of impairment
   2. Support the client's self-esteem through verbal interactions
   3. Teach the client biofeedback techniques to reduce anxiety
   4. Expose the client gradually to anxiety-provoking situations

8. When a nurse revises a client's nursing care plan based on the client's responses that show evidence that goals were not attained, the phase of the nursing process being applied would be:
   1. Planning
   2. Evaluation
   3. Assessment
   4. Implementation

9. After speaking with the parents of a child dying from leukemia, the physician gives a verbal DNR order but refuses to put it in writing. The nurse should:
   1. Follow the order as given by the physician
   2. Refuse to follow the order, unless the nursing supervisor OKs it
   3. Ask the physician to write the order in pencil on the client's chart before leaving
   4. Determine whether the family is in accord with the physician and follow hospital policy

10. A young client, who is a mother for the first time, is very anxious about her new parenting role. With the nurse's encouragement, she has joined the new mothers support group at the local "Y." This part of the plan is an example of:
    1. Tertiary prevention
    2. Primary prevention
    3. Secondary prevention
    4. Therapeutic prevention

11. The nurse manager who is helping a nurse with "burnout" should facilitate confrontation of the problem by urging the nurse to:
    1. Work on a primary nursing care unit
    2. Choose a nursing position on a low-stress unit
    3. Attend educational programs as often as possible
    4. Identify her personal responses to daily work stresses

PERSONALITY DEVELOPMENT (PD)

12. One afternoon the nurse on the unit overhears a young female client having an argument with her boyfriend. A while later the client complains to the nurse that dinner is always late and the meals are terrible. The nurse recognizes that the defense mechanism the client is using is:
    1. Projection
    2. Dissociation
    3. Displacement
    4. Intellectualization

13. Although upset by a young client's continuous complaints about all aspects of care, the nurse ignores them and attempts to divert the conversation. Immediately following this exchange with the client, the nurse discusses with a friend the various stages of development of young adults. The defense mechanism the nurse is using is:
    1. Substitution
    2. Sublimation
    3. Identification
    4. Intellectualization

14. During an interview with the parents of an adolescent female, the nurse notices that her father continually defends and makes excuses for all of his daughter's actions whereas her mother seems to feel her daughter is just lazy and that there is nothing wrong with her that she couldn't change with some effort. The nurse recognizes that the dynamic used by this family is known as:
    1. Coalition
    2. Resignation
    3. Scapegoating
    4. Reaction formation

15. The nurse is aware that according to Erikson, a young child's increased vulnerability to anxiety in response to separations or pending separations from significant others results from failure to complete the developmental task called:
    1. Trust
    2. Identity
    3. Initiative
    4. Autonomy

16. The nurse knows that Erikson identified the developmental tasks of the preschool child from 3 to 5 years as:
    1. Initiative versus guilt
    2. Industry versus inferiority
    3. Breaking away versus staying at home
    4. Sexual impulses versus psychosexual development

17. According to Erikson, a young adult must accomplish the tasks associated with the stage known as:
    1. Initiative versus guilt
    2. Intimacy versus isolation
    3. Industry versus inferiority
    4. Generativity versus stagnation

18. A 23-year-old female client is admitted to a psychiatric unit after several episodes of uncontrolled rage at her parents' home. She is diagnosed as having a borderline personality disorder. While watching a television newscast describing an incident of violence in the home, the client states, "People like that need to be put away before they kill someone." The nurse recognizes that the client is using:
    1. Denial
    2. Projection
    3. Introjection
    4. Sublimation

19. A 65-year-old who emigrated from Cuba 25 years ago is admitted to the hospital with a history of depression. The client, who speaks little English and has few outside interests since retiring, states, "I feel useless and unneeded." According to Erikson, the client is in the developmental stage of:
    1. Initiative versus guilt
    2. Integrity versus despair
    3. Intimacy versus isolation
    4. Identity versus role confusion

20. A 7-year-old hospitalized boy wakes up crying because he has wet his bed. It would be most appropriate for the nurse to:
    1. Allow him to change his bed and pajamas
    2. Change his bed while he changes his pajamas
    3. Take him to the bathroom and change his pajamas
    4. Remind him that he must call for the nurse the next time

21. The mother of an 18-year-old comes to the local mental health center. She is extremely upset because her son has returned from his freshman year at college and is uncontrollable. He takes his brother's clothing, comes in at all hours, and refuses to get a job. Sometimes he is happy and outgoing, and other times he is withdrawn. The mother asks why her son is like this and speculates that college has done this to him. While contemplating this situation, the nurse understands that adolescents are usually:
    1. Anxious and unhappy
    2. Angry and irresponsible
    3. Impulsive and self-centered
    4. Hyperactive and self-destructive

22. According to Erikson, an individual who fails to master the maturational crisis of adolescence will most often:
    1. Rebel at parental orders
    2. Experience role confusion
    3. Be interpersonally isolated
    4. Use drugs and alcohol to escape

23. A constructive and lengthy method of confronting the stress of adolescence and preventing a negative and unhealthy developmental outcome would be:
    1. Role experimentation
    2. Adherence to peer standards
    3. Sublimation through schoolwork
    4. Development of dependency on parents

24. The parents of an overweight adolescent female tell the nurse that they are concerned that their daughter feels inferior to her sister who is an attractive, successful college senior. They ask the nurse what they can do about this problem. The nurse should:
    1. Suggest that they seem to be creating a problem where none exists
    2. Tell them to avoid talking about their older child's accomplishments
    3. Encourage them to give the adolescent recognition for her strong points
    4. Advise them to tell the adolescent to view her sister's success as a challenge

25. The nurse, along with an adolescent and the adolescent's parents, set bolstering the adolescent's self-esteem as a high-priority goal. The nursing action that would contribute to the achievement of this goal would be:
    1. Urging the adolescent to join a neighborhood social group
    2. Suggesting that the mother give the adolescent lots of hugs and cuddling
    3. Supporting the adolescent's interest in enrolling in a babysitting course
    4. Encouraging the adolescent to talk about feelings of pride in successful siblings

26. The nurse recognizes that a father's sexual abuse of a 13-year-old daughter was probably motivated by his:
    1. Need to control
    2. Feelings of anger
    3. Unfulfilled sexual need
    4. Unmet emotional needs

27. The nurse would evaluate that the plan for bolstering an overweight adolescent's self-esteem was effective when, three months later, the adolescent's mother reports that the adolescent:
    1. Asks her to prepare a favorite dessert
    2. Seems to be doing average work in school
    3. Joined a dirt bicycle club that meets at the school
    4. Imitates an older sibling's manner of speech and dress

28. According to Erikson, a person's adjustment to the period of senescence will depend largely on the adjustment the individual made to the developmental stage of:
    1. Intimacy versus isolation
    2. Industry versus inferiority
    3. Generativity versus stagnation
    4. Identity versus identity diffusion

29. When helping the older adult (age 65 to 75 years) successfully complete Erikson's task of this stage, the nurse should assist the client to:
    1. Invest creative energies in promoting social welfare
    2. Redefine a role in society and offer something of value
    3. Look to recapture opportunities that were not started or completed
    4. Feel a sense of satisfaction when reflecting back on past achievements

30. The nurse's role in maintaining or promoting the health of the older adult should be based on the principle that:
    1. Some of the physiologic changes that occur as a result of aging are reversible
    2. There is a strong correlation between successful retirement and good health
    3. Older adults can better accept the dependent state chronic illness often causes
    4. Thoughts of impending death are frequent and depressing to most older adults

31. When planning care for an older client, the nurse is aware that normal aging has little effect on a client's:
    1. Sense of taste or smell
    2. Gastrointestinal motility
    3. Muscle or motor strength
    4. Ability to handle life's stresses

32. Survivors of a major earthquake are being interviewed on admission to the hospital. The nurse notes that they exhibit a flattened affect, make minimal eye contact, and speak in a monotone voice. This would be indicative of the defense mechanism known as:
    1. Splitting
    2. Isolation
    3. Introjection
    4. Compensation

THERAPEUTIC RELATIONSHIPS (TR)

33. The nurse at the crisis intervention center asks a new female client, who has come because her husband is planning a divorce, her reasons for seeking help. The client responds by describing her first meeting with her husband when they were both teenagers. When doing crisis intervention, the nurse's most therapeutic response would be:
    1. "You're avoiding talking about the divorce."
    2. "What does this have to do with your divorce?"
    3. "And now your husband is asking for a divorce."
    4. "Would you like to tell me more about the early years?"

34. The nurse enters the room of an agitated, angry client to administer an ordered antipsychotic medication. The client shouts, "Get out of here!" The nurse's best approach would be to:
    1. Say, "I'll be back in 15 minutes and we can talk."
    2. Get assistance and give the client the medication by injection
    3. Explain why it is necessary that the client take the medication
    4. Say, "You must take the medicine that has been ordered for you."

35. An older female who has been a widow for 20 years comes to the community health center with a vague list of complaints. Her only child, a son, died at birth. She has lived alone since her husband's death and performs all of her own daily tasks of living. She had a very active social life in the past but has outlived many of her friends and family members. When taking this client's health history, it is important for the nurse to ask:
    1. "Do you feel all alone?"
    2. "Do you still miss your husband?"
    3. "What unfulfilled hopes do you have?"
    4. "How did you feel when your son died?"

36. A client with the diagnosis of panic disorder is placed on alprazolam (Xanax), which the client refuses to take because of fear of addiction. Initially the nurse should:
    1. Provide the client with information about Xanax
    2. Further assess the client's knowledge and feelings about Xanax
    3. Have the physician speak to the client about the safety of this drug
    4. Speak with the physician regarding a change in the client's medication

37. In addition to hallucinating, a client yells and curses throughout the day. The nurse should:
    1. Isolate the client until the behavior stops

2. Ignore the behavior exhibited by the client

3. Become aware of what the behavior means to the client

4. Be willing to explain the meaning of the behavior to the client

38. At times a client's anxiety level is so high it blocks attempts at communication and the nurse is unsure of what is being said. To clarify understanding, the nurse states, "Let's see whether we both mean the same thing." This is an example of the technique of:

1. Reflecting feelings
2. Making observations
3. Seeking consensual validation
4. Attempting to place events in sequence

39. To establish an open and trusting relationship with a client who has been hospitalized with severe anxiety, the nurse should:

1. Share an activity with the client
2. Give the client feedback about behavior
3. Respect the client's need for personal space
4. Encourage the staff to have frequent interaction with the client

40. The psychotherapeutic theory that uses hypnosis, dream interpretation, and free association as methods to release repressed feelings is the:

1. Behaviorist model
2. Psychoanalytic model
3. Psychobiologic model
4. Social-interpersonal model

41. The nurse recognizes that the focus of environmental (milieu) therapy is to:

1. Role-play life events to meet individual needs
2. Use natural remedies rather than drugs to control behavior
3. Manipulate the environment to bring about positive changes in behavior
4. Allow the clients freedom to determine whether or not they will be involved in activities

42. A 55-year-old widow of 6 months is brought to a psychiatric hospital. During the assessment interview, the client avoids eye contact, responds in a low voice, and is tearful. The best initial approach by the nurse would be:

1. "You'll find that you'll get better faster if you try to help us to help you."
2. "I know that this is difficult, but as soon as we are finished, I'll take you to your room."
3. "Hold my hand. I know you are frightened, but I will not allow anyone to harm you."

4. "I am Ms. Rose, your nurse. I'll take you to the day room as soon as I get some information."

43. The nurse is aware that in the working phase of the nurse-client relationship, clients:

1. Often focus the conversation on the nurse
2. Accept limits and initiate topics for discussion
3. Commonly exhibit testing behaviors such as flirtation and lateness
4. May repress emotionally charged material to avoid shocking the nurse

44. A client in a psychiatric unit is to be discharged after several weeks of being hospitalized. The client anxiously tells the nurse, "I don't know what I will do when I can't see you anymore." The nurse's most appropriate interpretation of this statement would be that the client is:

1. Saying "Thank you" to the nurse
2. Reacting to the planned discharge
3. Attempting to manipulate the nurse
4. Indicating a need for further hospitalization

45. A male client is preparing to leave the hospital and return to college. When saying good-bye, he hugs and kisses the nurse on the cheek. The nurse's most appropriate response would be to:

1. Hug the client in return
2. Wish him well with his studies
3. Smile at the client but say nothing
4. Encourage him to come back and say hello periodically

46. Three days after a stressful incident a client can no longer remember what there was to worry about. The nurse, in relating to this client, can be most therapeutic by recognizing that the inability to recall the situation is an example of the defense mechanism of:

1. Denial
2. Repression
3. Regression
4. Dissociation

47. The parents of a female client in a psychiatric hospital send an unwrapped birthday gift to the unit for their daughter but do not stay to visit with her. The client responds to this situation by crying. The best response by the nurse would be to:

1. Limit contact with her parents
2. Discuss her parent's behavior with her
3. Distract her by engaging her in an activity
4. Take her to the coffee shop for a birthday treat

48. A goal for a client with the nursing diagnosis of impaired verbal communication related to psychologic barriers would be that the client will:
    1. Be free of injury
    2. Demonstrate decreased acting-out behavior
    3. Interact with others in the external environment
    4. Identify the consequences of acting-out behavior

49. A 15-year-old is admitted to an adolescent unit for evaluation. The adolescent has a long history of drug abuse, stealing, refusal to comply with rules, and an inability to get along in any setting. When collecting data related to the adolescent's lifestyle, the nurse may be prevented from accurately listening to what the client is saying by:
    1. Personal cultural beliefs
    2. The client's disease process
    3. The pressure of time to complete care
    4. A personal need to secure information

50. Before effectively responding to a sexual assault victim on the phone, it is essential that the nurse in the rape crisis center:
    1. Get the client's full name and address
    2. Call for assistance from the psychiatrist
    3. Know some myths and facts about rape
    4. Be aware of any personal bias about rape

51. The nurse is aware that value clarification is a technique useful in therapeutic communication in that it helps:
    1. Make clients aware of their personal values
    2. Provide information related to clients' needs
    3. Assist clients in making correct decisions related to their health
    4. Alter clients' value systems to make them more socially acceptable

52. A reasonable short-term goal for clients who are functioning below the optimum level of mental health would be to help them become better able to:
    1. Understand the dynamics behind the inadequate interpersonal relations
    2. Confront their inadequacies in interpersonal relations and be more sociable
    3. Discuss their feelings regarding significant others and their life experiences
    4. Take actions that will increase their satisfaction with their relationships with others

53. A terminally ill client is moving gradually toward resolution of feelings about impending death. Basing the plan of care on the research of Elizabeth Kübler-Ross, the nurse should use nonverbal interventions after having assessed that the client is in the:
    1. Anger stage
    2. Denial stage
    3. Bargaining stage
    4. Acceptance stage

54. A terminally ill client tells the nurse, "I would love to learn to speak German before I die." The nurse's response to the client's desire to learn a foreign language should be based on an awareness that:
    1. Conversations and activities should focus on pleasant experiences
    2. Clients should be encouraged to set meaningful goals for themselves
    3. Activities that support the client's denial should not be encouraged
    4. The energies expended on such an activity would not justify the outcome

55. It is most helpful to the nurse who is attempting to apply the principles of positive mental health to understand that:
    1. Emotionally ill people can empathize easily with others
    2. Psychologically healthy people function optimally in all settings
    3. A sense of mastery of self and environment is crucial to emotional health
    4. Mental illness is characterized by observable signs of socially inappropriate behavior

56. The nurse should always take the time to keep a client's family informed about what is happening to the client. The main reason for this action is that informed families:
    1. Decrease the client's anxiety
    2. Commonly cause fewer nursing problems
    3. Appear more relaxed and at ease with the client
    4. Are better equipped to undertake necessary family role changes

57. The nurse must recognize that when a client is a member of a different ethnic community it is important to:
    1. Ensure that the nurse's biases are understood by the family
    2. Offer a therapeutic regimen compatible to the lifestyle of the family
    3. Recognize that the client's responses will be different from other clients' responses
    4. Make plans to counteract both the client's and the family's misconceptions of family practice

58. After working with an older male client for a period of time, the client tells the nurse he always enjoyed working and playing with children. During discharge planning the nurse recommends that the client look into the volunteer

foster grandparent program in his area. The nurse recognizes that this type of activity may help the client to:
1. Be able to find new acquaintances with similar interests
2. Take better care of himself if he feels needed by someone
3. Forget his problems when he sees the problems of others
4. Become motivated to become involved with younger people

59. The nurse is scheduled to be the co-leader of a therapy group to be formed in the mental health clinic. When planning for the first meeting, it is of primary importance that the nurse first consider the:
1. Number of clients in the group
2. Needs of the clients being included
3. Diagnoses of the clients being included
4. Socioeconomic status of the clients in the group

60. A newly admitted client with schizophrenia has a treatment plan that includes a physical activity group for several days before being assigned to an analytic group. The basis for this decision is that the client will:
1. Develop skills in dealing with leisure time
2. Have time to develop insight into personal problems
3. Be disruptive and unable to benefit from group therapy at this time
4. Learn to develop trust before moving into a potential anxiety-producing group

61. When planning therapeutic group sessions for regressed long-term clients, the nurse should take into consideration that these clients need:
1. A structured group experience
2. To feel in control of the group
3. Unorganized group experiences
4. Protection from interpersonal conflict

62. When leading a newly formed group of clients in a mental health clinic, the nurse notices that the group members frequently assume self-serving roles. The nurse understands that:
1. Certain subgroups may be emerging to control attention seekers
2. Some of the group members will need to be placed in another group
3. These behaviors usually occur in the early phase of group development
4. The group is attempting to reconcile conflicting viewpoints among its members

63. During the first session of a therapy group one of the clients asks, "What is supposed to happen in this group?" The most appropriate response by the nurse leader would be:
1. "Before I answer that, I'd like for you to tell me what you want to happen."
2. "This is your group and your participation will largely determine what happens."
3. "The purpose of this group is to examine the way each of you interacts with the other."
4. "You and the others are supposed to discuss any reality-based concerns you have about your illness."

64. A client with an ileostomy, who has been discharged from the hospital, decides to join a newly formed ostomy group. During the beginning phase of group development, the nurse should expect to observe the members:
1. Scapegoating other members
2. Satisfied with the group's help
3. Committed to identifying group goals
4. Avoiding the expression of their feelings

65. The best initial approach to take with a self-accusatory, guilt-ridden client would be to:
1. Contradict the client's persecutory delusions
2. Accept the client's statements as the client's beliefs
3. Medicate the client when these thoughts are expressed
4. Redirect the client whenever a negative topic is mentioned

66. The initial intervention strategy that is of primary importance when counseling an older female client who desires to remain independent but is having difficulty maintaining her independent living status would be:
1. Maintaining routines and supporting her usual habits
2. Helping her secure assistance with cleaning and shopping
3. Writing down and repeating important information for her use
4. Setting clear goals and time limitations for her visits with the nurse

67. The nurse plans to use family therapy as a means of assisting a family to cope with their child's terminal illness. The nurse's basis for this choice is that:
1. It is more time-efficient to deal with the whole family together
2. The entire family is involved, since what happens to one member impacts all
3. The nurse can control manipulation and alliances better by using this mode of intervention
4. It will prevent the parents from deceiving each other about the true nature of their child's condition

68. A client who has recently been diagnosed with AIDS comments to the nurse, "There are so many rotten people around. Why couldn't one of them get AIDS instead of me?" The nurse could best respond:
1. "I can understand why you're afraid of death."
2. "It seems unfair that you should have this disease."
3. "I'm sure you really don't wish this on someone else."
4. "Have you thought of speaking with a minister?"

69. The parents of an autistic child begin family therapy with a nurse therapist. The father states that the family members wish to share their religion with the therapist. The nurse should:
1. Limit the father's discussion of religion
2. Plan for a mutual discussion of religious beliefs
3. Invite the family's minister to a therapy session
4. Keep the sessions focused on the family's concerns

70. A 17-year-old, admitted to the hospital because of weight loss and malnutrition, is diagnosed as having anorexia nervosa. After the client's physical condition is stabilized, the psychiatrist, in conjunction with the client and the parents, decides to institute a behavior modification program. The nurse is aware that a major component of behavior modification is that it:
1. Rewards positive behavior
2. Decreases necessary restrictions
3. Deconditions fear of weight gain
4. Reduces anxiety-producing situations

71. When caring for a client with a major depressive disorder, the nurse's first priority should be to help the client to:
1. Feel comfortable with the nurse
2. Investigate new leisure activities
3. Participate in small group activities
4. Initiate conversations about feelings

72. A client with a bipolar mood disorder, manic phase, had been hyperactive and sarcastic to the nurse and other clients. This behavior has been decreasing and the client tells the nurse, "My husband and I have problems getting along sometimes. We see things differently." The response by the nurse that would be the least therapeutic would be:
1. "Explain what you mean by seeing things differently."

2. "Not getting along with one's spouse can be upsetting."
3. "You are calmer today. What has made the difference?"
4. "Tell me about a specific time when you and your husband had problems."

73. The nurse is planning a discharge conference with a psychiatric client and the client's family. The priority nursing action that should be included in the discharge plan is:
1. Obtaining a more complete family history
2. Teaching the client about the medication to be taken
3. Discussing new issues that could be worked on at home
4. Exploring what has been learned from this hospitalization

74. In an attempt to remain objective and support a client during a crisis, the nurse uses imagination and determination to project the self into the client's emotions. The nurse accomplishes this by using the technique known as:
1. Empathy
2. Sympathy
3. Projection
4. Acceptance

75. After a traumatic event a client is extremely upset and exhibits pressured and rambling speech. A therapeutic technique that the nurse can use when a client's communication rambles would be:
1. Touch
2. Silence
3. Focusing
4. Summarizing

76. When a client with paranoid ideation tells the nurse about people coming through the doors to commit murder, the nurse should:
1. Listen to what the client is saying
2. Refuse to listen to the client's stories
3. Tell the client that no one can get through the door
4. Ask the client to explain where this information came from

77. When communicating with a client with a psychiatric diagnosis, the nurse uses silence. When silence is used in therapeutic communication, clients should feel:
1. Unhurried to answer
2. It is their turn to talk
3. The nurse is thinking
4. There is nothing more to say

78. When speaking with a client diagnosed with schizophrenia, the nurse notices that the client keeps interjecting sentences that have nothing to do with the main thoughts being expressed. The client asks whether the nurse understands. The nurse should reply:
    1. "You aren't making any sense; let's talk about something else."
    2. "I'd like to understand what you are saying, but you are too confused now."
    3. "Why don't you take a rest and then we can talk again later this afternoon."
    4. "I'd like to understand what you are saying, but I'm having difficulty following you."

79. A mother visiting her hospitalized teenage daughter gets into an argument with her. Leaving her daughter's room in tears, the mother meets the nurse and relates the argument, stating, "I can't believe I got so angry I could have hit her." The most therapeutic response by the nurse would be:
    1. "Sometimes we find it difficult to live up to our own expectations of ourselves."
    2. "Why don't you bring a surprise for your daughter. It will make you both feel better."
    3. "You can't compare yourself to an abusing parent. After all, you didn't beat your child."
    4. "You're a wonderful mother. Everything will be OK. Teenagers can really drive you to distraction."

80. A husband is upset that his wife's delirium tremens have persisted for the second day. The initial response by the nurse that would be most appropriate is:
    1. "I see that you are very worried. Medications are being used to lessen your wife's discomfort."
    2. "This is totally normal. I suggest that you go home because there is nothing you can do to help at this time."
    3. "Are you afraid that your wife may die? I assure you that very few alcoholics die during the detoxification process."
    4. "The staff is making your wife comfortable while she is undergoing the withdrawal process. Your wife will not feel pain."

81. At a staff meeting discussing the return of one of the staff nurses from a drug rehabilitation program, one nurse states, "I don't know why we are wasting time on this. We all know that those people go back to using drugs as soon as the pressures increase." The nurse manager's best response would be:
    1. "It's important for us to share our feelings about staff members with problems."
    2. "I guess you feel somewhat guilty that you failed to recognize that this nurse was addicted."
    3. "I know it's hard, but it's our professional obligation to work with these individuals."
    4. "Since you have such strong negative feelings, I don't think you should be assigned to work with this staff member."

82. A newly admitted client looks at but does not respond to the nurse. The nurse's most appropriate action would be to state:
    1. "I guess you would rather be alone for now; I will return later so we can talk."
    2. "I am talking to you. Are you having trouble understanding what I am saying?"
    3. "I am here to tell you about the services available to you on the mental health unit and to offer you my help."
    4. "This is the mental health unit of the hospital. We have many services to offer. Let me tell you about them."

83. A newly admitted client quietly listens to a nurse's explanation of the services and activities available on the mental health unit. When the nurse is finished, the client looks around and states, "So this is where they keep the crazies." The nurse's most appropriate initial response would be:
    1. "These people are sick. They are not crazy."
    2. "Some people feel that way. Let's talk about mental health."
    3. "Are you feeling that a person has to be crazy to need mental health services?"
    4. "No, that is not correct. Let me explain the purpose of a mental health unit."

84. A 24-year-old male psychiatric client has been talking with the nurse regularly for 1 week. He has expressed that he sometimes has a problem with people. He has lost three jobs and four roommates in the last 6 months. When exploring the issue of the client's relationships with people, the nurse's most appropriate response would be:
    1. "Let's not focus on those past experiences; let's focus on the future."
    2. "That's a lot of changes. What happened in those jobs and with those roommates?"
    3. "It must be distressing to have had to adapt to these changes; tell me how you did it."
    4. "Tell me more about some of the specific problem situations you've experienced with these people."

85. The nurse tells a client that talking with the staff members is part of the therapy program. The client responds, "I don't see how talking to you can possibly help." The nurse's most appropriate response would be:
    1. "I can see how you would feel that way now, but hopefully you'll change your mind."
    2. "You will never know whether or not it is helpful unless you are willing to give it a try."
    3. "The one-to-one relationship has proven itself very helpful for others. Why don't you give it a try?"
    4. "Hopefully, I can help you sort out your thoughts and feelings so you can better understand them."

86. The nurse can best handle the answering of personal questions asked by the client in any phase of the nurse-client relationship by:
    1. Reviewing the positive and negative aspects of the subject
    2. Providing brief, truthful answers and redirecting the focus of conversation
    3. Offering an honest, brief expression of personal views on the subject raised
    4. Gently reminding the client that the nurse's feelings are not the client's concern

87. After admitting a confused 80-year-old client to the mental health unit, the nurse considers the aging process. The nurse recognizes that of the following factors, the one not symptomatic of aging would be:
    1. Slowing of responses
    2. Changing of personality
    3. Lowering of intelligence
    4. Prolonging of ability to learn

88. A male client with dementia due to Parkinson's disease has been placed in a nursing home. His wife appears tired and angry on her first visit with her husband. As she is leaving she says to the unit nurse in a sarcastic tone, "Let's see what you can do with him." The nurse's most therapeutic response would be:
    1. "It must have been very difficult to care for him."
    2. "I don't understand what you mean by that comment."
    3. "We have experience in caring for clients such as your husband."
    4. "It's too bad you didn't realize you needed help to care for him."

89. An overweight, 12-year-old male is brought to the clinic by his parents. The father states, "You've got to do something to help him. Just

look at his size." The child tells the nurse that he dislikes school because his classmates tease him about his weight. He states rather sadly, "I'm always last when they choose up sides in gym." The nurse's most therapeutic response would be:
    1. "That hurts a lot when you want to be liked."
    2. "Not everybody's a great athlete. You have other strengths."
    3. "Have you tried letting them know how that makes you feel?"
    4. "Won't it be great when you lose weight and can do better in gym?"

90. During a group therapy session occasionally silence will occur. To deal with this situation in a growth-promoting way, the leader should:
    1. Call on specific members to talk when silence occurs
    2. Be willing to sit indefinitely to wait the silence out
    3. Go around the group, requiring each member to talk in turn
    4. Comment on the silence or nonverbal behavior related to the silence

91. At a therapy group session a group member, using a teasing manner, makes several negative remarks about the nurse's appearance and behavior. The nurse could best respond by saying to:
    1. The group, "What do you think this client is trying to tell me?"
    2. The group, "Do you think this client's behavior is appropriate today?"
    3. The client, "You seem very interested in my appearance and behavior. What's this all about?"
    4. The client, "I cannot just sit here and let you talk about me this way. What have I done to make you angry?"

92. A registered nurse, who is a beginning group leader in a community mental health center, has been assigned to start a new group with regressive, long-term clients. The nurse manager should explain that in the beginning new group leaders are expected to:
    1. Talk extensively about their own experiences
    2. Confront group members about a variety of issues
    3. Have difficulty handling conflicts between members of the group
    4. Have less difficulty with long-term clients without acute problems

93. A nurse-group leader in a mental health center has used a variety of techniques in an effort to promote group cohesion. The nurse would

recognize the presence of group cohesion if the group members:
1. Readily accept new members
2. Withdraw from disliked members
3. Socialize more when productivity decreases
4. Use the phrase "our group" during discussions

94. During a therapy group session, after one of the members relates a traumatic incident that happened during the week, another client with a smile states, "Things haven't gone well in my life this week either." It would be most appropriate for the nurse to:
1. Ask the client to share what has been happening during this week
2. Make a note of the incongruity of the client's message but remain silent
3. Say to the client, "You say things have been bad this week, yet you are smiling."
4. Comment, "This seems to have been a bad week for a number of group members."

95. As a young male client is receiving a dialysis treatment, the nurse notes he is not talking with the other clients and his eyes are lowered and his jaw is clenched. The nurse states, "You look discouraged." The client replies, "I'm a bother. Not much good to anyone anymore. My wife would at least get some insurance money if I died." The nurse's most therapeutic response would be:
1. "I can understand how you feel."
2. "You feel so bad you wish you were dead."
3. "We all have days we feel like that. Let's talk about your diet."
4. "I know it's hard, but don't let it get you down or let your wife hear you."

96. When the behavior of a visiting family member agitates a depressed client, the nurse should:
1. Take the client to the coffee shop for a treat
2. Distract the client by providing another activity
3. Limit the client's contact with the family member
4. Discuss the family member's behavior with the client

97. A client in a psychiatric hospital requests an unaccompanied pass and it is denied. The client vocalizes anger toward the staff for this decision. The nurse should recognize that this anger is resulting from feelings of:
1. Hopelessness
2. Worthlessness
3. Powerlessness
4. Indecisiveness

EMOTIONAL DISORDERS RELATED TO PHYSICAL HEALTH AND CHILDBEARING (ED)

98. A 3-year-old child's parents have been unable to visit since the child was admitted to the hospital. The toddler has become quiet and withdrawn. To best help the child at this time, the nurse should:
1. Bring the child a doll or stuffed animal to cuddle
2. Encourage the child to play games with the other children
3. Assign the same nurse to care for the child whenever possible
4. Contact the child's parents and tell them to come immediately to visit

99. A 9-year-old boy has just been told he must stay in the hospital in traction for at least two weeks. The nurse finds him crying and unwilling to talk. At this time, the nurse should give the highest priority to:
1. Giving him privacy and allowing him to cry
2. Trying to distract him to prevent embarrassment
3. Telling him that his injury will not be permanent
4. Arranging for him to have a tutor begin immediately

100. A 16-year-old high school student is referred to the Health Center by a local hotline because she fears she has contracted herpes. The teenager is upset and shares this with the nurse. An appropriate initial response would be:
1. "Let me get a brief health history now."
2. "Try not to worry until you know if you have herpes."
3. "Herpes has received too much attention in the media; let's be realistic."
4. "You sound worried; let me make arrangements to have the doctor examine you."

101. A 15-year-old adolescent tearfully states that her father has been sexually assaulting her for the past eight years. Initially the nurse should:
1. Attempt to determine what type of incidents preceded the abuse
2. Explain that this must be reported immediately to the Child Protective Services
3. Tell the adolescent that sharing this information is a positive step in getting help
4. Determine whether the adolescent understands what is involved in sexual intercourse

102. A client with a history of hypertension comes to the clinic, where the intake physical reveals a blood pressure of 180/102 mm Hg. When the nurse asks whether the client has been taking any medications, the client replies, "I took the pills the doctor prescribed for a few weeks, but I didn't feel any different. So, I decided I'd just take them if I felt sick." The best initial response by the nurse would be:
    1. "I'm glad to hear you felt well enough to stop the medication."
    2. "You must be quite frightened about having high blood pressure."
    3. "You really should try to take your medication; the physician felt it was needed."
    4. "I think we should talk to the physician about a plan of treatment you can follow."

103. A male client with a history of ulcerative colitis is admitted to the hospital because of severe rectal bleeding. He appears to be an angry, demanding person. One day the nursing assistant tells the nurse, "I've had it with that client and all his demands. I'm not going in there again." The nurse's best response to this statement would be:
    1. "You need to try to be patient with him. He's going through a lot right now."
    2. "I'll talk with him and see whether I can figure out the best way for us to handle this."
    3. "Just ignore him and get on with the rest of your work. Let someone else take a turn."
    4. "He's frightened and taking it out on the staff. Let's think how we can approach him."

104. A client calls out to every nursing staff member who passes by the door and asks them to do or get something. The nurse can best manage this behavior by:
    1. Closing the door to the room so the client cannot see the staff members as they pass by
    2. Assigning one staff member to approach the client regularly and spend time talking with the client
    3. Informing the client that one staff member will come in frequently to see whether the client has any requests
    4. Arranging for a variety of staff members to take turns going into the room to see whether the client has any requests

105. A client having presurgical testing prior to a possible colon resection and colostomy says to the nurse, "If I have to have this surgery, I know my husband will never come near me." The nurse's best initial response would be, "You're:
    1. Probably underestimating his love for you."
    2. Concerned that your husband will reject you."
    3. Wondering about the effect on your sexual relations."
    4. Worried that the surgery will change how others see you."

106. A client requiring surgery because of mitral valve incompetence is admitted to the hospital and states, "I need a new valve, and do an oil change, too!" The most therapeutic response by the nurse would be:
    1. "You really don't need to hide your anxieties."
    2. "You sure came to the right place for a valve job."
    3. "I'm glad to see you're handling the situation so well."
    4. "I'm sure you have a great deal to ask about your surgery."

107. A female client, who has been told by her physician that she has untreatable metastatic carcinoma, tells the nurse that she believes the physician has made an error, she does not have cancer, and she is not going to die. The nurse evaluates that the client is experiencing the stage of death and dying known as:
    1. Anger
    2. Shock
    3. Bargaining
    4. Acceptance

108. A 68-year-old has metastatic carcinoma and has been told by the physician that death will occur within a month or two. The nurse enters the client's room after the physician leaves and finds the client crying. The nurse's action should take into consideration that:
    1. Crying relieves depression and helps the client face reality
    2. Crying releases tension, which frees psychic energy for coping
    3. Nurses should not interfere with a client's behavior and defenses
    4. Accepting a client's crying maintains and strengthens the nurse-client bond

109. A terminally ill 76-year-old client is very quiet and unwilling to have visitors. During the initial contact with the client, the nurse should:
    1. Attempt to understand what the death and dying process means to the client
    2. Avoid talking about the client's condition unless the client initiates the discussion
    3. Ascertain how much pain the client is experiencing and what medications have been ordered

4. Explore the extent to which the client is aware of the prognosis and the client's feelings about the situation

110. A female client terminally ill with cancer says to the nurse, "My husband is avoiding me. He doesn't love me anymore because of this damn tumor!" The nurse's most appropriate response would be:
   1. "What makes you think he doesn't love you?"
   2. "Avoidance is a defense; he needs your help to cope."
   3. "He is probably having difficulty dealing with your illness."
   4. "You seem very upset. Tell me how your husband is avoiding you."

111. The major improvement in the body image of clients following early fitting with prostheses after amputation is usually related to:
   1. The improvement of functional abilities
   2. The feeling that they look more "whole"
   3. The acceptance they receive from others
   4. The fact that something is being done to help

112. A pregnant client, who has type 2 diabetes and a history of three spontaneous abortions, is scheduled for a contraction stress test. Before the test she begins to cry when answering the nurse's questions about her previous pregnancies. She states, "I know it's my diabetes. This baby will never live. It's all my fault." The nurse's best response would be:
   1. "I understand that this must be very stressful for you."
   2. "Diabetes and pregnancy are difficult to deal with together."
   3. "This baby will live because it is being very closely monitored."
   4. "I know you're worried, but getting upset can alter test findings."

113. The nurse identifies that a client who has had a myocardial infarction is struggling with an alteration in self-concept. The nurse intervenes to promote client autonomy. The behavior that would demonstrate an increase in client autonomy would be when the client:
   1. Actively participates in planning self-care
   2. Verbalizes realistic expectations of caregivers
   3. Discusses necessary lifestyle changes with family members
   4. States the conditions for recovery following a myocardial infarction

114. An adult woman, who has severe rheumatoid arthritis, becomes depressed. The nurse begins to work with her in one-to-one sessions to help her deal with her depressive episode. The best long-term goal for this client would be that the client will:
   1. Eat at least two meals per day with other clients
   2. Decrease negative thinking about herself, others, and life
   3. Make one positive verbal comment to another client daily
   4. Maintain hygiene and grooming, and attend structured activities

115. Before signing a consent for a total laryngectomy, a client asks, "Nurse, the doctor says he's going to take part of my throat out and put a hole in my neck to breathe. Will I be able to talk like before?" The nurse's best response would be:
   1. "Would you like to talk to the doctor again to answer your questions?"
   2. "We have lots of clients with this operation. You'll talk again. You'll see."
   3. "Not like before but there is nothing to worry about. This procedure is done often."
   4. "Why don't you tell me what you know about your surgery? You seem very concerned."

DISORDERS FIRST EVIDENT BEFORE ADULTHOOD (BA)

116. The nurse is aware that a child's emotional problems usually occur as a result of:
   1. Rejection by the parents
   2. Family pathologic factors
   3. Authoritarian parenting style
   4. Overbearing overprotectiveness

117. The nurse would expect a child with a diagnosis of reactive attachment disorder to:
   1. Have been physically abused
   2. Cling to the mother and cry on separation
   3. Be able to develop only superficial relationships with others
   4. Have a more positive relationship with the father than with the mother

118. The nurse is aware that a child experiencing emotional problems would probably exhibit:
   1. Impaired ability to test reality
   2. Passive and deliberate behavior
   3. Overinvolvement with peer groups
   4. A mild to moderate level of anxiety

119. When assessing disturbed children, the clue that the nurse would find most indicative of severe emotional problems would be the child's:
    1. Physical complaints
    2. Behavioral outbursts
    3. Poor school performance
    4. Lack of response to the environment

120. A school-age child is brought to the clinic by the mother, who states, "Something is very wrong. My child never seems happy and refuses to play." When assessing this child for depressed behavior, the nurse should initially begin with the statement:
    1. "Tell me about yourself."
    2. "Let's talk about what you do after school."
    3. "Can you tell me what is making you so unhappy?"
    4. "Why does your mother think that you are unhappy?"

121. When teaching parents about childhood depression the nurse should say, "It:
    1. May appear as acting-out behavior."
    2. Is short in duration and resolves easily."
    3. Looks almost identical to adult depression."
    4. Does not respond to conventional treatment."

122. When implementing a tertiary preventive program for the mentally challenged, the nurse should:
    1. Teach mentally challenged children how to feed themselves
    2. Refer children for evaluation if they fail to meet developmental milestones
    3. Encourage the use of birth control methods by women who are mentally challenged
    4. Utilize the Denver Developmental Screening Test to evaluate children attending well-child clinics

123. A toddler has a history of frequent temper tantrums. The mother asks how to limit this acting-out behavior. The nurse's most therapeutic response would focus on:
    1. Restraining the child whenever a tantrum begins
    2. Moving the child to a quiet area before the tantrum begins
    3. Telling the mother to ignore the tantrum whenever possible
    4. Asking the physician to order medication for behavioral control

124. With the diagnosis of a possible pervasive developmental autistic disorder, the nurse would find it most unusual for a 3-year-old to demonstrate:
    1. Ritualistic behavior
    2. An interest in music
    3. An attachment to odd objects
    4. Responsiveness to the parents

125. A 3-year-old child is admitted to a mental health facility with a diagnosis of autistic disorder. It is essential for the nurse planning care for this toddler to know the child's:
    1. Use of language
    2. Body boundaries
    3. Mother and father
    4. Method of reality testing

126. The nurse is aware that language development in the autistic child resembles:
    1. Echolalia
    2. Stuttering
    3. Speech lag
    4. Scanning speech

127. A 7-year-old girl is brought to the clinic by her mother, who tells the nurse that her child has been having trouble in school, has difficulty concentrating, and is falling behind in her schoolwork since she and her husband separated six months ago. The mother reports that lately her daughter has not been eating her dinner and she often hears her crying in her room. The nurse realizes that the child:
    1. Feels different from her classmates
    2. Is working through her feelings of loss
    3. Would probably be happier living with her father
    4. Probably blames herself for her parents' breakup

128. When assessing the mental status of a 7- or 8-year-old child, it is most important for the nurse to:
    1. Engage the child in a discussion about feelings
    2. Use direct questions to determine the child's mental ability
    3. Listen to the parents' description of the child's behavior
    4. Compare the child's functioning from one time to another

129. An only child who lives with the mother (the custodial parent) begins demonstrating school and emotional problems after the parents' marital breakup. It is decided that the child would probably benefit most from family therapy. The nurse plans that the first group session will include:
    1. The parents

2. The mother and the child

3. The parents and the child

4. The mother, the child, and the child's teacher

130. A 10-year-old child who has a history of school failure and destructive acting out is admitted to a child psychiatric unit with the diagnosis of attention-deficit/hyperactivity disorder (ADHD). The youngest of three children, the child is identified by both the parents and the siblings as the family problem. The parents tell the nurse that the child's behavior has resulted in severe marital problems. The nurse would be correct in identifying the family's pattern of relating to the child as:
   1. Controlling
   2. Patronizing
   3. Scapegoating
   4. Overburdening

131. To help a disturbed, acting-out child develop a trusting relationship, the nurse should:
   1. Inquire as to the child's feelings about the parents
   2. Implement 30-minute one-to-one interactions daily
   3. Offer periodic support and emphasize safety in play activities
   4. Initiate limit-setting and explain the rules that must be followed

132. A 6-year-old child recently started school but has been refusing to go for the past three weeks. The nurse is aware that an appropriate intervention for this child would be to:
   1. Enroll the child in a special education program
   2. Delay the return to school for several months
   3. Convince the child that school is a place to have fun
   4. Develop a behavior modification program with the child

133. The school nurse is requested to present an educational program on attention deficit disorder to the teaching staff of an elementary school. The nurse should emphasize that:
   1. This problem usually is evident before 4 years of age
   2. This disorder occurs more frequently in lower socioeconomic groups
   3. It is estimated that this problem affects around 3% to 7% of the school-age population
   4. Children with this disorder sleep more than others because of their high activity level

134. An acting-out, hyperactive 9-year-old boy is started on a behavior modification program. One day he is playing a game with his peers and becomes frustrated when he begins to lose. He begins to kick the other children under the table and to call them names. The nurse, using the most appropriate behavior modification technique, should:
   1. Negatively reinforce the child by taking two of his tokens
   2. Require the child to have a time-out to regain control
   3. Ignore the child's behavior with the intent of extinguishing it
   4. Engage the child in a conversation about good sportsmanship

135. After one month in a special school, a hyperactive 10-year-old is asked to leave the group therapy session because of disruptiveness. The child begins to cry when being led out. The nurse's best approach at this time would be to:
   1. Send the child for a time-out in a quiet room
   2. Engage the child in a talk about the school day
   3. Offer an interpretation of the child's self-defeating behavior
   4. Provide nurturance by sharing a snack and a glass of milk with the child

136. A hyperactive, self-destructive child is to be discharged from an inpatient setting in a few weeks. In preparation for the child's discharge, it is most important for the nurse to plan to:
   1. Establish, maintain, and/or enforce limits on behavior
   2. Meet with the child's teacher to review the child's needs
   3. Help the child begin to terminate relationships with the staff
   4. Schedule a home visit and a community trip with the child's family

ANXIETY, SOMATOFORM, FACTITIOUS, AND DISSOCIATIVE DISORDERS (AX)

137. Some clients repeatedly perform ritualistic behaviors throughout the day to limit anxious feelings. The nurse recognizes that these behaviors are:
   1. Obsessions
   2. Compulsions
   3. Under personal control
   4. Related to rebelliousness

138. The nurse can evaluate that a client has successfully achieved the long-term goal of mobilizing effective coping responses when the client states, "When I feel myself getting anxious I will:
1. Use meditation and relaxation exercises."
2. Get involved in some type of quiet activity."
3. Avoid the situation that precipitated the anxiety."
4. Carefully examine what precipitated my anxiety."

139. When the nurse considers a client's placement on the continuum of anxiety, a key in determining the degree of anxiety being experienced is the client's:
1. Memory state
2. Creativity level
3. Perceptual field
4. Delusional system

140. An older adult who lives alone tells the nurse at the community health center, "I really don't need anyone to talk to. The TV is my best friend." The nurse recognizes that the client is using the defense mechanism known as:
1. Denial
2. Projection
3. Sublimation
4. Displacement

141. When working with a client who has a phobia about black cats, the nurse should anticipate that a problem for this client would be:
1. Denying that the phobia exists
2. Anger toward the feared object
3. Anxiety when discussing the phobia
4. Distortion of reality when completing daily routines

142. The nurse is aware that the therapy that has the highest success rate for people with phobias would be:
1. Systematic desensitization using relaxation techniques
2. Insight therapy to determine the origin of the anxiety and fear
3. Psychotherapy aimed at rearranging maladaptive thought processes
4. Psychoanalytical exploration of repressed conflicts of an earlier developmental phase

143. The nurse is aware that the symptoms that distinguish post-traumatic stress disorders from other anxiety disorders would be:
1. Lack of interest in family and others
2. Reexperiencing the trauma in dreams or flashbacks
3. Avoidance of situations and certain activities that resemble the stress
4. Depression and a blunted affect when discussing the traumatic situation

144. A 27-year-old female accountant, who recently completed graduate school, has come to the health clinic for a preemployment physical. During the health history, the new employee frequently states, "I feel so nervous about starting this job." She is able to connect with her feelings, thoughts, and actions but constantly focuses her attention on starting the new job. The nurse determines that the client is exhibiting:
1. A moderate level of job-related anxiety
2. An inappropriate response to handling new situations
3. A severe level of anxiety related to new situations
4. An ineffective coping mechanism in handling job-related stress

145. A client with a generalized anxiety disorder is hospitalized. The nurse realizes that an environment conducive to reducing emotional stress and providing psychologic safety is one in which:
1. Needs are a primary concern
2. All the client's needs are met
3. Realistic limits and controls are set
4. The physical environment is kept in order

146. A client comes to the hospital because of intense feelings of unrest, inability to sleep, and frequent episodes of panic. The client tells the nurse, "I admitted myself because I think I'm going crazy." The nurse should recognize the client's remark as a:
1. Plea for support
2. Symptom of depression
3. Reflection of insightfulness
4. Test of the nurse's trustworthiness

147. A client, who is to begin a physical therapy regimen after orthopedic surgery, verbally expresses anxiety about starting this new therapy. The nurse should acknowledge that some of this apprehension can be an asset because it will:
1. Slow down physiologic functioning
2. Increase alertness to the environment
3. Mobilize automatic behavioral responses
4. Promote the use of ego defense mechanisms

148. A nurse is accompanying a client with a diagnosis of substance-induced anxiety disorder

who is pacing the halls and crying. When the client's pacing and crying increase, the nurse suddenly feels uncomfortable and experiences a strong desire to leave. The probable reason for this feeling would be:
1. A desire to go off duty after a busy day
2. A fear of the client becoming assaultive
3. An empathic communication of anxiety
4. An inability to tolerate any more bizarre behavior

149. The nurse is aware that nursing intervention for client with anxiety disorder should include:
1. Supporting the verbalization of feelings by the client
2. Promoting the suppression of anger/hostility by the client
3. Insisting that the client accept the role of psychologic factors
4. Limiting the involvement of the client's family during the acute phase

150. The husband of a young mother who has attempted suicide asks if he may bring their 26-month-old daughter to visit his wife. The nurse's best response would be:
1. "Of course, children of all ages are welcome to visit relatives."
2. "Probably so, but you better check this with her physician first."
3. "It may be very upsetting for your child to see her mother so depressed."
4. "Tell me what your wife said when you offered to bring your child for a visit."

151. A client is pacing the floor and appears extremely anxious. The nurse approaches in an attempt to alleviate the client's anxiety. The most therapeutic question by the nurse would be:
1. "Are you feeling upset right now?"
2. "Would you like me to walk with you?"
3. "Shall we sit and talk about your feelings?"
4. "Would you like to go to the gym and work out?"

152. A 15-year-old client with the diagnosis of panic disorder jumps when spoken to, complains of feeling uneasy, and states, "It's as though something bad is going to happen." It would be most therapeutic for the nurse to:
1. Stay with the client to be a calming presence
2. Encourage the client to communicate with the staff
3. Allow the client to set the parameters for the interaction

4. Help the client to understand the cause of the feelings described

153. A client with a diagnosis of panic disorder, who had a panic attack on the previous day, says to the nurse, "That was a terrible feeling I had yesterday. I'm so afraid to talk about it." The nurse's most therapeutic response would be:
1. "It's best that you try to talk about it."
2. "OK, we don't have to talk about it now."
3. "What were you doing yesterday when you first noticed the feeling?"
4. "I understand, but don't be concerned; that feeling probably won't come back."

154. A female client is admitted to the acute care psychiatric unit with a diagnosis of panic disorder with agoraphobia. During the initial assessment phase the nurse should focus on:
1. Learning about the client's home life to facilitate planning care
2. Reducing the client's level of anxiety so that further interviewing can occur
3. Helping the client identify the source of her anxiety so the source can be avoided
4. Suggesting to the client that she rest for a while and informing her that they will talk later

155. When talking with a female client who displays many of the emotional and physiologic symptoms associated with a panic disorder, the nurse should:
1. Describe for her the possible reasons for her anxiety
2. Use short simple sentences and a firm authoritative voice
3. Ask many questions, because she probably is not going to volunteer much information
4. Suggest that she refrain from crying, because most of the time crying makes matters worse

156. A client is admitted to the hospital because of incapacitating obsessive-compulsive behavior. The statement that best describes how clients with obsessive-compulsive behavior view this disorder would be:
1. "It's not my fault that I act this way; the devil makes me do it."
2. "I know there's no reason to do these things, but I can't help myself."
3. "The things I do take a little time, but they make me a productive person."
4. "I don't know why everyone is upset with me; I'm doing nothing wrong."

157. A female client with a compulsive need to wash her hands many times during the day states that she feels she must get along better with her coworkers, but she has to be able to have unconditional access to the bathroom. When addressing the need for change, the nurse's most appropriate response would be:
    1. "Let's see what you can arrange with your coworkers."
    2. "What things can you change to get along better with your coworkers?"
    3. "What things need to change for you to get along better with your coworkers?"
    4. "I don't see how that approach will work to promote a working relationship with your coworkers."

158. The nurse plans to teach a client to use healthier coping behaviors that consciously can be used to reduce anxiety. These include:
    1. Eating, dissociation, fantasy
    2. Sublimation, fantasy, rationalization
    3. Exercise, talking to friends, suppression
    4. Repression, intellectualization, smoking

159. The nurse could evaluate that the staff's approach to setting limits for a demanding, angry client was effective if the client:
    1. No longer calls the nursing staff for assistance
    2. Understands the reasons why frequent calls to the staff were made
    3. Apologizes for disrupting the unit's routine when something is needed
    4. Discusses concerns regarding the emotional condition that required hospitalization

160. The change in an older adult client's behavior that would indicate that the nurse should reassess the client's needs and current plan of care, which was attempting to maintain the client's independent living style, would be the development of:
    1. Confusion
    2. Hypochondriasis
    3. Additional complaints
    4. Increased socialization

161. During the first meeting of a therapy group, the members become quite uncomfortable. The nurse notes frequent periods of silence, tense laughter, and a good deal of nervous movement in the group. The nurse would assess that these responses:
    1. Require active leader intervention to relieve symptoms of obvious stress
    2. Indicate unhealthy group processes with an unwillingness to relate openly

    3. Are expected group behaviors because relationships are not yet established
    4. Should be pointed out and discussed so members will not become too uncomfortable

162. During the working phase of a therapy group, a female group member becomes tearful after being told by another member that she needs to change her behavior. The nurse evaluates that the client:
    1. Feels too fragile to be challenged at this time
    2. Has been depressed about this aspect of her behavior
    3. Has had her feelings hurt by this response
    4. Is angry about the confrontation with another member

CRISIS SITUATIONS (CS)

163. A crisis can best be defined as:
    1. An imbalance of life
    2. A threat to equilibrium
    3. The perception of the problem by the client
    4. A situation requiring help other than personal resources

164. When working with families encountering problems, it is most important that the nurse have a:
    1. Good memory for details
    2. Common social background
    3. Warm nature and loving personality
    4. Sense of self and empathy for others

165. An adolescent client seeks help at a crisis intervention clinic. The client relates, "I dropped out of college because the instructors were dumb and the kids acted like babies. I was a psychiatric aide for six weeks. I got into trouble because the staff's thinking was archaic. I tried waiting on tables but got fired. The boss said I was nasty to the customers. They were the nasty ones. Now I can't even pay my rent. If people were nicer, I wouldn't be in this mess." In relation to crisis theory, this client's stressful events can be seen as:
    1. Experiential
    2. Age-related and frequent
    3. Usually noncrisis producing
    4. Situational and maturational

166. Situational crises are usually resolved in a time period of:
    1. 1 to 4 days

2. 2 to 3 weeks

3. 1 to 2 months

4. 2 to 6 months

167. The most critical factor for the nurse to determine during crisis intervention would be the client's:
    1. Developmental history
    2. Available situational supports
    3. Underlying unconscious conflict
    4. Willingness to restructure the personality

168. A young mother of three children, each born one year apart, has been hospitalized after attempting to hang herself. The client is being treated with milieu therapy. The nurse is aware that this therapeutic modality consists of:
    1. Using positive reinforcement to reduce guilt
    2. Uncovering unconscious conflicts and fantasies
    3. Providing individual, group, and family therapy
    4. Manipulating the environment to benefit the client

169. The nurse suggests a crisis intervention group to a client experiencing a developmental crisis. These groups are successful because the:
    1. Client is encouraged to talk about personal problems
    2. Crisis group supplies a workable solution to the client's problems
    3. Crisis intervention worker is a psychologist and understands behavior patterns
    4. Client is assisted to investigate alternative approaches to solving the identified problem

170. A nurse is taking calls at a local crisis center hotline and receives a telephone call from a suicidal adolescent. The nurse can safely terminate the call when the client:
    1. Wishes to terminate the conversation
    2. Has responded to the nurse's initial assessment of suicidal risk
    3. Begins to repeat the same information that has already been discussed
    4. Can state a preventive plan of action for dealing with self-destructive behaviors

171. A young college student tells the nurse in the school's health service that his girlfriend's period is late and they both think she is pregnant. The client, with a broad smile on his face, states loudly and angrily, "If she is pregnant I will drop out of school, marry her, and get a full-time job." The nurse's best initial assessment of the client's verbal and nonverbal behavior would be that they are:
    1. Uniform
    2. Consistent
    3. Incongruent
    4. Appropriate

172. When talking to the nurse about his decision to drop out of school and marry his girlfriend who is pregnant, a young college student says, "It's really the best decision. It is important for a child to have two parents." The nurse recognizes that the client is using the defense mechanism known as:
    1. Projection
    2. Introspection
    3. Displacement
    4. Intellectualization

173. A 24-year-old secretary, pregnant for the first time, receives a letter from her boyfriend with a check for $500 and the news that he has left. The client, who is very upset and feels at the end of her rope, calls the crisis intervention center for help. The nurse recognizes that the client is experiencing a crisis because the:
    1. Client is under a great deal of stress
    2. Client is going to have to raise her child alone
    3. Client's boyfriend left her when she was pregnant
    4. Client's past methods of adapting are ineffective for this situation

174. An unmarried, pregnant client who is attending a crisis intervention group has decided to continue the pregnancy and keep the baby. Now the crisis intervention nurse's primary responsibility would be to:
    1. Support the client for making a wise decision
    2. Explore other problems the client may be experiencing
    3. Make an appointment for the client to see a physician for prenatal care
    4. Provide information about other health resources where the client may receive additional assistance

175. An unmarried, pregnant client, who has been attending a crisis intervention clinic, has decided to keep the baby and is looking forward to motherhood. The nurse recognizes that the decision to attend prenatal child-care classes is an example of:
    1. Intrinsic motivation
    2. Extrinsic motivation
    3. Operant conditioning
    4. Behavior modification

176. A client who has been pregnant for five months spontaneously aborts after an accident. The client tells the nurse she feels depressed over the loss of her son. She describes how he would have looked and how bright he would have been. The nurse assesses that the client is demonstrating symptoms of:
1. The panic level of anxiety
2. A pathologic grief reaction
3. The typical grief syndrome
4. A diminished ability to test reality

177. A client who has just experienced her second spontaneous abortion expresses anger toward her physician, the hospital, and the "rotten nursing care." When assessing the situation, the nurse recognizes that the client may be using the coping mechanism of:
1. Denial
2. Projection
3. Displacement
4. Reaction formation

178. A couple in their late twenties were happy to be expecting a child. The client has a cesarean birth and is disappointed that the baby is a boy. The husband is pleased. On the second postpartum day, when the baby is brought to the client, she seems far away, as though she is daydreaming. The nurse calls the client's name and the client states, "I don't have a baby." She proceeds to rock her empty arms. The nurse recognizes that the precipitating factor for the client's emotional reaction is probably her:
1. Alteration in role
2. Husband's behavior
3. Religious upbringing
4. Desire for a baby girl

179. The parents of an 11-month-old infant diagnosed with failure to thrive are referred to the crisis intervention clinic. The nurse is aware that the first aspect of crisis intervention that should be employed would be:
1. Analytic therapy
2. Problem solving
3. Prescriptive work
4. Exploratory therapy

180. The nurse, suspecting that a newly admitted infant is the victim of child abuse, assesses the parents' interaction with their baby. The typical parental behavior that might confirm child abuse would be:
1. Displaying sensitivity about their child-care ability
2. Taking the initiative in meeting their child's needs
3. Having difficulty in showing concern for their child
4. Demonstrating heightened interest in their child's welfare

181. Child physical maltreatment is suspected in a 3-year-old girl admitted to the hospital with many poorly explained injuries. During a conversation, the statement by the mother that would further this suspicion would be:
1. "When I get angry, I take her for a walk."
2. "I send her to her room alone when she misbehaves."
3. "I make her stand in the corner when she doesn't eat her dinner."
4. "The other children were no problem; this one is stubborn and whiny."

182. An experienced mental health nurse who is on duty in a community mental health center assesses a 30-year-old male client brought in by a law enforcement officer. The recent history notes that the client was in jail and attempted to hang himself with his shirt. He was found by a guard and immediately cut down and brought in for a suicidal assessment. Physically the client is stable but emotionally he continues to state he "wants to die." The nurse uses a standardized tool to assess high-risk suicidal factors. The risk factor that is considered to be most "lethal" would be:
1. History of alcohol and drug abuse
2. Previous high-risk suicide attempts
3. History of isolation and withdrawal from friends and coworkers
4. Recent family disorganization due to wife's unemployment and his incarceration

183. When counseling the 20-year-old parents of a 13-month-old, the nurse is aware that the defense mechanism most often used by the physically abusive parent is:
1. Idealization
2. Transference
3. Manipulation
4. Displacement

184. When speaking with a mother accused of physical child abuse, the nurse should expect her to:
1. Attempt to rationalize and explain her behavior
2. Offer a detailed explanation of how her son was injured
3. Ask how she may get permission to visit her son on the pediatric unit
4. Reveal an overwhelming feeling that her child needed corrective discipline

185. When a diagnosis of child abuse is established, a nursing care priority would be:
    1. Staying with the parents while they visit
    2. Protecting the total well-being of the child
    3. Teaching the parents methods of discipline
    4. Promoting parental attachment to the child

186. The nurse may best assist an abusing parent to alter behavior toward an abused 2-year-old child by helping the client to:
    1. Recognize what behavior is appropriate for a 2-year-old child
    2. Learn appropriate ways of punishing the child's inappropriate behavior
    3. Identify the specific ways in which the child's behavior provokes frustration
    4. Ignore the child's negative, nondestructive behavior and support acceptable behavior

187. A nurse on the pediatric unit is assigned to care for a 2-year-old child with a history of being physically abused. The nurse should expect the child to:
    1. Smile readily at anyone who enters the room
    2. Be wary of physical contact initiated by anyone
    3. Begin to cry and scream as the nurse nears the bedside
    4. Pay little attention to the nurse standing at the bedside

188. When working with children who have been sexually abused by a family member it is important for the nurse to understand that these victims usually are overwhelmed with feelings of:
    1. Hatred and revenge
    2. Self-blame and guilt
    3. Humiliation and anger
    4. Confusion and disbelief

189. When the pediatric nurse practitioner examines the genital area of a 5-year-old child suspected of being sexually abused, the primary nurse can be most therapeutic by:
    1. Explaining the procedure and remaining with the child during the examination
    2. Telling the child that the practitioner wants to see if there is "anything wrong down there"
    3. Helping the mother explain the examination and the findings in terms the child will understand
    4. Asking whether the child would prefer the nurse or the mother to be present during the examination

190. A young child suspected of being sexually abused says to the nurse, "Did I do something bad?" The nurse's most therapeutic reply would be:
    1. "Who said you did something bad?"
    2. "What do you mean something bad?"
    3. "Do you think that you did something bad?"
    4. "I'm not sure I would say it was something bad."

191. A 13-year-old female student tearfully reveals to the school nurse that her brother has been forcing her to have intercourse. The nurse should:
    1. Suspect that this revelation is a cry for help related to some other crisis
    2. Recognize that this revelation is an attention getting method to meet unmet needs
    3. Assume that this revelation is true and follow the school's protocol for investigation
    4. Accept that this revelation may be a way to explain a suspected pregnancy and refer her for a pregnancy test

192. Before helping a client who has been sexually assaulted, the nurse should recognize that the rapist is motivated by feelings of:
    1. Passion
    2. Hostility
    3. Inadequacy
    4. Incompetence

193. During a nurse's interview with a client who has been sexually assaulted, the woman states that she should have fought back. The most therapeutic response by the nurse would be:
    1. "You are feeling guilty about submitting."
    2. "You may have submitted, but you are alive."
    3. "It's over; let's not explore what you could have done."
    4. "It is hard to know, but it's all right now; you are alive."

194. A recently married 22-year-old is brought to the trauma center by the police. She had been robbed, beaten, and sexually assaulted. The client, although very anxious and tearful, appears in control. The physician orders diazepam (Valium) 5 mg po prn for agitation. The nurse should administer this medication when the:
    1. Client requests something to calm her
    2. Physician is ready to do a vaginal examination
    3. Client's crying and trembling seem to increase
    4. Nurse determines the client's anxiety is increasing

195. The husband of a woman who has been sexually assaulted arrives at the hospital after being called by the police. After reassuring him about his wife's condition, the nurse should give priority to:
1. Discussing with him his own feelings about the situation
2. Calling the rape counselor in immediately to meet with the wife
3. Helping him to understand how his wife feels about the situation
4. Making him comfortable until the physician has completed examining his wife

196. A 15-year-old female is brought to the high school health office by two of her friends, who state, "We think she just took a handful of pills." The adolescent appears alert and refuses to speak. The school nurse's initial response should be to:
1. Ask the adolescent if she took any pills
2. Ask her friends where the adolescent got the pills
3. Call the rescue squad to stand by for an emergency
4. Call the adolescent's parents and tell them they must come immediately

197. The biggest problem for an older female client to cope with immediately after the death of her husband will probably be her:
1. Anger
2. Finances
3. Loneliness
4. Estrangement

198. A male client is brought to the psychiatric emergency room after attempting to jump off a bridge. The client's wife states that he lost his job several months ago and has been unable to find another job. The primary nursing intervention at this time would be to assess for:
1. Feelings of excessive failure
2. A past history of depression
3. Current plans to commit suicide
4. The presence of marital difficulties

199. In response to a parent's question about childhood suicide, the nurse's most appropriate response would be:
1. "Children do not have readily available means to kill themselves."
2. "Suicide threats and gestures in children should be taken seriously."
3. "Children younger than age 6 may threaten but do not attempt suicide."
4. "Suicide in young children is manipulative rather than self-destructive acting out."

200. A 7-year-old child has been diagnosed as having acute myelogenous leukemia. The physician has discussed the diagnosis and prognosis with the parents. While the parents are sitting in the lounge after visiting their child, they have a severe argument over something trivial. The nurse should recognize that they are using the defense mechanism of:
1. Denial
2. Projection
3. Displacement
4. Compensation

201. An 8-year-old child with a terminal illness is demanding of the staff. The child asks for many privileges that other children on the unit do not have, such as staying up later to watch TV and eating candy. The staff members know the child does not have long to live. The nurse can best help the staff members cope with the child's demands by encouraging them to:
1. Give as many extra treats as possible since the child is dying
2. Set reasonable limits to help the child become more secure and content
3. Give the child some extra treats so they will feel less anxiety after the child dies
4. Recognize that the dying child has unique needs, and special privileges can provide the necessary security

202. A 7-year-old child dies after an explosion at school. The parents arrive at the hospital a few minutes later and are told what had happened. The parents ask the nurse whether they can see their child. The best response by the nurse would be:
1. "It's best to wait a while."
2. "I will take you in to see your child now."
3. "Would you like to wait until the physician can be with you?"
4. "It will be less traumatic if you wait to see your child at the funeral home."

203. A 35-year-old woman is brought to a mental health hospital by her husband. The client is in a stupor and the husband states that her drinking has intensified in the three years since their son died. Taking this history into consideration, the nurse makes a tentative nursing diagnosis of:
1. Dysfunctional grieving
2. Disabled family coping
3. Disturbed personal identity
4. Disturbed thought processes

204. A mother whose daughter is killed in a school bus accident tells the nurse that her daughter

was just getting over the chickenpox and did not want to go to school, but she insisted that she go. The mother cries bitterly and says her child's death is her fault. The nurse should realize that perceiving a death as preventable will most often influence the grieving process in that:
1. The loss may be easier to understand and to accept
2. Bereavement may be of greater intensity and duration
3. The grieving process may progress to a psychiatric illness
4. It causes the mourner to experience a pathologic grief reaction

205. The initial nursing intervention for the significant others during the shock phase of a grief reaction should be focused on:
1. Staying with the individuals involved
2. Mobilizing the individuals' support systems
3. Directing the individuals' activities at this time
4. Presenting full reality of the loss to the individuals

206. Shortly after the death of her husband following a long illness, the wife visits the mental health clinic complaining of malaise, lethargy, and insomnia. The nurse, knowing that it is most important to help the wife cope with her husband's death, should attempt to determine the:
1. Age of the wife
2. Timing of the husband's death
3. Socioeconomic status of the client
4. Adequacy of the wife's support system

207. A female client's stream of consciousness is occupied exclusively with thoughts of her mother's death. The nurse should plan to help the client through this stage of grieving, which is known as:
1. Restitution
2. Resolving the loss
3. Shock and disbelief
4. Developing awareness

208. When an individual successfully completes the grieving process after the death of a significant other, the individual will be able to:
1. Accept the inevitability of death
2. Go on with life and forget the past
3. Remember the significant other realistically
4. Focus mainly on the good qualities of the person who died

209. The nurse discusses the plan of care with a depressed client whose husband has recently died. The nurse recognizes it would be most helpful to:
1. Encourage the client to talk about and plan for the future
2. Involve the client in group outdoor games each morning
3. Motivate the client to interact with male clients and the staff
4. Talk with the client about her husband and the details of his death

210. After completing the assessment of a female client who cannot function because of an impending divorce, the nurse recognizes that the most effective nursing intervention for this client would be to:
1. Help her to identify any precipitating factors
2. Assist her to explore and try out new coping skills
3. Develop the care plan to fit her perception of the events
4. Reduce her support systems to make her more independent

211. A depressed client, whose spouse recently died, attends an inpatient group therapy session in which the nurse is a co-leader. Toward the end of the session another client talks about being divorced and the resulting feelings of abandonment. As the members are leaving the session, the nurse notices that tears are running down the depressed client's face. Considering this client's depressed state, the nurse should:
1. Ask another client to stay and spend time talking with the client
2. Request that group members return and discuss this client's feelings
3. Observe the client's behavior carefully during the next several hours
4. Go to the client's room and encourage a discussion of thoughts and feelings

212. An older female comes to the mental health clinic. Assessment reveals that the client feels depressed and vaguely anxious and is unable to sleep at night. The client states, "I haven't felt right since my husband died eight months ago." The nurse makes the nursing diagnosis of dysfunctional grieving associated with the loss of the husband. The nurse identifies this diagnosis because of the client's:
1. Inability to talk about her loss
2. Difficulty in expressing her loss
3. Lack of sleep and the presence of symptoms of depression
4. Prolonged period of grief and mourning after her husband's death

213. A client with an inoperable occipital lobe tumor has been experiencing frightening visual hallucinations, especially when alone. The nurse can best help the client cope with these hallucinations by planning to:
    1. Move the client to a four-bed room closer to the nurse's station
    2. Suggest that the client turn on the radio or television when alone
    3. Have family or friends remain with the client until hallucinations stop
    4. Suggest that the client not be alone and work out a schedule for visitors

214. An older widow with lung cancer is now in the terminal stage of her illness. Her family is puzzled by her mood changes and apparent anger at them. The nurse should plan to explain to the family that the client is:
    1. Working through her situation
    2. Frightened by her impending death
    3. Attempting to reduce family dependence on her
    4. Hurt that the family will not take her home to die

215. A 76-year-old widower is terminally ill. He is very quiet, not talking much, and is unwilling to have visitors. During the initial contact with this client, the nurse should:
    1. Assess what the client knows about death and the dying process
    2. Avoid talking about his condition unless he initiates the discussion
    3. Encourage him to at least accept phone calls from those who wish to visit him
    4. Explore the extent to which he knows of his condition and what it means to him personally

216. A client who has been sexually abused tearfully states, "I'm no good now; there is nothing to live for." The most therapeutic response by the nurse would be:
    1. "Tell me more about your feelings."
    2. "I can understand why you feel worthless."
    3. "Why do you feel there is nothing to live for?"
    4. "You feel this way now because of what has happened."

217. The nurse recognizes that to help a couple work through their feelings about the husband's terminal illness, it would be important to:
    1. Assist the couple to express their feelings about his terminal illness to each other
    2. Refer the husband to the psychotherapist for assistance in dealing with his anger about death
    3. Place the couple in a couple's therapy group that addresses the terminal illness of one partner
    4. Encourage the couple to verbalize their feelings to a therapist during their individual therapy sessions

218. The husband of a client who is dying tells the nurse that he knows that his wife is asking the nurses to leave her pain medication on the bedside table and fears she is saving it up for a suicide attempt. The nurse knows that many of the staff members have mixed feelings about the client's terminal status and prolonged pain. The nurse uses an approach that is ethically sound by:
    1. Reporting the information to the nurse manager responsible for the unit
    2. Speaking to all of the nurses and telling them not to leave the medication at the bedside
    3. Suggesting a nursing conference be held to discuss staff feelings as well as the medication problem
    4. Asking the head nurse to handle the problems of the client's medication and the staff's feelings

219. An older female client, whose husband had been ill for a prolonged period of time, is visited by her husband's hospice nurse several weeks after the funeral for her husband. The nurse recognizes that the wife's biggest problem at this time will probably be her:
    1. Loneliness and feelings of isolation
    2. Anger at the husband for abandoning her
    3. Financial worries about maintaining her lifestyle
    4. Guilt over feelings of relief that her husband has died

220. The grieving wife of a client who has just died says to the nurse, "We should have spent more time together. I always felt the children's needs came first." The nurse recognizes that the wife is experiencing:
    1. Displaced anger
    2. Expected feelings of guilt
    3. Shame for past behaviors
    4. Ambivalent feelings about her husband

221. The nurse is aware that benzodiazepines should not be ordered for individuals undergoing acute grief because they:
    1. Magnify depression and increase the risk of suicide
    2. Suppress the brain activity needed to prevent depression

3. Extend the period of denial and suppress the grieving process
4. Cause lethargy and prevent the return to interpersonal activity

222. A female client is readmitted to the hospital in the terminal stage of cancer. When talking with the nurse the client states, "I don't understand why my husband won't tell me what's going on at home. His telling me not to worry, that everything is being taken care of, doesn't help." The most realistic interpretation of the husband's behavior is that he is:
1. Attempting to stop the client from worrying
2. Expressing his unacknowledged anger with her dying
3. Acting out his need for dominance in their relationship
4. Attempting to deal with his needs and trying to cope without her input

DEMENTIA, DELIRIUM, AND OTHER COGNITIVE DISORDERS (DD)

223. A 70-year-old retired man has had difficulty remembering his daily schedule and finding the right words to express himself. He is diagnosed as having dementia of the Alzheimer's type. The nurse is aware that symptoms of this disorder:
1. Have periods of remission
2. Develop over a long period
3. Usually occur fairly rapidly
4. Begin after a loss of self-esteem

224. An 84-year-old widow with dementia, who had been living with her daughter before hospitalization, is being discharged with a referral to the visiting nurse. When the nurse visits, the client is in bed sleeping at 10 AM. Her daughter states that she gives her mother sleeping pills to stop her wandering at night. The nurse should:
1. Discuss the possibility of placing the client in a nursing home
2. Explore the use of a home health aide to sit with the client at night
3. Suggest moving the client among family members on a monthly basis
4. Empathize with the daughter but suggest that wrist restraints would be better

225. When the nurse is communicating with a client with substance-induced persisting dementia, the client cannot remember facts and fills in the gaps with imaginary information. The nurse is aware that this is typical of:
1. Concretism
2. Confabulation

3. Flight of ideas
4. Associative looseness

226. When taking a health history from a client who has a moderate level of cognitive impairment due to dementia, the nurse would expect to note the presence of:
1. Hypervigilance
2. Increased inhibition
3. Enhanced intelligence
4. Accentuated premorbid traits

227. An 84-year-old woman is admitted to the hospital with a diagnosis of dementia of the Alzheimer's type. The nurse recognizes that this disorder is a:
1. Functional disorder that occurs in the later years of life
2. Problem that first emerges in the third decade of life
3. Disorder that is easily diagnosed through laboratory and psychologic tests
4. Cognitive problem that is a slow, relentless, diffuse deterioration of the mind

228. An older client is admitted to the hospital with the diagnosis of dementia of the Alzheimer's type and depression. The client has all of the following symptoms. The symptom that is unrelated to the depression would be:
1. Shallow or labile affect
2. Neglect of personal hygiene
3. "I don't know" answers to questions
4. Apathetic response to the environment

229. When planning activities for an older nursing home resident with a diagnosis of vascular dementia, the nurse should:
1. Plan varied activities that will keep the resident occupied
2. Provide familiar activities that the resident can successfully complete
3. Offer challenging activities to maintain the resident's contact with reality
4. Make sure that the resident actively participates in the unit's daily activities

230. An older client's family tells the nurse that the client has suffered some memory loss in the last few years. They say that the client is sensitive about not being able to remember and tries to cover up this loss to avoid embarrassment. When attempting to increase the client's self-esteem, the nurse should try to avoid discussing events that require memory of the client's:
1. Work years
2. Married life
3. Recent days
4. Young adulthood

231. During the first month in a nursing home, a client demonstrates numerous behaviors related to disorientation and cognitive impairment. The nurse's plan for care should continue to take into consideration the:
    1. Ability of the client to perform tasks without becoming frustrated
    2. Assessment of the client's orientation to time, place, and person
    3. Identification of stressors that appear to precipitate the client's disruptive behavior
    4. Fact that the client's cognitive impairment will increase until adjustment to the home is accomplished

232. An older female client, who is confused and often does not recognize her children, is admitted to a nursing home. The client appears slovenly in attire, often soiling her clothing with feces and urine. The nurse can best manage this problem by:
    1. Putting the client into orientation therapy
    2. Supervising the client's bathroom activities closely
    3. Toileting the client at least once every 2 hours
    4. Explaining to the client how offensive her behavior is to others

233. A 65-year-old retired baker is admitted to the hospital with the diagnosis of dementia. The client is frequently agitated, confused, incontinent of urine and feces, and at times, unaware of the presence of others. The question by the nurse that would best test the client's ability for abstract thinking would be:
    1. "Can you give me today's complete date?"
    2. "How are a television set and a radio alike?"
    3. "What would you do if you fell and hurt yourself?"
    4. "Can you repeat the following numbers: 8, 3, 7, 1, and 5."

234. When checking memory impairment in a client with dementia, the nurse should first assess for:
    1. A disorientation of self
    2. The recall of past events
    3. The recall of recent events
    4. An impaired ability to name objects

235. An older nursing home resident with the diagnosis of early onset dementia likes to talk about olden days and at times has a tendency to confabulate. The nurse should recognize that this behavior serves to:
    1. Prevent regression

2. Increase self-esteem
3. Attract the attention of others
4. Reminisce about achievements

236. A priority of care for a client with a dementia resulting from AIDS would be:
    1. Assessing for pain frequently
    2. Planning for remotivational therapy
    3. Arranging for long-term custodial care
    4. Providing basic intellectual stimulation

237. When planning care for a 72-year-old client who has been admitted to the hospital because of bizarre behavior, forgetfulness, and confusion, the nurse should give priority to:
    1. Preserving the dignity of the client
    2. Promoting a structured environment
    3. Determining or ruling out an organic etiology
    4. Limiting the acceleration of symptomatology

238. An older nursing home resident with the diagnosis of dementia of the Alzheimer's type hoards leftover food from the meal tray and other seemingly valueless articles and stuffs them into pockets "so the others won't steal them." The nurse should plan to:
    1. Remove unsafe and soiled articles from the resident's belongings during the night
    2. Give the resident a small bag in which to place selected personal articles and food
    3. Tell the resident that the staff is required to keep harmful objects out of reach in the resident's closet
    4. Explain to the resident why the nursing home's policy for cleanliness and safety must be followed

239. A 54-year-old client has demonstrated increasing forgetfulness, irritability, and antisocial behavior. After being found disoriented and semi-naked walking down a street, the client is admitted to the hospital, and a diagnosis of dementia of the Alzheimer's type is made. The client expresses fear and anxiety. Considering the client's diagnosis, the best approach would be for the nurse to:
    1. Explore in depth the reasons for the client's concerns
    2. Initiate a program of planned interaction and activity
    3. Reassure the client by the frequent presence of staff members
    4. Explain the purpose of the unit and why admission was necessary

240. Nursing management of a forgetful, disoriented client with behaviors signifying dementia should be directed toward:
1. Rechanneling the client's excessive energies
2. Restricting gross motor activity to prevent injury
3. Managing the client's somewhat bizarre behaviors
4. Preventing further deterioration in the client's condition

241. An older adult resident of a nursing home, with the diagnosis of dementia of the Alzheimer's type, frequently talks about the good old days at the ranch. On the basis of an understanding of the resident's diagnosis, the nurse's most appropriate action at this time would be to:
1. Involve the resident in interesting diversional activities in a small group
2. Allow the resident to reminisce about the past and listen with interest to the stories
3. Gently remind the resident that those "good old days" are past and thinking should focus on the present
4. Introduce the resident to other residents of the same age so that they can mutually share their past experiences

242. A 79-year-old widow with dementia living in a nursing home is to join a group in recreational therapy. The nurse identifies that the client has laid out several dresses on her bed but has not changed from her nightgown. The approach by the nurse that would be most appropriate is:
1. Reminding her to dress more quickly to avoid delaying the other clients
2. Allowing her as much time as she needs but explaining that she will be very late
3. Helping her select appropriate attire and offering her assistance in getting dressed
4. Assisting her to dress while telling her what time she is expected in the activity room

243. A client with dementia has an alteration in the expression of emotions. An unusual emotional behavior would be:
1. Lability
2. Passivity
3. Curiosity
4. Withdrawal

EATING AND SLEEP DISORDERS (ES)

244. The nurse has just admitted a young client with anorexia nervosa. When obtaining the client's history and physical assessment, it would be unlikely that the client's condition would reveal:
1. Alopecia
2. Amenorrhea
3. Constipation
4. Hypertension

245. The nurse, working in a mental health facility, determines that the priority nursing intervention for a newly admitted client with bulimia nervosa would be to:
1. Monitor the client continuously
2. Observe the client during meals
3. Teach the client to measure intake and output
4. Involve the client in developing a daily meal plan

246. A teenage girl has been diagnosed with bulimia nervosa and is currently seeing a community mental health nurse weekly on an outpatient basis. The treatment approach that appears to be most helpful and leads to the greatest improvement for these clients is to engage them in:
1. Family therapy
2. Supportive group therapy
3. Cognitive-behavior therapy
4. Eclectic therapy with emphasis on crisis intervention

247. A young woman was hired as an assistant editor of a small magazine in another area of the state. Her new colleagues at work were friendly but did not socialize with her. The client turned to food for comfort and began inducing vomiting to prevent a gain in weight. When the binge-purge behaviors began to interfere with her ability to meet her job responsibilities, she made an appointment at the local mental health clinic. The priority assessment during this initial appointment would be the client's level of:
1. Anxiety
2. Boredom
3. Loneliness
4. Depression

248. A major recognizable difference between clients with anorexia nervosa and clients with bulimia nervosa is that clients with anorexia usually:
1. Tend to be more extroverted than clients with bulimia nervosa
2. Seek intimate relationships while clients with bulimia avoid them
3. Are at greater risk for fluid and electrolyte imbalances than are clients with bulimia
4. Deny the problem while clients with bulimia generally recognize that their eating pattern is abnormal

249. An adolescent, who is extremely underweight, talks constantly about being fat, eats very little food, and disappears into the bathroom after meals, angrily says to the nurse, "I don't need to be here. I don't have any problems. Stop watching me." To reduce the client's feeling of being threatened, the nurse would be most therapeutic by responding:
1. "I hear how frustrated you are to be here."
2. "If you do not follow the rules you will lose your privileges."
3. "Your feelings are part of your illness. You will feel different."
4. "I'll get you the medication your physician ordered for anxiety."

250. The nurse is aware that the signs and symptoms that would be most specific for diagnosing anorexia nervosa are:
1. Slow pulse, 10% weight loss, and alopecia
2. Compulsive behaviors, excessive fears, and nausea
3. Excessive activity, memory lapses, and an increased pulse
4. Excessive weight loss, amenorrhea, and abdominal distention

251. A 5-foot, 5-inch tall 15-year-old female who weighs 80 pounds is admitted to a mental health facility with a diagnosis of anorexia nervosa. The nurse recognizes that her problem most likely is caused by:
1. Her wish to be accepted by her peers
2. A desire to control her life and her environment
3. A delusion in which she believes she must be thin
4. The media's emphasis on the beauty of thinness

252. A characteristic that would suggest to the nurse that an adolescent may have bulimia would be:
1. Badly stained teeth
2. A positive body image
3. A previous history of gastritis
4. Frequent regurgitation and re-swallowing of food

253. Clients with eating disorders often exhibit similar symptoms. The nurse would expect an adolescent client with anorexia to exhibit:
1. Affective instability
2. Repetitive motor mechanisms
3. Depersonalization and derealization
4. Disheveled, unkempt physical appearance

254. The nursing intervention that should receive the highest priority in the period immediately following an emaciated 13-year-old's admission to the hospital for starvation secondary to anorexia nervosa would be:
1. Providing adequate rest and nutrition
2. Monitoring the client's fluid and electrolyte balance
3. Completing an assessment of the client's mental status
4. Obtaining more data about the client's diet and exercise program

255. While planning care for a client who appears very thin, verbalizes a fear of eating, and has a diagnosis of anorexia nervosa, the nurse determines that a realistic goal would be that the client will:
1. Eat 100% of the diet within two days
2. Gain 5 pounds by the end of the week
3. Assist with meal plans within five days
4. Consume a diet high in fat and calories

256. The nurse is aware that the major health complication associated with intractable anorexia nervosa would be:
1. Endocrine imbalance causing amenorrhea
2. Decreased metabolism causing cold intolerance
3. Cardiac dysrhythmias resulting in cardiac arrest
4. Glucose intolerance resulting in protracted hypoglycemia

257. While admitting a young client with anorexia nervosa to the unit, the nurse finds a bottle of assorted pills in the client's luggage. The client tells the nurse they are antacids for stomach pains. The best initial response by the nurse would be:
1. "Let's talk about your drug use."
2. "These pills don't look like antacids."
3. "Tell me more about these stomach pains."
4. "Some adolescents take pills to lose weight."

258. When planning care for a teenager with anorexia nervosa, nursing intervention should include:
1. Rewarding weight gain by increasing privileges
2. Discussing the importance of eating a balanced diet
3. Encouraging the client to include high-caloric foods in the diet
4. Family therapy focusing on the influence of the client's behavior on the family

259. The parents of an adolescent female are very upset about their daughter's diagnosis of anorexia nervosa and the treatment plan

proposed. The best intervention by the nurse when the client's parents ask to bring food in for the client would be to state:
1. "Your concerns about food contribute to her problem."
2. "While in the hospital, she should eat the hospital food."
3. "For now, allow the hospital staff to handle her food needs."
4. "It is important that you bring in whatever you think she'll eat."

260. When distinguishing whether a client may have anorexia nervosa or bulimia nervosa, the nurse should recognize those adaptations that relate only to anorexia nervosa. Check all those that apply.
1. _____ Cachexia
2. _____ Binge eating
3. _____ Constipation
4. _____ Decreased blood pressure
5. _____ Increased body temperature
6. _____ Delayed psychosexual development

261. When interacting with an adolescent client with the diagnosis of anorexia nervosa, the nurse should:
1. Show empathy
2. Maintain control
3. Set and maintain limits
4. Focus on dietary nutrition

262. The multidisciplinary team decides to employ a behavior modification approach to a young female's problem with anorexia nervosa. A planned nursing intervention that would follow this approach would be to:
1. Have the client role-play interactions with her parents
2. Restrict the client to her room until she gains 2 pounds
3. Provide the client with a high-calorie, high-protein diet
4. Force the client to talk about her favorite foods for 1 hour a day

263. When an adolescent female client with the diagnosis of anorexia nervosa starts to discuss food and eating, the nurse should plan to:
1. Use her current interest in food to encourage her to increase her intake
2. Tell her gently but firmly to direct her discussion of food to the nutritionist
3. Listen closely to determine her favorite foods and secure these foods for her
4. Let her talk about food as long as she wants, but limit discussion about her eating

264. When talking with one of the day nurses, a client with the diagnosis of anorexia nervosa states that the day nurses give better care and are nicer than the night nurses. The client also asks a question that the day nurse is aware was answered by one of the night nurses. The nurse should recognize that the client:
1. Needs assistance in exploring and verbalizing feelings about the night nurses
2. Is trying to develop a bond of trust with a staff member that should be supported
3. Is attempting to divide the staff, and the behavior should be reported to the other staff members
4. Has negative feelings about the night nurses, and the nurses should be informed of these feelings

265. The nurse notes that a young female with anorexia nervosa telephones home just before each mealtime. She ignores reminders to eat and continues talking until the other clients are finished eating. She then refuses to eat "cold food." The nurse should:
1. Insist that the client eat the cold food
2. Remove the client's telephone privileges
3. Hang the telephone up when meals are served
4. Schedule a family meeting to discuss the problem

266. A young male client with anorexia nervosa telephones home just before mealtime. The client uses the phone calls to avoid eating. The nurse could evaluate that the nursing plan to set limits on this avoidance behavior was effective when the client:
1. Organizes an aerobic group for the clients
2. Arrives on time for meals without being called
3. Begins reading and clipping recipes from magazines
4. Contacts his family frequently by telephone between meals

267. The parents of a male adolescent diagnosed with anorexia nervosa ask the nurse how long their son's treatment will take. The most therapeutic response by the nurse would be:
1. "Treatment of anorexia nervosa takes a long time and setbacks are common."
2. "Most anorectic adolescents respond favorably to treatment within a few weeks."
3. "Your son's prognosis depends on your willingness to become involved in therapy."
4. "Your son's progress depends on determining what triggered his desire to lose weight."

DISORDERS OF MOOD (MO)

268. A client's methods of coping are maladaptive. The nurse can best help the client develop healthier coping mechanisms by:
    1. Promoting interpersonal relationships with peers
    2. Providing a stress-free environment for the client
    3. Allowing the client to assume responsibility for decisions
    4. Setting realistic limits on the client's maladaptive behavior

269. The nurse can minimize agitation in a disturbed client by:
    1. Ensuring constant client and staff contact
    2. Increasing appropriate sensory stimulation
    3. Discussing the reasons for suspicious beliefs
    4. Limiting unnecessary interactions with the client

270. The nurse is aware that aside from feeling sad and having difficulty concentrating and sleeping, other common signs of depression include:
    1. Rigidity and a narrowing of perception
    2. Alternating episodes of fatigue and high energy levels
    3. Diminished pleasure in activities and alteration in appetite
    4. Fleeting participation and interest in activities of daily living

271. The nurse understands that extremely depressed clients seem to do best in settings where they have:
    1. Varied activities
    2. Multiple stimuli
    3. Routine activities
    4. Minimal decision making

272. When caring for a client with a major depression, the nurse usually has the most difficulty dealing with the:
    1. Client's lack of energy
    2. Negative nonverbal responses
    3. Client's psychomotor retardation
    4. Pervasive quality of the depression

273. When working with a client who is depressed, the nurse should initially:
    1. Accept what the client says
    2. Attempt to keep the client occupied
    3. Try to keep the client from talking too much
    4. Keep the client's surroundings bright and gay

274. When planning continuing care for the depressed client, the nurse should include:
    1. Offering the client an opportunity to make some decisions
    2. Encouraging the client to decide how to spend leisure time
    3. Making all decisions to relieve the client of this responsibility
    4. Allowing the client time to be alone to decide in which activities to engage

275. The nurse identifies establishing trust as a major nursing goal for a depressed client. This goal can best be accomplished by:
    1. Spending the day with the client
    2. Asking the client at least one question daily
    3. Waiting for the client to initiate conversation
    4. Spending short periods of time with the client every day

276. A client in an acute mental health unit appears severely depressed. The client does not initiate conversation or perform personal care. Questions are answered with a barely audible one- or two-word response. The nurse sits with the client and makes no demands. The nurse's intervention is based on the premise that:
    1. The nurse should spend time with all assigned clients
    2. This demonstrates that the client is worthy of attention
    3. One-to-one interaction is expected in an acute care unit
    4. The depressed client needs stimulation from the environment

277. One day, the nurse sits by a depressed client's bed and states, "I will be spending some time with you today." The client responds angrily, "Go talk to someone else. They need you more." The most therapeutic response by the nurse would be:
    1. "Why are you angry with me?"
    2. "I'll go, but I will be back tomorrow."
    3. "Don't say that. You are important, too."
    4. "I will be spending the next 15 minutes with you."

278. One morning a client with the diagnosis of acute depression states, "God is punishing me for my past sins." The nurse's best response would be:
    1. "Why do you think that?"

2. "God is punishing you for your sins?"

3. "You really must feel upset about this."

4. "If you feel this way, you should talk to your clergyman."

279. An older widower in a nursing home, who is sitting by himself in a lounge, states, "I am all alone; no one has any use for me." The response by the nurse that would be most appropriate is:
1. "You seem upset. Let's talk about what is bothering you"
2. "We need to be alone sometimes. It helps to get to know ourselves better."
3. "You should focus on ways to change this. Let's play some games to improve your morale."
4. "Have you done anything to avoid feeling lonely? I think you should socialize more with others."

280. The nurse has been working with a suicidal client for three weeks, on the inpatient unit. One morning the client greets the nurse cheerfully and states, "Everything is looking up. I am not going to have problems for very long." The nurse realizes that the client's behavior and statement may indicate:
1. An increased risk of suicide
2. Resolution of suicidal ideation
3. A positive response to treatment
4. Decreased levels of stress since hospitalization

281. As a client's depression begins to lift, the nurse encourages involvement with unit activities, primarily because this type of activity:
1. Provides for and encourages group interaction
2. Supports the client's self-esteem and builds self-confidence
3. Allows the client to verbalize repressed feelings of hostility
4. Keeps the client in view of the staff to limit suicide opportunities

282. On the fifth hospital day, the nurse observes that a depressed client remains lying on the bed when the clients are called to the dining room for lunch. To encourage the client to eat, the nurse should:
1. Simply state, "I will accompany you to the dining room."
2. Bring a tray to the client's room and leave it without comment

3. Provide information about the importance of eating to maintain health
4. Firmly state, "All clients are expected to go to the dining room for meals."

283. A 50-year-old homemaker is brought to the hospital with a history of weight loss, crying spells, restlessness, early morning insomnia, sitting in one place just staring into space, and picking at her skin. During the last 6 months, her husband of 30 years has been made president of his company and their children have both married. From the history, the nurse should realize the client is demonstrating the classic symptoms associated with:
1. Bipolar mood disorders
2. Major depressive episodes
3. Involutional induced reactions
4. Mood-incongruent manic disorders

284. The primary nursing diagnosis for a client with a medical diagnosis of major depression would be:
1. Spiritual distress related to depression
2. Situational low self-esteem related to altered role
3. Powerlessness related to the loss of idealized self
4. Impaired verbal communication related to depression

285. A depressed female client appears to show sadness in her nonverbal behavior. The nurse should plan to help the client to:
1. Increase her structured physical activity
2. Decide which activities of daily living she can perform
3. Deal with painful feelings by sharing and expressing them
4. Improve her ability to communicate with significant others

286. A depressed client is very resistive and complains about inabilities and worthlessness. The best approach by the nurse would be to:
1. Involve the client in activities in which success can be ensured
2. Listen to the client and delay any planned activity for another time
3. Encourage the client to select an activity in which there is some interest
4. Schedule activities for the client that can be implemented independently

287. A 34-year-old mother of a 28-month-old child has attempted suicide and is brought to a mental health facility. She says to the nurse, "I am a bad mother and have mistreated my child." The husband indicates he and his wife have been alienated since the child's birth and that he plans to seek a divorce soon. The nurse is aware that the most probable basis for this client's depression is her:
   1. Use of withdrawal as a defense in an attempt to survive in a relationship with a man who wishes to desert her
   2. Unmet dependency needs that have aroused unacceptable, hostile feelings that are turned inward against the self
   3. Child-abusing behavior that has resulted in feelings of guilt and shame that are being relieved by a punitive superego
   4. Basic feeling of loneliness that has resulted in the use of self-abasement to evoke love, sympathy, and compliments from others

288. When finding a depressed client crying, the most therapeutic response by the nurse to help the client explore feelings would be:
   1. "Does crying help?"
   2. "I know you are upset."
   3. "Tell me what has upset you."
   4. "Do you want to tell me why you are crying?"

289. A client remains depressed even after an 8-week trial on several antidepressant medications. A decision to initiate electroconvulsive therapy (ECT) is being considered by the treatment team. A contraindication for administering electroconvulsive therapy even with the use of a medication such as succinylcholine chloride (Anectine) would be:
   1. The presence of a brain tumor
   2. A current urinary tract infection
   3. The presence of diabetes mellitus
   4. A history of hypothyroid disorder

290. A client scheduled to begin electroconvulsive therapy to treat a severe depression that has not responded to any of the antidepressant medications tells the nurse, "I am frightened that there will be a permanent loss of memory after the treatment." The most therapeutic response by the nurse would be:
   1. "Your memory loss may be permanent, but it is usually just temporary."
   2. "You will not experience a permanent memory loss so there is no need to be frightened."
   3. "You will experience a temporary loss of memory and it is normal to feel frightened about this."
   4. "Your memory loss will be temporary, and it will help block out many of your painful past experiences."

291. An older man has not responded to an adequate trial of antidepressant drugs for treatment of major depression with suicidal ideation. The physician schedules electroconvulsive therapy (ECT). The client is able to discuss the advantages and disadvantages with the primary nurse. The client understands that a major disadvantage of ECT is that:
   1. Relief of symptoms requires weeks of treatment
   2. Fractures of bones can result from the precipitated seizure
   3. Both anterograde and retrograde memory impairment can occur
   4. Substantial loss of mental function occurs and continues a long time

292. To further assess a client's suicidal potential, the nurse should be especially alert to the client's expression of:
   1. Anger and resentment
   2. Anxiety and loneliness
   3. Frustration and fear of death
   4. Helplessness and hopelessness

293. A client whose wife recently died appears extremely depressed. The client states, "What's the use in talking? I'd rather be dead. I can't go on without my wife." The best response by the nurse would be:
   1. "You'd rather be dead?"
   2. "Tell me, what does death mean to you?"
   3. "I can understand why you feel that way."
   4. "Are you thinking about killing yourself?"

294. A hospitalized depressed client has been taking a mood-elevating drug for several weeks. The client's energy is returning and the client no longer talks about suicide. In response to this client's behavior, the nurse should:
   1. Keep the client under closer observation
   2. Engage the client in preliminary discharge planning
   3. Observe the client for side effects of the medication
   4. Help the client to plan for an unaccompanied 2-hour pass

295. The nurse becomes aware of an older client's feeling of loneliness when the client states, "I

only have a few friends. My daughter lives in another state and couldn't care whether I live or die. She doesn't even know I'm hospitalized." The nurse recognizes that the client's communication is probably a:
1. Clue to depression that is blocking motivation
2. Call for help to prevent acting on suicidal thoughts
3. Manipulative attempt to persuade the nurse to call the daughter
4. Request for information about community social support groups

296. A female client, who is clinically depressed, reports that she has not experienced sexual orgasm in the past 3 years. The nurse is aware that this condition is best described as:
1. Diminished libido
2. Dysfunctional hypo-orgasmia
3. Primary orgasmic dysfunction
4. Situational orgasmic dysfunction

297. A female client, who was admitted to the hospital because she attempted suicide, reveals that her desire for sex has diminished since her child's birth 3 years ago. The most accurate nursing diagnosis would probably be sexual dysfunction related to:
1. Decreased sexual desire associated with depression
2. Decreased sexual desire associated with dependency
3. Inadequate sexual desire associated with marital stress
4. Inadequate sexual desire associated with identity confusion

298. A clinically depressed female client, on a psychiatric unit of a local hospital, uses embroidery scissors to cut her wrists. After treatment, when the nurse approaches, the client is tearful and silent. The best initial intervention by the nurse would be to:
1. Sit quietly next to the client and wait until she begins to speak.
2. Note the client's behavior, record it, and notify the attending physician
3. Say, "You are crying; does that mean you feel badly about attempting suicide and really want to live?"
4. State, "I notice you are tearful and seem sad. Tell me what it's like for you and perhaps we can begin to work it out together."

299. A male client with the diagnosis of bipolar disorder, depressed type, is found lying on the floor in his room in the psychiatric unit. He states, "I don't deserve a comfortable bed; give it to someone else." The nurse should best respond:
1. "Everyone has a bed and this one is yours."
2. "You are not allowed to sleep on the floor."
3. "I don't understand why you are on the floor."
4. "You're too valuable a person to be lying on the floor."

300. A client is admitted with a bipolar disorder, depressed type, episode. The nursing history indicates a progressive increase in depression over the past month. The nurse should expect the client to display:
1. Elated affect related to reaction formation
2. Loose associations related to a thought disorder
3. Physical exhaustion related to decreased physical activity
4. Paucity of verbal expression related to slowed thought processes

301. A client with a bipolar mood disorder, manic type, says to the nurse, "I don't know what I'm doing here. I never felt better in my life; I've got the world on a string around my finger." The most therapeutic response to this comment would be:
1. "Have you ever felt this way before?"
2. "You are feeling pretty high right now."
3. "You've got the whole world on a string!"
4. "Why do you think you're feeling so good?"

302. When selecting a room for a client with the diagnosis of bipolar I disorder, who is hyperactive and talking nonstop in a loud demanding voice, the nurse recognizes that a most important factor would be that the:
1. Room has a pleasant view
2. Atmosphere be quiet and restful
3. Location be close to the nurses' station
4. Roommates have similar behavioral responses

303. When developing an initial nursing care plan for a female client with a bipolar I disorder (manic episode) the nurse should plan to:
1. Increase her gym time
2. Isolate her from her peers
3. Provide food, fluids, and rest
4. Encourage her active participation in unit programs

304. When a client, who has a bipolar mood disorder, is hyperactive it is difficult to entice the client to sit still long enough to eat a complete meal. A care plan states, "Provide finger foods such as carrots, celery, and cheese sticks at 10 AM, 2 PM, and 7 PM." Recent assessment of this client indicates that all of the food at mealtime is eaten but snacks have been refused. The nursing staff should:
1. Change the plan based on the evaluation
2. Revise the nursing diagnosis based on the present analysis of behavior
3. Continue to implement the plan so that the client's nutritional status will improve
4. Reassess the client's nutritional status in 1 week and make changes based on that assessment

305. A nursing care plan for a client with a bipolar I disorder should include:
1. Providing a structured environment
2. Touching the client to provide reassurance
3. Engaging the client in conversation about current affairs
4. Designing activities that will require the client to maintain contact with reality

306. A female client is hospitalized for a bipolar mood disorder, manic type. She is hyperactive, obnoxious, calls the nurse names, is sarcastic to the staff, and taps the nurse playfully on the buttocks. When caring for this client, it is most important for the nurse to:
1. Spend extra time with the client
2. Place the client alone in a quiet room
3. Disregard this behavior when the client acts out
4. Be aware of own feelings toward the client

307. A female client is admitted to the psychiatric unit wearing evening clothes and bright facial makeup. During the first 24 hours the client paces continually and laughs loudly. When approached by the nurse, the client refuses to cooperate with any requests, shouting, "I am in charge. I give the orders!" The nurse recognizes that in addition to neurotransmitter alterations, the client's manic symptoms can be viewed as:
1. A fulfillment of innate desires
2. A response to an imagined loss
3. An uncontrollable urge to relate
4. An attempt to ward off depression

308. A 32-year-old woman is hospitalized with a diagnosis of bipolar disorder, manic episode. She becomes loud and vulgar and disturbs the other clients. The nurse should:
1. State, "You are bothering the other clients."
2. Segregate the client until this phase of her illness passes
3. Realize that vulgar talk is part of the illness and ignore it
4. State, "We don't like that kind of talk around here."

309. A client who has been diagnosed with bipolar disorder, manic episode, has been sleeping very little and has not eaten for 2 weeks prior to hospitalization. The nurse is aware that in the overactive client, feeding problems frequently result from the client's:
1. Feeling of unworthiness
2. Inability to take the time to eat
3. Unconscious desire for punishment
4. Preoccupation with ritualistic behavior

310. The nurse realizes that the environment is very important when caring for a client with a diagnosis of bipolar II disorder with hypomanic episodes. The nurse should therefore:
1. Put bright drapes in the client's room to cheer up the client
2. Place the client in a private room to provide a quiet atmosphere
3. Assign the client to a room with other clients to provide company
4. Locate the client in a room near the day-room to provide access to activities

311. A client demonstrating manic behavior is elated and sarcastic. The client is constantly cursing and using foul language and has the other clients on the unit terrified. The nurse should:
1. Demand that the client stop the behavior immediately
2. Firmly tell the client that the behavior is unacceptable
3. Ask the client to identify what is precipitating the behavior
4. Increase the client's medication or get additional medication ordered

312. Nursing care for a client with a bipolar mood disorder, manic phase, is sometimes difficult. An important fact for the nurse to remember when planning care is that these clients are:
1. Aware of reality
2. Out of contact with the environment
3. Quite embarrassed by their symptoms
4. Able to control the acting-out behavior

313. Encouragement and praise should be given to hyperactive clients to help them increase their feelings of self-esteem. When they have behaved well, the best way to let them know the staff is aware of their improvement is for the nurse to say:
   1. "You behaved well today."
   2. "I knew you could behave."
   3. "Everyone likes you better when you behave like this."
   4. "Your behavior today was much better than yesterday."

314. A male client with cyclothymic disorder with hypomanic symptoms is admitted to the psychiatric unit. He has progressively lost weight and does not take the time to eat his food. The nurse can best respond to this situation by:
   1. Providing a tray for him in his room
   2. Assuring him that he is deserving of food
   3. Pointing out that the energy he is burning up must be replaced
   4. Ordering food that he can hold in his hand to eat while moving around

315. A client with a diagnosis of bipolar disorder with rapid cycling is readmitted 4 months after discharge. The client has become increasingly hyperverbal, loud, and intrusive. The most therapeutic response by the nurse who had cared for the client during the previous hospitalization would be:
   1. "Tell me about the medicine you take."
   2. "You seem to have a need to interrupt me."
   3. "I have a feeling that you are under great stress."
   4. "How is your relationship with your spouse?"

DISORDERS OF PERSONALITY (PR)

316. The desensitization method that has been used successfully with clients experiencing phobias focuses on:
   1. Imagery
   2. Role-playing
   3. Assertiveness training
   4. Modeling or imitation

317. A client comes to the psychiatric clinic for treatment of a phobia about cats. The nurse at the clinic should anticipate that this client will demonstrate:
   1. Fear of discussing the phobia
   2. Anger toward the feared object
   3. Poor impulse control when threatened
   4. Distortion of reality when completing daily routines

318. A hospitalized psychiatric client with the diagnosis of personality disorder demands a sleeping pill before going to bed. After being refused the sleeping pill, the client hurls a book at the nurse. The nurse recognizes this behavior as:
   1. Ego alien
   2. Exploitive
   3. Acting out
   4. Manipulative

319. A 30-year-old female client, who has an obsessive-compulsive disorder, asks the nurse to change her room, stating that she hates her roommate and can't stand to be in the same room with her. Just as she finishes speaking, her roommate enters and the client tells her she missed her and has been all over the unit looking for her. The nurse recognizes that the client is using:
   1. Projection
   2. Sublimation
   3. Displacement
   4. Reaction formation

320. The mother of a 17-year-old female, hospitalized for extremely disturbed acting-out behavior, leaves a shopping bag at the desk saying, "This is for my daughter's birthday. I'm too busy to visit today." The gift is an unwrapped expensive pocketbook with the price tags attached. The daughter becomes upset and tearful after being given the message and opening the package. The mother's behavior is an example of:
   1. Maternal rejection
   2. Projective behavior
   3. A double-bind message
   4. Passive-aggressive behavior

321. A nurse on a mental health unit has developed a therapeutic relationship with an acting-out, manipulative client. One day as the nurse is leaving, the client says, "Please stay. I'm afraid the evening staff doesn't like me. They often punish me." The nurse can best assist this client by saying:
   1. "I'll ask the staff not to punish you."
   2. "Tell me more about what you're feeling now."
   3. "Don't worry, I told you everything would be all right."
   4. "You know I leave at this time. We'll talk about this in the morning."

322. To maintain a therapeutic relationship with a client diagnosed as having a borderline personality disorder, the nurse on the psychiatric unit should:
1. Be firm, consistent, and understanding and focus on specific behaviors
2. Provide an unstructured environment for the client to promote self-expression
3. Use an authoritarian approach because this type of client needs to learn to conform to the rules of society
4. Record but ignore marked shifts in mood, suicidal threats, and temper displays because they last only a few hours

323. After a conference with the psychiatrist, a client with a borderline personality disorder cries bitterly, pounds the bed in frustration, and threatens suicide. It would be most helpful for the nurse to:
1. Leave the client for a short period until the client regains control
2. Pat the client reassuringly on the back and say, "I know it is hard to bear."
3. Sit down and listen attentively if the client wishes to talk about the problem
4. Ask about the client's troubles and point out that other people also have problems

324. A client is exhibiting withdrawn patterns of behavior. The nurse is aware that this type of behavior eventually produces feelings of:
1. Anger
2. Paranoia
3. Loneliness
4. Repression

325. The nurse recognizes that a client's withdrawn behavior may temporarily provide a:
1. Defense against anxiety
2. Basis for emotional growth
3. Time for internal problem solving
4. Delay to collect personal resources

326. The nursing team has a conference to develop goals for the care of a withdrawn, shy, male client with low self-esteem, who is afraid to talk to members of the opposite sex. The objective that should be given priority would be, "The client will:
1. Increase his self-esteem."
2. Examine his feelings toward females."
3. Understand the cause of his sexual disorder."
4. Increase his knowledge of sexual functioning."

327. A female client with severe incapacitation because of obsessive-compulsive behavior has

been admitted to the hospital. The client's compulsive ritual involves changing her clothing 8 to 12 times a day. She continually asks the nurse for advice regarding her problems but then ignores it. This is an example of the conflict of:
1. Apathy versus anger
2. Trust versus mistrust
3. Intimacy versus isolation
4. Dependence versus independence

328. A client misses breakfast because of an elaborate handwashing ritual. During the early stage of the client's hospitalization, it would be most therapeutic for the nurse to:
1. Prevent the client from beginning the ritual until after breakfast is served
2. Encourage the client to interrupt the ritual for meals at the scheduled times
3. Allow the client to choose between eating breakfast or completing the ritual
4. Wake the client early so the ritual can be completed before breakfast is served

329. A 38-year-old mother with obsessive-compulsive disorder has become immobilized by her elaborate handwashing and walking rituals. The nurse recognizes that the basis of obsessive-compulsive disorder is often:
1. Feelings of guilt and inadequacy
2. Problems with anger and remorse
3. Problems with being too conscientious
4. Feelings of unworthiness and hopelessness

330. An executive secretary experiences an overwhelming impulse to count and arrange the rubber bands and paper clips in the desk. The client feels something dreadful will occur if the ritual is not carried out. In regard to the client's symptoms, the nurse is aware that:
1. Compulsive rituals are useful in our society as long as they can be controlled
2. Compulsive rituals serve to control anxiety resulting from unconscious impulses
3. The symptoms are a displacement of general anxiety onto an unrelated specific fear
4. The client is consciously controlling the symptoms, although this raises anxiety

331. A client who uses a ritual of counting paper in the computer printer tells the nurse, "I am spending 30 minutes counting each time and my boss is getting very upset. What should I do?" The nurse could best suggest that the client:
1. Arrive at work 30 minutes early each morning for counting

2. Limit the counting activity to only 20 minutes each time

3. Substitute another activity at home such as counting shoes or other objects

4. Talk with the boss and ask for tolerance until the psychiatric treatments help

332. A client who uses a complex ritual says to the nurse, "I feel so guilty. None of this makes any sense. Everyone must really think I'm crazy." The most therapeutic response by the nurse would be:
1. "Your behavior is bizarre, but it serves a useful purpose in your life."
2. "You are concerned about what other people are thinking about you."
3. "Guilt serves no useful purpose. It just helps you stay stuck where you are."
4. "I am sure people understand that you cannot help this behavior right now."

333. A female client with obsessive-compulsive disorder takes a lot of time each day to wash her hands. She is frequently late for appointments. The most therapeutic intervention by the nurse would be to:
1. Encourage her to speed up her ritual so that she can meet her appointments on time
2. Let her know how angry others become when she holds up activities to wash her hands
3. Verbally discourage her from washing her hands so frequently to prevent skin breakdown
4. Accept her ritualistic behavior in a matter-of-fact manner without displaying amusement or criticism

334. When planning care for a client using ritualistic behavior, the nurse must realize that the ritual:
1. Is under the client's conscious control
2. Helps the client control the anxiety level
3. Is used by the client primarily for secondary gains
4. Helps the client focus on the inability to deal with reality

335. It is observed that at times a client with a personality disorder clings to the nurse and at other times maintains a noticeable distance. The nurse realizes that this pattern of behavior illustrates that the client has conflicting fears of:
1. Shame versus rejection
2. Lost self-esteem versus hostility
3. Abandonment versus identity loss
4. Engulfment versus interdependence

336. At 10 PM a client with a personality disorder is in the hospital's lounge playing cards. When the nurse enters, the client requests a sleeping pill. The nurse responds, "First go to bed and attempt to sleep." The nurse's response was directed toward:
1. Setting limits
2. Reality testing
3. Routinizing care
4. Conditioning behavior

337. A client with a personality disorder is playing cards with another person in the hospital's lounge. When the other person cheats at cards, the client responds by aggressively scattering the deck of cards around the room. The nurse assesses that the client has:
1. Poor reality testing
2. A violent personality
3. An antisocial personality
4. Inadequate impulse control

338. An adolescent with a long history of drug abuse, stealing, refusal to comply with rules, and an inability to get along in any setting is admitted to an adolescent unit for evaluation. The most appropriate plan of care for the adolescent at this time would be for the nurse to:
1. Allow as much freedom as possible, setting few rules and minimum structure
2. Act as a role model for mature behavior while providing a very structured setting
3. Provide activities that ensure immediate gratification as well as social stimulation
4. Behave in a moralistic, punitive manner toward the adolescent when rules are not followed

339. A 22-year-old male is admitted to the psychiatric unit for observation for an antisocial personality disorder. He has been in repeated legal difficulty since he was a teenager and was recently arrested on charges of falsifying police records. As the client and the nurse are discussing his upcoming court date, the client states, "I know that everything has already been set. I don't have any witnesses so how can I prove I didn't do it. I know they'll convict me. I think I'll get out of town." Based on this statement the most appropriate nursing assessment would be that the client is using:
1. Escape ideation
2. Projective denial
3. Impaired judgment
4. Distorted reality testing

340. A male adolescent with the diagnosis of antisocial personality disorder spends a great deal of time with a female adolescent client on the unit. One day the nursing assistant enters the female client's room and finds them in her bed. Later the nursing assistant reports the incident to the nurse. The nurse should:
    1. Arrange a discussion with both adolescents
    2. Lock the bedroom doors to keep the clients within view of the staff
    3. Assign a staff member to observe both clients every 15 minutes
    4. Call a unit meeting to talk about sexual activity among all of the clients

341. An adolescent female with an antisocial personality disorder plans to live with her parents after discharge. The parents request advice on how to respond to their daughter's behavior. The nurse tells them it would be most therapeutic for them to:
    1. Discuss her behavior with her and encourage her to develop self-control
    2. Avoid setting expectations for her behavior and react to each situation as it arises
    3. Help her find new friends and encourage her to get a job and assume responsibility for herself
    4. Set clear limits, explain the consequences of disregarding them, and firmly and consistently apply them

342. A client with an antisocial personality disorder has been remanded to the inpatient psychiatric unit for approximately 1 week. The client refuses to discuss any problems with the nursing staff and the team has decided an appropriate intervention would be to use confrontation. One morning the nurse asks the client how things went the day before. The client states, "I didn't do much. I watched TV and read a little." The most appropriate confrontational response by the nurse would be:
    1. "It seems that you're expecting us to wave a magic wand and cure you."
    2. "That's not much for someone who wants to get out of the hospital soon."
    3. "It seems that you're having difficulty facing up to your part in all your problems, and I wonder why that is."
    4. "It doesn't sound to me like you've been doing much work on the problems that brought you into the hospital."

343. One afternoon a male client on the inpatient psychiatric service complains to the nurse that he has been waiting for over an hour for someone to accompany him to activities. The nurse replies, "We're doing the best we can. There are a lot of other people on the unit who need attention too." This response demonstrates the nurse's use of:
    1. Impulse control
    2. Defensive behavior
    3. Reality reinforcement
    4. Limit-setting behavior

344. Windows in the recreation room of the adolescent unit have been found broken on numerous occasions, and after group discussion, one of the adolescents provides facts indicating that a male adolescent client has broken them. The nurse, using assertive intervention, should:
    1. Knock on the door of the adolescent's room and ask whether he would like to come out and talk about the situation
    2. Approach the adolescent when he is alone and, after making eye contact, inquire about his involvement in these incidents
    3. Confront the adolescent openly in the group, using a controlled voice and maintaining direct eye contact with him
    4. Use a trusting approach to the adolescent, implying that the staff doubts his involvement but requests his denial for the record

345. An 18-year-old is admitted to the hospital after taking 20 tablets of an anxiolytic. The client's diagnosis is antisocial personality disorder. When obtaining the history the nurse learns that the client had been arrested for drug use and is out on bail. During visiting hours, the nurse discovers the client and visitors smoking. By the odor, the nurse knows they are smoking marijuana. When confronted, the client responds, "I'm celebrating. Didn't you hear? I went to trial today and just got put on probation." The nurse's best response would be:
    1. "You were lucky you just got probation, so don't get right back into trouble."
    2. "I understand your relief about the trial, but pot smoking is against the rules."
    3. "Why don't you and your friends come out and join the other clients and their visitors."
    4. "If you can't follow the rules against pot smoking, your visiting privileges will be canceled."

346. An adolescent client with an antisocial personality disorder was admitted to the hospital because of drug abuse and repeated sexual acting-out behavior. The nurse could evaluate

that nursing actions directed toward modifying the behavior of this client had been successful when the client:
1. Promises never to take drugs again
2. Discusses the need to seduce other adolescents
3. Recognizes the need to conform to society's norms
4. Identifies the feelings underlying the acting-out behavior

347. A nurse in an outpatient mental health setting has been assigned to care for a new client who has been diagnosed with an antisocial personality disorder. During assessment the nurse would expect to observe that the client:
1. Pays great attention to detail and demonstrates high levels of anxiety
2. Has scars from self-mutilation and a history of many negative relationships
3. Demonstrates suspiciousness, avoids eye contact, and engages in limited conversation
4. Is charming, has an above average intelligence, and demonstrates a tendency to manipulate

348. A nursing diagnosis for a client with a multiple personality disorder is chronic low self-esteem probably related to childhood abuse. The most appropriate short-term client outcome would be:
1. Engaging in object-oriented activities
2. Recognizing each existing personality
3. Eliminating defense mechanisms and fears
4. Verbalizing the need for antianxiety medications

349. A client with a multiple personality disorder is to be discharged after a 2-week hospitalization. The nurse evaluating the effectiveness of the short-term therapy would expect the client to verbalize:
1. That many of the personalities can be ignored
2. That the personalities serve no protective purpose
3. The ability to deal openly with feelings and fears
4. The need for long-term outpatient psychotherapy

SCHIZOPHRENIC DISORDERS (SD)

350. The nurse has just completed a mental status examination on a newly admitted male psychiatric client and goes back to the nurses' station to write up the report. The nurse reflects on the client's long-drawn-out explanation of why he was admitted and notes that he used excessive detail to answer relevant questions, until finally arriving at a reasonable answer. The nurse notes on the record that this client used:
1. Flight of ideas
2. Circumstantiality
3. Tangential thoughts
4. Thought-blocking process

351. A newly admitted client is apathetic and exhibits an inappropriate affect. A diagnosis of acute schizophrenic reaction is made. Considering the diagnosis, a symptom the nurse would expect to observe in the client's communication or behavior is:
1. Suicidal preoccupation
2. Absence of self-criticism
3. Autistic magical thinking
4. Abstract and logical deductions

352. A 30-year-old female graduate student, who has become increasingly withdrawn and neglectful of her studies and personal hygiene, is brought to the psychiatric hospital by her roommate. After a detailed assessment, a diagnosis of schizophrenia is made. It is unlikely that the client will demonstrate:
1. A weak ego
2. A low self-esteem
3. Concrete thinking
4. Effective self boundaries

353. A client who has been admitted with a diagnosis of schizophrenia says to the nurse, "Yes, it's March. March is *Little Women*. That's literal you know." These statements illustrate:
1. Echolalia
2. Neologisms
3. Flight of ideas
4. Loosening of associations

354. When assessing a client with the diagnosis of an acute schizophrenic reaction, the nurse recognizes that the potential for recovery is better in a client whose history reveals the:
1. Occurrence of a precipitating event
2. Slow and insidious onset of the illness
3. Presence of a family history of schizophrenia
4. Presence of many poorly defined prepsychotic symptoms

355. A 20-year-old male is admitted to a mental health facility because of inappropriate behavior. The client has been hearing voices, responding to imaginary companions, and withdrawing to his room for several days at a time. The nurse understands that the withdrawal is a defense against the client's fear of:
1. Rejection
2. Punishment
3. The unknown
4. Powerlessness

356. When asking the family about the onset of problems in a young client with the diagnosis of schizophrenia, the nurse would expect that they would relate the client's difficulties began in:
1. Puberty
2. Adolescence
3. Late childhood
4. Early childhood

357. A female client, recently admitted to the hospital, is pacing the floor and acting aloof and suspicious. According to her husband she laughed in a silly manner when told her father was critically injured, and she has had difficulty with her colleagues at work, accusing them of sabotage. The client has stated that she is being controlled by others. The nurse, to be most helpful, should first:
1. Obtain a complete copy of the client's history
2. Review a textbook description of the schizophrenic client
3. Observe and evaluate the behavior in terms of the client's needs
4. Meet with the client's husband to learn more about the client

358. A young woman, who is admitted to the hospital with a diagnosis of schizophrenia, is actively hallucinating and delusional. When planning care, the nurse should be aware that hallucinations are:
1. Usually triggered by unknown factors
2. Misinterpretations of environmental stimuli
3. Generally related to the client's thought processes
4. Always extremely frightening and upsetting to the client

359. A client with schizophrenia repeatedly says to the nurse, "No moley, jandu! No moley, jandu." The nurse understands that this is called:
1. Echolalia
2. Concretism
3. Neologisms
4. Paleologic thinking

360. After 2 days on the unit, a female client with the diagnosis of schizophrenic reaction refuses to take a shower. It would be most appropriate for the nurse to:
1. Have the staff give her a shower
2. Simply state the client must shower now
3. Tell her she can shower when she feels more comfortable
4. Point out that her appearance is upsetting the other clients

361. A client is admitted to a psychiatric unit with the diagnosis of schizophrenia, undifferentiated type. When assessing the client, the nurse identifies the presence of the characteristics related to this disorder. Check all that apply.
1. _____ Bizarre behavior
2. _____ Extreme negativism
3. _____ Disorganized speech
4. _____ Vague hallucinations
5. _____ Persecutory delusions
6. _____ Psychomotor retardation

362. A client who has been hospitalized with schizophrenia tells the nurse, "My heart has stopped and my veins have turned to glass!" The nurse recognizes this as an example of:
1. Echolalia
2. Hypochondriasis
3. Somatic delusions
4. Depersonalization

363. A female client with acute schizophrenia tells the nurse, "Everyone hates me." The best response by the nurse would be:
1. "Tell me more about this."
2. "Everyone does not hate you."
3. "That feeling is part of your illness."
4. "You may be doing something to promote this feeling"

364. Breaks with reality, such as those experienced by clients with schizophrenia, necessitate that the nurse first realize that:
1. Extended institutional care is a necessary part of the treatment modality
2. Clients believe what they feel they have undergone and are experiencing
3. Electroconvulsive therapy produces remission in most clients with schizophrenia
4. The clients' families must cooperate in the maintenance of the psychotherapeutic plan

365. An adult male is admitted to the psychiatric unit after attempting suicide. The client's history reveals that his first child died of SIDS two years ago, he has been unable to work since the death of the child, and he attempted suicide before but was never hospitalized. When talking with the nurse he states, "I hear my son telling me to come over to the other side." The nurse recognizes that this statement would be most reflective of a:

1. Fixed delusion
2. Somatic delusion
3. False hallucination
4. Command hallucination

366. By recognizing common behaviors exhibited by the client who has a diagnosis of schizophrenia, the nurse can anticipate:
    1. Disorientation, forgetfulness, and anxiety
    2. Grandiosity, arrogance, and distractibility
    3. Withdrawal, regressed behavior, and lack of social skills
    4. Slumped posture, pessimistic outlook, and flight of ideas

367. The nurse is aware that a common nursing diagnosis for clients with a schizophrenic disorder is:
    1. Social isolation related to impaired ability to trust
    2. Risk for other-directed violence related to hallucinations
    3. Disturbed sleep pattern related to impaired thinking ability
    4. Impaired physical mobility related to fear of loss of control of hostile impulses

368. On admission a disturbed, unkempt female client refuses to remove her clothing. To best meet the client's needs the nurse should:
    1. Get assistance and remove her clothing to meet her basic hygiene needs
    2. Provide her with two outfits to assist the client to make a simple decision
    3. Tell her she will look more attractive in clean clothes to increase her self-esteem
    4. Wait and allow her to undress when she is ready, to help the client maintain her identity

369. A long-term goal for a paranoid male client who has unjustifiably accused his wife of having many extramarital affairs would be to help the client develop:
    1. Faith in his wife
    2. Better self-control
    3. Feelings of self-worth
    4. Insight into his behavior

370. A 25-year-old male client is being treated for a schizophrenic disorder. The client accuses the nurses and the physicians of being homosexuals. This behavior indicates that the client is:
    1. Attempting to keep the focus off his own problems

2. Trying to embarrass those perceived as authority figures
3. Having difficulty handling unacceptable feelings about himself
4. Exploring emotionally charged reactions to threatening situations

371. The most appropriate intervention for the nurse to take after finding an acting-out, disturbed client in the fetal position would be to:
    1. Tap the client gently on the shoulder and say, "I'm here to spend time with you."
    2. Sit down beside the client on the floor and say, "I'm here to spend time with you."
    3. Go to the client and say, "I'll be waiting for you by the table and chairs so please get up and join me."
    4. Leave the client alone because the behavior demonstrates the client is too regressed to benefit from talking with the nurse

372. The treatment team plans a schedule for a newly admitted client with schizophrenia that is believed will be nonthreatening and meet the client's needs. The plan is explained to the client and a written copy is posted in the client's room. When it is time to go for a walk, the nurse should approach the client and say:
    1. "It's time to go for your walk."
    2. "When would you like to go for your walk?"
    3. "Do you want to take your scheduled walk now?"
    4. "You are supposed to be going for your walk now."

373. The nurse believes an emotionally disturbed client is ready to begin participating in therapeutic activities. The nurse initially should suggest:
    1. Attending a class on medications
    2. Participating on the softball team
    3. Drawing or painting with the nurse
    4. Watching television in the dayroom

374. A female client with schizophrenia is going to occupational therapy for the first time. She tells the nurse she doesn't want to go. The nurse's reply that would be of most help to the client would be:
    1. "I will go with you to occupational therapy."
    2. "It is only for an hour, then you will be back."
    3. "Try it once; if you don't like it you need not go back."
    4. "The doctor ordered it as part of your treatment. You should go."

375. A client with a long history of disturbed behavior is unable to cope with the slightest change in the environment. To enhance the client's coping skills, the nurse should plan to:
1. Allow time for compulsive behavior
2. Maintain a low level of environmental stimuli
3. Provide ample opportunities for intellectual activities
4. Schedule short independent tasks that are achievable

376. To deal with a client's hallucinations therapeutically, the nurse plans to:
1. Reinforce the perceptual distortions until the client develops new defenses
2. Provide an unstructured environment and assign the client to a private room
3. Avoid helping the client make connections between anxiety-producing situations and hallucinations
4. Distract the client's attention by providing a competing stimulus that is stronger than the hallucinations

377. When managing interpersonal relationships with a client with schizophrenia, the nurse should first:
1. Allow the client to be alone when desired but provide quiet activities
2. Insist that the client join group activities and functions with other clients
3. Establish a one-to-one relationship before bringing the client into group activities
4. Encourage the client to become dependent but set limits on the extent of this behavior

378. To plan care for a client with undifferentiated schizophrenia, the nurse should recognize that the client's delusions are a defense against underlying feelings of:
1. Guilt
2. Inferiority
3. Aggression
4. Persecution

379. A male client diagnosed with schizophrenia, undifferentiated type, is currently admitted to a psychiatric inpatient unit. The client's medical record indicates he has been in and out of hospitals for 17 years. The nurse and the client plan for realistic outcomes before discharge. A realistic outcome for this client would be that the client will:
1. No longer believe that people are following him
2. Refrain from acting upon delusions or hallucinations

3. Avoid a relapse by taking his neuroleptic medication, so as not to be admitted for at least 9–12 months
4. Learn methods of coping with hallucinations by the use of distraction and not paying attention to the thoughts

380. A male client claims the voices he hears are clearly telling him what actions and decisions to make. It would be most therapeutic for the nurse to:
1. Play soft music when the client starts hearing voices
2. Begin talking to the client when he is hearing the voices
3. Demonstrate to the client that his perceptions are wrong
4. Recognize that the client is probably frightened by the voices

381. When a client with the diagnosis of schizophrenia talks about being controlled by others, the nurse should:
1. Express disbelief about the client's delusion
2. Arrange an interesting daily schedule for the client
3. Respond to the verbal content of the client's delusion
4. Acknowledge the feeling tone or theme of the client's delusion

382. A client on the psychiatric unit sits alone most of the day. No other clients ever seem to go near the client. The nurse, deciding to establish a relationship, approaches the client. As the nurse gets approximately 3 feet away, the client lets out a string of profanity and says, "Leave me alone; I don't want to talk to you!" The most appropriate response for the nurse to make at this time would be:
1. "I'll leave for now, but I'll be back later."
2. "Why do you feel the need to greet me in this way?"
3. "Do not talk to me like that. I am here to spend time with you."
4. "I don't like it when you talk like that. Are you trying to push me away?"

383. One afternoon the nurse observes a male client rushing down the hall of the unit rapidly, hitting his fist against the wall as he goes. The best nursing action at this time would be to:
1. Forcefully use additional staff members to subdue the client and stop his acting-out behavior
2. Attempt to approach the client in a nonthreatening manner to determine the basis for his agitation

3. Observe the client to see whether this behavior escalates and may involve harm to other clients or staff

4. Immediately summon staff assistance to enable administration of medication prescribed for the client's agitation

384. At mealtime, a client with schizophrenia moves to the counter to choose food but is unable to decide what to do next. The nurse, recognizing the client's ambivalence, assists by using:
    1. Nonverbal communication
    2. Clear, simple declarative statements
    3. Basic questions requiring simple choices
    4. A reward system for each food item chosen

385. A client with the diagnosis of schizophrenia watches the nurse pour juice for the morning medication from an almost empty pitcher and screams, "That juice is no good! It's poisoned." The nurse should:
    1. Remark, "You sound frightened."
    2. Pour the client a glass of juice from a full pitcher
    3. Assure the client that the juice is not poisoned
    4. Take a drink of the juice to show the client that it is OK

386. When a disturbed acting-out client's condition improves, the physician suggests giving a 1-day pass. The client's family is very nervous about the pass and is worried about what they will do if the client starts to act out. The nurse's best intervention at this time would be to:
    1. Have the social worker talk with the family
    2. Cancel the pass until the family is reassured
    3. Have the client promise the family that acting out will not occur
    4. Discuss this concern at a meeting with the client and the family present

387. One morning the nurse finds a disturbed client curled up in the fetal position in the corner of the dayroom. The most accurate initial evaluation of the behavior would be that the client is:
    1. Feeling more anxious today
    2. Attempting to hide from the nurse
    3. Tired and probably did not sleep well last night
    4. Physically ill and experiencing abdominal discomfort

388. An extremely agitated male client hospitalized in a mental health unit begins to pace around the dayroom. The nurse should:
    1. Lock the client in his room to limit external stimuli
    2. Let the client pace in the hall away from other clients
    3. Encourage the client to work with another client on a unit task
    4. Get the client involved in a card game to distract his thoughts

389. The nurse notices a male client sitting alone in the corner smiling and talking to himself. Realizing that the client is hallucinating, the nurse should:
    1. Ask the client why he is smiling
    2. Leave the client alone until he stops talking
    3. Invite the client to help to decorate the dayroom
    4. Tell the client it is not good for him to talk to himself

390. To increase the self-esteem of a client with schizophrenia, the nurse should plan to:
    1. Reward healthy behaviors
    2. Identify various means of coping
    3. Encourage good hygiene and grooming
    4. Explain the diagnosis and treatment plan

391. A young client with schizophrenia states, "I am starting to hear voices." The nurse could best respond:
    1. "What are the voices saying, and what do they mean to you?"
    2. "You are the only one hearing the voices. Are you sure you hear them?"
    3. "The health team will observe your behavior and we will not leave you alone."
    4. "I understand you are hearing voices talking to you, and that they are very real to you."

392. When being admitted to a mental health facility, a young male adult tells the nurse that the voices he hears frighten him. The nurse understands that clients tend to hallucinate more vividly:
    1. Before meals
    2. After going to bed
    3. During group activities
    4. While watching television

393. One morning a client tells the nurse, "My legs are turning to rubber because I have an incurable disease called schizophrenia." The nurse recognizes that this is an example of:
    1. An hallucination
    2. Paranoid thinking
    3. Depersonalization
    4. Autistic verbalization

394. A young male college student, who has a history of schizophrenia, paranoid type, is admitted for psychiatric treatment. He asserts that his professors are forcing him to fail and withdraw from school. He is guarded and withdrawn. A few hours after admission, another client sits down beside him. He jumps up and runs down the hall angrily shouting, "Leave me alone! Don't touch me!" The most accurate assessment of this behavior is that he:
1. Fears close contact with people
2. Is having an hallucinatory experience
3. Is responding to his delusional thoughts
4. Has confused the other client with one of his professors

395. When interacting with a confused, acting-out female client with a diagnosis of schizophrenia, the most therapeutic nursing intervention would be to:
1. Reassure the client that she will get better
2. Direct the client's daily activities on the unit
3. Help the client to clarify her experience and gain insight into her behavior
4. Provide the client with solutions to past and current problems she is experiencing

396. A male client in a mental health facility is tugging on his ear during a unit meeting. When the nurse comments about it, the client replies, "You know, it's that microcomputer those foreign agents implanted in my ear. They're trying to control my every thought and deed." Based on this statement the nurse should recognize that the client is experiencing:
1. Illusions
2. Hallucinations
3. Delusional thoughts
4. Neologistic thinking

397. The nurse recognizes that paranoid delusions usually are related to the defense mechanism of:
1. Projection
2. Regression
3. Repression
4. Identification

398. A client with schizophrenia tells the nurse, "There are foreign agents conspiring against me; they're out to get me at every turn." The verbal intervention that would be most appropriate is:
1. "These people you call foreign agents are out to do you in. What else is happening?"
2. "It must be frightening to believe that people are out to trick you at every opportunity."

3. "What's happened to make you believe these people you call foreign agents are after you?"
4. "I can understand how frightening your thoughts are; however, your thoughts do not seem factual to me."

399. When establishing a nursing care plan, the nurse should understand that a male client's delusion that he is an important government adviser is most likely related to:
1. A psychotic loss of touch with his real identity
2. An attempt at wish fulfillment created to manipulate others
3. A need to feel a sense of importance and control over his environment
4. An attempt to compensate for feelings of depression about his problems

400. During the admission procedure, a client who has paranoid ideation refuses to answer the nurse's questions, stating, "You are in a conspiracy to kill me." The nurse understands these feelings are related to the client's:
1. Low self-esteem
2. Need to be alone
3. Need for attention
4. Lack of acceptance

401. When planning care for a client using paranoid ideation, the nurse should realize the importance of:
1. Not placing any demands on the client
2. Removing stress so that the client can relax
3. Giving the client difficult tasks to provide stimulation
4. Providing the client with activities in which success can be achieved

402. During a one-to-one interaction with a client with schizophrenia, paranoid type, the client says to the nurse, "I figured out how foreign agents have infiltrated the news media. They want to shut me up before I spill the beans." This statement can best be described as:
1. A nihilistic delusion
2. A delusion of grandeur
3. An auditory hallucination
4. An overevaluation of the self

403. A disturbed client is admitted to the hospital for psychiatric evaluation. When taking the nursing history, the nurse asks why the client came to the hospital. The client states, "They lied about me. They said I murdered my mother. You killed her. She died before I was born." The nurse recognizes that the client is experiencing:
1. Ideas of grandeur

2. Confusing illusions
3. Persecutory delusions
4. Auditory hallucinations

404. In addition to being honest and matter-of-fact, a nursing approach that may be helpful when planning the care of clients diagnosed with schizophrenia of the paranoid type would be:
1. Exploring prominent life events
2. Limiting exploration to recent situations
3. Providing a nonthreatening environment
4. Ascertaining the content of their delusions

405. The nurse planning to establish a trusting relationship with a client who is using paranoid ideation should begin by:
1. Seeking the client out frequently to spend long blocks of time together
2. Sitting in the unit and observing the client's behavior throughout the day
3. Being available on the unit frequently but waiting for the client to approach
4. Calling the client into the office to establish a contract for regular therapy sessions

406. A client with schizophrenia, paranoid type, is delusional, withdrawn, and negativistic. The nurse should plan to:
1. Explain to the client the benefits of a group activity
2. Matter-of-factly invite the client to play ping–pong
3. Encourage the client to become involved in group activities
4. Mention to the client that the psychiatrist has ordered increased activity

407. A client refuses to eat, stating, "The food is poisoned." The nurse should:
1. Ask the client what foods are desired so they can be ordered
2. Encourage the client's family to bring favorite foods from home
3. Suggest going to the cafeteria and selecting foods the client feels safe eating
4. Go with the client to the cafeteria and taste the food to show that it is not poisoned

408. Lunch is being served, and the clients must walk to the dining room. The nurse finds one client sitting alone with the head slightly tilted as if listening to something. The nurse should state:
1. "I know you're busy but it's lunchtime."

2. "Lunchtime, let's go! We don't want to miss it!"
3. "Are those voices bothering you again? I'll help you get ready for lunch."
4. "It's lunchtime. I'll walk with you to the dining room and sit with you there."

SUBSTANCE ABUSE (SA)

409. A factor that might place a young person in a high-risk category for substance abuse would be:
1. Curiosity and daring attitude
2. Occasional periods of depression
3. Loss of a parent through death or separation
4. Typical stresses associated with adolescence

410. A 20-year-old carpenter falls from a roof and incurs fractures of the right femur and left tibia. The client reveals a history of substance abuse. A primary consideration for the nurse who is caring for this client would be to:
1. Confront the client about substance abuse
2. Communicate in the same speech pattern that the client uses
3. Avoid upsetting the client by calling attention to the drug abuse
4. Realize that this client will need more pain medication than a nonabuser

411. The nurse is aware that the defense mechanism commonly used by clients who are alcoholics is:
1. Denial
2. Projection
3. Displacement
4. Compensation

412. A client, with the diagnosis of alcoholism, explains to the nurse that alcohol has a calming effect and states, "I function better when I'm drinking than when I'm sober." The nurse recognizes that the client is using the defense mechanism of:
1. Sublimation
2. Suppression
3. Compensation
4. Rationalization

413. Within a few hours of alcohol withdrawal, the nurse should assess a client for the presence of:
1. Yawning, anxiety, convulsions
2. Tremors, fever, profuse diaphoresis
3. Disorientation, paranoia, tachycardia
4. Irritability, heightened alertness, jerky movements

414. A client is admitted to an alcohol rehabilitation center. On the fourth day after admission, the nurse detects a strong odor of alcohol on the client's breath. The first action by the nurse should be to:
1. Locate and remove the alcoholic substance
2. Ask directly where the client got the alcohol
3. Convey the staff's disappointment in this behavior
4. Notify the physician that the client has been drinking

415. A 42-year-old with a long history of alcohol abuse seeks help with the problem in one of the local hospitals. The nurse is aware that the major underlying factor for success in an alcohol treatment program will be the client's:
1. Family
2. Motivation
3. Psychiatrist
4. Self-esteem

416. A 65-year-old male is admitted to a mental health facility with a diagnosis of substance-induced persisting dementia resulting from chronic alcoholism. When conducting the admitting interview, the nurse determines that the client is using confabulation. The nurse recognizes that this is caused by the client's:
1. Ideas of grandeur
2. Marked memory loss
3. Need to get attention from others
4. Difficulty in accepting the diagnosis

417. The nurse's plan of care for a client with substance-induced persisting dementia resulting from chronic alcohol ingestion should take into consideration that this disorder is thought to be caused by:
1. An increase in serotonin
2. A reduction in iron intake
3. The malabsorption of riboflavin
4. A deficiency of thiamine in the diet

418. A male client who has a long history of alcohol abuse is informed that he has extensive liver damage. The client, whose father was an alcoholic and died of cirrhosis, lives with his mother. The client, when told that he has approximately 1 year to live if alcohol abuse persists, becomes intensely depressed and one evening leaves the hospital and returns drunk. The nurse is aware that the client's behavior suggests that he:
1. Believes he inherited the disease of alcoholism from his father and cannot stop drinking

2. Does not trust the judgment of the health professionals because he feels well physically
3. Wants to punish his mother for his physical and emotional discomfort and cause her pain
4. Cannot associate his increasing depression and lack of fulfillment to his heavy use of alcohol

419. When planning care for a client, who has a long history of heavy drinking, the nurse must be aware that the most serious, life-threatening symptoms from alcohol withdrawal usually occur:
1. 8 to 12 hours after the last drink
2. 12 to 24 hours after the last drink
3. 24 to 72 hours after the last drink
4. 72 to 96 hours after the last drink

420. A salesman with a history of heavy drinking is on a detoxification unit. He asks the nurse's permission to skip the Alcoholics Anonymous (AA) meeting held daily. The nurse's initial response should be:
1. "What are your feelings about going to AA?"
2. "What is it that you dislike about going to AA?"
3. "It's all right to wait until you feel like going to AA."
4. "Attending AA meetings is an important part of your treatment."

421. A client with a history of heavy drinking is brought to a psychiatric facility in a stupor. On the day after admission the client is confused, disoriented, and delusional. The nurse should be aware that the client may be developing alcoholic:
1. Amnesia
2. Hallucinations
3. Withdrawal delirium
4. Uncomplicated dementia

422. The nurse is aware that the reason some alcoholics are unable to stop drinking even though they begin to attend AA meetings is that they:
1. Enjoy the feeling caused by drinking alcohol
2. Physiologically require the substance in their body
3. Are trying drastically to alter a long-standing habit
4. Often have a character defect that defeats their willpower

423. When working with a client who is in an alcohol detoxification program, it would be most important for the nurse to:

1. Accept the client as a worthwhile person
2. Provide nurturing since the client needs it
3. Discuss the ill effects of alcohol with the client
4. Promote compliance by gently prodding the client

424. To give clients with long histories of alcohol abuse greater responsibility for self-control, the nurse initially should plan to:
1. Tell them about detoxification programs
2. Confront them with their substance abuse
3. Administer their medications according to the prescribed schedule
4. Assist them to identify and adopt more healthful coping patterns

425. Two days after admission to the detoxification program, a client with a long history of alcohol abuse tells the nurse, "I don't know why I came here." The nurse's best response would be:
1. "You feel you don't need this program?"
2. "You did admit yourself into the program."
3. "You realize you are trying to avoid your problem."
4. "Don't you remember why you decided to come here?"

426. A 40-year-old client has a long history of alcohol abuse. After an automobile accident the client is arrested for driving while intoxicated and is admitted to the hospital. When the client becomes angry and blames others, the nurse can be most therapeutic by stating:
1. "You know you are to blame for your alcohol abuse."
2. "You need help now or you are going to get even sicker."
3. "I can see that you are irritable and I want to help you feel better."
4. "I will talk to your family and friends about their behavior if you want me to."

427. On the third day of hospitalization a client with a history of heavy drinking develops delirium tremens. When the client is experiencing hallucinations, it would be most appropriate for the nurse to:
1. Do nothing because the client may just be having vivid dreams or nightmares
2. Pretend to see the imaginary things the client is talking about and do what the client asks
3. Tell the client that others do not sense or perceive the same things that seem to be so frightening

4. Ask the client to describe the sensation, then assure the client that the sensation is caused by alcohol withdrawal

428. A client has been in the alcohol detoxification unit for 5 days. One evening the client complains of numbness and tingling in the feet and legs. At this time it would be most appropriate for the nurse to:
1. Gently massage the client's lower extremities with lotion
2. Emphasize the need to rest and to keep the lower extremities elevated
3. Use mechanical aids to keep bed sheets off the client's lower extremities
4. Observe for the progression of symptoms and monitor the pedal pulses frequently

429. The family of a client who has completed alcohol detoxification relates that they are concerned about the client's behavior if drinking occurs. They state, "When the drinking starts, it really disrupts family life and we're not sure how to handle it." The nurse's best response would be:
1. "Try to maintain a pleasant home environment for your family."
2. "Include the client in the family's activities even when drinking has occurred."
3. "Search the house regularly for hidden alcohol and accompany the client outside."
4. "Help avoid embarrassment by making excuses for the client when functioning is impossible."

430. A 19-year-old waitress is admitted to the emergency department with a fractured femur. The client's history reveals multiple drug abuse for the last 8 months. When caring for this client, the nurse is aware that the most serious life-threatening symptoms during withdrawal usually result from:
1. Heroin
2. Methadone
3. Barbiturates
4. Amphetamines

431. When planning care for a client who has just finished withdrawal from multiple drug abuse, the nurse should take into consideration that this client probably is:
1. Unable to give up drugs
2. Unconcerned with reality
3. Unable to delay gratification
4. Unaware of the danger of drug addition

432. A 37-year-old male high school principal has been remanded by the court to the drug rehabilitation unit of a psychiatric facility for treatment of cocaine addiction. When obtaining a history from this client, the nurse expects that he would report that he:
1. Sleeps a great deal
2. Has lost considerable weight
3. Noted recent speech difficulties
4. Has very quiet and sedentary habits

433. As a client addicted to cocaine withdraws from the drug, the nurse should expect to observe:
1. Delirium
2. Suspicion
3. Depression
4. Hyperactivity

434. The nurse is aware that a serious effect of inhaling cocaine would be:
1. Esophageal varices
2. Extrapyramidal-tract symptoms
3. Deterioration of the nasal septum
4. Acute fluid and electrolyte imbalances

435. With a tentative diagnosis of opiate addiction, the nurse should assess a recently hospitalized client for signs of opiate withdrawal. These signs would include:
1. Lacrimation, vomiting, drowsiness
2. Nausea, dilated pupils, constipation
3. Muscle aches, pupillary constriction, yawning
4. Rhinorrhea, convulsions, subnormal temperature

436. After a binge with cocaine, a young male is found unconscious and is admitted to the hospital with acute cocaine toxicity. Initial nursing action should be directed toward:
1. Giving support and understanding
2. Maintaining a drug-free environment
3. Providing the necessary physical care
4. Establishing a therapeutic relationship

437. After a visit from several friends the nurse finds a client with a known history of opiate addiction in a deep sleep and unresponsive to attempts at arousal. The nurse assesses the client's vital signs and evaluates that an overdose of opiates had occurred if the findings showed a blood pressure of:
1. 70/40 mm Hg, a pulse of 120, and respirations of 10
2. 120/80 mm Hg, a pulse of 84, and respirations of 20
3. 140/90 mm Hg, a pulse of 76, and respirations of 28

4. 180/100 mm Hg, a pulse of 72, and respirations of 18

438. The nurse, when planning care for a client recovering from an opiate overdose, should take into consideration that the client's underlying problem is probably a feeling of:
1. Guilt with a rejection of reality
2. Hostility with a need for acceptance
3. Inferiority with strong dependency needs
4. Anger caused by an overwhelming need for independence

439. The nurse is aware that opiates are most commonly used because the individual:
1. Desires to become independent
2. Wants to fit in with the peer group
3. Attempts to blur reality and reduce stress
4. Enjoys the social interrelationships that occur

440. The nurse should know that the most common side effects of regular cocaine use include:
1. Nausea, fatigue, and extreme hunger
2. Anxiety, dysphoria, and suspiciousness
3. Seizures, hoarseness, and electrolyte imbalance
4. Lethargy, sexual arousal, and hormone imbalance

441. A client with a known history of opiate addiction is treated for multiple stab wounds to the abdomen. After surgical repair the nurse notes that the client's pain is not relieved by the prescribed morphine injections. The nurse recognizes that the failure to achieve pain relief from the morphine injections indicates that the client is probably experiencing the phenomenon of:
1. Tolerance
2. Habituation
3. Physical addiction
4. Psychologic addiction

442. At a staff meeting the question of a staff nurse returning to work after a drug rehabilitation program is discussed. The nurse manager helps the staff to decide that the most therapeutic way to handle the nurse's return would be to:
1. Offer the nurse support in a direct, straightforward manner
2. Avoid mentioning the problem unless the nurse brings up the topic
3. Assign another staff member to keep the nurse under close observation
4. Make certain the nurse is assigned to administer only non-narcotic medications

443. It is determined that a staff nurse has a drug abuse problem. As an initial intervention the staff nurse should be:
1. Counseled by the staff psychiatrist
2. Dismissed from the job immediately
3. Forced to promise to abstain from drugs
4. Referred to the employee assistance program

444. The nurse manager in the surgical intensive care unit notes that a number of clients do not seem to be responding to morphine that has been administered for pain. Later that evening the nurse manager finds a staff nurse in the nurses' lounge dozing. When awakened, the staff nurse appears somewhat uncoordinated and has slurred speech. The nurse manager should:
1. Ask the other staff members whether they have noticed anything unusual
2. Arrange to observe covertly the next time this staff nurse administers morphine
3. Tell the staff nurse that everyone now knows who has been stealing the opiates
4. Call the nursing director and have the director present before confronting the staff nurse

445. A client with the dual diagnosis of major depression and polysubstance abuse has been attending group therapy. One day the client tells the nurse, "The things they talk about in group don't really pertain to me." At this time it would be most appropriate for the nurse to:
1. Confront the client with realistic feedback
2. Identify the client's stress-coping tolerance
3. Communicate that the client needs to get involved
4. Question what the client means by the statement

446. A client who has been drinking heavily since the death of a child 3 years ago is brought to the mental health unit in a stupor by the spouse. Taking the client's history into consideration, the nurse makes a tentative nursing diagnosis of:
1. Dysfunctional grieving
2. Disabled family coping
3. Substance abuse, alcohol
4. Disturbed personal identity

447. A client with a long history of alcohol abuse is placed on a diet high in vitamin B₁ (thiamine). The nurse would know that the diet is understood when the client states, "I will select something for each meal from among:
1. Fish, aged cheese, and breads."

2. Poultry, milk products, and eggs."
3. Lean pork, organ meat, and nuts."
4. Leafy and green vegetables and citrus fruits."

448. A client being admitted for alcoholism reports having had alcoholic blackouts in the past. The nurse recognizes that an alcoholic blackout is best described as:
1. A fugue state resembling absence seizures
2. Fainting spells followed by loss of memory
3. Absence of memory in relation to drinking episodes
4. Loss of consciousness lasting less than 10 minutes

449. A client with a long history of alcohol abuse who has been in the hospital for 1 week tells the nurse, "I feel much better and will probably not require any further treatment." When evaluating the client's progress the nurse should recognize that:
1. The client has accepted the illness and now needs to use willpower to resist the alcohol
2. As long as the client's family remains supportive, the client will probably not use alcohol again
3. The client lacks insight about the emotional aspects of the illness and most likely needs continued supervision
4. The physician must be notified of the client's statement so that aversion therapy can be started before the client's discharge

DRUG-RELATED RESPONSES (DR)

450. Methylphenidate (Ritalin) is prescribed to treat a 7-year-old child's attention-deficit/hyperactivity disorder (ADHD). Ritalin is used in the treatment of this disorder in children for its:
1. Diuretic effect
2. Synergistic effect
3. Paradoxical effect
4. Hypotensive effect

451. A high-powered executive, who has been admitted to a mental health facility because of anxiety and physical symptoms related to work pressures, improves and is able to go home for short visits. The physician orders alprazolam (Xanax) 0.25 mg po tid. The most common side effect of this medication is:
1. Drowsiness
2. Bradycardia
3. Agranulocytosis
4. Tardive dyskinesia

452. The nurse understands that after starting the administration of alprazolam (Xanax) it is important to assess for potential side effects. Initially the nurse should:
    1. Measure urinary output
    2. Monitor the blood pressure
    3. Assess for abdominal distention
    4. Check the size of the pupils frequently

453. A client's family asks about the treatment of schizophrenia. The nurse, before responding, recalls that:
    1. Electroconvulsive therapy is more effective in treating schizophrenia than mood disorders
    2. Family therapy has not proven to be effective in the treatment of clients with schizophrenia
    3. Insight therapy has proven to be highly successful in the treatment of clients with schizophrenia
    4. Drug therapy, while not eliminating the underlying problem, reduces the symptoms of acute schizophrenia

454. A young adult being treated for substance abuse asks the nurse about methadone. The nurse responds that methadone is useful in the treatment of narcotic addiction because it:
    1. Is a nonaddictive drug
    2. Has an effect of longer duration
    3. Has no cumulative effect in the body
    4. Carries little risk of psychologic dependence

455. To prevent life-threatening complications from the administration of the neuroleptic drug chlorpromazine (Thorazine) to a disturbed, acting-out client, it is important that the nurse:
    1. Provide adequate restraint
    2. Monitor the client's vital signs
    3. Protect against exposure to direct sunlight
    4. Watch the client for extrapyramidal side effects

456. On the psychiatric unit, a client has been receiving high doses of haloperidol (Haldol) for 2 weeks. The client states, "I just can't sit still and I feel jittery." The nurse suspects that the client may be experiencing the side effect known as:
    1. Akathisia
    2. Torticollis
    3. Tardive dyskinesia
    4. Parkinsonian syndrome

457. In addition to hydration during delirium tremens, the physician prescribes parenteral administration of lorazepam (Ativan) for the client. The nurse understands that this drug is given during detoxification primarily to:
    1. Prevent physical injury to the client when seizures occur
    2. Enable the client to sleep and eat better during periods of agitation
    3. Quiet the client and encourage cooperation and acceptance of treatment
    4. Reduce the anxiety-tremor state and prevent more serious withdrawal symptoms

458. A male client has been receiving lithium for the past 2 weeks for treatment of a bipolar disorder, manic phase. When planning teaching, the nurse understands that it is important for this client to know that:
    1. A low-sodium diet must be followed every day
    2. He will need to take lithium for the rest of his life
    3. It will be necessary to take a diuretic with the lithium
    4. Lithium blood levels must be checked every 2 to 3 months

459. When lithium levels are scheduled to be done, the nurse should remember that serum lithium concentration is most stable:
    1. 2 to 4 hours after the last dose
    2. 4 to 6 hours after the last dose
    3. 6 to 8 hours after the last dose
    4. 8 to 12 hours after the last dose

460. A depressed client is receiving paroxetine (Paxil). The nurse monitors this client for the side effects associated with Paxil. Check all that apply.
    1. _____ Sexual dysfunction
    2. _____ Depressed respirations
    3. _____ Insomnia and restlessness
    4. _____ Hypertension or hypotension
    5. _____ Irregular menses or secondary amenorrhea
    6. _____ Hypertensive crisis when it interacts with foods containing tyramine

461. After a client has been receiving a new neuroleptic drug, the nurse observes extrapyramidal symptoms and anticipates that the physician will limit these side effects by prescribing:
    1. Zolpidem (Ambien)
    2. Hydroxyzine (Atarax)
    3. Dantrolene (Dantrium)
    4. Benztropine mesylate (Cogentin)

462. The nurse is aware that haloperidol (Haldol) is most effective for clients who exhibit:
    1. Manic-assaultive behavior

REVIEW QUESTIONS **311**

2. Excited-depressed behavior
3. Excited-overactive behavior
4. Withdrawn-secretive behavior

463. A client who is taking lithium arrives at the mental health center for a routine visit. The client has slurred speech, has an ataxic gait, and complains of nausea. The nurse recognizes that these adaptations are:
1. Related to low lithium levels
2. Associated with cyclic mood disorders
3. Often associated with therapeutic lithium levels
4. Probably associated with toxic levels of lithium

464. The immediate treatment for a client who has ingested a tricyclic antidepressant in an amount that is 20 to 30 times the daily recommended dose would include:
1. Dialysis or forced diuresis
2. Administration of physostigmine
3. IM or IV administration of an anticholinergic
4. Closer monitoring to prevent further suicidal attempts

465. A noncompliant, suspicious client with schizophrenia is to be discharged. The client will live with an aging mother and attend an outreach group. The nurse recognizes that the medication most appropriate for this client would be:
1. Amitriptyline (Elavil)
2. Tranylcypromine (Parnate)
3. Fluphenazine hydrochloride (Prolixin)
4. Fluphenazine decanoate (Prolixin Decanoate)

466. A client is started on fluphenazine decanoate (Prolixin Decanoate). When teaching about this drug, the nurse should emphasize that:
1. Driving is forbidden while taking this drug
2. There will be a feeling of increased energy while on this drug
3. A sunscreen must be used for all outdoor activity on a year-round basis
4. The client's essential hypertension will indirectly be controlled by this drug

467. For a client suspected of and demonstrating the symptoms associated with opiate overdose, the nurse would expect the physician to prescribe:
1. Naloxone
2. Methadone
3. Epinephrine
4. Amphetamine

468. The nurse should teach a client receiving tranylcypromine (Parnate) that failure to adhere to the dietary restrictions can result in:
1. Syncope
2. Bradycardia
3. Hypertensive crisis
4. Hyperglycemic episodes

469. A client has been placed on disulfiram (Antabuse) and will be discharged tomorrow. The nurse recognizes that teaching regarding this medication has been effective when the client states:
1. "I must be careful to check over-the-counter medications."
2. "This medication should never be combined with antibiotics."
3. "I will not be able to eat cheese or aged products with this medication."
4. "It's important to wait at least 8 hours after taking this pill before drinking any alcohol."

470. An antipsychotic, haloperidol (Haldol), is ordered three times a day for a male client who has been admitted to the psychiatric service because he has become delusional, more argumentative, and physically and verbally abusive to his wife. The nurse would be aware that the client is responding favorably to the medication when his behavior changes and he becomes more:
1. Enthusiastic about eating the hospital diet
2. Aware of his behavior and its consequences
3. Involved with the activities of others on the unit
4. Preoccupied with his delusions, but less physically abusive

471. A client who is going home on a weekend pass has been receiving risperidone (Risperdal) 3 mg tid. The nurse should inform the client that:
1. The dosage can be reduced if the client feels better at home
2. The medication does not need to be taken during the time spent at home
3. Alcoholic beverages should not be consumed while taking this medication
4. All the medication should be taken early in the day to be sure it is not forgotten

472. When talking with a client who has been receiving paroxetine (Paxil), an antidepressant medication, the nurse diagnoses the presence of a knowledge deficit when the client states:
1. "I notice I'm a little drowsy in the mornings."
2. "I'm expecting to feel somewhat better in 3 weeks."
3. "I've been on the medication for 8 days now and I don't feel any better."
4. "I know I will probably have to take this medication for at least a few months."

473. A client has been taking amoxapine (Asendin) for the last 3 months with no improvement. The physician orders phenelzine (Nardil) 15 mg tid. The nurse should:
1. Question the order and not administer the medication
2. Withhold the medication until CBC and enzymes have been drawn
3. Ask the client about allergies to feathers before giving the first dose
4. Remind the client this medication must be taken with meals and all milk products must be avoided

474. The physician prescribes a tricyclic medication to decrease a client's depression. A precaution that the nurse must keep in mind when initiating treatment with this group of drugs is that:
1. Eating cheese or drinking wine may cause a hypertensive crisis
2. The blood level may not be sufficient to cause noticeable improvement for 2 to 3 weeks
3. They must be given with milk and crackers to avoid hyperacidity and abdominal discomfort
4. Blood levels will need to be obtained weekly for 3 months to check for appropriate therapeutic levels

475. A 50-year-old divorced mother has become increasingly depressed and the physician prescribes an antidepressant. After 20 days of therapy, she returns to the clinic. She appears relaxed, smiles at the nurse, and the most significant conclusion the nurse can draw from this behavior would be that the client:
1. Wants to please the staff
2. Has resolved her conflicts
3. Is responding to the antidepressant therapy
4. May have an increased potential for suicide

476. A client is extremely depressed, and the physician orders a tricyclic antidepressant, imipramine hydrochloride (Tofranil). The client asks the nurse what the medication will do. The nurse's best response would be:
1. "This medication will help you forget why you are depressed."
2. "The medication will help increase your appetite and make you feel better."
3. "When you take this along with phenelzine (Nardil), you'll feel less depressed."
4. "You will begin to feel much better after taking this medication for 2 to 3 days."

477. A client with an organic mental disorder becomes increasingly agitated and abusive. The physician orders haloperidol (Haldol). The nurse should assess the client for untoward effects including:
1. Jaundice and vomiting
2. Tardive dyskinesia and nausea
3. Hiccups and postural hypotension
4. Parkinsonism and agranulocytosis

478. A client with schizophrenia is given antipsychotic drugs. The nurse is aware that of all the extrapyramidal effects associated with these drugs the one causing the most concern would be:
1. Akathisia
2. Tardive dyskinesia
3. Parkinsonian syndrome
4. An acute dystonic reaction

479. A 46-year-old mechanic has been hospitalized with schizophrenia, paranoid type. The physician has prescribed a phenothiazine drug. The hospital recreation department has planned a fishing trip. It is important that the nurse:
1. Provide the client with a solar defensive ointment
2. Give the client a single dose of medication to take after lunch
3. Caution the client about limiting undue exertion during the trip
4. Take the client's blood pressure before allowing participation in the activity

480. A client with schizophrenia, undifferentiated type, is receiving a typical antipsychotic/neuroleptic. The nurse should be alert for extrapyramidal signs and symptoms, which include:
1. Shuffling gait, tremors, and restlessness
2. Nausea, vomiting, and muscular cramps
3. Drowsiness, disorientation, and slurred speech
4. Tachycardia, urinary retention, and constipation

481. The physician orders haloperidol (Haldol) concentrate 10 mg po bid for a client who is also receiving phenytoin (Dilantin) for control of epilepsy. When planning the client's care, the nurse should be aware that anticonvulsants may interact with Haldol to:
1. Mask its therapeutic effect
2. Interfere with its absorption
3. Enhance its rate of metabolism
4. Potentiate its CNS depressant effect

482. An older female client residing in a long-term care facility has been receiving lithium 600 mg twice a day for three weeks to reduce her manic behavior. Presently, she is experiencing nausea, vomiting, diarrhea, thirst, polyuria, slurred speech, and muscle weakness. The nurse should:

1. Withhold the next dosage of lithium and draw blood for toxicity levels
2. Obtain an order from the doctor for an antidote for lithium toxicity and administer stat
3. Assess for coarse hand tremors and if absent give the daily dosage with a small amount of water
4. Suggest the doctor change the lithium to an antiepileptic such as carbamazepine (Tegretol) which has the ability to control mania within two weeks

483. The nurse has completed a teaching session with a client starting mood-stabilizing medications. The client comment that indicates to the nurse that further teaching is needed would be:

1. "I realize that I will need to keep in touch with my doctor."
2. "I know I won't have to stay on this medication for too long."
3. "Taking medication without using other forms of therapy may not be as effective."
4. "Taking the medication is better than experiencing the highs and lows I have been having."

484. A client who is receiving an MAO inhibitor is going home on a weekend pass. Considering this drug, the nurse plans to caution the client to avoid:

1. Pork, spinach, and fresh oysters
2. Milk, peanut butter, and meat tenderizers
3. Cheese, beer, and products with chocolate
4. Orange drinks, fresh apples, and ice cream

485. A client is receiving haloperidol (Haldol) for agitation. When observing the client for side effects, the nurse would recognize that the side effect that is unrelated to extrapyramidal-tract symptoms would be:

1. Akathisia
2. Opisthotonos
3. Oculogyric crisis
4. Hypertensive crisis

486. The blocking of dopamine by antipsychotic drugs can cause extrapyramidal side effects such as akathisia. The nurse understands that client behaviors that reflect akathisia include:

1. Acute muscle spasms and torticollis
2. Bizarre facial and tongue movements
3. Motor restlessness, foot tapping, and pacing
4. Tremor, shuffling gait, drooling, and rigidity

487. A client who has schizophrenia is receiving a phenothiazine antipsychotic medication. The nurse should withhold this medication if the client experiences:

1. Akathesia
2. Yellow sclerae
3. A shuffling gait
4. Photosensitivity

488. A client is started on fluphenazine decanoate (Prolixin Decanoate). The nurse is aware that the primary advantage of this medication is that:

1. There are no side effects
2. It has a long-lasting effect
3. It is safe to use during pregnancy
4. The need for laboratory monitoring is reduced

489. A client receiving buspirone hydrochloride (BuSpar) is admitted to the hospital with the diagnosis of possible hepatitis. The nurse notices that the client's sclerae look yellow. The nurse's initial action regarding this medication should be to:

1. Withhold the BuSpar
2. Give the BuSpar with milk
3. Reduce the dosage of the BuSpar
4. Assure the client that the BuSpar can be given parenterally

490. A female client who is taking clozapine (Clozaril) calls the nurse to say she has suddenly developed a sore throat and has a high fever. The nurse, recognizing the drug's effects, evaluates the client's complaints and tells her to:

1. Stay in bed, force fluids, take aspirin, and skip the next two scheduled doses of Clozaril
2. Stop the medication immediately and see her physician when an appointment is available
3. Continue the medication, drink fluids, take aspirin, and see her physician if not improved in a few days
4. Skip the medication and, if her physician cannot see her today, go to the emergency department for evaluation

491. The physician plans to have a client continue on lithium after discharge. The nurse would recognize that the teaching about the medication plan was understood when the client states, "I know that this medication:

1. Should be stopped if illness is suspected."
2. May need to be taken for the rest of my life."
3. Must be increased at the first sign of a manic episode."
4. Rarely causes serious side effects when taken correctly."

492. An antianxiety medication is prescribed for an extremely anxious client. The client states, "I'm afraid to take these pills because I heard they're addicting." The nurse's response is based on the knowledge that antianxiety medications:
1. Rarely causes dependence when dosage is controlled
2. May result in psychologic but not physiologic dependence
3. May require increased dosage but rarely cause dependence
4. Have the potential for physiologic and psychologic dependence

493. A client is admitted to the hospital with a diagnosis of depression that has not responded to tricyclic antidepressants or outpatient ECT. The physician orders tranylcypromine (Parnate). The nurse would be aware that the teaching about the drug was understood when the client states, "While taking this medicine I should avoid eating:
1. Red meat."
2. Fresh fish."
3. Chocolate."
4. Citrus fruit."

494. Forty-eight hours after starting on haloperidol (Haldol), a male client is observed standing by the nurse's station with his head arched sharply backward. The nurse should recognize that the client:
1. Needs to have the dosage increased since his psychotic behavior is not lessening
2. Is experiencing temporary side effects that usually disappear after several days
3. Is having pseudoparkinsonian side effects and needs to have the dosage adjusted
4. Needs immediate treatment because he is experiencing an acute dystonic reaction to the drug

495. A neuromuscular blocking agent is administered to a client before ECT therapy. The nurse should carefully observe the client for:
1. Seizures
2. Loss of memory
3. Nausea and vomiting
4. Respiratory difficulties

496. Considering the anticholinergic-like side effects of many of the psychotropic drugs, the nurse should encourage clients taking these drugs to:
1. Suck on hard candy
2. Restrict their fluid intake
3. Eat a diet high in carbohydrates

4. Avoid products that contain aspirin

497. A young adult client with schizophrenia is started on haloperidol (Haldol). When the nurse gives the client the medication, the client asks, "What's this for?" The nurse could best respond, "This medication:
1. Will help you to relax and think more clearly."
2. Fights 'the blues' and keeps your thoughts together."
3. Will raise your seizure threshold, letting you think more clearly."
4. Maintains an even mood while keeping your temper under control."

498. When administering hydroxyzine hydrochloride (Vistaril), the nurse should monitor the client for the common side effects of this drug, which include:
1. Ataxia and confusion
2. Drowsiness and dry mouth
3. Vertigo and impaired vision
4. Slurred speech and headache

499. The nurse is aware that the psychiatrist is concerned that one of the clients receiving haloperidol (Haldol) may be developing neuroleptic malignant syndrome. The nurse should carefully assess the client for symptoms that would include:
1. Jaundice, malaise, and pruritus
2. Sore throat, seizures, and tremors
3. Diaphoresis, muscle rigidity, and hyperpyrexia
4. Loss of visual acuity, dry skin, and hyperbilirubinemia

500. An antidepressant is prescribed for a depressed client. After 1 week, a member of the client's family comes to speak with the nurse and expresses concern that there does not seem to be much improvement after taking the medication. When responding to the family member the nurse explains that:
1. As the client's physical condition improves, the antidepressant medication will act more effectively
2. The client may require other drugs in addition to the antidepressants before behavioral changes are noted
3. In clients who have been depressed for a prolonged period, the drug takes additional time to be effective
4. Antidepressants are slow-acting drugs, and it may take 3 to 4 weeks until therapeutic effectiveness is achieved

Mental Health Nursing Answers and Rationales

NURSING PRACTICE (NP)

1. 4 **Legally, it is the responsibility of the staff to notify law enforcement officers so that the client can be returned. (3) (PI; LE; IM)**
1 Although this will be done eventually, law enforcement officers should be notified first.
2 This is not a priority.
3 Same as answer 1.

2. 2 **Talking with colleagues who face or who have faced the same problems may provide constructive help with the situation. (3) (PI; MR; IM)**
1 This is an avoidance technique; feelings must be addressed.
3 This avoids feelings and may make the nurse more uncomfortable.
4 This does not address the needs of the nurse and may interfere with a productive nurse-client relationship.

3. 3 **An understanding and supportive approach to a colleague with burnout allows the individual to identify the problem; this intervention points out behavior. (3) (SE; MR; IM)**
1 This interferes with self-identification of the problem; also, the individual may get defensive.
2 This moves right into trying to solve a problem before the individual has an opportunity to share feelings or identify the problem.
4 This is an accusatory approach; this does not give the individual an opportunity to address the overtime or to express feelings.

4. 3 **The type of care needed by the client requires trust in the caregiver; trust develops more rapidly when there is a cooperative relationship. (2) (PI; MR; PL)**
1 Limiting staff time may place the client in jeopardy.
2 The staff should not be put in the position of punishing the client; positive reinforcement is more therapeutic.
4 Rewards may be used to provide incentive for changes in behavior; punishment is inappropriate.

5. 2 **When the nurse and client agree to work together, a contract should be established; the length of the relationship should be discussed in terms of its ultimate termination. (2) (PI; CJ; PL)**
1 The client may discuss termination during the working phase; however, the subject should initially be discussed during the orientation phase.
3 Termination and discharge plans may be discussed more thoroughly during this phase, but the subject should initially be discussed during the orientation phase.
4 Same as answer 3.

6. 4 **This will ensure that a thorough assessment of the family's needs is made and the appropriate assistance initiated. (3) (SE; MR; IM)**
1 This is inadequate; in addition, household objects can serve as well as store-bought toys.
2 This could frighten the client and precipitate feelings of guilt; in addition, the word retardation is not accepted terminology.
3 This is premature; this may or may not be necessary.

7. 1 **Assessment is the first step of the nursing process and must be done before planning care. (1) (SE; CJ; AS)**
2 Nursing interventions follow assessment; high levels of anxiety interfere with interactions.
3 This technique may be used once the anxiety is reduced; assessment is the priority at this time.
4 Same as answer 3.

8. 2 **Evaluation includes assessing the client's response to care, judging the effectiveness of the nursing care plan, and changing the plan as necessary. (1) (SE; CJ; NP)**
1 Planning includes the development of a plan that focuses on specific goals and actions unique to the client's needs.
3 Assessing entails collecting and reviewing objective and subjective data about the client's health status.
4 Implementation includes performing specific actions designed to achieve the stated goals.

9. 4 **This verifies family and physician agreement and uses institutional policy developed by the ethics committee. (2) (SE; MR; IM)**
1 The nurse should not accept this inappropriate burden.
2 Same as answer 1.
3 The order must be in ink on the written record.

10. 2 **Primary prevention is directed towards health promotion and prevention of problems. (3) (SE; MR; AN)**
1 Tertiary prevention is focused on rehabilitation and the reduction of residual effects of illness.
3 Secondary prevention is related to early detection and treatment of problems.
4 There is no category of prevention called therapeutic prevention.

11. 4 **To confront burnout, the individual must first identify stressors, coping strategies used, and effectiveness of these strategies. (1) (PI; MR; PL)**
1 This may help, but prevention begins with knowing oneself and the effectiveness of one's coping strategies.
2 This may help prevent burnout, but it is not the first step in confronting the problem after it occurs.
3 Same as answer 2.

PERSONALITY DEVELOPMENT (PD)

12. 3 **Displacement reduces anxiety by transferring the emotions associated with an object or person to another, emotionally safer object or person. (2) (PI; CJ; AS)**
1 Projection is the attempt to deal with unacceptable feelings by attributing them to another.
2 Dissociation is an attempt by the person to detach emotional involvement or the self from an interaction or the environment.
4 Intellectualization is the use of facts or other logical reasoning rather than feelings to deal with the emotional impact of a problem; this is a form of denial.

13. 4 **The nurse is using facts and knowledge to detach the self from the emotional impact of the client's problem and decrease the anxiety it is causing. (3) (SE; CJ; AS)**
1 Substitution is similar to displacement; this reduces anxiety by transferring the emotions associated with an object or person to another, safer object or person.
2 Sublimation is the channeling of unacceptable thoughts or feelings into acceptable activity.

3 Identification is the unconscious imitation of the behavior of another who is considered important, in an attempt to incorporate this important other into the self.

14. 1 **The father is siding with his daughter and supports her whereas the mother accuses her of negative behavior; this is an example of a coalition or alliance; both the mother and the father may be in denial. (3) (SE; CJ; AS)**
2 Resignation is evident when someone gives up.
3 Scapegoating is when an individual is labeled or blamed by other family members as the cause of the family's problems.
4 Reaction formation is a defense mechanism that causes individuals to overtly behave in a manner that is exactly opposite to what they really feel in an attempt to conceal unacceptable feelings.

15. 1 **Without the development of trust, the child has little confidence that the significant other will return; separation is considered abandonment by the child. (1) (PM; CJ; AN)**
2 Without identity, the individual will have a problem forming a social role and a sense of self; this results in identity diffusion and confusion.
3 Without initiative, the individual will experience the development of guilt when curiosity and fantasies about sexual roles occur.
4 Without autonomy, the individual has little self-confidence, develops a deep sense of shame and doubt, and learns to expect defeat.

16. 1 **This is the developmental task of the preschool child; the child will feel guilty if initiative is stifled by others. (2) (PM; CJ; AN)**
2 This is the task of the school-age child.
3 This is not a developmental task identified by Erikson.
4 Same as answer 3.

17. 2 **The major tasks of young adulthood are centered around human closeness and sexual fulfillment; lack of love results in isolation. (1) (PM; CJ; AN)**
1 This stage is associated with early childhood.
3 This stage is associated with middle childhood.
4 This stage is associated with middle adulthood.

18. 2 **Projection is the process of attributing one's own thoughts about one's self to others. (3) (PI; CJ; AN)**
1 Denial involves pushing out of awareness one's own thoughts, wishes, or feelings that are unacceptable to one's self.
3 Introjection is the process of taking in someone else's values, beliefs, attitudes, or qualities.

4 Sublimation is the process of substituting a socially acceptable activity for one that is less so.

19. 2 **This is the task of the older adult; this client has not adapted to triumphs and disappointments, so there is no acceptance of what life is and was; this results in feelings of despair and disgust. (2) (PI; CJ; AN)**
    1 This is the task of the preschool child.
    3 This is the task of the young adult.
    4 This is the task of the adolescent.

20. 2 **This action would not call attention to the accident and would minimize the child's embarrassment. (2) (SE; CJ; IM)**
    1 The child would probably be unable to accomplish this task without assistance; failure to complete the task would add to embarrassment.
    3 This would add to the child's embarrassment.
    4 Same as answer 3.

21. 3 **Adolescence is a time of great upheaval and maturation; before this maturational process is completed, adolescents act without thinking things through and are more concerned with their own needs, rather than the needs of others. (1) (PM; CJ; AN)**
    1 The rapid and complex biologic, social, and emotional changes during adolescence do not necessarily lead to these psychologic responses.
    2 Same as answer 1.
    4 Same as answer 1.

22. 2 **According to Erikson, adolescents are struggling with identity versus role confusion. (2) (PI; CJ; AN)**
    1 This reflects part of the struggle for independence; it does not indicate failure to achieve the developmental task of adolescence.
    3 Adolescents tend to be group oriented, not isolated; they struggle to belong, not to escape.
    4 Most adolescents do not use drugs and alcohol to escape.

23. 1 **Adolescents learn about who they are by assuming and experiencing a variety of roles; experimentation results in the retention or rejection of behavior and roles. (2) (PM; CJ; EV)**
    2 This is not constructive; this would not allow for experimentation with a variety of roles.
    3 Sublimation would not be constructive and would delay and interfere with the successful completion of the struggle to formulate one's identity.
    4 This is not constructive; it does not allow for the development of independence.

24. 3 **This action would foster the development of an improved self-esteem. (2) (SE; CJ; IM)**
    1 A problem does exist; their child is overeating.
    2 Parents cannot avoid talking about the sibling, but should avoid any comparisons.
    4 The child already is doing this, and it has diminished her self-esteem.

25. 3 **This is an achievable goal that will bolster the adolescent's self-esteem. (2) (PM; CJ; PL)**
    1 This may not improve the adolescent's self-esteem.
    2 Same as answer 1.
    4 Same as answer 1.

26. 4 **Sexually abusing fathers usually are emotionally dependent and have feelings of inferiority; the child represents a less threatening sex object. (3) (PI; CJ; AN)**
    1 Power is more of a factor in rape, not incest.
    2 Rape, rather than incest, involves feelings of anger; violence rarely accompanies the incestuous act.
    3 Incest meets emotional, not physical, needs.

27. 3 **This would demonstrate a movement toward peer group activity and interests; exercise would demonstrate an interest in an improved physical condition. (2) (PM; CJ; EV)**
    1 This would not demonstrate an increase in self-esteem.
    2 There are no data to indicate that school was a problem.
    4 Same as answer 1.

28. 3 **Erikson theorized that how well people adapt to the present stage depends on how well they adapted to the stage immediately preceding it, in this instance adulthood. (2) (PM; CJ; AN)**
    1 This is the developmental task of an earlier stage of development; although Erikson believed that the strengths and weaknesses of each stage are present in some form in all succeeding stages, their influence decreases with time.
    2 Same as answer 1.
    4 Same as answer 1.

29. 4 **This encourages the client to accept what life is or was and helps avoid feelings of despair. (3) (PM; CJ; IM)**
    1 This could require a reversal in the client's past lifestyle; this is unlikely, if not impossible, for the client at this age.
    2 This would be impossible to accomplish and denies the reality of what was or is in life.
    3 This desire must come from the client.

30. 2 **The individual who can reflect back on life and accept it for what it was and is and who can adjust to and enjoy the changes retirement brings is less likely to develop health problems, especially stress-related health problems. (2) (PM; CJ; AN)**
 1 These changes may not be reversible.
 3 Dependency is often threatening to this age group.
 4 Most emotionally healthy older individuals do not focus on these thoughts.

31. 4 **An individual's ability to handle stress develops through experience with life; aging does not reduce this ability but often strengthens it. (1) (PM; CJ; PL)**
 1 The senses of taste and/or smell are often diminished in the older individual.
 2 Gastrointestinal motility is slowed in the older individual.
 3 Muscle or motor strength is diminished in the older individual.

32. 2 **Isolation is the separation of thought or memory from feeling. (3) (PI; CJ; AN)**
 1 Splitting is the polarizing of positive and negative feelings.
 3 Introjection is integrating the beliefs and values of another into one's own ego.
 4 Compensation is making up for a real or imagined lack in one area by overemphasizing another.

THERAPEUTIC RELATIONSHIPS (TR)

33. 3 **This response brings the client back to the current concern; in crisis therapy, time is limited and refocusing helps to use it in the most therapeutic manner. (2) (PI; CJ; IM)**
 1 This statement is too pointed; although it is important to focus on reality, it should be done in a manner that does not belittle the client.
 2 This statement is too blunt; the aim is to refocus the client on the current problem without being demeaning.
 4 This statement encourages descriptions of material not directly related to the crisis.

34. 1 **This allows the agitated, angry client time to regain self-control; telling the client that the nurse will return will decrease possible guilt feelings and implies to the client that the nurse cares enough to return. (3) (PI; CJ; IM)**
 2 This shows no respect for the client's feelings; it may decrease trust and increase feelings of anger, helplessness, and hopelessness.
 3 An agitated, angry client will not be able to accept a logical explanation.

 4 Continued insistence may provoke increased anger and further loss of control.

35. 3 **The answer to this question will provide the nurse with an idea of the client's hopes and frustrations without being threatening or probing. (3) (PI; CJ; AS)**
 1 This question is probing, disregards the client's statement, and provides little information for the nurse to use when planning care.
 2 Same as answer 1.
 4 Same as answer 1.

36. 2 **Before deciding how to decrease the client's fears of addiction, the nurse must explore the full extent of the client's knowledge and feelings about taking the drug. (1) (PI; CJ; AS)**
 1 Information may or may not be helpful; the client's feelings are what must be addressed.
 3 It is too early; exploration to find the basis of the fear is necessary first.
 4 Same as answer 3.

37. 3 **All behavior has meaning; before planning intervention, the nurse must try to understand what the behavior means to the client. (3) (PI; CJ; AS)**
 1 Isolation may increase anxiety and precipitate more acting-out behavior.
 2 Ignoring behavior does little to alter it, and it may even cause further acting out.
 4 The nurse cannot explain the meaning of the client's behavior; only the client can.

38. 3 **This is a technique that prevents misunderstanding so that both the client and the nurse can work toward a common goal in the therapeutic relationship. (2) (PI; CJ; AN)**
 1 This would not provide for clarification or understanding.
 2 Same as answer 1.
 4 Same as answer 1.

39. 3 **Moving into a client's personal space increases feelings of threat, which increases anxiety. (2) (PI; CJ; IM)**
 1 The client in crisis is usually unable to concentrate on an activity.
 2 This will increase anxiety at this time and may convey a lack of acceptance.
 4 This would increase anxiety until a trusting relationship has been developed.

40. 2 **The psychoanalytic model studies the unconscious and uses the strategies of hypnosis, dream interpretation, and free association as a means of releasing repressed feelings. (1) (PI; CJ; AN)**

1 The behaviorist model subscribes to the belief that the self and mental symptoms are viewed as learned behaviors that persist because they are consciously rewarding to the individual; this model deals with behaviors on a conscious level of awareness.

3 The psychobiologic model views emotional and behavioral disturbances as stemming from a physical disease; abnormal behavior is directly attributed to a disease process; this model deals with behaviors on a conscious level of awareness.

4 The social-interpersonal model affirms that crucial social processes are involved in the development and resolution of disturbed behavior; this model deals with behavior on a conscious level of awareness.

41. 3 **Environmental (milieu) therapy aims at having everything in the client's surroundings geared toward helping the client. (3) (PI; MR; AN)**
1 Role-playing is not a necessary ingredient of any type of therapy.
2 Neither natural treatments nor drugs are a necessary part of environmental therapy.
4 Clients are strongly encouraged to be involved in various types of activities.

42. 2 **This response should limit anxiety; it identifies feelings and tells the client what will happen in the immediate future. (3) (PI; CJ; IM)**
1 This is threatening and provides false reassurance; it puts responsibility on the client and does not allow for the expression of feelings.
3 This could lead the client to think that the environment is unsafe, which would increase insecurity and anxiety.
4 Being with other people in a strange environment will add more stress to the new and already frightening experience of hospitalization.

43. 2 **This is a correct description of the working phase of a relationship; trust has been established and a relationship has been developed based on mutual respect. (2) (SE; CJ; AN)**
1 This behavior would occur during the orientation phase before trust is established.
3 Same as answer 1.
4 Same as answer 1.

44. 2 **The stress of termination may precipitate fears of abandonment and the client may regress. (3) (PI; CJ; AN)**
1 The client is expressing fear, not thanks.
3 No data suggest that the client is manipulating

the nurse; the client's expression of apprehension is typical of someone in this situation.
4 The client's statement is not indicative of anything that should cause a delay in discharge but rather indicates anxiety over termination.

45. 2 **An explicit termination statement is most appropriate; offering an expression of well-wishes sets an optimistic, positive tone while maintaining the nurse-client relationship. (2) (PI; CJ; IM)**
1 A return of the physical contact should be avoided because it may precipitate anxiety in the client or may be interpreted as a desire to change the relationship from professional to personal.
3 Smiling and saying nothing may indicate acceptance of the physical exchange and blurs boundaries.
4 This response is nontherapeutic because it indicates an ongoing rather than a terminating relationship.

46. 2 **The client's inability to recall is an example of repression, which is the unconscious and involuntary forgetting of painful events, ideas, and conflicts. (2) (PI; CJ; AN)**
1 There is nothing to demonstrate that denial, an unconscious refusal to admit an unacceptable behavior or idea, has occurred.
3 There is nothing to demonstrate that regression, a return to an earlier, more comfortable developmental level, has occurred.
4 There is nothing to demonstrate that dissociation, the separation and detachment of emotional affect and significance from a particular idea, situation, or incident, has occurred.

47. 2 **Helping the client to understand the meaning of the parent's behavior can reduce the parent's emotional control over her. (2) (PI; CJ; IM)**
1 This is a temporary measure and does not reduce the emotional conflict with the parents.
3 Distraction is not a therapeutic way to deal with realistic feelings.
4 This ignores the necessity of clarifying her parent's behavior.

48. 3 **This goal is related to the nursing diagnosis and is appropriate and measurable. (1) (SE; CJ; AN)**
1 This is not related to the nursing diagnosis; this is true for everyone but the priority for this client is to facilitate interaction with others.
2 This is not related to the nursing diagnosis; acting-out behavior is not inherent in the situation.
4 Same as answer 2.

49. 1 **Without an awareness of personal beliefs, the nurse unconsciously may stop listening if the client expresses deviant beliefs. (1) (PB; CJ; AN)**
   2 Although this may create some anxiety, it usually does not interfere with accurate listening.
   3 Same as answer 2.
   4 Same as answer 2.

50. 4 **If nurses are unaware of their biases about sexual assault, they will be unprepared to evaluate objectively and meet the client's needs. (1) (PB; CJ; AN)**
   1 This would interrupt communication; information can be solicited later.
   2 The nurse should be able to deal with this client without assistance.
   3 It is not necessary to know these to effectively respond to the client in a therapeutic manner.

51. 1 **Value clarification is a technique that uncovers individuals' values so that the individuals can be more aware of them and their effect on others. (2) (PI; CJ; AN)**
   2 This is not an outcome of values clarification.
   3 Same as answer 2.
   4 Same as answer 2.

52. 3 **The ability to discuss feelings about others and life situations is necessary for positive mental health. (2) (PI; CJ; AN)**
   1 This is a long-term, not a short-term, goal.
   2 Same as answer 1.
   4 Same as answer 1.

53. 4 **When acceptance is reached the individual is beginning to withdraw; communication is simple, concise, and most often nonverbal. (3) (PI; CJ; PL)**
   1 Kübler-Ross's research has shown that this stage usually needs verbal interventions and communication.
   2 Same as answer 1.
   3 Same as answer 1.

54. 2 **The client's goal is meaningful, and the nurse should do everything possible to help the client achieve it. (2) (SE; MR; AN)**
   1 There is no reason to attempt to move the client away from a meaningful goal.
   3 The evidence does not demonstrate that the client is using denial.
   4 If the client wants to work toward a goal, the energy expenditure is justified.

55. 3 **An individual must feel a sense of control over self and the environment to feel secure, reduce anxiety, and function at an optimal level. (3) (PM; CJ; AN)**
   1 Most emotionally ill people are too introspective to empathize with others.
   2 No one functions optimally in all settings; the healthy individual can accept and handle temporary periods of confusion and loss of control.
   4 Many individuals with mental illness do not demonstrate observable signs of socially inappropriate behavior.

56. 4 **Early notification provides an opportunity to prepare for change. (3) (SE; MR; PL)**
   1 This may be a secondary gain but is not the primary purpose.
   2 Same as answer 1.
   3 Same as answer 1.

57. 2 **The client cannot be expected to accept or even respond to a plan that would be incompatible with the family's lifestyle. (1) (SE; MR; PL)**
   1 The family should not have to adjust to the nurse's biases; the nurse must accept biases before they interfere with care.
   3 All individuals respond differently to situations.
   4 There is no documentation that misconceptions are present.

58. 2 **Clients usually respond with better motivation for self-care if they feel someone is depending on them and they are needed. (2) (PM; MR; PL)**
   1 Clients need to feel needed, not just to establish new social contacts.
   3 Emotionally healthy individuals do not feel better simply because others have more problems.
   4 Same as answer 1.

59. 2 **When planning a group, the nurse must ensure that clients have similar needs to promote relationships and interactions; diverse needs do not foster group process. (2) (PI; CJ; PL)**
   1 Although important, this is not a primary consideration.
   3 Behavior and needs, rather than diagnoses, are of primary importance.
   4 This has little effect on group process.

60. 4 **The development of trust is the first step in developing a nurse-client relationship. (1) (SE; CJ; AN)**
   1 This is not the purpose; it provides a less stressful environment for the client to develop the belief that the staff is concerned and supportive.
   2 This cannot be achieved in several days; the ability to develop insight may take a lifetime or may never be accomplished.

3 Not all clients with schizophrenia have bizarre, agitated behavior.

61. 1 **Regressed, long-term clients need structure and external controls to help organize their thought processes. (2) (PI; CJ; PL)**
2 Most regressed long-term clients would be very anxious if they were placed in a leadership role.
3 Such experiences are beyond the capability or psychologic tolerance of these clients and may lead to decompensation.
4 These clients need gentle assistance to deal with conflict situations.

62. 3 **This is a necessary phase of group development in that it helps members discover what they can expect from the leader and other members. (3) (PI; CJ; AN)**
1 Group factions are unlikely to emerge in the first session; moreover, factions seldom emerge to control disruptive group behavior.
2 It is inappropriate to make this assumption at the first meeting.
4 The group has not yet developed to this phase; conflict resolution and management occur only in operating groups.

63. 1 **To achieve the greatest therapeutic value from a group session, the members must be involved in deciding what will be discussed. (3) (SE; MR; PL)**
2 By this response the nurse leader abdicates the leadership role and places the entire responsibility for the success of the group on its members.
3 This response presents an extremely structured view of the purpose of a therapy group; the members must be involved in the selection of the topics to be discussed.
4 Same as answer 3.

64. 4 **Feelings are discussed after individuals feel secure in the group. (3) (PI; MR; EV)**
1 This occurs at a later phase, after emotions and feelings have been stimulated by group interaction.
2 In the initial phase the members are not yet helping each other.
3 This commitment does not occur in the beginning phase; it occurs when the group becomes a cohesive unit.

65. 2 **The nurse must accept the client's statement and beliefs as real to the client to develop trust and move into a therapeutic relationship. (2) (PI; CJ; PL)**
1 Clients cannot be argued out of delusions.

3 These feelings and thoughts are constant; this would result in an overdose.
4 Redirecting the client's conversation whenever negative topics are brought up adds to the client's feelings that negative thoughts are correct.

66. 1 **The client has been able to function well up to this time, and the client's usual behavior and routines should be supported. (2) (PM; CJ; PL)**
2 At this time the data presented do not identify this as a need.
3 Same as answer 2.
4 Same as answer 2.

67. 2 **Family therapy views the whole (Gestalt) within the context in which the emotional problems are occurring. (3) (SE; MR; PL)**
1 Time efficiency is not an adequate rationale for choosing this therapeutic approach.
3 This may or may not be true; an astute nurse can control manipulation and alliance within any group.
4 Promotion of truthfulness is a secondary gain achieved through this mode of therapy.

68. 2 **The client is in the anger or "why me" stage of grieving; encouraging the client to express feelings will help resolve them while moving him toward acceptance. (2) (PI; CJ; IM)**
1 This response does not reflect what the client said; introducing the topic of death is not therapeutic at this time.
3 This is a judgmental response that may create a rift in the nurse-client relationship.
4 Suggesting that the client speak with a minister may precipitate guilt feelings and ignores the present concern.

69. 4 **If religion is a family concern, then the nurse should allow discussion of the family's thoughts and feelings on the subject. (2) (SE; MR; PL)**
1 If religion is a family concern, its discussion should be encouraged, not limited.
2 The role of the nurse is to facilitate and listen, not to have a mutual discussion.
3 The minister is not part of the family unit; the minister would be invited only if requested by the family.

70. 1 **In behavior modification, positive behavior is reinforced and negative behavior is punished or not reinforced. (2) (SE; MR; PL)**
2 This may be a part of the program, but it is not a major component.
3 Same as answer 2.
4 Same as answer 2.

71. 1 **Before therapy can begin, a trusting relationship must develop. (2) (PI; CJ; PL)**
    2 A client with major depression would not have the impetus or energy to investigate new leisure activities.
    3 This is not appropriate initially; a trusting one-to-one relationship must be developed first.
    4 This would not be successful unless the client had developed a trusting, comfortable relationship with the nurse.

72. 3 **With this response the nurse has changed the subject; it would be better to continue discussing the same subject. (2) (PI; CJ; IM)**
    1 This is a therapeutic response because it asks the client to clarify and elaborate.
    2 This is an acceptable response because it focuses on the client's implied feelings.
    4 This is a therapeutic response because it asks the client to focus on more specific details.

73. 4 **Evaluation and termination are the foci of a discharge planning conference; it is important for the nurse to assist the family in viewing the hospitalization as a learning experience. (3) (SE; MR; PL)**
    1 This should have been done before the discharge conference, where evaluation and future planning are the foci.
    2 Same as answer 1.
    3 Same as answer 1.

74. 1 **Empathy is the projection of self into another's emotions to share the emotions and the other's state of mind; this technique helps the nurse understand the meaning and significance of the experience to the client. (1) (PI; CJ; IM)**
    2 Sympathy is a shared expression of sorrow over a real or imagined loss.
    3 Projection is an unconscious defense, not a therapeutic technique.
    4 This does not require the nurse to project the self into the client's emotions but rather to accept the client and the emotions.

75. 3 **Focusing is indicated when communication is vague; the nurse attempts to concentrate or focus the client's communication on one specific aspect. (2) (PI; CJ; IM)**
    1 Touch would invade the client's space and would do nothing to help focus the client's communication.
    2 Silence would prolong the rambling communication; the client needs to be focused.

    4 Until the concern is identified and explored, summarizing would be impossible.

76. 1 **This demonstrates that the nurse believes that what the client has to say is important; this also encourages verbalization. (2) (PI; CJ; IM)**
    2 This would increase feelings of worthlessness and persecution and would cut off communication.
    3 This would accomplish little; individuals cannot be talked out of feelings.
    4 Feelings cannot always be explained; this forces the client to further develop the delusional system.

77. 1 **Silence is a tool employed during therapeutic communication that indicates that the nurse is listening and receptive; it allows the client time to collect thoughts, gain control of emotions, or speak without hurrying. (2) (PI; CJ; IM)**
    2 Silence should be comfortable and should not create a feeling of pressure to break it by talking.
    3 The nurse's facial expression should be projected outward, not inward.
    4 This would close communication.

78. 4 **This lets the client know the nurse is trying to understand; it increases the client's feeling of self-esteem and points out reality. (3) (PI; CJ; IM)**
    1 Clients with schizophrenia have problems with associative links, and these same problems will occur regardless of the topic.
    2 This statement cuts off communication and tells the client that the nurse will speak only if the client's communication makes sense.
    3 Same as answer 2.

79. 1 **This response reflects the feelings being expressed at this time. (2) (PI; CJ; IM)**
    2 This does not address the real concern; the mother's argument may have been justified and the daughter's behavior should not be rewarded.
    3 This avoids the issue; the fear may be that next time control may be lost and abuse may occur.
    4 False reassurance avoids the real issue.

80. 1 **Recognizing the spouse's feelings and giving simple factual information help to allay anxiety. (2) (PI; CJ; IM)**
    2 This discourages further verbalization of concerns and promotes feelings of isolation and helplessness.
    3 This is an inappropriate statement, especially during this time of stress; it also gives little assurance to the family.

4 This is false reassurance and does not allow the spouse to verbalize anxieties or fears.

81. **1 Unless staff can share both positive and negative feelings, resentment, anger, and frustration will develop. (3) (SE; MR; IM)**
    2 This response attacks the speaker and cuts off communication in the group.
    3 This response does little to foster communication and positive relationships among staff members.
    4 Same as answer 2.

82. **3 This statement addresses the reality that the client is on the mental health unit and offers assistance. (2) (PI; CJ; IM)**
    1 On the basis of the information available, it would be too early to make this decision.
    2 This is a hostile statement that assumes the client is unable to follow the conversation.
    4 This statement assumes the client is disoriented as to place; it sounds like the beginning of a lecture.

83. **3 This response addresses the client's misconceptions about mental health services and the specific fear of being crazy. (2) (PI; CJ; IM)**
    1 This response ignores the feeling tones behind the client's statement and focuses on facts.
    2 Same as answer 1.
    4 Same as answer 1.

84. **4 This invites the client to explore interpersonal problems more fully, while showing interest in what the client is communicating. (2) (PI; CJ; IM)**
    1 Experiences may provide data about the nature of the problem.
    2 This question is too direct and does not allow the client a choice of selecting those problems that are of particular concern.
    3 This implies that the client is coping adequately and does not focus on the client's difficulties with interpersonal relationships.

85. **4 This response is optimistic and supportive and clarifies the purpose of the relationship. (2) (PI; CJ; IM)**
    1 This statement diminishes the client's response and sets up a challenge; it does not foster a therapeutic relationship.
    2 Same as answer 1.
    3 Same as answer 1.

86. **2 Unless the nurse answers the question, the client will continue to focus on the nurse rather than on the self; the nurse can best redirect after a brief answer. (2) (PI; MR; IM)**
    1 This moves the focus to the nurse's opinions rather than the client's feelings.
    3 Same as answer 1.
    4 This is not therapeutic; the client is being asked to share, and the nurse should also be willing.

87. **3 There is no loss of intellectual ability unless there is a pathologic problem. (1) (PM; CJ; AN)**
    1 Neurologic responses are slowed because of reduced sensorireceptor sensitivity.
    2 Excluding pathologic processes, the personality will be consistent with that of earlier years.
    4 Short-term memory is reduced because of a shortened attention span, delayed transmission of information to the brain, and perceptual deficits.

88. **1 This response recognizes problems of the caregiver without a hint of blame for admission; it opens the channel of communication. (2) (PI; CJ; IM)**
    2 This is a hostile response that would place the caregiver on the defensive.
    3 Same as answer 2.
    4 Same as answer 2.

89. **1 This response identifies the child's feelings and lets the child know the nurse can understand them. (3) (PI; CJ; IM)**
    2 This denies the child's feelings and does not offer support.
    3 This is an unrealistic response; the child would probably be unable to express his feelings to peers.
    4 This is unrealistic and the nurse cannot be sure that weight loss will improve the child's ability in gym.

90. **4 Commenting on the silence will encourage exploration of what is happening in the group and the member's thoughts and feelings about it. (3) (PI; MR; IM)**
    1 Calling on specific members limits growth potential of the members; allowing the group to respond spontaneously increases growth potential.
    2 Waiting indefinitely can result in increased anxiety and a power struggle between members and the leader, each determined to outwait the other.
    3 Forcing responses instead of allowing spontaneous responses will decrease thoughtful exploration of what is happening.

91. 3 This response focuses the client on the behavior and what the client is trying to achieve by such behavior; it also helps the client to see how such behavior affects others. (3) (SE; MR; IM)

1 The group would not know what the client was trying to tell the nurse; only the client would know and should be asked directly.

2 This response uses a nondirect approach to attack the client.

4 This is an attacking, defensive response made without really knowing what the client was attempting to accomplish.

92. 3 New group leaders experience anxiety and insecurity, which limit their ability to mediate conflicts between members. (2) (PI; MR; AN)

1 This behavior is self-serving and disruptive to group process.

2 This is often counterproductive, especially with regressed long-term clients who may decompensate when confronted with their behavior.

4 Long-term regressed clients need more help with communication than clients with acute problems.

93. 4 The use of pronouns *we*, *us*, and *our* often indicates that group members experience a sense of belonging. (2) (PI; CJ; EV)

1 Cohesive groups tend to resent new members.

2 Cohesive groups tend to accept and sometimes even protect disliked members.

3 This reflects lack of group cohesion; socialization may be superficial.

94. 3 This is an open-ended, nonjudgmental response that points out incongruity between the client's verbal and nonverbal communication. (2) (SE; MR; IM)

1 This would not help the client recognize the incongruity.

2 Same as answer 1.

4 Same as answer 1.

95. 2 This response uses paraphrasing to restate the content of the client's statement; it encourages further communication. (1) (PI; CJ; IM)

1 Feelings are personal and can really not be understood by others; this is an ineffective attempt to empathize and refocuses the attention on the nurse.

3 This response negates the client's feelings and changes the subject; the client needs to talk, and this response cuts off communication.

4 This response negates the client's feelings, makes the feelings impossible to share, may make the client feel guilty for the feelings, and tells the client how to behave and feel.

96. 4 Helping the client to understand the meaning of the family member's behavior reduces the family member's emotional control over the client. (2) (PI; MR; IM)

1 This ignores the necessity of clarifying the family member's behavior.

2 Distraction is not a therapeutic way to deal with realistic feelings.

3 This is a temporary measure and does not reduce the emotional conflict with the family member.

97. 3 Anger is a common feeling when people do not have control over decisions that affect them. (1) (PI; CJ; AN)

1 There is no information that indicates this conclusion.

2 Same as answer 1.

4 Same as answer 1.

EMOTIONAL DISORDERS RELATED TO PHYSICAL HEALTH AND CHILDBEARING (ED)

98. 3 This action would provide the child with a constant caregiver with whom the child could relate. (1) (PM; CJ; IM)

1 Although this may provide some comfort, the child needs to receive love and attention from an adult.

2 Same as answer 1.

4 This would increase the parents' guilt and anxiety; data given assume parents have been unable, not unwilling, to visit the child.

99. 1 The 9-year-old needs an opportunity to express emotions in private; talking about feelings after the child has regained control would be therapeutic. (2) (PM; CJ; AN)

2 This action would give the child a feeling that crying was wrong.

3 This is not of great concern to the child at this moment.

4 Same as answer 2.

100. 4 This response immediately recognizes the client's fear as real and offers a service to meet the identified need for information about the client's physical status. (2) (PI; MR; IM)

1 This ignores the client's concern and focuses on the nurse's need to complete the task of obtaining a health history.

2 This response minimizes the client's real concern about having a sexually transmitted disease.

3 This minimizes the client's concern and implies that the client is being unrealistic.

101. 3 **This is an emotionally supportive response; it demonstrates that sharing this information is acceptable and provides hope that she will get help. (1) (PI; CJ; IM)**
    1 The client may draw the conclusion that her actions precipitated the father's behavior; the client needs support and this response could increase feelings of guilt.
    2 This is not a priority at this time and may interfere with future sharing; the client needs immediate emotional support.
    4 This implies that the client does not know what she is talking about; the client needs support whether the act is real or imagined.

102. 4 **This is a nonjudgmental response that does not pressure the client but does clearly indicate that treatment is necessary. (2) (SE; MR; IM)**
    1 This is an unrealistic response that gives approval to the client's behavior.
    2 This response is not supported by the client's statement.
    3 This nonsupportive response tells the client that the physician knows best.

103. 4 **This response interprets the client's behavior without belittling the nursing assistant's feelings; it encourages the assistant to get involved with plans for future care. (3) (SE; MR; IM)**
    1 Although this response recognizes the client's feelings, it does not help the nursing assistant to deal with the client.
    2 This assumes the nursing assistant has nothing to contribute and only the nurse can deal with the problem.
    3 This does not help the nursing assistant, nor does it demonstrate an understanding of the client's feelings.

104. 2 **This action provides continuity and demonstrates to the client that the nursing staff is concerned; frequent contact reduces the client's need to call staff members. (2) (SE; MR; PL)**
    1 This would increase the client's anxiety and need for contact with staff.
    3 Telling the client is not the same as doing it; the client would not believe that the staff members would come in frequently.
    4 This would not provide continuity of care.

105. 4 **This is an open-ended response that encourages further discussion without focusing on an area that the nurse, not the client, feels is the problem. (3) (PI; CJ; IM)**
    1 This response denies the client's feeling and can cause feelings of guilt for questioning the partner's love.
    2 This is too specific; the nurse does not have enough information to come to this conclusion.
    3 Same as answer 2.

106. 4 **This response fosters open lines of communication with the client. (2) (PI; CJ; IM)**
    1 This response would put the client on the defensive because it exposes the defensive behavior being used.
    2 This response does not recognize the client's concern and cuts off further communication.
    3 This could be interpreted as a sarcastic response that may cut off further communication.

107. 2 **The client has difficulty accepting the inevitability of death and attempts to deny the reality of it. (1) (PI; CJ; AN)**
    1 In the anger stage the client strikes out with the "why me" and the "how could God do this" type of statements; the client is angry at life and still angrier to be removed from it by death.
    3 In this stage the client attempts to bargain for more time; the reality of death is no longer denied, but the client attempts to manipulate and extend the remaining time.
    4 In the acceptance stage the client accepts the inevitability of death and peaceably awaits it.

108. 2 **Crying is an expression of an emotion that, if not expressed, increases anxiety and tension; the increased anxiety and tension use additional psychic energy and hinder coping. (2) (PI; CJ; AN)**
    1 Crying does not relieve depression, nor does it help a client face reality.
    3 This is not universally true; in most instances the client's defenses should not be taken away until they can be replaced by more healthy defenses; the nurse must interfere with behavior and defenses that may place the client in danger; the client's current behavior creates no threat to the client.
    4 This is not always true; many clients are embarrassed by what they consider to be a "show of weakness" and have difficulty relating to the individual who witnessed it; the nurse must do more than just accept the crying to strengthen the nurse-client relationship.

109. 4 A starting point for working with all clients is ascertaining what is known, their understanding of their particular situation, and its meaning to them. (2) (PI; CJ; AS)

1 It is not merely understanding what death and the dying process mean to the client, which is a philosophical discussion, but how the individual feels about the situation.

2 Encouraging conversation about the situation tends to decrease anxiety.

3 This is part of the plan of care, but it is secondary; the coping behavior is a priority according to the data provided.

110. 4 This response recognizes the client's feelings and encourages the client to look at the basis or reality of the expressed concern. (2) (PI; CJ; IM)

1 This response ignores the client's statement; the client has already told the nurse the basis for the feelings.

2 This puts the responsibility for the husband's behavior on the client, who may not be able to handle it.

3 This is a weak excuse for the behavior of the husband and may or may not be true.

111. 1 Improved functioning relates most to improved body image, even if the prosthesis is not at all like the original body part. (3) (PI; CJ; AN)

2 A slight improvement in body image occurs with a "normal" look, but the "normal" look usually occurs only when the prosthesis is covered by clothing.

3 Acceptance by others does not necessarily guarantee acceptance by self.

4 Although mood may be improved with an aggressive rehabilitation program, this in itself does not improve body image.

112. 1 The nurse empathizes with the client and keeps the lines of communication open without being judgmental. (2) (PB; CJ; IM)

2 This response does not address the client's feelings and may increase anxiety.

3 This is false reassurance; close monitoring does not guarantee a live baby.

4 This response denies the client's right to emotions and may evoke more feelings of guilt about her past obstetrical history.

113. 1 Planning self-care demonstrates decision making by the client; participating in care enhances feelings of self-worth and autonomy. (1) (PI; CJ; EV)

2 Expectations do not reflect autonomy.

3 This does not reflect autonomy; it may be intellectualization.

4 Same as answer 3.

114. 2 The best long-term goal would be that the client attains a positive attitude about the self, others, and life in general; this would indicate that treatment has been effective and discharge should occur. (3) (PI; CJ; EV)

1 This is a short-term goal associated with a therapeutic milieu.

3 This is an intermediate goal that helps the client focus on others; this goal would be a step toward achieving long-term goals.

4 This is a short-term goal and an expected behavior on an inpatient unit.

115. 4 The nurse should strive to clarify misconceptions and fears; this response promotes further communication and begins where the client is. (3) (PI; CJ; AS)

1 This avoids assuming the responsibility of answering the client's question; the client needs an immediate clarification.

2 The fact that others have had the surgery provides little solace; the remainder of the response is false reassurance and does not truthfully answer the client's question.

3 This denies the client's feelings and cuts off communication.

DISORDERS FIRST EVIDENT BEFORE ADULTHOOD (BA)

116. 2 A child usually assumes a role in the family, and the child's problems reflect the pathologic factors that develop to fill that role. (3) (PI; CJ; AN)

1 This may create problems, but these problems usually develop later in life.

3 Same as answer 1.

4 Same as answer 1.

117. 3 Children who have experienced attachment difficulties with primary caregivers are not able to trust others and therefore relate superficially. (3) (PI; CJ; AS)

1 This is a possibility, but not a necessity for this diagnosis.

2 The child probably will not cling or react when separated from the mother.

4 Attachment will not occur with either parent.

118. 1 Children with emotional problems usually have difficulty dealing with reality and tend to withdraw; they are afraid to use reality testing. (2) (PI; CJ; AS)

2 Behavior is more often disorganized rather than deliberate and aggressive rather than passive.

3 There is usually a withdrawal from the peer group.

4 The anxiety level usually is severe, often approaching the panic level.

119. 4 **Unresponsiveness to the environment may be an indicator of severe childhood depression, autism, or possibly schizophrenia; all three are serious disorders. (3) (PI; CJ; AS)**
1 This may be seen in children without emotional problems as well as in those with emotional problems; this behavior alone would not indicate severe emotional problems.
2 Same as answer 1.
3 Same as answer 1.

120. 2 **This structured but nonthreatening statement avoids beginning with problems and may put the child at some ease, producing information that may be useful. (3) (PI; CJ; AS)**
1 This statement is too open and global; the child would probably not know how to answer this question or know where to begin.
3 This question can produce a "yes" or "no" answer; also, the child may not know the answer to this question.
4 This question would probably produce an "I don't know" response; the focus should be on the child, not the mother.

121. 1 **Children have difficulty verbally expressing their feelings; acting-out behaviors, such as temper tantrums, may indicate an underlying depression. (3) (PI; CJ; AS)**
2 Childhood depression is serious and requires treatment.
3 Adult and childhood depression may be manifested in different ways.
4 Many conventional therapies, including medication, are effective.

122. 1 **Tertiary prevention focuses on interventions that prevent complete disability or reduce the severity of a disorder or its associated disabilities. (3) (SE; MR; PL)**
2 This would be secondary prevention aimed at case-finding and early intervention.
3 This would be primary prevention.
4 Same as answer 2.

123. 2 **This helps the child gain control by reducing stimuli while helping limit and prevent the use of tantrums by the child as an attention-getting behavior. (3) (PM; CJ; IM)**
1 This would probably increase the behavior associated with the tantrum.
3 Although ignoring the temper tantrum may sometimes help, it often forces the child to act out further; using time-out is more

successful because the child is removed and both the parent and child have a "cooling-off" period.
4 Medication is not the treatment of choice.

124. 4 **One of the symptoms an autistic child displays is a lack of responsiveness to others; there is little or no extension to the external environment. (2) (PI; CJ; AS)**
1 Repetitive behavior provides comfort.
2 Music is nonthreatening, comforting, and soothing.
3 Repetitive visual stimuli, such as a spinning top, are nonthreatening and soothing.

125. 2 **The autistic child's world is an internal one; the child does not interact with the environment. (2) (PI; CJ; AS)**
1 Autistic children rarely communicate verbally.
3 Although this would be beneficial, it is not essential for providing care.
4 Autistic children do not interact with the environment; they have blocked out reality.

126. 1 **The autistic child repeats sounds or words spoken by others. (2) (PI; CJ; AN)**
2 Stuttering is a speech disorder in which the same syllable is repeated, usually at the beginning of a word.
3 This is associated with neurologic disorders, not autism.
4 Same as answer 3.

127. 4 **Children usually blame themselves for their parents' marital problems, believing that they are the reason one parent leaves. (2) (PI; CJ; AN)**
1 No data are presented to lead to this conclusion.
2 The child's response is not typical of grief work.
3 Same as answer 1.

128. 4 **Comparison over time is the only way for the nurse to accurately assess the mental status of a child. (2) (PM; CJ; AS)**
1 This would not be an accurate method because the child's ability to discuss feelings is limited.
2 This would be threatening and may precipitate anxiety.
3 This may be unrealistic and biased; the nurse should take the parents' description of behavior into consideration but should rely on personal assessment and observation over time.

129. **2 This is the family constellation as it is now constructed; without prior discussion and permission, an invitation to anyone else would be an intrusion of privacy. (3) (SE; MR; AN)**
   1 In addition to needing the mother's permission to invite the father, the nurse must also include the child in family therapy.
   3 The father cannot be invited without prior discussion with and permission of the mother.
   4 The teacher is not part of the family constellation.

130. **3 When all the members of a family blame one member for all their problems, scapegoating is occurring. (2) (PI; CJ; AN)**
   1 There are no data to support identifying this pattern of relating.
   2 Same as answer 1.
   4 Same as answer 1.

131. **3 This action would set a foundation for trust because it allows the child to see that the nurse cares. (2) (PI; CJ; IM)**
   1 This would be threatening at this stage of the relationship.
   2 This would be too infrequent to develop trust.
   4 Although this is necessary, limit-setting does not support the development of a trusting relationship.

132. **4 A behavior modification program tailored for and developed with the individual child is the most appropriate approach at this time. (3) (PI; CJ; IM)**
   1 There are no data to indicate that the child is in need of special education.
   2 This would serve no purpose and could be viewed by the child as a reward for behavior.
   3 This may not be true; the child may not like school and may not think it is fun; having fun is not the purpose of school.

133. **3 The DSM-IV-TR reports an incidence of ADHD in about 3% to 7% of school-age children. (3) (SE; MR; IM)**
   1 This problem usually becomes evident around 6 to 7 years of age and is noted in at least two different settings (school and home).
   2 Socioeconomic factors do not play a major role in the occurrence of this disorder.
   4 These children have less need for sleep.

134. **2 This intervention would be most successful because it provides a time period for the hyperactive child to regain control; it is neither a** positive nor a negative reinforcement of acting-out behavior. (3) (PI; CJ; IM)
   1 The child would interpret removal of tokens as a punishment.
   3 Ignoring the behavior may force the child to act out even more to gain attention.
   4 This action would reward acting-out behavior by providing special attention.

135. **3 This would help the child develop insight into reasons for the acting-out behavior. (3) (PI; CJ; IM)**
   1 This denies that the child's problem behavior is continuing and does not help the child develop insight.
   2 Same as answer 1.
   4 Same as answer 1.

136. **4 This would provide a trial opportunity for the child and the family to reunite outside the confines of the hospital. (2) (SE; MR; PL)**
   1 It is too late; this should have been done much earlier.
   2 This is not the responsibility of the nurse.
   3 Same as answer 1.

ANXIETY, SOMATOFORM, FACTITIOUS, AND DISSOCIATIVE DISORDERS (AX)

137. **2 A compulsion is an uncontrollable, persistent urge to perform an act repetitively to relieve anxiety. (2) (PI; CJ; AN)**
   1 An obsession is a persistent idea, thought, or impulse that cannot be eliminated from consciousness by logical effort.
   3 The urge to perform a compulsive act is not under the client's control because avoiding the act increases anxiety.
   4 Clients are compelled to perform these ritualistic behaviors; they are not trying to rebel.

138. **1 These are effective coping mechanisms to reduce stress. (2) (PI; CJ; EV)**
   2 This is not always possible; forced quiet activity may increase stress and anger rather than reduce it.
   3 This is not always possible; stress can develop from a variety of feelings stimulated by many situations.
   4 This is not easy to identify; it is better to learn to deal with feelings once they develop.

139. **3 Perceptual fields are a key indicator of anxiety level because the perceptual fields narrow as anxiety increases. (2) (PI; CJ; AS)**
   1 This is not related directly to anxiety levels.

2 Same as answer 1.

4 Same as answer 1.

140. 1 The client's statement is an example of the use of denial, a defense that blocks problems by unconsciously refusing to admit they exist. (2) (PI; CJ; AS)

2 Projection is a defense that is used to deny unacceptable feelings and emotions and attribute them to others.

3 Sublimation is a defense that is used to substitute socially acceptable behavior for unacceptable instincts.

4 Displacement is a defense that is used to allow the shifting of feeling from an emotionally charged person or object to a safe, substitute person or object.

141. 3 Discussion of the feared object triggers an emotional response to the object. (2) (PI; MR; AS)

1 People with phobias generally acknowledge their existence.

2 Extreme fear would be more of a problem than anger.

4 Distortion of reality related to the daily routine usually is not a problem for a person with a phobia.

142. 1 The most successful therapy for people with phobias involves behavior modification techniques using desensitization. (3) (PI; MR; PL)

2 Insight into the origin of the phobia will not necessarily help the client overcome the problem.

3 This may increase understanding of the phobia, but may not help the client to deal with the fear; there is no maladaptive thought process associated with phobias.

4 Psychoanalysis may increase understanding of the phobia, but may not help the client deal successfully with the unreasonable fear.

143. 2 Experiencing the actual trauma in dreams or flashbacks is the major symptom that distinguishes post-traumatic stress disorders from other anxiety disorders. (2) (PI; CJ; AN)

1 This symptom is not usually associated with anxiety disorders.

3 This symptom would be more common in phobic disorders.

4 Although depression may be generated by discussion of the traumatic situation, the affect is usually exaggerated, not blunted.

144. 1 The ability to connect feelings, thoughts, and actions, plus inattention for all but the

anxiety-causing subject, are associated with a moderate level of anxiety. (2) (PI; CJ; AN)

2 The development of mild or moderate anxiety is common in new situations because of apprehension related to the unknown.

3 Severe anxiety is related to dissociation, selective inattention, and an inability to connect feelings, thoughts, and actions.

4 There is insufficient information to come to this conclusion.

145. 3 These actions make the environment as emotionally nonthreatening as realistically possible. (2) (PI; CJ; PL)

1 All needs cannot be met; the person must learn how to deal with delaying gratification.

2 It is not possible or realistic to meet all of a person's needs.

4 Order in the environment is of less importance; providing a nonthreatening environment is the priority action.

146. 1 Anxiety is a threat to the identity of the individual; the client is seeking assurance that the fear and panic being experienced will not mean loss of control. (2) (PI; CJ; AN)

2 The client is not exhibiting depression but severe anxiety and panic.

3 This is not evidence of insightfulness but a plea for help in reducing the anxiety.

4 The client is not testing the nurse; the client is asking for help.

147. 2 Mild and moderate levels of anxiety can be beneficial because they focus attention on the environment by attempting to ward off additional anxiety. (2) (PI; CJ; AN)

1 Initially, anxiety increases physiologic functioning; these functions decrease after prolonged anxiety because of exhaustion.

3 Automatic behavioral responses may hinder, rather than increase, an individual's awareness.

4 Ego defense mechanisms may hinder, rather than increase, an individual's awareness.

148. 3 Because anxiety can be an interpersonal experience, it is contagious; the nurse then has a strong urge to get away. (2) (SE; CJ; AN)

1 The desire to go off duty would not suddenly make the nurse uncomfortable.

2 This is possible, but not probable; the client is exhibiting anxiety, not hostility, at this time.

4 There is no indication that this or any other behavior encountered has been bizarre.

149. 1 **Freedom to ventilate feelings acts as a safety valve to reduce the anxiety. (1) (PI; CJ; PL)**
    2 The suppression of anger or hostility would add to clients' anxiety.
    3 This would not be therapeutic; it might add to the anxiety clients are feeling.
    4 This may or may not be helpful; clients' families may provide support to the clients.

150. 4 **The nurse should clarify if the spouse has discussed the child's visiting with the client before commenting further. (3) (PI; MR; AS)**
    1 This response assumes that the client has consented to the visit; this assumption may be incorrect.
    2 Same as answer 1.
    3 This response makes an assumption that requires more data and discussion to validate.

151. 2 **The nurse's presence may provide the client with support and feelings of control. (2) (PI; CJ; IM)**
    1 It is evident that the client is upset; this question is not therapeutic and may lead to anger, which would interfere with the development of a therapeutic nurse-client relationship.
    3 The client is too distraught to sit; to be therapeutic, the nurse should walk with the client, thus demonstrating concern.
    4 The client is in a panic; anger is not primary; there is no need to work off aggression.

152. 1 **Fear can be overwhelming; the nurse's presence provides protection from possible danger. (2) (PI; CJ; IM)**
    2 The client's anxiety level is interfering with the ability to communicate; anxiety must be reduced first.
    3 The client's anxiety level is so high that sufficient emotional energy to set parameters would not be available.
    4 This would add to the client's anxiety at this time.

153. 3 **This response helps the client focus on situations that precipitate frightening feelings. (2) (PI; CJ; AS)**
    1 This response would not help the client to focus on feelings.
    2 The nurse cannot be certain what the client means about being afraid to talk about it; this response would not help the client to focus on feelings.

    4 This is false reassurance; the nurse cannot guarantee that the feelings will not come back.

154. 2 **The client will be unable to concentrate or focus on the interview if anxiety is not reduced. (2) (PI; CJ; AS)**
    1 This is not the priority at this time; anxiety must be reduced and the client's level of comfort increased.
    3 Same as answer 1.
    4 The client could not rest until anxiety is reduced.

155. 2 **The attention span is shortened, making it difficult to follow long sentences; an authoritative voice lets the client know that the nurse is in control of the situation; the client is unable to set controls because of the anxiety level. (2) (PI; CJ; IM)**
    1 This could increase the client's anxiety level further.
    3 Same as answer 1.
    4 Crying is an outlet and should not be discouraged; telling someone not to cry usually increases the crying and adds to anxiety.

156. 2 **Intellectually the person knows the compulsive acts are senseless but is unable to stop doing them because they control anxiety. (2) (PI; CJ; AN)**
    1 This is an example of delusional thinking.
    3 This is rationalization; obsessive-compulsive behavior is usually counterproductive, time consuming, and interferes with functioning.
    4 This is an example of denial.

157. 2 **This focuses on desired relationships with others and assists the client to focus on possible solutions. (3) (PI; CJ; IM)**
    1 This focuses on how others can accommodate the client's needs rather than how the client can bring compulsive acts under control.
    3 This does not focus on how the client can bring compulsive acts under control.
    4 This is a negative response that is discouraging and probably would curb discussion about the problem.

158. 3 **These are positive coping behaviors that can be used consciously to promote mental health. (1) (SE; MR; PL)**
    1 These are not healthy coping behaviors, and their frequent use can lead to distortions of reality.

2 Same as answer 1.

4 Same as answer 1.

159. 4 **This would document that the client feels comfortable enough to discuss the problems that have motivated the behavior. (3) (PI; CJ; EV)**

1 This does not demonstrate a resolution of problems underlying the behavior.

2 Without discussion of the problems underlying the behavior, little would be accomplished.

3 Same as answer 1.

160. 1 **The development of confusion would indicate that the client's ability to maintain equilibrium has not been achieved and that further disequilibrium was occurring. (2) (PM; CJ; EV)**

2 This would not indicate the plan needed to be changed unless the client's history demonstrates no prior use of this defense.

3 Same as answer 2.

4 This would be a positive response to any plan of care but is not directly related to independence.

161. 3 **Members have not established trust and are hesitant to discuss problems; the behaviors observed reflect anxiety and insecurity. (2) (PI; CJ; AS)**

1 This would add to the anxiety and insecurity of group members.

2 These behaviors are expected in the early stage of group interaction.

4 Same as answer 1.

162. 1 **The client's response demonstrates an inability to deal with the other member's confrontational approach at this time. (2) (PI; CJ; EV)**

2 There is not enough information to make this evaluation.

3 The group has reached the working stage, and if the client were able to deal with this confrontation, the nurse would expect the client to state the feeling generated by the statement.

4 Same as answer 3.

CRISIS SITUATIONS (CS)

163. 2 **Caplan's theory states that a crisis is an internal disturbance caused by a stressful event that alters the usual way of coping with a threat to the self; this temporarily disturbs the equilibrium of the person involved. (3) (PI; CJ; AN)**

1 This is not the definition of a crisis.

3 This is not the definition of a crisis; it is the assessment the nurse must make in the first phase of crisis intervention.

4 This is not the definition of a crisis but how a crisis is resolved.

164. 4 **Awareness of limitations and the ability to place oneself in another's situation are essential to be able to intervene effectively. (1) (SE; MR; AN)**

1 This is not a necessary characteristic to help families with problems and many times would be impossible to achieve; this is not a prerequisite for understanding.

2 Although this may be helpful, it is not a priority.

3 Same as answer 2.

165. 4 **The data presented indicate developmentally related struggles and specific situations that are extremely stressful; multiple stresses can produce a crisis situation for the individual when past coping mechanisms are ineffective. (1) (PM; CJ; AS)**

1 It is not the experience but the individual's response to the experience that determines a crisis.

2 A crisis is not an age-related problem; a crisis results when the individual's past coping mechanisms are no longer effective for dealing with a present stressful situation.

3 The individual's inability to cope indicates a crisis.

166. 3 **A situational crisis is a sudden, unexpected event with which the individual is unable to cope using past coping behaviors; this time frame provides an opportunity for the individual to learn new coping behaviors. (2) (PI; CJ; AN)**

1 This would be too short a period of time for the individual to develop new, successful coping mechanisms.

2 Same as answer 1.

4 This would be a longer than expected time period.

167. 2 **Personal internal strengths and supportive individuals are critical factors that can be employed to assist the individual to cope with a crisis. (2) (PI; CJ; AS)**

1 Although this information may be helpful, it is not essential; factors concerning the present situation are paramount.

3 Identifying unconscious conflicts takes a long time and is inappropriate for crisis intervention.

4 This is a goal of psychotherapy, not crisis intervention.

168. 4 Any aspect of the treatment environment can be used to benefit the client in milieu therapy. (3) (PI; CJ; AN)

1 This is part of behavioral modification, not milieu therapy.

2 This is part of psychoanalytic, not milieu, therapy.

3 These are separate treatment modalities, not part of milieu therapy.

169. 4 A crisis intervention group helps clients reestablish psychologic equilibrium by assisting them to explore new alternatives for coping; it considers realistic situations using rational and flexible problem-solving methods. (1) (SE; MR; AN)

1 This is not an immediate goal of crisis intervention.

2 Clients are never given a solution; they are assisted in arriving at their own acceptable, workable solutions.

3 It is not necessary for crisis intervention workers to be psychologists.

170. 4 The client should be able to state specific behaviors that can be used to decrease self-destructive thoughts and actions; the client must be empowered. (1) (PI; LE; EV)

1 This is ineffective because the client may end the conversation and remain suicidal.

2 The nurse may gather data through the suicidal risk assessment tool, but the client may not have attained a catharsis; therefore, the dialogue should continue until a contract has been set or self-destructive behaviors have diminished.

3 This is an indication that the nurse should help the client focus on life and not on suicide; the client has not yet attained a catharsis.

171. 3 Although the client's facial expression suggests happiness, the client's tone of voice gives the message of anger; the behaviors are not congruent. (1) (PI; CJ; AS)

1 The data given do not support this assessment.

2 Same as answer 1.

4 Same as answer 1.

172. 4 The client is using intellectual reasoning to block confronting the unconscious conflict and the stress of having to deal with his girlfriend's pregnancy. (2) (PI; CJ; AS)

1 There are no data that demonstrate that the client is projecting blame on anyone else.

2 There are no data that demonstrate that the client is concentrating thoughts and emotions on his inner self.

3 There are no data that demonstrate the shifting of emotions from an emotionally charged object or person to a neutral one.

173. 4 A crisis is defined as a situation in which the client's previous methods of adaptation are inadequate to meet present needs. (2) (PI; CJ; AN)

1 A crisis is not necessarily related to the degree of stress; it occurs when past coping mechanisms are ineffective.

2 This is not the immediate stress for which the client has no coping mechanism.

3 This is not causing the crisis; the client's lack of coping mechanisms is the cause.

174. 4 The crisis center nurse's main responsibility is to assist the client in using the problem-solving process; the client should be helped to explore alternative solutions and be given information regarding other agencies, facilities, and services. (2) (SE; MR; PL)

1 Although the client's decision should be supported, this is a judgmental response.

2 This is not part of the immediate intervention during the crisis; the client may be encouraged to seek help later for other problems.

3 This is one of many instructions for which the client must take primary responsibility.

175. 1 Intrinsic motivation is motivation that is stimulated from within the learner; it is most effective because the learner recognizes the need to know, is self-directed, and is ready to learn. (2) (PM; CJ; EV)

2 This is stimulation from outside sources and is often ineffective; desire must come from within.

3 There is no external reward for attending classes.

4 This is a new behavior based on a new situation; there is no external reward for attending classes.

176. 3 The client is grieving the loss of a fantasized child; talking about it is part of the typical grief reaction. (3) (PI; CJ; AS)

1 The client is sad, not out of control or immobilized.

2 The client is coping with the loss effectively.

4 The client recognizes the loss but is lamenting what could have been.

177. 3 The client's anger over the abortion is shifted to the staff and the hospital because she is unable to deal with the abortion at this time. (2) (PI; CJ; AN)
    1 The client is neither ignoring nor refusing to recognize reality.
    2 The client is not attributing unacceptable or undesirable thoughts or feelings to another.
    4 The client is not using a behavior pattern opposite to what she feels.

178. 1 Emotionally immature individuals are often unable to deal with the role changes associated with parenthood. (2) (PI; CJ; AN)
    2 This may have contributed to the crisis but did not precipitate it.
    3 Same as answer 2.
    4 Same as answer 2.

179. 2 The parents must be involved with exploring alternative methods to cope with the present crisis; this involves problem-solving techniques. (3) (PI; MR; IM)
    1 This is aimed at insight and subsequent change in behavior and is not focused specifically on one problem.
    3 This dictates to the parents rather than adding to their self-esteem by having them contribute to the solution.
    4 The parents' feelings may be explored, but this is supplemental to the work of problem solving.

180. 3 Abusive parents seek gratification for their own needs; they may project blame for the abuse on their child and find it difficult to conceal their hostility. (1) (PI; CJ; AS)
    1 Abusive parents typically have an ill-developed nurturing role with little perception of their parenting inability.
    2 Abusive parents are more concerned with their own needs than their child's.
    4 Same answer as 2.

181. 4 If one child in the family is identified as being different by the parents or siblings, coupled with other signs of abuse, physical abuse should be suspected and further investigation is warranted. (1) (PI; CJ; AS)
    1 Taking a walk would be helpful for both the mother and the child and would not indicate abuse.
    2 This is an acceptable punishment for misbehaviors.
    3 Although this is demeaning, it is not physical abuse.

182. 2 A history of high-lethality attempts at suicide indicates that the individual attempted suicide in the past and therefore may attempt to commit suicide again in the future. (1) (PI; CJ; AN)
    1 Although the correlation between substance abuse, particularly alcohol, and suicide is high, this is of lesser concern at this time because of the client's incarceration.
    3 Isolation from friends and coworkers would be of less significance than having an unstable, dissatisfying life with family members or having a history of prior suicide attempts.
    4 Although both of these events may cause stress, numerically, they would receive a lesser rating than having a history of multiple high-risk suicide attempts.

183. 4 Displacement is a defense mechanism in which one's pent-up feelings toward others who are a threat are discharged on less threatening others. (3) (PI; CJ; AN)
    1 Idealization is attributing overstated positive characteristics to others.
    2 Transference is a mechanism by which affects or emotional tones are shifted from one individual to another.
    3 Manipulation is a mechanism by which individuals attempt to manage, control, or use others to suit their own purpose or to gain an advantage.

184. 4 These underlying feelings commonly precipitate trying to improve the child's behavior by beating. (2) (PI; CJ; AS)
    1 These parents usually do not admit their behavior, so they do not have a need to rationalize it.
    2 These parents offer many vague explanations of how the child was injured; rarely is the explanation detailed.
    3 This would be an unusual request because the abusing parent usually does not ask to see the child.

185. 2 Management of the abused child places protection of the child's total being above consideration for parents' rights or wishes. (2) (PI; MR; IM)
    1 Supervision may be necessary, but staying with them the entire time would not help to build trust.
    3 Teaching methods of discipline is not appropriate at this time.
    4 Protecting the child, not promotion of parental attachment, is the priority at this time.

186. **3** **By learning how the child's behavior provokes frustration, parents may develop more acceptable ways of responding. (3) (PI; MR; IM)**
    1 Although these parents need to learn what behavior is appropriate for a given age level, they must first learn how to respond correctly to less appropriate behavior.
    2 Punishment is an act of retribution, not an act of discipline.
    4 Negative behavior cannot be ignored, but should be handled appropriately.

187. **2** **This child would distrust any approach because approaches commonly result in pain; abused children remain alert in an attempt to ward off an attack. (2) (PI; CJ; AS)**
    1 This child would not be open to an approach by a stranger; basic trust of others has not developed in abused children.
    3 This child usually would not cry out; abused children learn not to expect comforting or soothing of pain by others.
    4 This child would be acutely aware of anyone coming near; abused children attempt to defend themselves by keeping alert to the possibility of attack.

188. **2** **These children often have nonsexual needs met by this individual and are powerless to refuse; ambivalence results in self-blame and guilt. (2) (PI; CJ; AN)**
    1 These feelings may exist, but they are not the overwhelming feelings reported.
    3 Same as answer 1.
    4 Same as answer 1.

189. **1** **This would provide reassurance and support for the child. (2) (SE; MR; IM)**
    2 Using the phrase "anything wrong down there" could cause the child to have negative feelings about the self.
    3 Depending on the mother's involvement, this might be threatening rather than supportive to the child.
    4 Asking the child to make this decision at this time would be nontherapeutic and may be threatening.

190. **2** **This response would elicit further clarification of what the child means by "bad." (3) (PI; CJ; AS)**
    1 This would not be helpful; it would do nothing to clarify the child's idea of what "bad" means or the child's feelings about what happened.

    3 The nurse must determine what the child means by the word "bad" before reflecting the term back to the child.
    4 This would be a nontherapeutic response because the uncertainty implied by the nurse could increase the child's feelings of guilt.

191. **3** **This revelation should be accepted as truthful and it should be investigated immediately so that emotional and physical care can be instituted; the student needs to feel safe and supported. (1) (PI; MR; IM)**
    1 Accusations of incest rarely are used in this way.
    2 Although lying may be a way of calling attention to unmet needs, this particular type of lie is rare.
    4 Blaming a family member is not the usual way that teenagers attempt to explain a pregnancy.

192. **2** **Rapists are believed to harbor and act out hostile feelings toward all women through the act of rape. (2) (PI; CJ; AN)**
    1 This is never the cause; passion is not a part of rape.
    3 This may be an unconscious feeling, but it is not the motivating factor.
    4 Fears about incompetence or impotency may be present, but they are not the motivating factors in a rape.

193. **4** **Whatever action the client took to save her life was the right action; this statement supports the woman. (3) (PI; CJ; IM)**
    1 This is nontherapeutic; the word "submit" in any form is emotionally charged and increases feelings of guilt.
    2 Same as answer 1.
    3 This leaves the client with the thought she could have done something else.

194. **1** **Because rape is a threat to the sense of control over one's life, some control should be given back to the client as soon as possible. (3) (PI; MR; PL)**
    2 This takes control away from the client; the client could view this as an additional assault on the body that increases feelings of vulnerability and anxiety and does not restore control.
    3 This is an expected form of ventilating emotions; the client should be told that medication is available if desired.
    4 Same as answer 2.

195. 1 **Partners may themselves feel angry and abused; these feelings should be rapidly and openly discussed. (3) (SE; CJ; AN)**
   2 This should not be done yet; rape counselors work with the victim and partner together.
   3 The partner's feelings must be resolved before the partner can help the client.
   4 This may be reassuring, but it leaves the partner alone to deal with feelings.

196. 1 **This is the most direct approach to ascertain if pills were ingested; the client usually will respond to this type of direct question. (2) (PI; CJ; AS)**
   2 This would not provide useful information.
   3 This is not an initial response; a determination must first be made regarding the number of pills taken.
   4 This would be appropriate later but is not an initial priority.

197. 1 **Anger at her husband for leaving her may make her feel guilty for having these feelings. (3) (PI; CJ; AS)**
   2 Financial security may or may not be a problem for this client.
   3 Loneliness will be something she will have to cope with later, depending on her support system; it is not an immediate problem.
   4 Estrangement may be something she will have to cope with later; it is not an immediate problem.

198. 3 **Whether there is a suicide plan is a major criterion when assessing the client's determination to make another attempt. (1) (SE; MR; AS)**
   1 Although this may be important for planning future therapeutic approaches, this does not explore the potential for suicide, the priority at this time.
   2 Same as answer 1.
   4 Same as answer 1.

199. 2 **Suicide threats and gestures are a means of communicating anger, frustration, hopelessness, and despair to significant others and should always be taken seriously. (1) (PI; CJ; IM)**
   1 Children have many means readily available; there are many common objects around the home and playground that could be used to commit suicide.
   3 Although suicide is the second leading cause of death in the 15- to 24-year-old age group, children younger than age 6 do attempt suicide and some succeed.

   4 A suicidal gesture usually is a cry for help, but a suicide attempt usually is self-destructive; a suicide attempt may be carried out with the belief that death will result; neither a suicidal gesture nor a suicide attempt is manipulative; an impulsive act that is a rage response designed to punish others may be manipulative.

200. 3 **The parents are focusing their feelings about their child's prognosis on someone or something else, in this case each other. (1) (PI; CJ; IM)**
   1 Denial is ignoring, avoiding, or refusing to recognize painful realities.
   2 Projection is the attribution of one's own feelings to another person.
   4 Compensation is making up for a perceived deficiency by emphasizing another feature perceived as an asset.

201. 2 **Reasonable limits are necessary because they provide security and help to keep the child's behavior within acceptable bounds. (3) (SE; MR; PL)**
   1 This is an unrealistic approach that allows the child to manipulate the total situation.
   3 Care should be directed to help the child, not the staff members.
   4 Relationships, not special privileges, should provide the necessary security.

202. 2 **Seeing their child as soon as possible will validate the death for them and initiate the grieving process. (2) (SE; MR; IM)**
   1 This will delay and prolong the grieving process; the response offers no explanation for waiting.
   3 This is unnecessary; the parents have asked to see their child now.
   4 It would be more traumatic to wait and delay the reality of the death.

203. 1 **An unsuccessful adaptation to loss is a major defining characteristic of this diagnosis; the history of the loss of a son and the intensity of the client's drinking since his death should lead to this nursing diagnosis. (1) (PI; CJ; AN)**
   2 There is no documentation that the family has not attempted to provide support.
   3 There is no documentation that the client is unable to distinguish between self and others.
   4 There is no documentation that the client is misinterpreting internal or external stimuli.

204. 2 Deaths that are perceived as preventable cause more guilt for the mourners and therefore increase the intensity and length of the grieving process. (2) (PI; CJ; AN)

1 The opposite usually is true.

3 It may prolong and intensify the mourning process but will not necessarily result in a pathologic reaction.

4 Same as answer 3.

205. 1 This provides support until the individuals' coping mechanisms and personal support systems can be mobilized. (3) (PI; CJ; IM)

2 The individuals, not the nurse, must mobilize their support systems.

3 This is not the role of the nurse.

4 The individuals need time before the full reality of the death can be accepted.

206. 4 Support is most important when dealing with the crisis of death; the support system must be relied on for coping with the loss. (2) (SE; MR; AS)

1 The client's age may play a role in coping, but it is not the most important factor.

2 The timing may be important if death is just one of a multiplicity of stresses, but it is not the most important factor in helping a client cope.

3 The socioeconomic status may be important in long-term planning, but it is not the most important factor in the grieving process.

207. 2 Resolving a loss is a slow, painful, continuous process until a mental image of the dead person, almost devoid of negative or undesirable features, emerges. (3) (PI; CJ; PL)

1 The various rituals of the funeral help to initiate the recovery or restitution stage.

3 This stage usually is dominated by a refusal to accept or comprehend the fact that a loved one has died.

4 The reality of the death and its meaning as a loss, plus anger, dominate this stage.

208. 3 Successful resolution means being able to remember the good as well as the bad qualities of the deceased and accepting them as part of being human. (1) (PI; CJ; EV)

1 Resolution involves working through feelings, not just accepting what occurred.

2 Resolution does not mean forgetting but rather realistically remembering the past.

4 This is an unhealthy response that can become pathologic because of the unresolved feelings about the other person's qualities.

209. 4 Discussing the partner and the partner's death will help the client work through the grief process. (3) (PI; CJ; PL)

1 The client must deal with the past and present before addressing the future.

2 This would refocus the client's attention away from dealing with feelings; the client would probably not have the physical or emotional energy to get involved with group activities.

3 Same as answer 2.

210. 2 Intervention is aimed at restoring equilibrium by helping the client develop new ways to cope and assisting with the exploration of available support systems. (2) (PI; CJ; IM)

1 Identification of the precipitating factors should have taken place during the assessment phase.

3 The client's perception may be distorted; the nurse should strive to help maintain a realistic perception.

4 Decreasing support systems will not lead to independence but will increase the client's vulnerability and precipitate feelings of abandonment.

211. 4 Helping a client deal with unresolved grief involves assisting the client to express thoughts and feelings about the lost object or person as a necessary part of grief work. (1) (PI; CJ; IM)

1 This is the responsibility of the nurse; another client would not have the expertise to help the client.

2 This would be too threatening; at this point the client needs therapeutic one-to-one interaction.

3 The current nonverbal behavior indicates that the client is dealing with feelings; an opportunity should be provided for a verbal exploration.

212. 3 These are the defining characteristics of dysfunctional grieving. (3) (PI; CJ; AS)

1 The client's communication does not lead to this conclusion.

2 Same as answer 1.

4 Eight months does not constitute a prolonged period of mourning.

213. 2 Such stimuli encourage the client to remain reality oriented; research has shown that competing stimuli are useful in controlling hallucinations.

(2) (PB; CJ; PL)

1 This does not ensure that the client's needs will be met.

3 This is not realistic and fosters greater dependency; it focuses on the client's inability to deal with the problem and increases the client's fear of being alone.

4 Same as answer 3.

214. 2 **Anger is associated with one of the stages of dying; understanding the stages leading to the acceptance of death may help the family to accept the client's moods and anger. (2) (PI; MR; PL)**

1 This may not be true unless stated by the client.

3 The client's anger is one of the stages of accepting death.

4 Same as answer 1.

215. 4 **A starting point for working with all clients is ascertaining what is known, their understanding of their particular situation, and its meaning to them. (2) (PI; CJ; AS)**

1 It is not merely understanding what death and the dying process means, but how the individual feels about the situation.

2 Encouraging conversation about the condition tends to decrease anxiety and would be desirable.

3 This would meet the needs of others rather than the client, who is the priority concern.

216. 1 **This response is on a feeling level and encourages the client to explore how she feels. (1) (PI; CJ; IM)**

2 This statement supports the negative feelings of worthlessness.

3 This response focuses on negative feelings.

4 This argumentative statement denies the client's feelings.

217. 1 **It is important for the couple to discuss their feelings to maintain open communication and support each other. (2) (PI; CJ; PL)**

2 This action would not meet the needs of this couple; it focuses only on the client's needs and ignores the partner's needs.

3 This may be useful in the future but probably is premature; they need to share their feelings with each other first.

4 This may elicit feelings but will not improve communication between the couple.

218. 3 **This approach is positive because it attempts to deal with the staff's feelings as well as** the problem; the nurse therefore is taking an ethically sound action without being moralistic or authoritarian. (1) (SE; MR; PL)

1 This abdicates the nurse's responsibility and may create anger and guilt in the staff members.

2 Same as answer 1.

4 Same as answer 1.

219. 1 **The client has lost a companion and a purpose in life; these feelings can be overwhelming until new activities are developed. (2) (PI; CJ; AS)**

2 Anger should not be a major problem for this client; anger may have been a factor when the terminal nature of the illness was diagnosed.

3 Data do not address the financial status of this client.

4 If there is guilt over feelings of relief about the husband's death, they would be transitory and not a major problem.

220. 2 **The spouse is expressing the expected feelings of guilt associated with the death of a loved one; there usually is initial guilt over what might have been. (1) (PI; CJ; AN)**

1 No evidence supports this conclusion.

3 The spouse is expressing guilt, not shame.

4 Same as answer 1.

221. 3 **With this sedating medication, the individual does not face the reality of the loss and merely delays the onset of the pain associated with it; because most support is available at the time of the death and the funeral, benzodiazepines at this time deny the individual the opportunity to use this assistance. (2) (PI; CJ; AN)**

1 This classification of drugs does not magnify the risk of suicide.

2 Brain activity does not cause a reactive depression.

4 Although sedation and muscle relaxation initially may occur with these drugs, these are not the reasons they are not ordered.

222. 4 **The nurse should recognize that the husband's behavior represents anticipatory grieving. (3) (PI; CJ; AN)**

1 Although this may be true, the husband is involved with his own needs at this time.

2 The husband is beginning the grieving process; the husband's actions do not appear to be an expression of anger but rather an attempt to cope with the situation.

3 There are no data to substantiate this conclusion.

DEMENTIA, DELIRIUM, AND OTHER COGNITIVE DISORDERS (DD)

223. **2 Dementias, such as that of the Alzheimer's type, result from pathologic changes of CNS cells producing symptoms that are long-term and progressive. (2) (PI; CJ; AN)**
   1 Once CNS neurons are destroyed, remissions are uncommon.
   3 Symptoms of delirium, not dementia, develop rapidly as a result of derangements of cerebral metabolism and of neurotransmission.
   4 Environmental or interpersonal events do not precipitate dementias.

224. **2 This action will reduce the need for sleeping pills, which frequently add to the older client's confusion. (2) (PI; MR; IM)**
   1 The family is not asking that the client be moved from the home; the nurse's focus should be to help reduce the confusion the client experiences at night, keep the client safe, and ease the burden on the family.
   3 Same as answer 1.
   4 Restraints add to the client's confusion and tend to increase bizarre behavior.

225. **2 Confabulation, or the filling in of memory gaps with imaginary facts, is a defense mechanism used by people experiencing memory deficits. (1) (PI; CJ; AS)**
   1 Concretism is demonstrated by speech in which the major or salient point being made by the speaker is lost because it is buried in excessive verbal detail.
   3 Flight of ideas is demonstrated by speech that jumps from one topic to another with no obvious connection for either the speaker or the listener.
   4 Associative looseness is demonstrated by speech that is difficult to follow because the connections between the speaker's statements or train of thoughts are so loose that they are not obvious to the listener.

226. **4 A moderate level of cognitive impairment due to dementia is characterized by increasing dependence on environmental and social structure and by increasing psychologic rigidity with accentuated previous traits and behaviors. (3) (PI; CJ; AS)**
   1 Although paranoid attitudes may be exhibited, the decrease in cognitive functioning, disorientation, and loss of memory usually do not lead to hypervigilance.

   2 With the decrease in impulse control that is associated with dementia, decreased, not increased, inhibition would be present.
   3 An enhancement of intelligence would not occur in dementia; initially, intellectual deterioration is subtle.

227. **4 Dementia of the Alzheimer's type accounts for 80% of dementias in older adults; it may be due to a neurotransmitter deficiency and it is characterized by a steady decline in intellectual functioning, including memory deficits, disorientation, and decreased cognitive ability. (1) (PI; CJ; AN)**
   1 It is an organic, not functional, disorder.
   2 Over 90% of people with dementia of the Alzheimer's type are over the age of 50.
   3 Dementia of the Alzheimer's type is difficult to diagnose and often is made when other etiologies for the dementia have been ruled out.

228. **1 With a depression, there is little or no emotional involvement and therefore little alteration in affect. (3) (PI; CJ; AS)**
   2 This is associated with depression because of low self-esteem.
   3 People who are depressed do not have physical or emotional energy; "I don't know" answers require little thought and/or decision making.
   4 This is associated with depression because a sense of futility leads to a lack of response to the environment.

229. **2 Routines and familiarity with activities or the environment provide for a sense of security. (2) (PI; CJ; PL)**
   1 Change is poorly tolerated; frustration and the inability to accomplish tasks lead to lowered self-esteem.
   3 Challenging activities can be frustrating and can lead to hostility or withdrawal.
   4 Decreased physical capacity and attention span limit active participation; frustration can result.

230. **3 Clients with dementia have the greatest loss in the area of recent memory. (2) (PI; CJ; PL)**
   1 Memory of remote events usually remains fairly intact.
   2 Same as answer 1.
   4 Same as answer 1.

231. **1 When the client is unable to perform a task, frustration occurs and results in more disorganized behavior. (3) (PI; CJ; PL)**

2 The client's disorientation is documented and will not change, although some day-to-day variations may occur; most important is the assessment of the client's ability to function.

3 There is no documentation of disruptive behavior; frustration must be avoided.

4 The client probably will never adjust any further.

232. **3 This client needs toileting every 2 hours to prevent soiling; physically seating the client on the toilet often prevents accidents and negates the use of diapers. (3) (PB; CJ; IM)**

1 The client needs to be physically placed on the toilet; confusion limits effectiveness of other actions.

2 Same as answer 1.

4 Same as answer 1.

233. **2 This forces the client to find a common characteristic of two things, an ability that is the criterion for abstract thinking. (3) (PI; CJ; AS)**

1 This tests orientation, not abstract thinking.

3 This tests judgment, not abstract thinking.

4 This tests short-term memory, not abstract thinking.

234. **3 A common sign of dementia is the loss of memory for recent events. (3) (PI; CJ; AS)**

1 Disorientation of self is not a common sign of dementia; disorientation to time and place are more common.

2 Recall of past events is less impaired than that of recent events.

4 This is not as common as recent memory loss; if there were speech or language disturbances then this ability should be assessed.

235. **2 Confabulation is used as a defense mechanism against embarrassment caused by a lapse of memory; the client fills in the blanks in memory by making up details. (2) (PI; CJ; AN)**

1 Regression is a defense mechanism in which the individual moves back to earlier developmental defenses.

3 Although older adults fear being forgotten or losing others' affection, this is not the reason for confabulation.

4 Confabulation is not used to reminisce about past achievement.

236. **4 This action maintains, for as long as possible, the client's remaining intellectual functions by providing an opportunity to use them. (3) (SE; CJ; PL)**

1 Although pain syndromes can occur in clients with dementia from AIDS, frequent pain assessment is not a priority; providing cognitive stimulation facilitates the use of nonpharmacologic treatments for pain management as long as possible.

2 Remotivation is not always possible with extensive organic damage.

3 There are no data to indicate that the client needs custodial care at this time.

237. **2 This client would require a structured environment, regardless of the cause of the behavior; this would help provide a safe environment. (2) (SE; CJ; PL)**

1 This is important but is secondary to promotion of an environment conducive to safety and security.

3 A battery of screening tests probably will be used in an attempt to determine the cause of the dementia; however, provision for safety is necessary first.

4 Same as answer 1.

238. **2 This allows the client to exercise the right to decide which articles to keep and provides for safety and cleanliness. (2) (SE; CJ; PL)**

1 This deceives the client, limits judgment, and creates mistrust toward the staff.

3 This does not help because all of the objects the client is hoarding are not harmful.

4 Explanations alone will not provide for safety or meet this client's needs because of a decreased attention span and memory.

239. **3 The client needs constant reassurance because forgetfulness blocks previous explanations; frequent presence of staff members serves as a continual reminder. (2) (PI; MR; PL)**

1 The client needs continual reassurance and would not remember times for planned interactions or activities.

2 This client would be unable to explain the reasons for concern.

4 This client will not remember the explanation from one moment to the next.

240. **3 This client requires external controls to minimize danger of injury and to preserve human dignity. (2) (PI; CJ; PL)**

1 The staff cannot prevent all gross motor activity; the client needs to use muscles or atrophy will occur.

2 The client will not have excessive energy.

4 Further deterioration usually cannot be prevented in this disorder.

241. 2 **This encourages verbalization, gives the client a feeling of security, and decreases the sense of isolation. (1) (PI; CJ; IM)**
    1 This action discourages verbalization between client and nurse; the client may be unable to function in a small group because of increased anxiety.
    3 This discourages verbalization of feelings and will lead to feelings of being unwanted.
    4 Same as answer 1.

242. 3 **This approach assists the client with decision making; new situations may be stressful and lead to ambivalence. (2) (PI; CJ; IM)**
    1 This will increase stress and possible feelings of guilt.
    2 The client may perceive this as punishment; the client may not have the psychic energy or decision-making ability to get dressed without help.
    4 This is not sharing decision making, and hurrying the client may lead to feelings of frustration and resentment.

243. 3 **Intellectual deterioration decreases interest in the environment. (1) (PI; CJ; AS)**
    1 Diffuse impairment of brain tissue function results in fluctuations in the extremes of emotions; lability of mood is common.
    2 These clients usually fluctuate between aggressive acting out and passive acceptance.
    4 Intellectual deterioration can result in behavior that mimics withdrawal.

EATING AND SLEEP DISORDERS (ES)

244. 4 **Hypotension, not hypertension, may occur because of dehydration. (2) (PI; CJ; AS)**
    1 Alopecia can result from malnutrition.
    2 Amenorrhea results from endocrine imbalances that occur when fat stores are depleted.
    3 Constipation may occur because of lack of fiber in the diet.

245. 1 **These clients often hide food or force vomiting; therefore, they must be carefully observed. (2) (PI; CJ; PL)**
    2 This is insufficient because these clients may induce vomiting after eating.
    3 Fluid and electrolyte balance can become a problem for these clients and monitoring is required, but at this time it is the responsibility of the nurse, not the client, to do this.

    4 These clients will not become involved in planning meals; this is a long-term goal.

246. 3 **Research indicates that cognitive-behavioral therapy has been shown to be most effective in the treatment of bulimia nervosa. (3) (PI; CJ; AN)**
    1 Although this therapy is important and may be helpful, it is not the most effective therapy for clients with bulimia nervosa.
    2 Same as answer 1.
    4 Although many nurses employ the use of an eclectic model when conducting psychotherapy, use of the crisis model is not the most effective therapy for clients with bulimia nervosa.

247. 4 **Depression commonly coexists with bulimia; it is essential to assess the client's level of depression to prevent self-harm. (3) (PI; CJ; AS)**
    1 Although this is important to assess, it is not the priority.
    2 Same as answer 1.
    3 Same as answer 1.

248. 4 **The client with anorexia nervosa denies the need for food or presence of hunger; the client with bulimia hides the behavior because there is recognition that the behavior is a problem. (3) (PI; CJ; AN)**
    1 Clients with anorexia nervosa are more introverted and tend to avoid relationships.
    2 Same as answer 1.
    3 Clients with bulimia are at a greater risk for fluid and electrolyte problems because of the purging; clients with anorexia nervosa are more at risk for severe nutritional deficiencies.

249. 1 **This is the best initial response; it encourages additional ventilation of feelings. (3) (PI; CJ; IM)**
    2 This is not necessarily true, and the response is somewhat threatening and nontherapeutic.
    3 Same as answer 2.
    4 This would not be therapeutic; the client is verbally expressing feelings, and the behavior does not require medication at this time.

250. 4 **These are the major signs of anorexia nervosa; weight loss is excessive (15% of expected weight) and nutritional deficiencies result in amenorrhea and a bloated abdomen. (3) (PB; CJ; AS)**
    1 Weight loss is greater than 10%.

2 These are not associated with anorexia nervosa.

3 Memory lapses are not associated with anorexia nervosa; the other symptoms are more associated with anxiety.

251. **2 Eating and weight loss become the means of control when independence is discouraged and overprotectiveness and intrusiveness are practiced. (2) (PI; CJ; AN)**
1 Controlling oneself within the family seems to be more important than peer group acceptance.
3 Although the client with anorexia nervosa's fear of weight gain sometimes reaches delusional proportions, it is based on a belief that being fat is the problem.
4 Although this is true, the response of the client with anorexia nervosa falls outside of the usual range.

252. **1 Dental enamel erosion occurs from repeated self-induced vomiting. (3) (PI; CJ; AS)**
2 Often body image is disturbed.
3 This is not associated with bulimia.
4 Habitual regurgitation of small amounts of undigested food (rumination) and re-swallowing of food are not associated with bulimia; emptying of the stomach contents through the mouth (vomiting) is associated with bulimia.

253. **1 Individuals with anorexia often display irritability, hostility, and a depressed mood. (3) (PI; CJ; AS)**
2 This is associated with individuals with autism.
3 These are associated with individuals with schizophrenia.
4 Clients with eating disorders usually are meticulous about dress and physical appearance.

254. **2 These clients usually are severely malnourished and have severe fluid and electrolyte imbalances; unless these imbalances are corrected, cardiac irregularities and death can occur. (2) (PB; CJ; PL)**
1 This is important, but it is not the highest priority at this time.
3 Same as answer 1.
4 Same as answer 1

255. **3 This client must assume responsibility for self-care for treatment to be successful; assisting with meal planning allows the client some control over the foods eaten while using healthy guidelines. (1) (PI; CJ; PL)**
1 This is an unrealistic goal because the client is afraid of eating and gaining weight.
2 Same as answer 1.
4 The client's anxiety level will increase if presented with high-fat foods and a large number of calories; anxiety about eating must be at manageable levels if the client is to progress in treatment.

256. **3 These clients have severely depleted levels of potassium and sodium because of their starvation diet and energy expenditure; these electrolytes are necessary for proper cardiac functioning. (2) (PB; CJ; AN)**
1 Although this may occur, it is not the major health problem.
2 Same as answer 1.
4 Same as answer 1.

257. **3 This is a nonthreatening, open-ended response that focuses discussion and leaves channels of communication open. (2) (PI; CJ; AS)**
1 Although this does not quite accuse the client of lying, it is a threatening response that questions the client's truthfulness.
2 Same as answer 1.
4 Same as answer 1.

258. **1 Behavior modification programs have been helpful treatment modes for many clients suffering from anorexia nervosa. (2) (PI; C; PL)**
2 This is ineffective; the person with anorexia nervosa is more concerned with losing weight than with eating a balanced diet.
3 A well-balanced diet should be encouraged.
4 Although family therapy may be helpful, placing emphasis on the anorexia may reinforce the negative behavior.

259. **3 It is most therapeutic for the staff to control food needs, thus removing the parents from the struggle. (3) (SE; CJ; IM)**
1 This may be interpreted as accusatory and increase the parents' guilt.
2 This is nontherapeutic; it cuts off the parents from future involvement.
4 This continues the struggle between the parents and the client.

260.

1 __x__ **A state of malnutrition with muscle wasting, weakness, and emaciation (cachexia) occurs with anorexia nervosa; clients usually are 15% to 30% below ideal body weight. (2) (PI; CJ; AS)**

2 _____ Recurrent episodes of the rapid consumption of a large amount of food in a discrete period of time (binge eating) are associated with bulimia nervosa.

3 _____ Constipation can occur with both anorexia nervosa and bulimia nervosa, usually because of a lack of adequate fluids and intestinal stimulating foods.

4 _____ Hypotension can occur with both anorexia nervosa and bulimia nervosa, usually because of dehydration.

5 _____ Hypothermia, not hyperthermia, occurs with anorexia nervosa, usually caused by decreased subcutaneous tissue.

6 __x__ **Many clients with anorexia nervosa exhibit psychologic symptoms, including a lack of age-appropriate interest in sex and relationships.**

261. 3 The client's security is increased by limit-setting; guidelines remove responsibility for behavior from the client and increase compliance with the regimen. (2) (SE; MR; PL)

1 The client needs limit setting, not empathy.

2 Simply maintaining control is not therapeutic and increases the power struggle.

4 Emphasis on dietary intake establishes a power struggle between the client and the nurse.

262. 2 This action would be neither a positive nor a negative reinforcement of specific behavior; it would provide rewards for achievement of specific goals. (2) (PB; CJ; PL)

1 This would not be included in a behavior modification program.

3 Same as answer 1.

4 Clients talk freely about food; the problem is with ingestion, not discussion.

263. 2 All food issues should be discussed with the nutritionist, thus removing a potential source of conflict between the nurse and client. (2) (PB; MR; PL)

1 This would increase the conflict between the nurse and client.

3 This would accomplish little because the client's failure to eat is not based on food likes or dislikes.

4 This may be self-defeating because discussion of food would be the major focus of all nurse-client interactions.

264. 3 Clients with anorexia nervosa use manipulation to divide the nursing staff; sharing this knowledge alerts health team members. (3) (PI; CJ; AN)

1 This would be counterproductive because it supports the client's manipulative behavior.

2 The client is attempting to manipulate the staff; this is not how trust is established.

4 Same as answer 1.

265. 4 By talking to the client on the telephone at mealtimes, the family is enabling the client to continue destructive behavior; the client and family must be included in discussion of and possible solutions to the problem. (2) (SE; MR; PL)

1 This would be a punitive approach that would not deal with the underlying problem.

2 Same as answer 1.

3 Same as answer 1.

266. 2 This would demonstrate a change in behavior as well as a positive approach to meals. (2) (PI; CJ; EV)

1 This would be typical behavior of a client with anorexia nervosa.

3 The problem is not a lack of interest about food but a deliberate refusal to ingest food.

4 This behavior is unrelated to the behavior that needed to be changed.

267. 1 Recovery necessitates major changes in self-esteem and body image, which require therapy over a long period of time. (2) (PI; CJ; IM)

2 Long-term therapy is required.

3 This is only one factor; the client must also be willing to work with the family and to accept the pain associated with change.

4 This is too simplistic a response; anorexia nervosa is not a desire merely to lose weight.

DISORDERS OF MOOD (MO)

268. 4 This provides structure and helps the client learn acceptable behavior. (2) (PI; CJ; PL)

1 The client may not be ready for this at the present time.

2 No environment will be stress free.

3 Same as answer 1.

269. 4 Limiting unnecessary interactions will decrease stimulation and thus agitation. (2) (PI; CJ; PL)

1 Constant client and staff contact increases stimulation and thus agitation.

2 This bombards the client's sensorium and increases agitation.

3 Not all disturbed clients are suspicious.

270. 3 Depression is characterized by feelings of hopelessness, helplessness, and despair, leaving little room for any pleasure; alteration in appetite (either decreased or increased) is common in depressed clients. (2) (PI; CJ; AS)

1 Although there is a narrowing of perception, rigidity would be uncommon.

2 Fatigue is continually present and does not alternate with high energy levels.

4 There is a loss of interest and little participation in activities of daily living.

271. 3 Depression usually is both emotional and physical, so a simple daily routine is the least stressful and least anxiety producing. (1) (SE; CJ; PL)

1 A depressed client has limited interest in any activity; offering many may increase the anxiety.

2 Too many stimuli increase anxiety in a depressed client.

4 An extremely depressed client may be incapable of making even simple decisions.

272. 4 Depression is "contagious"; it affects the nurse as well as the client. (2) (SE; CJ; AN)

1 The client's lack of energy should not make nursing care difficult.

2 These clients usually do not offer negative responses; they offer no response.

3 Same as answer 1.

273. 1 Because clients cannot be argued out of their feelings, it is best to initially accept them; it also encourages communication. (2) (PI; CJ; PL)

2 This delays discussing the client's feelings and has little value.

3 The depressed client does very little talking and needs to be encouraged to communicate.

4 This has little effect on the depressed client; it can increase depression.

274. 1 Allowing the client to make those decisions that can be handled helps improve confidence. (2) (PI; CJ; PL)

2 The client is depressed, and this could result in total inactivity.

3 This action would demoralize the client; also, it is impossible for one individual to make all the decisions for another.

4 Same as answer 2.

275. 4 This action demonstrates to the client that the nurse feels the client is worth spending time with, and it helps restore and build trust. (2) (PI; CJ; PL)

1 This action would be impossible to carry out on a regular basis unless the client was potentially suicidal.

2 This action does little to establish communication between the nurse and the client and might be threatening.

3 The depressed client may never get around to speaking to the nurse and, left alone, will withdraw even further.

276. 2 A severely depressed client not only has a low energy level, but also low self-esteem; this intervention demonstrates that the client is important and worthy of attention, which will help support self-esteem. (1) (PI; CJ; AN)

1 Although this is a true statement, this does not address the needs of this client specifically.

3 Same as answer 1.

4 Depressed clients do need stimulation; however, with severe depression the energy level is extremely low and care first must be provided on a basic level.

277. 4 The fact that the nurse spends time with the client conveys a feeling of importance and helps build the client's self-esteem. (3) (PI; CJ; IM)

1 This places the client on the defensive and does not respond to the feelings of worthlessness communicated by the client.

2 This infers agreement with the client's statement that the client is not worthy; the nurse should stay to convey a sense of self-worth to the client.

3 This response cuts off communication; the client responds better to actions than to words.

278. 3 This response focuses on the client's feelings rather than the statement, and it serves to open channels of communication. (2) (PI; CJ; IM)

1 This response asks the client to decide what is causing feelings; most people are unable to answer why they feel as they do.

2 This response simply echoes the client's statement and does not reflect feelings or stimulate further communication.

4 This response does nothing to stimulate further communication; in fact, it tells the client to talk about feelings with someone else.

279. 1 **This is a therapeutic approach that indicates an awareness of the client's feelings and encourages verbalization. (2) (PI; CJ; IM)**
  2 Moralizing is a barrier to effective communication.
  3 This is diverting the client's attention to something other than feelings.
  4 This conveys a judgmental or critical attitude toward the client.

280. 1 **Sudden lifting of mood may indicate an increased risk for suicide; the client may have the emotional energy to make the decision to act on suicidal ideas. (1) (PI; CJ; EV)**
  2 This conclusion does not consider the client's statement "I am not going to have problems for very long"; this may indicate continuing suicidal thoughts.
  3 Same as answer 2.
  4 Stress levels may be decreased; however, the client's statement may indicate that the decision to commit suicide has been made.

281. 1 **Group interaction provides a sense of belonging and fosters the assumption of responsibility. (2) (PI; CJ; AN)**
  2 The group is not the best arena for the expression of repressed hostility.
  3 This is not assured by group interaction.
  4 This is not the purpose of group interaction.

282. 1 **The client will be most likely to eat if accompanied and encouraged by an individual with whom a trusting relationship has been established. (1) (PI; CJ; IM)**
  2 This will not encourage the client to eat and will promote isolation.
  3 This is inappropriate at this time; the client is not interested in maintaining health, nor is the client ready for any teaching.
  4 This would be ineffective at this time; the client is too introspective to care.

283. 2 **This is a psychiatric problem in which there is no prior history of depression; it is related to age, changes in lifestyle, and feelings of not contributing and being worthless. (1) (PI; CJ; AS)**
  1 In bipolar disorders, depression alternates with periods of extreme restlessness, hyperactivity, and flamboyance in dress and behavior; this is not evident here.
  3 Involutional melancholia, which was usually characterized by depression with agitation, is no longer considered a specific disorder.

  4 There is no inconsistency between the behavior and the mood.

284. 4 **Depressed clients demonstrate decreased communication because of a lack of psychic or physical energy. (2) (PI; CJ; AN)**
  1 There is insufficient evidence to identify this as the primary nursing diagnosis.
  2 Same as answer 1.
  3 Same as answer 1.

285. 3 **Sharing painful feelings reduces the isolation and sense of uniqueness that feelings can cause; sharing of these feelings usually decreases depression. (2) (PI; CJ; PL)**
  1 This would do little to decrease the client's sadness and does not consider the client's low level of energy.
  2 Same as answer 1.
  4 This may be important for the future, if a problem exists, but the expression and sharing of painful feelings are more important than improving communication.

286. 1 **Some success is important to increase the client's self-esteem. (3) (PI; CJ; IM)**
  2 This would support the client's feelings of uselessness.
  3 The client, who is in a major depression, would not have the interest or energy to act independently.
  4 Same as answer 3.

287. 2 **Caring for her child refocuses unmet dependency needs of the mother resulting in resentment and anger; feelings cause ambivalence and guilt, which are turned inward. (3) (PI; CJ; AN)**
  1 There are no data to support this conclusion; the client's behavior appears to have provoked the spouse's response.
  3 There are no data to support the conclusion that child abuse occurred.
  4 Self-destructive behaviors do not usually evoke love, sympathy, or compliments from others.

288. 3 **This therapeutic response encourages expression of the client's feelings. (2) (PI; CJ; IM)**
  1 This response does not explore feelings, and the client may interpret it as a put-down.
  2 The nurse would not know the client is upset unless the client tells the nurse.
  4 The client may not know or may not wish to tell; in addition, the response asks for facts and does not elicit feelings.

289. 1 **A CT scan would identify pathology; the ECT would be contraindicated in the presence of a brain tumor because the treatment causes an increase in intracranial pressure. (2) (SE; CJ; AN)**
    2 There would be no contraindication to ECT with this health problem.
    3 Same as answer 2.
    4 Same as answer 2.

290. 3 **Giving the client simple facts and relating that it is normal to feel nervous help reduce the client's fears. (2) (PB; CJ; IM)**
    1 Memory loss affects recently learned information such as the ECT experience; this response would unnecessarily worry the client.
    2 Although true about the memory loss, this response would serve to negate the client's feelings.
    4 ECT does not selectively block out painful experiences.

291. 3 **This disadvantage is a side effect of the therapy and is expected. (3) (PI; MR; PL)**
    1 The therapy begins to demonstrate results in two to three treatments.
    2 Succinylcholine (Anectine) prevents the external manifestations of a tonic-clonic seizure, thus minimizing fractures and dislocations.
    4 There is no substantial loss of mental function after the treatment is completed.

292. 4 **The expression of these feelings may indicate that this client is unable to continue the struggle of life. (2) (SE; CJ; AS)**
    1 These are not indications of potential suicide; the client is still responding to the world, not attempting to leave it.
    2 These usually are not sufficient to precipitate a suicide attempt.
    3 The client attempting suicide usually sees death as a release.

293. 4 **This is the most important assessment to make because suicide is a possibility with every depressed client. (2) (SE; CJ; AS)**
    1 The client has already said this, and it responds to only part of the client's statement.
    2 This is a philosophic approach that would not encourage discussion of feelings.
    3 The nurse does not have enough information to have this understanding; this response does not encourage communication.

294. 1 **As the client's motivation and energy return, there is a greater threat that suicidal ideation will be acted out. (3) (PI; LE; EV)**
    2 Although this eventually will be done, the priority is to determine the potential for suicide.
    3 Although this should be done, the greater risk of suicide takes precedence.
    4 An unaccompanied pass should not be planned until the potential for suicide has been ruled out; an accompanied pass is a better action initially.

295. 1 **This statement provides clues that the client feels no one cares, so there is no reason the client should care. (2) (SE; CJ; AN)**
    2 The clues presented do not lead to this conclusion.
    3 Same as answer 2.
    4 Same as answer 2.

296. 4 **This is the correct description; the client had attained orgasm previously. (2) (PI; CJ; AN)**
    1 Libido is sexual desire; it usually does not influence physiologic response.
    2 This is a nonexistent term; it would be impossible to evaluate the quality of an orgasm.
    3 This defines the disorder whereby the female has never attained an orgasm.

297. 1 **Decreased sexual desire is a major symptom of clinical depression. (1) (PI; CJ; AN)**
    2 Although depression is often related to unmet dependency needs, decreased sexual desire is associated with the depression.
    3 The sexual difficulties are associated with the depression, and the depression may be the major cause of the marital stress.
    4 Role confusion, not identity confusion, is associated with the depression.

298. 4 **This recognizes feelings and behavior; it encourages the client to share feelings and promotes trust, which is essential for a therapeutic relationship. (2) (PI; CJ; IM)**
    1 Without verbal encouragement, the depressed client will not respond to this intervention.
    2 Although these are important actions, they are not enough; nursing intervention with the client must be included.
    3 This assumes too much and may be inaccurate; an indirect approach should be used.

299. 1 **A matter-of-fact approach helps avoid a cycle in which the nurse expresses concern to a client who feels unworthy, which increases feelings of unworthiness. (3) (PI; CJ; IM)**
   2 Citing a hospital policy focuses on rules and regulations, which may exacerbate the client's negative personal feelings because he is breaking the rules.
   3 This is a statement that the client may not be able to explain.
   4 This statement may increase feelings of unworthiness because it creates a gap between the nurse's estimate of the client and what the client feels.

300. 4 **As depression increases, thought processes become slower and verbal expression decreases due to lack of emotional energy. (2) (PI; CJ; AS)**
   1 The affect of a depressed person usually is one of sadness or it may be blank; elation is related to a bipolar disorder, manic episode.
   2 Loose associations are associated with schizophrenia, not depression.
   3 Decreased physical activity would not produce physical exhaustion; physical exhaustion is associated with a bipolar disorder, manic episode.

301. 2 **This response demonstrates empathy; in addition, it focuses on the client's feelings. (2) (PI; CJ; IM)**
   1 This can be answered by a "yes" or "no"; an open-ended response would allow for more self-expression.
   3 This response reflects only part of the content; it may be the least significant part of the client's statement.
   4 "Why" questions should be avoided because people often do not know why they feel or behave the way they do; this question may cause defensiveness.

302. 2 **During the manic phase of the illness, the client responds to everything in the environment; therefore, it is important that the room be quiet and restful to decrease stimulation. (2) (SE; CJ; PL)**
   1 This is not an important consideration at this time for this client.
   3 This room would be too stimulating because of its location.
   4 This would tend to increase both the client's and the roommate's behavioral acting out.

303. 3 **The client in a manic episode of the illness often neglects basic needs; these needs are a priority to ensure adequate nutrition, fluid, and rest. (3) (PB; CJ; PL)**

   1 Although the client needs to expend excess energy, physical exhaustion and dehydration are real possibilities during the manic episode of the illness.
   2 This would be counterproductive.
   4 The client is unable to actively participate in structured activities at this time.

304. 1 **Because the plan does not meet the client's needs, it should be changed. (3) (PI; MR; EV)**
   2 This nursing diagnosis should be changed based on more than one behavior.
   3 Continuing the plan will be frustrating for the client and the staff because the client's behavior indicates that snacks are not wanted.
   4 When the client's needs are not being met, the plan should be changed.

305. 1 **Structure tends to decrease agitation and anxiety and to increase the client's feelings of security. (1) (SE; CJ; PL)**
   2 Touching can be threatening for many clients and should not be used indiscriminately.
   3 Conversations should be kept simple; the client with a bipolar disorder, either depressed or manic phase, may have difficulty following involved conversations about current affairs.
   4 Clients with bipolar disorders are in contact with reality, so this activity would serve little purpose.

306. 4 **These individuals are acutely aware of others' feelings; perceived negative feelings may increase the client's hostility and inappropriate behavior. (2) (PI; CJ; PL)**
   1 If the nurse's feelings are negative, increasing the time spent with the client will exaggerate problems for both the nurse and the client.
   2 Placing the client in isolation may appear punitive rather than therapeutic.
   3 Ignoring the behavior toward the nurse may be beneficial; however, limits may need to be set to protect other clients' rights.

307. 4 **The client expends a great amount of energy running headlong into reality in an attempt to ward off or avoid facing feelings of depression. (3) (PI; CJ; AN)**
   1 The behavior is not an expression of innate desires but an attempt to avoid feelings of depression.
   2 This client is not attempting to compensate for an imagined loss but is trying to avoid feelings of depression.

3 The client has no difficulty relating to others; this behavior is an attempt to avoid feelings of depression.

308. **2 During the manic phase clients are unable to control their behavior and should be protected from embarrassing themselves or harming others. (2) (SE; CJ; IM)**

1 These clients are unable to deal with others' or their own feelings; the client's own feelings are primary at this time.

3 Behavior cannot be ignored because the client or others could be hurt if limits are not set.

4 This statement is critical of the client, who is unable to respond differently at this time.

309. **2 During a manic episode clients attempt to keep active to prevent the feeling of depression from overtaking them; avoidance of their feelings, not food, is their priority, and they do not take the time to eat. (2) (PI; CJ; AN)**

1 Feelings of grandeur have replaced unconscious feelings of unworthiness at this phase of the illness.

3 These clients would not be aware of unconscious feelings; the manic phase is not characterized by a desire for punishment.

4 Clients in the manic phase do not control anxiety by the use of ritualistic behavior; ritualistic behavior is common in clients with an obsessive-compulsive disorder.

310. **2 The excited, overactive client needs a calm environment; external stimulation serves to cause further excitation. (2) (SE; MR; IM)**

1 The client needs reduced, not increased, external stimulation.

3 Same as answer 1.

4 Same as answer 1.

311. **2 A firm voice is most effective; the statement tells the client that it is the behavior, not the client, that is upsetting to others. (2) (PI; CJ; IM)**

1 Demanding that the client stop the current behavior is a useless action; the client is out of control and needs external control.

3 The client does not know what is precipitating the behavior, and the question would be frustrating.

4 This should be done only when there is real danger from exhaustion; external controls must be set.

312. **1 These individuals are acutely aware of what is happening and react strongly to environmental stimuli. (2) (PI; CJ; AN)**

2 These clients are not out of contact with reality; in fact, they are continually reacting to it.

3 These clients' symptoms are an attempt to avoid anxiety and do not cause embarrassment.

4 These individuals are unable to control acting-out behavior.

313. **1 This response simply states a fact and delivers praise without making demands. (3) (PI; CJ; EV)**

2 This puts the total responsibility for control on a client who needs external controls set.

3 This does not help the client separate the self from the behavior; it tells the client that acting-out behavior will result in rejection.

4 The client may not recall what happened yesterday and would not be able to compare the differences.

314. **4 The client with hypomanic symptoms cannot tolerate sitting long enough to eat an adequate meal; handheld foods will help to meet the client's nutritional needs and do not require the client to sit down. (2) (PB; CJ; PL)**

1 This client will most likely ignore the tray.

2 Unworthy feelings are related to a depressive, not manic, episode.

3 It is unlikely that this client would understand or care about this information.

315. **1 Antidepressants can induce rapid cyclic behaviors; this statement elicits information in a nonchallenging, nonthreatening manner. (3) (PB; CJ; EV)**

2 This statement is challenging and is not focused on assessing the problem.

3 This statement would do little to promote discussion with this client.

4 This question is not focused on the symptoms manifested.

DISORDERS OF PERSONALITY (PR)

316. **1 Imagery is a therapeutic approach used to facilitate positive self-talk; mental pictures under the control of and initiated by the client may correct faulty cognitions. (3) (PI; CJ; AN)**

2 This is a useful general behavioral approach but is not a specific desensitization technique.

3 Same as answer 2.

4 These are useful general behavioral approaches but are not specific desensitization techniques.

317. 1 A discussion of the feared object will trigger an emotional response to the object. (2) (PI; CJ; AN)
2 Extreme fear would be more of a problem than anger.
3 Clients with phobias generally have rigid impulse control.
4 Distortion of reality related to daily routines usually is not a problem for a client with a phobia.

318. 3 Acting out is the process of expressing feelings behaviorally. (1) (PI; CJ; AN)
1 The action is not in conflict with the basic personality and is therefore not ego-dystonic.
2 The action is not exploitative, since no evidence is provided to demonstrate that anyone has been used to get what the client wants.
4 The action is not manipulative, since no evidence is provided to demonstrate that anyone has been influenced against his or her wishes.

319. 4 The client's expressed feelings are opposite and are an acceptable substitute for repressed antisocial feelings when facing the roommate. (2) (PI; CJ; AN)
1 The client's feelings are expressed to the nurse, not projected or attributed to others.
2 The client expressed real feelings to the nurse and made no attempt to make them socially acceptable.
3 The client's feelings for the roommate are not directed toward or displaced on any other person or object.

320. 3 The mother's behavior sends two conflicting messages; one says "I care" and the other says "I don't care"; this behavior is often demonstrated by people with personality disorders. (3) (PI; CJ; AS)
1 If the mother were rejecting the daughter, she would not have brought a gift.
2 No evidence of a projection of feelings is given.
4 Passive-aggressive behavior is an indirect, rather than direct, expression of angry or hostile feelings.

321. 4 This response demonstrates acceptance of the client and sets limits on the client's manipulative behavior. (3) (PI; CJ; IM)
1 This is false reassurance and it assists in the attempt to manipulate the ensuing staff members.
2 The nurse would be allowing further manipulation by the client by not leaving when the shift was over.

3 This is false reassurance; the nurse cannot make everything all right.

322. 1 Consistency, limit-setting, and supportive confrontation are essential nursing interventions to provide a secure, therapeutic environment for this client. (1) (PI; CJ; PL)
2 To be therapeutic the environment needs structure and the staff must assist the client to set short-term goals for behavioral changes.
3 The use of an authoritarian approach will increase anxiety in this type of client, resulting in feelings of rejection and withdrawal.
4 Ignoring the client's behavior would be nontherapeutic and would reinforce the client's underlying fears of abandonment.

323. 3 Sitting with the client indicates acceptance and demonstrates that the nurse feels the client is worthy of the nurse's time. (2) (PI; CJ; IM)
1 It would be better to stay with the client quietly until control is regained; staying prevents a follow-through on the client's threat.
2 This would have the effect of closing off further communication.
4 This would provide little comfort for the client.

324. 3 The withdrawn pattern of behavior prevents the individual from reaching out to others for sharing; the isolation produces feelings of loneliness. (2) (PI; CJ; AN)
1 Feelings of anger may result in withdrawal, but withdrawal does not produce feelings of anger.
2 Feelings of paranoia may result in withdrawal, but withdrawal does not produce these feelings.
4 Repression is an unconscious defense whereby the individual excludes ideas, feelings, or situations from the conscious level of thought; this is not the result of withdrawal.

325. 1 Withdrawal provides a temporary defense against anxiety because it limits contact with reality and decreases the client's world. (2) (PI; CJ; AN)
2 Withdrawal does not accomplish this because feelings and anxieties are still present and little attempt is made to work through problems.
3 Same as answer 2.
4 Same as answer 2.

326. 1 **If this goal is met, the client's relationship with others should improve in all aspects, including sexual, as self-esteem and self-confidence improve. (3) (PI; MR; PL)**
2 This goal is not appropriate at this time; examining these feelings would be nonproductive until the client's self-esteem improves.
3 Increasing insight may be helpful, but should not receive priority.
4 Increasing the client's knowledge of sexual functioning is important, but improving self-esteem should receive priority.

327. 4 **A conflict exists between wanting to be taken care of and wanting to be self-reliant; ambivalence fosters lowered self-esteem. (3) (PI; CJ; AN)**
1 These do not relate to the behavior described; people usually do not alternate these emotions, which are at opposite ends of the spectrum.
2 This is the developmental task of the infant, according to Erikson; it is not related to the behavior described.
3 This is the developmental task of the young adult, according to Erikson; it is not related to the behavior described.

328. 4 **In the early part of treatment, before new defenses are developed, enough time must be allowed for the client to complete the ritual to keep anxiety under control. (2) (PI; CJ; IM)**
1 The ritual is a defense that cannot be interrupted or delayed; it is used until new defenses are developed.
2 Same as answer 1.
3 Same as answer 1.

329. 1 **Ritualistic behavior seen in this disorder is aimed at controlling guilt and inadequacy by maintaining an absolute set pattern of action. (3) (PI; CJ; AN)**
2 Although the person with an obsessive-compulsive disorder may be angry and remorseful, the basic problem is usually guilt.
3 The behavior and attitudes of clients with this disorder are contradictory; they are conscientious about some things and lax about others.
4 Although the person with an obsessive-compulsive disorder may feel unworthy and hopeless, guilt is considered the basic problem.

330. 2 **This is the psychoanalytic explanation for the development of obsessive-compulsive symptomatology. (2) (PI; CJ; AN)**
1 Compulsive rituals commonly result in interference with activities of daily living and the individual becomes dysfunctional; rituals cannot be controlled.
3 This is not related to rituals but rather to phobias.
4 The client is unable to consciously stop the behavior because anxiety would become overwhelming if the defense were not used.

331. 2 **This limits the time and still allows the ritual; until the underlying cause of anxiety can be dealt with, rituals should be allowed as much as possible. (2) (PI; CJ; PL)**
1 This provides for only one time period and probably would result in increased anxiety.
3 One ritual cannot be substituted for another; this would interfere with the performance of the original ritual and could result in overwhelming anxiety.
4 This is the client's decision; the nurse should not recommend this action.

332. 2 **Paraphrasing encourages further ventilation by the client. (2) (PI; CJ; IM)**
1 This is a negative response that may increase the client's fears about being "crazy."
3 This response denies the client's feelings.
4 This provides false reassurance and implies that the client is out of control, which may increase fears.

333. 4 **Responding to the ritualistic behavior in a matter-of-fact way avoids reinforcing the behavior; allowing time for rituals avoids increasing the anxiety level. (2) (PI; CJ; IM)**
1 Attempts to speed up ritualistic behavior will increase the level of anxiety.
2 Disparaging the client will decrease self-esteem, increase anxiety and guilt, and may increase symptoms.
3 Attempts to discourage ritualistic behavior often increase anxiety levels and increase symptoms.

334. 2 **The rituals used by a client with obsessive-compulsive disorder help control the anxiety level by maintaining a set pattern of action. (2) (PI; CJ; AN)**
1 The client cannot consciously control the ritual.
3 Rituals are used primarily to handle feelings of anxiety and are generally seen by the client as illogical; they provide few secondary gains.
4 Rituals are used primarily to handle feelings of anxiety and are a means of diverting attention from these feelings.

335. 3 **This reflects a reenactment of the mother/child relationship; behavior vacillates between distancing to avoid engulfment and clinging to avoid being rejected. (3) (PI; CJ; AN)**

1 Shame often results from a struggle, but is not the focus of a conflicting fear.

2 Self-esteem and fear of hostility are outcomes, not the focus of a conflict.

4 Engulfment is part of the conflict, but interdependence is not a conflicting fear and may be a healthy balance of dependence and independence.

336. 1 **The expectation is communicated that before the medication is given the client must first try to sleep before indicating the need for it. (3) (PI; CJ; PL)**

2 No data are given to indicate that the client is out of touch with reality, nor would this be a form of reality testing.

3 No data are given to substantiate that the nurse is enforcing a rule to preserve the routine; in addition, it does not individualize care.

4 This is not an attempt to condition behavior; it merely communicates an expectation.

337. 4 **The client is angry and reacts impulsively; the action is unplanned and is not under the client's control. (2) (PI; CJ; AN)**

1 No data are provided to suggest that the client is out of contact with reality; the client is reacting to a real situation with anger.

2 There is no identifiable cluster of behaviors to suggest that the client has a violent personality.

3 There is no pattern of behavior to suggest an antisocial personality, which may or may not involve impulse control.

338. 2 **The client is unable to control impulses at this time, so controls must be provided for the client; the nurse's behavior provides a role model. (2) (PI; CJ; PL)**

1 The client is not able to establish self-controls; freedom could prove frightening to a client who is not in control.

3 This is nontherapeutic; this would probably provoke more acting-out behavior.

4 Same as answer 3.

339. 1 **The client's comments indicate a desire to escape from the situation by the use of a loosely conceived, poorly developed plan. (2) (PI; CJ; AS)**

2 There is nothing in the client's statement to indicate that this problem is occurring.

3 Same as answer 2.

4 Same as answer 2.

340. 1 **Both clients must be included in a discussion about this behavior to make certain that limits on future behavior are understood by both of them; this action also places controls on the manipulative behavior often used by clients with an antisocial personality disorder. (2) (SE; MR; PL)**

2 This action would cause the clients to find another place to meet; the response sets no limits on behavior but only addresses location.

3 This action would not set any limits on behavior and puts staff members in the policing role.

4 Although this may be necessary, the nurse must respond directly to the clients involved in this situation.

341. 4 **These would be the most therapeutic parental actions; the client must be made accountable for behavior and must know that manipulation and acting out will not be tolerated. (2) (SE; MR; PL)**

1 This would probably be a continuation of the parents' previous response to the client and would prove to be of little value.

2 This could cause the client to continue to act out to test the limit of the parents' endurance.

3 Same as answer 1.

342. 4 **This response confronts the client with the fact that the client has not been working on personal problems. (2) (PI; CJ; IM)**

1 This response is not confrontational but is sarcastic, judgmental, and attacking; this would tend to put the client on the defensive.

2 Same as answer 1.

3 This response requires insight from the client; insight would be uncommon with this client's diagnosis.

343. 2 **The nurse's response is not therapeutic because it does not recognize the client's needs but tries to make the client feel guilty for being demanding. (3) (PI; CJ; AN)**

1 Impulse control would refer to a sudden driving force being constrained or held back.

3 Nothing in the nurse's statement would achieve this; the nurse is defensive, not therapeutic.

4 Same as answer 3.

344. 2 **Private confrontation with reported facts provides for verification; a calm, direct manner is most assertive. (2) (PI; CJ; IM)**
 1 This action places control in the hands of the client rather than the nurse, which could lead to aggressive confrontation.
 3 This is aggressive confrontation, not assertive intervention.
 4 This is not assertive intervention; it is manipulation and is not truthful.

345. 4 **This client needs firm, realistic limits set on behavior; this statement permits the client to make the choice and clearly states the consequences of behavior. (2) (PI; CJ; IM)**
 1 Clients with this diagnosis do not learn from past errors.
 2 This client would care very little about rules.
 3 The client and visitors do not want to socialize with other clients and visitors.

346. 4 **The expression of feelings by this individual would demonstrate the development of some insight and a willingness to at least begin to look at underlying causes of behavior. (2) (PI; CJ; EV)**
 1 These words probably would have little meaning to the client.
 2 Same as answer 1.
 3 Same as answer 1.

347. 4 **A client with an antisocial personality disorder is charming on first contact; this charm is a manipulative ploy; these clients usually are bright and use their intelligence for self-gain. (2) (PI; CJ; AS)**
 1 This behavior more closely applies to an individual with an obsessive-compulsive personality disorder.
 2 The client with a borderline personality disorder self-mutilates when under stress; there is a fear of abandonment so that any relationship is better than no relationship.
 3 This resembles the behavior of an individual with a paranoid personality, which includes suspiciousness and lack of trust.

348. 2 **The client must recognize the existence of the subpersonalities so that interpretation can occur. (3) (PI; CJ; AN)**
 1 This is not relevant to clients with multiple personality disorders; this outcome relates to clients with obsessive-compulsive behaviors.
 3 This is not realistic; integration of the personalities generates fear and defensiveness in the client, and defense mechanisms will be used.

 4 This is inappropriate; anxiety serves as a motivator for behavioral change, and antianxiety medications must be used judiciously.

349. 4 **A multiple personality disorder is a complex, multifaceted problem that requires long-term therapy to achieve integration of the personalities. (3) (PI; CJ; EV)**
 1 None of the personalities can be ignored because their presence must be dealt with before integration can occur.
 2 If they did not serve a protective purpose, they would be abandoned.
 3 Each personality has the ability to deal openly with feelings and fears, but the personalities need to be integrated.

SCHIZOPHRENIC DISORDERS (SD)

350. 2 **Circumstantial thought process is noted when thoughts and speech are associated with excessive and unnecessary detail that is usually relevant to a question and an answer is ultimately given. (3) (PI; CJ; AS)**
 1 Flight of ideas is the overproductive speech characterized by rapid shifting from one topic to another with fragmentation of ideas.
 3 Tangential thoughts are similar to circumstantial thought processes but the person never answers the question or returns to the central point of the conversation.
 4 This is noted when there is a sudden stopping in the train of thought or in the middle of the sentence.

351. 3 **These clients are threatened by reality; withdrawal from reality and the use of magical thinking reduce anxiety. (2) (PI; CJ; AS)**
 1 Clients with schizophrenia are not preoccupied with suicidal thoughts.
 2 Clients with schizophrenia have low self-esteem and a low self-image and usually have feelings of guilt and self-blame.
 4 The loosening of associative links that occurs in schizophrenia makes these impossible.

352. 4 **A person with this disorder would not have adequate self-boundaries. (3) (PI; CJ; AS)**
 1 A weak ego is seen in a person with schizophrenia.
 2 Low self-esteem is associated with people with schizophrenia because they have inadequate ego defenses, lack of ego strengths, and distortions of reality.
 3 Concrete thinking is symptomatic of schizophrenia.

353. 4 Loose associations are thoughts that are presented without the logical connections usually necessary for the listener to interpret the message. (2) (PI; CJ; AS)
   1 Echolalia is the purposeless repetition of words spoken by others or repetition of overheard sounds.
   2 Neologisms are new meaningless words coined by the client, or new unique meanings given to old words.
   3 Flight of ideas is the rapid skipping from one thought to another; thoughts usually have only superficial or chance relationships.

354. 1 The presence of ego strengths is demonstrated by some level of adjustment before the occurrence of the precipitating event; these ego strengths can be used to help the client reorganize the personality. (1) (PI; CJ; AS)
   2 This would tend to contribute to a poor prognosis.
   3 Same as answer 2.
   4 Same as answer 2.

355. 1 An aloof, detached, withdrawn posture is a means of protecting the self by withdrawing and maintaining a safe, emotional distance. (3) (PI; CJ; AN)
   2 Withdrawal is not the usual response to fear of punishment.
   3 Fear of the unknown usually results in anxiety and panic, not withdrawal.
   4 Fear of powerlessness usually results in anger and aggression, not withdrawal.

356. 2 The usual age of onset of schizophrenia is adolescence or early adulthood. (2) (PI; CJ; AS)
   1 Symptoms usually do not appear this early.
   3 Same as answer 1.
   4 Same as answer 1.

357. 3 By observing the client, the nurse is able to adjust care and communications to reflect assessment of individual needs. (1) (PI; CJ; AS)
   1 This initially is not vital to help the client; the nurse should try to meet the client's needs at this point in time.
   2 Same as answer 1.
   4 Same as answer 1.

358. 3 Hallucinations are sensory experiences unrelated to external stimuli; they usually follow a client's thought processes. (1) (PI; CJ; PL)
   1 Hallucinating experiences are triggered by high levels of anxiety and usually follow the client's thought processes.

   2 Misinterpretations of environmental stimuli are illusions.
   4 Hallucinations are not always frightening; sometimes they are somewhat pleasurable.

359. 3 Neologisms are words that are invented and understood only by the person using them. (1) (PI; CJ; AN)
   1 Echolalia is the verbal repeating of exactly what is heard.
   2 Concretism is a pattern of speech characterized by the absence of abstractions or generalizations.
   4 Paleologic thinking is a disturbed system of logic in which subjects are made identical if two variables about them are the same.

360. 3 The client needs to feel comfortable in the environment before establishing enough trust to undress for showering; the nurse's statement allows the client to make the decision. (2) (PI; CJ; IM)
   1 This action would add to the client's anxiety and feelings of loss of control; it could also add to any delusional thoughts the client may have.
   2 Same as answer 1.
   4 This statement would not help the client's self-image, and it does not matter what other clients think.

361.
   1 _x_ **Bizarre behavior is associated with undifferentiated schizophrenia. (3) (PI; CJ; AS)**
   2 _____ Extreme negativism is associated with catatonic schizophrenia.
   3 _x_ **Disorganized speech is associated with undifferentiated schizophrenia.**
   4 _x_ **Vague hallucinations are associated with undifferentiated schizophrenia.**
   5 _____ Persecutory delusions are associated with paranoid schizophrenia.
   6 _____ Psychomotor retardation is associated with catatonic schizophrenia.

362. 3 A somatic delusion is a fixed false belief about one's body. (2) (PI; CJ; AN)
   1 Echolalia is the automatic and meaningless oral repetition of another's words or phrases.
   2 Hypochondriasis is a severe, morbid preoccupation with an unrealistic interpretation of real or imagined physical symptoms.
   4 Depersonalization is a feeling of unreality and alienation from oneself.

363. 1 This explores more fully the client's ideas, experiences, or relationships; this response promotes communication. (2) (PI; CJ; IM)

2 Arguing about delusions increases anxiety and diminishes trust.

3 This denies feelings and implies the client is wrong; it may cause the client to defend feelings further.

4 This puts the blame on the client and implies the feelings are based on reality.

364. 2 Failure to accept the client and the client's fears establishes a barrier to effective communication. (1) (PI; CJ; AN)

1 Today, mental health therapy is directed toward returning the client to the community as rapidly as possible.

3 Electroconvulsive therapy (ECT) is not the treatment of choice for clients with schizophrenia.

4 Family cooperation is helpful but not an absolute necessity.

365. 4 Command hallucinations are auditory hallucinations that give verbal messages to do harm either to the self or others; giving an identity to the hallucinated voice increases the risk of compliance. (3) (PI; CJ; AN)

1 A delusion is a false belief held to be true even with evidence to the contrary.

2 A somatic delusion is a belief that the body is changing in an unusual way.

3 There are no false hallucinations; a hallucination is always real to the client.

366. 3 These are classic behaviors exhibited by clients with a diagnosis of schizophrenia. (2) (PI; CJ; AS)

1 This behavior is more commonly associated with dementia, not schizophrenia.

2 This behavior is more commonly associated with bipolar disorder, manic phase, not schizophrenia.

4 This behavior is more commonly associated with depression, not schizophrenia.

367. 1 The client cannot reach out to others because of lack of trust; withdrawal is used to defend against interpersonal threats and results in isolation. (2) (PI; CJ; AN)

2 Most clients with schizophrenic disorders are not violent.

3 Sleep disturbances are not common because clients tend to use sleep to withdraw from reality.

4 This usually is not associated with this disorder.

368. 4 Any other approach would be threatening, increase anxiety, and probably result in a physical confrontation. (3) (PI; CJ; PL)

1 This would increase the client's anxiety and probably result in a physical confrontation.

2 This would increase anxiety, not foster decision making.

3 This would increase anxiety, not self-esteem.

369. 3 Helping the client to develop feelings of self-worth would reduce the client's need to use pathologic defenses. (2) (PI; CJ; PL)

1 Faith or the lack of faith is not the basic underlying problem but merely a symptom of it.

2 Self-control or the lack of self-control is not the basic underlying problem but merely a symptom of it.

4 Insight can develop only when the need to use the defense is reduced.

370. 3 Using the defense mechanism of projection, the client is attributing to others those personal feelings that are objectionable to the self. (2) (PI; CJ; AN)

1 No evidence is given to support an interpretation that redirection is being used.

2 There is no evidence to support this interpretation.

4 The client is not exploring emotionally charged reactions.

371. 2 This response accepts the client at the client's present level and, in addition, allows the client to set the pace of the relationship. (3) (PI; CJ; IM)

1 This approach to any client can be misinterpreted and may precipitate an aggressive response.

3 This response asks the client to reach out to the nurse; in the therapeutic relationship the nurse must reach out to the client.

4 Even if the client is too withdrawn to respond, the nurse's physical presence can be reassuring.

372. 1 This is a declarative statement that adheres to the treatment plan; it presents the attitude that the client is expected to go for the walk and does not require the client to make a decision that may be impossible to make at this time. (3) (PI; MR; IM)

2 This requires a decision that the client may or may not be able to make.

3 This requires a decision that the client may or may not be able to make; also, the client may say no.

4 This is an accusatory statement that could jeopardize the nurse-client relationship.

373. 3 Participating with one trusted individual gradually diminishes the need for withdrawal. (2) (PI; CJ; PL)
1 This would not increase socialization but rather would promote withdrawal.
2 This activity fosters competition, which would not be helpful at this time.
4 Same as answer 1.

374. 1 This statement lets the client know the nurse sees her as a person and is willing to help her face a new experience. (2) (PI; CJ; IM)
2 This will do nothing to allay the client's anxiety about facing a new situation.
3 This is untrue; even if the client does not like it, as part of the therapy program, she should be encouraged to go.
4 Same as answer 2.

375. 4 Providing opportunities to experience success in activities enhances coping abilities. (2) (PI; CJ; PL)
1 This reinforces disturbed coping skills.
2 A change in activities, not the level of stimuli, is what causes stress for this client.
3 Success with tasks, not intellectual activities, enhances coping skills.

376. 4 This is very helpful in decreasing hallucinations because it provides another stimulus to compete for the client's attention. (2) (PI; CJ; PL)
1 This would foster and support the hallucinations.
2 Same as answer 1.
3 Connections should be made to decrease the use of hallucinations.

377. 3 To function interpersonally with a group, these individuals must first develop a trusting one-to-one relationship. (2) (PI; CJ; PL)
1 These individuals need interaction to increase trust; they will not seek interactions without encouragement.
2 If forced, these individuals will be too fearful of the group to function in it or benefit by it.
4 Dependency could have an adverse effect on individuals with schizophrenia.

378. 2 The delusional system contains grandiose ideation that allows the client to feel important rather than inferior. (2) (PI; CJ; AN)
1 Although these individuals often feel guilty, feelings of inferiority, not guilt, precipitate delusions.
3 These individuals usually are able to express aggressive feelings without difficulty.

4 Delusions of persecution are not usually present in clients with undifferentiated schizophrenia.

379. 4 Psychoeducation should center around symptom management and techniques for dealing with hallucinations to empower the client as one of the keys to preventing relapse; this involves identifying symptom triggers and strategies for management. (3) (PI; MR; EV)
1 This type of delusion is not characteristic of clients experiencing undifferentiated schizophrenia; this delusion would be noted in clients with paranoid schizophrenia.
2 This action is expected in the acute phase when client safety is of the greatest concern; this is a short-term, not long-term, goal.
3 Although this would be ideal, a relapse is likely to occur whether or not medication compliance occurs, particularly if the client has inadequate health practices and an unreliable support system.

380. 4 The client truly believes the voices are real because the voices reflect the client's thoughts; the voices are usually accusatory and derogatory and therefore very frightening. (2) (PI; CJ; IM)
1 Playing soft music after hallucinations have started will not be strong enough to compete for the client's attention.
2 This would be too late; competing stimuli must be present to block the occurrence.
3 This is incorrect; the client cannot be talked out of a hallucination.

381. 4 This helps the client explore underlying feelings and allows the client to understand the message the verbalizations are communicating. (3) (PI; CJ; IM)
1 This denies the client's feelings rather than accepting and working with them.
2 Attempting to divert the client denies feelings rather than accepting and working with them.
3 This focuses on the delusion itself rather than the feeling causing the delusion.

382. 1 This response accepts the client's behavior (desires) but lets the client know the nurse is not going to give up attempts to establish a relationship. (2) (PI; CJ; IM)
2 This response requests insight that the client does not have at this point.
3 This does not respect the client's wish for space at the present time.

4 This response on an initial encounter does not show respect for the client's space and is inappropriately interpreted.

383. **2 Attempting to approach the client in a nonthreatening manner and using a calm, consistent, nonviolent approach often helps the agitated client to gain more self-control. (2) (PI; CJ; IM)**
1 This action would increase, not decrease, agitation.
3 Action should not be postponed; escalation must be prevented.
4 This is premature; medication should not be used before trying to verbally calm the client.

384. **2 Ambivalence makes decision making difficult if not impossible; simple, easy-to-follow declarative statements limit the choices available for the indecisive client. (2) (PI; CJ; IM)**
1 The client would be unable to interpret nonverbal communication and would experience increased confusion and indecision.
3 This is inappropriate because the pressure to make choices may increase the client's ambivalence and discomfort.
4 Same as answer 3.

385. **1 This response reflects the client's feelings and avoids focusing on the delusion. (2) (PI; CJ; IM)**
2 This will not change the client's feelings because the other pitcher could also be perceived as poisoned.
3 This will not change the client's feelings because the belief is real to the client.
4 This will not change the client's feelings; the client would believe that the nurse was not really drinking the juice.

386. **4 This approach gives the client and family an opportunity to discuss their feelings together and clarifies their expectations. (2) (SE; MR; IM)**
1 This is the nurse's responsibility and should not be passed to someone else.
2 This is not the nurse's role; the family may never be reassured.
3 This would do little to reassure the family.

387. **1 The fetal position represents regressed behavior; regression is a way of responding to overwhelming anxiety. (1) (PI; CJ; EV)**
2 This interpretation assumes that the nurse controls the client's behavior; the client is not responding to the nurse any differently than to anyone else who tries to establish reality contact.

3 There are no data to substantiate this; further assessment is necessary to make this interpretation.
4 Same as answer 3.

388. **2 This allows the client to work off energy without upsetting other clients. (1) (PI; CJ; IM)**
1 This causes isolation and should be used only as a last resort if the client presents an actual danger to himself or others.
3 The client's present emotional state would limit concentration and prevent interaction with others.
4 Same as answer 3.

389. **3 This provides a stimulus that competes with and reduces hallucinations. (2) (PI; CJ; IM)**
1 This is a direct question that the client probably could not answer; it would also increase anxiety.
2 If the nurse waits for the client to stop hallucinating, there may be no chance for contact with this client.
4 In addition to setting unrealistic standards, this response fails to recognize that the client believes the hallucinations are real.

390. **1 By realistically rewarding the healthy behaviors, the nurse provides secondary gains and encourages their continued use. (1) (PI; CJ; PL)**
2 This would be important but would do little to increase the client's self-esteem.
3 Same as answer 2.
4 Same as answer 2.

391. **4 This response validates the presence of the client's hallucinations without agreeing with them, which communicates acceptance, and can form a foundation for trust; it may help the client return to reality. (3) (PI; CJ; IM)**
1 This would be inappropriate because the client's contact with reality is too tenuous to explore this kind of analysis.
2 This response demeans the client, which blocks a trusting relationship and future communication.
3 This meets the staff members' needs, not the client's needs; this response is condescending and impairs future communication.

392. **2 Auditory hallucinations are most troublesome when environmental stimuli are diminished and there are few competing distractions. (1) (PI; CJ; AN)**
1 This is a time of relatively high, competing environmental stimuli.
3 Same as answer 1.
4 Same as answer 1.

393. 3 **The state in which the client feels unreal or believes that parts of the body are distorted is known as depersonalization or loss of personal identity. (1) (PI; CJ; AN)**
  1 This is not an example of an hallucination; an hallucination is a sensory experience for which there is no external stimulus.
  2 The client's statement does not indicate any feelings that others are out to do harm, are responsible for what is happening, or are in control of the situation.
  4 The statement is not an example of autistic verbalization.

394. 1 **Clients with schizophrenia, paranoid type, usually become very anxious in social situations; the other client's closeness may have triggered latent homosexual feelings. (2) (PI; CJ; AN)**
  2 This is an invalid interpretation given the data presented.
  3 Same as answer 2.
  4 Same as answer 2.

395. 3 **Clients must be helped to develop insight into their behavior before the behavior can be altered; insight is an essential part of treatment. (1) (PI; CJ; PL)**
  1 This is false reassurance.
  2 Deciding on and directing activities for the client are self-defeating and may precipitate aggression.
  4 This is not therapeutic and does not assist the client to develop insight.

396. 3 **This statement depicts the cognitive disturbance called a delusion, which is a fixed set of false beliefs that cannot be corrected by reason. (2) (PI; CJ; AN)**
  1 An illusion is a misperception of an actual environmental stimulus.
  2 An hallucination is a sensory experience, unrelated to external stimuli.
  4 Neologisms are made-up words understood only by the maker.

397. 1 **Projection is a mechanism in which inner thoughts and feelings are projected onto the environment, seeming to come from outside the self rather than from within. (2) (PI; CJ; AN)**
  2 Regression is the use of a behavioral characteristic appropriate to an earlier level of development.
  3 Repression is the involuntary exclusion of painful or conflicting thoughts from awareness.

  4 Identification is the taking on of the thoughts and mannerisms of an individual who is admired or idealized.

398. 4 **This statement recognizes the client's feelings and points out reality. (3) (PI; CJ; IM)**
  1 This response is inappropriate because it reinforces the client's delusional system.
  2 Although this is an empathic response, it does not point out reality; the word "trick" does not have the same connotation as "do me in."
  3 This does not recognize feelings and places the client on the defensive.

399. 3 **The client is fearful and suspicious; the feeling of being in a powerful position helps the client deal with anxiety. (2) (PI; CJ; AN)**
  1 The client is not out of touch with self-identity; the real identity has been given an important role.
  2 This is incorrect; the client is compensating for feelings of inadequacy.
  4 Same as answer 2.

400. 1 **Clients use a structured delusional system to justify and compensate for their feelings of worthlessness and low self-esteem. (2) (PI; CJ; AN)**
  2 Clients experiencing delusions of a paranoid nature are isolated and need contact with people to increase their contact with reality.
  3 This is not the purpose of the delusional system.
  4 There are no data to indicate this client is not accepted by others.

401. 4 **This will help the client develop self-esteem and reduce the use of paranoid ideation. (2) (PI; CJ; AN)**
  1 Because people must function in a social environment, it is almost impossible to avoid placing some demands on others.
  2 It is impossible to remove all stress in the environment.
  3 This could succeed in supporting the client's ideas of persecution and will lower the client's self-esteem.

402. 2 **Thoughts of being pursued by some powerful agent or agents because of one's special attributes or powers are fixed false beliefs and referred to as delusions of grandeur. (3) (PI; CJ; AN)**
  1 There is no evidence to indicate that a delusion of total or partial nonexistence is being used.

3 There is no evidence to indicate that a sensory-perceptual disturbance is present.

4 Delusions of grandeur are usually used to deny unconscious feelings of low self-esteem.

403. 3 **The client's verbalization reflects feelings that others are blaming the client for negative actions. (1) (PI; CJ; AN)**

1 There are no data that demonstrate the client has feelings of greatness or power.

2 There are no data that demonstrate the client is experiencing confusing misinterpretations of stimuli.

4 There are no data that demonstrate the client is hearing voices at this time.

404. 3 **These clients are hypersensitive to external stimuli and respond with less anxiety to a minimally threatening environment. (2) (PI; CJ; PL)**

1 This is too threatening an approach and interferes with the goals of therapy.

2 This is not therapeutic and limiting; it would tend to trigger suspiciousness and hostile outbursts.

4 Focusing on delusional material tends to reinforce the delusional system.

405. 3 **The recommended approach for working with suspicious clients is to allow them to set the pace for the relationship. (3) (PI; CJ; PL)**

1 This would be threatening and add to feelings of paranoia.

2 Same as answer 1.

4 Same as answer 1.

406. 2 **Activities that require limited interpersonal contact are less threatening. (3) (PI; CJ; PL)**

1 Group activities require interaction with other people, which is threatening to individuals with paranoid feelings.

3 Same as answer 1.

4 Individuals with schizophrenia, paranoid type, usually do not respond to an authoritarian approach because they do not trust others, particularly those who act in an aggressive manner.

407. 3 **Clients with paranoia often feel safer selecting foods from a cafeteria-type display that is prepared for the general population rather than eating from a tray specifically prepared for them. (3) (PI; CJ; IM)**

1 This would not provide security because part of the food could still be poisoned.

2 Same as answer 1.

4 Same as answer 1.

408. 4 **This approach sets limits and provides support; hallucinations can be frightening and the nurse's presence provides support while not actually focusing on the hallucination. (2) (PI; CJ; IM)**

1 This is nontherapeutic because it does not recognize the client's need for support and direction.

2 Same as answer 1.

3 This approach is nontherapeutic; it makes a judgment with insufficient evidence and focuses on the hallucination; it fails to recognize the client's need for support and direction.

SUBSTANCE ABUSE (SA)

409. 3 **Parental loss or separation has an association with the onset of addiction because initially the drugs are used to relieve anxiety or unpleasant feelings or to sustain a pleasant existence outside the realm of reality. (3) (PI; CJ; AN)**

1 Curiosity may be a factor in experimenting with drugs, but not abusing them.

2 Depression would have to be more than occasional, in addition to other contributing factors.

4 The period of adolescence alone would not place a person in a high-risk category for substance abuse.

410. 4 **Because of cross-tolerance the client may need large doses of analgesia for pain relief. (1) (PI; CJ; IM)**

1 Confronting the client is not the nurse's responsibility at this time.

2 The nurse should serve as a role model to raise the client to a more acceptable level of behavior.

3 The client must be helped to recognize that a problem with drugs exists.

411. 1 **Denial is a method of resolving conflict or escaping unpleasant realities by ignoring their existence. (1) (PI; CJ; AN)**

2 With projection the person faults another person for having unacceptable impulses, thoughts, or behaviors that are too uncomfortable to accept as one's own.

3 With displacement the person transfers an emotion from one object, person, or situation to another, usually safer, object, person, or situation.

4 With compensation the person makes up for personal inadequacies by emphasizing attributes to gain social approval.

412. **4 The attempt to justify a behavior by giving it acceptable motives is an example of rationalization. (2) (PI; CJ; AN)**
1 Sublimation is the substitution of a socially acceptable behavior for one that is less acceptable.
2 Suppression is the intentional excluding of things, people, feelings, or events from consciousness.
3 Compensation is the attempt to emphasize a characteristic viewed as an asset to make up for a real or imagined deficiency.

413. **4 Alcohol is a central nervous system depressant; these symptoms are the body's neurologic adaptation to the withdrawal of alcohol. (2) (PB; CJ; AS)**
1 Convulsions are not early signs of alcohol withdrawal; they would not occur before 48 to 72 hours of abstinence.
2 Fever and diaphoresis may be seen during prolonged periods of delirium and are a result of autonomic overactivity.
3 These are late signs of severe withdrawal that occur with delirium tremens; tachycardia results from autonomic overactivity.

414. **1 The nurse should remove the substance before the client has an opportunity to consume more alcohol. (3) (PI; CJ; IM)**
2 The primary concern is not where the alcohol was obtained, but protecting the client from consuming more.
3 Making the client feel guilty can increase the desire for more alcohol.
4 The client may drink the remaining alcohol while the nurse notifies the physician.

415. **2 Motivation is necessary to assist the client in withstanding the pain of giving up a defense; motivation is more influential in facilitating change than any external factor. (2) (PI; CJ; AN)**
1 Although having family support is important, motivation to change is the most important factor.
3 This can be of assistance, but internal factors will have a greater impact on rehabilitation than will external factors.
4 Self-esteem will be useful if it precipitates abstinence behavior; however, people who are alcoholics commonly have low self-esteem.

416. **2 Clients with this disorder have a loss of memory and adapt to this by filling in areas that cannot be remembered with false information. (3) (PI; CJ; AN)**

1 This does not occur with this type of dementia.
3 This is not attention-seeking behavior; the individual is not aware of the confabulation.
4 These people are not coping with the diagnosis; when confabulating, the individual believes that everything that is said is accurate and truthful.

417. **4 This disorder is caused by a prolonged deficiency of vitamin B$_1$ (thiamine) and the direct toxic effect of alcohol on brain tissue. (2) (PI; CJ; PL)**
1 This is unrelated to substance-induced persisting dementia caused by alcoholism.
2 Same as answer 1.
3 Same as answer 1.

418. **4 This behavior indicates that the client lacks insight and is denying that alcohol is the problem. (1) (PI; CJ; AN)**
1 There are no data to support this conclusion.
2 Same as answer 1.
3 Same as answer 1.

419. **3 Delirium tremens, a life-threatening CNS response to alcohol withdrawal, occurs in 1 to 3 days when blood alcohol levels drop as alcohol is detoxified and excreted. (2) (PB; CJ; PL)**
1 Jitteriness, nervousness, and insomnia may occur at this time; these are not life threatening.
2 Nervousness, insomnia, nausea, vomiting, and increased BP and pulse may occur at this time; these are not life threatening.
4 Withdrawal symptoms will begin to subside at this time; the risk for complications is diminished.

420. **1 This response forces the client to face what going to AA means to the client. (3) (PI; CJ; IM)**
2 This focuses the client on negative aspects; also, the client may be unable to answer.
3 This reinforces avoidance; the client may never feel like going; it avoids dealing with the client's problem.
4 Although this is true, it does not explore the client's feelings; the nurse should try to identify why the client does not want to go.

421. **3 The central nervous system is affected by the abrupt withdrawal of alcohol intake resulting in**

the classic responses indicated; they occur within a week after the cessation or reduction of alcohol intake. (2) (PI; CJ; EV)

1 The information presented does not demonstrate the presence of impaired short-term or long-term memory.

2 The information presented does not demonstrate the presence of auditory hallucinations; these usually develop within 48 hours of cessation or reduction of alcohol intake.

4 There are insufficient data to identify dementia; impairment of thought processes, judgment, and intellectual abilities would have to continue for 3 weeks or longer.

422. 3 **To maintain sobriety, alcoholics must forever totally alter patterns of behavior that have been reinforced and used for prolonged periods of time. (2) (PI; CJ; AN)**

1 Although drinking helps to reduce the pain of reality, it does not make the abuser feel good.

2 There is no known physiologic need for alcohol.

4 Alcoholics do not have character defects; drinking helps to blunt the pain of reality.

423. 1 **Clients who abuse alcohol characteristically have lowered self-esteem; therefore, it is important for the nurse to accept the person as an individual with value. (1) (PI; CJ; PL)**

2 Although nurturing is important, this client must learn self-reliance.

3 This probably would be an old story to this client and would have little positive effect.

4 This action would not provide an atmosphere that would help the client withstand the stress of the detoxification program.

424. 4 **The client must learn to develop and use more healthful coping mechanisms if drinking is to be stopped; the responsibility is with the client because the client must do the changing. (2) (PI; MR; PL)**

1 This would tell the client what to expect but would not instill responsibility for change.

2 This will increase guilt and place the client on the defensive; it usually does not foster the development of a trusting relationship.

3 Medications do not provide the motivation for change; this must come from within the client.

425. 1 **This statement recognizes the feeling of ambivalence associated with admitting that a problem with alcohol exists; this occurs early in treatment. (2) (PI; CJ; IM)**

2 This places the client on the defensive and interferes with communication.

3 Same as answer 2.

4 Same as answer 2.

426. 3 **This focuses on the client's feelings with a supportive, helpful approach. (2) (PI; CJ; IM)**

1 This is a judgmental approach that alienates the client from the therapeutic process and prevents the establishment of rapport.

2 Same as answer 1.

4 This intervention reinforces the client's denial and avoidance of the problem.

427. 3 **This strengthens the client's link with reality and reassures the client of safety because the hallucinations are usually frightening. (2) (PI; CJ; IM)**

1 The nurse must respond to the client's behavior by attempting to point out reality and reduce anxiety.

2 Validation reinforces the client's distorted perceptions of reality, is not helpful, and may be unsafe.

4 It is not helpful to argue or try to explain the hallucinations away because they are real to the client.

428. 3 **Peripheral neuropathy is present, and this measure will limit tactile stimulation. (2) (PB; CJ; IM)**

1 This would do little to relieve discomfort or reduce the occurrence of neurologic symptoms.

2 Same as answer 1.

4 This may be done periodically; however, these symptoms are not caused by impaired circulation but rather by peripheral neuropathy.

429. 1 **This supports the family of the addicted individual and allows the family to continue on with life by reducing guilt. (2) (SE; CJ; IM)**

2 The family has already stated that this is impossible when drinking occurs.

3 This places the burden for preventing drinking on the family and will create feelings of resentment and guilt.

4 This is enabling behavior, which does not help the abuser or the family.

430. 3 Withdrawal from central nervous system depressants is associated with more severe morbidity and mortality; adaptations begin with anxiety, shakiness, and insomnia; within 24 hours convulsions, delirium, tachycardia, and death can occur. (3) (PI; CJ; AN)

1 Withdrawal from this substance is rarely life threatening, but it does cause severe discomfort such as abdominal cramping and diarrhea.

2 Same as answer 1.

4 Amphetamine withdrawal is not life threatening, but it causes severe exhaustion and depression.

431. 3 A person with an addictive personality is unable to adequately deal with reality; drugs help to blur reality and reduce frustrations. (3) (PI; CJ; PL)

1 It is possible, but not easy; it requires a change in attitude and a deconditioning process.

2 Users of drugs are concerned with reality and their drug use is an attempt to blur the pains of reality.

4 Intellectually people may be aware of the dangers of drug addiction but emotionally cannot buy into the reality that it could happen to them.

432. 2 The loss of appetite and increased metabolic rate associated with cocaine addiction both promote weight loss. (2) (PI; CJ; AS)

1 This behavior is associated with barbiturate addiction.

3 This behavior is associated with alcohol addiction.

4 Same as answer 1.

433. 3 There is no set of symptoms associated with cocaine withdrawal, only the depression that follows the high caused by the drug. (2) (PI; CJ; AS)

1 This is more commonly associated with alcohol or amphetamine withdrawal.

2 This is commonly associated with alcohol withdrawal.

4 This is more commonly associated with withdrawal from opiates or antianxiety drugs.

434. 3 Cocaine is a chemical that, when inhaled, causes destruction of the mucous membranes of the nose. (1) (PI; CJ; AN)

1 This problem is associated with alcoholic cirrhosis.

2 These problems are associated with typical antipsychotic medications.

4 These problems are associated with alcoholic cirrhosis and are related to malnutrition, dehydration, and ascites.

435. 3 These adaptations are associated with opiate withdrawal, which occurs after cessation or reduction of prolonged moderate or heavy use of opiates. (2) (PB; CJ; AS)

1 Lacrimation and vomiting are present, but insomnia, not drowsiness, occurs with opiate withdrawal.

2 Nausea is present, but diarrhea, not constipation, and constricted pupils, rather than dilated pupils, occur with opiate withdrawal.

4 Rhinorrhea is present, but fever, rather than a subnormal temperature, and muscle aches, rather than convulsions, occur with opiate withdrawal.

436. 3 The client is unconscious and unable to meet physical needs; a patent airway, breathing, and circulation are essential needs. (2) (PB; CJ; PL)

1 Support and understanding are important once the client's physical condition has stabilized.

2 Maintaining a drug-free environment will be a priority later in the treatment program.

4 Establishing a therapeutic relationship will increase in importance once the client's physical condition has stabilized.

437. 1 Opiates cause central nervous system depression, resulting in severe respiratory depression, hypotension, and unconsciousness. (2) (PB; CJ; AS)

2 These findings, particularly the respirations, are not indicative of an overdose of an opiate.

3 Same as answer 2.

4 Same as answer 2.

438. 3 Addicted individuals often use a substance to increase their feelings of worth; the substance helps them appear bigger in their own eyes; they have strong unmet dependency needs. (2) (PI; CJ; AN)

1 Although guilt about breaking society's code may be present, there is no rejection of reality, just an inability to deal with it.

2 Although there is a need for acceptance, there is no underlying feeling of hostility.

4 Although anger is present and internalized, there is no struggle for independence.

439. 3 Individuals often take drugs because they cannot deal with the pain of reality; the drug blurs the pain. (1) (PI; CJ; AN)

1 Drugs increase dependency rather than foster independence.

2 Although this factor may encourage initial use by some adolescents, it is not the most common reason for use.

4 The use of drugs fosters social isolation rather than social relationships.

440. **2 Stimulating the central nervous system with cocaine most commonly causes these responses, which can progress to fear, hallucinations, paranoid delusions, and violent behavior. (2) (PB; CJ; AS)**

1 Nausea is not a side effect; euphoria, rather than fatigue, and loss of appetite, rather than hunger, are side effects.

3 These are not common side effects.

4 An increase in energy, rather than lethargy, occurs; some cocaine users believe it maximizes sexual experiences, but there is no documentation of this physiologic response.

441. **1 Tolerance is a phenomenon that occurs in addicted individuals and increases the amount of drug needed to satisfy their need; the client should receive adequate analgesia postoperatively. (1) (PB; CJ; AN)**

2 The problem is not related to dependence and addiction; the failure to respond to an adult dose of an opiate is related to tolerance.

3 Same as answer 2.

4 Same as answer 2.

442. **1 This allows the individual to use staff members as a support system and removes an opportunity to deny the problem. (3) (SE; MR; PL)**

2 This supports and permits denial; both the individual and the staff know a problem exists, and the individual must deal with it.

3 This is a nonprofessional approach that would be nontherapeutic.

4 Although this may be part of a return-to-work contract, it is not necessarily therapeutic; it simply reduces legal risks.

443. **4 This is a nonpunitive approach that attempts to help the nurse as an individual and as a professional. (2) (SE; MR; IM)**

1 This may be necessary for long-term therapy but would not be the initial approach.

2 This is a punitive, nontherapeutic response that offers no chance for rehabilitation.

3 The client has an addiction problem; promises will not keep the client from abusing drugs.

444. **4 This is a serious charge, and confrontation should occur in the presence of a supervisor. (3) (SE; MR; IM)**

1 This is unnecessary; as a professional, the nurse manager has enough information to confront the other nurse.

2 This is not a professional approach; the nurse manager has a legal responsibility to intervene.

3 This is an assumption that may result in an altercation; a witness should be present.

445. **1 The client is using denial to separate from the group members and needs realistic feedback to prevent withdrawal. (3) (SE; MR; IM)**

2 This would not help the client to become involved with the group.

3 This is inadequate; the client first needs to recognize that the problems being discussed are applicable.

4 The client's meaning is clear; questioning the client at this point would be nontherapeutic.

446. **1 The history of the loss of a child and the intensity of the client's drinking since the child's death should lead to this nursing diagnosis. (3) (PI; CJ; AN)**

2 There is no documentation that the family has not attempted to provide support; it is the family who has brought the client for help.

3 This is a medical, not nursing, diagnosis.

4 There is no documentation that the client is unable to distinguish between the self and nonself.

447. **3 These provide high levels of thiamine; other sources include legumes, whole and enriched grains, and lean beef. (2) (PB; CJ; EV)**

1 In this list, only fish is considered a source of thiamine.

2 In this list, only eggs are considered a source of thiamine; this list contains sources of protein.

4 Most vegetables contain only traces of thiamine; citrus fruits provide vitamin C.

448. **3 Although unclear, alcoholic blackouts appear to result from adaptations that central nervous system cells have made to the substance. (3) (PB; CJ; AN)**

1 The individual does not have any type of seizure during the blackout.

2 Fainting is not associated with the blackout.

4 The individual loses memory but not consciousness.

449. 3 The client is still denying the illness and has not resolved the basic problem that led to the alcoholism. (2) (PI; CJ; EV)

1 This is incorrect because the client is still denying the illness; willpower alone will not keep the client away from alcohol.

2 This may be true, but it does not ensure compliance or successful rehabilitation.

4 This is not helpful unless the client understands the basis of the conflicts and how to resolve them.

DRUG-RELATED RESPONSES (DR)

450. 3 Methylphenidate (Ritalin), a stimulant, has an opposite effect on hyperactive children; this action is as yet totally unexplained. (3) (PI; CJ; AN)

1 Ritalin does not have this effect.

2 Same as answer 1.

4 Although Ritalin has a hypotensive effect, this is not why it is given to hyperactive children.

451. 1 Alprazolam (Xanax), a benzodiazepam, potentiates the actions of GABA, enhances presympathetic inhibition, and inhibits spinal polysynaptic afferent pathways; drowsiness, dizziness, and blurred vision are common side effects. (3) (PB; CJ; EV)

2 Xanax may cause tachycardia, not bradycardia.

3 Agranulocytosis usually is a side effect of the antipsychotics in the phenothiazine group.

4 This occurs after prolonged therapy with antipsychotic medications; Xanax is an antianxiety medication, not an antipsychotic.

452. 2 Hypotension is a major side effect of alprazolam (Xanax) that occurs early in therapy; (1) (PB; CJ; EV)

1 An alteration in urinary output is not a common side effect; retention may occur after prolonged use.

3 This is not a common side effect; distention from constipation may occur after prolonged use.

4 Blurred vision, not dilated pupils, would occur more commonly; dilated pupils due to CNS depression is not a common side effect, although it may occur with overdose or prolonged use.

453. 4 Psychoactive drugs have been shown to be capable of interrupting the acute psychiatric process, making the client more amenable to other therapies. (1) (PB; MR; AN)

1 ECT is effective in treating depressed clients.

2 Family therapy is effective but is a long-term, costly therapy; symptoms must be reduced before the client can participate.

3 Clients with schizophrenia usually have little insight into their problems; confronting the client through insight therapy would increase anxiety.

454. 2 The duration of effect is 12 to 24 hours compared to other opiates, which have a 3 to 6 hour duration of effect. (2) (PI; MR; IM)

1 It is just as addictive but controls addiction and keeps the client out of the illicit drug market.

3 Methadone does have a cumulative effect in the body.

4 The physical as well as the psychologic dependence is high, just as in other opiates.

455. 2 A hypotensive reaction can be a common adverse effect of chlorpromazine; vital signs should be assessed before and after each dose. (2) (PB; CJ; AS)

1 Restraints of any type may increase the client's anxiety and result in struggling and increased agitation.

3 Photosensitivity occurs most commonly when clients are taking large doses and are spending time outdoors in the sun.

4 Tardive dyskinesia usually results from prolonged large doses of phenothiazines in susceptible clients.

456. 1 Akathisia, a side effect of haloperidol (Haldol), develops early in therapy and is characterized by restlessness and agitation. (2) (PB; CJ; EV)

2 Torticollis is characterized by a stiff neck and is not a side effect of this drug.

3 Tardive dyskinesia is characterized by gross involuntary movements of the extremities, tongue, and facial muscles that develop after prolonged therapy.

4 Pseudoparkinsonism is characterized by motor retardation, rigidity, and tremors; the reaction resembles Parkinson's syndrome but usually responds to medications or stopping the haloperidol.

457. 4 Lorazepam potentiates the actions of GABA, which reduces the anxiety and irritability associated with withdrawal. (3) (PB; CJ; AN)

1 This drug helps to reduce the risk of seizures but does not prevent physical injury if a seizure occurs.

2 Although these benefits may occur, they are not the primary objective for using the drug.

3 The ability of the client to accept treatment depends on readiness to accept the reality of the problem.

458. **4 Lithium's therapeutic window is very narrow, and toxic levels could occur unless there is routine monitoring of the blood's drug level; during the acute phase of mania the therapeutic blood level of lithium should be between 1.0 to 1.5 mEq/L; maintenance therapeutic blood levels of lithium should be between 0.5 to 1.2 mEq/L. (2) (PB; MR; PL)**

1 A low-sodium diet can lead to hyponatremia, which must be avoided because it limits the excretion of lithium resulting in toxicity.

2 This may or may not be true.

3 Diuretics reduce sodium and should be avoided; lithium is not excreted when sodium levels are decreased resulting in toxicity.

459. **4 Lithium concentration is most stable at this time; absorption and excretion occurs 8 to 12 hours after the last dose. (3) (PB; CJ; PL)**

1 Absorption and excretion rates vary; concentrations may be falsely higher at this time affecting the reliability of the readings.

2 Same as answer 1.

3 Same as answer 1.

460.

1 __x__ **Genitourinary side effects of Paxil include ejaculatory disorders, male genital disorders, and urinary frequency. (3) (PB; CJ; EV)**

2 _____ This is associated with opiates, that depress the central nervous system.

3 __x__ **Central nervous system side effects of Paxil include insomnia, restlessness, dizziness, tremors, nervousness, and headache.**

4 __x__ **Cardiovascular side effects of Paxil include hypertension, orthostatic hypotension, palpitations, and vasodilation.**

5 _____ This is associated with tiagabine hydrochloride, an antiepileptic used for bipolar disorders.

6 _____ This is associated with monoamine oxidase inhibitors used for depression.

461. **4 Benztropine mesylate (Cogentin), an anticholinergic, helps balance neurotransmitter activity in the CNS and helps control extrapyramidal-tract symptoms. (2) (PB; MR; AN)**

1 Zolpidem (Ambien) is a sedative, hypnotic drug used for short-term insomnia.

2 Hydroxyzine (Atarax) is a sedative that depresses activity in the subcortical areas in the CNS; it is used to reduce anxiety.

3 Dantrolene (Dantrium) has a direct effect on skeletal muscle by acting on the excitation-contraction coupling of muscle fibers and not at the level of the CNS as do most other muscle relaxation drugs.

462. **3 Haloperidol (Haldol) reduces emotional tensions, excessive psychomotor activity, panic, and fear. (2) (PB; CJ; AN)**

1 Clients exhibiting manic behaviors do not respond well to Haldol, and it can exacerbate their underlying feelings of depression.

2 Clients exhibiting excited-depressed behavior do not respond well to Haldol because it tends to increase the depression.

4 Haldol appears to have few stimulating effects and, in fact, increases feelings of lassitude and fatigue.

463. **4 The classic signs and symptoms that indicate lithium toxicity include slurred speech, ataxia, nausea, and vomiting. (1) (PB; CJ; AS)**

1 When lithium levels are low the client would present with recurring signs and symptoms of the mood disorder.

2 These are not signs and symptoms of a mood disorder.

3 If lithium levels were within the therapeutic range, the client's mood would be more stable; the client may experience GI symptoms, but would not experience slurred speech or an ataxic gait.

464. **2 The drug physostigmine (Antilirium) may be used to manage an overdose of a tricyclic antidepressant; it increases acetylcholine at cholinergic nerve terminals and reverses central and peripheral anticholinergic effects. (3) (PB; CJ; PL)**

1 Dialysis or forced diuresis is an ineffective treatment for an overdose of a tricyclic antidepressant.

3 Acetylcholine levels are depressed from the tricyclic antidepressant; anticholinergics are most effective in managing the side effects of antipsychotic/neuroleptic drugs.

4 Prevention of suicidal behavior is always advantageous; however, in this case, immediate emergency intervention is necessary.

465. 4 **Prolixin Decanoate is effective for noncompliant clients; it is an injectable form of Prolixin and lasts 3 to 4 weeks. (3) (PB; CJ; AN)**
   1 Elavil is a tricyclic antidepressant and would not be appropriate for this client; it is administered to clients who are depressed.
   2 Parnate is a monoamine oxidase inhibitor (MAOI) and would not be appropriate for this client; it is administered to clients with mood disorders.
   3 Prolixin is a short-acting medication; it is not as effective as Prolixin Decanoate for a noncompliant client.

466. 3 **Extreme photosensitivity is a common side effect of Prolixin; use of sunscreens and avoidance of tanning are essential. (3) (PB; MR; PL)**
   1 Once the client's medication is adjusted and CNS response is noted, driving may be permitted; drowsiness usually subsides after the first few weeks.
   2 This is untrue; energy is usually decreased.
   4 Although this drug can cause postural hypotension, it does not consistently lower blood pressure.

467. 1 **This drug is a narcotic antagonist that displaces narcotics from receptors in the brain, reversing respiratory depression. (2) (PB; MR; PL)**
   2 This is a synthetic opiate that causes CNS depression; it would add to the problem of overdose.
   3 This drug would have no effect on respiratory depression related to the presence of an overdose of a narcotic.
   4 Same as answer 2.

468. 3 **Monoamine oxidase uptake is inhibited by the medication, increasing concentrations of endogenous epinephrine, norepinephrine, serotonin, and dopamine in CNS storage sites; high levels of these transmitters in the presence of tyramine can cause hypertensive crisis. (2) (PB; MR; PL)**
   1 This may be an adverse reaction to the drug but is not related to drug-food interaction.
   2 Same as answer 1.
   4 This is not related to drug-food interaction.

469. 1 **Some over-the-counter medications contain alcohol and could trigger a reaction. (3) (PB; MR; EV)**
   2 Antabuse and antibiotics generally can be administered concurrently.
   3 This would be appropriate for clients receiving monoamine oxidase inhibitors (MAOIs), not Antabuse.

   4 If alcohol is taken with this drug it will cause severe nausea, vomiting, hypotension, headache, tachycardia, tachypnea, flushed face, and bloodshot eyes; Antabuse is aversion therapy for clients who abuse alcohol.

470. 2 **As the therapeutic level is reached and maintained, the client's psychotic symptoms decrease and insight increases. (2) (PB; CJ; EV)**
   1 This does not indicate that the client is responding therapeutically to the medication.
   3 Same as answer 1.
   4 This behavior may be an indication that the client is not responding to the medication because some of the symptoms are increasing.

471. 3 **Risperdal potentiates the action of alcohol and can cause oversedation if the drug and alcohol are taken together. (1) (SE; MR; IM)**
   1 This medication should be taken consistently to prevent recurrence of symptoms and maintain blood drug levels.
   2 Same as answer 1.
   4 Medications should be taken as ordered; taking them all at one time can interrupt the maintenance of a constant therapeutic blood level.

472. 3 **This is too short a period of time; clients usually begin to feel a lightening of depression in approximately 14 to 20 days, with the full antidepressant effects being felt between 3 and 4 weeks. (1) (PB; MR; EV)**
   1 Drowsiness usually occurs early in treatment but passes with time.
   2 It usually takes this long before the full effects of the antidepressant are experienced.
   4 Clients usually remain on these medications for several months.

473. 1 **Asendin is a tricyclic antidepressant and Nardil is a monoamine oxidase inhibitor (MAOI); antidepressants are contraindicated in concomitant use with MAOIs. (3) (PB; MR; IM)**
   2 Blood tests are not done specifically before administering MAOIs.
   3 Although checking for allergies is important, an allergy to feathers is not specific to MAOIs.
   4 Nardil does not have to be taken with food; milk products, with the exception of aged cheeses and yogurt, may be eaten; products containing tyramine must be avoided.

474. 2 **These drugs do not produce an immediate effect; nursing measures must be continued to decrease the chance of suicide. (2) (SE; CJ; IM)**
1 These food precautions are taken with MAO inhibitors.
3 These precautions are unnecessary.
4 Toxicity is not as prevalent a problem with tricyclics as it is with lithium.

475. 4 **A therapeutic response can be seen at this time; the client may have more energy to act out suicidal ideation. (2) (PI; CJ; EV)**
1 There are insufficient data to draw this conclusion.
2 It is unlikely that conflicts have resolved in such a short time.
3 Although true, it is not the most significant conclusion.

476. 2 **This drug creates a general sense of well-being, increases appetite, and helps lift depression. (2) (PB; CJ; EV)**
1 The client might not know the reason for depression, and the drug does not cause amnesia.
3 Concomitant use of MOAIs and tricyclic antidepressants is contraindicated.
4 Symptomatic relief usually begins after 2 to 3 weeks of therapy.

477. 4 **The parkinsonian symptoms are related to extrapyramidal-tract effects, and agranulocytosis is related to bone marrow depression. (2) (PB; CJ; EV)**
1 Jaundice is an adverse reaction; vomiting is not.
2 Tardive dyskinesia is an adverse reaction; nausea is not.
3 The rate of orthostasis is low; hiccups usually are not noted.

478. 2 **Tardive dyskinesia, an extrapyramidal symptom characterized by vermicular movements of the tongue, protrusion of the tongue, chewing and puckering movements of the mouth, and a puffing of the cheeks, is often irreversible even when antipsychotic medication is withdrawn. (2) (PB; CJ; AN)**
1 Motor restlessness (akathisia) can be treated with an antiparkinsonian or anticholinergic drug while antipsychotic medication continues.
3 Parkinsonian-like symptoms can be treated with antiparkinsonian or anticholinergic drugs while antipsychotic medication is continued.
4 An acute dystonic reaction can be treated with antiparkinsonian or anticholinergic drugs while the antipsychotic medication is continued.

479. 1 **Phenothiazines frequently cause a photosensitivity that can be controlled with sunscreens. (1) (SE; CJ; IM)**
2 The medication must be administered as prescribed.
3 Limiting activity is not a necessary precaution when taking phenothiazines.
4 Participating in the outing should not affect the client's blood pressure negatively.

480. 1 **These are common extrapyramidal signs (pseudoparkinsonism), which occur as side effects of neuroleptics; they usually are controlled with antiparkinsonian drugs. (2) (PI; CJ; EV)**
2 These are common side effects that occur with antidepressants.
3 These are common side effects that occur with CNS depressants.
4 These are signs of lithium toxicity.

481. 4 **Anticonvulsants and Haldol exert a synergistic CNS depressant effect. (2) (PB; MR; EV)**
1 The effect is potentiated.
2 Anticonvulsants do not affect absorption or metabolism of Haldol.
3 Same as answer 2.

482. 1 **These are signs and symptoms of early lithium toxicity; older clients should be monitored carefully and given smaller doses of lithium because its excretion from the kidneys is slower than in younger adults. (1) (PB; CJ; IM)**
2 There is no antidote for lithium toxicity; the lithium should be withheld.
3 A coarse hand tremor is an indication of advanced lithium toxicity; the lithium should be withheld.
4 Although antiepileptics work in 25% to 50% of clients with treatment-resistant bipolar disorder, this is not the appropriate treatment for lithium toxicity.

483. 2 **This comment reveals that the client does not understand that the medication is necessary to prevent mood swings; the client should recognize the importance of long-term medication compliance. (1) (PB; MR; EV)**
1 Regular medical visits are needed to assure the best management of the illness.
3 Various cognitive and behavioral therapies provide support in coping with life's stressors.
4 Compliance with medication regimens should eliminate the mood swings for most people with bipolar disorder.

484. 3 These foods are high in tyramine, which in the presence of an MAO inhibitor, such as Marplan, can cause an excessive epinephrine-type response that can result in a hypertensive crisis. (2) (SE; CJ; PL)
  1 There is no relationship between these foods and this medication.
  2 Same as answer 1.
  4 Same as answer 1.

485. 4 A hypertensive crisis would not be associated with extrapyramidal-tract symptoms. (2) (PB; CJ; EV)
  1 Akathisia, characterized by restlessness and twitching or crawling sensations in muscles, is an extrapyramidal side effect.
  2 Opisthotonos, characterized by hyperextension and arching of the back, is an extrapyramidal side effect.
  3 Oculogyric crisis, characterized by the uncontrolled upward movement of the eyes, is an extrapyramidal side effect.

486. 3 These are signs of akathisia, which is an involuntary movement disorder characterized by an inability to sit still. (2) (PB; CJ; AS)
  1 Muscle spasms and pulling of the head to the side by neck muscles (torticollis) are related to acute dystonia.
  2 These are associated with tardive dyskinesia.
  4 These are signs of pseudoparkinsonism.

487. 2 Yellow sclerae are a sign of toxicity that has damaged the liver and would necessitate withholding the drug. (2) (PI; CJ; PL)
  1 This is a common side effect that usually is alleviated by anti-Parkinson agents.
  3 Same as answer 1.
  4 Photosensitivity is an expected side effect of the drug; the medication does not have to be withheld.

488. 2 This medication can be taken every 2 weeks instead of every day. (1) (PB; CJ; AN)
  1 The side effects are the same as most other antipsychotic drugs.
  3 The action of this drug during pregnancy is uncertain; animal studies have demonstrated an adverse effect on the fetus.
  4 Same as answer 1.

489. 1 The medication should be stopped immediately because the jaundice indicates possible liver damage, which would prolong elimination of the drug and may result in toxic accumulation. (1) (SE; CJ; EV)
  2 Milk does not change the effect of the drug.
  3 The drug must be stopped, not reduced.

  4 The drug is available only in an oral form; in addition, the route of administration would not influence the occurrence of toxic accumulation.

490. 4 Infection can indicate agranulocytosis, a serious side effect that can occur with therapy and can cause death. (3) (PB; CJ; EV)
  1 This is not advisable because the client may be developing agranulocytosis, a potentially life-threatening side effect that needs immediate treatment.
  2 Same as answer 1.
  3 Same as answer 1.

491. 2 For clients with bipolar disorders, it has been shown that long-term lithium therapy flattens the highs of the euphoric episode and the lows of the depressed episode. (1) (PB; MR; EV)
  1 The physician should be notified before medication is stopped.
  3 Clients should never adjust their own dosage of medication.
  4 The therapeutic level and the toxic level are very close, and serious side effects do occur.

492. 4 Antianxiety medications have the potential for physiologic and/or psychologic dependence; the nurse should teach the client about both the advantages and disadvantages of taking this drug. (2) (PB; CJ; AN)
  1 Physiologic and/or psychologic dependence can develop even when the dosage is controlled.
  2 Both psychologic and physiologic dependence can develop.
  3 Tolerance does not develop.

493. 3 Foods such as chocolate, aged cheese, and pickled herring and those with excessive caffeine have high levels of tyramine and cause dangerous hypertension in clients taking MAO inhibitors. (2) (SE; MR; EV)
  1 There is no need to limit intake of this food while taking MAO inhibitors.
  2 Same as answer 1.
  4 Same as answer 1.

494. 4 This acute dystonic reaction is a severe side effect of Haldol and requires intramuscular or intravenous administration of antiparkinsonian medication. (2) (PB; CJ; EV)
  1 The dosage would not be increased but discontinued, and antiparkinsonian medication should be administered.
  2 At this point symptoms are so severe that this medication must be discontinued.

3 These symptoms are more severe than pseudoparkinsonism and require more than an adjustment in this medication.

495. 4 **A neuromuscular blocker, such as succinylcholine (Anectine), produces respiratory depression because it inhibits contractions of respiratory muscles. (1) (PB; CJ; EV)**

1 As a muscle relaxant, the neuromuscular blocking agent prevents seizures.

2 The loss of memory results from the ECT treatment, not from the neuromuscular blocking agent.

3 Because the client is not permitted anything by mouth for 8 to 10 hours before the treatment, this is not a major problem.

496. 1 **Hard candy may produce salivation, which helps alleviate the anticholinergic-like side effect of dry mouth that is experienced with some psychotropics. (2) (PB; CJ; PL)**

2 Fluids should be encouraged, not discouraged; fluids may alleviate the dry mouth.

3 This is unnecessary.

4 Same as answer 3.

497. 1 **This is an accurate and concise explanation of Haldol's effects; it blocks postsynaptic dopamine receptors in the brain. (1) (PB; CJ; IM)**

2 This is a neuroleptic; it does not alter mood.

3 This drug lowers the seizure threshold.

4 Same as answer 2.

498. 2 **This drug suppresses activity in key regions of the subcortical area of the CNS; it also has antihistaminic and anticholinergic effects. (1) (PB; CJ; EV)**

1 These symptoms are not associated with Vistaril.

3 Same as answer 1.

4 Same as answer 1.

499. 3 **These are the classic signs of neuroleptic malignant syndrome, which is caused by neuroleptic-induced blockage of dopamine receptors. (3) (PB; CJ; EV)**

1 These are side effects of Haldol, but they are not signs of neuroleptic malignant syndrome.

2 Same as answer 1.

4 Same as answer 1.

500. 4 **The effects of antidepressants are cumulative; it may be some time before improvement is noted. (2) (PB; MR; IM)**

1 Antidepressants help relieve the physical and mental discomforts of the depressed client.

2 It is too early to arrive at this conclusion.

3 Antidepressants are effective regardless of the length of the depression.

Mental Health Nursing Quiz 1

1. The nurse evaluates that a client has understood the teaching about the side effects and precautions associated with the neuroleptic drug haloperidol (Haldol) when the client states:
   1. "I will immediately report any diarrhea or vomiting to my doctor."
   2. "I will not eat any tyramine-containing foods while I'm taking Haldol."
   3. "I'll maintain an adequate fluid intake, since I may urinate more than usual."
   4. "I'll avoid direct sunlight and use sunburn preventatives when I go outdoors."

2. When caring for a middle-age female client who has lost about 20 pounds over the last 2 months, cries easily, sleeps poorly, and refuses to participate in any family or social activities that she previously enjoyed, it is very important for the nurse to:
   1. Provide the client with a high-calorie, high-protein diet
   2. Set firm consistent limits to reduce the client's crying episodes
   3. Assure the client that she will regain her usual function in a short time
   4. Allow the client to externalize her feelings, especially anger, in a safe manner

3. A client recently admitted to the hospital with the diagnosis of schizophrenia, paranoid type, says to the nurse, "I know they're spying on me in here, too. I'm not safe anywhere!" The most therapeutic response by the nurse would be:
   1. "Nobody's spying on you in here."
   2. "Why do you feel they'd want to follow you here?"
   3. "You don't feel safe anywhere, not even in the hospital."
   4. "You are safe in the hospital; nothing can happen to you here."

4. To foster a therapeutic relationship with a deeply depressed, unresponsive client who stares into space, remains curled up in bed, and refuses to talk, the nurse must first break through the client's withdrawal. Initially, this can best be achieved by:
   1. Sitting quietly next to the client for set periods of time each hour
   2. Urging the client to participate in simple games with other clients
   3. Gently touching the client on the arm when the opportunity arises
   4. Informing the client that dressing and going to the dayroom is required

5. When assessing an adolescent client with the diagnosis of schizophrenia, undifferentiated type, the nurse should expect to observe:
   1. Paranoid delusions, hallucinations, and hyperactivity
   2. Ritualistic behavior, inappropriate affect, and paranoia
   3. Depression, disorders of thought, and loosened associations
   4. Loosened associations, bizarre behavior, and hallucinations

6. The nurse counselor in the mental health clinic is working with a couple and their two sons, ages 14 and 16. One son has been in trouble at school because of truancy and poor grades. The other son appears quiet and withdrawn, and the parents report no problems. The father has been unemployed, and the mother works as a waitress. They have had severe marital problems for the past 10 years. The priority nursing diagnosis for this family at this time would be:
   1. Impaired parenting related to marital problems
   2. Impaired adjustment related to the children growing older
   3. Disabled family coping related to the son's school problems
   4. Impaired social interaction related to an inability to form relationships

7. A teenage client is admitted to the hospital with a history of increasingly bizarre behavior. The client states, "I am wired to the television and it informed me that my family is out to kill me." The initial action by the admitting nurse that would be most therapeutic for this client would be:
   1. Taking the client to the dayroom and introducing the other clients on the unit
   2. Reassuring the client that the unit is safe and that the client will be protected from the family
   3. Telling the client that the door is locked and no one is permitted to enter the unit to harm any client
   4. Introducing the client to the primary nurse who will be assigned to work on a one-to-one basis with the client

8. When a disturbed client who has a history of using neologisms says to the nurse, "My lacket hss kelong mon," the nurse should respond by:
   1. Trying to learn the language of the client
   2. Telling the client that these words are not understood
   3. Communicating in simple terms directed toward the client
   4. Recognizing that the client needs a nurse who can understand the fantasies expressed

9. A disturbed client, unprovoked, attacks another client. A short-term goal for this client would be to:
   1. Get the client to apologize for the attack to the other client
   2. Have a staff member whom the client trusts stay with the client
   3. Protect others from the client's impulsive acts by secluding the client
   4. Keep the client actively participating in activities and in contact with reality

10. The nurse is aware that the medication used to prevent symptoms of withdrawal in clients with a long history of alcohol abuse would be:
    1. Lorazepam (Ativan)
    2. Phenobarbital (Luminal)
    3. Chlorpromazine (Thorazine)
    4. Methadone hydrochloride (Methadone)

11. An adolescent is arrested for shoplifting and is brought to the psychiatric unit. Although describing her child as intelligent, witty, entertaining, and friendly, the mother states, "My child is somewhat unreliable, untruthful, and insincere." The client is diagnosed as having a personality disorder. The most accurate nursing diagnosis for the client would be:
    1. Ineffective coping
    2. Antisocial personality disorder
    3. Risk for introverted and mature behavior
    4. Impairment of common sense, feelings of guilt and remorse

12. An older individual, accompanied by family members, is admitted to the hospital with the symptoms of dementia. During the admission procedures, the initial approach by the nurse that would be most helpful to this client would be:
    1. "You are somewhat disoriented now, but do not worry. You will be all right in a few days."
    2. "I am the nurse on duty today. You are at the hospital. Your family can stay with you for a while."

3. "Let me introduce you to the staff here before you get acquainted with our ward policy and routine."
4. "Do not be frightened. I am the nurse, and everyone here in the hospital will help you get well."

13. The nurse is aware that a 6-year-old with normal psychosocial development would have achieved Erikson's developmental tasks of trust, autonomy, and:
    1. Identity
    2. Intimacy
    3. Initiative
    4. Belonging

14. The daycare treatment team decides it would be therapeutic for a client with an obsessive-compulsive personality disorder to get a part-time job. On the day of the job interview, the client comes to the center very anxious and displays an increase in compulsive behaviors. The nurse could best respond to these behavioral changes by stating:
    1. "I know you're anxious, but make yourself go and try to conquer your fear."
    2. "If going to an interview makes you this anxious, it seems to me that you're not ready to work."
    3. "Going for your interview triggered some feelings in you. Describe what you're feeling at this time."
    4. "It must be that you really don't want that job after all. I think you should think more about it."

15. A group of clients from a psychiatric unit are going to a professional ball game accompanied by staff members. The purpose of visits into the community under the supervision of staff members is to:
    1. Assist the clients in adjusting to anxieties in the community
    2. Help the clients return to reality under controlled conditions
    3. Observe the clients' abilities to cope with a more complex society
    4. Broaden the clients' experiences by providing exposure to cultural activities

16. To foster a healthy grieving response to the birth of a stillborn child, the nurse's best acknowledgment of an expression of anger from the mother would be:
    1. "You may be wondering if something you did caused this."
    2. "You are young; wait and see, you'll have other children."

3. "It's God's will; we have to have faith that it was for the best."
4. "This often happens when something is wrong with the baby."

17. One day the nurse and a client sit together and draw. The client draws a face with horns on top of the head and says, "This is me. I'm a devil." The nurse should respond:
    1. "I don't see a devil. Why do you see a devil?"
    2. "Let's go to the mirror and see what you look like."
    3. "You are not a devil. Don't talk about yourself like that."
    4. "When I look at you, I see an attractive young person, not a devil."

18. The nurse is aware that most clients with phobias use the defense mechanisms of:
    1. Dissociation and denial
    2. Projection and displacement
    3. Introjection and sublimation
    4. Substitution and reaction formation

19. The nurse manager recognizes that one of the nurses in ICU may be experiencing burnout. The nurse manager should plan to help this nurse begin to confront the problem by:
    1. Transferring to a primary nursing care unit
    2. Identifying personal responses to daily work stresses
    3. Attending educational programs as often as possible
    4. Choosing a nursing position on a low-stress unit

20. A client is admitted to a psychiatric unit with a history of sleeplessness, lack of interest in eating, and charging of excessive purchases to charge accounts. The symptoms that the nurse should expect the client to exhibit in the hospital would include:
    1. Depressed mood and crying
    2. Increased insight into behavior
    3. Decreased psychomotor activity
    4. Increased interest in the environment

21. A client leaves group therapy in the middle of the session. The nurse finds the client obviously upset and crying. The client tells the nurse that the group's discussion was too much to tolerate. The most therapeutic nursing action would be to:
    1. Request kindly but firmly that the client return to the group to work out conflicts

2. Suggest that the client accompany the nurse to a quiet place so that they can talk about the situation
3. Ask the group leader what happened in the group session and base intervention on this additional information
4. Respect the client's right to decline therapy at this time and report the incident to the rest of the health team members

22. A client sits huddled in a chair and leaves it only to let out a scream, run to the end of the hallway, and crouch in a corner. The nurse, observing this, realizes that this behavior is classified as:
    1. Reactive
    2. Regressive
    3. Dissociative
    4. Hallucinatory

23. Caring for a withdrawn, reclusive, psychotic client, the priority goal would be for the client to develop:
    1. Trust
    2. Self-worth
    3. A sense of identity
    4. An ability to socialize

24. When a client is receiving valproate (Depacon), it is important for the nurse to monitor:
    1. Weight
    2. Visual acuity
    3. Bowel sounds
    4. Potassium level

25. A client has been experiencing delusions. The nurse understands that according to psychodynamic theory, delusions are:
    1. A defense against anxiety
    2. Precipitated by external stimuli
    3. The result of paleologic thinking
    4. Subconscious expressions of anger

26. A nurse on the psychiatric unit is assigned to work with a client who appears reclusive and mistrustful of everyone. The nurse can help the client to develop trust by:
    1. Attempting to be prompt for their scheduled meetings
    2. Stating simply and sincerely that the nurse cares about the client's feelings
    3. Listening attentively to the client's positive feelings and ignoring negative feelings
    4. Handing the client medication and not watching to see whether it is swallowed

27. A female client in the terminal stage of cancer is admitted to the hospital in severe pain. The client refuses medication for the pain because it puts her to sleep and she wants to be awake. One day, despite the client's objection, a nurse administers the pain medication saying, "You know that this will make you more comfortable." The nurse in this situation could be charged with:
    1. Battery
    2. Assault
    3. Invasion of privacy
    4. Lack of informed consent

28. The nurse, recognizing the possible cause of alcohol-induced amnestic disorder, should take into consideration when planning a client's care that the client is probably experiencing:
    1. A deficiency in thiamine
    2. An increase in serotonin
    3. An iron intake reduction
    4. A riboflavin malabsorption

29. The day following the birth of their baby, the parents are very upset to learn that the baby has a heart defect. At this time it would be most helpful for the nurse to:
    1. Allow the parents to express their anger
    2. Explain the diagnosis in a variety of ways
    3. Encourage the parents to talk with other parents
    4. Assure the parents that surgery will correct the problem

30. An older client with vascular dementia has difficulty following simple directions and selecting clothes to be worn for the day. The nurse recognizes that these problems are the result of:
    1. Impaired judgment
    2. Decreased attention span
    3. Clouding of consciousness
    4. Loss of abstract thinking ability

31. A 16-year-old female client is admitted to the adolescent psychiatric unit with a diagnosis of anorexia nervosa. The adolescent has lost 40 pounds during the last 6 months and her current weight is 75 pounds. When approaching this client, the nurse should initially:
    1. Point out how bad she looks
    2. Refrain from discussing her appearance
    3. Recognize that she is deliberately trying to kill herself
    4. State the rules about eating in a matter-of-fact manner

32. In addition to suicide, an awareness of serious health problems in adolescents requires that the school nurse teach the faculty that adolescents are at risk for:
    1. Rubella and mononucleosis
    2. Heroin abuse and malnutrition
    3. Genital herpes and alcohol abuse
    4. Diabetes and the use of marijuana

33. During the admission interview of a client with a diagnosis of bipolar I disorder, manic episode, the nurse would expect the client to demonstrate:
    1. Flight of ideas
    2. Ritualistic behaviors
    3. Associative looseness
    4. Delusions of persecution

34. To therapeutically relate to parents who are known to have maltreated their child, the nurse must first:
    1. Identify personal feelings about child abusers
    2. Recognize the emotional needs of the parents
    3. Call authorities to report the suspected incident
    4. Gather information about the child's home environment

35. A young woman who has just lost her first job comes to the mental health clinic very upset and states, "Without warning, I just start crying without any reason." The nurse's initial response should be:
    1. "Do you know what makes you cry?"
    2. "Most of us need to cry from time to time."
    3. "Crying unexpectedly must be very upsetting."
    4. "Are you having any other problems at this time?"

36. A client who is receiving haloperidol (Haldol), 5 mg tid, complains of twitching of the fingers. The nurse should respond:
    1. "This is a temporary situation until your body adjusts to the medication."
    2. "You need the medication that we are giving you. You will soon get used to the side effects."
    3. "Let's wait a few days and see whether the side effects of the drug you are receiving go away."
    4. "I will get the doctor to order a medication that will help overcome this. It is a side effect of the drug you are taking."

37. The nurse, finding a client with schizophrenia lying under a bench in the hall, could best respond to the client's statement, "God told me to lie here," by stating:

1. "I didn't hear anyone talking. Come with me to your room."
2. "What you heard was in your head; it was your imagination."
3. "Come to the dayroom and watch television. You will feel better."
4. "God would not tell you to lie in the hall. God would want you to behave reasonably."

38. One day as the nurse sits next to a depressed client, the client states, "I want to tell you something but you must promise not to tell anyone." The best response by the nurse would be:
    1. "OK, I won't. It's good for you to talk about what's bothering you."
    2. "You can tell me if you want to, but I cannot give you that promise."
    3. "You have my promise not to tell. What's the secret you want to tell me?"
    4. "You seem to be more depressed today. Why don't you tell me what you are thinking?"

39. A male client with a history of marginally socially acceptable behavior is admitted to the hospital for evaluation. The client tells the nurse he has been married multiple times but never loved, nor would he support any of the women or the children he produced. The nurse could identify that the client's behavior, according to the psychoanalytic model, demonstrates a defect in:
    1. Id development
    2. Ego development
    3. Sexual development
    4. Superego development

40. When working with clients who use manipulative, socially acting-out behaviors, the nurse should be:
    1. Strict, punishing, and restrictive
    2. Sincere, cautious, and consistent
    3. Supportive, accepting, and friendly
    4. Sympathetic, motherly, and encouraging

41. A male client with the diagnosis of antisocial personality disorder takes a female nurse by the shoulder, suddenly kisses her, and shouts, "I like you." The most appropriate response by the nurse would be:
    1. "Thank you, I like you too."
    2. "I wish you wouldn't do that."
    3. "Don't ever touch me like that again."
    4. "I like you too, but please don't do that again."

42. A client with schizophrenia is started on an antipsychotic/neuroleptic medication. The nurse is aware that these drugs are used primarily to:
    1. Keep the client quiet and relaxed
    2. Reduce the need for physical restraints
    3. Control the client's behavior and reduce stress
    4. Make the client more receptive to psychotherapy

43. The nurse is aware that the major defense mechanism used by an individual with a phobic disorder is:
    1. Avoidance
    2. Regression
    3. Repression
    4. Conversion

44. A young adult client is admitted to the hospital with a diagnosis of schizophrenia, paranoid type. The client's family is concerned about the client's safety and well-being because the client has been stating, "The voices are telling me to kill myself." The priority nursing diagnosis for this client should be:
    1. Chronic low self-esteem
    2. Disturbed sensory perception
    3. Risk for self-directed violence
    4. Impaired verbal communication

45. On a visit to the clinic, the husband of an alcohol abuser confides to the nurse that he and his wife are experiencing marital difficulties. He states, "After all the years of her drinking, I can't believe this is happening now that she's been sober for 6 months." An appropriate nursing diagnosis for the husband at this time would be:
    1. Impaired adjustment related to altered communication patterns
    2. Ineffective role performance related to changes in wife's needs
    3. Situational low self-esteem related to wife's increased independence
    4. Compromised family coping related to altered marital relationships

46. The nurse notices that each time the physician or nurse manager visits a disturbed female client, she becomes extremely anxious. Today, after visiting with the physician, the client sits wringing her hands. The best initial response by the nurse would be:
    1. "How do you handle your anxiety?"
    2. "I notice that you are wringing your hands."
    3. "Do you realize why you are wringing your hands?"
    4. "Tell me why you are afraid of authority figures."

47. A female client is admitted to the psychiatric unit with the diagnosis of obsessive-compulsive disorder that is demonstrated by an increasing, consuming obsession with dirt. The client feels her hands are dirty and has a need to wash them about 70 to 80 times a day. The client's hands are red and raw with some bleeding. An immediate nursing goal for this client would be to get the client to:
1. Understand that her hands are not dirty
2. Stop washing her hands so the skin will heal
3. Develop insight into her emotional problems
4. Limit the number of times she washes her hands

48. The nurse, when assessing the behavior of the parents of a physically maltreated child, would expect that they:
1. Become irritable about having the history taken
2. Show concern about the child's medical condition
3. Give contradictory explanations about what happened
4. Present many details related to how the trauma occurred

49. An inpatient therapy group on a psychiatric unit has as its goal helping clients participate in life more fully by gaining insight and changing behavior. The nurse leader can best help the group achieve this goal by using a leadership style that is:
1. Stimulating and guiding
2. Autocratic and directing
3. Laissez-faire and observing
4. Democratic and controlling

50. The nurse recognizes that behavior is usually viewed and accepted as normal if it:
1. Fits within standards accepted by one's society
2. Helps the person to reduce the use of defense mechanisms
3. Expresses the individual's feelings and thoughts accurately
4. Helps the individual to achieve short-term and long-term goals

Mental Health Nursing Quiz 1 Answers and Rationales

1. 4 **Photosensitivity is a side effect of many antipsy-chotic medications. (3) (PB; CJ; EV; DR)**
  1 These symptoms are side effects of lithium, not of Haldol.
  2 Avoiding tyramine-containing foods is a precaution associated with MAO inhibitors, not with Haldol.
  3 This is a precaution associated with lithium, not with Haldol.

2. 4 **The greatest danger associated with depression is self-inflicted injury when feelings, especially anger, are internalized. (2) (PI; CJ; PL; MO)**
  1 There are not enough data to determine if the weight loss resulted in malnutrition.
  2 The client is unable to control or regulate this behavior at this time.
  3 This is false reassurance; this is not supportive of the client's feelings.

3. 3 **Rephrasing allows for further communication, expresses understanding, and does not belittle the client's feelings. (3) (PI; CJ; IM; SD)**
  1 Presenting reality to the client at this time only raises anxiety and leads the client to defend the delusion.
  2 "Why" questions make a client defensive, and the wording implies the client's delusion could be true.
  4 This is false reassurance; in any event, a suspicious client would not believe the nurse.

4. 1 **Sitting quietly with a severely withdrawn client can provide an opportunity for nonthreatening interaction. (2) (PI; CJ; PL; MO)**
  2 The client is unable to deal with a one-to-one relationship at this time.
  3 Entering a withdrawn client's body space is intrusive and stressful; it often precipitates a need for further withdrawal.
  4 Placing demands on the withdrawn client causes a sense of threat, increased anxiety, and a need for additional withdrawal.

5. 4 **These are the primary behaviors associated with a thought disorder, such as schizophrenia. (2) (PI; CJ; AS; SD)**
  1 These symptoms are more common in paranoid-type schizophrenia than in the undifferentiated type.

  2 Ritualistic behavior is generally associated with obsessive-compulsive disorders, not schizophrenia.
  3 Depression is not characteristic of schizophrenia.

6. 1 **The parents' ongoing marital problems appear to have interfered with their parental roles, with resulting behavior problems in their children. (3) (SE; MR; AN; BA)**
  2 There are no data to support this diagnosis.
  3 Same as answer 2.
  4 Same as answer 2.

7. 4 **This is extremely important because the disturbed client can be assisted back to reality by a nurse who is involved in the client's environment and is interested in the client as an individual and in the client's feelings. (2) (PI; MR; IM; SD)**
  1 This would be a later action.
  2 The nurse does not know the client will not be frightened; this would be false reassurance.
  3 This would have no effect since the client is involved with a strong delusional pattern.

8. 2 **This is a simple statement that the client is not understood; it provides feedback and points out reality. (2) (PI; CJ; IM; SD)**
  1 Neologisms have symbolic meaning only for the client.
  3 This will be of limited help and does not present reality.
  4 There is no one other than the client who can understand the fantasies.

9. 2 **The client needs someone with whom there is a working and trusting relationship; this individual must observe, protect, anticipate, and prevent the client from acting out on destructive impulses. (3) (PI; MR; PL; SD)**
  1 At this time the client cannot be held responsible for this behavior.
  3 It may be necessary to do this, but staying with the client is a more appropriate immediate action.
  4 The client may not be ready for participation, though there is a need to be kept in touch with reality.

10. 1 **This drug is most effective in preventing delirium tremens. (2) (PB; CJ; PL; SA)**
   2 This drug is used to prevent withdrawal symptoms associated with barbiturate use.
   3 This antipsychotic medication can be used to combat the physiologic effects of amphetamine use.
   4 This drug is used to prevent withdrawal symptoms associated with opiate use.

11. 1 **History demonstrates that the client has had a difficult time controlling impulsive behavior and has consistently exhibited poor judgment; this indicates ineffective coping. (1) (PI; CJ; AN; PR)**
   2 This is a psychiatric, not a nursing, diagnosis.
   3 This is not an acceptable nursing diagnosis.
   4 Same as answer 3.

12. 2 **Familiarity with the environment and orientation to the staff may help promote security and feelings of trust. (2) (PI; CJ; IM; DD)**
   1 This denies the client's feelings and provides false reassurance.
   3 A person under stress cannot assimilate much information; verbiage could lead to more confusion.
   4 This statement denies feelings and is false reassurance because all personnel are not involved with the client.

13. 3 **A 6-year-old should have resolved the developmental task of initiative versus guilt. (1) (PM; CJ; AN; PD)**
   1 Resolution of identity versus role confusion occurs at adolescence.
   2 Resolution of intimacy versus isolation occurs at adulthood.
   4 This is part of Maslow's hierarchy of needs; the need for love and belonging arises once physical and safety needs are met.

14. 3 **These symptoms are a defense against anxiety resulting from decision making, which triggers old fears; the client needs support. (2) (PI; CJ; EV; PR)**
   1 This denies the client's overwhelming anxiety and lacks realistic support.
   2 This is judgmental; the client should be encouraged to work through the symptoms, not to avoid risk.
   4 This is judgmental; an increase in anxiety does not necessarily mean the client does not want to attain the goal.

15. 3 **The nurse's observations can help identify those clients who are ready to cope with outside** stress and those who are not. (3) (SE; MR; EV; SD)
   1 Attendance at a ball game would not accomplish this.
   2 Same as answer 1.
   4 There is nothing to indicate that any of these clients needed to broaden their cultural experiences.

16. 1 **The mother must be helped to identify feelings. (1) (PI; CJ; IM; CS)**
   2 This is false reassurance; it does not encourage the client to explore feelings.
   3 This answer is based on the nurse's religious beliefs; there is no indication that the client has the same beliefs; this closes off communication.
   4 Many stillborn children are apparently free of any defects.

17. 4 **This response points out reality while attempting to let the client understand that the nurse sees the client as a person of worth. (3) (PI; CJ; IM; SD)**
   1 This asks the client to explain feelings, which may be an unrealistic goal.
   2 The client may indeed view the self as a devil.
   3 This is a somewhat punitive response; it cuts off communication.

18. 2 **Clients with phobias deal with anxiety by placing it on specific persons, objects, or situations through the process of displacement and/or projection. (3) (PI; CJ; AS; AX)**
   1 The person with a phobia recognizes and admits the exaggerated fear as a real part of the self.
   3 Neither introjection, whereby a person internalizes and incorporates the traits of another, nor sublimation, whereby socially acceptable behavior is substituted for unacceptable instincts, is related to phobic activity.
   4 A less-valued object is not substituted for one more highly valued (substitution) nor are the expressed feelings opposite to the experienced feelings of fear (reaction formation).

19. 2 **Identification of work stressors in the environment, coping strategies used, and evaluating the effectiveness of these strategies is the first step. (2) (SE; MR; PL; NP)**
   1 This may help, but prevention begins with knowing oneself and the effectiveness of one's coping strategies.
   3 Attending continuing education programs can help alleviate burnout, but this is not the

first step in confronting the problem when it occurs.

4 Choosing a nursing position on a low-stress unit can help alleviate burnout, but it is not the first step in confronting the problem when it occurs.

20. **4 In an attempt to ward off depression, the client in the hyperactive phase of bipolar I disorder runs headlong into reality, becoming totally involved in everything that goes on in the environment. (2) (PI; CJ; AS; MO)**
1 This would be more indicative of the depressive episode.
2 During this phase, there is no insight into behavior.
3 The opposite occurs; psychomotor activity is greatly increased.

21. **2 This approach incorporates the principles of starting where the client is and helping the client verbalize feelings; it also provides for additional data collecting. (2) (PI; CJ; IM; TR)**
1 The client is not ready to do this.
3 This would be a later step, after the more appropriate nursing action was completed.
4 This accepts the client's right not to be forced back into the group; however, direct nursing intervention should be attempted at this time.

22. **2 This behavior reflects the early fetal position; the individual curls up for both protection and security. (3) (PI; CJ; AN; SD)**
1 The client's behavior is not in response to an observable stimulus.
3 The client's behavior does not indicate dissociation or depersonalization.
4 The client's behavior gives no indication of an hallucinatory pattern.

23. **1 Trust is basic to all therapies; without trust a therapeutic relationship cannot be established. (2) (PI; CJ; PL; SD)**
2 The development of self-worth is a long-term goal; developing trust is the priority.
3 There is nothing to indicate that the client does not have a sense of identity.
4 Although helping the client relate to others is a part of the treatment, it is not a priority goal at this time.

24. **1 Common side effects include anorexia, dyspepsia, nausea, and vomiting. (3) (PB; CJ; EV; DR)**

2 This has no relationship to the administration of lithium.
3 Same as answer 2.
4 Same as answer 2.

25. **1 Delusions are a way the unconscious defends the individual from real or imagined threats. (2) (PI; CJ; AN; SD)**
2 Illusions are false interpretations of actual external stimuli.
3 This is logical thinking that is formulated from an illogical base.
4 Delusions are precipitated by feelings of anxiety, not anger.

26. **1 This helps the client to feel important enough for the nurse to remember their meeting and be on time. (2) (PI; CJ; IM; TR)**
2 The client is mistrustful of others and will probably not believe the nurse; caring is best demonstrated through behavior.
3 Feelings should never be ignored but should be accepted as important to the client.
4 This would not only be an unsafe practice but may make the client feel that the nurse does not care enough to stay.

27. **1 This is the intentional touching of one person by another without permission of the person being touched. (2) (SE; LE; EV; NP)**
2 This is an intentional act without touching that makes a person fearful or produces reasonable apprehension of bodily harm.
3 This refers to the right of clients to have their private affairs protected.
4 This applies to written permission for procedures and treatments to be performed.

28. **1 The deficiency of thiamine (vitamin B₁) is thought to be a primary cause of alcohol-induced amnestic disorder. (3) (PB; CJ; PL; SA)**
2 This is unrelated to alcohol-induced amnestic disorder.
3 Same as answer 2.
4 Same as answer 2.

29. **1 Parents need to express and deal with their feelings; then perhaps they can move toward other coping strategies. (2) (PI; CJ; IM; TR)**
2 This does not focus on the need presented by the parents.
3 This does not focus on their present concern but could be useful sometime in the future.
4 This is premature, possibly false, reassurance.

30. 4 Impairment of abstract thinking interferes with interpreting and defining words in addition to following directions and selecting clothes. (3) (PI; CJ; AN; DD)
  1 Following directions does not require skill in judgment or decision making.
  2 The selection of clothes does not require an intact attention span.
  3 Dementia does not cause a clouding of consciousness; delirium does.

31. 2 Initially, the nurse should not discuss the client's appearance because this focuses on an observation rather than on feelings. (2) (PI; CJ; IM; ES)
  1 This is a judgmental statement; in addition, the client does not believe she looks "bad."
  3 The client's objective is not suicide; the client has a need to control her eating.
  4 Stating the rules would be ineffective and would not convince the client to eat.

32. 3 Adolescence is the period of development characterized by experimentation with risky behaviors; this experimentation often leads to unprotected sex and alcohol abuse. (2) (PM; CJ; AN; BA)
  1 Mononucleosis is a problem for adolescents, but rubella is a health risk for young children and pregnant women, not adolescents.
  2 Malnutrition is not a particular risk for adolescents unless other problems are present; heroin is not the drug of choice for adolescents.
  4 Marijuana use continues to present some risks in adolescents, but the development of diabetes is not a particular risk for this age group.

33. 1 This is a fragmented, pressured, nonsequential pattern of speech typically used during a manic episode. (1) (PI; CJ; AS; MO)
  2 These are repetitive, purposeful, and intentional behaviors that are carried out in a stereotyped fashion; they are found in clients with obsessive-compulsive disorders.
  3 This is the pattern of speech found in clients with schizophrenia; usual connections between words and phrases are lost to the listener and meaningful only to the speaker.
  4 These are fixed false beliefs that others are plotting to do harm; they are found in clients with paranoid-type schizophrenia.

34. 1 Self-awareness is an essential element in providing support, understanding, and empathy to others. (1) (PI; CJ; AS; NP)
  2 Meeting the emotional needs of these parents cannot be accomplished until an interpersonal relationship is established; to establish an interpersonal relationship with clients the nurse must first be aware of personal feelings.
  3 Although this eventually will be done, the nurse must first be aware of personal feelings.
  4 Although important, these data do not take priority at this time.

35. 3 This response identifies the client's feelings. (1) (PI; CJ; IM; AX)
  1 This is an unrealistic question; the cause of anxiety may not be known.
  2 This response moves the focus away from the client.
  4 This disregards the client's comment; it is a direct question that may impede communication.

36. 4 This response assures the client that the staff member is able to help and that the client's concerns are accurate. (2) (PB; MR; EV; DR)
  1 It is a reversible condition that can be treated with benztropine (Cogentin) or diphenhydramine (Benadryl).
  2 It is not a symptom that requires adjusting to, rather one that must be treated.
  3 Early treatment to reverse the symptom is important.

37. 1 The nurse is focusing on reality and trying to distract and refocus the client's attention. (3) (PI; CJ; IM; SD)
  2 This statement is too blunt and belittling; this approach rarely is effective.
  3 This is false reassurance; the nurse does not know that the client will feel better.
  4 This may be interpreted as belittling or an attempt to convince the client that the behavior is irrational; it usually is ineffective.

38. 2 By being honest, if a client tells the nurse something that should be shared, the nurse would not have to break a promise or risk harm to the client or others. (2) (SE; LE; IM; NP)
  1 Encouraging discussion is helpful, but putting oneself in the position of possibly having to break a promise is not therapeutic.
  3 This puts the nurse in the position of having to break a promise, which could destroy rapport and decrease trust.
  4 This response ignores the client's statement and avoids the issue.

39. 4 Superego development reflects the internalized norms of the family and society; the antisocial personality has never achieved this internalization. (2) (PI; CJ; AN; PR)

1 A person with this behavior has an overdeveloped need to seek pleasure.

2 The ego is not the problem; the defect is in the superego.

3 There may be a defect in sexual attitudes but not in sexual development.

40. **2 A sincere, cautious, and consistent attitude limits this individual's ability to manipulate both situations and staff members. (3) (PI; CJ; PL; PR)**

1 An attitude such as this would allow the client to rationalize the manipulative behavior to deal with the response of the nurse.

3 In accepting the person, the nurse should not support negative behavior; a friendly attitude may encourage further problem behavior.

4 This would encourage clients to continue in their lifestyle rather than learn appropriate ways to relate to their environment.

41. **4 This accepts the client while rejecting and setting limits on the behavior the client is using. (2) (PI; CJ; IM; PR)**

1 This encourages this type of behavior instead of setting limits.

2 This sends a confusing message to the client because it is unclear what the nurse did not like.

3 This rejects the client instead of the behavior.

42. **4 Antipsychotic/neuroleptic medications help control anxiety and acting-out behavior, making the client more approachable. (3) (PB; CJ; AN; DR)**

1 Although the medication may produce this effect, it is not the primary purpose of administration.

2 Same as answer 1.

3 Same as answer 1.

43. **1 The person transfers anxieties to activities or objects, usually inanimate objects, which are then avoided to decrease anxiety. (1) (PI; CJ; AN; AX)**

2 Regression, the return to an earlier, more comfortable level of development, is not the defense mechanism used by someone with a phobia.

3 Repression, the pushing of unacceptable impulses or ideas into the unconscious, is not the defense mechanism used by someone with a phobia.

4 Conversion, the transferring of a mental conflict into a physical symptom, is not the defense mechanism used by someone with a phobia.

44. **3 Client safety always has the highest priority over any other client needs. (1) (SE; CJ; PL; SD)**

1 Although important, this diagnosis is not a priority at this time.

2 Same as answer 1.

4 Same as answer 1.

45. **2 Sobriety may alter how the alcoholic perceives the self and others, which can influence relationships; people who need to feel needed or who have assumed the role of the enabler may find this role altered as the alcohol abuser begins to change during recovery. (3) (PI; CJ; AN; SA)**

1 There are no data to support this nursing diagnosis.

3 There is no indication that there are negative feelings about the self or self-capabilities.

4 Same as answer 1.

46. **2 The nurse is making an observation; bringing it to the attention of the client is an initial step in understanding that behavior. (1) (PI; CJ; IM; TR)**

1 This is premature because the client may not even be aware of anxiety.

3 This is requesting a response that the client probably is incapable of explaining.

4 This is premature and does not allow for self-recognition of feelings.

47. **4 This action still permits the client to deal with feelings of anxiety while aiming to reduce skin damage. (2) (PB; CJ; AN; PR)**

1 The anxiety is too great for the client to understand why handwashing is not necessary.

2 This will not allow the client any outlet for dealing with extreme anxiety, which is the priority need at this time.

3 Recognition must precede the development of insight; neither can be done until the level of anxiety is reduced.

48. **3 In an attempt to block the hospital staff from discovering what happened, abusing parents often provide inconsistent accounts. (3) (PI; CJ; AS; CS)**

1 This may or may not occur.

2 Abusing parents tend to show more concern about how the child's condition affects them than about how the child is affected.

4 Abusing parents tend to be vague about the details of the accident but maintain the child was accidentally injured.

49. **1 This type of leader stimulates, guides, and assists the group to develop its maximum potential by facilitating and balancing group forces. (2) (SE; MR; AN; TR)**

2 This type of leader makes most of the decisions and controls the group, thus limiting group growth potential.

3 This type of leader allows group members to take over the group; if there are no members with leadership skills, little is gained from the group.

4 Democratic leadership allows for group growth, but controlling leadership limits it.

50. **1 An accepted practice in some parts of the world may well be considered abnormal behavior in others. (2) (SE; CJ; AN; PD)**

2 People need relief from tension from time to time and make use of defense mechanisms to accomplish this.

3 Thoughts and feelings are under unconscious control and are seldom accurately expressed by behavior; they may be expressed in dreams.

4 If the behavior were aggressive or destructive, even though it helped reach a goal, it could not be considered normal.

1. A client, who is admitted to the hospital for an elective prostatectomy, is extremely anxious and has hand tremors. The client's wife informs the nurse that the client has been drinking heavily for the last 5 years. While the client is unpacking his suitcase, the nurse notices him hiding a bottle of whiskey in the rear of the drawer. The nurse's responsibility in relation to the alcohol includes:
   1. Trying to catch the client drinking the alcohol
   2. Confiscating the alcohol when the client is not looking
   3. Waiting for the client to bring up the subject of drinking
   4. Asking the client how much alcohol he drinks in a week

2. When a female client who has pressured speech mumbles incoherently, the most appropriate intervention would be for the nurse to:
   1. Set limits on the client's behavior by refusing to talk with her unless she speaks clearly
   2. Ignore the client's mumbling since she is using this pathologic manner of speech to get attention
   3. Consistently ask the client to repeat what she said, so she will learn to recognize she is mumbling
   4. Indicate to the client that she needs to slow down because what she says is important and cannot be understood

3. A 16-year-old, arrested for assault and robbery, has a history of truancy and prostitution. The client demonstrates little emotion and is unconcerned that this behavior has caused emotional distress to others. The diagnosis of antisocial personality disorder is made. According to psychoanalytic theory, the client's lack of remorse and repetitive behavior is probably related to an underdeveloped:
   1. Id
   2. Ego
   3. Superego
   4. Limbic system

4. The nurse can be most therapeutic when approaching an autistic toddler who is sitting in a corner rocking and spinning a top by:
   1. Gently stroking the toddler's arm to gain the child's attention

2. Sitting down and staring at the spinning top with the toddler
   3. Holding the toddler to provide a sense of support and security
   4. Waiting for the toddler to make the initial contact before moving close

5. When developing a plan of care for a client who is using ritualistic behavior, the nurse must recognize that the ritual:
   1. Is under conscious control
   2. Is used primarily for secondary gains
   3. Helps the client control the level of anxiety experienced
   4. Helps the client to focus on the inability to deal with reality

6. The nurse is aware that the level of achievement at 20 years of age, according to Erikson's developmental stages, should be:
   1. Having the capacity for love and a commitment to work
   2. Being creative and productive and having concern for others
   3. Having a coherent sense of self and plans for self-actualization
   4. Accepting the worth, integrity, and uniqueness of one's past and present life

7. A depressed client is brought to the emergency department after taking an overdose of a sedative. After a lavage, the client states, "Let me die. I'm no good." The nurse's most appropriate response would be:
   1. "Do you feel like telling me why you did this?"
   2. "Of course you're good; we'll take care of you."
   3. "You must have been upset to try to take your life."
   4. "You have been through a rough time; let me take care of you."

8. Clients receiving electroconvulsive therapy are usually given a muscle relaxant just before the treatment. The major disadvantage of this drug is that it inhibits the:
   1. Biceps and triceps muscles
   2. Facial and thoracic muscles
   3. Intercostal and diaphragmatic muscles
   4. Sternocleidomastoid and abdominal muscles

9. When planning care for a confused or delusional client, it is most important for the nurse to:
   1. Maintain quiet, dim surroundings to minimize stimuli
   2. Encourage realistic activity considering the client's ability
   3. Recognize that the client is unable to differentiate fantasy from reality
   4. Provide physical hygiene and comfort to demonstrate that the client is worthy of receiving care

10. A client is receiving an antipsychotic drug bid. Two thirds of the daily dose is given in the evening, one third in the morning. This is done to:
    1. Maintain diurnal rhythms
    2. Help the client sleep at night
    3. Reduce sedation during the daytime
    4. Decrease assaultiveness in the evening

11. In her eighth month of pregnancy, a 24-year-old client is brought to the hospital by the police, who were called when she barricaded herself in a ladies restroom of a restaurant. During the admission, the client shouts, "Don't come near me! My stomach is filled with bombs, and I'll blow up this place if anyone comes near me." This is an example of:
    1. Ideas of reference
    2. Loose associations
    3. Delusional thinking
    4. Tactile hallucinations

12. A client who appears dejected, barely responds to questions, and walks very slowly about the mental health unit tells the nurse in a barely audible voice that life is no longer worth living. The nurse's most therapeutic response to this statement would be:
    1. "Have you been thinking about suicide?"
    2. "What could be so bad to make you feel that way?"
    3. "We'll talk about your feelings after you have rested."
    4. "Let's talk about something pleasant, and you'll feel better."

13. A client with a diagnosis of bipolar I disorder, manic episode, is started on a regimen of an antipsychotic agent and lithium carbonate. The nurse is aware that the rationale behind this regimen is that the antipsychotic:
    1. Potentiates the action of lithium for more effective results
    2. Interacts with lithium to prevent progression to the depressive phase
    3. Acts to quiet the client while allowing time for the lithium to take effect
    4. Helps decrease the incidence of lithium toxicity in the first week of therapy

14. After detoxification, a client with a long history of alcohol abuse has agreed to attend Alcoholics Anonymous meetings at the hospital. On the day of the second meeting, the client states, "I cannot attend the AA meeting today because I am expecting an important phone call." The nurse's most therapeutic response would be:
    1. "You are expected to go to the meeting."
    2. "Is your phone call really that important?"
    3. "Go to the meeting after you receive the call."
    4. "You can wait for the call and skip the meeting."

15. A client describes delusional material in minute detail to the nurse. The nurse should:
    1. Get the client involved in a repetitive project
    2. Accept this as the client's reality without argument
    3. Encourage the client to continue to discuss the delusional material
    4. Change the topic as soon as the client begins to discuss delusional material

16. A disturbed client who has been out of touch with reality has been hospitalized for several weeks. One day the nurse notes the client's hair is dirty and asks whether the client would like to wash it. The client answers, "Yes, and I'd like to shower and change my clothes, too." The nurse uses this information to assess that the client:
    1. Is open to suggestions
    2. Has some feelings of self-worth
    3. May be entering a hyperactive phase
    4. Has a need for social reassurance and approval

17. A hyperactive client becomes loud and insulting and says to a staff member, "Get lost, you old buzzard!" The nurse could best handle this situation by:
    1. Telling the client that it is not necessary to be so rude
    2. Saying, "Here is something I feel you might be interested in."
    3. Pointing out that the staff member is neither old nor a buzzard
    4. Asking the client, "Could you please tell me why you are so angry?"

18. Thirty minutes after administering fluphenazine (Prolixin) to a client, the nurse notices the client's jaw is rigid, the tongue is thick, the client is drooling, and speech is slurred. There are a number of prn orders in the client's chart. The nurse should administer:
    1. Haloperidol (Haldol), 2 mg IM
    2. Diazepam (Valium), 10 mg PO
    3. Benztropine (Cogentin), 2 mg IM
    4. Trihexyphenidyl (Artane), 1 mg PO

19. The nurse understands that the unconscious basis of an obsessive-compulsive disorder is often:
    1. Feelings of guilt and inadequacy
    2. Problems with anger and remorse
    3. Problems with being too conscientious
    4. Feelings of unworthiness and hopelessness

20. A client with an obsessive-compulsive disorder continually walks up and down the hall, touching every other chair. If unable to do this, the client becomes upset. The nurse should:
    1. Keep talking to distract the client, which will help the client forget about touching the chairs
    2. Allow the client to continue to touch the chairs as long as desired and wait until fatigue sets in
    3. Remove all chairs from the hall, thereby relieving the client of the necessity to touch every other one
    4. Allow the behavior to continue for a specified time, letting the client help set the time limits to be imposed

21. To begin to establish a therapeutic relationship with a withdrawn, reclusive client, the nurse must:
    1. Obtain a complete history from the family
    2. Plan to keep the client's anxiety at a minimum
    3. Ascertain what topics are of interest to the client
    4. Protect the client from self-destructive tendencies or injury

22. The nurse understands that vascular dementia results from:
    1. A long history of poor nutrition and associated avitaminosis
    2. Disruptions in the cerebral blood flow resulting in thrombi or emboli
    3. A delayed response to severe emotional trauma in early adulthood
    4. Anatomic changes in the brain that produce acute but transient symptoms

23. The parents of an infant born with a unilateral cleft lip and palate are very concerned about the defect and ask the nurse, "What caused our baby to be born deformed?" The nurse should reply:
    1. "Are you feeling guilty?"
    2. "I'm glad that you are able to ask these kinds of questions."
    3. "I don't know, but you don't need to worry because surgery can correct it."
    4. "It sounds as if you are wondering what you might have done to cause this situation."

24. When caring for a client with a somatoform disorder, conversion-type paralysis, the nurse should:
    1. Avoid discussing the paralysis
    2. Explain the reason for the paralysis
    3. Ask how the client feels about being paralyzed
    4. Encourage the client to get up, pointing out that walking is possible

25. A client with bulimia nervosa eats two sandwiches, two salads, and four desserts for lunch. After the meal the nurse would expect to observe the client:
    1. Performing excessive exercises
    2. Hoarding more food for a later binge
    3. Withdrawing from the group to the bathroom
    4. Actively socializing with small groups of clients

26. A client who has been sexually assaulted and is aware of the possible legal implications decides to prosecute the rapist. The nurse carefully listens and documents all observations. This is done because with a charge of rape the burden of proof:
    1. Rests with the rape victim
    2. Rests with the health team
    3. Is on the defendant to prove innocence
    4. Must be established before the case will be heard

27. When the nurse enters the room to administer medication to an agitated and angry client with schizophrenia, paranoid type, the client shouts, "Get out of here!" The nurse should:
    1. State, "You must take your medicine now."
    2. Say, "I'll be back in 15 minutes and we can talk."
    3. Explain why it is necessary to take the medication
    4. Get assistance and give the medication by injection

28. When talking with the nurse, a client with a mood disorder states, "I feel rotten and useless. I cannot think straight. I feel overwhelmed by everything. I don't know if I can go on." When recording this encounter in the client's record, the most objective description of the client's mood would be:
    1. Client is not able to cope with problems and this hospitalization; states, "I cannot think straight."
    2. Client appeared to be very depressed for most of the morning. Little interest in self or environment
    3. Client stated, "I feel rotten and useless. I feel overwhelmed by everything. I don't know if I can go on."
    4. Client expressed suicidal thoughts about not being able to go on and has decreased ability to think clearly

29. A client who is going to occupational therapy for the first time tells the nurse, "I do not want to go." The nurse, taking the client's diagnosis of schizophrenia into consideration, could best help the client by stating:
    1. "I will go with you to occupational therapy."
    2. "It is only for 1 hour, then you will be back."
    3. "Try it once; if you don't like it, you need not go back."
    4. "The doctor ordered it as part of your treatment. You should go."

30. A client is to begin lithium carbonate therapy. The nurse should ensure that prior to the drug's administration the client should have baseline:
    1. Renal studies
    2. Enzyme studies
    3. Neurologic studies
    4. Fluid and electrolyte studies

31. After lunch one afternoon, the nurse notes that a client with the symptoms of dementia is alone in the dayroom away from other clients. When the nurse approaches, the client says, "I am all alone. No one has any use for me." The response by the nurse that would be most appropriate at this time would be:
    1. "You seem upset. Would you like to tell me what is bothering you?"
    2. "We need to be alone sometimes. It helps us get to know ourselves better."
    3. "You should focus on ways to change this. Let's play some games to improve your morale."
    4. "Have you done anything to avoid feeling lonely? I think you should socialize more with others."

32. A 5-year-old with an attention-deficit/hyperactivity disorder (ADHD) exhibits a short attention span and demonstrates intermittent head banging, hair pulling, and excessive motor activity. The most important nursing diagnosis for this child at this time would be:
    1. Anxiety related to shortened attention span
    2. Disturbed sleep pattern related to hyperactivity
    3. Disturbed body image related to acting-out behavior
    4. Risk for self-directed violence related to self-destructive behavior

33. An older male is widowed suddenly when his wife is killed in an automobile accident. The first action by the nurse in the emergency department to best help the client at this time would be:
    1. Asking a member of the clergy to visit him
    2. Having the physician order a sedative for him
    3. Referring him to a support group that meets near his home
    4. Assuring him that everything possible was done for his wife

34. The nurse should be aware that the statement by a client that would indicate an irreversible adverse response to long-term therapy with an antipsychotic medication would be:
    1. "My mouth is always dry."
    2. "I'm not eating like I should."
    3. "I can't seem to sleep at night."
    4. "My tongue and lips move themselves."

35. The staff of the psychiatric unit conducts a biweekly orientation meeting for newly admitted clients. When planning for this meeting, the nurse recognizes that the beginning of the meeting should be directed toward defining the:
    1. Rules for client behavior
    2. Purpose of the group meeting
    3. Clients' role and the leader's expectations
    4. Development of trust between staff and clients

36. A disturbed client remains aloof and ridicules and is sarcastic to other clients. The client identifies with and only will respond to the staff. The care plan at this time should include:
    1. Encouraging group participation with withdrawn clients
    2. Assigning the client activities to be carried out with the staff
    3. Explaining that the client should be more accepting of others
    4. Accepting the client's negative behavior; praising positive responses

37. When a therapy group is achieving its objective, the nurse leader would expect to observe that all members:
    1. Now attend every session of the group
    2. Comment on each topic discussed by the group
    3. Follow through on obeying rules governing behavior
    4. Make an effort to include each other in the discussion

38. During crisis intervention therapy, it is most important for the nurse to assume the:
    1. Passive listener role
    2. Friendly adviser role
    3. Active participant role
    4. Participant observer role

39. The assessment that would cause the nurse to stop giving haloperidol (Haldol) to a client until further laboratory work was done would be:
    1. Grimacing
    2. Shuffling gait
    3. Yellow sclerae
    4. Photosensitivity

40. A client, who is to have a mastectomy for cancer of the breast, tells the nurse that she is worried about what she will look like after the surgery. The nurse's most appropriate initial response would be:
    1. "Try not to think about the surgery now."
    2. "I can understand that you'd be concerned."
    3. "Everyone having this surgery feels the same way."
    4. "Why don't you discuss this with your husband?"

41. A client comes to the mental health clinic complaining about feelings of extreme terror when attempting to ride in an elevator and feeling very uneasy in large crowds. The client feels uncomfortable about these fears and is beginning to experience difficulty concentrating at work. When assessing the situation, the nurse should understand that the client's symptoms are probably associated with:
    1. The development of an obsession as a result of conflicts with society
    2. Depression about life events, which frequently leads to unreasonable fears
    3. A terrifying incident in an elevator in the past that has been repressed but unresolved
    4. Generalized anxiety about conflicts that has been displaced into specific unreasonable fears

42. A husband and wife are admitted to the trauma unit with gunshot wounds sustained in a robbery. Shortly after admission, the husband dies from his wounds. A potential nursing diagnosis for the wife, related to the death of the husband, would be:
    1. Ineffective coping
    2. Impaired adjustment
    3. Disturbed personal identity
    4. Interrupted family processes

43. A 30-year-old high school dropout, who is employed as a dishwasher, and his 37-year-old wife of 9 years have five children between the ages of 2 months and 8 years. He has a long history of drinking heavily, especially on weekends, and it takes little or no provocation to send him into a rage, yelling obscenities, throwing and breaking furniture, and occasionally hitting his wife and the older children. The nurse recognizes that this abusive behavior is probably related to the client's:
    1. Feeling trapped in a marriage
    2. Living in the culture of poverty
    3. Low socioeconomic background
    4. Long-standing problem with alcohol

44. A client with symptoms of manic behavior has pressured speech punctuated with profanity. It would be most therapeutic for the nurse to deal with this client's behavior by:
    1. Thoroughly explaining the type of behavior allowed in the facility
    2. Encouraging interaction with another client who is exhibiting similar behavior
    3. Quietly stating that the use of profanity is unbecoming and will not be tolerated
    4. Allowing for the expression of hostility in a safe manner without being judgmental

45. A 3-year-old child is admitted to a children's mental health unit with a diagnosis of infantile autism. The major goal of therapy for a child with this pervasive developmental disorder would be, the child will:
    1. Develop language skills
    2. Limit the use of regressive behavior
    3. Be mainstreamed into a regular preschool group
    4. Recognize the self as an independent person of worth

46. A client with the diagnosis of an antisocial personality disorder responds to a rebuff by a nurse by saying, "You sure do look messy today." The most appropriate response by the nurse would be:
    1. "Don't you feel well today?"
    2. "That's not a nice thing to say."
    3. "I get the feeling you're angry with me."
    4. "I really didn't think anyone would notice."

47. A nurse who has been working with a client with the diagnosis of borderline personality disorder is leaving for vacation in 2 weeks and tells the client. The nurse would recognize progress in the ability to maintain more mature relationships if the client:
    1. States, "I must get well enough by then so I can also leave."
    2. Wishes the nurse a safe trip and offers thanks for the help received
    3. Responds, "I guess your leaving is just another loss I must adjust to."
    4. Informs the nurse that there is no sense in waiting 2 weeks; the relationship can end today.

48. When a 4-year-old child is admitted to the hospital with traumatic injuries, a common clue that physical maltreatment has occurred is that the child:
    1. Does not cry during painful procedures
    2. Shows no expectation of being comforted
    3. Cries for long periods and has large hematomas
    4. Ignores offers of toys and favors and cries when picked up

49. The nurse's first action when a schizophrenic client, who was admitted to a psychiatric facility involuntarily, runs away would be to notify the:
    1. Law enforcement officers of the client's elopement
    2. Client's family that the client has left the hospital
    3. Client's psychiatrist after discovering the client has gone
    4. Physicians who certified the client's need for hospitalization

50. A client receiving risperidone (Risperdal) is going on an all-day fishing outing with family members. It is important that the nurse:
    1. Provide the client with sunscreen ointment
    2. Caution the client to avoid excessive activity and overexertion
    3. Give the client an additional dose of medication to take after lunch
    4. Take the client's blood pressure before allowing the family to leave with the client

Mental Health Nursing Quiz 2 Answers and Rationales

1. 4 **This assesses the client's level of alcohol abuse by direct questioning. (2) (SE; MR; AS; SA)**
   1 This is a judgmental approach that uses manipulation and decreases the client's self-esteem.
   2 This is not straightforward and will decrease trust.
   3 The client probably would not bring up the subject because denial is often used to cope with alcohol abuse.

2. 4 **This response provides feedback, which helps communication stay focused and demonstrates an interest in the client as a person. (2) (PI; CJ; IM; MO)**
   1 This response would not set limits but would create feelings of rejection.
   2 Ignoring the client communicates the nurse's lack of interest and concern.
   3 This response would only increase the client's anxiety and anger; it may precipitate acting-out behavior.

3. 3 **Lack of remorse indicates a weak superego, the aspect of personality concerned with prohibitions. (2) (PI; CJ; AN; PR)**
   1 This aspect of personality is not underdeveloped in this person; the id acts to achieve self-gratification.
   2 The ego is not related to acting-out behavior.
   4 This is not underdeveloped; it is related to achieving pleasure.

4. 2 **Autistic children relate best with objects, which can be used as a bridge in interpersonal relationships; this begins at the child's level. (2) (PI; CJ; IM; BA)**
   1 Autistic children usually have difficulty tolerating being touched.
   3 Autistic children often become agitated when movement is restricted and personal space is invaded.
   4 Autistic children will not initiate contact or interactions.

5. 3 **The rituals help control anxiety by maintaining a set pattern of action. (2) (PI; CJ; PL; PR)**
   1 The reason for the ritual is under unconscious control.
   2 Rituals generally are seen by the client as illogical; they provide few secondary gains.

4 Rituals are a means of diverting attention from this anxiety-producing inability.

6. 1 **Young adults, ages 18 to 35, should be developing meaningful relationships and establishing themselves in a career. (1) (PM; CJ; AN; PD)**
   2 The stage of adulthood (generativity versus stagnation) is concerned with productivity, nurturance, and support of the next generation.
   3 Having a coherent sense of self is a task of adolescence.
   4 From age 65 to death, the individual should experience a feeling of the worth of one's life.

7. 3 **Showing understanding of and identifying the client's feelings by giving feedback helps in establishing a therapeutic relationship. (2) (PI; CJ; IM; MO)**
   1 This is too direct; it does not allow the client time to reflect and explore feelings.
   2 This negates the person's feelings and cuts off any further communication of feelings.
   4 This encourages dependence; it does not allow for exploration of feelings.

8. 3 **Succinylcholine (Anectine) causes paralysis of muscles, including the intercostals and diaphragm, so artificial support of respirations is required to sustain life. (1) (PB; CJ; AN; DR)**
   1 This is the purpose of the drug, not a disadvantage.
   2 Same as answer 1.
   4 Same as answer 1.

9. 2 **These clients need sensory stimulation to maintain orientation and should be encouraged to do as much as possible for themselves, depending on their ability. (3) (PI; CJ; PL; SD)**
   1 Surroundings should be bright to minimize confusion.
   3 These clients are usually not completely out of contact with reality; it is important to differentiate fantasy from reality, but this would not take top priority in care.
   4 Although it is important to make certain that clients receive physical hygiene and comfort, they should be encouraged to help themselves as much as possible.

10. 3 **Antipsychotic drugs tend to make the client listless or drowsy and can interfere with the ability to participate in the therapeutic regimen. (2) (PB; CJ; AN; SD)**
   1 Antipsychotic drugs do not appreciably affect diurnal rhythms.
   2 Antipsychotic drugs do not induce sleep, just listlessness.
   4 Assaultiveness is associated with increased anxiety and is unrelated to time.

11. 3 **Delusions are false fixed beliefs that have a minimal reality base. (1) (PI; CJ; AN; SD)**
   1 Ideas of reference are false beliefs that every statement or action of others relates to the individual.
   2 Loose associations are verbalizations that sound disjointed to the listener.
   4 Tactile hallucinations are false sensory perceptions of touch without external stimuli.

12. 1 **It is important to determine whether the client is thinking about suicide; the direct approach is most appropriate. (1) (PI; MR; AS; MO)**
   2 This response not only denies feelings but also tells the client it is not right to feel that way.
   3 This response indicates that the client's feelings do not have top priority.
   4 This response denies the client's feelings and offers false reassurance.

13. 3 **Antipsychotics usually are prescribed to calm agitated clients during the three-week period it takes for the lithium to become effective. (3) (PB; CJ; AN; DR)**
   1 Antipsychotic drugs have a different, not a potentiating, mechanism of action.
   2 The drugs are used to control symptoms of mania, not to prevent depression.
   4 The neuroleptic drug has no effect on lithium toxicity.

14. 1 **This helps the client recognize and adhere to established limits and goals. (2) (PI; CJ; IM; SA)**
   2 This response can be degrading and reinforces the client's manipulative behavior.
   3 This reinforces the client's pattern of manipulation.
   4 Same as answer 3.

15. 2 **The delusional client can never be argued out of a delusion because it serves as a defense against reality and is the client's reality; it is best to accept the delusion without discussion. (3) (PI; CJ; IM; SD)**
   1 The client would have difficulty getting involved in a repetitive activity; the activity would not stop the delusion.

   3 Encouraging discussion would give validity to the delusion.
   4 This action can lead to increased feelings of guilt about the delusion because the client will not understand why the nurse is changing the topic.

16. 2 **When individuals express interest in physical appearance, it demonstrates a rebuilding of the self-image and the return of feelings of worth and concern for how others see them. (1) (PI; CJ; EV; SD)**
   1 The client's response goes further than the nurse's implied suggestion; this is an expression of the client's needs, not the nurse's.
   3 The client's response is well within the normal range; it does not indicate the beginning of a hyperactive phase.
   4 The information provided does not demonstrate a need for social reassurance or approval.

17. 2 **Clients in the manic phase of a bipolar I disorder are easily distracted; rather than placing emphasis on their behavior, staff members should use the easy distractibility of these clients to redirect this behavior to more constructive channels. (1) (PI; CJ; IM; MO)**
   1 This focuses on the behavior; it is a punitive response that does not foster communication.
   3 This encourages the client to defend the statement; it does not foster communication about feelings.
   4 The client would be unable to explain the basis for the expressed anger to the nurse.

18. 3 **Cogentin is an anticholinergic, antiparkinsonian drug used to treat drug-induced extrapyramidal symptoms associated with phenothiazine therapy; the IM route would reduce symptoms more rapidly. (2) (PI; MR; IM; DR)**
   1 This medication would produce parkinsonism, not relieve it.
   2 This medication is not effective in reducing extrapyramidal adaptations.
   4 While Artane is an appropriate medication, swallowing pills would be difficult for the client; the oral medication should not be administered.

19. 1 **Ritualistic behavior is aimed at controlling guilt and inadequacy by maintaining an absolute set pattern of action. (2) (PI; CJ; AS; PR)**
   2 These are not the major bases for this disorder.
   3 The behavior and attitudes of clients with this disorder are contradictory; they are conscientious about some things and lax about others.
   4 Same as answer 2.

20. **4 It is important to set limits on the behavior, but it is also important to involve the client in the decision making. (3) (PI; CJ; IM; PR)**
  1 This would be nontherapeutic; rarely can a client be distracted from a ritual.
  2 This is a nontherapeutic approach; some limits must be set by the client and nurse together.
  3 This would increase anxiety because the client uses the ritual as a defense against anxiety.

21. **2 When a client who is unable to cope feels that someone is assuming control, it promotes a feeling of security; as this continues, a sense of trust in this individual is established. (3) (PI; CJ; IM; SD)**
  1 This would be important in planning care but not in establishing a therapeutic relationship.
  3 This is less important in the beginning phase of a relationship.
  4 The client does not exhibit self-destructive tendencies at this time.

22. **2 Vascular dementia results from the sudden closure of the lumen of arterioles, causing infarction of the brain tissue in the affected area. (3) (PB; CJ; AS; DD)**
  1 Inadequate nutrition may be one of the factors that brings about a general decline of health; however, there is no direct evidence that avitaminosis causes primary degenerative dementia.
  3 Severe emotional trauma may contribute to but does not necessarily cause primary degenerative dementia.
  4 Neural degeneration leads to permanent, not transient, changes.

23. **4 An almost universal reaction to the birth of an imperfect child is guilt; encouraging the parents to discuss such feelings, without actually asking whether they feel guilty, provides an opportunity to express such thoughts. (2) (PI; CJ; IM; CS)**
  1 This statement lacks sensitivity to the parents' feelings.
  2 This statement does not focus on the actual concern the parents are expressing.
  3 This statement cuts off the parents' expression of feelings.

24. **1 Discussion should not be initiated by the nurse; symptoms should be accepted but should not be the focus of discussion. (3) (PI; CJ; PL; AX)**
  2 This response would take away the client's unconscious defense and increase anxiety.

  3 This response would increase anxiety because it focuses on unconscious feelings about the paralysis.
  4 This response denies the client's symptoms; in reality this client cannot make the legs move to walk.

25. **3 Bulimia is characterized by the binge-purge cycle; most clients withdraw from others and vomit after an eating binge. (2) (PI; CJ; AS; ES)**
  1 Although some individuals with bulimia may perform excessive exercises, this is a more common finding with the diagnosis of anorexia nervosa.
  2 Although individuals with bulimia may hoard food, this behavior commonly occurs later, when limits are put on their intake.
  4 Most individuals with bulimia do not seek support or socialization after a binge, although they may socialize at other times.

26. **1 When the person who has been sexually assaulted chooses to prosecute the rapist, the victim must prove that rape occurred; the accused is innocent until proven guilty. (1) (SE; LE; AN; NP)**
  2 The medical team may be asked to provide evidence at the trial, but the victim must prove that the rapist is guilty.
  3 The perpetrator tries to establish innocence in a rape case; the victim must prove that the rapist is guilty.
  4 Guilt or innocence will be established by a jury, with the burden of proof placed on the victim.

27. **2 This allows the angry client time to regain self-control; announcing a plan to return decreases fear of abandonment or retribution. (3) (PI; CJ; IM; SD)**
  1 Staying and insisting that the client take the medication may provoke increased anger and further loss of control.
  3 Clients will not accept logical explanations when angry.
  4 This approach shows no respect for the client's feelings; it may decrease trust and increase anger.

28. **3 This statement directly quotes the client with no added value judgments. (2) (SE; LE; AS; NP)**
  1 This is a subjective judgment and an interpretation of what the client actually said.
  2 Same as answer 1.
  4 Same as answer 1.

29. 1 This statement indicates that the nurse sees the client as a person and is willing to help the client face a new experience. (2) (PI; CJ; IM; SD)

   2 This will do nothing to allay the client's anxiety about facing a new situation.

   3 Even if the client does not like it, it is part of the therapy program and the client should be encouraged to go.

   4 Same as answer 2.

30. 1 Because of the severity of side effects and the stress lithium places on the renal as well as the cardiovascular system, its administration is contraindicated in clients with renal or cardiovascular disease. (2) (PB; CJ; AS; DR)

   2 This is necessary after the start of lithium administration.

   3 This is not necessary; lithium does not alter neurologic functions.

   4 Same as answer 2.

31. 1 This is a therapeutic approach that indicates awareness of the client's feelings and encourages verbalizations. (1) (PI; CJ; IM; TR)

   2 Moralizing is a roadblock to effective communication.

   3 This is diverting the client's attention to something else and ignoring the client's attempt to verbalize.

   4 This conveys a judgmental or critical attitude toward the client's actions.

32. 4 Excessive motor activity with intermittent head banging and hair pulling is self-destructive behavior that can result in injury; prevention of self-injury has the highest priority. (1) (SE; CJ; AN; BA)

   1 This is not the most important nursing diagnosis according to the data presented; prevention of self-injury is primary.

   2 Same as answer 1.

   3 Same as answer 1.

33. 4 This assurance helps allay guilt, reduces anxiety, and assists with coping. (3) (PI; CJ; IM; CS)

   1 The client should be consulted before a clergyman is called.

   2 This could delay the grieving process.

   3 It is too soon for this intervention.

34. 4 This is characteristic of tardive dyskinesia, an irreversible, antipsychotic, drug-induced, neurologic disorder. (2) (PB; CJ; EV; DR)

   1 This is an anticholinergic-like side effect that is not considered serious.

   2 This is unrelated to antipsychotic medications.

   3 This drug would cause sedation, not insomnia.

35. 2 Clients should know why they are there, what to expect, and what is to be accomplished. (1) (SE; MR; PL; TR)

   1 This would come after the explanation of the purpose of the group.

   3 Same as answer 1.

   4 This is not necessary to define; this is a goal.

36. 4 When the client realizes that staff are not responding to negative behaviors but are providing praise for positive accomplishments, the client's behavior should change, since recognition and self-esteem will have been gained for socially acceptable behavior. (2) (PI; CJ; PL; SD)

   1 The withdrawn clients must be protected from the client's ridicule and sarcasm just as this client must be protected.

   2 This is unrealistic because a goal is to function again in society.

   3 This is expecting too much of the client at the present time.

37. 4 This shows an increase in socialization and an awareness of the behavior of others. (2) (SE; MR; EV; TR)

   1 Attendance alone is insufficient to evaluate the effectiveness of group therapy.

   2 The quantity and extent of comments are not what are significant.

   3 This may indicate a greater degree of impulse control on the part of the members, which is not the primary goal of group therapy.

38. 3 To intervene in a crisis the nurse must assume a direct, active role because the client's abilities to cope are lessened and help is needed to problem-solve. (2) (PI; CJ; PL; CS)

   1 This would be insufficient to help the client.

   2 The role of the nurse should not include giving advice; this promotes dependence.

   4 Same as answer 1.

39. 3 Yellow sclerae are a sign of jaundice, indicating an elevation of liver enzymes, which may be irreversible even if drug therapy is discontinued. (2) (PB; CJ; EV; DR)

   1 Although this may be a sign of a serious side effect, it may just be a behavioral response of the disorder; the nurse should notify the physician rather than withhold the drug.

   2 This is a Parkinson-type syndrome, which can be reversed with treatment; continuation of medication is permitted.

   4 Photosensitivity is not a problem as long as the client is cautioned to stay out of the sun.

40. 2 **Women facing breast surgery often have many feelings relating to their sexuality, change in body image, etc.; the nurse plays a vital role in helping the client verbalize feelings, and this response keeps channels of communication open. (2) (PB; CJ; IM; CS)**

1 The client's concerns are real, and such a statement will only block further communication.

3 This does not focus on the importance of the client as an individual; each person feels differently.

4 This can be interpreted as the nurse's reluctance to listen; the client may not be able to talk with the husband about this.

41. 4 **Phobias are specific fears that serve as a means of coping with generalized anxiety. (2) (PI; CJ; AN; AX)**

1 Anxiety, not obsession, is related to phobias.

2 Anxiety, not depression, is related to phobias; finding a direct connection to life events is often difficult.

3 A direct connection to life events is often difficult to determine.

42. 1 **Because of the shock and trauma associated with the death of her spouse, it is expected that the client may have an alteration in usual coping mechanisms. (2) (PI; CJ; AN; CS)**

2 There are no data that indicate that the wife has a change in health status, which is a major defining characteristic associated with this nursing diagnosis.

3 No information is presented to indicate that the client cannot distinguish between the self and nonself.

4 No family is mentioned in the situation.

43. 4 **Alcohol often reduces inhibitions and is one of the leading causes of violent behavior. (1) (PI; CJ; AS; SA)**

1 This factor alone rarely precipitates abusive behavior.

2 Same as answer 1.

3 Same as answer 1.

44. 4 **This shows acceptance and protects the client and others from possible aggressive behavior. (2) (PI; CJ; PL; MO)**

1 Explanations are not helpful because the client's easy distractibility interferes with understanding.

2 Both clients would be very responsive to external stimuli; therefore this action could lead to loss of control for both.

3 This is a threatening approach that increases feelings of inadequacy.

45. 4 **In autism, the child does not have a self-concept or view the self as separate; until this goal is attained other therapies will produce little or no positive outcomes. (2) (PI; CJ; AN; BA)**

1 The child with autism may have language skills but usually does not use them; nonverbal behavior is most generally associated with autism.

2 Regressive behavior should be anticipated as the child undergoes therapy, especially when working through earlier phases of development.

3 To be mainstreamed, the child must first have a developing independence.

46. 3 **This helps the client focus on feelings rather than pointing out that the current behavior is unacceptable. (2) (PI; CJ; IM; PR)**

1 This gives the client an alibi for unacceptable behavior.

2 This points out the behavior in a negative way.

4 The nurse is becoming defensive rather than dealing with the problem directly.

47. 2 **This demonstrates the client's acceptance of the professional role of the nurse as well as the ability to end dependent relationships. (2) (PI; CJ; EV; PR)**

1 This shows an inability to relate to other staff members involved with the client's care.

3 This still shows the existence of manipulation on the client's part.

4 This shows a childish need to punish the nurse for leaving.

48. 2 **Children who have been physically abused quickly learn that attention-seeking behavior such as crying for comforting provokes more abuse; therefore they learn to accept the maltreatment silently. (2) (PI; CJ; AS; CS)**

1 This may or may not occur.

3 Maltreated children seldom cry.

4 Maltreated children rarely cry; they tend to accept strangers.

49. 1 **Legally it is the responsibility of the staff to notify law enforcement officers so that the client can be returned. (2) (SE; LE; IM; NP)**

2 The staff should notify the family, but it is not the first intervention.

3 Although this would be done, it is not the priority at this time.

4 Although the physicians may appreciate being notified, it is not the first priority.

50. 1 **Risperidone causes photosensitivity, which can be controlled by the use of sunscreens and protective clothing. (1) (PB; CJ; IM; DR)**

2 This is not a necessary precaution when taking this atypical antipsychotic drug; the client should be allowed to participate fully.

3 The medication should be administered as prescribed; additional doses should not be administered.

4 Participating in an outing should not affect the client's blood pressure.

Chapter 5

NURSING PRACTICE (NP)

1. A married couple in their 80s, with grown children, is living independently. The husband has an enlarged prostate and is at times incontinent of urine. He is alert but forgetful. The wife has diabetes, is arthritic, and walks with difficulty. Both need some help with bathing, dressing, and meal preparation. The plan that would appear most suitable for this couple would be to:
   1. Admit them together to a nursing home
   2. Place them together in an assisted-living facility
   3. Keep them in their home with a home health aide
   4. Suggest that they move in with one of their children

2. A client is scheduled for a craniotomy to remove a brain tumor. To prevent the development of cerebral edema after surgery, the nurse should anticipate the use of:
   1. Steroids
   2. Diuretics
   3. Anticonvulsants
   4. Antihypertensives

3. The nurse caring for a client at night insists that the client cannot tolerate the ordered intermittent tube feedings. The primary nurse should first:
   1. Suggest that an antiemetic be prescribed
   2. Change the feeding schedule to omit nights
   3. Request that the type of solution be changed
   4. Gather more data from the night nurse about the technique used

4. Before administering preoperative medication to a client, the nurse should plan to:
   1. Verify the consent
   2. Have the client void
   3. Check the vital signs
   4. Remove the client's dentures

5. The nurse auscultates a client's lungs and hears a fine crackling sound in the left lower lobe during inspiration. If the nurse charts that crackles and rhonchi are heard in the left lower lobe, the notation would be a:
   1. Nursing diagnosis
   2. Wrong interpretation
   3. Accurate nursing assessment
   4. Correct statement if palpation ruled out crepitus

6. The home care nurse makes an initial visit to a 60-year-old widowed client with right ventricular failure who lives with her divorced, drug-addicted daughter and her seven grandchildren. The nurse finds the client feeding a 6-month-old granddaughter and preparing dinner for the rest of the family. A 14-year-old grandson, disabled and in a wheelchair, states his mother is sleeping. The nurse should proceed by:
   1. Sitting down with the client and exchanging identifying data and information
   2. Accepting coffee when offered by the client and socializing for a few minutes
   3. Asking the client whether it is all right to look around the apartment to evaluate environmental conditions
   4. Questioning the client to determine whether there is a private place to take a health history and perform an examination

7. A client refuses to go to the twice-a-day prescribed sessions in physical therapy. The nurse might best approach this problem by:
   1. Having the client observe the progress of a more cooperative client with the same problem
   2. Being the client's advocate and asking the physician whether therapy can be decreased to once daily
   3. Assuring the client that pain medication will be administered before the scheduled physical therapy sessions
   4. Planning a conference with the client, the physical therapist, and the nurse present to discuss the client's feelings

8. A 22-year-old male client with AIDS signs a "do not resuscitate" (DNR) order when he is admitted to the hospital. When respiratory arrest occurs three weeks later, the client is not resuscitated. A true statement about the legal aspects of a DNR order would be:
   1. Age is an important factor in the decision not to resuscitate
   2. The decision not to resuscitate resides with the client's physician
   3. The status of the DNR order is contingent on the policies of the institution
   4. Once the order has been signed, it remains in force for the entire hospitalization

9. A client is scheduled for surgery. Legally, the client may not sign the operative consent if:
   1. Ambivalent feelings regarding the operation are present
   2. Any sedative type of medication has recently been given
   3. A discussion of alternatives with two physicians has not occurred
   4. A complete history and physical has not been performed and recorded

10. A client with ascites is to have a paracentesis and has signed the consent. While the nurse is caring for him, he says that he has changed his mind and no longer wants the procedure. The best initial response by the nurse would be:
    1. "Why did you sign the consent?"
    2. "Can you tell me why you decided to refuse the procedure?"
    3. "You are obviously afraid about something concerning the procedure."
    4. "Although the procedure is very important, I understand why you changed your mind."

11. A nurse stops at the scene of an accident and finds a man with a deep laceration on his hand, a fractured arm and leg, and abdominal pain. The nurse wraps the man's hand in a soiled cloth and drives him to the nearest hospital. The nurse is:
    1. Negligent and can be sued for malpractice
    2. Practicing under guidelines of the Nurse Practice Act
    3. Protected for these actions, in most states, by Good Samaritan legislation
    4. Treating a health problem that can and should be addressed by a physician

12. When meeting the unique preoperative teaching needs of the older adult, the nurse plans a teaching program based on the principle that

learning:
1. Reduces general anxiety
2. Is negatively affected by aging
3. Requires continued reinforcement
4. Necessitates readiness of the learner

13. A client returns to the surgical unit after a liver biopsy. The nurse identifies a moderately large amount of bile-colored drainage on the dressing. The client also complains of right upper quadrant pain. The nurse should:
    1. Medicate the client for pain as ordered
    2. Ensure that the client remains in the supine position
    3. Monitor the client's vital signs every 15 minutes
    4. Notify the physician of the client's status immediately

14. A visitor from a room adjacent to a client asks the nurse what disease the client has. The nurse responds, "I will not discuss any client's illness with you. Are you concerned about it?" This response is based on the nurse's knowledge that to discuss a client's condition with someone not directly involved with that client is an example of:
    1. Libel
    2. Slander
    3. Negligence
    4. Breach of confidentiality

15. When approaching homosexual clients with AIDS, it is most important for nurses to:
    1. Have a strong sense of their own sexual identity
    2. Admit their feelings of uncomfortableness to the clients
    3. Become aware of their own attitudes regarding homosexuality
    4. Pay particular attention to establishing a meaningful rapport

16. During a home visit, the nurse discovers that a child in the household has a disability and has been experiencing convulsions. In addition the child's mother is unresponsive to the child's physical, emotional, or medical needs and seems to provoke convulsive episodes by harsh verbal exchanges with the child. The nurse believes that intervention by an appropriate community resource is indicated. A referral should be made to the:
    1. Outpatient clinic
    2. Hospital pediatric unit
    3. Bureau of child welfare
    4. Bureau of the handicapped

17. A client with AIDS is to receive palliative treatment. A palliative approach would involve planning measures to:
1. Restore the client's health
2. Promote the client's recovery
3. Relieve the client's discomfort
4. Support the client's significant others

GROWTH AND DEVELOPMENT (GD)

18. Developmentally, a 21-year-old male client who has sustained a spinal injury below the level of T6 will most likely have difficulty with:
1. Mastering his environment
2. Identifying with the male role
3. Developing meaningful relationships
4. Differentiating himself from the environment

19. An 82-year-old retired school teacher is admitted to a nursing home. During the physical assessment, the nurse identifies an ocular problem common to persons at this client's developmental level which is:
1. Tropia
2. Myopia
3. Hyperopia
4. Presbyopia

20. The nurse recognizes that a 70-year-old female can best limit further progression of osteoporosis by:
1. Taking supplemental calcium and vitamin D
2. Increasing the consumption of eggs and cheese
3. Increasing the consumption of milk and milk products
4. Taking supplemental magnesium and vitamin E

21. The nurse is aware that a common conflict experienced by the older adult is the conflict between:
1. Youth and old age
2. Retirement and work
3. Independence and dependence
4. The wish to die and the wish to live

22. A day after an explanation of the effects of surgery to create an ileostomy, a 68-year-old male client remarks to the nurse, "It will be difficult for my wife to care for a helpless old man." These comments by the client regarding himself are an example of Erikson's conflict of:
1. Initiative vs guilt
2. Integrity vs despair
3. Industry vs inferiority
4. Generativity vs stagnation

23. An 85-year-old client has just been admitted to a nursing home. The nurse should plan special measures to accommodate age-related sensory losses such as:
1. Difficulty in swallowing
2. Increased sensitivity to heat
3. Diminished sensation of pain
4. Heightened response to stimuli

24. When correcting myths about aging, the nurse should teach that older adults usually have:
1. Periods of confusion
2. An inflexible attitude
3. Some senile dementia
4. A slower reaction time

25. An 80-year-old female is admitted to the hospital because of complications associated with severe dehydration. The client's daughter asks the nurse how her mother could have become dehydrated because she is alert and able to care for herself. The nurse's best response would be:
1. "The body's need for fluid decreases with age because of a change in the body composition."
2. "Access to fluid may be limited and insufficient to meet the daily needs of the older adult."
3. "Memory declines with age, and the older adult may forget to ingest adequate amounts of fluid."
4. "The thirst reflex diminishes with age, and therefore the recognition of the need for fluid is decreased."

26. A 75-year-old female client tells the nurse that she read about a vitamin that may be related to aging because of its relationship to the structure of cell walls and wonders whether she should be taking it. The nurse should recognize that the client is probably referring to:
1. Vitamin A
2. Vitamin C
3. Vitamin E
4. Vitamin B_1

27. After the removal of a cast from a fractured arm, an 82-year-old client is to receive physical therapy. In an older adult, mild exercise is expected to cause respirations to:
1. Increase to 24 breaths per minute
2. Decrease in rate as depth increases
3. Become progressively more difficult
4. Become irregular but stay at 18 breaths per minute

28. Nursing actions for the older adult should include health education and promotion of self-care. When working with the older adult the nurse should:
    1. Encourage exercise and naps
    2. Strengthen the concept of ageism
    3. Reinforce the client's strengths and promote reminiscing
    4. Teach about a high-carbohydrate diet and focus on the present

29. A 90-year-old female resident of a nursing home falls and fractures the proximal end of her right femur. The physician plans to surgically reduce the fracture with an internal fixation device. The general fact about the older adult that the nurse should remember when caring for this client would be that:
    1. Aging causes a lower pain threshold
    2. Physiologic coping defenses are reduced
    3. Most confusional states result from dementia
    4. Older adults psychologically tolerate changes well

30. The nurse is aware that the mental process most sensitive to deterioration with aging seems to be:
    1. Creativity
    2. Judgment
    3. Intelligence
    4. Short-term memory

31. The nurse is preparing a community health program for senior citizens. The nurse teaches the group that physical findings that are typical in older people include:
    1. A loss of skin elasticity and a decrease in libido
    2. Impaired fat digestion and increased salivary secretions
    3. An increase in body warmth and some swallowing difficulties
    4. Increased blood pressure and decreased hormone production in women

32. An 89-year-old client with osteoporosis is admitted to the hospital with a compression fracture of the spine. The nurse understands that a factor of special concern when caring for this client is the client's:
    1. Irritability in response to deprivation
    2. Decreased ability to recall recent facts
    3. Inability to maintain an optimal level of functioning
    4. Gradual memory loss resulting from change in environment

33. When considering Erikson's psychosocial developmental tasks, a nurse should focus care for middle-aged adults around their need to be:
    1. Productive
    2. Controlling
    3. Independent
    4. Autonomous

34. When nurses are conducting health assessment interviews with older clients, they should:
    1. Leave a written questionnaire for clients to complete at their leisure
    2. Ask family members rather than the clients to supply the necessary information
    3. Keep referring to previous questions to ascertain that the information given is correct
    4. Spend time in several short sessions to elicit more complete information from the clients

EMOTIONAL NEEDS RELATED TO HEALTH PROBLEMS (EH)

35. The way individuals cope with an unexpected hospitalization depends on all of the following. The one that is most significant would be their:
    1. Age
    2. Basic personality
    3. Financial resources
    4. General physical health

36. One week after admission to the cardiac care unit a client displays an outburst of anger and tells the nurse to get out of the room. The most appropriate nursing action would be to:
    1. Administer the prescribed sedative
    2. Return when the client has had time to calm down
    3. Notify the physician of the client's behavior
    4. Gently point out that this behavior is inappropriate

37. A female client has just spent five minutes complaining to the nurse about numerous aspects of her hospital stay. The best initial nursing response would be to:
    1. Attempt to explain the purpose of different hospital routines to the client
    2. Explain to the client that becoming so upset dangerously blocks her need for rest
    3. Refocus the conversation on the client's fears, frustrations, and anger about her condition
    4. Permit the client to release feelings and then promptly leave to allow her to regain composure

38. A client with hypertension is scheduled for a scan and electrolyte studies. During an interview with the nurse, the client exclaims, "I don't know why the doctor doesn't just give me a prescription for high blood pressure pills, that probably is all it is. I'm missing work by being here." The nurse's best response would be:
1. "It might not be high blood pressure. We have to be sure."
2. "I know it's frustrating, but you need to have a diagnostic workup."
3. "It's frustrating to miss work and not know for sure what's wrong."
4. "Maybe you could ask your doctor if the tests could be done on separate days."

39. A client, who has recently had an abdominoperineal resection and colostomy, accuses the nurse of being uncomfortable during a dressing change because the "wound looks terrible." The nurse recognizes that the client is using the defense mechanism known as:
1. Projection
2. Sublimation
3. Intellectualization
4. Reaction formation

40. A female client who has had abdominal surgery asks if she can return to work after discharge. The most appropriate response by the nurse would be:
1. "No, not for at least two weeks."
2. "What type of work did you have in mind?"
3. "Yes, but do you know what it means to take it easy?"
4. "No, because you must get plenty of rest when you get home."

41. When planning discharge teaching for a client who has had an ileostomy, the nurse should place primary emphasis on:
1. Informing the client of the nearest ileostomy association
2. Telling the client whom to contact if assistance is needed
3. Encouraging the client to return to work as soon as possible
4. Teaching the client the importance of irrigations to regulate bowel movements

42. The left foot of a client with a history of intermittent claudication becomes increasingly cyanotic and numb. Gangrene of the left foot is diagnosed and, because of the high level of arterial insufficiency, an above-the-knee (AK) amputation is scheduled. The response that would demonstrate emotional readiness for the surgery would be that the client:
1. Explains the goals of the procedure
2. Displays few signs of anticipatory grief
3. Participates in learning perioperative care
4. Verbalizes acceptance of future dependence

43. When a client who had an above-the-knee amputation complains of phantom limb sensations, the nursing staff should:
1. Reassure the client that these sensations will pass
2. Encourage the client to get involved in diversional activities
3. Explain the psychological component involved to the client
4. Describe the neurological mechanisms in language that the client understands

44. Building confidence in one's worth is important for a client who is scheduled for a below-the-knee amputation because an amputation:
1. Alters a person's sexuality
2. Implies a lack of wholeness
3. Increases dependency needs
4. Affects an idealized self-image

45. A client who recently was diagnosed as having myelocytic leukemia discusses the diagnosis by referring to statistics, facts, and figures. The nurse recognizes that the client is using the defense mechanism known as:
1. Projection
2. Sublimation
3. Intellectualization
4. Reaction formation

46. A client with newly diagnosed multiple myeloma, being treated with chemotherapy, asks, "How long do you think I have to live?" The most appropriate response by the nurse would be:
1. "Let me ask your physician for you."
2. "I can understand why you are worried."
3. "Tell me about your concerns right now."
4. "It depends on whether the tumor has spread."

47. A female client who is dying jokes about the situation even though she is becoming sicker and weaker. The nurse's most therapeutic response would be:
1. "Why are you always laughing?"
2. "Your laughter is a cover for your fear."
3. "Does it help to joke about your illness?"
4. "She who laughs on the outside, cries on the inside."

48. A male client is dying. Hesitatingly, his wife says to the nurse, "I'd like to tell him how much I love him, but I don't want to upset him." The nurse could best reply:
    1. "I think he'd have difficulty dealing with that now."
    2. "You must keep up a strong appearance for him."
    3. "Don't you think he knows that without your telling him?"
    4. "It's best to share your feelings with him while you can."

49. The nurse notes that a female client seems to be depressed after a thymectomy for treatment of myasthenia gravis. The nursing action that would be most appropriate at this point would be:
    1. Recognizing that depression often occurs after surgery
    2. Asking her physician to arrange for a psychologic consultation
    3. Reassuring the client that she will feel better when her discharge date is set
    4. Talking with the client about her prognosis, emphasizing things that she can do

50. A client who has sustained damage to the bladder is being prepared for diagnostic tests. The client asks, "If I have my bladder removed, how will I ever be able to urinate?" The most therapeutic answer by the nurse would be:
    1. "You can still function normally without a bladder."
    2. "I am sure this is very upsetting to you, but it will be over soon."
    3. "The tests will help to determine if your bladder has to be removed."
    4. "I know you're upset, but there are alternatives to removing your bladder."

51. A client is taught how to change the dressing and how to care for a recently inserted nephrostomy tube. On the day of discharge the client states, "I hope I can handle all this at home; it's a lot to remember." The best response by the nurse would be:
    1. "I'm sure you can do it!"
    2. "Oh, a family member can do it for you."
    3. "You seem to be nervous about going home."
    4. "Perhaps you can stay in the hospital another day."

52. A psychologic problem that frequently occurs when a client is on hemodialysis would be:
    1. Reactive depression
    2. Postpump psychosis
    3. Superego constriction
    4. Dialysis disequilibrium

53. An 83-year-old client with type 2 diabetes is admitted to the ambulatory surgery unit for elective cataract surgery. Before surgery the client asks the nurse, "How will my diabetes be managed while I am here?" The best response by the nurse would be:
    1. "The anesthesiologist will take care of it."
    2. "What did your surgeon or the anesthetist tell you?"
    3. "Your surgeon will write orders for fluids and insulin."
    4. "I'm not quite certain I understand what you are asking."

54. A client's discouragement with the diagnosis of nodular poorly differentiated lymphocytic lymphoma (NLPD) continues during radiation therapy because of the long time required for treatment and its side effects. When assisting the client to plan for the future, the nurse should emphasize that:
    1. Antidepressant medication can be prescribed
    2. The client's feelings are expected and will lessen with time
    3. A positive outlook can influence the outcome of cancer therapy
    4. The prognosis for NLPD is more favorable than for other types of lymphoma

55. A client has just been diagnosed with multiple sclerosis. The client is obviously upset with the diagnosis and asks, "Am I going to die?" The nurse's best response would be:
    1. "Most individuals with your disease live a normal life span."
    2. "Is your family here? I would like to explain your disease to all of you."
    3. "The prognosis is variable; most individuals experience remissions and exacerbations."
    4. "Why don't you speak with your physician who can give you more details about your disease."

56. The physician orders airborne precautions for a client with tuberculosis. After being taught about the details of airborne precautions, the client is seen walking down the hall to get a glass of juice from the kitchen. The most effective nursing intervention would be to:
    1. Ensure regular visits by staff members
    2. Explore what the precautions mean to the client

3. Report the situation to the infection control nurse

4. Reteach the entire airborne precautions to the client

57. A 60-year-old widow living with her daughter, who has seven children, develops heart failure and is referred for home health care. On the first visit by the nurse, the client is feeding a grandchild and preparing dinner for the family. The other children are playing in the area. The best way for the nurse to proceed would be to:

1. Socialize for a few minutes with the client
2. Sit down with the client in the living room
3. Make an appointment with the client on a different day
4. Ask the client if there is a private place to perform the physical assessment

58. The nurse should suspect that a male client who has had a recent myocardial infarction is experiencing denial when he:

1. Attempts to minimize his illness
2. Lacks an emotional response to his illness
3. Expresses displeasure with his activity program
4. Refuses to discuss his condition with his wife

59. The major improvement in body image following early fitting with a prosthesis after amputation usually is related to the:

1. Acceptance received from others
2. Client's improved functional abilities
3. Fact that something is being done to help
4. Feeling that the client looks more "whole"

60. Teaching for clients who have sustained a sudden, traumatic, major loss is often most satisfactorily done during the acceptance or adaptation stage of coping. The nurse is aware that the rationale for this fact is that clients in this stage are:

1. Ready for discharge and therefore in need of preparation
2. At the peak of mental anguish and therefore open to change
3. Less angry and therefore more compliant and easier to deal with
4. Less anxious and more aware of reality and therefore ready to learn

61. On the fourth day after surgery for a fractured hip, a client appears angry and very restless and says, "I can't stand this another minute. There's a wrinkle in my sheet, and my water is warm." The client changes position frequently and does not maintain eye contact with the nurse. The best initial interpretation of the client's behavior is that it indicates:

1. Severe discomfort in the hip
2. An increased level of anxiety
3. Anger at the poor nursing care
4. Frustration with the need for leg abduction

62. The nurse, caring for a male client after head and neck surgery, has been concerned with the client's anger and depressive episodes about the effects of surgery. The action by the client that would indicate that the client is reaching acceptance would be:

1. Smiling and becoming more extroverted
2. Performing self care of the tracheal stoma
3. Ambulating in the hall and sitting in the lounge
4. Allowing a family member to participate in care

63. A young married woman, who has been hospitalized with partial- and full-thickness burns over 30% of the total body surface area, is to be discharged. She asks the nurse, "How will my husband be able to care for me at home?" The nurse should interpret this statement as:

1. Readiness to discuss her deformities
2. Indication of a change in family relations
3. A need for more time to think about the future
4. Beginning realization of implications for the future

64. A client in thyrotoxic crisis tells the nurse, "I know I'm going to die. I'm very sick." The best response by the nurse would be:

1. "You must feel very sick and frightened."
2. "Tell me why you feel you are going to die."
3. "I can understand how you feel, but people do not die from this problem."
4. "If you would like, I will call your family and tell them to come to the hospital."

65. The nurse should be aware that sensory restriction in a client who is blind can:

1. Heighten the client's ability to make decisions
2. Decrease the client's restlessness and lethargy
3. Increase the use of daydreaming and fantasy
4. Lead to the use of permanent neurotic behaviors

66. A young female client is diagnosed as having stage IIIA Hodgkin's disease with a grossly involved spleen and is scheduled for a splenectomy. After the nurse performs preoperative teaching the client appears very anxious. The best approach for the nurse to use at this time would be to:
1. Allow the client to regress at this time and let her rest quietly
2. State that she seems anxious and ask her whether she would like to talk for a while
3. Consider her reaction an unconscious response and inquire about her relations with her mother
4. Recognize that anxiety prevented the client from understanding, and repeat the information in simpler terms

67. A female client with chronic renal failure has been on hemodialysis for two years. She relates to the nurse in the dialysis unit in an angry, critical manner and is frequently noncompliant with medications and diet. The nurse can best intervene by first understanding that the client's behavior is most likely:
1. An attempt to punish the nursing staff
2. A constructive method of accepting reality
3. A defense against underlying depression and fear
4. An effort to maintain life to the fullest extent possible

68. Before major abdominal surgery for cancer the client says to the nurse, "I really don't think this is cancer at all. I'll bet they won't find anything." The nurse's most appropriate initial response would be:
1. "I can understand why you'd like to believe that."
2. "I hope you're right, but the tests do indicate cancer."
3. "It must be difficult to be facing such serious surgery."
4. "You think the physician may have made a wrong diagnosis?"

69. A female client is diagnosed as having cancer of the breast and is admitted to the hospital for a lumpectomy to be followed by radiation. While being admitted to ambulatory surgery by the nurse, the client has tears in her eyes and her chin is quivering. In a shaky voice the client says, "I can't believe this is happening." The nurse's best response would be:
1. "You can't believe this is happening?"
2. "This must be a very scary time for you."

3. "Do you have any questions at this time?"
4. "Cancer of the breast has a high cure rate."

70. After a laryngectomy is scheduled, the most important factor for the nurse to include in the preoperative teaching plan would be:
1. Establishing a means for communicating postoperatively
2. Explaining that there will be a feeding tube postoperatively
3. Demonstrating how to care for a permanent laryngeal stoma
4. Teaching how to cough and expectorate bronchial secretions

71. The nurse identifies that a client who had extensive abdominal surgery appears depressed. The most appropriate nursing action would be:
1. Talk with the client, encouraging exploration of feelings
2. Ask the client's physician to prescribe an antidepressant medication
3. Recognize that the client's depression is an expected response to surgery
4. Reassure the client that feelings of depression will lift after returning home

72. A male client is hospitalized following a major automobile accident. As the client is describing the accident to a friend, he becomes very restless, and his pulse and respirations increase sharply. It is most important for the nurse to recognize that these symptoms are probably related to:
1. Bleeding from undiscovered injury
2. Delayed psychologic response to trauma
3. The client's method of seeking sympathy
4. A parasympathetic nervous system response to anxiety

73. A male client with a parotid tumor tells the nurse that he is anxious to undergo surgery to remove the tumor. He states that he is not too sure about delaying surgery until preoperative radiotherapy is completed. The best response by the nurse would be:
1. "You are concerned about the delay of surgery?
2. "You are anxious about the effects of radiotherapy?"
3. "I think you do not have confidence in the doctor's decision."
4. "I can understand your anxiety concerning the delay of surgery."

74. A 54-year-old male police officer, who has just had surgery for oral carcinoma, indicates to the

nurse that he wants only his wife to visit. To support him at this time, the nurse should first:
1. Comply with the client's wishes
2. Ask the client why he does not want others to visit
3. Have the wife explain to the client that everything will be OK
4. Promote communication to find out how the client really feels

75. A male client with pancreatic cancer is aware of the terminal nature of the illness. Behaviors that would indicate that he is accepting the fact of his impending death are:
1. Alternately crying and talking openly about death
2. Getting second, third, and fourth medical opinions
3. Making out his will and planning a visit to a good friend
4. Refusing to follow treatments and stating, "I'm going to die anyway."

76. A female client with a terminal illness decides to donate her eyes for organ transplantation after she dies. Statutes that address organ transplantation attempt to prevent abuse by:
1. Permitting active euthanasia when necessary
2. Preventing children from giving organs to others
3. Allowing physicians to control both donor and recipient
4. Requiring participating institutions to have review boards

77. To be most effective when teaching colostomy care to a client, the nurse must first:
1. Wait until a family member is present
2. Assess barriers to learning colostomy care
3. Wait until the client has accepted the change in body image
4. Begin with simple written instructions concerning the care

78. During the evening after a paracentesis, the nurse notices that the client, although denying any discomfort, seems very anxious. The best nursing approach would be to:
1. Offer the client a back rub
2. Administer the prescribed opiate
3. Reinforce the physician's explanation of the procedure
4. Explore the client's concerns and administer the ordered anxiolytic

79. A client with recently diagnosed diabetes states, "I feel bad. I don't seem to get along with my husband. He does not care about my diabetes." The nurse's most appropriate response would be:
1. "You don't get along with your husband."
2. "I'm sorry, what can I do to make you feel better?"
3. "It's probably just temporary; he needs more time to adjust."
4. "You are unhappy. I wonder, have you tried to talk to your husband?"

80. A 38-year-old administrative assistant visits a neurologist after experiencing a tonic-clonic seizure. The physician suspects a brain tumor, and a CT scan is scheduled. Before the test the nurse should:
1. Describe the equipment involved
2. Provide the prescribed pre-scan sedative
3. Explain that no radiation will be involved
4. Advise the client to withhold routine medications

81. A client with AIDS comments to the nurse, "There are so many rotten people around. Why couldn't one of them get AIDS instead of me?" The nurse could best respond:
1. "It seems unfair that you should be so ill."
2. "I can understand why you're afraid of death."
3. "Have you thought of speaking with a minister?"
4. "I'm sure you really don't wish this on someone else."

82. A client is to be transferred from the coronary care unit to a progressive care unit. The client asks the nurse, "Are you sure I'm ready for this move?" From this statement the nurse ascertains that the client is most likely experiencing:
1. Fear
2. Depression
3. Dependency
4. Ambivalence

83. A 65-year-old widower becomes aware that a portion of his peripheral vision is impaired. The ophthalmologist diagnoses a retinal detachment and schedules surgery. The client appears apprehensive when he arrives at the hospital for the cryosurgical examination and interview. When explaining what is to be expected during hospitalization, the nurse should include:
1. Familiarizing the client with his surroundings
2. Explaining to the client that his surgery will be very brief
3. Teaching the client coughing and deep breathing exercises
4. Reassuring the client that repair of the retina has a good prognosis

84. A 47-year-old woman with jaundiced skin and abdominal pain is diagnosed with biliary obstruction. She is refusing all visitors. The nurse should:
    1. Listen to her fears
    2. Grant her request about visitors
    3. Encourage her to visit with relatives
    4. Darken the room by pulling the drapes

85. A carpenter with full-thickness burns of the entire right arm confides the fears that, "I'll never be able to use my arm again and I'll be scarred forever." The nurse's best initial response would be:
    1. "The staff is taking steps to minimize scarring."
    2. "Think about how lucky you are. You are alive."
    3. "I know you're worried, but it is too early to tell how much scarring will occur."
    4. "Try not to worry for now; concentrate on your range-of-motion exercises."

BLOOD AND IMMUNITY (BI)

86. The nurse is aware that nutritional support of a client's natural defense mechanisms would indicate the need for a diet high in:
    1. The essential fatty acids
    2. Dietary cellulose and fiber
    3. The amino acid, tryptophan
    4. Vitamins A, C, E, and selenium

87. Twelve hours after a female client is admitted to the critical care unit following a motorcycle injury, she begins to complain of increased abdominal pain in the left upper quadrant. A ruptured spleen is diagnosed, and she is scheduled for an emergency splenectomy. When preparing the client for surgery the nurse should emphasize the:
    1. Complete safety of the procedure
    2. Expectation of postoperative bleeding
    3. Risk of the procedure with the other injuries
    4. Presence of abdominal drainage for several days after the surgery

88. After abdominal surgery a client develops internal hemorrhaging. During further assessments, the nurse should expect the client to exhibit:
    1. Polyuria
    2. Bradypnea
    3. Tachycardia
    4. Hypertension

89. When assessing for hemorrhage after a client has a total hip replacement, the most important nursing action would be to:
    1. Measure the girth of the thigh
    2. Check the vital signs every four hours
    3. Examine the bedding under the client
    4. Observe for ecchymosis at the operative site

90. A client is brought to the emergency service after an automobile accident. The client's blood pressure is 100/60 mm Hg, and the physical assessment suggests a ruptured spleen. Based on this information, the nurse should assess the client for an early sign of decreased arterial pressure, such as:
    1. Warm, flushed skin
    2. Confusion and lethargy
    3. Increased pulse pressure
    4. Reduced peripheral pulses

91. When a client is experiencing hypovolemic shock with decreased tissue perfusion, the nurse recognizes the body initially attempts to compensate by:
    1. Producing less ADH
    2. Producing more red blood cells
    3. Maintaining peripheral vasoconstriction
    4. Decreasing mineralocorticoid production

92. After sustaining multiple internal injuries from being hit by a car, the client's blood pressure suddenly drops to 80/60 mm Hg. The nurse should realize that this is probably caused by:
    1. A reduction in the circulating blood volume
    2. Diminished vasomotor stimulation to the arterial wall
    3. Vasodilation resulting from diminished vasoconstrictor tone
    4. Cardiac decompensation resulting from electrolyte imbalance

93. The nurse is aware that shock associated with a ruptured abdominal aneurysm is called:
    1. Vasogenic shock
    2. Neurogenic shock
    3. Cardiogenic shock
    4. Hypovolemic shock

94. A client has emergency surgery for a ruptured appendix. After assessing that the client is manifesting symptoms of shock, the nurse should:
    1. Prepare for a blood transfusion
    2. Notify the physician immediately
    3. Elevate the head of the bed 30 degrees
    4. Increase the liter flow of the oxygen being administered

95. During the progressive stage of shock, anaerobic metabolism occurs. The nurse must be aware that initially this causes:
1. Metabolic acidosis
2. Metabolic alkalosis
3. Respiratory acidosis
4. Respiratory alkalosis

96. A client who is in hypovolemic shock has a hematocrit value of 25%. The nurse should anticipate that the physician will order:
1. Ringer's lactate
2. Serum albumin
3. Blood replacement
4. High molecular dextran

97. Polycythemia is frequently associated with chronic obstructive pulmonary disease (COPD). When assessing for this complication, the nurse should observe for:
1. Pallor and cyanosis
2. Dyspnea on exertion
3. A decreased hematocrit
4. An elevated hemoglobin

98. The physician orders 2 units of blood to be infused into a client who is bleeding. Before blood administration the nurse's highest priority should be:
1. Obtaining the client's vital signs
2. Monitoring the hemoglobin and hematocrit levels
3. Allowing the blood to reach room temperature
4. Determining proper typing and cross-matching of blood

99. A client who is scheduled for a modified radical mastectomy decides to have family members donate blood in the event it is needed. The client has type A negative blood. Blood could be used from relatives whose blood is:
1. Type O positive
2. Type AB negative
3. Type A or O negative
4. Type A or AB negative

100. The physician orders a blood transfusion for a client. When administering blood, the priority nursing intervention would be to:
1. Warm the blood to body temperature to prevent chills
2. Use an infusion pump to increase accuracy of infusion
3. Infuse the blood at a slow rate during the first 5 to 10 minutes

4. Draw blood samples from the client after each unit is transfused

101. A client with esophageal varices is admitted with hematemesis, and two units of blood are ordered. Halfway through the first unit of blood the client complains of flank pain. The nurse's first action should be to:
1. Stop the transfusion
2. Obtain the vital signs
3. Assess the pain further
4. Monitor the hourly urinary output

102. Halfway through the administration of a unit of blood, a client complains of lumbar pain. After stopping the transfusion, the nurse should:
1. Obtain vital signs
2. Notify the blood bank
3. Assess the pain further
4. Increase the flow of normal saline

103. A male client with chronic liver disease reports that his gums bleed spontaneously. In addition, the nurse notes small hemorrhagic lesions on his face. The nurse recognizes that the client needs additional:
1. Bile salts
2. Folic acid
3. Vitamin A
4. Vitamin K

104. A client comes to the clinic complaining of weight loss, fatigue, and a low-grade fever. Physical examination reveals a slight enlargement of the cervical lymph nodes. When the nurse is assessing possible causes for the fever, it would be most appropriate initially for the nurse to ask:
1. "Have you been sexually active lately?"
2. "Do you have a sore throat at the present time?"
3. "Have you been exposed recently to anyone with an infection?"
4. "When did you first notice that your temperature had gone up?"

105. The nursing staff has a team conference on AIDS and discusses the routes of transmission of the human immunodeficiency virus (HIV). The discussion reveals that an individual has no risk of exposure to HIV when that individual:
1. Has intercourse with just the spouse
2. Makes a donation of a pint of whole blood
3. Uses a condom each time there is sexual intercourse
4. Limits sexual contact to those without HIV antibodies

106. The nurse knows that a positive diagnosis for HIV infection is made based on:
    1. Positive ELISA and Western blot tests
    2. A history of high-risk sexual behaviors
    3. Evidence of extreme weight loss and high fever
    4. Identification of an associated opportunistic infection

107. Blood screening tests of the immune system of a client with AIDS would indicate:
    1. A decrease in CD4 T cells
    2. An increase in thymic hormones
    3. An increase in immunoglobulin E
    4. A decrease in the serum level of glucose-6-phosphate dehydrogenase

108. When taking the blood pressure of a client who has AIDS, the nurse must:
    1. Wear clean gloves
    2. Use barrier techniques
    3. Wear a mask and gown
    4. Wash the hands thoroughly

109. A client with acquired immunodeficiency syndrome (AIDS) and *Cryptococcus* pneumonia is incontinent of feces and urine and is producing copious sputum. When providing care for this client the nurse's priority should be to:
    1. Wear goggles when suctioning the client's airway
    2. Use gown, mask, and gloves when bathing the client
    3. Use gloves to administer oral medications to the client
    4. Wear a gown when assisting the client with the bedpan

110. In addition to *Pneumocystis carinii*, a client with AIDS also has an ulcer 4 cm in diameter on the leg. Considering the client's total health status, the most critical nursing diagnosis would be:
    1. Social isolation
    2. Impaired skin integrity
    3. Impaired gas exchange
    4. Imbalanced nutrition: less than body requirements

111. A Schilling test is ordered for a client who is suspected of having pernicious anemia. The nurse recognizes that the primary purpose of the Schilling test is to determine the client's ability to:
    1. Store vitamin B_{12}
    2. Digest vitamin B_{12}
    3. Absorb vitamin B_{12}
    4. Produce vitamin B_{12}

112. When discussing the therapeutic regimen of vitamin B_{12} for pernicious anemia with a client, the nurse should explain that:
    1. Weekly Z-track injections provide needed control
    2. Daily intramuscular injections are required for control
    3. Intramuscular injections once a month will maintain control
    4. Oral tablets of vitamin B_{12} taken daily will control the symptoms

113. The nurse knows that the teaching regarding the use of vitamin B_{12} injections to treat pernicious anemia is understood when a client states, "I must take the drug:
    1. When feeling fatigued."
    2. Until my symptoms subside."
    3. Monthly, for the rest of my life."
    4. During exacerbations of anemia."

114. A client with Hodgkin's disease enters a remission period and remains symptom-free for 6 months, when a relapse occurs. The client is diagnosed at stage IV. The therapy option the nurse should expect to be implemented at this time would be:
    1. Radiation therapy
    2. Combination chemotherapy
    3. Radiation with chemotherapy
    4. Surgical removal of the affected nodes

115. The treatment regimen for a female diagnosed with Hodgkin's disease, Stage III$_2$ will start with nodal irradiation. The client and her husband have been trying to have a child, and she expresses concern when she learns that the radiation therapy includes the pelvic nodal area. When questioned about this, the nurse should refer the client to the physician, since the nurse is aware that:
    1. Ovaries can be surgically moved and placed in a shielded area
    2. Radiation used is not radical enough to destroy ovarian function
    3. Intermittent radiation to the area does not cause permanent sterilization
    4. Ovarian function will be temporarily destroyed but will return in about six months

116. A young woman is admitted to the oncology unit with a diagnosis of Hodgkin's disease. Staging is done and the client's spleen is found to be grossly involved, and it is surgically removed. A complication specifically related to a splenectomy for which the nurse

should monitor the client would be:
1. Pulmonary embolism
2. Inadequate lung aeration
3. Hypoactive bowel sounds
4. Postoperative hemorrhage

117. A client receiving chemotherapy (cyclophosphamide [Cytoxan]) and a steroid (prednisone) has a white blood cell count of 12,000/cu mm and a red blood cell count of 4.5 million/cu mm. The instructions that should receive the priority by the nurse would be to:
1. Omit the daily dose of prednisone
2. Avoid large crowds and persons with infections
3. Shave with an electric rather than a safety razor
4. Increase the intake of high-protein foods and red meats

118. An older adult develops severe bone marrow depression from chemotherapy for cancer of the prostate. The nurse should:
1. Monitor for signs of alopecia
2. Increase daily intake of fluids
3. Monitor intake and output of fluids
4. Use a soft toothbrush for oral hygiene

119. The laboratory results of a client following chemotherapy for cancer indicate bone marrow depression. The nurse should encourage the client to:
1. Use an electric razor when shaving
2. Drink citrus juices frequently for nourishment
3. Increase activity levels and ambulate frequently
4. Sleep with the head of the bed slightly elevated

120. A client has received three courses of chemotherapy and is admitted for tests before continuing with the fourth in the series. The physician decides to omit the treatment because the client demonstrates myelosuppression. When discussing this with the client, the nurse should explain that:
1. Calcium must be increased in the diet because of the effects of myelosuppression
2. Eating a balanced diet, resting, and trying to avoid bleeding and infections are appropriate at this time
3. The development of myelosuppression explains why the client has nausea, vomiting, anorexia, and alopecia
4. Frequent testing for restlessness, muscle control, and pupillary response will be necessary because the meninges may be irritable

121. A client who is suspected of having leukemia has a bone marrow aspiration. Immediately following the procedure, the nurse should:
1. Apply brief pressure to the site
2. Ask the client to lie on the affected side
3. Swab the site with an antiseptic solution
4. Monitor the vital signs every hour for four hours

122. On admission, the blood work of a young adult with leukemia indicates an elevated blood urea nitrogen (BUN) and uric acid. The nurse is aware that these laboratory results may be related to:
1. Lymphadenopathy
2. Thrombocytopenia
3. Hypermetabolic state
4. Hepatic encephalopathy

123. When obtaining a health history from a young client with probable acute lymphocytic leukemia (ALL), the clinical manifestations the nurse should expect to be present are:
1. Petechiae, alopecia
2. Anorexia, insomnia
3. Anorexia, petechiae
4. Alopecia, bleeding gums

124. A retired farmer has been admitted with a diagnosis of acute lymphoblastic leukemia. When the client is receiving chemotherapy, the nurse should assess for the development of life-threatening thrombocytopenia by monitoring the client for:
1. Fever
2. Diarrhea
3. Headache
4. Hematuria

125. A client who has had bone pains of insidious onset for four months is suspected of having multiple myeloma. The nurse understands that one of the diagnostic findings specific for multiple myeloma would be:
1. Low serum calcium levels
2. Bence-Jones protein in the urine
3. Occult and frank blood in the stool
4. Positive bacterial culture of sputum

126. The nurse understands that the most definitive test to confirm a diagnosis of multiple myeloma is:
1. Bone marrow biopsy
2. Serum test for hypercalcemia
3. Urine test for Bence-Jones protein
4. X-ray films of the ribs, spine, and skull

127. A client with multiple myeloma is scheduled to have a chest x-ray examination and a bone scan. For this client, the primary responsibility of the nursing and radiology staff is to:
    1. Explain the procedure and its purpose
    2. Observe the client for shortness of breath
    3. Provide for rest periods during the procedure
    4. Handle the client with supportive movements

128. A client, diagnosed with multiple myeloma, asks the physician about what treatment will be administered. The nurse would expect the physician to reply:
    1. "Alpha-interferon therapy."
    2. "Radiation therapy on an outpatient basis."
    3. "Surgery to remove the lesion and lymph nodes."
    4. "Chemotherapy employing a combination of drugs."

129. A client with multiple myeloma, who is receiving chemotherapy, has a temperature that has risen three degrees during a six-hour period and is now 102.2° F. The nurse should:
    1. Administer the prescribed antipyretic and notify the physician
    2. Obtain the other vital signs and recheck the temperature in one hour
    3. Assess the amount and color of urine and obtain a specimen for a urinalysis
    4. Note the consistency of respiratory secretions and obtain a specimen for culture

130. A client with multiple myeloma asks how the disease may progress. When teaching this client, the nurse should discuss the possibility that:
    1. Blood transfusions may be necessary
    2. Frequent urinary tract infections may result
    3. IV fluid therapy may be administered in the home
    4. The disease is exacerbated by exposure to ultraviolet rays

131. The nurse is aware that a client is receiving azathioprine (Imuran), cyclosporine, and prednisone before kidney transplant surgery to:
    1. Stimulate leukocytosis
    2. Provide passive immunity
    3. Prevent iatrogenic infection
    4. Reduce antibody production

132. A client has an exacerbation of systemic lupus erythematosus. The dosage of steroid medication is increased, and a home health care nurse is to provide health teaching. To reduce the frequency of exacerbations, the nurse should teach the client:
    1. Techniques to reduce stress
    2. Principles of proper hygiene
    3. Measures to improve nutrition
    4. Signs of an impending exacerbation

133. A farmer steps on a rusty nail and the puncture site becomes swollen and painful. Tetanus antitoxin is prescribed. The nurse explains that this is used because it:
    1. Provides antibodies
    2. Stimulates plasma cells
    3. Produces active immunity
    4. Facilitates long-lasting immunity

134. A tuberculin skin test with purified protein derivative (PPD) tuberculin is performed as part of a routine physical examination. The nurse should instruct the client to make an appointment so the test can be read in:
    1. 3 days
    2. 5 days
    3. 7 days
    4. 10 days

135. A client is admitted with cellulitis of the left leg and a temperature of 103° F. The physician orders IV antibiotics. Before instituting this therapy, the nurse should:
    1. Determine whether the client has allergies
    2. Apply a warm, moist dressing over the area
    3. Measure the amount of swelling in the client's leg
    4. Obtain the results of the culture and sensitivity tests

136. After multiple bee stings a client has an anaphylactic reaction. The nurse is aware that the symptoms the client is experiencing are caused by:
    1. Respiratory depression and cardiac arrest
    2. Decreased cardiac output and dilation of major blood vessels
    3. Bronchial constriction and decreased peripheral resistance
    4. Constriction of capillaries and decreased peripheral circulation

137. The plan of care for a postoperative client who has developed a pulmonary embolus includes monitoring and bed rest. The client asks why all activity is restricted. The nurse's response is based on the principle that bed rest:
    1. Prevents further platelet aggregation
    2. Enhances the peripheral circulation in the deep vessels

3. Decreases the potential for further dislodgement of emboli
4. Maximizes the amount of blood available to damaged tissues

138. A client comes to the clinic for a physical and asks to be tested for AIDS. The nurse explains that the initial screening for AIDS will be done via the:
1. Western blot test
2. CD4 T cell count
3. Polymerase chain reaction test
4. Enzyme-linked immunosorbent assay (ELISA)

139. A Schilling test is ordered for a client suspected of having cobalamin deficiency because of pernicious anemia. The nurse must plan to:
1. Give all medications on time
2. Order foods low in vitamin B$_{12}$
3. Keep an accurate intake and output
4. Collect a 24- to 48-hour urine specimen

CARDIOVASCULAR (CV)

140. To determine the status of a client's carotid pulse, the nurse should palpate:
1. Below the mandible
2. In the lateral neck region
3. At the anterior neck, lateral to the trachea
4. Along the clavicle at the base of the neck

141. During auscultation of the heart, the nurse would expect the first heart sound (S1) to be the loudest at the:
1. Base of the heart
2. Apex of the heart
3. Left lateral border
4. Right lateral border

142. When auscultating a client's heart, the nurse understands that the first heart sound is produced by the closure of the:
1. Mitral and tricuspid valves
2. Aortic and tricuspid valves
3. Mitral and pulmonic valves
4. Aortic and pulmonic valves

143. When assessing an 85-year-old client's vital signs, the nurse should remember that a number of expected changes in cardiac output results from the aging process. The finding that would be consistent with a pathologic condition rather than the aging process would be:
1. A pulse-rate irregularity
2. A pulse rate of 60 beats per minute

3. An equal apical and radial pulse
4. An apical rate obtainable at fifth intercostal space, midclavicular line

144. Thrombus formation is a danger for all postoperative clients. The nurse should act independently to prevent this complication by:
1. Assisting the client to exercise in bed
2. Urging the client to drink adequate fluids
3. Applying elastic stockings to the client's legs
4. Massaging the client's extremities gently with lotion

145. Oxygen by nasal cannula is prescribed for a client. The nurse plans to use safety precautions in the room because oxygen:
1. Is flammable
2. Supports combustion
3. Has unstable properties
4. Converts to an alternate form of matter

146. An electrocardiogram is ordered for a client complaining of chest pain. An early finding in the lead over an infarcted area would be:
1. Flattened T waves
2. Absence of P waves
3. Elevated ST segments
4. Disappearance of Q waves

147. A client has a Swan-Ganz catheter inserted for monitoring cardiovascular status. With the Swan-Ganz catheter the most accurate measurement of the client's left ventricular pressure would be the:
1. Right atrial pressure
2. Cardiac output by thermodilution
3. Pulmonary artery diastolic pressure
4. Pulmonary capillary wedge pressure

148. A thallium scan is scheduled for a client who has had a myocardial infarction to:
1. Monitor the action of the heart valves
2. Establish the viability of myocardial muscle
3. Visualize the ventricular systole and diastole
4. Determine the adequacy of electrical conductivity

149. After a traumatic accident, a client is admitted to the hospital's emergency department with a blood pressure of 100/60 and the physician suspects a ruptured spleen. The nurse should assess the client for an early sign of decreased arterial pressure, such as:
1. Weak radial pulses
2. Warm, flushed skin
3. Increased pulse pressure
4. Lethargy with confusion

150. A male client has a discectomy and fusion for a herniated disk. When getting out of bed for the first time, with assistance from two nurses, the client complains of feeling faint and light-headed. The nurses should have the client:
1. Sit on the edge of the bed, so they can hold him upright
2. Lie down immediately, so they can take his blood pressure
3. Slide slowly to the floor, so he will not fall and hurt himself
4. Bend forward, because it will increase the blood flow to his brain

151. A client has a right upper lobectomy to remove a cancerous lesion. After this surgery the nurse should monitor the client for the most life-threatening complication, which would be:
1. Decreased cardiac output due to mediastinal shift
2. Dyspnea due to increased intrathoracic pressure
3. Pneumothorax due to increased abdominal pressure
4. Hemothorax due to decreased thoracic drainage

152. A client with a family history of atherosclerosis is advised to follow a diet based on the U.S. Department of Agriculture's Food Guide Pyramid. The nurse should teach the client to eat:
1. 4 to 6 servings of fruit daily
2. 5 to 7 servings of vegetables daily
3. 3 to 5 servings of meat, poultry, or fish daily
4. 6 to 11 servings of bread, rice, or pasta daily

153. A female client tells the nurse that the physician just told her that her triglycerides and cholesterol are excessively elevated. The client appears discouraged and says, "Well, I guess I'd better cut out all the fat and cholesterol in my diet." The nurse's most appropriate response would be:
1. "Well yes, that would certainly lower the amount of your blood fats."
2. "That's good, but be sure to compensate by adding more proteins and carbohydrates."
3. "You need some fat to supply the necessary fatty acids, so it's mainly just a need for cutting down the amount."
4. "You need some cholesterol in your diet because your body cannot manufacture it, so just avoid excessive amounts."

154. The nurse is aware that the gradual occlusion of the internal or common carotid arteries, manifested by transient ischemic attacks, may occur because of:
1. Acquired valvular heart disease
2. Atherosclerosis of the vascular system
3. Emboli associated with atrial fibrillation
4. Developmental defects of the arterial wall

155. To help reduce a client's risk factors for heart disease, the nurse, when discussing dietary guidelines, should teach the client to:
1. Avoid eating between meals
2. Limit the amount of unsaturated fat
3. Decrease the amount of fat-binding fiber
4. Increase the ratio of complex carbohydrates

156. A client's diet is modified to eliminate foods that act as cardiac stimulants. The nurse should teach this client to avoid:
1. Yogurt
2. Red meat
3. Club soda
4. Chocolate

157. A steam fitter is brought to the emergency department by coworkers and is admitted with a possible myocardial infarction. The client is experiencing severe chest pain. He is diaphoretic, and his pulse rate is 110 beats per minute. The nurse should immediately:
1. Increase the oxygen flow
2. Take a 12-lead electrocardiogram
3. Administer nitroglycerin until the pain subsides
4. Notify the physician and administer morphine

158. The nurse plans to teach a client receiving a 2-gram sodium-restricted diet that the foods lowest in sodium are:
1. Meat and fish
2. Milk and cheese
3. Fruits and juices
4. Dry cereals and grains

159. A 60-year-old client with a long history of cardiovascular problems, including angina and hypertension, is to have a cardiac catheterization. During precardiac catheterization teaching, the nurse should explain to this client that the major purpose for this procedure is to:
1. Obtain the pressures in the heart chambers
2. Determine the existence of congenital heart disease
3. Visualize the disease process in the coronary arteries
4. Measure the oxygen content of various heart chambers

160. A client returns from a cardiac catheterization and is to remain in the supine position for six hours with the affected leg straight. These measures prevent:
1. Orthostatic hypotension
2. Headache and disorientation
3. Bleeding at the arterial puncture site
4. Infiltration of radiopaque dye into tissue

161. After a cardiac catheterization, the client complains of tingling sensations in the affected leg. The nurse should first:
1. Assess for bleeding at the catheter insertion site
2. Evaluate the affected leg for heat, edema, and pain
3. Compare the femoral, popliteal, and pedal pulses in both legs
4. Obtain the temperature, pulse, respirations, and blood pressure

162. After a cardiac catheterization the nurse should assess the client for the expected response of:
1. A marked increase in the volume of urine output
2. A decrease in BP of 25% from precatheterization BP
3. Respiratory distress and an increase in respiratory rate
4. Complaints of heart pounding with mild chest discomfort

163. For the first several hours after a cardiac catheterization, it would be most essential for the nurse to:
1. Keep the head of the client's bed elevated 45 degrees
2. Monitor the client's apical pulse and blood pressure frequently
3. Encourage the client to cough and deep-breathe every two hours
4. Check the client's temperature every hour until it returns to normal

164. When developing a plan of care for a client who has had a cardiac catheterization, the nurse should include:
1. Ambulating the client 2 hours after the procedure
2. Keeping the client NPO for 4 hours after the procedure
3. Checking the vital signs every 15 minutes for 8 hours
4. Maintaining the supine position for a minimum of 4 hours

165. A 56-year-old housewife, who has a history of angina, is scheduled for a cardiac catheterization. Catheter entry will be through the femoral artery. The nurse should inform the client that she will:
1. Be fully alert and awake during the procedure
2. Be able to ambulate shortly after the procedure
3. Experience a feeling of warmth during the procedure
4. Have to remain in the semi-Fowler's position for 12 hours after the procedure

166. The nurse understands that the most common characteristic of anginal pain is that it is:
1. Unchanged by rest
2. Precipitated by light activity
3. Described as sharp or knifelike
4. Relieved by sublingual nitroglycerin

167. A client with continuous blood loss becomes increasingly diaphoretic, clammy, and pale. The client's blood pressure falls to 90/60. The nursing action that is of primary importance is to:
1. Place the client in a reclining position
2. Delay repositioning of the client for a few hours
3. Allow the client to determine the position of comfort
4. Assist the client to assume the semi-Fowler's position

168. An early finding that would indicate that a client is hypertensive is:
1. An extended Korotkoff's sound
2. A regular pulse of 92 beats per minute
3. A diastolic blood pressure that remains greater than 90 mm Hg
4. An achy, throbbing headache over the left eye when arising in the morning

169. An 82-year-old client, whose baseline blood pressure was 140/90 mm Hg has the blood pressure taken by the home health nurse. The nurse obtains a sitting blood pressure of 160/100 mm Hg in the left arm. The nurse should initially:
1. Advise the client to restrict fluid and sodium intake and avoid stress
2. Call the physician and report the elevated blood pressure reading immediately
3. Take the client's blood pressure in the right arm and then in both arms while standing
4. Conclude that this is an expected reading for an older person and record the information

170. A businessman makes many long airplane trips. He confides to the nurse at his place of business that he is concerned because his legs swell on these long flights. The nurse should advise him to:
    1. Relax in a reclining position
    2. Sit upright with legs extended
    3. Walk about the cabin at least once every hour
    4. Sit in any position that relieves pressure on the legs

171. A client with a history of hypertension develops pedal edema and demonstrates dyspnea on exertion. The nurse recognizes that this probably is:
    1. Caused by cor pulmonale
    2. The result of right atrial failure
    3. A result of left ventricular failure
    4. Associated with wheezing and coughing

172. A high school football coach is admitted to the coronary care unit with a tentative diagnosis of myocardial infarction. When assessing the client's pain, the nurse would probably expect him to describe it as:
    1. Severe, intense chest pain
    2. A burning sensation of short duration
    3. Mild chest pain, radiating to the fingers
    4. A squeezing chest pain, relieved by nitroglycerin

173. A hospitalized client complains of chest pain that feels like a pressure or weight on the chest. The client also states, "I feel nauseated and very weak." The nurse should:
    1. Perform a nutritional assessment
    2. Summon medical help for a potential emergency
    3. Explore and then discuss possible sources of stress
    4. Provide reassurance while helping the client to focus on pleasant topics

174. A client who has been admitted to the cardiac care unit with a myocardial infarction complains of chest pain. The nursing intervention that would be most effective in relieving the client's pain would be to administer the ordered:
    1. Morphine sulfate 2 mg IV
    2. Oxygen per nasal cannula
    3. Nitroglycerin sublingually
    4. Lidocaine hydrochloride 50 mg IV bolus

175. The nurse is teaching a client who has recovered from a myocardial infarction how to

prevent a future one. The nurse evaluates that further teaching is needed when the client states, "I will:
    1. Restrict my physical activity."
    2. Take one baby aspirin every day."
    3. Continue my smoking cessation program."
    4. Try to lose the extra weight I'm carrying around."

176. A client is admitted to the coronary care unit complaining of "vicelike" chest pain radiating to the neck. Assessment reveals a blood pressure of 124/64, an irregular apical pulse of 64 beats per minute, and diaphoresis. Cardiac monitoring is instituted, and morphine sulfate 15 mg q4h prn is ordered. The priority nursing care for this client should be directed toward:
    1. Relief of pain
    2. Client teaching
    3. Cardiac monitoring
    4. Maintenance of bed rest

177. A male client who is hospitalized following a myocardial infarction asks the nurse why he is receiving morphine. The nurse replies that morphine:
    1. Dilates coronary blood vessels
    2. Relieves pain and prevents shock
    3. Decreases anxiety and restlessness
    4. Helps prevent fibrillation of the heart

178. A client who is diagnosed with a myocardial infarction is admitted to the coronary care unit with orders for bed rest and medication for chest pain. Within an hour after admission, the nurse finds the client walking around the unit. The nurse's best initial response would be:
    1. "Tell me what you are doing out of bed."
    2. "It must be frustrating to be confined in bed."
    3. "You need to rest; therefore, you should get back into bed."
    4. "Please get back in bed immediately. The doctor wants you to rest."

179. A client, who is being monitored in the coronary care unit because of a myocardial infarction, has to have a bowel movement. The nurse should:
    1. Place the client onto a bedpan
    2. Help the client into the bathroom
    3. Roll the client onto a fracture pan
    4. Assist the client to a bedside commode

180. A client with a recent myocardial infarction is admitted to the cardiac care unit. The nurse can best determine the effectiveness of the client's ventricular contractions by:
1. Observing anxiety levels
2. Evaluating enzyme results
3. Monitoring urinary output hourly
4. Assessing breath sounds frequently

181. Isoenzyme laboratory studies are ordered for a client following a myocardial infarction. The most reliable early indicator of myocardial insult would be:
1. AST
2. Myoglobin
3. Troponin T and I
4. CK-MB and CPK totals

182. A client who has had a myocardial infarction develops cardiogenic shock despite treatment in the emergency department. When assessing this client the nurse would not expect to find:
1. Tachycardia
2. Restlessness
3. Warm moist skin
4. Decreased urinary output

183. When a client has a myocardial infarction, one of the major manifestations is a decrease in the conductive energy provided to the heart. When assessing this client the nurse understands that the existing action potential is in direct relationship to the:
1. Heart rate
2. Refractory period
3. Pulmonary pressure
4. Strength of contraction

184. The possibility of death from complications always accompanies an acute myocardial infarction. The complication the nurse should monitor the client for during the first 48 hours is:
1. Pulmonary edema
2. Pulmonary embolism
3. Ventricular tachycardia
4. Failure of the right ventricle

185. Because a client with a myocardial infarction can develop left ventricular failure, the nurse should assess this client for:
1. Distended neck veins
2. Anorexia and weight loss
3. Paroxysmal nocturnal dyspnea
4. Right upper quadrant tenderness

186. A client who has had a myocardial infarction experiences a noticeably decreased pulse pressure. The nurse should recognize this as a possible indication of:
1. Increased blood volume
2. Hyperactivity of the heart
3. Increased cardiac sufficiency
4. Decreased force of contraction

187. A client has mitral valve insufficiency (regurgitation). Which area should be used specifically when auscultating the heart to determine the presence of this problem?

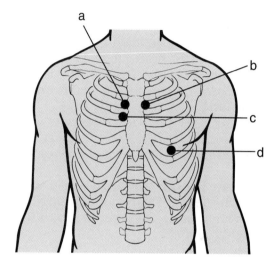

1. a
2. b
3. c
4. d

188. The nurse notes premature ventricular contractions (PVCs) on a client's cardiac monitor and recognizes that these complexes are a sign of:
1. Atrial fibrillation
2. Cardiac irritability
3. Impending heart block
4. Ventricular tachycardia

189. The wife of a client who has had emergency coronary artery bypass surgery asks why her husband has a dressing on his left leg. The nurse explains that:
1. This is the access site for the heart-lung machine
2. A filter is inserted in the leg to prevent embolization
3. The saphenous vein was used to bypass the coronary artery
4. The arteries in distal extremities are examined during surgery

190. The nurse is discussing discharge instructions with a client who has had coronary bypass surgery (CABG) and his wife. The client states, "My wife is afraid to have sex with me. When will it be safe to have sex again?" The most appropriate response by the nurse would be:
    1. "You should wait at least six weeks, but check with your doctor."
    2. "You will need to talk that over with your doctor before you leave."
    3. "When you feel you have recovered enough to resume sexual activity."
    4. "As soon as you can climb one flight of stairs without fatigue or discomfort."

191. It is determined that a client with heart block will require implantation of a permanent pacemaker to assist heart function. In response to the client's inquiries as to why this is necessary, the nurse's best response would be that it will:
    1. "Initiate a normal heartbeat."
    2. "Shock the AV node to contract."
    3. "Slow the heart to a more normal rate."
    4. "Synchronize the action of the heart valves."

192. A client has had a ventricular demand pacemaker inserted. The priority nursing intervention immediately after the pacemaker insertion would be to:
    1. Encourage fluids
    2. Assess the implant site
    3. Monitor the heart rate and rhythm
    4. Encourage turning and deep breathing

193. A client's wife arrives at the cardiac care unit and is informed that her husband needs a pacemaker. The wife expresses the concern that her husband could accidentally become electrocuted. The nurse's best response would be:
    1. No one has been electrocuted yet by a pacemaker."
    2. New technology prevents electrocution from occurring."
    3. The voltage emitted is not strong enough to electrocute him."
    4. Pacemakers are pretested for safety before they are inserted."

194. While obtaining a health history the nurse would expect a 78-year-old client admitted to the hospital with chronic heart failure to report a:
    1. Tingling in the hands and arms
    2. Feeling of being "bloated" after eating
    3. Need to use three pillows at night to sleep
    4. Swelling of the ankles more apparent in the morning than at night

195. A client with a history of hypertension and left ventricular failure arrives for a scheduled clinic appointment and tells the nurse, "My feet are killing me. These shoes got so tight." The nurse's best initial action would be to:
    1. Weigh the client
    2. Notify the physician
    3. Take the client's pulse rate
    4. Listen to the client's breath sounds

196. A client is admitted with early heart failure. The statement by the client that is uniquely related to heart failure that the nurse would expect is:
    1. "I see spots before my eyes."
    2. "I am tired at the end of the day."
    3. "I feel bloated when I eat a large meal."
    4. "I have trouble breathing when I climb a flight of stairs."

197. When performing a physical assessment of a client with heart failure, the adaptation that would be unexpected is:
    1. Dependent edema
    2. Progressive fatigue
    3. Moist, clammy skin
    4. Collapsed neck veins

198. The nurse understands that heart failure can best be described as:
    1. A cardiac condition caused by inadequate circulating blood volume
    2. An acute state in which the pulmonary circulation pressure decreases
    3. An inability of the heart to pump blood in proportion to metabolic needs
    4. A chronic state in which the systolic blood pressure drops below 90 mm Hg

199. A 76-year-old client is admitted with the diagnosis of mild chronic heart failure. The sounds indicative of chronic heart failure that the nurse expects to hear when listening to the client's lungs would be:
    1. Stridor
    2. Crackles
    3. Wheezes
    4. Friction rubs

200. When assessing a client with a diagnosis of left ventricular failure, the nurse should expect to find:
    1. Crushing chest pain
    2. Dyspnea on exertion
    3. Jugular vein distention
    4. Extensive peripheral edema

201. The teaching plan for a client receiving digoxin for left ventricular failure should include having the client:
    1. Sleep flat in bed
    2. Rest during the day
    3. Follow a low-potassium diet
    4. Take the pulse three times a day

202. A client is admitted to the intensive care unit with pulmonary edema. When performing the admission assessment, the nurse should expect:
    1. A decreased blood pressure
    2. Radiating anterior chest pain
    3. A pulse that is weak and rapid
    4. Crackles at the base of each lung

203. The physician orders "bathroom privileges only" for a client with pulmonary edema. The client becomes irritable and asks the nurse whether it is really necessary to stay in bed so much. The nurse's best reply would be:
    1. "Why do you want to be out of bed?"
    2. "Yes. Bed rest plays a role in most therapy."
    3. "Rest helps your body direct energy to healing."
    4. "Not always. Ask your physician to change the order."

204. When assessing a client for signs of right ventricular failure the nurse should expect to note:
    1. A slowed pulse rate
    2. Neck vein distention
    3. A pleural friction rub
    4. Increasing hypotension

205. The nurse suggests that a client with right ventricular failure should:
    1. Take a hot bath before bedtime
    2. Avoid sleeping in an air-conditioned room
    3. Avoid emotionally stressful situations when possible
    4. Exercise daily until the pulse rate exceeds 100 beats per minute

206. A client is admitted to the medical unit with a diagnosis of right ventricular heart failure. The nursing assessment that supports this medical diagnosis would be:
    1. Dyspnea on exertion
    2. Nocturnal orthopnea
    3. Distended jugular veins
    4. Decreased arterial blood pressure

207. The home health care nurse is assessing a client with cardiac insufficiency. The nurse notes that the client's pulse rate increases from 70 to 92 beats per minute while climbing the stairs. The nurse should instruct the client to:
    1. Continue climbing
    2. Stand still and rest
    3. Walk down the stairs
    4. Climb at a slower rate

208. The client that would be considered at the highest risk for a dissecting aneurysm is:
    1. A 50-year-old white male with moderate hypertension
    2. A 55-year-old Black male with uncontrolled hypertension
    3. A 42-year-old Black female with peripheral vascular disease
    4. A 40-year-old white female with uncontrolled hypertension

209. During a routine physical examination, an abdominal aortic aneurysm is diagnosed. The client is immediately admitted to the hospital, and surgery is scheduled for the next morning. When performing the admission assessment the nurse should expect:
    1. Severe radiating abdominal pain
    2. Cyanosis and symptoms of shock
    3. A pattern of visible peristaltic waves
    4. A palpable pulsating abdominal mass

210. On the morning of surgery a client is admitted for resection of an abdominal aortic aneurysm. While awaiting surgery, the client suddenly develops symptoms of shock. The nurse should:
    1. Prepare for blood transfusions
    2. Notify the physician immediately
    3. Give the client nothing by mouth
    4. Administer the prescribed sedative

211. To prevent thrombus formation after most surgeries, the nurse should plan to:
    1. Keep the bed gatched to elevate the client's knees
    2. Have the client dangle the legs off the side of the bed
    3. Have the client use an incentive spirometer every hour
    4. Encourage the client to ambulate with assistance as needed

212. The sign or symptom the nurse should expect when assessing a client with severe varicosities of both legs would be:
    1. Increased sensitivity to cold
    2. Pallor of the lower extremities
    3. Increasing ankle edema over the day
    4. Calf pain when the foot is dorsiflexed

213. A client who had injection sclerotherapy for varicose veins has been advised to wear compression (support) stockings. The nurse should explain that:
    1. The best length is to the middle of the knees
    2. It is best to apply them before getting out of bed
    3. They should be applied at the first sign of discomfort
    4. Elastic bandages may be substituted because they are more economical

214. When collecting data from a client with varicose veins who is to have sclerotherapy, the nurse should expect the client to report:
    1. A feeling of heaviness in both legs
    2. Intermittent claudication of the legs
    3. Calf pain on dorsiflexion of the foot
    4. Hematomas of the lower extremities

215. Before having sclerotherapy for varicose veins, a female client who states she is fearful of a chemical injection asks the nurse to explain what would be involved if she insisted on a ligation and stripping to correct the problem. The nurse should explain that this surgery involves:
    1. Removing the dilated saphenous veins
    2. Cleaning out plaque from within the vessels
    3. Anastomosing superficial veins to deep veins
    4. Placing an umbrella filter in the large affected veins

216. A client with a history of thrombophlebitis and varicosities is to have a herniorrhaphy for an incarcerated hernia. The client's past medical history and present diagnosis indicate to the nurse that a primary responsibility following surgery is to:
    1. Raise the foot of the bed
    2. Get the client out of bed twice daily
    3. Maintain body alignment with firm support of the extremities
    4. Encourage the client to turn often and to exercise the legs regularly

217. After a long history of recurrent thrombophlebitis in extensive varicose veins of the lower extremities, surgical intervention is suggested to the client. When asked about the procedure, the nurse should explain that this surgery involves:
    1. Removing the dilated superficial vein
    2. Bypassing the varicosities with artificial veins
    3. Stripping the cholesterol deposits from the vein
    4. Creating fistulas between superficial and deep veins

218. Before discharging a client who has had an inguinal herniorrhaphy, the nurse teaches the client about exercising to prevent venous stasis. For best results the nurse should:
    1. Demonstrate specific exercises
    2. Suggest frequent moving of the legs
    3. Advise against sitting for prolonged periods
    4. Suggest that the client change position frequently

219. A client with extensive bone and soft-tissue injuries to the right leg is on bed rest. When positioning the affected extremity, the nurse should:
    1. Keep the right leg resting straight on the bed, parallel to the left leg
    2. Elevate the entire right leg with pillows, keeping the foot higher than the knee
    3. Maintain both legs on the bed while using an abduction pillow to keep them separated
    4. Attach a padded ankle sling to a Balkan frame to support the right foot and elevate the leg

220. A client with a history of thrombophlebitis is scheduled for a left incarcerated hernia repair with insertion of a mesh graft to reinforce the area. Preoperatively, the nurse should specifically assess the client for:
    1. Edema of the left leg
    2. Mobility of the left leg
    3. A positive left-sided Babinski reflex
    4. Presence of peripheral arterial pulses

221. A client reports a history of bilateral blanching and pain in the fingers on exposure to cold. When rewarmed the fingers become bright red and "tingly" with a slow return to normal color. The client smokes one to two packs of cigarettes per day. The nurse recognizes that the client has Raynaud's disease and not Raynaud's phenomenon because of the:
    1. Tingling sensation
    2. Skin color changes
    3. Bilateral involvement
    4. Changes in skin temperature

222. The nurse encourages a client with Raynaud's disease to stop smoking because it causes:
    1. Pain and tingling
    2. Cyanosis and necrosis
    3. Peripheral vasoconstriction
    4. Excessive blood oxygen content

223. A 60-year-old farmer, who has been smoking two packs of cigarettes daily for 40 years, comes to the outpatient clinic with an ischemic

left foot. It is determined the cause is arterial insufficiency. The client needs to understand that the pain in his foot is a result of inadequate blood supply, which may be further diminished by:

1. Drinking alcohol
2. Lowering the limb
3. Smoking cigarettes
4. Consuming excessive fluid

224. A client with arterial insufficiency of both lower extremities is visited by the home health care nurse. An essential nursing intervention would be to teach the client to:

1. Massage the legs when painful
2. Maintain elevation of both legs
3. Apply a hot water bottle to the legs
4. Check arterial pulses in the legs regularly

225. A 55-year-old bank teller, with a history of occasional pain in the left foot when walking, has now developed pain at rest. The left foot is cyanotic, numb, and painful. The suspected cause is arteriosclerosis. The nurse should teach the client that the pain in the foot is more likely to decrease if he:

1. Keeps the left foot cool
2. Crosses his legs with the left one on top
3. Complies with the prescribed exercise program
4. Keeps the left foot elevated at a 30-degree angle

226. When supporting vasodilation by the use of warmth for a client with peripheral arterial insufficiency, the nurse should caution the client to avoid:

1. Turning the room thermostat below 78° F
2. Applying a hot water bottle to the abdomen
3. Drinking a warm cup of tea when feeling chilly
4. Using a heating pad to wrap the extremities

227. A client develops a nonhealing ulcer of the right lower extremity and complains of leg cramps after walking short distances. The client asks the nurse what causes these leg pains. The nurse's best response would be:

1. "Muscle weakness occurs in the legs because of a lack of exercise."
2. "Edema and cyanosis occur in the legs because they are dependent."
3. "Pain occurs in the legs while walking because there is a lack of oxygen to the muscles."

4. "Pressure occurs in the legs because of vasodilation and pooling of blood in the extremity."

228. The physician prescribes a progressive exercise program that includes walking for a client with a history of diminished arterial perfusion to the lower extremities. The nurse should explain to the client that if leg cramps occur while walking, the client should:

1. Take one aspirin twice a day
2. Stop and rest until the pain resolves
3. Walk more slowly while pain is present
4. Take one nitroglycerin tablet sublingually

229. A client with peripheral arterial insufficiency is to have surgery. Upon admission, the client complains of discomfort and aches in the legs and feet. To safely position this client the nurse should take into consideration that the feet and legs should be:

1. Placed dependent to the torso
2. Dependent by using a fully extended knee gatch
3. Raised to a two-pillow height above the buttocks
4. Elevated by raising the foot of the bed on blocks

230. A client comes to the outpatient clinic with a painful leg ulcer. The symptom that supports the diagnosis of arterial ulcer is:

1. Pain at the ulcer site
2. Bleeding around the ulcer area
3. Dependent edema of the extremities
4. Stasis dermatitis on affected extremity

231. A client is admitted to the hospital with a large leg ulcer, and a femoral angiogram is performed. After this procedure the nurse should:

1. Provide passive ROM to all extremities
2. Elevate the foot of the bed for 36 hours
3. Apply pressure to the catheter insertion site
4. Assist the client to stand if unable to void

232. A client with an occlusion of the left femoral artery is scheduled for an arteriogram. When assessing the extremity prior to the arteriogram, the nurse would note as most significant:

1. A mottling of the left leg
2. An absence of the left pedal pulse
3. An unexplained coolness of the left foot
4. A thickening of the toenails on the left foot

233. Before a femoral arteriogram is started, the nurse should plan to teach the client that:
    1. Radioactive dye will be injected into the femoral vein
    2. A local anesthetic will be given to lessen any pain at the site
    3. Contrast media will be injected into a small vessel of the foot
    4. Medication will be administered intravenously to induce sleep

234. Six hours after a femoral-popliteal bypass graft, the client's blood pressure becomes severely elevated. The nurse should notify the physician primarily because the client's:
    1. Hypervolemia needs to be corrected immediately
    2. Blood pressure could cause the graft to occlude
    3. Intraabdominal pressure could compromise the viability of the graft
    4. Cardiovascular status could precipitate a cerebrovascular accident

235. A client with a history of severe intermittent claudication has a femoral-popliteal bypass graft. An appropriate postoperative intervention on the day after surgery would be to:
    1. Keep the client on bed rest
    2. Have the client sit in a chair
    3. Assist the client with ambulation
    4. Encourage the client to keep the legs elevated

236. A client with peripheral arterial insufficiency tells the nurse that sometimes walking causes severe pain in the calf muscles. When preparing a teaching plan, the nurse should recognize that this pain is called:
    1. Rest pain
    2. Phantom limb sensation
    3. Raynaud's phenomenon
    4. Intermittent claudication

237. The nurse provides discharge teaching for a client with a history of hypertension who has had a femoral-popliteal bypass graft. The nurse is aware that the teaching is effective when the client says, "I should:
    1. Massage my calves gently every day."
    2. Keep my foot elevated when I am in bed."
    3. Sit in a hot bath for 25 minutes twice a day."
    4. Assess the color and pulses of my legs every day."

238. The nurse is aware that during the early postoperative period after open heart surgery adequate oxygenation is essential because:
    1. Clients have closed chest drainage in place
    2. Hypoxia can precipitate respiratory alkalosis
    3. Hypoxia can stimulate dangerous dysrhythmias
    4. An increased respiratory rate adds to postoperative pain

239. The nurse in the ICU is monitoring a client who has had an aortic valve replacement. The nurse is aware that a slow pulse rate during the early postoperative period following open heart surgery can indicate:
    1. Shock
    2. Hypoxia
    3. Heart block
    4. Heart failure

ENDOCRINE (EN)

240. When obtaining a health history from a client recently diagnosed with type 1 diabetes, the nurse should expect the client to mention symptoms associated with the classic signs of diabetes, such as:
    1. Polydipsia, polyuria, irritability
    2. Polydipsia, polyphagia, polyuria
    3. Polydipsia, nocturia, weight loss
    4. Polyphagia, diaphoresis, polyuria

241. When obtaining the history of a 24-year-old graduate student recently diagnosed with type 1 diabetes, the nurse would expect to identify the presence of:
    1. Edema
    2. Anorexia
    3. Weight loss
    4. Hypoglycemic episodes

242. A client has recently been diagnosed with type 1 diabetes. A glucose tolerance test is ordered. The order reads, "Administer glucose 1.0 g/kg." The client weighs 240 pounds. The nurse should administer:
    Answer: _____.

243. The physician orders daily determinations of fasting blood glucose levels for a client with diabetes mellitus. The goal of treatment is that the client will have glucose levels within the range of:
    1. 40 to 65 mg/dl of blood
    2. 70 to105 mg/dl of blood
    3. 110 to 145 mg/dl of blood
    4. 150 to 175 mg/dl of blood

244. A 50-year-old male with a history of type 1 diabetes has had progressive problems with venous stasis. He tells the nurse in the clinic that he bumped his leg a week ago and now has an open draining area just above the ankle. When exploring this client's health history, the most important assessment by the nurse would be to ascertain:
    1. Whether he uses Humulin N insulin or Humulin R insulin
    2. How many times a day the client voids and how often he moves his bowels
    3. The type of treatment the client is receiving and how he has managed his care
    4. How many children the client has and whether they are having similar problems

245. When assessing the laboratory values of a client with type 2 diabetes, the nurse should expect the results to reveal:
    1. Ketones in the blood but not the urine
    2. Glucose in the urine but not in the blood
    3. Urine negative for ketones and glucose in the blood
    4. Urine and blood positive for both glucose and ketones

246. The nurse should explain to a client with diabetes that self-monitoring of blood glucose is preferred to urine glucose testing because it is:
    1. More accurate
    2. Easier to perform
    3. Done by the client
    4. Not influenced by drugs

247. A client is diagnosed as having type 2 diabetes. A priority teaching goal would be, "The client will be able to:
    1. Perform foot care daily."
    2. Administer insulin as ordered."
    3. Test urine for sugar and acetone."
    4. Identify signs of hypoglycemia/hyperglycemia."

248. The nurse teaches a client with type 2 diabetes how to provide self-care to prevent infections of the feet. The nurse recognizes that the teaching was effective when the client says, "I should:
    1. Massage my feet and legs with oil or lotion."
    2. Apply heat intermittently to my feet and legs."
    3. Eat foods high in protein and carbohydrate kilocalories."
    4. Control my diabetes through diet, exercise, and medication."

249. A 25-year-old physical fitness instructor has been feeling increasingly tired and seeks medical care. Type 1 diabetes is diagnosed. The nurse explains that the increased fatigue is the result of
    1. Increased metabolism at the cellular level
    2. Increased glucose absorption from the intestine
    3. Decreased production of insulin by the pancreas
    4. Decreased glucose secretion into the renal tubules

250. A client, newly diagnosed as having type 1 diabetes, is encouraged to exercise on a regular basis primarily because exercise has been shown to:
    1. Decrease insulin sensitivity
    2. Stimulate glucagon production
    3. Improve the cellular uptake of glucose
    4. Reduce metabolic requirements for glucose

251. A client with type 2 diabetes is taking one oral tablet daily. The client asks whether an extra pill should be taken before exercise. The nurse should reply:
    1. "You will need to decrease your exercise."
    2. "Your diet and medicine will not be affected by exercise."
    3. "An extra pill will help your body use glucose correctly."
    4. "No, but observe for signs of hypoglycemia while exercising."

252. A client who is taking an oral hypoglycemic daily for type 2 diabetes develops the flu and is concerned about the need for special care. The nurse should advise the client to:
    1. Avoid food, drink clear liquids, take a daily temperature, and stay in bed
    2. Skip the oral hypoglycemic pill, drink plenty of fluids, and stay in bed
    3. Eat as much as possible, increase fluid intake, and call the office again the next day
    4. Take the oral hypoglycemic pill, drink warm fluids, and perform a serum glucose test ac and hs

253. An obese client with type 2 diabetes asks about the use of alcohol or special "dietetic" food in the diet. The client should be taught that:
    1. Unlimited amounts of sugar substitutes can be used as desired
    2. Alcohol can be used, with its calories accounted for in the diet
    3. Alcohol should not be used in cooking because it adds too many calories
    4. Special "dietetic" foods are needed because many regular foods cannot be used

254. A client with type 2 diabetes travels frequently and asks how to plan meals during trips. The nurse's most appropriate response would be:
1. "You can order diabetic foods on most airlines and in restaurants."
2. "You should plan your food ahead and carry it with you from home."
3. "Make regular food choices, wherever you are, following your food plan."
4. "You can monitor your blood glucose level frequently and can eat accordingly."

255. A client with newly diagnosed diabetes indicates a hatred for asparagus, broccoli, and mushrooms. When reviewing the exchange list with the client, the nurse would know that the teaching about the exchange list was understood when the client states, "Instead of these foods I can eat:
1. String beans, beets, or carrots."
2. Corn, lima beans, or dried peas."
3. Baked beans, potatoes, or parsnips."
4. Corn muffins, corn chips, or pretzels."

256. While hospitalized, a client with diabetes is observed picking at calluses on the feet. The nurse should immediately:
1. Warn the client of the danger of infection
2. Suggest that the client wear white cotton socks
3. Check the client's shoes for proper fit in the area of the calluses
4. Demonstrate and teach the importance of proper foot care to the client

257. After a surgical procedure for cancer of the pancreas that included the removal of the stomach, the head of the pancreas, the distal end of the duodenum, and the spleen, the postoperative manifestation by the client that would require immediate attention by the nurse would be:
1. Jaundice
2. Indigestion
3. Weight loss
4. Hyperglycemia

258. Four hours after surgery, the blood glucose level of a client who has type 1 diabetes is elevated. The nurse should expect to:
1. Administer an oral hypoglycemic
2. Institute urine glucose monitoring
3. Give supplemental doses of regular insulin
4. Decrease the rate of the intravenous infusion

259. A client who has type 1 diabetes is admitted to the hospital for major surgery. Prior to surgery the client's insulin requirements are elevated but well controlled. Postoperatively the nurse would anticipate that the client's insulin requirements will:
1. Fluctuate widely
2. Increase sharply
3. Remain elevated
4. Decrease immediately

260. A client is admitted to the hospital with diabetic ketoacidosis. The nurse understands that the elevated ketone level present with this disorder is caused by the incomplete oxidation of:
1. Fats
2. Protein
3. Potassium
4. Carbohydrates

261. The serum potassium level of a client who has diabetic ketoacidosis is 5.4 mEq/L. When monitoring the ECG tracing, the nurse would expect to observe:
1. Abnormal P waves and depressed T waves
2. Peaked T waves and widened QRS complexes
3. Abnormal Q waves and prolonged ST segments
4. Peaked P waves and increased number of T waves

262. A client with type 1 diabetes is placed on an insulin pump. The most appropriate short-term goal when teaching this client to control the diabetes is: "The client will:
1. Adhere to the medical regimen."
2. Remain normoglycemic for three weeks."
3. Demonstrate the correct use of the insulin pump."
4. List three self-care activities necessary to control the diabetes."

263. When the nurse plans to teach a client with type 1 diabetes about the use of an insulin pump, it is of major importance that the client understand that the:
1. Needle should be changed every day
2. Glucose monitoring will be monitored once daily
3. Pump is an attempt to mimic the way a healthy pancreas works
4. Pump will be implanted in a subcutaneous pocket near the abdomen

264. For proper foot care, the nurse should instruct a client with type 2 diabetes to:
1. Remove all corns and stop smoking
2. Always wear shoes and use natural fiber socks
3. Wear nylon socks and wash feet in warm water

4. Wear shoes that are slightly larger and avoid using corn removers

265. A client with type 1 diabetes of long duration takes Humulin N and Humulin R insulin every morning. At noon, before eating lunch, the client is admitted to the emergency department with an acute myocardial infarction. Two hours later, the client's serum glucose level drops to 30 mg/dl, and insulin coma is diagnosed. The nurse understands the reason for the development of acute hypoglycemia in this client is that:
1. Glycogenolysis increased when lunch was not eaten after taking Humulin N insulin
2. The stress brought on by the chest pain increases the use of serum glucose available to the client
3. Glucose levels that are controlled by insulin drop more quickly than those controlled by oral antidiabetics
4. The client's body became sensitive to the prescribed dose of insulin after long use, and the blood glucose level dropped erratically

266. When assisting a client with type 1 diabetes, the nurse notes a 5 cm nodule on the upper arm where the client states she has been injecting her insulin at home. The nurse is aware that the nodule, which is neither warm nor painful, is a result of:
1. Keratosis
2. An allergy
3. An infection
4. Lipodystrophy

267. When assessing a client who is experiencing hypoglycemia, the nurse should expect to find:
1. Lethargy
2. Tachycardia
3. Warm, dry skin
4. Increased respirations

268. A client with diabetic ketoacidosis who is receiving intravenous fluids and insulin complains of tingling and numbness of the fingers and toes and shortness of breath. The cardiac monitor shows the appearance of a U wave. The nurse should recognize that these symptoms indicate:
1. Hypokalemia
2. Hyponatremia
3. Hypoglycemia
4. Hypercalcemia

269. The nurse recognizes that a client with diabetes understands the teaching about the treatment of hypoglycemia when the client says, "If I become hypoglycemic I should initially eat:

1. Sugar and a slice of bread."
2. Hard candy and fruit juice."
3. Chocolate candy and a banana."
4. Peanut butter crackers and a glass of milk."

270. A 62-year-old client is admitted for hypertension and serum electrolyte studies have yielded abnormal results. The scheduled workup includes a scan for an aldosteronoma. The nurse recognizes that this scan is ordered to rule out disease of the:
1. Kidney cortex
2. Thyroid gland
3. Adrenal cortex
4. Pituitary gland

271. A client with an aldosterone-secreting adenoma is scheduled for surgery to remove the tumor. The client wonders what will happen if surgery is canceled. The nurse would base a response on the fact that:
1. Surgery will prevent the tumor from metastasizing to other organs
2. The tumor must be removed to prevent heart and kidney damage
3. Chemotherapy is as reliable as surgery to treat adenomas of this type
4. Radiation therapy can be just as effective as surgery if the tumor is small

272. Late in the postoperative period after resection of an aldosterone-secreting adenoma, the nurse would expect the client's blood pressure to:
1. Rise quickly above preoperative levels
2. Gradually return to near normal levels
3. Fluctuate greatly during this entire period
4. Drop very low, then rise rapidly to normal levels

273. The wife of a client who has had a resection of an aldosterone-secreting tumor of the adrenal glands says, "I hope this is the end of the problem and that my husband will be back to work soon." Based on an understanding of the health problem, the nurse should:
1. Explain that surgery will effect a cure, and the left adrenal gland is functioning to meet the body's needs
2. Caution the wife against setting her expectations too high, since the outcome for this problem is variable
3. Advise the wife to investigate other occupational alternatives for her husband if he plans to return to work
4. Tell her that although her husband will require hormone supplements for the rest of his life, he should be able to work

274. The nurse would expect the diagnostic studies of a client with Cushing's syndrome to show:
1. Moderately increased serum potassium levels
2. Increased numbers of eosinophils in the blood
3. High levels of 17-ketosteroids in a 24-hour urine test
4. Normal to low levels of adrenocorticotropic hormone (ACTH)

275. A female client has a tentative diagnosis of Cushing's syndrome. The nurse's physical assessment of this client will probably include the findings of:
1. Fever and tachycardia
2. Lethargy and constipation
3. Hypertension and moon-face
4. Hyperactivity and exophthalmos

276. A 49-year-old female is admitted to the hospital with a possible diagnosis of Addison's disease. An important nursing responsibility during a 24-hour-urine collection for the client suspected of having Addison's disease would be to:
1. Assess the client for signs of edema
2. Keep the client quiet and reduce stress
3. Monitor the client for an elevation of blood pressure
4. Restrict the client's fluid intake for the 24 hours

277. A female college freshman visits the health center because she feels nervous, irritable, and extremely tired. She complains that, although she eats large amounts of food, she has frequent bouts of diarrhea and is losing weight. The nurse observes a fine hand tremor, an exaggerated reaction to external stimuli, and a wide-eyed expression. The laboratory tests that might be ordered to determine what may be causing this client's symptoms are the:
1. PTT and PT
2. T_3, T_4, and TSH
3. VDRL and CBC
4. Serum barbiturate levels

278. During a home visit to a client, the nurse notices tremors of the client's hands. When discussing this assessment the client reveals being nervous, having difficulty sleeping, and feeling as if the collars of shirts are getting tight. The nurse recognizes that the physician should be notified immediately when the client also mentions:
1. Feelings of warmth
2. A recent weight loss
3. An increased appetite

4. Fluttering in the chest

279. A client visits the clinic because of concerns about insomnia and recent weight loss. A tentative diagnosis of hyperthyroidism is made. In addition to the adaptations noted, the nurse should further assess this client for:
1. Fatigue
2. Dry skin
3. Anorexia
4. Bradycardia

280. Before obtaining blood for protein-bound iodine, T_3, and T_4 tests the nurse should ask a client suspected of having a hyperactive thyroid if the client has had:
1. An allergy to seafood or iodine
2. More protein intake than usual
3. Anything to eat or drink recently
4. X-rays using radiopaque dye recently

281. When assessing a client with Graves' disease, the nurse should expect to find:
1. Constipation, dry skin, and weight gain
2. Lethargy, weight gain, and forgetfulness
3. Weight loss, exophthalmos, and restlessness
4. Weight loss, protruding eyeballs, and lethargy

282. When assessing a client with Graves' disease (hyperthyroidism) the nurse would expect to find a history of:
1. Diaphoresis
2. Menorrhagia
3. Dry, brittle hair
4. Sensitivity to cold

283. The nurse teaches a client with exophthalmos how to reduce discomfort and prevent corneal ulceration. The nurse recognizes that the teaching is understood when the client states, "I should:
1. Eliminate excessive blinking."
2. Not move my extraocular muscles."
3. Elevate the head of my bed at night."
4. Avoid using a sleeping mask at night."

284. A client is scheduled to have a thyroidectomy for cancer of the thyroid. Preoperative instructions for the postoperative period should include teaching the client to:
1. Cough and deep breathe every two hours
2. Perform range-of-motion exercises of the head and neck
3. Support the head with the hands when changing position

4. Apply gentle pressure against the incision when swallowing

285. A client is diagnosed with hyperthyroidism and surgery is scheduled because the client refuses ablation therapy. While awaiting the surgical date, the nurse should plan to instruct the client to:
1. Consciously attempt to calm down
2. Eliminate coffee, tea, and cola from the diet
3. Keep the home warm and use an extra blanket at night
4. Schedule activities during the day to overcome lethargy

286. When planning for a client's return from the operating room after a subtotal thyroidectomy, the nurse should understand that with this surgery:
1. The entire thyroid gland is removed
2. A small part of the gland is left intact
3. One parathyroid gland is also removed
4. A portion of the thyroid and four parathyroids are removed

287. A client with cancer of the thyroid is scheduled for a thyroidectomy. Postoperatively the nurse should plan to have:
1. A tracheostomy set at the client's bedside
2. A quiet, dimly lit room ready for the client
3. A large soft pillow for use under the client's head
4. An intermittent suction apparatus at the client's bedside

288. A client with malignant hot nodules of the thyroid gland has a thyroidectomy. Immediately after the thyroidectomy, the nurse's priority action should be to:
1. Elevate the client's head to limit edema of the neck
2. Monitor the client's intake and output to assess for fluid overload
3. Encourage the client to cough and deep-breathe to prevent atelectasis
4. Assess the client's level of consciousness to determine recovery from anesthesia

289. Immediately after a subtotal thyroidectomy the nurse plans to assess a female client for unilateral injury of the laryngeal nerve every 30 to 60 minutes by:
1. Checking her throat for edema
2. Observing her for signs of tetany
3. Asking her to state her name out loud
4. Palpating the side of her neck for blood seepage

290. When planning care for a client who has had a thyroidectomy, the nursing action that should be given highest priority during the first 24 hours postoperatively is:
1. Humidifying the room air continuously
2. Performing range-of-motion neck exercises q4h
3. Assessing for hoarseness and voice weakness every two hours
4. Checking vital signs every two hours after they have stabilized

291. When planning care for a client in the first 24 hours after a thyroidectomy, the nurse should include:
1. Checking the back and sides of the operative dressing
2. Supporting the head during mild range-of-motion exercises
3. Encouraging the client to ventilate feelings about the surgery
4. Advising the client that regular activities can be resumed immediately

292. During the early postoperative period after a subtotal thyroidectomy, the observation that has the highest priority would be:
1. Hemorrhage
2. Thyrotoxic crisis
3. Airway obstruction
4. Hypocalcemic tetany

293. After a client has a thyroidectomy the nurse should observe for possible complications. The nurse should be aware that if tingling and numbness of the fingers and toes, muscle twitching, or muscle spasms occur, the client may be:
1. Hypokalemic
2. Hypocalcemic
3. In thyrotoxic crisis
4. In hypovolemic shock

294. On the third postoperative day after a subtotal thyroidectomy for a tumor, the client complains of a "funny, jittery feeling." On the basis of this statement, the nurse's best action would be to:
1. Explain that this type of reaction is expected after thyroid surgery
2. Take the vital signs and place the client in a high Fowler's position
3. Request STAT serum calcium and phosphorus levels and chart the results
4. Test for Chvostek's and Trousseau's signs and notify the physician of the complaints

295. After a thyroidectomy, a client should be monitored for thyrotoxic crisis, which would be evidenced by:
1. An increased pulse deficit
2. A decreased blood pressure
3. A decreased heart rate and respirations
4. An increased temperature and pulse rate

296. After treatment with propylthiouracil for hyperthyroidism, a client has the thyroid ablated with ^{131}I. On a visit to the endocrine clinic, the client exhibits signs and symptoms of thyrotoxic crisis (thyroid storm). The nurse is aware that this is often associated with:
1. An iodine deficiency
2. A decreased serum calcium
3. Increased sodium retention
4. Excessive thyroid replacement

297. When preparing a client for discharge after a thyroidectomy, the nurse should teach the signs of hypothyroidism. The nurse would be aware that the client understands the teaching when the client says, "I should call my physician if I develop:
1. Muscle cramping and sluggishness."
2. Fatigue and an increased pulse rate."
3. Dry hair and an intolerance to cold."
4. Tachycardia and an increase in weight."

298. A client who has had a subtotal thyroidectomy does not understand how hypothyroidism could develop when the problem was hyperthyroidism. The nurse should base a response on the knowledge that:
1. Hypothyroidism is a gradual slowing of the body's function
2. There will be a decrease in pituitary thyroid-stimulating hormone
3. There may not be enough thyroid tissue left to supply adequate thyroid hormone
4. Atrophy of tissue remaining after surgery reduces secretion of thyroid hormones

299. The nurse should teach a client, who had a thyroidectomy for thyroid cancer, to observe for signs of surgically induced hypothyroidism. Check all that should be included in the teaching plan.
1. _____ Dry skin
2. _____ Lethargy
3. _____ Insomnia
4. _____ Tachycardia
5. _____ Sensitivity to cold
6. _____ Increasing restlessness

FLUIDS AND ELECTROLYTES (FE)

300. A 74-year-old client comes to the emergency room complaining of weakness and dizziness. The blood pressure is 90/60, pulse is 92 and weak, and body weight reflects a three-pound loss in two days. The weather has been very warm and the client's fluid intake has not increased. The most appropriate nursing diagnosis for this client would be:
1. Deficient fluid volume related to insufficient fluid intake
2. Feeding self-care deficit, related to altered thought processes
3. Ineffective tissue perfusion related to decreased cardiac strength
4. Imbalanced nutrition: less than body requirements related to aging

301. An older female adult who lives alone had not answered her phone for several days. She was found unconscious on the bathroom floor by her family and was admitted to the hospital with the diagnoses of a fractured hip and renal failure due to dehydration. In the 24 hours since she has been hospitalized, she has received 1500 mL of intravenous fluid. Her next serum electrolyte series reflects hyponatremia. The nurse recognizes that this may result from an increase in:
1. Salt intake
2. Fluid intake
3. Sodium absorption
4. Glomerular filtration

302. During an eight-hour shift a client drinks two 6-ounce cups of tea and vomits 125 mL of fluid. Intravenous fluids absorbed equaled the urinary output. During this eight-hour period the client's fluid balance would be:
Answer: _____.

303. A client weighed 210 pounds on admission to the hospital. After two days of diuretic therapy the client weighs 205.5 pounds. The nurse could estimate that the amount of fluid the client has lost is:
1. 0.5 L
2. 1.0 L
3. 2.0 L
4. 3.5 L

304. A male client with a history of heart failure and atrial fibrillation comes to the clinic for his regular two-week visit. The client is nine pounds heavier than his usual weight. The nurse

interprets that the most likely cause of this sudden weight gain would be:
1. Fluid retention
2. Urinary retention
3. Renal insufficiency
4. Abdominal distention

305. The dietary practice that will help a client reduce the dietary intake of sodium would be:
1. Increasing the use of dairy products
2. Using steak sauce for flavoring foods
3. Restricting the use of artificial sweeteners
4. Avoiding the use of carbonated beverages

306. An ECG is performed before a client is to have a cardiac catheterization, and hypokalemia is suspected. To confirm the presence of hypokalemia, the nurse would expect the physician to order:
1. Blood cultures × 3
2. A complete blood count
3. A serum electrolyte level
4. An x-ray film of long bones

307. The physician has ordered 1000 mL TPN in 12 hours to be infused via a subclavian catheter. When preparing the equipment it would be most important for the nurse to obtain:
1. A steady IV pole
2. An infusion pump
3. An infusion set delivering 60 gtt/mL
4. A set of clamps (hemostats) taped at the bedside

308. A client is to receive an intravenous solution containing potassium chloride. When starting this IV infusion the nurse should select:
1. The antecubital space in the client's arm
2. The largest possible vein in the client's arm
3. A vein in the back of the client's dominant hand
4. A vein in the back of the client's nondominant hand

309. When evaluating a client's response to fluid replacement therapy, the observation that indicates adequate tissue perfusion to vital organs would be:
1. Urinary output of 30 mL per hour
2. Central venous pressure reading of 2 cm H_2O
3. Pulse rates of 120 and 110 in a 15-minute period
4. Blood pressure readings of 50/30 and 70/40 mm Hg within 30 minutes

310. The physician orders total parenteral nutrition for a client with cancer of the pancreas. A right subclavian catheter is inserted by the physician. The nurse knows that the most important reason for using a central line is that:
1. It prevents the development of phlebitis
2. It is more convenient so clients can use their hands
3. There is less chance of this infusion infiltrating
4. The amount of blood in a major vein helps to dilute the solution

311. When administering albumin intravenously, the nurse is aware that body water will shift from the:
1. Interstitial compartment to the extracellular compartment
2. Extracellular compartment to the intracellular compartment
3. Intravascular compartment to the interstitial compartment
4. Intracellular compartment to the intravascular compartment

312. The nurse is aware that the shift of body fluids associated with the intravenous administration of albumin occurs by the process of:
1. Osmosis
2. Filtration
3. Diffusion
4. Active transport

313. The nurse teaches a client with chronic renal failure that salt substitutes cannot be used in the diet because:
1. A person's body tends to retain fluid when a salt substitute is included in the diet
2. Limiting salt substitutes in the diet prevents a buildup of waste products in the blood
3. Salt substitutes contain potassium, which must be limited to prevent abnormal heartbeats
4. A substance in the salt substitute interferes with the transfer of fluid across capillary membranes, resulting in anasarca

314. The nurse is aware that total parenteral nutrition is a more desirable therapy than just intravenous fluids for clients with gastrointestinal problems. The nurse understands that clients receiving only IV fluids lose weight because of:
1. Lack of bulk in the diet
2. Deficient carbohydrate intake
3. Insufficient intake of water-soluble vitamins
4. Increased concentrations of electrolytes in cells

315. If the electrolyte, potassium, is not added to a basic total parenteral nutrition solution, hypokalemia results. The nurse knows that the signs of hypokalemia include:
    1. Hyperventilation
    2. Metabolic alkalosis
    3. Dysrhythmias such as heart block
    4. A decreased serum potassium of 5.5 mEq/L

316. When a client is receiving total parenteral nutrition, it is important for the nurse to assess the:
    1. Blood for glucose
    2. Stool for occult blood
    3. Urine for specific gravity
    4. Abdomen for bowel sounds

317. The nurse knows that one of the complications of total parenteral nutrition would be:
    1. Infection
    2. Hepatitis
    3. Anorexia
    4. Dysrhythmias

318. A client's clinical symptoms indicate a possible gastric ulcer. Considering the symptoms of epigastric pain, vomiting, dehydration, weakness, lethargy, and shallow respirations, and the laboratory results that demonstrate metabolic alkalosis, the primary nursing diagnosis for this client would be:
    1. Impaired gas exchange related to pain
    2. Deficient fluid volume related to vomiting
    3. Risk for injury related to increased weakness
    4. Chronic pain related to hypersecretion of gastric acids

319. A client with hypertension is being taught to restrict the intake of sodium. The nurse would know that the teaching about foods low in sodium was understood when the client states, "I can eat:
    1. Broiled scallops."
    2. Bologna on rye bread."
    3. Shredded wheat cereal."
    4. Carrot and celery sticks."

320. A 79-year-old male resident of a nursing home has been refusing to eat or drink for the past few days, and his urinary output has dropped to less than 300 mL/day. He is confused and hypotensive. He is diagnosed as having renal failure secondary to dehydration. The physician orders 50% glucose and regular insulin. The nurse understands that this is ordered for a client in renal failure to:
    1. Prevent cardiac arrest
    2. Increase urinary output

    3. Prevent respiratory acidosis
    4. Decrease serum calcium levels

321. A client has a decreased serum sodium level. The nurse should assess for signs of hyponatremia, which include:
    1. Dry skin
    2. Confusion
    3. Tachycardia
    4. Pale coloring

322. A young, male client with a history of ulcerative colitis had been admitted to the hospital with severe abdominal pain and loose, bloody stools. Two months after leaving the hospital against medical advice, the client is readmitted for an exacerbation of the illness. At this time he is weak, thin, and irritable and is now willing to consider surgery. To best assist the client at this time, the nurse should attempt to:
    1. Replace his lost fluids and electrolytes
    2. Help him regain his former body weight
    3. Teach him how to use an ileostomy appliance
    4. Encourage his interaction with other post-ileostomy clients

323. A client with an acute episode of ulcerative colitis is admitted to the hospital. Blood studies reveal that the chloride level is low. This electrolyte deficiency can best be corrected by:
    1. A low-residue diet
    2. Intravenous therapy
    3. Total parenteral nutrition
    4. An oral electrolyte solution

324. When assessing a client with diabetes mellitus, the nurse expects that the primary fluid shift that occurs would be:
    1. Intravascular to interstitial because of glycosuria
    2. Intracellular to intravascular because of hyperosmolarity
    3. Extracellular to interstitial because of hypoproteinemia
    4. Intercellular to intravascular because of increased hydrostatic pressure

325. The nurse is reviewing an arterial blood gas report for a client with type 1 diabetes. The nurse understands that the result that reflects diabetic ketoacidosis would be:
    1. pH – 7.28, PCO_2 – 28, HCO_3 – 18
    2. pH – 7.30, PCO_2 – 54, HCO_3 – 28
    3. pH – 7.50, PCO_2 – 49, HCO_3 – 32
    4. pH – 7.52, PCO_2 – 26, HCO_3 – 20

326. A client with a history of cardiac dysrhythmias is admitted to the hospital with the diagnosis of dehydration. The nurse should anticipate that the physician will order:
1. A glass of water every hour until hydrated
2. Small, frequent intake of juices, broth, or milk
3. Short-term NG replacement of fluids and nutrients
4. A rapid IV infusion of an electrolyte and glucose solution

327. A client is diagnosed as having renal failure. During the oliguric phase the nurse should assess the client for:
1. Alkalosis
2. Hyperkalemia
3. Hypocalcemia
4. Hypernatremia

328. The physician prescribes a protein-, sodium-, and potassium-restricted diet for a client with end stage renal disease who is receiving dialysis. The nurse would know that the dietary teaching was effective when the client says, "I:
1. Must exclude meat from my diet."
2. Cannot add seasoning to my food."
3. Can eat canned, no-salt vegetables."
4. Should avoid using salt substitutes."

329. Before administering a prescribed intravenous solution that contains potassium chloride, the assessment by the nurse that should be brought to the physician's attention would be:
1. Poor skin turgor with "tenting"
2. Behaviors indicating irritability and confusion
3. A urinary output of 200 mL during the previous shift
4. An oral intake of 300 mL of fluid during the previous shift

330. A client with hyperpyrexia who has just been started on IV antibiotics has a diminished urine output. The nurse should recognize that this is probably the result of:
1. A declining blood pressure
2. Bacterial invasion of the kidneys
3. A compensatory response to fever
4. Nephrotoxicity from antimicrobial agents

331. A client is hospitalized with 50% of the body surface area burned. At the beginning of the 48-hour postburn period (acute or diuretic phase) the client's urine specific gravity is 1.015, urine output is 50 mL, hematocrit is 32, albumin is 3.6 g/dL, and the pulmonary arterial wedge pressure is 10 mm Hg. These data indicate that:
1. Albumin is critically low
2. Hemoconcentration is occurring
3. Fluid therapy has been successful
4. Replacement has been too aggressive

332. A client with partial- and full-thickness burns over 25% of the total body surface area (TBSA) is hospitalized in the burn unit. A large-bore central venous line is inserted to permit rapid administration of fluids and electrolytes. The large amounts of lactated Ringer's solution and 5% dextrose in saline are administered to:
1. Prevent fluid shifts
2. Expand the plasma
3. Maintain blood volume
4. Replace electrolytes lost

333. The sign that would be an indication of adequate fluid replacement for a client with a 30% total body surface area burn is a:
1. Urinary output of 15 to 20 mL /hr
2. CVP falling from 5 to 1 mm water
3. Slowing of a previously rapid pulse
4. Hematocrit level rising from 50 to 55

334. During the first 48 hours following a thermal injury, the nurse should assess for:
1. Hypokalemia and hyponatremia
2. Hyperkalemia and hyponatremia
3. Hypokalemia and hypernatremia
4. Hyperkalemia and hypernatremia

335. A client's extensive burns are being treated with silver nitrate 0.5% dressings. A week after treatment is begun, the nurse notes that the client's sodium level is 135 mEq/L and the potassium level is 3.0 mEq/L. The nurse should notify the physician and expect to:
1. Add KCl to current IV of Ringer's lactate
2. Add NaCl to current IV of Ringer's lactate
3. Change the NaCl with 20 mEq KCl to 5% D$_5$W
4. Change the 5% D$_5$W with 40 mEq KCl to 5% D$_5$W

336. The laboratory findings of a 40-year-old man with burns are BUN, 30 mg/dL; serum potassium 6.3, mEq/L; pH, 7.1; PO$_2$, 90 mm Hg; and Hgb, 7.4 g/dL. The nurse is aware that these findings indicate:
1. Azotemia
2. Hypokalemia
3. Metabolic alkalosis
4. Respiratory alkalosis

337. Thirty-six hours after a young male is admitted with severe burns he is placed on a fluid diet. Considering his potassium level is still 6.0 mEq/L, the nurse should recommend:
1. Milk
2. Jell-O
3. Orange juice
4. Tomato juice

338. A client is receiving a 2-g sodium diet. The family asks whether they can bring some snacks from home. The nurse suggests that they bring foods low in sodium such as:
1. Ice cream
2. Celery sticks
3. Fresh oranges
4. Peanut butter cookies

339. A client with ascites has a paracentesis, and 1500 mL of fluid is removed. Immediately following the procedure it is most important for the nurse to observe for:
1. Decreased peristalsis
2. A rapid, thready pulse
3. Respiratory congestion
4. An increase in temperature

340. A client is receiving an IV infusion. The priority nursing observation to identify a complication of IV therapy would be:
1. Bleeding at the infusion site
2. Shortness of breath and wheezing
3. A feeling of warmth throughout the body
4. An infiltration at the catheter insertion site

341. A 79-year-old client is admitted for dehydration, and an IV infusion of normal saline at 125 mL/hr is started. One hour later the client begins screaming, "I can't breathe." The nurse should:
1. Call the physician to order a sedative
2. Discontinue the IV and call the physician
3. Elevate the head of the bed and obtain vital signs
4. Assess for allergies and change the IV to an intermittent infusion device

342. A client has been receiving 2500 mL of IV fluid and 300 to 400 mL of oral intake daily for two days. The client's urine output has been decreasing and now has been less than 40 mL per hour for the past three hours. The nurse should initially:
1. Catheterize the client to empty the bladder
2. Assess breath sounds and obtain the client's vital signs
3. Check for dependent edema and continue to monitor I&O

4. Decrease the IV flow rate and increase oral fluids to compensate

343. A hospitalized client on a 2 g sodium, 1600 calorie ADA diet complains about the bland food and refuses to eat dinner. The nurse should first:
1. Ask the client what foods are usually eaten at home
2. Explain to the client that the diet will eventually have to be accepted
3. Provide the client with several packets of lemon juice and one packet of salt
4. Urge the client to eat to become accustomed to the diet that must be eaten at home

344. After abdominal surgery a client should be encouraged to turn from side to side and to carry out deep breathing exercises. These activities are essential to prevent:
1. Metabolic acidosis
2. Metabolic alkalosis
3. Respiratory acidosis
4. Respiratory alkalosis

345. Nasogastric tube irrigations are ordered for a client after surgery. The nurse instills 30 mL of saline solution and 10 mL is returned. The nurse should:
1. Record 20 mL as intake
2. Increase the amount of suction
3. Reposition the nasogastric tube
4. Irrigate the tube more frequently

346. A client has a nasogastric tube attached to continuous low suction after major abdominal surgery. The nurse caring for the client is monitoring for signs of hypokalemia. Check all that would apply.
1. _____ Irritability
2. _____ Dysrhythmias
3. _____ Muscle weakness
4. _____ Abdominal cramps
5. _____ Tingling of the fingertips

347. A client's arterial blood gases (ABGs) show the following values: a PO_2 of 89 mm Hg, a PCO_2 of 35 mm Hg, and a pH of 7.37. These findings indicate that the client is experiencing:
1. Fluid balance
2. Acid-base balance
3. Oxygen depletion
4. Metabolic acidosis

348. A client is diagnosed as having metabolic acidosis. The nurse understands that in metabolic acidosis the:
1. Blood pH level is increased

2. Plasma bicarbonates are increased
3. Excess hydrogen ions are excreted in the urine
4. Respiratory center in the medulla is depressed

349. A client appears very anxious, with 40 shallow respirations per minute. The client complains of feeling dizzy and lightheaded and of having tingling sensations of the fingertips and around the lips. The nurse should recognize that the client's complaints are probably related to:
1. Eupnea
2. Hyperventilation
3. Kussmaul's respirations
4. Carbon dioxide intoxication

350. Nursing intervention for a client who is hyperventilating should focus on providing reassurance and:
1. Administering oxygen
2. Using an incentive spirometer
3. Having the client breathe into a paper bag
4. Administering an IV containing bicarbonate ions

351. The physician orders serum electrolytes. To determine the effect of persistent vomiting, the nurse should be most concerned with monitoring the:
1. Sodium and chloride levels
2. Bicarbonate and sulfate levels
3. Magnesium and protein levels
4. Calcium and phosphate levels

352. A client is hospitalized with epigastric pain, nausea, and vomiting of four days' duration. The following laboratory values are noted: a plasma pH of 7.51; a PCO_2 of 50 mm Hg; a bicarbonate of 58 mEq/L; a chloride of 55 mEq/L; a sodium of 132 mEq/L; and a potassium of 3.8 mEq/L. The nurse recognizes that the collected data indicate:
1. Hyperkalemia
2. Hypernatremia
3. Hyperchloremia
4. Metabolic alkalosis

353. A 32-year-old woman is brought to the emergency service with complaints of epigastric pain and prolonged vomiting. Her respirations are rapid and shallow, her skin is dry and flushed, and she appears weak and lethargic. As a result of the client's data base, the nurse makes a nursing diagnosis of:
1. Risk for injury related to weakness
2. Acute pain related to duodenal ulcer
3. Deficient fluid volume related to vomiting

4. Ineffective breathing patterns related to pain

354. After a gastrectomy a client has a nasogastric tube to low continuous suction. The client begins to hyperventilate. The nurse should be aware that this pattern will alter the client's arterial blood gases by:
1. Increasing the PO_2 level
2. Decreasing the pH level
3. Decreasing the PCO_2 level
4. Increasing the HCO_3 level

355. A client with systemic lupus erythematosus is taking prednisone. The nurse is aware that steroids can cause hypokalemia. Taking into consideration food preferences, the nurse should encourage the client to eat:
1. Oatmeal
2. Broccoli
3. Cooked rice
4. Cooked carrots

356. When a client is in profound (late) hypovolemic shock, the nurse should assess the client's laboratory values, especially the arterial blood gases, because people in late shock will develop:
1. Hypokalemia
2. Metabolic acidosis
3. Respiratory alkalosis
4. A decreased PCO_2 level

357. The physician orders additional diagnostic studies to assess a client's acid-base status. The laboratory value that would indicate metabolic acidosis is:
1. Urine pH of 8.4
2. Gastric content pH of 6.0
3. Venous serum pH of 7.28
4. Arterial plasma pH of 7.40

358. The physician determines that a client has metabolic acidosis from severe dehydration. The characteristic respiration that the nurse would expect with metabolic acidosis is:
1. Dyspnea
2. Hyperpnea
3. Kussmaul's breathing
4. Cheyne-Stokes breathing

359. When a client develops respiratory alkalosis, the nurse should expect the laboratory values to reflect:
1. An elevated pH, elevated PCO_2
2. A decreased pH, elevated PCO_2
3. An elevated pH, decreased PCO_2
4. A decreased pH, decreased PCO_2

360. A client with chronic obstructive pulmonary disease (COPD) has a blood pH of 7.25 and PCO_2 of 60. These blood gases require nursing attention because they indicate:
1. Metabolic acidosis
2. Metabolic alkalosis
3. Respiratory acidosis
4. Respiratory alkalosis

361. A client has an order for lactated Ringer's solution to run at 150 mL per hour with an administration set that delivers 15 gtt/mL. An IV pump is not available. The nurse should set the IV to run at:
1. 26 drops per minute
2. 34 drops per minute
3. 38 drops per minute
4. 42 drops per minute

362. Surgery is performed on a client with a parotid tumor. The postoperative arterial blood gas values are pH 7.32; PCO_2 53 mm Hg; HCO_3 25 mEq/L. The nurse should:
1. Have the client breathe into a rebreather bag at a slow rate
2. Obtain a medical order for the administration of a diuretic
3. Encourage the client to cough productively and take deep breaths
4. Obtain a medical order for the administration of sodium bicarbonate

363. After surgical clipping of a ruptured cerebral aneurysm, a client develops the syndrome of inappropriate secretion of antidiuretic hormone (ADH). The nurse is aware that manifestations of excessive levels of antidiuretic hormone are:
1. Increased BUN and hypotension
2. Hyperkalemia and poor skin turgor
3. Hyponatremia and decreased urine output
4. Polyuria and increased specific gravity of urine

364. A client with a history of alcoholism and cirrhosis is admitted with severe dyspnea as a result of ascites. The nurse should understand that the ascites is most likely the result of increased:
1. Secretion of bile salts
2. Pressure in the portal vein
3. Interstitial osmotic pressure
4. Production of serum albumin

365. Because of delayed treatment, a client with hepatitis B (HBV) developed cirrhosis and is admitted to a medical unit. One potential sequela of chronic liver disease is fluid and electrolyte imbalance. The nurse recognizes this may be attributed to a decrease in serum albumin level, which leads to:
1. Hemorrhage and subsequent anemia
2. Diminished resistance to bacterial insult
3. Malnutrition of cells, especially hepatic cells
4. Reduction of colloidal osmotic pressure in the blood

366. The physician orders intravenous serum albumin for a client with advanced cirrhosis of the liver. The expected outcome from this treatment will be a decrease in:
1. Urinary output
2. The abdominal girth
3. Hepatic encephalopathy
4. The serum ammonia level

367. An agitated, hyperventilating, semicomatose client is brought to the emergency service. The family indicates that they found empty bottles of 100 aspirin tablets and 50 cold tablets and assumes the client took them several hours ago. The client's vital signs are BP 160/100, pulse 140, respirations 40, and temperature 101.5° F. An oral airway is in place. The test considered the most vital in providing information that will guide the emergency treatment for this client would be:
1. A 24-hour urine
2. A blood glucose
3. Serum electrolytes
4. Liver function tests

368. The physician orders a client's IV fluids to be delivered at 80 mL /hour. To adjust the drip rate when administering the IV via gravity, the nurse must know the:
1. Total volume of fluid in the IV bag
2. Size of the needle or catheter in the vein
3. Drops per milliliter delivered by the infusion set
4. Diameter of the tubing being used to instill the fluid

369. The physician orders IV fluids and gentamicin sulfate (Garamycin) 100 mg IVPB q8h for a client. The nurse, using gravity to instill the IV, hangs the piggyback gentamicin higher than the primary IV bag. When the piggyback bag is empty, the client observes air in the tubing of the IVPB and becomes frightened. The nurse should explain that:
1. Air in the tubing, even if it got into the vein, would not be fatal unless it were a large amount

2. The gentamicin and now the air are flowing into the large IV bag, not into the venous system directly

3. The solution from the large IV bag will begin to flow when the solution from the smaller bag ceases to flow

4. The clamps on the tubing leading from both bags can be closed for a few minutes to prevent air from entering the vein

370. A client is receiving total parenteral nutrition through a subclavian vein. The nurse should:
    1. Place the client in the supine position before changing the tubing
    2. Monitor the blood pressure frequently to assess for hypovolemia
    3. Administer IV antibiotics through this central line to prevent infection
    4. Determine blood glucose levels routinely and decrease the infusion rate if they are elevated

371. A client is receiving total parenteral nutrition. The adaptation that would indicate that the client was hyperglycemic would be:
    1. Polyuria
    2. Paralytic ileus
    3. Hypoventilation
    4. A serum glucose of 105 mg/100mL

GASTROINTESTINAL (GI)

372. After surgical implantation of radon seeds for oral cancer, the nurse should observe the client for the side effects of the radiation including:
    1. Nausea and/or vomiting
    2. Hematuria and/or occult blood
    3. Hypotension and/or bradycardia
    4. Abdominal cramping and/or diarrhea

373. A client with cancer of the tongue has radon seeds implanted. The plan of care states that the client is to receive meticulous oral hygiene. This plan can best be implemented by:
    1. Offering a firm-bristled toothbrush
    2. Providing an antiseptic mouthwash
    3. Using a gentle spray of normal saline
    4. Swabbing the mouth with a moistened gauze square

374. When teaching a client how to prevent constipation, the nurse recognizes that the client understands what has been taught when the client states that a preferred breakfast cereal would be:
    1. Cheerios
    2. Corn Flakes
    3. Froot Loops
    4. Rice Krispies

375. A client has decided to become a vegan (total vegetarian) and wishes to plan a diet to ensure adequate protein quality. To provide guidance, the nurse should instruct this client to:
    1. Add milk to grains to provide complete proteins
    2. Use eggs with plant foods to provide essential amino acids
    3. Plan a careful mixture of plant proteins to provide a balance of amino acids
    4. Add cheese to grains and beans to increase the quality of the protein consumed

376. To motivate an obese client to eventually include aerobic exercises in a weight-reduction program, the nurse should discuss exercise and its relationship to weight loss. The nurse would know that this teaching was effective when the client states, "I know that exercise will:
    1. Raise my heart rate."
    2. Decrease my appetite."
    3. Lower my metabolic rate."
    4. Increase my lean body mass."

377. A client is admitted to the hospital with complaints of frequent loose, watery stools; anorexia; malaise; and a considerable weight loss during the past month. Laboratory findings indicate leukocytosis and an elevated sedimentation rate. The nurse recognizes that the presenting symptoms in conjunction with the laboratory findings could be indicative of:
    1. The consistent, long-term use of an irritant-type laxative
    2. An emotional response that has resulted in physical symptoms
    3. Systemic responses of the body to a localized inflammatory process
    4. Poor dietary practices that have resulted in an alteration of bowel function

378. When assessing a client's abdomen, the nurse palpates the area directly above the umbilicus. This area is known as the:
    1. Iliac area
    2. Epigastric area
    3. Hypogastric area
    4. Suprasternal area

379. A client is scheduled for a barium swallow; the nurse should:
    1. Ask the client about allergies to iodine
    2. Ensure a laxative is ordered after the test
    3. Give only clear fluids on the day of the test
    4. Administer cleansing enemas before the test

380. A 79-year-old client is admitted to the hospital with painful abdominal spasms and severe diarrhea of two days' duration. The order of physical skills the nurse should follow when performing an admitting examination of this client should be "inspection" followed by:
   1. Percussion, palpation, auscultation
   2. Palpation, auscultation, percussion
   3. Percussion, palpation, auscultation
   4. Auscultation, palpation, percussion

381. Routine postoperative intravenous fluids are designed to supply hydration and electrolytes and only limited energy. Since 1 L of a 5% dextrose solution contains 50 g of sugar, 3 L/day would supply approximately:
   1. 400 kilocalories
   2. 600 kilocalories
   3. 800 kilocalories
   4. 1000 kilocalories

382. After abdominal surgery a client is placed on a progressive postsurgical diet. This diet is characterized by progressive alterations in the:
   1. Caloric content of food
   2. Nutritional value of food
   3. Texture and digestibility of food
   4. Variety of food and fluids included

383. The diet ordered for a client permits 190 g of carbohydrates, 90 g of fat, and 100 g of protein. The nurse understands that this diet contains approximately _____ calories.

384. A client's serum albumin value is 2.8 g/dl. The nurse should evaluate client teaching as successful when the client says, "For lunch I am going to have:
   1. Fruit salad."
   2. Sliced turkey."
   3. Spinach salad."
   4. Clear beef broth."

385. The most effective method for the nurse to assess a client's response to ongoing serum albumin therapy for biliary cirrhosis is to monitor the client's:
   1. Weight daily
   2. Vital signs frequently
   3. Urine output every half hour
   4. Urine albumin level every shift

386. A male client who is a heavy smoker is placed on a high-calorie, high-protein diet. In light of the history of smoking the client should be encouraged to eat foods high in:
   1. Niacin
   2. Thiamin
   3. Vitamin C
   4. Vitamin B_{12}

387. A client is cautioned to avoid vitamin D toxicity while increasing protein intake. The nurse would know that the teaching was understood when the client states, "I must increase my intake of:
   1. Tofu products."
   2. Fruit and eggnog."
   3. Powdered whole milk."
   4. Cottage cheese custard."

388. When helping a client plan a therapeutic diet, the nurse is aware that an excellent food source of vitamin C is:
   1. Apples
   2. Lettuce
   3. Broccoli
   4. Apricots

389. The physician tells a client that an increase in vitamin E and beta-carotene is important for healthier skin. The nurse teaches the client that excellent food sources of both of these substances are:
   1. Spinach and mangoes
   2. Fish and peanut butter
   3. Oranges and grapefruits
   4. Carrots and sweet potatoes

390. Because of multiple physical injuries and emotional concerns, a hospitalized client is at high risk to develop a stress (Curling's) ulcer. The nurse should know that stress ulcers usually are evidenced by:
   1. Unexplained shock
   2. Melena for several days
   3. Sudden massive hemorrhage
   4. A gradual drop in the hematocrit value

391. A client should be instructed to avoid straining on defecation to prevent bleeding after pelvic surgery. The nurse is aware that the related teaching has been understood when the client states, "I must increase my intake of:
   1. Ripe bananas."
   2. Milk products."
   3. Green vegetables."
   4. Creamed potatoes."

392. A client with Parkinson's disease complains about a problem with elimination. The nurse should encourage the client to:
   1. Eat a banana daily
   2. Decrease fluid intake

3. Take cathartics regularly
4. Increase residue in the diet

393. The physician orders three stool specimens for occult blood from a client who complains of blood-streaked stools and a 10-pound weight loss in one month. To ensure valid test results the nurse should instruct the client to:
1. Avoid eating red meat before testing
2. Test the specimen while it is still warm
3. Discard the first stool of the day and use the next three stools
4. Take three specimens from different sections of the fecal sample

394. When a client develops steatorrhea, the nurse should describe this stool as:
1. Dry and rock-hard
2. Clay colored and pasty
3. Bulky and foul smelling
4. Black and blood-streaked

395. Because of chronic crampy pain, diarrhea, and cachexia, a young adult is to receive total parental nutrition (TPN) via a central line. Before preparing the client for the insertion of the catheter, the nurse should understand that:
1. There will be a moderate amount of pain
2. The feeding will be administered intermittently
3. Fluoroscopy must be done before TPN is started
4. The jugular vein is the most commonly used insertion site

396. The physician orders total parenteral nutrition 1 L q12h. The primary nursing responsibility should be to monitor the client's:
1. Electrolytes
2. Urinary output
3. Administration rate
4. Serum glucose levels

397. When preparing a client to go home with total parenteral nutrition, the nurse should help the client plan:
1. Which days will be used for administration
2. For daily insertion of the circulatory access
3. For professional help to administer the TPN
4. A schedule of administration around regular activity

398. A client has symptoms associated with salmonellosis. Relevant data to gather from this client include a history of:
1. Rectal cancer in the family

2. All foods eaten in the past 24 hours
3. Any recent extreme emotional stress
4. An upper respiratory infection in the past 10 days

399. A client is admitted to the hospital with the diagnosis of acute salmonellosis. The nurse would expect that the client will be receiving:
1. Antacids
2. Electrolytes
3. Antidiarrheics
4. Antispasmodics

400. During a health symposium, a nurse teaches the group how to prevent food poisoning. The nurse evaluates that the teaching has been understood when one of the participants states:
1. "All meats and cream-based foods need to be refrigerated."
2. "Once most food is cooked it does not need to be refrigerated."
3. "Poultry should be stuffed and then refrigerated before cooking."
4. "Cooked food should be cooled before being put into the refrigerator."

401. The nurse should teach the client with gastroesophageal reflux disease that after meals the client should:
1. Take a short walk
2. Drink 8 oz of water
3. Lie down for at least 20 minutes
4. Rest in a sitting position for one-half hour

402. The laboratory values of a client with cancer of the esophagus show a hemoglobin of 7 g/dl, hematocrit of 25%, and RBC count of 2.5 million/mm^3. Considering these data, an appropriate nursing diagnosis for the client at this time would be:
1. Ineffective airway clearance related to tumor growth and metastasis
2. Imbalanced nutrition: less than body requirements related to dysphagia
3. Acute pain related to pressure of the tumor on surrounding tissues and nerves
4. Risk for injury related to possible metastasis and subsequent airway obstruction

403. Immediately after esophageal surgery the priority nursing assessment concerns the client's:
1. Incision
2. Respirations
3. Level of pain
4. Nasogastric tube

404. A client with achalasia is to have bougienage to dilate the lower esophagus and cardiac sphincter. After the procedure the nurse should assess the client for esophageal perforation, which is indicated by:
1. Faintness and feelings of fullness
2. Diaphoresis and cardiac palpitations
3. Elevated heart rate and abdominal pain
4. Increased blood pressure and urinary output

405. A 54-year-old obese bachelor arrives at the clinic complaining of epigastric distress and esophageal burning. During the health history, he admits to binge drinking and frequent bronchitis. After diagnostic studies, a diagnosis of hiatus hernia is made. The health problem that would most likely have contributed to the development of the hiatus hernia would be:
1. Obesity
2. Bronchitis
3. Esophagitis
4. Alcoholism

406. When discussing future meal plans with a client who has a hiatus hernia, the nurse asks what beverage the client usually enjoys with meals. The beverage that should be included in the diet when the client is discharged is:
1. Ginger ale
2. Apple juice
3. Orange juice
4. Cola beverages

407. A female client, who has a hiatal hernia, is 5 feet 3 inches tall, and weighs 140 pounds, asks the nurse how to best prevent esophageal reflux. The nurse's best response would be:
1. "Increase your intake of fat with each meal."
2. "Lie down after eating to help your digestion."
3. "Reduce your caloric intake to foster weight reduction."
4. "Drink several glasses of fluid during each of your meals."

408. A male client is diagnosed with acute gastritis secondary to alcoholism and cirrhosis. When obtaining this client's history, the nurse should give priority to the client's statement that:
1. His pain is increased after meals
2. He experiences nausea frequently
3. His stools have a tarry appearance
4. He recently joined Alcoholics Anonymous

409. When performing the initial history and physical examination of a client with a tentative diagnosis of peptic ulcer, the nurse would expect the client to describe the pain as:
1. Gnawing epigastric pain or boring pain in the back
2. Located in the right shoulder and preceded by nausea
3. Sudden, sharp abdominal pain, increasing in intensity
4. Heartburn and substernal discomfort when lying down

410. A client is suspected of having a peptic ulcer. When obtaining a history from this client, the nurse would expect the reported pain to:
1. Intensify when the client vomits
2. Occur one to three hours after meals
3. Increase when the client eats fatty foods
4. Begin in the epigastrium and radiate across the abdomen

411. An adaptation after a gastroscopy that indicates a major complication would be:
1. Increased GI motility
2. Difficulty swallowing
3. Nausea and vomiting
4. Abdominal distention

412. A traveling salesman develops gastric bleeding and is hospitalized. An important etiologic clue for the nurse to explore while taking this client's history would be:
1. Any recent foreign travel
2. The client's usual dietary pattern
3. Any change in status of family relationships
4. The medications that the client has been taking

413. After an acute episode of upper GI bleeding, a client vomits undigested antacids and complains of severe epigastric pain. The nursing assessment reveals an absence of bowel sounds, pulse rate of 134, and shallow respirations of 32 per minute. In addition to calling the physician, the nurse should:
1. Keep the client NPO in preparation for surgery
2. Start oxygen per nasal cannula at 3 to 4 L per minute
3. Place the client in the supine position with the legs elevated
4. Ask the client whether any red or black stools have been noted

414. Following a subtotal gastrectomy, a client begins to eat more food in varied forms. After meals the client experiences a cramping discomfort and a rapid pulse with waves of weakness,

which are often followed by nausea and vomiting. The nurse recognizes that this response is known as the dumping syndrome which is caused by:
1. A sluggish passage of food dumping into the small intestine
2. Rapid passage of dilute food mixture into the small intestine
3. Sudden passage of hyperosmolar food solution into the small intestine
4. Passage of food that is less concentrated than surrounding extracellular fluid into the small intestine

415. A client is diagnosed with cancer of the stomach and is scheduled for a partial gastrectomy. Preoperative preparation for this client should include an explanation about the postoperative:
1. Gastric suction
2. Oxygen therapy
3. Fluid restriction
4. Urinary catheter

416. A client with gastric cancer asks whether this cancer will spread. The nurse recognizes that the client is looking for reassurance but knows that gastric cancers are most likely to metastasize to the:
1. Liver and lung
2. Bone and brain
3. Pancreas and brain
4. Lymph nodes and blood

417. Twelve hours after a subtotal gastrectomy, the nurse notes large amounts of bloody drainage from the client's nasogastric tube. The nurse should:
1. Instill 30 mL of iced normal saline into the tube
2. Clamp the tube and call the physician immediately
3. Report the type and quantity of drainage to the physician
4. Continue to monitor the drainage and record the observations

418. The nurse should assess for the development of pernicious anemia when a client has a history of:
1. Hemorrhage
2. Diabetes mellitus
3. Poor dietary habits
4. Having had a gastrectomy

419. After a client has a total gastrectomy, the nurse should plan to include in the discharge teaching the need for:
1. Monthly injections of vitamin B_{12}
2. Regular daily use of a stool softener
3. Weekly injections of iron dextran (Imferon)
4. Daily replacement therapy of pancreatic enzymes

420. After two months of self-management for symptoms of gastritis is unsuccessful, a client goes to the physician and extensive carcinoma of the stomach is diagnosed. The client asks the nurse how the disease got so advanced. The nurse's explanation should be based on the knowledge that carcinoma of the stomach is:
1. Difficult to accurately diagnose until late in the disease process
2. Painful in early stages and often misdiagnosed as myocardial infarction
3. Usually diagnosed following the discovery of enlarged lymph nodes in the epigastric area
4. Rarely diagnosed early because the symptoms are usually nonspecific until late in the disease

421. A client with extensive gastric carcinoma is to be admitted to the hospital for an esophagojejunostomy. When preparing this client for surgery, the nurse should include information about the possibility that:
1. A chest tube will be in place in addition to a nasogastric tube
2. Liquids by mouth may be permitted the evening after surgery
3. Trendelenburg position will be used on the first day after surgery
4. Complete bed rest may be necessary for 48 hours after surgery

422. When teaching a client how to avoid the dumping syndrome following a gastrectomy, the nurse should emphasize:
1. Increasing activity after eating
2. Avoiding excess fluids with meals
3. Eating heavy meals to delay emptying
4. Providing carbohydrates with each meal

423. Immediately after a subtotal gastrectomy a client is brought to the post anesthesia care unit. The nurse identifies small blood clots in the gastric drainage. The nurse should:
1. Clamp the tube
2. Consider this a normal event
3. Instill the tube with iced saline
4. Notify the physician of this finding

424. On the third postoperative day after a subtotal gastrectomy, a client complains of severe abdominal pain. The nurse palpates the client's abdomen and notes rigidity. The nurse should first:
1. Assist the client to ambulate
2. Assess the client's vital signs
3. Administer the prescribed analgesic
4. Encourage the use of the spirometer

425. To determine when a client who has had a subtotal gastrectomy can begin oral feedings after surgery, the nurse must assess for the:
1. Presence of flatulence
2. Extent of incisional pain
3. Stabilization of hematocrit levels
4. Occurrence of dumping syndrome

426. A client who has had a gastric ulcer asks what to do if the epigastric pain occurs. The nurse would know that the teaching was effective when the client states, "I will:
1. Increase my food intake."
2. Take the aspirin with milk."
3. Eliminate fluids with meals."
4. Take an antacid preparation."

427. A 45-year-old divorced father of five is diagnosed with duodenal ulcer. He asks, "Now that I have an ulcer, what comes next?" The nurse's best response would be:
1. "Most peptic ulcers heal with medical treatment."
2. "Clients with gastric ulcers experience pain while eating."
3. "Early surgery is advisable, especially after the first attack."
4. "If ulcers are untreated, cancer of the stomach can develop."

428. A client is diagnosed as having a peptic ulcer. When teaching about peptic ulcers, the nurse should instruct the client to report any stools that appear:
1. Frothy
2. Ribbon shaped
3. Pale or clay colored
4. Dark brown or black

429. After abdominal surgery a client returns to the unit with a nasogastric tube to decompression. The physician has ordered an antiemetic q6h prn for nausea. When the client complains of nausea the first action by the nurse should be to:
1. Check for placement of the tube
2. Administer the ordered antiemetic

3. Irrigate the tube with normal saline
4. Notify the physician of the problem

430. Three hours after a subtotal gastrectomy a male client, who has a nasogastric tube to continuous low suction and IV fluids, complains of nausea and abdominal pain. His abdomen appears distended and there are no bowel sounds. The nurse should first:
1. Give the prn pain medication
2. Instill 30 mL of air into the tube
3. Check stools and gastric drainage for blood
4. Notify the physician of absent bowel sounds

431. A client who had a gastric resection for cancer of the stomach is admitted to the post anesthesia care unit with a nasogastric tube. The nurse should expect to observe:
1. Periodic vomiting
2. Intermittent bouts of diarrhea
3. Gastric distention after 6 hours
4. Bloody drainage for the first 12 hours

432. A client progresses to a regular diet after a gastrectomy for gastric cancer. After eating lunch he becomes diaphoretic and has palpitations. These symptoms are probably the result of:
1. An intolerance to fatty foods
2. Dehiscence of the surgical incision
3. An extracellular fluid shift in the bowel
4. Diminished peristalsis in the small intestine

433. After a subtotal gastrectomy a client develops the dumping syndrome. In addition, about two hours after the initial postmeal attack, the client experiences a second period of discomfort, feeling somewhat "shaky." The nurse recognizes that this latter follow-up effect, which is precipitated by the dumping syndrome, is caused by:
1. The increased use of simple carbohydrates in meals, creating a more prolonged glucose rise
2. The increased fat content and larger amount of seasoned food, creating digestive discomfort
3. Hyperglycemia from a rapidly absorbed glucose load, which overwhelms the insulin-adjusting mechanism
4. Mild hypoglycemia from an overproduction of insulin that occurs in response to the postprandial blood glucose rise

434. The group of characteristics that would alert the nurse that a client is at increased risk of developing gallbladder disease would be a female:
1. Over the age of 40, obese
2. Under the age of 40, history of high fat intake

3. Over the age of 40, low serum cholesterol level
4. Under the age of 40, family history of gallstones

435. A client with a tentative diagnosis of cholecystitis is discharged from the emergency department with instructions to make an appointment for a definitive diagnostic workup. The recommendation that would produce the most valuable diagnostic information would be:
1. "Keep a journal related to your pain."
2. "Save all stool and urine for inspection."
3. "Follow the doctor's orders exactly without question."
4. "Keep a record of the amount of fluid you drink daily."

436. The nurse asks a client to make a list of the foods that cause dyspepsia. If the client has cholecystitis, the foods that are most likely to be included on this list would be:
1. Nuts and popcorn
2. Meatloaf and baked potato
3. Chocolate and boiled shrimp
4. Fried chicken and buttered corn

437. A client is having surgery for a cholecystectomy and common bile duct exploration. The nurse understands that after surgery the client will:
1. Need to take oral bile salts
2. Be unable to concentrate bile
3. Be incapable of producing bile
4. Not be able to digest fatty foods

438. A client develops a gallstone that becomes lodged in the common bile duct. The physician schedules an endoscopic sphincterotomy. Preoperative teaching should include information that for the procedure the client will:
1. Have a spinal anesthetic
2. Receive an epidural block
3. Have a general anesthetic
4. Receive an intravenous sedative

439. A client has cholelithiasis with possible obstruction of the common bile duct. Before the scheduled cholecystectomy, nutritional deficiencies and excesses should be corrected. A nutritional assessment should be conducted to determine whether the client:
1. Is deficient in vitamins A, D, and K
2. Eats adequate amounts of dietary fiber
3. Consumes excessive amounts of protein
4. Has excessive levels of potassium and folic acid

440. A client undergoes an abdominal cholecystectomy with common duct exploration. In the immediate postoperative period, the nursing action that should assume the highest priority for this client is:
1. Irrigating the T-tube frequently
2. Changing the dressing at least bid
3. Encouraging coughing and deep breathing
4. Promoting an adequate fluid intake by mouth

441. A 40-year-old client is admitted with biliary cancer. The associated jaundice gets progressively worse. The nurse should be most concerned about the potential complication of:
1. Pruritus
2. Bleeding
3. Flatulence
4. Hypokalemia

442. After a cholecystectomy to remove a cancerous gall bladder, the client has a T-tube in place that has drained 300 mL of bile-colored fluid during the first 24 hours. The nurse should:
1. Increase fluid intake to compensate for this loss
2. Clamp the tube intermittently to slow drainage
3. Consider this an expected response after surgery and record the results
4. Empty the portable drainage system and reestablish negative pressure

443. An obese client with a history of gallstones has an abdominal cholecystectomy. After surgery the nurse plans to alleviate tension on the surgical wound by:
1. Limiting deep breathing
2. Maintaining T-tube patency
3. Maintaining nasogastric tube patency
4. Encouraging the right side-lying position

444. A client with cholelithiasis has a laser laparoscopic cholecystectomy. Postoperatively it is most appropriate for the nurse to:
1. Wait about 24 hours to begin clear liquids
2. Offer the client clear carbonated beverages
3. Monitor the abdominal incision for bleeding
4. Instruct the client to resume moderate activity in two to three days

445. Because of prolonged bile drainage from a T-tube, a client may develop symptoms related to a lack of fat-soluble vitamins such as:
1. Easy bruising
2. Muscle twitching
3. Excessive jaundice
4. Tingling of the fingers

446. A client with cholelithiasis is scheduled for a lithotripsy. Preoperative teaching should include the information that:
1. Opiates will be available for postoperative pain
2. A fever is a common response to this intervention
3. Heart palpitations commonly occur after the procedure
4. Analgesics and anesthetics are not necessary during the procedure

447. A client is to be discharged after a laser laparoscopic cholecystectomy. The nurse would recognize that the discharge instructions were understood when the client states:
1. "I can change the bandages every day."
2. "I should not bathe the surgical sites for a week."
3. "I may have mild shoulder pain for about a week."
4. "I should remain on a full liquid diet for three days."

448. After a cholecystectomy, a client asks whether there are any dietary restrictions that must be followed. The nurse would recognize that the dietary teaching was understood when the client tells a family member:
1. "I will need to avoid fatty foods for the rest of my life."
2. "Most people can tolerate a regular diet after this type of surgery."
3. "I should not eat those foods that upset me before I had surgery."
4. "Most people need to eat a high-protein diet for several months after surgery."

449. The nurse is aware that the laboratory test result that most likely would indicate acute pancreatitis is an elevated:
1. Blood glucose level
2. Serum amylase level
3. Serum bilirubin level
4. White blood cell count

450. A 50-year-old farmer is admitted to the hospital with severe back and abdominal pain, nausea and occasional vomiting, and an oral temperature of 101° F. He reports drinking six to eight beers a day. A diagnosis of acute pancreatitis is made. Based on the data presented, the nursing diagnosis that is of primary concern for this client would be:
1. Disturbed self-concept related to illness
2. Acute pain related to inflammation of the pancreas
3. Deficient fluid-volume related to inadequate fluid intake
4. Imbalanced nutrition less than body requirements related to vomiting

451. As a client's symptoms of acute pancreatitis subside, it is most important that the nurse instruct the client to:
1. Avoid eating hot spicy foods
2. Avoid ingesting alcoholic beverages
3. Eat a bland diet of six small meals a day
4. Eat a high-carbohydrate, low-fat, low-protein diet

452. When teaching a client about the diet following a pancreaticoduodenectomy (Whipple procedure) performed for cancer of the pancreas, the statement the nurse should include would be:
1. "There are no dietary restrictions; you may eat what you desire."
2. "Your diet should be low in calories to prevent taxing your diseased pancreas."
3. "Meals should be restricted in protein because of your compromised liver function."
4. "Low-fat meals should be eaten because of interference with your fat digestion mechanism."

453. A long-term complication that a client must be made aware of after a pancreaticoduodenectomy for cancer of the pancreas is hypoinsulinism. The nurse would know that the teaching about hypoinsulinism is understood when the client states, "I should seek medical supervision if I experience:
1. Oliguria."
2. Anorexia."
3. Weight gain."
4. Increased thirst."

454. After revision of the pancreas because of cancer, total parenteral nutrition is instituted via a central venous infusion route. During the fourth hour of the infusion the client complains of nausea, fatigue, and a headache. The hourly urine output is twice the amount of the previous hour. The nurse should call the physician and:
1. Stop the infusion and cover the insertion site
2. Slow the infusion and check the serum glucose level

3. Prepare the client for immediate surgery for possible bowel obstruction
4. Increase fluids via a peripheral IV route and give analgesics for the headache

455. After surgery for cancer of the pancreas, the client's nutritional and fluid regimen will be influenced by the remaining amount of functioning pancreatic tissue. Considering both the exocrine and the endocrine functions of the pancreas, the client's postoperative regimen would primarily include managing the intake of:
1. Alcohol and caffeine
2. Fluids and electrolytes
3. Vitamins and minerals
4. Fats and carbohydrates

456. A client with a 20-year history of excessive alcohol use is admitted to the hospital with jaundice and ascites. A priority nursing action during the first 48 hours after the client's admission will be to:
1. Monitor the client's vital signs
2. Increase the client's fluid intake
3. Improve the client's nutritional status
4. Identify the client's reasons for drinking

457. A male client with liver dysfunction reports that his gums bleed spontaneously. In addition, the nurse notes small hemorrhagic lesions on his face. The nurse recognizes that the client needs additional vitamin:
1. D
2. E
3. A
4. K

458. A client with ascites is scheduled for a paracentesis. To prepare the client for the abdominal paracentesis the nurse should:
1. Medicate the client for pain
2. Encourage the client to drink fluids
3. Shave and prep the client's abdomen
4. Instruct the client to empty the bladder

459. A client is diagnosed as having hepatitis A. The information from the health history that is most likely linked to hepatitis A is:
1. Working for a local plumber
2. Washing dishes at a local restaurant
3. Working in a hemodialysis unit of a hospital
4. Being exposed to arsenic compounds at work

460. The nurse instructs a client diagnosed with hepatitis type A about untoward signs and symptoms related to hepatitis that may develop. The one that should be reported to the physician would be:
1. Fatigue
2. Anorexia
3. Yellow urine
4. Clay-colored stools

461. A client with jaundice associated with hepatitis expresses concern over the change in skin color. The nurse should recognize that this color change is a result of:
1. Stimulation of the liver to produce an excess quantity of bile pigments
2. Increased destruction of red blood cells during the acute phase of the disease
3. Inability of the liver to remove normal amounts of bilirubin from the blood
4. Decreased prothrombin levels, leading to multiple sites of intradermal bleeding

462. A mother whose son has hepatitis A states that there is only one bathroom in their home and she is worried that other members of the family could get hepatitis. The nurse's best reply would be:
1. "I suggest that you buy a commode exclusively for your son's use."
2. "There is no problem with your son sharing the same bathroom with everyone."
3. "Your son may use the bathroom, but you need to use disposable toilet covers."
4. "It is important that your son and all family members wash their hands after using the bathroom."

463. The physician orders contact precautions for a client with hepatitis A. In addition to standard precautions, the isolation procedures that must be followed are:
1. A private room is required, and the door must be kept closed
2. Persons entering the room must wear a gown, a mask, and gloves
3. Gowns and gloves must be worn only when handling the client's soiled linen, dishes, or utensils
4. A gown and gloves must be worn when handling articles possibly contaminated by urine or feces

464. When performing the physical assessment of a client admitted to the hospital with a diagnosis of biliary cirrhosis, the skin change the nurse may expect to observe would be:
1. Vitiligo
2. Hirsutism
3. Melanosis
4. Telangiectasis

465. A 64-year-old client is suspected of having carcinoma of the liver and a liver biopsy is scheduled. The nurse understands that a liver biopsy may be contraindicated in certain situations. Therefore, it is important for the nurse to assess the client for:
1. Confusion and disorientation
2. The presence of any infectious disease
3. A prothrombin time of less than 40% of normal
4. An inclusion of foods high in vitamin K in the client's diet

466. When preparing a client for a liver biopsy, the nurse explains that during the test the client will be placed:
1. On the right side, with the left arm stretched up over the head
2. In the prone position, with both arms extended over the head
3. On the left side, with the right arm extended out in front across the bed
4. In a dorsal recumbent position, with the right arm raised and behind the head

467. When discussing a scheduled liver biopsy with a client, the nurse should explain that for several hours after the biopsy the client will have to remain in:
1. The left side-lying position with the head of the bed elevated
2. A high Fowler's position with both arms supported on pillows
3. The right side-lying position with pillows placed under the costal margin
4. Any comfortable recumbent position as long as the client remains immobile

468. Immediately after a liver biopsy, the client is placed on the right side. The nurse explains that this position should be maintained because it will:
1. Help stop bleeding if any occurs
2. Restore circulating blood volume
3. Be the position of greatest comfort
4. Reduce the fluid trapped in the biliary ducts

469. The nurse identifies a small amount of bile-colored drainage on the dressing of a client who has had a liver biopsy. The nurse should recognize that:
1. The pancreas has been lacerated
2. Fluid is leaking into the intestine
3. This is a typical, expected response
4. A biliary vessel has been penetrated

470. The serum ammonia level of a client with hepatic cirrhosis and ascites is elevated. The priority nursing intervention should be to:
1. Weigh the client daily
2. Restrict the client's oral fluid intake
3. Measure the client's urine specific gravity
4. Observe the client for increasing confusion

471. A client with a long history of alcohol abuse is admitted to the hospital with ascites, jaundice, and confusion. A diagnosis of hepatic cirrhosis is made. A nursing priority would be to:
1. Institute safety measures
2. Monitor respiratory status
3. Measure abdominal girth daily
4. Test stool specimens for blood

472. A client with a history of gastrointestinal varices develops severe hematemesis, and the physician inserts a Sengstaken-Blakemore tube. The nurse is aware that this tube is a:
1. Single-lumen tube for gastric lavage
2. Double-lumen tube for intestinal decompression
3. Triple-lumen tube used to compress the esophagus
4. Multi-lumen tube for gastric and intestinal decompression

473. A client with Laënnec's cirrhosis has a Sengstaken-Blakemore tube in place. The client becomes increasingly confused and tries to climb out of bed. The breath has become fetid. The nursing priority should be to:
1. Apply a safety jacket
2. Notify the physician immediately
3. Administer the prn sedative as ordered
4. Administer oxygen via a nasal catheter

474. A client with cirrhosis of the liver and malnutrition begins to develop slurred speech, confusion, drowsiness, and tremors. With these symptoms the diet would be limited to:
1. 20 g protein, 2000 calories
2. 80 g protein, 1000 calories
3. 100 g protein, 2500 calories
4. 150 g protein, 1200 calories

475. A client develops peritonitis and sepsis following the surgical repair of a ruptured diverticulum. The nurse should expect an assessment of the client to reveal:
1. Bradycardia
2. Hypertension
3. Abdominal rigidity
4. Increased bowel sounds

476. When assessing a client who has had abdominal surgery, the nurse knows that the first indicator for return of peristalsis would be when

the client:
1. Passes flatus
2. Has bowel sounds
3. Tolerates clear liquids
4. Has a bowel movement

477. One month after abdominal surgery a client is readmitted to the hospital with recurrent abdominal pain and fever. The diagnosis is fistula formation with peritonitis. The nurse should place the client in the:
1. Supine position
2. Right Sims' position
3. Semi-Fowler's position
4. Position that is most comfortable

478. The nurse is performing a physical assessment of a client with ulcerative colitis. The finding most often associated with a serious complication of this disorder would be:
1. Decreased bowel sounds
2. Loose, blood-tinged stools
3. Distention of the abdomen
4. Intense abdominal discomfort

479. A client with colitis inquires as to whether surgery will ever be necessary. When teaching about the disease and its treatment, the nurse should emphasize that:
1. Surgery for colitis is considered only as a last resort for most clients
2. Medical treatment for colitis is curative, and surgery is not required
3. Surgery for colitis is done early in the course of the disease for most clients
4. Medical treatment is all that will be needed if the client can acquire some emotional stability

480. When caring for a client who has had abdominal intestinal surgery, it is important for the nurse to remember that:
1. Air swallowing can cause gastric dilation
2. Preoperative enemas prevent a postoperative ileus
3. Rectal intubation will relieve nausea and vomiting
4. Clear liquids within 24 hours after surgery stimulate peristalsis

481. When discussing nutrition with a client who has inflammatory bowel disease of the ascending colon, the most appropriate suggestion by the nurse concerning food to include in the diet would be:
1. Scrambled eggs and applesauce
2. Bar-B-Q chicken and sweet potatoes
3. Fresh fruit salad with cheddar cheese
4. Chunky peanut butter on whole wheat bread

482. A client with colitis has a hemicolectomy performed. After surgery these observations are noted: increasing abdominal distention; vomited 300 mL dark green, viscous fluid; bowel sounds absent. Immediate care should be directed toward:
1. Replacing fluid losses
2. Decreasing the vomiting
3. Decompressing the bowel
4. Restoring electrolyte balance

483. After surgery for creation of an ileostomy, the client is to be discharged. Before discharge, the primary nursing intervention should be to:
1. Coax the client into caring for the ileostomy alone
2. Evaluate the client's ability to care for the ileostomy
3. Have the client change the dry sterile dressing on the incision without assistance
4. Ensure that the client understands the dietary limitations that must be followed

484. After the surgical creation of an ileostomy, a client is transferred to a rehabilitation unit. The client asks for help in selecting breakfast. The nurse should encourage the client to eat:
1. Hot coffee and oranges
2. Shredded wheat and milk
3. A western omelet and toast
4. Cream of wheat and bananas

485. When teaching a client about the signs of colorectal cancer, the nurse stresses that the most common complaint of persons with colorectal cancer is:
1. Rectal bleeding
2. Abdominal pain
3. Change in bowel habits
4. Change in caliber of stools

486. A 50-year-old executive reports a loss of 20 pounds in three months. The stools are black and tarry, and the physician schedules a colonoscopy. The nurse should prepare the client for the test by:
1. Administering an oil retention enema just before the test
2. Instructing that a bland diet be eaten the night before the test
3. Explaining that the pretest cathartic will cause diarrhea after the test
4. Advising the client not to eat or drink anything the morning of the test

487. A middle-age male client has an adenocarcinoma of the colon. The physician suspects that this has metastasized and orders a CAT scan of the liver. When preparing the client for the CAT scan the nurse should explain that:
1. After the procedure, he will need to rest in bed for about six hours to prevent complications
2. There will be some discomfort during the procedure but the physician will administer an analgesic
3. He will be in a twilight type of sleep during the procedure but may be able to hear people talking in the same room
4. He will be given an IV infusion containing a contrast medium before the procedure and must lie as still as possible for a period of time

488. A client diagnosed with cancer of the sigmoid colon is to have an abdominoperineal resection with a permanent colostomy. Before surgery a low-residue diet is ordered. The nurse explains that this is necessary to:
1. Lower the bacterial count in the GI tract
2. Limit production of flatus in the intestine
3. Prevent irritation of the intestinal mucosa
4. Reduce the amount of stool in the large bowel

489. A client with carcinoma of the colon is scheduled for an abdominoperineal resection. Preparation of this client should include:
1. Medications to promote diuresis
2. Restriction of fluids to 1500 mL daily
3. Antibiotics to reduce intestinal bacteria
4. Abdominal exercises to facilitate recovery

490. An abdominoperineal resection with a colostomy is scheduled for a client with cancer of the rectum. The nurse recognizes that the physician will need the client to sign a consent for a:
1. Permanent sigmoid colostomy
2. Permanent ascending colostomy
3. Temporary double-barrel colostomy
4. Temporary transverse loop colostomy

491. On the second day following an abdominoperineal resection, the nurse anticipates that the colostomy stoma will appear:
1. Dry, pale pink, and flush with the skin
2. Moist, red, and raised above the skin surface
3. Dry, purple, and depressed below the skin surface
4. Moist, pink, flush with the skin, and painful when touched

492. The nurse plans to teach a client to irrigate a new sigmoid colostomy when the:
1. Stool starts to become formed
2. Client can lie on the side comfortably
3. Abdominal incision is closed and contamination is no longer a danger
4. Perineal wound heals and the client can sit comfortably on the commode

493. A client returns from surgery with a permanent colostomy. During the first 24 hours the colostomy does not drain. The nurse should realize this is a result of:
1. Intestinal edema following surgery
2. A presurgical decrease in fluid intake
3. The absence of gastrointestinal motility
4. Proper functioning of nasogastric suction

494. When observing a return demonstration of a colostomy irrigation, the nurse knows that more teaching is required if the client:
1. Clamps off the flow of fluid when feeling uncomfortable
2. Lubricates the tip of the catheter prior to inserting it into the stoma
3. Discontinues the insertion of fluid after only 500 mL of fluid has been instilled
4. Hangs the irrigation bag on the bathroom door clothes hook during fluid insertion

495. A client has a colostomy because of cancer of the colon. Postoperatively it would be most therapeutic for the nurse to:
1. Empty the colostomy bag when it is three-fourths full
2. Allow one-half inch between the stoma and the colostomy bag
3. Help the client to remove the bag on the first day postoperatively
4. Apply stoma adhesive around the stoma before attaching the bag

496. The nurse would know that dietary teaching for a client with a colostomy had been effective when the client states, "It is important that I eat:
1. Food low in fiber so that there is less stool."
2. Bland foods so that my intestines do not become irritated."
3. Everything I ate before the operation, while avoiding foods that cause gas."
4. Soft foods that are more easily digested and absorbed by my large intestine."

497. Part of discharge teaching for a client with a sigmoid colostomy includes the use of appliances and dressings to protect clothing. When the client asks the nurse about these appliances,

the most appropriate response would be:
1. "Appliances will have to be used to avoid soiling your clothing."
2. "Special appliances are expensive but they provide for better bowel control."
3. "I will give you a large supply that will last until your next visit to the physician."
4. "Many people do not need appliances once they regulate their bowels by periodic irrigations."

498. A client is admitted for repair of bilateral inguinal hernias under a general anesthetic. Before surgery the nurse would assess the client for signs that strangulation may have occurred. An early sign of strangulation would be:
1. Increased flatus
2. Projectile vomiting
3. Sharp abdominal pain
4. Decreased bowel sounds

499. An 80-year-old male client had surgery for a strangulated hernia. One hour after surgery his blood pressure drops from 134/80 to 114/76. Assessment reveals that he does not have postoperative bleeding. The nurse should:
1. Turn him on his left side
2. Call his physician immediately
3. Encourage him to move his legs
4. Administer his pain medication as ordered

500. After a bilateral herniorrhaphy a male client should be observed for the development of:
1. Hydrocele
2. Paralytic ileus
3. Urinary retention
4. Thrombophlebitis

501. A client receiving a 1500 calorie ADA diet eats these foods for breakfast: 1 cup of milk (12 g carbohydrate, 8 g protein, 10 g fat); three-fourths of a cup corn flakes (15 g carbohydrate, 2 g protein); and a half of an orange (5 g carbohydrate). How may calories has this client ingested?
Answer: _____

INTEGUMENTARY (IT)

502. A 40-year-old male client, who is receiving combination chemotherapy for stage II Hodgkin's disease, is at risk for stomatitis. The nurse's teaching plan should include instructions to:
1. Brush his teeth once daily and use dental floss after each meal
2. Rinse his mouth three times a day with lemon juice and water

3. Vigorously clean his mouth with toothpaste and a firm toothbrush
4. Frequently cleanse his mouth with a soft toothbrush or a gentle spray

503. A client with multiple abrasions and lacerations to the trunk and all four extremities says, "I can't eat all this food." The food that the nurse should suggest be eaten first would be:
1. Meat loaf and tea
2. Meat loaf and strawberries
3. Tomato soup and baked apple
4. Tomato soup and buttered bread

504. When assessing the skin of an older adult, a normal change that the nurse might identify would be:
1. Signs of ecchymosis
2. Marked flaking of skin
3. Hyperpigmented patches
4. Scaling associated with dryness

505. A client has been in a coma for two months and is maintained on bed rest. The nurse understands that to prevent the effects of shearing force, the head of the bed should be at an angle of:
1. 30 degrees
2. 45 degrees
3. 60 degrees
4. 90 degrees

506. The physician orders bed rest for a client after surgery. The nurse is aware that the most beneficial method of preventing skin breakdown while the client is confined to bed is to:
1. Massage the skin with cream
2. Use a sheepskin pad on the bed
3. Promote passive range of motion
4. Encourage independent movement

507. The physician orders bed rest for a client with cellulitis of the leg. The nurse understands that the primary purpose of bed rest for this client is to:
1. Decrease catabolism to promote healing at the site of injury
2. Lower the metabolic rate in an attempt to help reduce the fever
3. Reduce the energy demands on the body in the presence of infection
4. Limit muscle contractions that may force causative organisms into the bloodstream

508. The nurse should caution a client with peripheral vascular disease that minor foot problems easily can become serious. The teaching plan should include the importance of:
    1. Trimming toenails so that they are short and rounded
    2. Checking bath water temperature by putting the toes in first
    3. Using alcohol to rub hands, feet, legs, and arms at least two times a day
    4. Securing professional treatment for any minor injuries to the extremities

509. A client who has had an above-the-knee amputation is fitted for a prosthesis. Two days after using the prosthesis, a small blister develops on the residual limb near the healed incision. The nurse should anticipate that the client will be advised to:
    1. Increase the frequency of limb-toughening exercises
    2. Discontinue using the prosthesis until the blister heals
    3. Clean and bandage the blister before putting the prosthesis back on
    4. Change the type of limb covering being used to avoid irritation

510. When planning a teaching session about care of the residual limb after a client had a below-the-elbow amputation, the nurse should include:
    1. Wearing a sling to bed every night
    2. Applying skin lotion at least twice a day
    3. Washing and drying the residual limb at least once a day
    4. Soaking the residual limb in warm water for 20 minutes daily

511. The nurse is preparing to change a client's dressing. The statement that best explains the basis of surgical asepsis that the nurse will perform in this procedure is:
    1. Keep the area free of microorganisms
    2. Protect self from microorganisms in the wound
    3. Confine the microorganisms to the surgical site
    4. Keep the number of opportunistic microorganisms to a minimum

512. The equipment that will be used by the nurse during central venous catheter site care for a client receiving total parenteral nutrition is:
    1. Double sterile gloves
    2. Mask and sterile gloves
    3. Gown and sterile gloves
    4. Mask, gown, and sterile gloves

513. An extremely obese client must self-administer insulin with an insulin syringe. The nurse should teach the client to:
    1. Pinch the tissue and inject at a 45-degree angle
    2. Pinch the tissue and inject at a 60-degree angle
    3. Spread the tissue and inject at a 45-degree angle
    4. Spread the tissue and inject at a 90-degree angle

514. A client develops an infection at a catheter insertion site. The nurse uses the term iatrogenic when describing this infection because it resulted from:
    1. Poor personal hygiene
    2. A therapeutic procedure
    3. Inadequate dietary patterns
    4. The client's developmental level

515. A client develops an infection of an abdominal incision and overhears the nurses say that it is a nosocomial infection. The client asks the nurse what this means. The nurse should reply:
    1. "The infection you had prior to hospitalization has flared up."
    2. "You acquired the infection after being admitted to the hospital."
    3. "This is a highly contagious infection requiring protective isolation."
    4. "As a result of medical treatment, you have developed a secondary infection."

516. When reestablishing a portable wound drainage system after emptying its contents, the nurse squeezes the collection container and replaces the stopper to:
    1. Establish positive pressure
    2. Decrease negative pressure
    3. Maintain atmospheric pressure
    4. Increase the difference in pressure

517. A client has surgery for invasive cancer of the head of the pancreas. The physician inserts a permanent biliary drainage tube (T-tube). After surgery, it is most important for the nurse to:
    1. Cleanse the area around the T-tube to prevent skin breakdown
    2. Maintain intermittent low suction on the T-tube to limit trauma
    3. Reposition the client from side to side every two hours to facilitate bile flow
    4. Attach the T-tube to a negative pressure drainage system to promote drainage

518. A male client is admitted to the hospital for intravenous antibiotic therapy and an incision and drainage of an abscess that developed at the site of a puncture wound. The nurse should begin teaching wound care to the client:
1. In the preoperative period
2. A few days before discharge
3. On the first postoperative day
4. During the first dressing change

519. The primary nurse tells a client with an infected wound that the nurse epidemiologist will visit daily. The client asks what the nurse epidemiologist does. The nurse could correctly explain the role by saying, "The nurse epidemiologist:
1. Helps providers of care to control infections."
2. Works in the laboratory to identify bacteria causing infection."
3. Is responsible for doing cultures of all infections and drainages."
4. Decides what antibiotics should be prescribed for infections."

520. After a choledocholithotomy, a client complains that the skin around the T-tube is raw and excoriated. After assessing the skin, the nurse should plan to:
1. Reinforce the dressings when they are wet
2. Cleanse the area with an antiseptic solution
3. Use a skin barrier around the T-tube exit site
4. Change the type of adhesive tape used on the dressing

521. A 35-year-old adult is admitted with multiple injuries because of an accident. The right foot has extensive bone and soft-tissue injuries and sterile dressings are applied. Two days later, when removing the dressing, the nurse finds it has adhered to the tissue in several places. The nurse should:
1. Apply diluted hydrogen peroxide to loosen the dressings
2. Loosen the dressings by pulling with gentle but steady traction
3. Soak the foot in a solution of Betadine until the dressings come off
4. Moisten the dressings with sterile saline until they can be removed easily

522. A client has a deep soft-tissue injury that is open and oozing blood. When managing this wound the nurse should:
1. Replace the dressing when it is completely saturated
2. Reinforce the dressing several times before changing it

3. Change the dressing each time the blood has oozed through to the outside
4. Pack the wound with antimicrobial gauze each time the dressing is changed

523. A client arrives at the emergency room after being bitten by a stray dog. The bite involved tearing of skin and deep soft tissue injury. The client says the dog was foaming at the mouth and afterward ran away. The first nursing action is to:
1. Ask the client about horse serum allergy
2. Notify the police department to capture the dog
3. Assess the client's injury, vital signs, and past history
4. Inoculate the client with human rabies immune globulin

524. A client comes to the clinic after being bitten by a raccoon in the woods in an area where rabies is endemic. The nurse recalls that rabies is:
1. A bacterial infection characterized by encephalopathy and opisthotonos
2. An acute bacterial septicemia that results in convulsions and a morbid fear of water
3. A nonspecific immunoresponse to organisms deposited under the skin by an animal bite
4. An acute viral infection, characterized by convulsions and difficulty swallowing, that affects the nervous system

525. A 30-year-old female dancer notices that a mole on her ankle has turned dark brown and seeks medical attention. A diagnosis of malignant melanoma is made. This client has increased her chance of survival by early treatment because melanoma spreads quickly. The nurse recognizes that melanoma spreads:
1. By seeding across membranes of body tissues
2. By runner-like chains of cells to satellite tumors
3. Through invasion of the lymphatic system and bloodstream
4. Through direct extension into subcutaneous tissue and to bone

526. A client who is to receive radiation says to the nurse, "My family and friends say that I will get a radiation burn." The best response by the nurse would be:
1. "It will be no worse than a sunburn."
2. "A localized skin reaction usually occurs."
3. "Have they had experience with this type of radiation?"
4. "Daily application of an emollient will prevent the burn."

527. A client is scheduled for radiation treatments Monday through Friday. The client asks why the treatments will not be given on Saturday and Sunday. The nurse's best response would be:
1. "The department operates Monday through Friday."
2. "This schedule gives normal cells time to recover."
3. "Your energy level will be increased greatly by a five-day schedule."
4. "Side effects are eliminated when treatment is administered for five rather than seven days."

528. A client is receiving radiation therapy. When teaching about skin care to the irradiated area, the nurse should instruct the client to:
1. Apply no lotions or powders to the area
2. Cover the area with a sterile gauze bandage
3. Put warm compresses on the site once a day
4. Lie on the back and unaffected side when sleeping

529. Irradiation to the chest wall on an outpatient basis is prescribed for a client after removal of a tumor in the right lung. When teaching skin care to the client, the nurse should emphasize:
1. Frequent washing to remove desquamated cells
2. Massaging four times a day to increase circulation
3. Keeping the skin dry and protected from abrasions
4. Using skin lotion twice daily to keep the skin supple

530. A client with scleroderma complains of having difficulty chewing and swallowing. When providing dietary counseling, the nurse should advise the client to:
1. Puree all foods before eating
2. Liquefy the food in a blender
3. Take frequent sips of water with meals
4. Use a local anesthetic mouthwash before eating

531. A female client with scleroderma tells the nurse that she often has numbness and tingling in her hands followed by blanching of her fingers. The nurse recognizes that the client has Raynaud's phenomenon, a condition commonly associated with scleroderma. The nurse should advise the client to:
1. Bathe her hands frequently in hot water
2. Keep her hands warm by wearing gloves
3. Briskly rub her hands to increase circulation
4. Take the anticoagulants that will be prescribed to prevent attacks

532. As part of the teaching plan for a client with scleroderma, the nurse should include the need for special skin care. The nurse should plan to advise the client to:
1. Keep the skin well lubricated
2. Use calamine lotion for pruritus
3. Apply warm soaks to the inflamed areas
4. Take frequent baths to remove scaly lesions

533. The physician orders a regimen of daily exercises for a client with scleroderma. The nurse understands that with this client exercises are performed to:
1. Preserve muscle strength
2. Support tissue regeneration
3. Prevent spread of the disease
4. Maintain a sense of well-being

534. A client, who has just had a colostomy, has an uneventful 24-hour postoperative course. Seventy-two hours after surgery, the primary nursing intervention for this client would be:
1. Keeping an accurate record of vital signs and oral intake
2. Emphasizing the importance of regulating the diet to form stool
3. Teaching care of the incision and how to perform colostomy irrigations
4. Observing and reporting drainage and the condition of the abdominal incision

535. When performing colostomy care, it is important for the nurse to teach the client to care for the skin around the stoma by:
1. Avoiding the use of soap or irritating agents
2. Rinsing with hydrogen peroxide and applying a gauze pad
3. Pouring saline over the stoma and wiping away fecal matter
4. Washing the area gently with soap and water before applying an appliance

536. A young male client is admitted to the burn center after incurring electrical burns to both hands while playing golf during a lightning storm. When assessing the entrance and exit wounds, the nurse is aware that electrical injury:
1. Causes severe nervous tissue destruction along a path of least resistance
2. Results in severe tissue destruction when the burn is incurred by direct current
3. Causes a line of destruction beginning at the grounding point to the point of contact
4. Results in visible dermal wounds that denote the internal electrical current destruction

537. The shirt of a young man starting a barbecue fire ignites. The most effective method for putting out the flames would be:
1. Slapping at the flames
2. Removing the burning clothes
3. Log-rolling the man in the grass
4. Pouring cold liquid over the flames

538. During a first-aid class, a student asks what should be done when a person rushes out of a house with burning clothes. The nurse explains that, after the flames are extinguished, it is most important to:
1. Give the person sips of water
2. Assess the person's breathing
3. Cover the person with a warm blanket
4. Calculate the extent of the person's burns

539. A family member suggests that butter be applied to the burns of a relative who experienced extensive burns during a house fire. An appropriate response by a neighbor who is a registered nurse would be, "We should just:
1. Apply ice."
2. Use first aid cream."
3. Wait for the ambulance."
4. Cover the area with a bed sheet."

540. A worker is involved in an explosion of a steam pipe and receives a scalding burn to the chest and arms. The burned areas are painful, mottled red, weeping, and edematous. These burns would be classified as:
1. Eschar
2. Full-thickness burns
3. Deep partial-thickness burns
4. Superficial partial-thickness burns

541. A client is seen in the emergency department after a barbecue accident. The physician diagnoses superficial partial-thickness burns. The family asks what is involved with this type of burn. The most accurate response by the nurse would be that the:
1. Epidermis has been damaged
2. Dermis has been partially damaged
3. Epidermis and dermis have been destroyed
4. Structures beneath the skin have been destroyed

542. A burn victim has waxy white areas interspersed with pink and red areas on the chest and all of both arms. The nurse calculates that the percentage of total body surface area (TBSA) that has sustained burns would be:
1. 20
2. 25

3. 30
4. 35

543. When a female client who has partial-thickness burns on her chest, abdomen, and right leg from a fire at her workplace arrives in the emergency department, the nurse's first responsibility should be to:
1. Carefully remove all of the client's clothing
2. Apply sterile saline dressings on all burned surfaces
3. Evaluate whether heat inhalation had occurred
4. Calculate total body surface area that has been burned

544. When a nurse is evaluating the condition of a client with burns of the upper body, an assessment that would indicate potential respiratory obstruction is:
1. Deep breathing
2. Hoarse quality to the voice
3. Rapid abdominal breathing
4. Pink-tinged, frothy sputum

545. During the first 48 hours after a thermal injury, the nurse should assess the client for:
1. Hypokalemia and hyponatremia
2. Hyperkalemia and hyponatremia
3. Hypokalemia and hypernatremia
4. Hyperkalemia and hypernatremia

546. A client is admitted to the hospital with burns on the trunk and arms. When oral intake is resumed on the fourth day after the injury, the nurse helps the client plan the menu for the next day. Discussion should focus on the need for a diet that includes:
1. High caloric intake, liberal potassium intake, and 3 g protein/kg/day
2. Moderate caloric intake, liberal potassium intake, and 3 g protein/kg/day
3. Moderate caloric intake, restricted potassium intake, and 1 g protein/kg/day
4. High caloric intake, restricted potassium intake, and 1 g protein/kg/day

547. A severely burned client has been hospitalized for two days. Until now recovery has been uneventful, but the client begins to exhibit extreme restlessness. The nurse recognizes that this most likely indicates that the client is developing:
1. Renal failure
2. Hypervolemia
3. Cerebral hypoxia
4. Metabolic acidosis

548. A client's partial-thickness burns differ from full-thickness burns in that with partial-thickness burns the burned area will:
   1. Require grafting before it can heal
   2. Be painful, reddened, and have blisters
   3. Have destruction of the epidermis and dermis
   4. Take months of extensive treatment before healing

549. A client with burns develops a wound infection. The nurse knows that local wound infections are primarily treated with:
   1. Oral antibiotics
   2. Topical antibiotics
   3. Intravenous antibiotics
   4. Intramuscular antibiotics

550. The nurse identifies that a client in the acute phase of burns has eaten only a small portion of each meal. Aware that malnutrition can have a variety of consequences, the nurse should assess the client for:
   1. Dehydration
   2. Dry, brittle hair
   3. Prolonged wound healing
   4. "Clubbing" of the finger tips

551. The method of treatment chosen for a client's burns is the exposure method with application of mafenide (Sulfamylon) bid. When applying this medication the nurse should plan to:
   1. Use medical asepsis
   2. Apply a dry sterile dressing
   3. Monitor liver function studies
   4. Give ordered pain medication

552. When the exposure method of treatment is used in caring for burns, the nurse should explain to the client that:
   1. Bathing will not be permitted
   2. Dressings will be changed daily
   3. Isolation precautions are required
   4. Room temperature must be kept at 72° F

553. When dressing the deep partial-thickness burns on a client's hands the nurse should use:
   1. Cotton-backed gauze and fully extend the fingers with thumb in opposition
   2. Non-cotton-backed gauze and place a hand roll with gauze between each finger
   3. Non-cotton-backed gauze and extend fingers fully with gauze between each finger
   4. Cotton-backed gauze and a hand roll, with fingers completely flexed and thumb in opposition

554. A client tells the nurse that the doctor mentioned doing skin grafts after a burn and asks when they will be done. The most appropriate response by the nurse would be:
   1. "Within seven days."
   2. "What did your doctor tell you?"
   3. "As soon as scar formation occurs."
   4. "As soon as signs of infection disappear."

555. A client, with burns over 35% of the body, complains of chilling. To promote the client's comfort, the nurse should:
   1. Limit the occurrence of drafts
   2. Keep the room temperature at 80°
   3. Place a sterile top sheet over the client
   4. Maintain the room humidity below 40%

556. The physician determines that a client's burn wounds need to be mechanically debrided and informs the client of this fact. Later the nurse should reinforce the physician's discussion by explaining that:
   1. The surgeon will surgically remove the dead tissue
   2. Enzymatic agents will be applied daily to the wounds
   3. Incisions will be made along the length of the eschar
   4. Mechanical devices will continually move the client's extremities

557. The nurse is aware that a temporary heterograft (pig skin) is used to treat burns because this graft will:
   1. Débride necrotic epithelium
   2. Be sutured in place for better adherence
   3. Relieve pain and promote rapid epithelialization
   4. Commonly be used concurrently with topical antimicrobials

558. A client with a full-thickness burn receives an allograft. Several days later the client points out that the graft is coming off at the edges. The nurse's best response would be:
   1. "It is not a permanent graft. I'll notify your physician."
   2. "You must have pulled it loose. I'll notify your physician."
   3. "An infection may be starting. Your physician will be here shortly."

4. "That was a permanent graft. Your physician probably will replace it."

559. When planning care to prevent deformities and contractures in a client with burns, the nurse should expect to begin range-of-motion exercises when the client's:
1. Pain has lessened
2. Vital signs are stable
3. Skin grafts are healed
4. Emotional status stabilizes

560. A client returns from surgery with an incisional dressing and a catheter that is attached to a portable wound drainage system exiting from the operative site. The nurse recognizes that the principle underlying the function of a portable drainage system is:
1. Gravity
2. Osmosis
3. Active transport
4. Negative pressure

561. After surgery for cancer, a client is to receive adjuvant chemotherapy. When teaching the client about the side effects of chemotherapy, the nurse should emphasize that the occurrence of alopecia is:
1. Usually rare
2. Never permanent
3. Frequently prolonged
4. Sometimes preventable

NEUROMUSCULAR (NM)

562. When preparing to assess the vagus nerve (cranial nerve X) of a client, the nurse will need:
1. A tuning fork
2. A tongue depressor
3. An ophthalmoscope
4. Cotton and a straight pin

563. The nurse in the neurologic clinic assesses for damage to the glossopharyngeal (ninth cranial) and vagus (tenth cranial) nerve by testing the client's ability to:
1. Shrug
2. Smell
3. Smile
4. Swallow

564. When assessing trigeminal nerve function the nurse should evaluate:
1. Corneal sensation
2. Smiling and frowning

3. Ocular muscle movement
4. Shrugging of the shoulders

565. A client, recently diagnosed with Bell's palsy, has many questions about the course of the disease. The nurse should explain that:
1. Pain occurs with transient ischemic attacks
2. Cool compresses decrease facial involvement
3. Most clients recover within three to five weeks
4. Body changes should be expected with residual effects

566. The nurse explains to a client with trigeminal neuralgia that a treatment that is effective on a temporary (6 to 18 months) basis is:
1. An intravenous injection of cobra venom
2. Microvascular decompression of the blood vessels at the nerve root
3. A lidocaine injection of the ventral root of the eleventh spinal nerve
4. An alcohol injection of the peripheral branch of the fifth cranial nerve

567. A client with pain and paresis of the left leg is scheduled for electromyography. Before the test, the nurse should explain that:
1. The involved area will be shaved immediately before testing
2. The client's heart rate and rhythm will be monitored frequently
3. Needles will be inserted into the affected muscles during the test
4. The client will be kept in a recumbent position after the procedure

568. The nurse is aware that the teaching about myasthenic and cholinergic crises is understood when a client who has been diagnosed with myasthenia gravis states that a symptom common to both is:
1. Diarrhea
2. Salivation
3. Difficulty breathing
4. Abdominal cramping

569. When assessing the progress of a client being treated for myasthenia gravis, the nurse would expect:
1. Partial improvement of muscle strength with mild exercise
2. Fluctuating weakness of muscles innervated by the cranial nerves
3. Dramatic worsening in muscle strength with anticholinesterase drugs
4. Little or no change in muscle strength regardless of therapy initiated

570. A 30-year-old homemaker with a five-year history of myasthenia gravis is admitted to the hospital. When assessing the client, the nurse identifies ptosis, dysarthria, dysphagia, and muscle weakness. Based on this client's diagnosis and status, the nurse should expect that the client's muscle:
1. Weakness will decrease with hot baths
2. Weakness will decrease with muscle use
3. Strength will decrease with repeated muscle use
4. Strength will improve immediately after meals

571. When assisting a client who has myasthenia gravis with a bath, the nurse notices that the client's arms become weaker with sustained movement. The nurse should:
1. Encourage the client to rest for short periods of time
2. Gradually increase the client's activity level each day
3. Continue the bath while supporting the client's arms
4. Administer a dose of pyridostigmine bromide (Mestinon)

572. A client with myasthenia gravis comes to the neurology clinic at 4 PM for a routine visit. During an assessment the nurse should expect the client to report:
1. Blurred vision and episodes of vertigo
2. Tremors of the hands when attempting to lift objects
3. Partial improvement of muscle strength with mild exercise
4. Involvement of the distal muscles rather than the proximal muscles

573. During a routine clinic visit of a client who has myasthenia gravis, the nurse reinforces previous teaching about the disease and self-care. The nurse would evaluate that the teaching was effective when the client recognizes that it is important to:
1. Plan activities for later in the day
2. Eat meals in a semirecumbent position
3. Avoid people with respiratory infections
4. Take muscle relaxants when under stress

574. The nurse is teaching a client with myasthenia gravis how to prevent a myasthenic crisis. The nurse knows health teaching has been effective if the client says:
1. "I'll take an antihistamine at the first sign of a cold."

2. "I can skip a dose of Mestinon if it upsets my stomach."
3. "We've told our daughter not to let her cold keep her from visiting us."
4. "The doctor may need to adjust the dosage of my medication if I'm more active."

575. A client is scheduled to have a series of diagnostic studies for myasthenia gravis, including a Tensilon test. The nurse should explain to the client that the diagnosis of myasthenia gravis will be confirmed if the administration of Tensilon produces a:
1. Brief exaggeration of symptoms
2. Prolonged symptomatic improvement
3. Rapid but brief symptomatic improvement
4. Symptomatic improvement of just the ptosis

576. The physician has ordered a diagnostic workup for a client who may have myasthenia gravis. The initial nursing goal for the client during the diagnostic phase would be that, "The client will:
1. Adhere to a teaching plan."
2. Achieve psychologic adjustment."
3. Maintain present muscle strength."
4. Prepare for the appearance of myasthenic crisis."

577. The most significant initial nursing observations that should be made about a client who is suspected of having myasthenia gravis, include the:
1. Ability to chew and speak distinctly
2. Capacity to smile and close the eyelids
3. Effectiveness of respiratory exchange and ability to swallow
4. Degree of anxiety and concern about the suspected diagnosis

578. A 50-year-old widow with myasthenia gravis has been living in a nursing home. She is receiving pyridostigmine bromide (Mestinon) to control symptoms but is beginning to experience increased difficulty in swallowing. The nursing intervention that would be most effective in preventing aspiration of food would be to:
1. Place an emergency tracheostomy set in her room
2. Assess her respiratory status before and after meals
3. Change her diet order from soft foods to clear liquids
4. Coordinate her meals with the peak effect of her medication

579. A client with myasthenia gravis, who is living in a nursing home, experiences inadequate

symptomatic control with pyridostigmine bromide (Mestinon) and the physician begins long-term steroid therapy. When this type of therapy is being initiated, it is especially important for the nurse to ensure that the client:
1. Increases sodium intake
2. Is placed on protective isolation
3. Decreases fluid intake to 1000 mL daily
4. Is monitored for an exacerbation of symptoms

580. A client newly diagnosed with myasthenia gravis is concerned about fluctuations in physical condition and generalized weakness. When planning for this client's care it would be most important for the nurse to plan to:
1. Space activities throughout the day
2. Restrict activities and encourage bed rest
3. Teach the limitations imposed by the disease
4. Have a member of the family stay with the client

581. The nurse identifies that a client exhibits the characteristic gait associated with Parkinson's disease. When recording on the client's chart, the nurse should describe this gait as:
1. Ataxic
2. Spastic
3. Shuffling
4. Scissoring

582. While performing the history and physical examination of a client with Parkinson's disease, the nurse should assess the client for:
1. Frequent bouts of diarrhea
2. Hyperextension of the neck
3. A low-pitched, monotonous voice
4. A recent increase in appetite and weight gain

583. While assessing a client with Parkinson's disease, the nurse identifies bradykinesia when the client exhibits:
1. Muscle flaccidity
2. An intention tremor
3. Paralysis of the limbs
4. A lack of spontaneous movement

584. An older adult with a history of parkinsonism has some rigidity and tremors despite medication. At this time the client has been admitted to the hospital with pneumonia. In view of the current medical problem and the rigidity, the nursing plan should include:
1. Gait training in the physical therapy department

2. Isometric exercises every two hours while awake
3. Active range-of-motion exercise every four hours
4. Passive range-of-motion exercises at least once every eight hours

585. A retired mailman with parkinsonism has been taking an anticholingeric medication for morning stiffness and tremors in the right arm. During a visit to the clinic, the client complains of some numbness in the left hand. The nurse should:
1. Make arrangements immediately for further medical evaluation
2. Refer the client to a physician if other neurologic deficits are present
3. Stress the importance of calling the family physician as soon as possible
4. Have the physician increase the dosage of the anticholinergic medication

586. The nurse might expect a client with multiple sclerosis to complain about the most common initial symptom, which is:
1. Diarrhea
2. Headaches
3. Skin infections
4. Visual disturbances

587. A client with multiple sclerosis is informed that it is a chronic progressive neurologic condition. The client asks the nurse, "Will I experience pain?" The nurse's best response would be:
1. "Tell me about your fears regarding pain."
2. "Analgesics will be ordered to control the pain."
3. "Let's make a list of the things you need to ask the physician."
4. "Pain is not a characteristic symptom of this disease process."

588. A 28-year-old woman has known for the past six years that she has multiple sclerosis. She has two children, one of whom is an active 2½-year-old. The client is currently in remission. At the present time, it would be most important for the nurse to encourage the client to:
1. Schedule periodic quality time with her child
2. Provide support to other people with multiple sclerosis
3. Develop a flexible schedule for completion of routine daily activities
4. Meet with the psychotherapy group for people with multiple sclerosis

589. Two weeks after experiencing a 48-hour episode of chills, fever, and upper respiratory symptoms, the client is admitted to the hospital with numbness of the hands and feet that has progressed upward and now involves the arms, legs, and lower trunk. The tentative diagnosis is Guillain-Barré syndrome. The nurse should continue to assess the client for the major clinical features of Guillain-Barré syndrome including:
1. Ptosis and dysphagia
2. Paresthesias and paralysis
3. Atrophy and fasciculations
4. Muscle weakness and drooling

590. During the neurological assessment of a client with a tentative diagnosis of Guillain-Barré syndrome, the nurse should expect that the client will manifest:
1. Diminished visual acuity
2. Increased muscular weakness
3. Pronounced muscular atrophy
4. Impairment in cognitive reasoning

591. A client who has Guillain-Barré syndrome asks, "Will I ever get better?" The most appropriate answer by the nurse would be:
1. "You'll notice your strength will improve each day."
2. "We are doing everything we can to provide the best care."
3. "You seem concerned about getting better. What do you think?"
4. "Your chances for recovery are very good but recovery is slow."

592. A client asks for an explanation about glaucoma. The nurse explains that with glaucoma there is:
1. An increase in the pressure within the eyeball
2. An opacity of the crystalline lens or its capsule
3. A curvature of the cornea that becomes unequal
4. A separation of the neural retina from the pigmented retina

593. When obtaining the nursing history from a client who has open-angle (chronic) glaucoma, a complaint that the nurse should expect is:
1. Flashes of light
2. Intolerance to light
3. Seeing floating specks
4. Loss of peripheral vision

594. A client who has open-angle (chronic) glaucoma is scheduled for eye surgery to promote aqueous humor outflow. The nurse would know that the client understands the preoperative teaching about the first 24 hours after surgery when the client states, "I should:
1. Cough and deep-breathe."
2. Lie on my unaffected side."
3. Move around freely in bed."
4. Elevate the head of my bed."

595. An older adult has cataracts in both eyes. The left cataract is scheduled to be extracted in several days. The nurse should plan to instruct the client that:
1. "Both eyes will be bandaged for 24 hours after surgery."
2. "You must remember to take deep breaths and cough several times an hour."
3. "You may have to remain on bed rest for three to four days after your surgery."
4. "At night you will be wearing a hard patch over your operated eye for a month or so."

596. After cataract surgery a client complains of feeling nauseated. The nurse should:
1. Give the client some dry crackers to eat
2. Administer the antiemetic drug as ordered
3. Explain that this is expected following surgery
4. Instruct the client to deep-breathe until the nausea subsides

597. After a left cataract extraction, a client complains of severe discomfort in the operated eye. The nurse recognizes that this is a problem that may be caused by:
1. Hemorrhage into the eye
2. Expected postoperative discomfort
3. Isolation related to sensory deprivation
4. Pressure on the eye from the protective shield

598. A client is being prepared for discharge from an ambulatory surgical unit following a cataract removal with an intraocular lens implant. The statement by the client that suggests to the nurse that discharge teaching was effective would be:
1. "I'm driving home since I feel so good."
2. "I can't wait until I get home to wash my hair."
3. "I can expect to see bright flashes of light for awhile."
4. "I'll call the surgeon if the analgesic doesn't relieve the pain."

599. After cataract surgery, a client is taught how to self-administer eyedrops before discharge. The nurse approves the technique when the client:
1. Holds the dropper tip above the eye
2. Places the drops on the cornea of the eye
3. Raises the upper eyelid with gentle traction
4. Squeezes the eye shut after instilling the eyedrops

600. After an automobile accident, a client complains of seeing frequent flashes of light. The nurse should suspect:
   1. Scleroderma
   2. Acute glaucoma
   3. A detached retina
   4. A cerebral concussion

601. After surgery to repair a retinal detachment, the client returns to the post anesthesia care unit with the affected eye patched. During the first four hours after surgery, the nurse should notify the physician if the client:
   1. Has not voided
   2. Cannot open the eye
   3. Becomes confused and restless
   4. Complains of sharp pain in the eye

602. A client who has had a retinal detachment has a scleral buckling procedure to attempt to reattach the retina. Before the client is discharged home, the nurse should:
   1. Instruct the client to wear dark glasses after the patch is removed
   2. Tell the client that usual activities can be resumed within two weeks
   3. Explain to the client that reading will help strengthen the eye muscles
   4. Reassure the client that the glasses worn before surgery can still be worn

603. When performing a neurologic check on a client with a head injury, the nurse identifies a diminished corneal reflex. Appropriate nursing care for an absent corneal reflex includes:
   1. Irrigating the eye every four hours
   2. Checking the corneal reflex every hour
   3. Instilling artificial tears whenever necessary
   4. Alternately taping the eyelids open and closed every two hours

604. After an automobile accident a client, who is unconscious and exhibiting decerebrate posturing, is brought to the emergency department. When assessing this client the nurse should expect to observe:
   1. Hyperextension of both the upper and lower extremities
   2. Spastic paralysis of both the upper and lower extremities
   3. Hyperflexion of the upper extremities and hyperextension of the lower extremities
   4. Flaccid paralysis of the upper extremities and spastic paralysis of the lower extremities

605. A client is admitted to the hospital from the emergency department for observation because of an accident. Assessment reveals a sutured laceration on the scalp, stable vital signs, orientation to person, place, and time, and an intravenous line for circulatory access. When performing an assessment the nurse identifies a clear, watery drainage oozing from the client's right ear. Before notifying the physician, the best nursing action to take would be:
   1. Testing the fluid for glucose and applying a sterile dressing
   2. Positioning the client so that the unaffected ear is dependent
   3. Covering the area with sterile gauze and applying slight pressure
   4. Cleaning the outer ear with normal saline and inserting a clean cotton ball

606. A client is admitted to the hospital after sustaining a head injury. The most reliable sign that this client is experiencing an increase in intracranial pressure would be a slowly:
   1. Rising respiratory rate
   2. Narrowing pulse pressure
   3. Decreasing level of consciousness
   4. Increasing diastolic blood pressure

607. During the immediate post-trauma period after injury to the frontal lobe of the brain, the nurse should place a client in the:
   1. Supine position
   2. Side-lying position
   3. Low-Fowler's position
   4. Trendelenburg position

608. The nurse in the emergency department prepares a checklist prior to transferring an unconscious client with a head injury to the neurologic trauma unit. The nursing action that would be of primary importance would be:
   1. Notifying the receiving unit of the transfer
   2. Having all the records and x-ray films ready for transfer
   3. Verifying that the family has been notified of the transfer
   4. Checking that a bag-valve mask is available during the transfer

609. A client who has sustained a severe head injury in a diving accident remains unconscious. In addition, the nurse observes bleeding from the left ear, as well as rhinorrhea. The nurse is aware that the drainage from the ear and nose indicates:
   1. Contusion
   2. Concussion
   3. Nose fracture
   4. Basilar fracture

610. A client with a severe head injury is being observed by the nurse for increasing intracranial pressure. The finding most indicative of increasing intracranial pressure would be:
1. Polyuria
2. Tachypnea
3. Increased restlessness
4. Intermittent tachycardia

611. A 28-year-old is brought to the emergency department unconscious after an accident. The client's pupils are equal and responsive to light. As part of the neurologic assessment, the nurse applies a painful stimulus to the client's left lower leg. An expected response would be to:
1. Extend the leg
2. Withdraw the leg
3. Make no movement
4. Plantar-flex the left foot

612. A client has had spinal anesthesia for surgery. On the second day after surgery the client complains of a headache. The nurse should:
1. Begin an early ambulation program
2. Supply the client with several containers of juice
3. Remove any elastic antiembolism stockings being worn
4. Assist the client to sit at the bedside and dangle the feet

613. A 26-year-old, admitted with the diagnosis of subarachnoid hemorrhage, exhibits aphasia and hemiparesis. These neurologic deficits, which may be present immediately after a subarachnoid hemorrhage, are primarily caused by:
1. Blood loss
2. Tissue death
3. Vascular spasms
4. Electrolyte imbalance

614. The nurse should plan to position a client who has experienced a subarachnoid hemorrhage:
1. In the supine position
2. On the unaffected side
3. With the head of the bed elevated
4. With sandbags on either side of the head

615. After an anterior fossa craniotomy, a client is placed on controlled mechanical ventilation. To ensure adequate cerebral blood flow the nurse should:
1. Clear the ear of draining fluid
2. Monitor the serum carbon dioxide
3. Discontinue anticonvulsant therapy
4. Elevate the head of the bed 30 degrees

616. When caring for an unconscious client with increasing intracranial pressure, the nursing intervention that is contraindicated would be:
1. Lubricating the skin with baby oil
2. Suctioning the oropharynx routinely
3. Elevating the head of the bed 20 degrees
4. Cleansing the eyes every four hours with normal saline

617. A client who had an infratentorial craniotomy is admitted to the intensive care unit after discharge from the post anesthesia care unit. Frequent assessments reveal that the client's intracranial pressure is increasing. The nurse should first:
1. Elevate the head of the bed
2. Administer an osmotic diuretic
3. Reduce the flow rate of IV fluid
4. Notify the physician of the finding

618. A client has a supratentorial craniotomy for a tumor in the right frontal lobe of the cerebral cortex. Postoperatively, the position that would be most appropriate for this client would be:
1. High Fowler's with knee gatch raised
2. Flat with a small pillow under the nape of the neck
3. Head of the bed elevated 20 degrees with the head turned to the operative side
4. Head of the bed elevated 45 degrees with a large pillow under the head and shoulders

619. A client has surgery for the creation of burr holes after sustaining a head trauma from a fall and is at risk for developing an infection. An early clinical manifestation of meningeal irritation for which the nurse should assess the client is:
1. Sunset eyes
2. Kernig's sign
3. Homans' sign
4. The plantar reflex

620. After three months of rehabilitation after a craniotomy, a female client is still having some motor speech difficulty. To promote the client's use of speech the nurse should:
1. Correct her mistakes immediately
2. Support her efforts to communicate
3. Reexplain why she is having difficulty speaking
4. Address her in simple words and short sentences

621. A client with a history of hypertension is admitted to the hospital with aphasia. A bruit is heard over the left carotid artery, the pulse is irregular, and there is a pulse deficit. The nurse

is aware that complete occlusion of the branches of the middle cerebral artery resulting in aphasia may occur because of:
1. A history of hypertensive disease
2. Emboli associated with atrial fibrillation
3. Developmental defects of the arterial wall
4. Inappropriate paroxysmal neural discharge

622. A client has a history of progressive carotid and cerebral atherosclerosis and transient ischemic attacks (TIAs). The nurse understands that TIAs are:
1. Temporary episodes of neurologic dysfunction
2. Transient attacks caused by multiple small emboli
3. Periods of alternating exacerbations and remissions
4. Ischemic attacks that result in progressive neurologic deterioration

623. A client has carotid atherosclerotic plaques, and a right carotid endarterectomy is performed. Two hours after surgery the client demonstrates progressive hypotension. The nurse should:
1. Increase the IV flow rate
2. Raise the head of the bed
3. Notify the physician immediately
4. Put the client in a slight Trendelenburg position

624. After a carotid endarterectomy, the client should be monitored for the complication of cranial nerve dysfunction. To monitor for this complication, the nurse should assess the client for:
1. Labored breathing
2. Edema of the neck
3. Difficulty in swallowing
4. Alteration in blood pressure

625. A client is admitted to the hospital with weakness in the right extremities and a slight speech problem. Vital signs are normal. During the first 24 hours, the nurse should give priority to:
1. Checking the client's temperature
2. Evaluating the client's motor status
3. Monitoring the client's blood pressure
4. Obtaining a urine specimen from the client

626. A client having a brain attack (CVA) is brought to the emergency department. The vital signs are: P, 78; R, 16; and BP, 120/80. The change in this client's vital signs that would indicate increasing intracranial pressure (ICP) requiring notification of the physician would be:
1. P 120, R 16, BP 80/60
2. P 50, R 22, BP 140/60
3. P 60, R 18, BP 126/96
4. P 56, R 20, BP 130/110

627. On the evening before discharge from the hospital, a client has a hypertensive crisis and a brain attack (CVA). Initially the nurse should place the client in a:
1. Supine position
2. Contour position
3. Side-lying position
4. Slight Trendelenburg position

628. Initially after a brain attack (CVA), a client's pupils are equal and reactive to light. Later the nurse assesses that the right pupil is reacting more slowly than the left and the systolic blood pressure is beginning to rise. The nurse recognizes that these adaptations are suggestive of:
1. Spinal shock
2. Hypovolemic shock
3. Transtentorial herniation
4. Increasing intracranial pressure

629. To prevent a client, who has had a brain attack (CVA) accident two days ago, from developing plantar flexion the nurse should:
1. Place a pillow under the thighs
2. Maintain the feet at right angles to the legs
3. Elevate the knee gatch to a 45-degree angle
4. Encourage active range of motion of all joints

630. A female client manifests right-sided hemianopia as a result of a brain attack (CVA). The nurse should:
1. Correct the client's misuse of equipment
2. Instruct the client to scan her surroundings
3. Provide tactile stimulation to the client's affected extremities
4. Teach the client to look at the position of her left extremities

631. The wife of a client who has had a brain attack (CVA) tells the home health nurse that her husband cries easily and without provocation. She asks why he is so emotionally labile. The nurse should explain that:
1. Her husband can remember only depressing events from the past
2. Her husband feels guilty about the demands he is making on his family
3. This is a way of getting attention, and the behavior should be ignored
4. This behavior is a common response over which he has very little control

632. The husband of a client with aphasia as a result of a brain attack (CVA) asks whether his wife's speech will ever return. The nurse should respond:
1. "You will have to ask your physician."
2. "It should return to normal in two or three months."
3. "It is hard to say how much improvement will occur."
4. "This will probably be the extent of her speech from now on."

633. When assisting the family to help an aphasic member regain as much speech function as possible, the nurse should instruct them to:
1. Speak louder than usual during visits
2. Tell the client to use the correct words when speaking
3. Give positive reinforcement for correct communication
4. Encourage the client to speak while being patient with all attempts

634. A client, employed as a carpenter, has trouble holding tools because of carpal tunnel syndrome. Because the client continues to work, the nursing diagnosis of most concern would be:
1. Anxiety
2. Chronic pain
3. Risk for injury
4. Situational low self-esteem

635. While walking in the hall a hospitalized client has a tonic-clonic seizure. During the seizure the nurse's priority should be to:
1. Protect the client's head from injury
2. Hold the client's arms and legs firmly
3. Move the client immediately to a soft surface
4. Attempt to insert an airway between the client's teeth

636. A client sustains a vertebral fracture at the T1 level as a result of diving into shallow water. On admission to the emergency department a detailed neurologic assessment is performed. The nurse should expect to find:
1. Inability to move the lower arms
2. Normal biceps reflexes in the arms
3. Loss of pain sensation in the hands
4. Difficulty breathing and a flaccid diaphragm

637. A client who sustained a spinal cord injury at the T2 level should be assessed for signs of autonomic dysreflexia because:
1. The injury results in loss of the reflex arc
2. There has been a partial transection of the cord

3. The injury is above the sixth thoracic vertebra
4. There is a flaccid paralysis of the lower extremities

638. The nurse is aware that a client with a spinal cord injury is developing autonomic dysreflexia when the client has:
1. Flaccid paralysis and numbness
2. Absence of sweating and pyrexia
3. Escalating tachycardia and shock
4. Paroxysmal hypertension and bradycardia

639. During the first week after a spinal cord injury at the T3 level, a male client and the nurse identify a short-term goal. An appropriate short-term goal for this client would be, "The client will:
1. Consider lifestyle changes."
2. Understand his limitations."
3. Perform independent ambulation."
4. Carry out personal hygiene activities."

640. A client who is recuperating from a spinal cord injury at the T4 level wants to use a wheelchair. In preparation for this activity the client should be taught:
1. Leg lifts to prevent hip contractures
2. Push-ups to strengthen arm muscles
3. Balancing exercises to promote equilibrium
4. Quadriceps-setting exercises to maintain muscle tone

641. A client whose vertebral column at the level of T6 and T7 was completely crushed and whose left leg was traumatically amputated above the knee is admitted to the ICU. When performing an assessment the nurse would expect to find that the client was experiencing:
1. Difficulty breathing
2. Pain in the residual limb
3. Pain at the level of compression
4. Spastic paralysis of the arms and legs

642. On the first postoperative evening after a lumbar laminectomy, a male client tells the nurse that his feet are as numb as they were before the operation. The nurse's best response would be:
1. "Let me elevate your feet so the numbness will decrease more quickly."
2. "That's important to know. I will inform your physician about your observation."
3. "Continue to let me know how you feel. It often takes time before this symptom subsides."

4. "There is no cause for concern because the numbness will subside when the anesthesia wears off."

643. A 48-year-old farmer is admitted for the repair and revision of a residual limb immediately after the traumatic amputation of the left hand in a corn picker accident. A week after surgery the client complains of constant throbbing in the affected limb. The most appropriate nursing intervention would be to:
1. Apply cool compresses to the limb
2. Secure an order for pain medication
3. Loosen the bandage around the limb
4. Elevate the extremity on two pillows

RESPIRATORY (RE)

644. An obese adult, who smokes 3 packs of cigarettes daily, is admitted for major abdominal surgery. Postoperatively, the most appropriate laboratory value that the nurse should monitor routinely that would reflect the client's respiratory status is the:
1. PO_2
2. PCO_2
3. Hemoglobin
4. Oxygen saturation

645. The description that should be used for the soft swishing sounds of normal breathing heard when the nurse auscultates a client's chest would be:
1. Fine crackles
2. Adventitious sounds
3. Vesicular breath sounds
4. Diminished breath sounds

646. A client who has a pneumonectomy is in the post anesthesia care unit. The nurse's primary concern at this time would be to maintain:
1. Blood replacement
2. Ventilatory exchange
3. Closed chest drainage
4. Supplementary oxygenation

647. When assessing the breath sounds of a client with chronic obstructive pulmonary disease (COPD), the nurse hears rhonchi. Rhonchi can best be described as:
1. Snorting during the inspiratory phase
2. Moist rumbling sounds that clear after coughing
3. Musical sounds more pronounced during expiration
4. Crackling inspiratory sounds unchanged with coughing

648. A client is brought to the hospital with deep partial-thickness burns on the face and full-thickness burns on the neck, entire anterior chest, and right arm. When assessing for heat inhalation, the nurse should first observe for:
1. Changes in the chest x-ray findings
2. Sputum that contains particles of blood
3. Nasal discharge containing carbon particles
4. Changes in the arterial blood gases consistent with acidosis

649. The nurse's physical assessment of a client with heart failure reveals tachypnea and bilateral crackles. The nurse should:
1. Initiate oxygen therapy
2. Assess for a pleural friction rub
3. Obtain a chest x-ray film immediately
4. Position the client in the Fowler's position

650. The best method to assess a client for stridor in the immediate postoperative period after a radical neck dissection is to:
1. Listen with a stethoscope over the trachea
2. Assess the client's ability to cough and deep breathe
3. Determine the client's ability to do neck exercises
4. Listen with a stethoscope over the base of the lungs

651. When discussing breathing exercises with a postoperative client, the nurse should include teaching the client to:
1. Take short frequent breaths
2. Exhale with the mouth open
3. Plan to do the exercises twice a day
4. Place a hand on the abdomen and feel it rise

652. A client is admitted to the intensive care unit with a diagnosis of acute respiratory distress syndrome. When assessing this client the nurse should expect to find:
1. Hypertension
2. Tenacious sputum
3. An altered mental status
4. A slowed rate of breathing

653. A client's respiratory status necessitates endotracheal intubation and positive pressure ventilation. The most immediate nursing intervention for this client at this time would be to:
1. Prepare the client for emergency surgery
2. Facilitate the client's verbal communication
3. Assess the client's response to the mechanical ventilation
4. Maintain sterility of the ventilation system the client is using

654. A client has been admitted to the emergency department with multiple injuries including fractured ribs. Because of the client's fractured ribs, the nurse should assess for signs of:
    1. Pneumonitis
    2. Hematemesis
    3. Pulmonary edema
    4. Respiratory acidosis

655. A client is placed on a ventilator. Because hyperventilation can occur when mechanical ventilation is used, the nurse should monitor the client for signs of:
    1. Hypoxia
    2. Hypercapnia
    3. Metabolic acidosis
    4. Respiratory alkalosis

656. A client is on a ventilator. One of the nurses asks what should be done when condensation resulting from humidity collects in the ventilator tubing. The best response to this question would be to:
    1. "Notify the respiratory therapist."
    2. "Empty the fluid from the tubing."
    3. "Decrease the amount of humidity."
    4. "Measure the fluid and record it on the I&O."

657. A 21-year-old male college student is admitted to the intensive care unit (ICU) after an accident in which he sustained multiple injuries. While the nurse is caring for this client, he coughs and his tracheostomy tube is expelled and falls onto the bed. The nurse should immediately:
    1. Hold the tracheostomy open with a tracheal dilator and call for assistance
    2. Insert an obturator into the tracheostomy and gently reinsert the tracheostomy tube
    3. Pick up the tracheostomy tube from his bed and replace it until a new tube is available
    4. Unwrap a new tracheostomy tube, prepare the new ties, and insert the tube using the obturator

658. After surgery in the inguinal area, the client complains of pain on the right side of the chest, becomes dyspneic, and begins to cough violently. The nurse suspects that a pulmonary embolus has occurred. The nurse immediately should:
    1. Auscultate the chest
    2. Obtain the vital signs
    3. Elevate the head of the bed
    4. Position the client on the right side

659. A client with a pulmonary embolus is intubated and placed on mechanical ventilation. When suctioning the endotracheal tube, the nurse should:
    1. Apply suction while inserting the catheter
    2. Hyperoxygenate with 100% oxygen before and after suctioning
    3. Use short, jabbing movements of the catheter to loosen secretions
    4. Suction two to three times in quick succession to remove all secretions

660. The respiratory status of a client with Guillain-Barré syndrome progressively deteriorates and a tracheostomy is performed. Nasogastric tube feedings are ordered. The nurse should:
    1. Deflate the tracheostomy cuff before starting tube feeding
    2. Inflate the tracheostomy cuff for one hour after each feeding
    3. Deflate the tracheostomy cuff after the tube feeding is completed
    4. Inflate the tracheostomy cuff before and for 30 minutes after each feeding

661. The nurse knows that when a client has a tracheostomy tube with a high-volume, low-pressure cuff, it is used primarily to prevent:
    1. Leakage of air
    2. Lung infection
    3. Mucosal necrosis
    4. Tracheal secretion

662. A 21-year-old aspiring actress is admitted for a rhinoplasty to improve her appearance and facilitate her breathing. When monitoring for hemorrhage after this surgery, the nurse should assess specifically for the presence of:
    1. Facial edema
    2. Excessive swallowing
    3. Pressure around the eyes
    4. Serosanguineous drainage on the dressing

663. A female college student who had a rhinoplasty is having the nasal packing removed several days after surgery. The nurse should recommend that the client:
    1. Avoid sneezing for 48 hours
    2. Brush her teeth after any intake
    3. Sleep on her back with one pillow
    4. Take food and fluids at a tepid temperature

664. A client with emphysema is short of breath and using accessory muscles of respiration. The nurse recognizes that the client's dyspnea is caused by:
    1. Spasm of the bronchi that traps the air

2. An increase in the vital capacity of the lungs
3. A too rapid expulsion of the air from the alveoli
4. Difficulty in expelling the air trapped in the alveoli

665. A client with an acute emphysemic episode is dyspneic and anxious. To decrease the dyspnea, the nurse's first action should be to:
1. Increase the oxygen to 6 L/min
2. Encourage rhythmical breathing
3. Check vital signs, including the BP
4. Have the client breathe into a brown bag

666. A client with a 10-year history of emphysema is admitted in acute respiratory distress. The nurse's assessment of this client will include observing for:
1. Pursed-lip breathing
2. Use of accessory muscles of respiration
3. Signs and symptoms of respiratory alkalosis
4. Prolonged inspiration with considerable effort

667. The client with chronic obstructive pulmonary disease (COPD) is predisposed to the development of CO_2 narcosis. Therefore, the nurse should:
1. Initiate pulmonary hygiene to clear air passages of trapped mucus
2. Encourage continuous rapid panting to promote respiratory exchange
3. Administer oxygen at a low concentration to maintain respiratory drive
4. Encourage slow, deep breathing with inhalation longer than exhalation to increase intake

668. A client with a history of emphysema is in acute respiratory failure with respiratory acidosis. Low level oxygen is administered by nasal cannula. Four hours later the nurse identifies that the client has increased restlessness and confusion followed by a decreased respiratory rate and lethargy. The nurse should:
1. Increase the oxygen by 2% increments
2. Question the client about the confusion
3. Percuss and vibrate the client's chest wall
4. Discontinue or decrease the oxygen flow rate

669. If a client undergoing peritoneal dialysis develops symptoms of severe respiratory difficulty during the infusion of the dialysate solution, the nurse should:
1. Slow the rate of the client's infusion
2. Place the client in a low Fowler's position
3. Auscultate the client's lungs for breath sounds
4. Drain the fluid from the client's peritoneal cavity

670. The nurse is aware that a client understands the instructions about an appropriate breathing technique for chronic obstructive pulmonary disease when the client:
1. Inhales through the mouth
2. Increases the respiratory rate
3. Holds each breath for a second at the end of inspiration
4. Progressively increases the length of the inspiratory phase

671. A client who is admitted with emphysema has a PCO_2 of 60. The nurse, noting this is excessively high, calls the physician to obtain an order for:
1. Mucolytics
2. Bronchodilators
3. Mechanical ventilation
4. Intermittent positive pressure breathing (IPPB)

672. The nurse is teaching a client diaphragmatic breathing. The client should be advised to:
1. Take rapid, deep breaths
2. Breathe with hands on the hips
3. Expand the abdomen on inhalation
4. Perform exercises in the orthopneic position

673. The statement by a male client with chronic obstructive pulmonary disease (COPD) that provides evidence that he is ready to quit smoking would be:
1. "I'll just finish this carton."
2. "I'll cut back to a half pack a day."
3. "I am quitting the only relaxation I have."
4. "I should find this easy because I don't drink when I smoke."

674. A client who has had emphysema for many years develops an enlarged liver. The nurse understands that this results from:
1. Liver hypoxia
2. Hepatic acidosis
3. Esophageal varices
4. Portal hypertension

675. When auscultating the chest of a client with chronic obstructive pulmonary disease, the nurse should usually expect to hear:
1. Diminished sounds
2. Crackles and gurgles
3. Expiratory wheezing
4. A pleural friction rub

676. A client with chronic obstructive pulmonary disease complains of a weight gain of 5 pounds in one week. The complication that may have precipitated this weight gain is:
1. Polycythemia
2. Cor pulmonale
3. Compensated acidosis
4. Left ventricular failure

677. A client with chronic obstructive pulmonary disease (COPD) complains of chest congestion especially in the morning. The nurse should suggest that the client:
1. Use a humidifier in the room
2. Sleep with two pillows at night
3. Cough even when it is nonproductive
4. Deep-breathe and cough before retiring

678. A client has chronic obstructive pulmonary disease (COPD) and cor pulmonale. When teaching about nutrition the nurse should instruct this client to:
1. Eat small meals six times a day to limit oxygen needs
2. Drink large amounts of fluid to help liquefy secretions
3. Lie down after eating to conserve energy needed for digestion
4. Increase the intake of protein to decrease intravascular hydrostatic pressure

679. A client with chronic obstructive pulmonary disease (COPD) is to use a nebulizer. The observation that indicates the nebulizer is being used incorrectly and additional teaching by the nurse is necessary would be that the client:
1. Positions the tip of the nebulizer beyond the lips
2. Holds the inspired breath for at least three seconds
3. Exhales slowly through the mouth with lips pursed slightly
4. Inhales with the lips tightly sealed around the mouthpiece

680. Assessment of a client with chronic obstructive pulmonary disease (COPD) reveals 32 shallow, labored respirations per minute with the involvement of accessory muscles of respiration. The client is lethargic and crackles and wheezes are heard on auscultation. Based on this assessment, the nurse should:
1. Encourage the client to take slow, deep breaths, and provide 5 L of oxygen via nasal cannula
2. Place the client in a side-lying position and perform chest physiotherapy using clapping and vibration

3. Place the client in a Fowler's position, suction the trachea, and administer 2 L of oxygen via nasal cannula
4. Suggest that the client assume a comfortable position, encourage rest, and then perform postural drainage exercises

681. A 70-year-old client with cancer of the right lung has a lobectomy. After surgery the client has a chest tube attached to suction. The observation that the nurse should report to the physician would be:
1. Clots in the tubing during the first 24 hours
2. Subcutaneous emphysema on the second day
3. Decreased bubbling in the water-seal chamber on the third day
4. Bloody fluid in the drainage-collection chamber in the first 24 hours

682. A 21-year-old client comes to the emergency department with the chief complaint of left-sided chest pain following a racquetball game. A chest x-ray examination reveals a left pneumothorax. When assessing the left side of the client's chest, the nurse would expect to find:
1. A dull sound on percussion
2. Vocal fremitus on palpation
3. Rales and rhonchi on auscultation
4. An absence of breath sounds on auscultation

683. A client with a pneumothorax asks, "Why did they put this tube into my chest?" The nurse should explain that the purpose of the chest tube is to:
1. Check for bleeding in the lung
2. Monitor the function of the lung
3. Drain fluid from the pleural space
4. Remove air from the pleural space

684. When evaluating the effectiveness of a chest tube inserted in a client with a pneumothorax, the nurse should assess for:
1. A productive cough
2. Return of breath sounds
3. Increased pleural drainage
4. Constant bubbling in the water-seal chamber

685. A client with extensive cancer of the upper right lobe of the lung has been informed that a lobectomy will be performed. The statement by the client that indicates adequate understanding of the intended surgery is:
1. "It shouldn't be that serious because the surgeon is going to use laser to destroy all the cells first."

2. "I really won't need this portion that they're cutting out, because I still have three parts on the left to help me breathe."

3. "I understand that several lung segments will be removed and that I'll have chest tubes in to help with drainage after surgery."

4. "I understand that the remaining lung tissue will fill in the empty space and that I'll have chest tubes in to help with drainage after surgery."

686. When inspecting a dressing following a partial pneumonectomy for cancer of the lung, the nurse observes some puffiness of the tissue around the area. When the area is palpated, the tissue feels spongy and crackles. When charting, the nurse should describe this assessment as:
1. Stridor
2. Crepitus
3. Pitting edema
4. Chest distention

687. On the first day following a right pneumonectomy a male client suddenly sits straight up in bed. His respirations are labored, and he is making a crowing sound. His skin is pale, cool, and moist. The nurse immediately should:
1. Notify the physician
2. Auscultate the left lung
3. Inspect the incision for bleeding
4. Check the chest tube for patency

688. A client in the post anesthesia care unit has just regained consciousness after a right pneumonectomy. The nurse should now:
1. Remove the airway
2. Assess the client for pain
3. Encourage deep breathing
4. Place the client on the left side

689. When turning a client following a right pneumonectomy, the nurse should plan to place the client in either the:
1. Right or left side-lying position
2. High Fowler's or supine position
3. Supine or right side-lying position
4. Left side-lying or low Fowler's position

690. The nurse should be vigilant for the unique complications associated with a pneumonectomy by observing the client for:
1. Signs of cardiac overload
2. Increased pulse and respirations
3. Cardiac irregularities with premature beats
4. Elevated BP, decreased temperature, and cold, moist skin

691. The most appropriate breathing and coughing routine for a client who has had a pneumonectomy would be every:
1. Hour for the first 24 hours and then every 2 hours
2. Two hours for the first 24 hours and then every 3 hours
3. Thirty minutes for the first 24 hours and then every 2 hours
4. Fifteen minutes for the first 24 hours and then every 2 hours

692. A client with oat cell lung cancer is scheduled for a mediastinoscopy and biopsy. The nurse should:
1. Tell the client that chest tubes will be present after the procedure
2. Explain that the procedure will visualize the lungs and the chest cavity
3. Advise the client of the NPO status after midnight the night before the test
4. Inform the client that some pleural fluid will be removed during the procedure

693. A client arrives in the emergency department and states, "I have a bad cold and chest pain that gets worse when I take a deep breath. In addition to obtaining the vital signs, the nurse auscultates the client's breath sounds. Where should the nurse place the stethoscope to determine the presence of a plural friction rub?

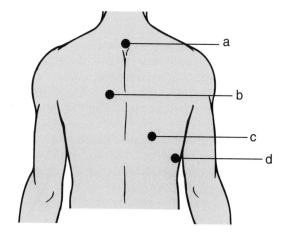

1. a
2. b
3. c
4. d

694. When assessing a client with pleural effusion, the nurse should expect to find:
    1. Moist crackles at the posterior of the lungs
    2. Reduced or absent breath sounds at the base of the lung
    3. Deviation of the trachea toward the involved side
    4. Increased resonance with percussion of the involved area

695. After a thoracentesis for pleural effusion a client returns to the physician's office for a follow-up visit. The nurse would suspect a recurrence of pleural effusion when the client says:
    1. "Lately I can only breathe well if I sit up."
    2. "During the night I sometimes have a fever and chills."
    3. "I get a sharp, stabbing pain when I take a deep breath."
    4. "I'm coughing up larger amounts of thicker mucus for the last two days."

696. A client with an exacerbation of a chronic inflammatory bowel disorder cannot tolerate food. A subclavian catheter is inserted. Immediately after insertion of the catheter, the priority nursing action would be to:
    1. Draw a blood sample to assess the blood glucose level
    2. Auscultate the client's lungs to evaluate breath sounds
    3. Obtain a chest x-ray to determine placement of the catheter
    4. Assess the arm and hand on the side of insertion for a motor or sensory deficit

697. A 40-year-old architect with a parotid tumor has been treated aggressively with radiotherapy and surgery. Postsurgical laboratory results indicate arterial blood gas values are pH 7.32; PCO$_2$ 53 mm Hg; HCO$_3$ 25 mEq. The action that should be taken by the nurse would be to:
    1. Have the client breathe into a rebreather bag at a slow rate
    2. Obtain a medical order for the administration of a diuretic
    3. Encourage the client to cough productively and take deep breaths
    4. Obtain a medical order for the administration of sodium bicarbonate

698. The nurse performs preoperative teaching related to a subtotal thyroidectomy. The nurse would know that the client understands the teaching about the local effects of a general anesthetic when the client states, "Immediately after surgery I will experience:
    1. Transient headaches."
    2. Feelings of chilliness."
    3. Paroxysmal hiccoughs."
    4. Discomfort swallowing."

699. After a gastroscopy the nurse should assess the client for the return of the gag reflex by:
    1. Touching the pharynx with a tongue depressor
    2. Observing for when the client spits the airway out
    3. Giving a small amount of water using a syringe
    4. Instructing the client to breathe deeply and cough gently

700. When caring for clients in the operating room, the nurse knows that the last physiologic function the client loses during the induction of an anesthetic is:
    1. Gag reflex
    2. Corneal reflex
    3. Consciousness
    4. Respiratory movement

701. When a client returns from a bronchoscopy, the nurse should withhold food and fluid for several hours to prevent:
    1. Aspiration
    2. Projectile vomiting
    3. Abdominal distention
    4. Dysphasia and dyspepsia

702. An 84-year-old client, with a history of hemoptysis and cough for the last six months, is suspected of having lung cancer. A bronchoscopy is performed. Two hours after the procedure the nurse notices an increase in the amount of bloody sputum. The nurse's first priority would be to:
    1. Notify the physician of the observation
    2. Continue to monitor the amount of sputum
    3. Monitor vital signs every hour for four hours
    4. Increase the client's coughing and deep breathing regimen

703. An older adult confined to bed in a nursing home develops bronchitis and atelectasis of the right lower lobe. When discussing the treatment regimen with the client, the nurse includes the need to:
    1. Lie on the affected side to relieve chest pain
    2. Lie on the unaffected side to promote drainage
    3. Sleep in the position of most comfort to promote rest

4. Sleep with the head elevated to stimulate deep breathing and coughing

704. A nursing diagnosis for a client with bronchial pneumonia is "Ineffective airway clearance related to retained secretions." Intervention to decrease retained secretions should include:
1. Administering oxygen as ordered
2. Gargling deeply with warm normal saline
3. Placing the client in a high Fowler's position
4. Increasing fluid intake to at least 2000 mL/day

705. After a laryngectomy a client becomes concerned about frequent coughing episodes and copious production of secretions. The nurse is aware that this increase of coughing and secretions is due to:
1. An upper respiratory infection caused by allergies
2. Inadequate turning, coughing, and deep breathing
3. An irritation of the stoma by the tracheostomy tube
4. The mucous membranes' reaction to unwarmed, dry air

706. An important nursing intervention that ensures adequate ventilatory exchange after surgery would be to:
1. Maintain humidified oxygen via nasal cannula
2. Position the client laterally with the neck extended
3. Assess for hypoventilation by auscultating the lungs
4. Remove the airway only when the client is fully conscious

707. During the immediate postoperative period after a laryngectomy, a nursing priority for the client should be to:
1. Provide emotional support
2. Observe for signs of infection
3. Keep the trachea free of secretions
4. Promote a means of communication

708. After surgery, the physician orders an incentive spirometer for a client. The nurse would know that the client was using the spirometer correctly when observing that the client:
1. Uses the incentive spirometer for 10 consecutive breaths an hour
2. Coughs twice before inhaling deeply through the mouthpiece
3. Inhales deeply, seals the lips around the mouthpiece, and exhales

4. Inhales deeply through the mouthpiece, holds the breath for two seconds, and then exhales

709. A 60-year-old male is returned to the surgical unit after a laryngoscopy. The nurse reminds the client not to take anything by mouth until instructed to do so. This nursing intervention generally would be considered:
1. Appropriate because these clients usually experience painful swallowing for several days
2. Appropriate because early drinking or eating after the client's laryngoscopy may result in aspiration
3. Inappropriate because the client is not unconscious and may be thirsty after being NPO
4. Inappropriate because the client is likely to be anxious and probably will not be aware of feeling thirsty

710. A total laryngectomy and radical neck dissection is scheduled for a client with cancer of the larynx. When reinforcing the physician's statements to the client, the nurse should review what the surgery entails and what abilities will be lost. The discussion also should focus on what abilities will be retained, such as the ability to:
1. Blow the nose
2. Sip through a straw
3. Chew and swallow food
4. Smell and differentiate odors

711. A client who has had a radical neck resection returns from surgery with two portable wound drainage systems at the operative site. Inspection of the neck incision reveals moderate edema of the tissues. Because of this problem, the nurse should assess the client for:
1. Loss of the gag reflex
2. Cloudy wound drainage
3. Restlessness and dyspnea
4. Dehiscence of the suture line

712. The physician orders a progressive diet as tolerated for a client who had head and neck surgery. The nurse should:
1. Keep suction apparatus readily available in case aspiration occurs
2. Administer the diet through a nasogastric tube until the suture line heals
3. Encourage the intake of pureed foods because they promote the swallowing reflex
4. Administer the prescribed pain medication 30 minutes before meals to limit discomfort

713. The nurse expects that the initial treatment for a client who has a leak of the thoracic duct following radical neck surgery would include inserting a:
1. Gastrostomy tube to drain the fluid, a high-fat diet, and bed rest
2. Rectal tube to prevent distention, a low-fat diet, and increased activity
3. Chest tube to drain the fluid, total parenteral nutrition, and bed rest
4. Nasogastric tube to drain the fluid, a moderate-fat diet, and increased activity

714. A 79-year-old pipe smoker is diagnosed as having cancer of the tongue. A hemiglossectomy and right radical neck dissection is performed. After surgery, the client is transferred to the post anesthesia care unit. When providing for a patent airway a primary nursing intervention should be to:
1. Suction frequently
2. Apply an ice collar
3. Maintain a high Fowler's position
4. Encourage coughing and expectoration

715. A half hour after awakening from anesthesia in the post anesthesia care unit (PACU) a 75-year-old client who has had radical head and neck surgery becomes agitated, disoriented, and confused. The nurse should:
1. Notify the physician immediately
2. Record the observations on the progress notes
3. Administer the prescribed oxygen by nasal cannula
4. Medicate the client with alprazolam (Xanax) as ordered

716. A client who has had a hemiglossectomy and right radical neck dissection arrives in the post anesthesia care unit with two portable drainage catheters in the area of the incision, which are attached to Hemovacs. Six hours later one Hemovac accumulates 180 mL of serosanguineous drainage. The priority nursing intervention should be to:
1. Turn the client on the right side
2. Chart the output as it is expected
3. Notify the physician immediately
4. Empty the container and reestablish negative pressure

717. A client is scheduled for coronary artery bypass surgery. The nurse explains to the client that chest tubes will be inserted during surgery to:
1. Prevent atelectasis postoperatively
2. Drain fluid from the pericardial sac

3. Reestablish negative intrapleural pressure
4. Monitor the amount of blood loss after surgery

718. When giving a client care on the second day after coronary artery bypass surgery, the nurse notes that the fluid in the water-seal chamber of the drainage device (Pleur-evac) stops fluctuating. The nurse should:
1. Increase the amount of suction
2. Add sterile water to the chamber
3. Look for obstructions of the tube
4. Consider this a normal occurrence

719. The nurse is instructed to measure and document the amount of drainage from a client's chest tube. The nurse should:
1. Aspirate fluid from the drainage collection chamber of the closed chest drainage system with a needle and syringe and measure the drainage
2. Connect a new closed chest drainage system, measure the fluid in the drainage collection chamber of the old system, and discard the old system
3. Mark the time and fluid level on the outside of the drainage collection chamber of the closed chest drainage system
4. Clamp the chest tube, empty the fluid from the drainage collection chamber of the closed chest drainage system into a measuring cup, and reconnect the system

720. A client who has had thoracic surgery has a chest tube connected to a water-seal drainage system attached to suction. When excessive bubbling is identified in the water-seal chamber, the nurse should:
1. Check the system for air leaks
2. "Strip" the chest tube catheter
3. Decrease the amount of suction pressure
4. Recognize that the system is functioning correctly

721. The nurse recognizes that a client who has had thoracic surgery needs further teaching when the client performs post-thoracotomy exercises by:
1. Extending the arm up and back and out to the side and back
2. Climbing a wall with the fingers until the arm is fully extended
3. Tying a rope to a doorknob and swinging the arm in wide circles
4. Extending the arm out and bringing it up to touch the nose with a finger

722. The nurse in the emergency department has been notified that a person, who has sustained a gunshot wound to the right side of the chest, would arrive soon. The nurse should plan to:
1. Reserve an operating room
2. Prepare equipment for a tracheostomy
3. Arrange for a portable x-ray examination
4. Obtain equipment for chest tube insertion

723. A chest tube is inserted after a crushing chest injury. The observation that indicates a desired response to treatment of the client's chest injury would be:
1. Increased breath sounds
2. Increased respiratory rate
3. Crepitus detected on palpation of the chest
4. Constant bubbling in the drainage collection chamber

724. On the way to an x-ray examination a client with a chest tube becomes confused and pulls the chest tube out. The nurse's immediate action should be to:
1. Place the client in the Trendelenburg position
2. Hold the insertion site open with a Kelly clamp
3. Obtain sterile Vaseline gauze to cover the opening
4. Cover the opening with the cleanest material available

725. A client has a chest tube for a pneumothorax. The nurse finds the client in respiratory difficulty with the chest tube separated from the drainage system. The nurse should:
1. Obtain a new sterile drainage system
2. Clamp the drainage tubing with two clamps
3. Reconnect the client's tube to the drainage system
4. Place the client in the high-Fowler's position immediately

726. To promote continued improvement in a client's respiratory status after a chest tube is removed, the nurse should:
1. Continue observing for dyspnea and crepitus
2. Encourage frequent coughing and deep breathing
3. Remind the client to turn from side to side at least every two hours
4. Encourage bed rest with active and passive range-of-motion exercises

727. A 60-year-old widow, who has had a myocardial infarction, lives with her drug-addicted daughter and her young child. The client confides to the home health care nurse that she receives no help from her daughter and they survive on her social security. She tells the nurse that her daughter coughs a great deal, does a lot of sleeping, and sometimes spits up blood. The nurse should pursue information about the daughter's condition for potential case finding because:
1. Death from tuberculosis has been generally on the increase
2. Children under the age of 14 are very susceptible to tuberculosis
3. The incidence of tuberculosis has dramatically decreased recently
4. Older adults with chronic illness are most adversely affected by tuberculosis

728. During a routine physical examination, a client's chest x-ray film reveals a lesion in the right upper lobe. When the nurse obtains a history from the client, the information that supports the physician's tentative diagnosis of pulmonary tuberculosis would be:
1. Frothy sputum and fever
2. Dry cough and pulmonary congestion
3. Night sweats and blood-tinged sputum
4. Productive cough and engorged neck veins

729. The nurse notes 12 mm of induration at the site of a Mantoux test when a client returns to the health office to have it read. The nurse should explain to the client that this:
1. Test result is negative, and no follow-up is needed
2. Test was used for screening and a tine test will now be given
3. Skin test is inconclusive and will have to be repeated in six weeks
4. Result indicates a need for further tests, including a chest x-ray film examination

730. To make a definitive diagnosis of tuberculosis, the nurse understands that the physician must order a:
1. Chest x-ray film
2. Tuberculin skin test
3. Pulmonary function test
4. Sputum for acid-fast testing

731. A client with pulmonary tuberculosis is being treated at home. To help control the spread of the disease, the client should be instructed to:
1. Have visitors sit at least 8 feet away
2. Keep personal articles away from the rest of the family
3. Open the windows slightly to allow air to circulate throughout the house
4. Avoid putting used dishes in the dishwasher with the rest of the family's dishes

732. A client's purified protein derivative (PPD) test and chest x-ray film results indicate pulmonary tuberculosis. The physician orders sputum specimens for acid-fast bacilli. The nurse knows that additional teaching is necessary when the client states that the sputum specimens must be:
    1. Coughed up from deep in the lungs
    2. Collected in the early morning hours
    3. Refrigerated until brought to the laboratory
    4. Brought to the clinic as soon as possible after collection

733. When teaching a client with tuberculosis about recovery after discharge from the hospital, the nurse should reinforce that the treatment measure with the highest priority is:
    1. Having sufficient rest
    2. Getting plenty of fresh air
    3. Changing the current lifestyle
    4. Consistently taking prescribed medication

734. A client with tuberculosis asks the nurse how long the chemotherapy must be continued. The nurse's most accurate reply would be:
    1. "1 to 2 weeks."
    2. "4 to 5 months."
    3. "At least 6 to 12 months."
    4. "Probably 3 years or longer."

REPRODUCTIVE AND GENITOURINARY (RG)

735. A client is scheduled for an intravenous pyelogram (IVP). The nurse explains that on the day before the IVP the client must:
    1. Eat a fat-free dinner
    2. Drink a large amount of fluids
    3. Omit dinner and limit beverages
    4. Take a laxative before going to bed

736. A 52-year-old woman is injured in a vehicular accident and is admitted for observation. Damage to her bladder is evident. The history that would indicate an increased risk of bladder rupture would be:
    1. Multiple bouts of cystitis
    2. Familial history of bladder cancer
    3. Failure to have voided before starting the trip
    4. Drinking two cups of coffee before the accident

737. A client has surgery to repair a bladder laceration. The routine nursing intervention that takes priority in postoperative care would be:
    1. Turning and positioning
    2. Range-of-motion exercises
    3. Lower back care three times daily
    4. Placing side rails in the up position

738. To facilitate micturition in a male client, the nurse should instruct him to:
    1. Use a urinal for voiding
    2. Drink cranberry juice daily
    3. Wash his hands after voiding
    4. Assume the normal position for voiding

739. The nurse instructs a client with a history of frequent urinary tract infections to drink cranberry juice to:
    1. Decrease the urinary pH
    2. Exert a bactericidal effect
    3. Improve glomerular filtration
    4. Relieve the symptom of dysuria

740. To help prevent a cycle of recurring urinary tract infections, the nurse should plan to instruct a female client to:
    1. Increase the daily intake of citrus juice
    2. Douche frequently with alkaline agents
    3. Urinate as soon as possible after intercourse
    4. Cleanse from the vaginal orifice to the urethra

741. A client complains of urinary problems. Cholinergic medications are prescribed. The nurse is aware that this type of medication is prescribed to prevent:
    1. Kidney stones
    2. A flaccid bladder
    3. A spastic bladder
    4. Urinary tract infections

742. Twenty-four hours after a penile implant the client's scrotum is edematous and painful. The nurse should:
    1. Assist the client with a sitz bath
    2. Apply warm soaks to the scrotum
    3. Elevate the scrotum using a soft support
    4. Prepare for a possible incision and drainage

743. A male client comes to the emergency room because he has a discharge from his penis. The physician suspects gonorrhea and asks the nurse to obtain a specimen and to send it for a culture. The nurse should:
    1. Instruct the client to provide a semen specimen
    2. Swab the discharge as it appears on the prepuce
    3. Obtain a specimen of the drainage from the anterior urethra
    4. Teach the client how to obtain a clean catch specimen of urine

744. A client comes to the infectious disease clinic because a sexual partner was recently diagnosed as having gonorrhea. The health history reveals that the client has engaged in receptive anal intercourse. The nurse should assess the client for:

1. Melena
2. Anal itching
3. Constipation
4. Ribbon-shaped stools

745. The nurse should ask the client with secondary syphilis about sexual contacts during the past:
1. 21 days
2. 30 days
3. 3 months
4. 6 months

746. A client is suspected of having late-stage (tertiary) syphilis. When obtaining a health history, the nurse recognizes that the statement by the client that would most support this diagnosis would be:
1. "I noticed a wart on my penis."
2. "I have sores all over my mouth."
3. "I've been losing a lot of hair lately."
4. "I'm having trouble keeping my balance."

747. A male client, age 56, is being worked up for possible cancer of the urinary bladder. Of the client's symptoms, the one that is most significant for cancer of the urinary tract is:
1. Dysuria
2. Retention
3. Hesitancy
4. Hematuria

748. A 64-year-old client has been diagnosed as having cancer of the bladder and is scheduled for a total cystectomy and the formation of an ileal conduit. When assessing the client eight hours after surgery, the nurse notes all of the following findings. The finding that should be promptly reported to the physician would be:
1. An edematous stoma
2. A dusky-colored stoma
3. Pink-tinged urinary drainage
4. The absence of bowel sounds

749. On the fourth postoperative day after a cystectomy and the formation of a continent diversion, the nurse notes mucus threads in a client's urine. The nurse should:
1. Send a specimen for culture and sensitivity
2. Report this to physician when making rounds
3. Increase the client's oral intake for the next 12 hours
4. Recognize this assessment as a normal occurrence

750. A client with an ileal conduit is being prepared for discharge. Before discharge the nurse should instruct the client to:
1. Abstain from beer and alcohol consumption
2. Maintain a daily fluid intake of at least 2000 mL
3. Notify the physician if the stoma size decreases
4. Avoid getting soap and water on the peristomal skin

751. A 45-year-old client develops acute glomerulonephritis following a streptococcal infection. When performing the health assessment the nurse would expect the client to report a history of:
1. Nocturia
2. Mild headache
3. A recent weight loss
4. An increased appetite

752. A client with acute glomerulonephritis complains of thirst. The nurse should offer:
1. Ginger ale
2. Hard candy
3. A milk shake
4. A cup of broth

753. To prevent future attacks of glomerulonephritis, the nurse planning discharge teaching should include instructions for the client to:
1. Take showers instead of bubble baths
2. Avoid situations that involve physical activity
3. Seek early treatment for respiratory infections
4. Continue the same restrictions on fluid intake

754. The nurse is aware that the most serious complication for a client with acute renal failure is:
1. Anemia
2. Infection
3. Weight loss
4. Platelet dysfunction

755. A male client with chronic renal failure is admitted because of a severe infection and anemia. The client is depressed and lethargic. The client's wife approaches the nurse and asks about the therapy and nursing care. The nurse explains the rationale of the client's treatment by stating:
1. "The staff must provide total care for your husband, because the infection makes him so fatigued."
2. "Your husband is irritable and depressed, so the physician may prescribe mood elevators to make him feel better."
3. "You may notice your husband's stools are dark because of all the iron he is receiving, but it is helping him overcome the anemia."
4. "The physician has restricted your husband's intake of meat, eggs, and cheese, so that his kidneys can clear the body of waste products."

756. The nurse is aware that the factor in a client's history that may have contributed to a present problem of renal calculi would be:
1. A high-cholesterol diet
2. Excess ingestion of antacids
3. An excessive exercise program
4. Frequent consumption of alcohol

757. When a client with ureteral colic voids, it may be characterized by:
1. Urgency and pain
2. Hematuria with sharp pain
3. A foul odor and dark urine
4. Frequency with small amounts of urine

758. When planning care for a client with ureteral colic, the nurse's goal should be based on the knowledge that most factors contributing to the development of renal stones can be overcome by:
1. Decreasing serum creatinine
2. Drinking 8 to 10 glasses of water daily
3. Excluding milk products from the diet
4. Excreting 2000 mL of urine per 24 hours

759. A male client is diagnosed as having phosphatic calculi. The nurse should teach the client that his diet may include:
1. Apples
2. Rye bread
3. Chocolate
4. Cheddar cheese

760. When taking the admitting history of a client with a left ureteral calculus who is scheduled for a transurethral ureterolithotomy, the nurse would expect the client to report:
1. A boring pain in the left flank
2. Pain that intensifies on urination
3. Spasmodic pain on the left side radiating to the suprapubis
4. Pain that is dull and constant in the costovertebral angle

761. The laboratory values of a client with renal calculi reveal a serum calcium within normal limits and an elevated serum purine. The nurse should recognize that the stone is probably composed of:
1. Cystine
2. Struvite
3. Oxalate
4. Uric acid

762. A client is transferred to the post anesthesia care unit after undergoing a pyelolithotomy. The client's urinary output is 50 mL/hr. The nurse should:
1. Chart the findings
2. Encourage oral fluids
3. Milk the nephrostomy tube
4. Notify the physician immediately

763. The most essential nursing care for a client with a nephrostomy tube would be to:
1. Ensure free drainage of urine
2. Milk the tube every two hours
3. Keep an accurate record of intake and output
4. Instill 2 mL of normal saline every eight hours

764. A female client is admitted to the hospital with severe renal colic caused by a ureteral calculus. Later that evening, the client's urinary output is much less than her intake. When it is noted that her bladder is not distended, the nurse should suspect the development of:
1. Oliguria
2. Hydroureter
3. Renal shutdown
4. Urethral obstruction

765. An obese client with calculi in the calyxes of the right kidney is admitted for their removal. The nurse prepares the client for the procedure by explaining that:
1. The right ureter will be removed
2. A suprapubic catheter will be in place
3. Surgery will be performed transurethrally
4. A small incision will be present in the right flank area

766. A male client who has had recurring renal calculi has a ureterolithotomy. Before discharge the nurse discusses the need to avoid urinary tract infections. The nurse knows that the signs of infection are understood when the client says he will report:
1. Urgency or frequency of urination
2. The inability to maintain an erection
3. Pain radiating to the external genitalia
4. An increase in alkalinity or acidity of urine

767. The nurse is aware that the person at highest risk of developing prostate cancer would be a:
1. 55-year-old Black male
2. 55-year-old Asian male
3. 45-year-old Hispanic male
4. 45-year-old Caucasian male

768. The nurse assesses a newly admitted client with kidney disease to determine symptoms

that may be present. A subjective symptom that the nurse should assess for is:
1. Uremia
2. Vomiting
3. Voiding at night
4. Flank discomfort

769. A 72-year-old male complaining of dysuria, nocturia, and difficulty starting the urinary stream is scheduled for a cystoscopy and biopsy of the prostate gland. After the procedure the client complains that he is unable to void. The nurse should:
1. Limit oral fluids until he voids
2. Assure him that this is expected
3. Insert a urinary retention catheter
4. Palpate above the pubic symphysis

770. When admitting a client with benign prostatic hyperplasia, the most relevant assessment would be:
1. Perineal edema
2. Urethral discharge
3. Flank pain radiating to the groin
4. Distention of the lower abdomen

771. A client is scheduled for a transurethral prostatectomy (TURP). He is concerned about the operation's effect on his sexual ability. The nurse should reply that he may:
1. Experience retrograde ejaculations
2. Have prolonged erections afterward
3. Be permanently impotent after the operation
4. Develop a decrease in libido after the surgery

772. A client who has had a transurethral prostatectomy (TURP) experiences dribbling after the indwelling catheter is removed. To alleviate this problem, the nurse should state:
1. "I know you are worried, but it will go away in a few days."
2. "Increase your fluid intake and urinate at regular intervals."
3. "Limit your fluid intake and urinate when you first feel the urge."
4. "The catheter will have to be reinserted until your bladder regains its tone."

773. After a transurethral resection of the prostate, the client's retention catheter is secured to his leg, causing slight traction of the inflatable balloon against the prostatic fossa. This is done to:
1. Limit discomfort
2. Provide hemostasis
3. Reduce bladder spasms
4. Promote urinary drainage

774. When planning care for a client with a continuous bladder irrigation after a transurethral vaporization of the prostate the nurse should:
1. Measure the output hourly
2. Monitor the specific gravity of the urine
3. Irrigate the catheter with saline three times daily
4. Exclude the amount of irrigant instilled from the output

775. After a transurethral vaporization of the prostate, the client complains that he needs to void. The nurse should first:
1. Assess the client's total intake and output for the day
2. Obtain the client's vital signs and notify the physician
3. Explain that the balloon inflated in the bladder causes this feeling
4. Check the tubing connected to the collection bag to see whether it is draining

776. The nurse would know that a client who has had a transurethral vaporization of the prostate understood his discharge teaching when he says, "I should:
1. Get out of bed into a chair for several hours daily."
2. Attempt to void every three hours when I'm awake."
3. Call the physician if my urinary stream decreases."
4. Avoid vigorous exercise for six months after surgery."

777. In the early postoperative period after a transurethral resection of the prostate, the most common complication the nurse should observe for would be:
1. Sepsis
2. Hemorrhage
3. Leakage around the catheter
4. Urinary retention with overflow

778. A 75-year-old male with a history of cancer of the prostate is admitted for a prostatectomy. The client's prostate specific antigen levels have become increasingly elevated. This finding should prompt the nurse to plan to:
1. Institute seizure precautions
2. Measure his intake and output
3. Monitor his plasma pH for acidosis
4. Handle him gently when turning him

779. A client, who had a transurethral prostatectomy, complains of painful bladder spasms. To limit these spasms the nurse should:
    1. Administer the ordered opiate every four hours
    2. Irrigate the indwelling catheter with 60 mL of isotonic solution
    3. Advance the catheter to relieve the pressure against the prostatic fossa
    4. Encourage the client to avoid contracting his muscles as if he were voiding

780. After prostate surgery a client's indwelling catheter and continuous bladder irrigation (CBI) are to be removed, and the nurse discusses the procedure with the client. The nurse recognizes that the teaching has been understood when the client states, "After the catheter is removed I probably will:
    1. Have dilute urine."
    2. Exhibit dark red urine."
    3. Be unable to pass my urine."
    4. Experience some burning on urination."

781. A client, who had a suprapubic prostatectomy for cancer of the prostate, returns to the post anesthesia care unit with a continuous bladder irrigation. The nurse realizes that the purpose of this irrigation is to:
    1. Promote continuous formation of urine
    2. Prevent the formation of clots in the bladder
    3. Facilitate the measurement of urinary output
    4. Provide continuous pressure on the prostatic fossa

782. After a suprapubic prostatectomy, the nurse understands that a client's plan of care must include the prevention of postoperative deep vein thrombosis. This can best be achieved by increasing the:
    1. Coagulability of the blood
    2. Velocity of the venous return
    3. Effectiveness of internal respiration
    4. Oxygen-carrying capacity of the blood

783. The nurse is aware that an early adaptation of clients with renal carcinoma would be:
    1. Flank pain
    2. Weight gain
    3. Periorbital edema
    4. Intermittent hematuria

784. An acute, life-threatening complication for which the nurse should assess a client in the early postoperative period after a radical nephrectomy for cancer of the kidney would be:
    1. Sepsis
    2. Hemorrhage
    3. Renal failure
    4. Paralytic ileus

785. The nurse's postoperative plan of care for a client who has had a radical nephrectomy should include:
    1. Giving the client a regular diet on the first postoperative day
    2. Clamping the nephrostomy tube when the client is out of bed
    3. Leaving the client's original dressing in place for at least the first 48 hours
    4. Turning the client from the back to the operated side every two to three hours

786. The nurse plans to teach a client who has been receiving hemodialysis for several months to be alert for signs of gastrointestinal bleeding. Bleeding into the GI tract is of particular significance to a client with chronic renal failure because:
    1. Hypovolemia can compromise renal function
    2. Blood is digested and increases the protein load
    3. Clotting problems make diagnosis of the bleeding site difficult
    4. The client in renal failure will not manifest the usual signs of blood loss

787. A client with chronic renal failure is on a restricted protein diet and is taught about high-biologic-value protein foods. An understanding of the rationale for this diet is demonstrated when the client states that high-biologic-value protein foods are:
    1. Needed to promote weight gain
    2. Necessary to prevent muscle wasting
    3. Used to increase urea blood products
    4. Responsible for controlling hypertension

788. The nurse would be aware that a client with chronic renal failure recognizes an adequate source of high-biologic-value protein when the food the client selected from the menu was:
    1. Apple juice
    2. Raw carrots
    3. Cottage cheese
    4. Whole wheat bread

789. The home health care nurse visits a 40-year-old housewife who has been placed on hemodialysis. When reviewing the diet with the client, the nurse encourages her to include:
    1. Rice
    2. Potatoes

3. Baked salmon
4. Barbecued beef

790. A male client with a history of chronic renal failure is hospitalized. The nurse assesses the client for signs of related renal insufficiency, which include:
1. Facial flushing
2. Edema and pruritus
3. Dribbling after voiding
4. Diminished force and caliber of stream

791. A client with uremic syndrome has the potential to develop many complications. The complication that the nurse should anticipate in such a client is:
1. Hypotension
2. Hypokalemia
3. Flapping hand tremors
4. An elevated hematocrit value

792. A young woman is admitted to the hospital in the oliguric phase of acute renal failure. The client estimates that the urine output for the last 12 hours to be less than 1 cup. The nurse realizes that the rationale for an order of 900 mL of water orally over the next 24 hours is that this amount of fluid will:
1. Equal the expected urinary output for the next 24 hours
2. Prevent the development of complicating hypostatic pneumonia
3. Prevent hyperkalemia, which could lead to serious cardiac dysrhythmias
4. Compensate for both insensible and expected urinary output over the next 24 hours

793. The nurse notes that the latest potassium level for a client in renal failure is 6.2 mEq. The first action by the nurse should be to:
1. Alert the cardiac arrest team
2. Call the laboratory and repeat the test
3. Take the vital signs and notify the physician
4. Obtain an ECG strip and have lidocaine available

794. While the nurse is at the bedside of a client in acute renal failure, the client states, "My doctor said that I will be getting some insulin. Do I also have diabetes?" The response that best demonstrates an understanding of the use of insulin in acute renal failure would be:
1. "No, the insulin will help your body handle a chemical called potassium."
2. "Why don't you ask that question when the doctor comes to see you today."

3. "You probably had an elevated blood sugar level, so your doctor is being cautious."
4. "No, but insulin will reduce the toxins in your blood by lowering your metabolic rate."

795. When teaching a client who has just started peritoneal dialysis about the procedure, the home health care nurse should inform the client that if drainage of dialysate from the peritoneal cavity ceases before the required amount has drained out, the client should:
1. Drink 8 oz of water
2. Turn from side to side
3. Deep-breathe and cough
4. Periodically rotate the catheter

796. The nurse teaches a client receiving peritoneal dialysis that the reason the dialysis solution is warmed to body temperature before it is instilled into the peritoneal cavity is to:
1. Force potassium back into the cells, thereby decreasing serum levels
2. Add extra warmth to the body because metabolic processes are disturbed
3. Help prevent cardiac dysrhythmias speeding up removal of excess serum potassium
4. Encourage removal of serum urea by preventing constriction of peritoneal blood vessels

797. A client with acute renal failure moves into the diuretic phase after one week of therapy. During this phase the client must be assessed for signs of developing:
1. Renal failure
2. Hypovolemia
3. Hyperkalemia
4. Metabolic acidosis

798. Diet instruction for a client who is being treated with continuous ambulatory peritoneal dialysis (CAPD) for chronic glomerulonephritis should include the need for:
1. Low-calorie foods
2. High-quality protein
3. Increased fluid intake
4. Foods rich in potassium

799. A client with chronic renal failure is to begin continuous peritoneal dialysis (CAPD). When assessing the client before the institution of CAPD, the nurse should be alert for the presence of:
1. Cardiac problems
2. Emotional lability
3. Client motivation
4. Pulmonary problems

800. When caring for a client on peritoneal dialysis, the nurse should:
1. Place the client in the side-lying position
2. Slightly warm the solution before instilling
3. Infuse the dialysate solution over two hours
4. Withhold medication until all solution is administered

801. If a client on peritoneal dialysis develops symptoms of severe respiratory difficulty during the infusion of the dialysate solution, the nurse should:
1. Slow the rate of infusion
2. Auscultate the lungs for breath sounds
3. Drain the fluid from the peritoneal cavity
4. Place the client in a low-Fowler's position

802. A client with end-stage renal disease is receiving continuous ambulatory peritoneal dialysis. The nurse is preparing to teach the client to monitor for signs of complications associated with peritoneal dialysis. Check all the complications that should be included in this teaching plan.
1. _____ Pruritus
2. _____ Oliguria
3. _____ Tachycardia
4. _____ Cloudy outflow
5. _____ Abdominal pain

803. Hemodialysis is planned for a client who has renal failure. The client is scheduled for the creation of an internal arteriovenous fistula and the placement of an external arteriovenous shunt to be used until the fistula heals. The nurse should keep in mind that:
1. Blood pressure readings will be higher in the arm with the fistula than in the arm with the shunt
2. The shunt is more subject to the complications of hemorrhage, clotting, and infection than the fistula
3. IV fluids should not be infused in the arm with the shunt, but they are permitted in the arm with the fistula
4. A light surgical dressing can be applied over the fistula incision, but the shunt should be thoroughly covered with a heavier dressing

804. A client has end-stage renal disease and is on hemodialysis. During dialysis, the client complains of nausea and a headache and appears confused. Operating on standing protocols, the nurse should:
1. Administer an antiemetic
2. Attempt to reorient the client
3. Decrease the rate of exchange
4. Monitor for changes in vital signs

805. A 62-year-old woman, who has been on hemodialysis for one year, asks the nurse what substances are being removed by the dialysis. The nurse identifies that one of the substances passing through the membrane would be:
1. RBCs
2. Sodium
3. Glucose
4. Bacteria

806. A client with chronic renal failure is accepted for a kidney transplant and attends a group educational program for potential transplant candidates. The client asks the nurse which kidney will be removed. The nurse's best response would be:
1. "Neither of your kidneys will be removed unless they are infected."
2. "It is up to the surgeon as to which kidney is replaced with the new one."
3. "The kidney that is the most diseased is removed and replaced with the new one."
4. "Your right kidney will be removed because it has a longer renal vein, making transplant easier."

807. A client has end-stage renal disease and is admitted for a kidney transplant. The nurse is aware that the donor must:
1. Have the same blood type
2. Be a member of the same family
3. Be approximately the same body size
4. Have matching leukocyte antigen complexes

808. When a client returns from the post anesthesia care unit after a kidney transplant, the nurse should plan to measure the client's urinary output every:
1. 1 hour
2. 2 hours
3. 3 hours
4. 15 minutes

809. After a successful kidney transplant for a client with end-stage renal disease, the nurse should anticipate that laboratory studies will demonstrate:
1. An increased specific gravity
2. A correction of hypotension
3. An elevated serum potassium
4. A decreasing serum creatinine

810. A client with a transplanted kidney is taught the signs of rejection. The nurse would know that the teaching was effective when the client says that a sign of rejection would be:
1. Weight loss
2. A subnormal temperature

3. An elevated blood pressure

4. An increased urinary output

811. A client who has had a kidney transplant develops leukopenia three weeks after surgery. The nurse should be aware that the leukopenia is probably caused by:
1. A bacterial infection
2. High creatinine levels
3. Rejection of the kidney
4. The antirejection medications

SKELETAL (SK)

812. The nurse recognizes that stimulation of calcium deposition in the bone after a distal femoral fracture is best achieved by:
1. Resting the extremity
2. Weight-bearing activity
3. The normal aging process
4. Ingesting foods high in calcium

813. A male college basketball player comes to the infirmary complaining of a "click" in his knee when walking. He states that it occasionally gives way when he is running and sometimes locks. He does not recall any specific injury. The nurse suspects that he may have:
1. Cracked the patella
2. A ruptured Achilles tendon
3. Injured the cartilage in the knee
4. A stress fracture of the tibial plateau

814. A client is scheduled for arthroscopic knee surgery and asks the nurse about the procedure. The statement by the nurse that best describes the procedure would be:
1. "You will be anesthetized and not remember anything about the procedure."
2. "It is surgical repair of a joint under direct visualization using an arthroscope."
3. "The procedure will determine the type of treatments the physician will prescribe."
4. "It is a radiologic procedure that will help diagnose the extent of the knee injury."

815. A client with cancer is scheduled for a bone scan to determine the presence of metastases. The nurse is aware that teaching prior to a scheduled bone scan was effective when the client states that:
1. "X-rays will be taken to identify where I may have lost calcium from my bones."
2. "A portion of my bone marrow will be removed and examined for cell composition."
3. "A radioactive chemical will be injected into my vein that will destroy cancer cells present in my bones."
4. "A substance of low radioactivity will be injected into my vein, and my body inspected by an instrument to detect where it is deposited."

816. Clients who have casts applied to an extremity must be monitored for complications. The most significant complication that the nurse should assess the extremity for is:
1. Warmth
2. Numbness
3. Skin desquamation
4. Generalized discomfort

817. After an open reduction and cast application for a compound fracture of the right ulna and radius as the result of a fall, the nurse should instruct the client to notify the physician immediately if there is:
1. Slight stiffness of the fingers
2. Increasing pain at the injury site
3. A small amount of bloody drainage on the cast
4. A bounding radial pulse in the affected extremity

818. A client's right tibia is fractured in an automobile accident, and a cast is applied. To assess for damage to major blood vessels from the fractured tibia, the nurse should monitor the client for:
1. Swelling of the right thigh
2. An increased blood pressure
3. Increased skin temperature of the foot
4. Prolonged reperfusion of the toes after blanching

819. Three days after a cast is applied to a client's fractured tibia, the client reports that there is a burning pain over the ankle. The cast over the ankle feels warm to the touch, and the pain is not relieved when the client changes position. The nurse's priority action should be to:
1. Obtain an order for an antibiotic
2. Explain that it is a typical response to a cast
3. Report the client's complaint to the physician
4. Administer the prescribed medication for pain

820. After a long leg cast is removed, the client should be instructed to:
1. Report any discomfort or stiffness of the ankle
2. Cleanse the leg by scrubbing with a brisk motion
3. Elevate the leg when sitting for long periods of time
4. Put the leg through a full range of motion once daily

821. The nurse performs full range of motion on a client's extremities. When putting an ankle through range of motion the nurse must perform:
1. Flexion, extension, and left and right rotation
2. Abduction, flexion, adduction, and extension
3. Pronation, supination, rotation, and extension
4. Dorsiflexion, plantar flexion, eversion, and inversion

822. The physician orders non-weight bearing with crutches for a client with a leg injury. The nurse understands that, before ambulation is begun, the most important activity to facilitate walking with crutches would be:
1. Sitting up in a chair to help strengthen back muscles
2. Keeping the unaffected leg in extension and abduction
3. Exercising the triceps, finger flexors, and elbow extensors
4. Using the trapeze frequently to strengthen the biceps muscles

823. The nurse would recognize that the demonstration of crutch walking with a tripod gait was understood when the client places weight on the:
1. Axillary regions
2. Palms of the hands
3. Feet, which are set wide apart
4. Palms of the hands and axillary regions

824. An x-ray film of a client's arm reveals a comminuted fracture of the radial bone. The nurse understands that with a comminuted fracture:
1. There is a break in the skin and the bone is protruding
2. The bone has broken into several fragments, but the skin is intact
3. Splintering has occurred on one side and bending on the other
4. The bone is broken into two parts, and the skin may or may not be broken

825. A client with osteomyelitis of the leg is to have a débridement of the infected bone. When planning for postoperative care the nurse knows that:
1. Frequent range-of-motion exercises are needed
2. The client's leg may be immobilized in a cast or splint
3. Septicemia is a common postoperative complication
4. The client will be allowed out of bed after the first day

826. While performing a physical assessment of a client with gout of the great toe, the nurse should assess for additional tophi (urate deposits) on the:
1. Chin
2. Ears
3. Buttocks
4. Abdomen

827. When teaching about the dietary control of gout, the nurse is aware that the dietary teaching was understood when the client states; "I will avoid eating:
1. Eggs."
2. Shellfish."
3. Fried poultry."
4. Cottage cheese."

828. An older female client is experiencing frequency and uses the bathroom often during the night. One night while attempting to go to the bathroom without assistance, she develops severe pain and is found to have a vertebral compression fracture. The nurse recognizes that this is a:
1. Collapse of vertebral bodies
2. Demineralization of the spinal cord
3. Wear and tear of the spinous processes
4. Bulging of the spinal cord from the vertebra

829. A client with painful swelling of a distal joint of the ring finger is diagnosed with rheumatoid arthritis. On the next clinic visit the client tells the nurse, "I am so confused. The doctor said I probably have arthritis, but my lab tests were negative. I don't see how that can be when I'm always so uncomfortable." The nurse's best response would be:
1. "It might help if you try not to think about your discomfort."
2. "Don't let that upset you; eventually the tests will be positive."
3. "Laboratory tests are often negative in the early stages of arthritis."
4. "Did the doctor say that they were going to repeat the laboratory tests?"

830. A client with rheumatoid arthritis asks the nurse about ways to decrease morning stiffness. The nurse should suggest:
1. Wearing loose but warm clothing
2. Avoiding excessive physical stress and fatigue
3. Taking a hot tub bath or shower in the morning
4. Planning a rest break periodically for about 15 minutes

831. When assessing a client experiencing an acute episode of rheumatoid arthritis, the nurse observes that the client's finger joints are

swollen. The nurse understands that this swelling is most likely related to:
1. Urate crystals in the synovial tissue
2. Inflammation in the joint's synovial lining
3. Formation of bony spurs on the joint surfaces
4. Escaped fluid from the capillaries, increasing interstitial fluids

832. As an acute episode of rheumatoid arthritis subsides, active and passive range-of-motion exercises are taught to the client's spouse. The nurse should teach that direct pressure not be applied to the client's joints because this may precipitate:
1. Pain
2. Swelling
3. Nodule formation
4. Ophaceous deposits

833. The physician orders bed rest for a client with acute arthritis who has bilateral, painful, swollen knee and wrist joints. To prevent flexion deformities during the acute phase, the client's positioning schedule should include placement in the:
1. Sims' position
2. Prone position
3. Contour position
4. Trendelenburg position

834. The physiotherapist in a nursing home develops an exercise program for an 82-year-old resident with rheumatoid arthritis. The nurse would recognize that the client understands the purpose of this program when the client states:
1. "I know the exercises are important, so I do them whenever I can."
2. "I do my exercises when I go to physical therapy in the morning and afternoon."
3. "Since I'm stiff in the morning, I do most of my exercises then, so I'm done for the day."
4. "After I eat breakfast, I do one set of exercises slowly. I space the rest of them throughout the day."

835. A client with rheumatoid arthritis states, "The only time I am without pain is when I lie perfectly still." During the convalescent stage, the nurse should encourage:
1. Active joint flexion and extension
2. Flexion exercises three times a day
3. Range-of-motion exercises once a day
4. Continued immobility until remission occurs

836. A client who has passed the acute phase of rheumatoid arthritis is now allowed out of bed as tolerated. After assisting the client out of bed, the nurse should place the client in a:
1. Low, soft lounge chair
2. Straight-back armchair
3. Wheelchair with footrests
4. Recliner chair with both legs elevated

837. The nurse teaches a client with rheumatoid arthritis techniques to reduce stress to the joints. The statement by the nurse that best describes a technique to reduce joint stress would be:
1. "Respond to pain in your joints."
2. "Use your smaller muscles most frequently."
3. "Do your heavy tasks all at once to reduce muscle strain."
4. "If your joints are warm or swollen, increase exercise to reduce swelling."

838. A 72-year-old client with osteoarthritis is admitted to the hospital for evaluation of a possible hip replacement. When teaching about ways to prevent disability the nurse suggests that when lying down the client should lie in a supine or prone position. The client states that these positions are uncomfortable for the knees and hips. The nurse should:
1. Tell the client to lie in whatever position is most comfortable
2. Encourage the client to maintain extension for set periods of time
3. Have the client place a pillow under the knees to relieve discomfort
4. Teach the client to remain in the semi-Fowler's position most of the time

839. A dock worker is admitted to the hospital with lower back pain and a tentative diagnosis of a herniated intervertebral disk. When assessing the client's back pain the nurse should ask:
1. "Is there any tenderness in the calf of your leg?"
2. "Have you had any burning sensation on urination?"
3. "Do you have any increase in pain during bowel movements?"
4. "Does the pain begin in your flank and move around to the groin?"

840. A client who is diagnosed as having a herniated intervertebral disc complains of pain. The nurse recognizes that the pain is caused by the:
1. Inflammation of the lamina of the involved vertebra
2. Shifting of two adjacent vertebral bodies out of alignment
3. Compression of the spinal cord by the extruded nucleus pulposus
4. Increased pressure of cerebrospinal fluid within the vertebral column

841. A client is awaiting surgery for a ruptured lumbar nucleus pulposus. The nurse's teaching should include that the pain will most likely increase if the client:
    1. Lies on the side
    2. Flexes the knees
    3. Coughs excessively
    4. Sits for long periods

842. A young adult with a herniated disk is scheduled for a discectomy with fusion. Preoperatively, the nurse should demonstrate the:
    1. Use of a trapeze
    2. Contour position
    3. Traction apparatus
    4. Log-rolling technique

843. After a client has spinal surgery, it is essential that the nurse:
    1. Encourage the client to drink fluids
    2. Log-roll the client to the prone position
    3. Assess the client's feet for circulation and sensation
    4. Observe the client for bowel movements and voiding patterns

844. The nurse teaches a male client, who developed degenerative joint disease of the vertebral column, to turn himself from his back to his side, keeping his spine straight. The least effort will be exerted if he does this by crossing his arm over his chest and:
    1. Bending his top knee to the side to which he is turning
    2. Pulling himself to one side by using his night table
    3. Crossing his ankles and turning with both his legs straight
    4. Flexing his bottom knee to the side to which he wishes to turn

845. A male client has a discectomy and fusion for a herniated disk. When getting out of bed for the first time, with assistance from two nurses, the client complains of feeling faint and lightheaded. The nurses should have the client:
    1. Sit on the edge of the bed, so they can hold him upright
    2. Lie down immediately, so they can take his blood pressure
    3. Slide slowly to the floor, so he will not fall and hurt himself
    4. Bend forward, because it will increase the blood flow to the brain

846. When preparing a client for discharge after a laminectomy, the nurse would know that further health teaching is necessary when the client says, "I should:
    1. Sleep on a firm mattress to support my back."
    2. Spend most of the day sitting in a straight-back chair."
    3. Put a pillow under my legs when sleeping on my back."
    4. Avoid lifting heavy objects until the doctor tells me I can."

847. A back brace is prescribed for a client who has had a laminectomy. The nurse should include in the teaching plan instructions to:
    1. Use the brace when the back feels tired
    2. Apply the brace before getting out of bed
    3. Put the brace on while in the sitting position
    4. Wear the brace when performing twisting exercises

848. After an amputation of a limb, a client begins to experience extreme discomfort in the area where the limb once was. An appropriate nursing diagnosis at this time would be:
    1. Ineffective coping related to surgery
    2. Hopelessness related to altered lifestyle
    3. Disturbed sensory perception related to bed rest
    4. Chronic pain related to phantom phenomenon

849. A client has an above-the-knee amputation because of a gangrenous leg ulcer. After the second postoperative day, to prevent deformities the nurse should:
    1. Keep the client's residual limb elevated on a pillow
    2. Place an abduction pillow between the client's legs
    3. Encourage the client to lie in the supine or prone position
    4. Teach the client to press the residual limb against a hard surface periodically

850. A client who has had an above-the-knee amputation has been fitted with a prosthesis. The finding that would indicate to the nurse that the prosthesis fits the residual limb correctly would be:
    1. Absence of phantom limb sensation
    2. Shrinkage of the end portion of the residual limb
    3. Uneven wearing down of the heels of the shoes
    4. Darkened skin areas surrounding the end of the residual limb

851. While a female ice skater with a fractured femur is being prepared for surgery, she exhibits cyanosis, tachycardia, dyspnea, and restlessness. Initially the nurse should:
    1. Call the physician
    2. Administer oxygen by mask
    3. Place her in a high-Fowler's position
    4. Lower her to the Trendelenburg position

852. A client with an above-the-knee amputation asks why the residual limb needs to be wrapped with an elastic bandage. The nurse explains that it:
    1. Limits the formation of blood clots
    2. Decreases phantom limb sensations
    3. Prevents hemorrhage and covers the incision
    4. Supports the soft tissue and minimizes edema

853. The nurse plans postoperative care for a client who is to have an above-the-knee amputation. The activity designed to aid in the use of crutches would be:
    1. Lifting weights
    2. Changing bed positions
    3. Caring for the residual limb
    4. Performing phantom limb exercises

854. The nurse is assisting a client with a full leg cast to use crutches. The nurse should interrupt the activity when the client exhibits:
    1. A pulse of 100 and deep respirations
    2. Flushed skin and slowed respirations
    3. Profuse diaphoresis and rapid respirations
    4. An increase in blood pressure and shallow respirations

855. A client requires a below-the-knee amputation. A major advantage of an immediate postoperative prosthesis is that it:
    1. Decreases phantom limb sensations
    2. Encourages a normal walking pattern
    3. Reduces the incidence of wound infection
    4. Allows for the fitting of the prosthesis before discharge

856. A 70-year-old client is scheduled for a below-the-knee amputation because of a 10-year history of poor arterial circulation to the lower extremities. The skill that the nurse has taught the client preoperatively that would be most helpful during the first several postoperative days would be to:
    1. Log-roll when turning in bed
    2. Toughen the distal residual limb
    3. Transfer from the bed to a wheelchair
    4. Stand on one leg for five minutes several times a day

857. A 30-year-old runner sustains multiple fractures of the left femur when hit by a car. At the scene of the accident, an immediate life-threatening systemic complication of injury to the long bones can be minimized by:
    1. Elevating the affected limb
    2. Encouraging deep breathing and coughing
    3. Handling and transporting the client gently
    4. Maintaining anatomic alignment of the client's limb

858. A 67-year-old widow fell while washing windows in her apartment. X-ray films indicate an intertrochanteric fracture of the left femur. She is to be placed in Buck's extension until surgery can be performed the next morning. Nursing care is based on the knowledge that the primary purpose of Buck's traction is to:
    1. Reduce the fracture
    2. Maintain abduction
    3. Immobilize the fracture
    4. Eliminate rotation of the femur

859. A client suffers a fracture of the left femur after jumping from the second story of a building during a fire. The client is placed in skeletal traction before open reduction and internal fixation is scheduled. The client keeps slipping down in bed. To alleviate this problem the nurse should:
    1. Elevate the foot of the bed
    2. Shorten the rope on the weights
    3. Release the traction and reposition the client
    4. Move the client toward the head of the bed every two hours

860. A 72-year-old male client has a total hip replacement for long-standing degenerative bone disease of the hip. When assessing this client postoperatively, the nurse should be aware that the most common complication of hip surgery is:
    1. Pneumonia
    2. Hemorrhage
    3. Wound infection
    4. Pulmonary embolism

861. A client has an open reduction and internal fixation for a fractured hip. Postoperatively, the nurse should position the client's affected extremity in:
    1. External rotation
    2. Slight hip flexion
    3. Moderate abduction
    4. Anatomic body alignment

862. After surgery for a fractured hip a client complains of pain. The nurse should:
1. Notify the physician
2. Use distraction techniques
3. Medicate the client as ordered
4. Perform a complete pain assessment

863. A client has an open reduction and internal fixation of a fractured hip. To prevent the most common complication following this type of surgery, the nurse should expect the physician's order to state:
1. "Turn from side to side q2h"
2. "Apply sequential compression stockings"
3. "Encourage isometric exercises to the extremities"
4. "Perform passive range of motion to the affected extremity"

864. The most appropriate action by the nurse when assisting a client, who has had a hip replacement, out of bed would be to:
1. Tell the client that weight-bearing must be on both legs equally
2. Advise the client that the legs must be kept wide apart at all times
3. Sit the client in a straight-back chair so that the hip is kept flexed at a 90-degree angle
4. Transfer the client using a mechanical lift because weight-bearing on the leg is not allowed

865. A client returns from surgery with a hip prosthesis. An abductor splint is in place. The nurse should remove the splint:
1. When the client gets up in a chair
2. If the client needs a change of position
3. Once the client's operative pain has ceased
4. To administer skin care and physical therapy

866. When assisting a client who has had a total hip replacement onto the bedpan on the first postoperative day, the nurse should instruct the client to:
1. Turn toward the operative side
2. Flex both knees and slowly lift the pelvis
3. Extend both legs and pull on the trapeze to lift the pelvis
4. Flex the unaffected knee and pull on the trapeze to lift the pelvis

867. The nursing care plan for a client who has had an open reduction and internal fixation (ORIF) of the left hip, includes observing for signs and symptoms of a fat embolism. These signs and symptoms probably would include:
1. Fever and chest pain
2. A positive Homans' sign
3. Loss of sensation in the operative leg
4. Tachycardia and petechiae over the chest

868. A client with a distal femoral shaft fracture is at risk for developing a fat embolus. A distinguishing sign that is unique to a fat embolus is:
1. Oliguria
2. Dyspnea
3. Petechiae
4. Confusion

869. When planning the discharge teaching for a client who has had a total hip replacement, the nurse should include encouraging the client to avoid:
1. Climbing stairs
2. Stretching exercises
3. Sitting in a low chair
4. Lying prone for at least 30 minutes

870. After a cervical neck injury a client is placed in a halo brace with a body cast. A statement by the client that indicates that the nursing diagnosis, body image disturbance, has been successfully resolved is:
1. "I just hate having everyone else do things for me."
2. "I've been staying under 800 calories daily most of the time."
3. "I've gotten used to the brace. I may even miss it when it's gone."
4. "I can't get to sleep, but I make up for it in the morning by sleeping later."

871. A client with a distal femoral fracture is placed in skeletal traction. The nurse is aware that the weights would only be removed if:
1. There is a life-threatening situation
2. The client complains of intense pain
3. There is evidence of external rotation
4. The cords have become twisted during turning

DRUG-RELATED RESPONSES (DR)

872. The physician orders 0.2 mg of cyanocobalamin (vitamin B_{12}) IM for a client with pernicious anemia. A vial of the drug labeled 1 mL = 100 mcg is available. The nurse should administer:
1. 0.5 mL
2. 1.0 mL

3. 1.5 mL
4. 2.0 mL

873. The client has an order for an antibiotic in an IV piggy-back of 50 mL of D₅W to run for 30 minutes. The micro-drip has a drop factor of 60 gtt/mL. The nurse should set the IV infusion to run at:
    1. 20 drops per minute
    2. 50 drops per minute
    3. 80 drops per minute
    4. 100 drops per minute

874. The physician orders lidocaine HCl, 1.5 mg per minute, for a client whose ECG tracing reveals multiple PVCs. The nurse adds 500 mg of lidocaine HCl to 100 mL of D₅W. The drop factor of the IV set is 60 gtt/mL. To administer the correct amount of medication the nurse should set the IV at:
    1. 10 gtt/minute
    2. 12 gtt/minute
    3. 14 gtt/minute
    4. 18 gtt/minute

875. The physician orders cefazolin sodium (Kefzol) 375 mg IVPB every eight hours. The vial of powder contains 500 mg of the drug. This must be reconstituted with 2 mL of 0.9% sodium chloride. In the resulting solution 1 mL equals 225 mg of Kefzol. The nurse should administer:
    1. 1.2 mL
    2. 1.4 mL
    3. 1.7 mL
    4. 2.2 mL

876. The physician orders aminocaproic acid (Amicar elixir) 4 g po for a client with an intracerebral hemorrhage. The bottle is labeled 250 mg/mL. The nurse should administer:
    1. 16 mL
    2. 1.6 mL
    3. 0.16 mL
    4. 0.016 mL

877. The physician orders 250 mg of an antibiotic IVPB. A vial containing 1 g of the powdered form of the drug must be reconstituted with 2.8 mL of diluent to form a withdrawable volume of 3 mL. Using this solution, the nurse should administer:
    1. 0.5 mL
    2. 0.7 mL
    3. 0.8 mL
    4. 1.1 mL

878. The physician orders 1000 micrograms of procainamide (Pronestyl) IV per minute. The directions state 500 mg of the drug should be added to 500 mL of D₅W. The IV set has a drop factor of 60 gtt/mL. To administer the medication correctly the nurse should set the flow rate at:
    1. 30 gtt/min
    2. 60 gtt/min
    3. 90 gtt/min
    4. 120 gtt/min

879. A client has an IV of D₅W 250 mL to which has been added 100 mg of morphine. The physician has ordered 14 mg of morphine per hour. The nurse should set the intravenous pump to deliver:
    1. 14 mL/hr
    2. 22 mL/hr
    3. 35 mL/hr
    4. 44 mL/hr

880. A client is receiving morphine for severe metastatic bone pain. To prevent complications from a side effect of morphine, the nurse should:
    1. Monitor for diarrhea
    2. Observe for an opiate addiction
    3. Wake the client every two hours
    4. Assess for altered breathing patterns

881. The pharmacy technician arrives on the nursing unit to deliver the requested opioids. A nurse is entering a client's room and not available to receive the medications. The most appropriate statement by the nurse to the pharmacy technician would be:
    1. "I'm sorry. Could you wait five minutes or come back?"
    2. "Leave the meds and sign out sheets by the secretary, please."
    3. "Bring them to me and I'll put them away in a couple of minutes."
    4. "Could you give them to the unit assistant? I'll be out in a few minutes."

882. A client is hospitalized with joint pain, loss of hair, yellow pigmentation of the skin, and an enlarged liver. The nurse should suspect and direct further assessment toward an excess intake of:
    1. Thiamin
    2. Vitamin A
    3. Vitamin C
    4. Pyridoxine

883. A client with tuberculosis is to begin isoniazid (INH), rifampin (Rifadin), and pyrazinamide therapy. The client says, "I've never had to take so much medication for an infection before." The nurse should explain:
    1. "Rifampin prevents side effects from INH."
    2. "This type of organism is difficult to destroy."
    3. "You'll need only one medication when you get better."
    4. "Your infection is well advanced and needs aggressive therapy."

884. A client with tuberculosis is started on a chemotherapy protocol that includes rifampin (Rifadin). The nurse knows the teaching about rifampin was effective when the client states:
    1. "I will have my hearing tested while I take this medicine."
    2. "I will drink large amounts of fluid while I take this medicine."
    3. "A skin rash is normal with rifampin and nothing to worry about."
    4. "It's normal for my urine to be orange colored from this medication."

885. The physician prescribes vitamin B_6 and isoniazid as part of the chemotherapy protocol for a client with tuberculosis. The nurse understands that vitamin B_6 is used because it:
    1. Improves the nutritional status of the client
    2. Enhances the tuberculostatic effect of isoniazid
    3. Accelerates destruction of dormant tubercular bacilli
    4. Counteracts the peripheral neuritis that isoniazid may cause

886. A client is diagnosed as having pulmonary tuberculosis, and one of the drugs the physician orders is pyrazinamide (PZA). The nurse evaluates that the teaching concerning the drug was effective when the client says, "I will:
    1. Drink at least two quarts of fluid a day."
    2. Report any changes in vision to the physician."
    3. Take the medication two hours after each meal."
    4. Expect a discoloration of urine, sweat, and tears."

887. A client is diagnosed with tuberculosis associated with HIV infection. The test results that are crucial for the nurse to review before starting antitubercular pharmacotherapy are:
    1. Liver function studies
    2. Pulmonary function studies
    3. Electrocardiogram and echocardiogram
    4. White blood cell counts and sedimentation rate

888. A client with HIV-associated *Pneumocystis carinii* pneumonia is to receive pentamidine isethionate (Pentam 300) IV once daily. To ensure client safety the nurse should:
    1. Mix the drug with sterile saline without a preservative
    2. Monitor the blood pressure for hypertension during therapy
    3. Administer the drug over a period of 20 to 30 minutes
    4. Assess blood glucose levels daily during therapy and several times after therapy

889. A client who is receiving mechanical ventilation begins to "fight" the respirator, and the physician orders atracurium (Tracrium). The most important nursing action for a client receiving Tracrium is to:
    1. Decrease anxiety
    2. Monitor skin integrity
    3. Promote urinary output
    4. Maintain mechanical ventilation

890. The physician orders 50 U of insulin to be added to an IV of glucose and water for a client with diabetes mellitus. The nurse understands that the only insulin that can be used is:
    1. Lente insulin
    2. Ultralente insulin
    3. Humulin R insulin
    4. Humulin N insulin

891. A client, newly diagnosed with type 2 diabetes, is receiving glyburide (Micronase) and asks the nurse how this drug works. The nurse answers the question about Micronase by telling the client it acts by:
    1. Stimulating the beta cells to produce insulin
    2. Accelerating the liver's release of stored glycogen
    3. Increasing glucose transport across the cell membrane
    4. Lowering blood sugar in the absence of beta cell function

892. A client is diagnosed as having type 2 diabetes and the physician prescribes glipizide (Glucotrol). While taking this medication, the client should be taught to observe for:
    1. Ketonuria
    2. Weight loss
    3. Ketoacidosis
    4. Hypoglycemia

893. A client with type 1 diabetes self-administers Humulin N insulin every morning at 8:00. The nurse recognizes that the client understands the action of this insulin when the client says, "I should be alert for signs of hypoglycemia between:
1. 1 PM and 3 PM."
2. 4 PM and 6 PM."
3. 8 PM and 10 PM."
4. 10 AM and noon."

894. A client with newly diagnosed type 1 diabetes is in a self-care teaching group. The nurse has confidence that the client is able to recognize hypoglycemia when the client states, "I will drink orange juice and eat a slice of bread when I feel:
1. Nervous and weak."
2. Flushed and short of breath."
3. Thirsty and have a headache."
4. Nauseated and have abdominal cramps."

895. A teaching program concerning diabetes and insulin therapy is begun for a client, newly diagnosed with type 1 diabetes. The client states, "I hate shots. Why can't I take the insulin in pill form?" The nurse's best response would be:
1. "Your diabetic condition is too serious for oral insulin."
2. "Insulin by mouth causes a high incidence of allergic reactions."
3. "Insulin is poorly absorbed and its action is erratic when given by mouth."
4. "Once your diabetes is controlled, your physician might consider an oral drug."

896. A client with hyperthyroidism is treated first with propylthiouracil (PTU). When teaching the client about this medication, the nurse should include the information that:
1. This medication will have to be taken for the remainder of life
2. Symptoms may not subside for several days or weeks after the start of therapy
3. Milk should be taken with the medication so that gastric irritation does not occur
4. The medication should be taken between meals so that it is more readily absorbed

897. A client with hyperthyroidism is to receive methimazole (Tapazole). The nurse should instruct the client that:
1. The drug has few side effects
2. Initial improvement will take two to four weeks
3. The medication may be taken at any time during the day

4. A large dose is used to decrease the length of time drug therapy is necessary

898. A client with arthritis is taking ibuprofen, a nonsteroidal antiinflammatory drug, and large doses of aspirin. The nurse, teaching about the symptoms of aspirin toxicity, advises the client to notify the doctor if the client develops:
1. Feelings of drowsiness
2. Disturbances in hearing
3. Intermittent constipation
4. A metallic taste in her mouth

899. A client with arthritis states that the aspirin which has been prescribed causes stomach irritation even when taken with food. The nurse should instruct the client to take the aspirin:
1. An hour before a meal
2. With sodium bicarbonate
3. With a full glass of liquid
4. At the same time as the other drugs

900. A client with arthritis asks the nurse if acetaminophen can be substituted for the aspirin that causes stomach irritation. The nurse's response should be based on the knowledge that acetaminophen:
1. Lacks anticoagulant action
2. Has the same action as aspirin
3. Lacks an antiinflammatory action
4. Has more severe side effects than aspirin

901. Dalteparin (Fragmin) 2500 IU subcutaneously daily is ordered for a client who has had abdominal surgery. The nurse explains the medication to the client based on the knowledge that this drug is given to:
1. Control expected postoperative fever
2. Provide a constant source of mild analgesia
3. Limit the inflammatory response associated with surgery
4. Provide prophylaxis against postoperative thrombus formation

902. The physician orders ibuprofen (Motrin) 800 mg po tid for a client with rheumatoid arthritis. The nurse would know that the teaching about the side effects of Motrin was effective when the client:
1. Recognizes that exercise must be balanced with rest
2. Makes an appointment for blood work in one month
3. Realizes that position changes should be made slowly
4. Understands that the drug must be taken between meals

903. A client who has had a long leg cast applied is to be discharged. When discussing pain management, the nurse should advise the client to take the prescribed prn Tylenol with codeine:
1. Just as a last resort
2. Before going to sleep
3. When the discomfort begins
4. As the pain becomes intense

904. A client had a laminectomy and is receiving a skeletal muscle relaxant that will be continued after discharge. After teaching the client about the skeletal muscle relaxant, the nurse recognizes that no further health teaching is necessary when the client says:
1. "If the medication makes me sleepy, I'll stop taking it."
2. "I'm going to take the medication three hours after meals."
3. "If the medication upsets my stomach, I'll take it with milk."
4. "I'll take an extra dose of the medication before I do anything active."

905. The physician orders a low dosage of an opioid to relieve the pain of a client with deep partial-thickness burns. The nurse recognizes that the preferred mode of administration is:
1. Oral
2. Rectal
3. Intravenous
4. Intramuscular

906. A female client is receiving ethylestrenol (Maxibolin), an anabolic steroid, for the treatment of the catabolic processes associated with a burn injury. The nurse should observe the client for signs of:
1. Lethargy
2. Virilization
3. Hyponatremia
4. Hyperglycemia

907. The nurse applies mafenide acetate cream (Sulfamylon) to a client's burns as ordered by the physician. This medication will:
1. Inhibit bacterial growth
2. Relieve pain from the burn
3. Prevent scar tissue formation
4. Provide chemical débridement

908. A client's burns are treated by the open exposure method and a topical antimicrobial is ordered. The nurse is aware that the statement that best explains the rationale for the use and side effects of the antimicrobial ordered by the physician would be:

1. Silvadene is easy to apply and has good bacteriocidal action but it can depress granulocyte formation
2. Sulfamylon causes no side effects and is effective for both gram-positive and gram-negative organisms
3. Silver nitrate paste has strong bacteriostatic properties and clients respond quickly to these dry dressings because they eliminate odors
4. Neomycin is a strong bacteriocidal agent effective against most organisms with the least number of toxic side effects for the client

909. The nurse attempts to give a male client with chronic arterial insufficiency of the legs the prescribed dose of aspirin but the client refuses it stating, "My legs are not painful." The nurse should:
1. Explain the reason for the medication and encourage the client to take it
2. Withhold the medication and tell the client to ask for it if his legs become uncomfortable
3. Withhold the medication at this time and return to check the client again in one-half hour
4. Request that the client take the medication to prevent him from being uncomfortable in the next few hours

910. The physician prescribes isosorbide dinitrate (Sorbitrate) 10 mg prn tid and a nitroglycerin transdermal disc once a day for a client with chronic angina pectoris. The client asks the nurse why the Sorbitrate is prescribed. The nurse's best response would be:
1. "It prevents the blood from clotting."
2. "It suppresses irritability in the ventricles."
3. "It allows more oxygen to get to heart tissue."
4. "It increases the force of contraction of the heart."

911. The physician orders atenolol (Tenormin) for a client with angina. When instructing the client about this medication, the nurse should teach the client about the potential side effect of:
1. Headache
2. Tachycardia
3. Constipation
4. Hypotension

912. The nurse teaches a client about the side effects of furosemide (Lasix), which has just been prescribed. The nurse assesses that the teaching was understood when the client states, "I should:
1. Wear dark glasses."
2. Avoid lying flat in bed."

3. Avoid eating citrus fruits."

4. Change my position slowly."

913. At each clinic visit, the nurse should assess a client taking furosemide (Lasix) for:
1. Tinnitus
2. Xanthopsia
3. Hyporeflexia
4. Bronchospasm

914. A client with a history of hypertension comes to the emergency department with double vision and a blood pressure of 260/120 mm Hg. In addition to other drugs, the physician orders a sodium nitroprusside (Nipride) infusion. The nurse recognizes that this drug decreases blood pressure by:
1. Decreasing the heart rate
2. Increasing cardiac output
3. Increasing peripheral resistance
4. Relaxing venous and arterial muscles

915. A client is receiving clonidine (Catapres) for hypertension. The nurse would recognize that the discharge instructions were understood when the client states, "I will call the doctor if I develop:
1. Pruritus."
2. Diarrhea."
3. Euphoria."
4. Photosensitivity."

916. A client with hypertensive heart disease who had an acute episode of heart failure is to be discharged on a regimen of propranolol HCl (Inderal) and digoxin (Lanoxin). The nurse should be aware that Inderal, when administered with Lanoxin, may:
1. Produce headaches
2. Precipitate bradycardia
3. Increase blood pressure
4. Stimulate nodal conduction

917. Digoxin (Lanoxin) is prescribed for a client with the diagnosis of heart failure. When planning care for this client, the nurse should include observations for digoxin toxicity and therefore should assess the client for:
1. Anuria
2. Constipation
3. Hypokalemia
4. Blurred vision

918. When administering warfarin (Coumadin) the nurse should know that the antidote for Coumadin is:
1. Vitamin K

2. Fibrinogen
3. Prothrombin
4. Protamine sulfate

919. The physician orders furosemide (Lasix) for a client with hypervolemia. The nurse understands that Lasix exerts its effects in the:
1. Distal tubule
2. Collecting duct
3. Glomerulus of the nephron
4. Ascending limb of Henle's loop

920. A client has been receiving a cardiac glycoside, a diuretic, and a vasodilator and is on bed rest. The client's apical pulse rate is 44 beats per minute. The nurse concludes that this pulse rate is most likely a result of the:
1. Diuretic
2. Vasodilator
3. Bed rest regimen
4. Cardiac glycoside

921. A client has been receiving digoxin (Lanoxin). The client calls the clinic and complains of "yellow vision." The nurse's best response would be:
1. "This is related to your illness, not your medication."
2. "Take this medication because this is not a serious side effect."
3. "This side effect is only temporary. You should continue the medication."
4. "The medication should be discontinued. Come to the clinic this afternoon."

922. A physician orders a tissue plasminogen activator to be administered intravenously over one hour for a client experiencing a myocardial infarction. The nursing priority that is specific to the use of this drug is the assessment of the client's:
1. Respiratory rate
2. Peripheral pulses
3. Level of consciousness
4. Intravenous insertion site

923. A 42-year-old client is admitted to the cardiac care unit with an anterior lateral myocardial infarction. The physician orders 500 mL of D_5W with 50 mg of nitroglycerin to be given intravenously to relieve pain. The nurse should monitor for the most common side effect of nitroglycerine which is:
1. Nausea
2. Syncope
3. Bradycardia
4. Hypotension

924. To hasten the absorption of a nitroglycerin tablet, the nurse should instruct the client to:
    1. Move the tablet around with the tip of the tongue
    2. Break up the tablet before placing it under the tongue
    3. Place the tablet under the tongue along with warm water
    4. Swallow saliva before placing the tablet under the tongue

925. The drug most commonly used to provide analgesia for the client who has had a myocardial infarction (MI) would be:
    1. Xanax
    2. Versed
    3. Morphine
    4. Neurontin

926. Nitroglycerin is prescribed for a client with a history of a myocardial infarction and atrial tachycardia. The nurse instructs the client about the prophylactic use of these tablets. The statement by the client that indicates the teaching was effective would be, "I should:
    1. Take one tablet at 9 AM, noon, and 4 PM."
    2. Not undertake any activity I consider strenuous."
    3. Have my wife take my pulse before I take a tablet."
    4. Take one tablet before climbing two flights of stairs."

927. When administering the ordered digoxin (Lanoxin) 0.25 mg po qd to a client with a history of type 1 diabetes who is now in heart failure, the nurse should:
    1. Give it with orange juice
    2. Monitor for dysrhythmias
    3. Administer it one hour after the morning insulin
    4. Withhold it if the apical pulse rate is 90 beats per minute

928. A client, admitted to the cardiac care unit (CCU) with a myocardial infarction, shows a series of premature ventricular contractions (PVCs) on the monitor. The nurse should anticipate that the client will be receiving:
    1. Atropine
    2. Epinephrine
    3. Sodium bicarbonate
    4. Lidocaine hydrochloride

929. The cardiac monitor indicates that a client's heart rate has increased to 150 beats per minute. Shortly after this increase, the nurse notices that the client is in ventricular tachycardia (VT). After reporting this to the physician, the nurse anticipates the physician will order:
    1. A bolus of lidocaine
    2. Intracardiac epinephrine
    3. Insertion of a pacemaker
    4. Manual cardiopulmonary resuscitation

930. A client is scheduled for an electrophysiology study (EPS) because of persistent ventricular tachycardia. Before the procedure the client is placed on a beta blocker. The client's response during the procedure that best indicates that the beta blocker is working effectively would be:
    1. Increased anxiety
    2. Sinus bradycardia
    3. Nausea and vomiting
    4. Ventricular fibrillation

931. When administering an intravenous titrated drip of lidocaine HCl to a client, a serious side effect that must be reported to the physician immediately is:
    1. Tremors
    2. Anorexia
    3. Tachycardia
    4. Hypertension

932. The physician prescribes furosemide (Lasix) 40 mg qd in conjunction with digoxin (Lanoxin) for a client. The nurse recognizes that potassium supplements are essential with this combination of drugs because:
    1. Digitalis causes significant potassium depletion
    2. Lasix requires adequate serum potassium to promote diuresis
    3. Potassium is destroyed by the liver as digoxin is detoxified
    4. Digitalis toxicity occurs rapidly in the presence of hypokalemia

933. The nurse would know that a client understands the side effects of hydrochlorothiazide (Esidrix) therapy when the client states, "I should call the physician if I develop:
    1. Insomnia."
    2. A stuffy nose."
    3. Increased thirst."
    4. Generalized weakness."

934. A client experiences cardiac standstill. In addition to cardiac stimulants, the nurse would expect to prepare:
    1. Aminophylline

2. Furosemide (Lasix)
3. Sodium bicarbonate
4. Phenytoin (Dilantin)

935. A client, who has had a brain attack (CVA), is unconscious with vital signs of P, 60; R, 16; and BP, 142/64. The medication order that should be questioned by the nurse would be:
1. Mannitol 140 mg IV
2. Dexamethasone 4 mg IV
3. Chlorpromazine 25 mg IM
4. Morphine sulfate 15 mg IM

936. A client is to have a pneumonectomy. For maximum effectiveness, the client's preanesthetic medication should be administered:
1. 2 hours before anesthesia
2. 15 minutes before anesthesia
3. 45 minutes before anesthesia
4. In conjunction with anesthesia

937. A 32-year-old women with stage III-B Hodgkin's disease is started on chemotherapy. The nurse should teach the client to report immediately the occurrence of:
1. A sore mouth
2. A fever of 100° F
3. Moderate diarrhea after treatment
4. Nausea for six hours after treatment

938. A client with cancer, who is receiving a chemotherapeutic regimen that includes vincristine (Oncovin), complains of numbness and loss of feeling in the legs below the knees. The client wants to know if the problem means the cancer is growing or if it is related to the medication. The nurse's answer should be based on the fact that:
1. Enlarged lymph nodes in the groin, related to the cancer, may cause these symptoms
2. Most chemotherapeutic regimens do not affect the nervous or peripheral vascular system
3. Vascular occlusion may cause this problem and immediate medical evaluation is indicated
4. Peripheral neuropathies can result from chemotherapy and usually are reversible if treated early

939. A client who has been taking enteric-coated aspirin for rheumatoid arthritis asks if acetaminophen (Tylenol) can be substituted because it is on sale. The nurse's response should be based on the fact that:
1. Both are analgesics

2. Both can cause gastritis
3. Aspirin is an antiinflammatory
4. Acetaminophen is an antipyretic

940. Specific nursing intervention for a client who is receiving doxorubicin (Adriamycin) for acute myelogenous leukemia should include:
1. Giving frequent oral hygiene and increasing oral fluids
2. Administering medications IM and encouraging activity
3. Serving hot liquids, such as broths or tea, with each meal
4. Emphasizing that the disease will be cured with this treatment

941. A client with small cell lung cancer is receiving chemotherapy. A complete blood count is ordered before each round of chemotherapy. The value in a complete blood count that the nurse should be most concerned about would be:
1. RBCs
2. WBCs
3. Platelets
4. Hematocrit

942. A client with cancer develops pancytopenia during the course of chemotherapy. The client asks the nurse why this has occurred. The nurse should explain that:
1. Steroid hormones have a depressant effect on the spleen and bone marrow
2. Normal cells are also susceptible to the effects of chemotherapeutic drugs
3. Lymph node activity is depressed by radiation therapy used prior to chemotherapy
4. Dehydration caused by nausea, vomiting, and diarrhea results in hemoconcentration

943. A client is receiving busulfan (Myleran) for chronic myelogenous leukemia. When assessing for complications of alkylating agents, the nurse should be alert for:
1. Stomatitis and nausea
2. Feminization or masculinization
3. Fluid retention and hyperglycemia
4. Leukopenia and thrombocytopenia

944. The nurse understands that the safe administration of high-dose methotrexate therapy should include:
1. Maintaining an acidic urine
2. Restricting IV fluids to 50 mL/hr
3. Providing a diet high in folic acid
4. Monitoring plasma levels of methotrexate

945. When a client, who is receiving methotrexate (Folex) for acute lymphocytic leukemia, develops a temperature of 101° F, the physician is notified. Aspirin 650 mg q4h prn is ordered. The nurse should:
1. Ask the physician for an antacid order
2. Question the type of antipyretic ordered
3. Question the dosage ordered by the physician
4. Withhold the aspirin until the temperature reaches 102° F

946. A client with multiple myeloma is treated with combination chemotherapy, including an alkylating agent. During the client's visit to the physician, the nurse notices petechiae and ecchymosis, and the client reports a small episode of epistaxis. This probably is related to:
1. Loss of sensation and signs of nerve trauma
2. Thrombocytopenia, a side effect of alkylating agents
3. Leukocytosis because of bone marrow involvement
4. Hypertension because of increased blood volume, a side effect

947. The physician prescribes finasteride (Proscar) for a 52-year-old client with benign prostatic hyperplasia. The nurse informs the client that:
1. Male pattern baldness can occur
2. Results can be expected in 6 to 12 weeks
3. Compliance will prevent the development of prostatic cancer
4. Protection should be worn during intercourse with a pregnant female

948. A client with cancer is receiving a multiple chemotherapy protocol. Included in the protocol is leucovorin calcium (Wellcovorin). The nurse recognizes that this drug is administered to:
1. Potentiate the effect of alkylating agents
2. Diminish the toxicity of folic acid antagonists
3. Limit the occurrence of nausea and vomiting associated with chemotherapy
4. Interfere with cell division at a different stage of cell division than the other drugs

949. A client who is receiving chemotherapy for cancer has nausea and vomiting because of the therapy. The client wants to know if it is true that smoking marijuana would help. Counseling by the nurse should include the fact that:
1. Smoking marijuana is illegal, and it is very difficult to obtain court permission to purchase it

2. Marijuana is more effective for nausea and vomiting if it is injected, but it can cause drowsiness
3. Smoking marijuana is not effective in the control of nausea and vomiting caused by chemotherapy
4. Tetrahydrocannabinol (THC), the ingredient in marijuana, can be taken in pill form and act as an antiemetic

950. A client with metastatic melanoma is being treated with interferon. The nurse is aware that the teaching about this drug is understood when the client states:
1. "I will increase my fluid intake to two to three liters daily."
2. "I need to discard any reconstituted solution at the end of the week."
3. "I can continue driving my car as before, as long as I have the stamina."
4. "I should be able to continue my usual activity while taking this medication."

951. A client with a parotid tumor that involves the lymph glands in the neck is being treated aggressively with radiotherapy, surgery, and chemotherapy. The physician prescribes vincristine (Oncovin), cyclophosphamide (Cytoxan), and prednisone. Before each chemotherapeutic dose, the client should be assessed for:
1. Peripheral paresthesia
2. Anginal-type chest pain
3. Ophthalmic papilledema
4. Coughing and/or pleurisy

952. A 21-year-old college student with diabetes mellitus requests additional information about the advantages of using pen-like insulin delivery devices. The nurse explains that the advantages of these devices over syringes includes:
1. Shorter injection time
2. Accurate dose delivery
3. Use of a smaller gauge needle
4. Lower cost with reusable insulin cartridges

953. The physician prescribes oral pancreatic enzymes for a client. The nurse would know that the teaching about the enzymes is understood when the client states, "I will take them:
1. At bedtime."
2. With meals."
3. One hour before meals."
4. On arising each morning."

954. After a course of doxorubicin hydrochloride (Adriamycin), the physician decides to prescribe

cisplatin (Platinol) for a client with metastatic cancer. To prevent toxic effects, the nurse should:
1. Administer the ordered leucovorin
2. Encourage regular vigorous oral care
3. Increase hydration to promote diuresis
4. Provide a high-protein, low-residue diet

955. The medication order that should be questioned by the nurse if it is prescribed for a client with acute pancreatitis is:
1. Zantac
2. Tagamet
3. Morphine
4. Phenergan

956. After an acute episode of GI bleeding, a peptic ulcer is confirmed by a gastroscopy and upper GI series. The physician orders ranitidine (Zantac) 150 mg bid with meals. The nurse should check this order with the physician because:
1. This is less than the recommended dose
2. Zantac is contraindicated for peptic ulcer
3. Zantac may be given by a variety of routes
4. This drug is usually given on an empty stomach

957. Prednisone, an adrenal steroid, is ordered for a client with an exacerbation of colitis. When administering the first dose, the nurse should stress that this drug:
1. Will protect the client from getting an infection
2. May decrease the client's appetite, causing weight loss
3. Is not curative but does cause a suppression of the inflammatory process
4. Is relatively slow in effecting a response but is effective in reducing symptoms

958. A client, who is scheduled for a bowel resection, is to receive antibiotics preoperatively. The nurse should teach the client that the purpose of the antibiotics is to help:
1. Prevent incisional infection
2. Avoid postoperative pneumonia
3. Eliminate bacteria from the GI tract
4. Limit the risk of a urinary tract infection

959. Immediately after a bilateral adrenalectomy, a client is receiving corticosteroids that are to be continued after discharge. The nurse should recognize a need for further teaching when the client states:
1. "I need to have periodic tests of my blood for glucose."

2. "I must take the pills between meals on an empty stomach."
3. "Hopefully, the dosage will be regulated so I can take them once or twice a day."
4. "I should tell the doctor if I am overly restless, depressed, or have trouble sleeping."

960. A client with hepatic cirrhosis develops hepatic encephalopathy. Neomycin is prescribed. The purpose of neomycin for a client with cirrhosis would be to:
1. Decrease intestinal edema
2. Reduce abdominal distention
3. Provide a prophylactic antibiotic
4. Diminish the blood ammonia level

961. A client with Graves' disease is to be treated with propylthiouracil (PTU). The nurse should teach the client to:
1. Drink a glass of milk daily
2. Observe for signs of infection
3. Take the drug through a straw
4. Limit exposure to bright sunlight

962. After radioactive iodine therapy, a female client becomes hypothyroid and is placed on levothyroxine (Synthroid). The client asks the nurse whether taking hormones will interfere with the ability to become pregnant. The nurse's best response would be:
1. "Do you think you won't be able to get pregnant?"
2. "Don't you think it's best to discuss this with your doctor?"
3. "While taking this medication, you should avoid becoming pregnant."
4. "If your thyroid function is controlled, the medicine should not interfere with your becoming pregnant."

963. The physician orders docusate sodium (Colace) every day for a client. The nurse recognizes that this drug is ordered specifically to:
1. Lubricate the feces and GI tract
2. Create an osmotic effect in the GI tract
3. Stimulate the motor activity of the GI tract
4. Lower the surface tension of feces in the GI tract

964. The physician prescribes bisacodyl (Dulcolax) for a client with cardiac disease. The nurse is aware that this drug acts by:
1. Softening feces
2. Producing bulk
3. Lubricating feces
4. Stimulating peristalsis

965. The physician orders Maalox by mouth and cimetidine (Tagamet) by IVPB for a client with crushing injuries caused by a train accident. The client asks why these medications are being administered. The nurse's best response would be:
    1. "They decrease irritability of the bowel."
    2. "They're ordered for all clients with multiple trauma."
    3. "They limit acidity in the stomach and intestine."
    4. "They're what your doctor ordered to calm your stomach."

966. The physician orders bed rest, Maalox, and esomeprazole (Nexium) for a client who has just had major surgery. After several days of this regimen, the client complains of diarrhea. The nurse recognizes that the diarrhea is most likely caused by:
    1. Bed rest
    2. The Maalox
    3. Diet alteration
    4. The esomeprazole

967. When caring for a client who has open-angle (chronic) glaucoma, the eyedrops the nurse should expect to administer would be:
    1. Tetracaine (Pontocaine)
    2. Cyclopentolate (Cyclogyl)
    3. Pilocarpine hydrochloride (Pilocar)
    4. Atropine sulfate (Atropisol Ophthalmic)

968. A client has a tonic-clonic seizure that involves all extremities. The nurse anticipates that the physician will order the IV administration of:
    1. Atropine
    2. Epinephrine
    3. Naloxone (Narcan)
    4. Diazepam (Valium)

969. When a client's condition is assessed after a tonic-clonic seizure caused by an overdose of acetylsalicylic acid, the most appropriate nursing action would be to:
    1. Insert a Foley catheter
    2. Check reflexes every hour
    3. Prepare a setup for a CVP line
    4. Monitor vital signs every 15 minutes

970. The physician prescribes phenytoin (Dilantin) for a young mother who has had a tonic-clonic seizure of unknown etiology. The nurse should instruct the client to:
    1. Take the medication on an empty stomach
    2. Brush her teeth and gums three times daily
    3. Stop taking the drug if abdominal pain occurs
    4. Note any change in her pulse and respiratory rates

971. A 60-year-old client is admitted with a tentative diagnosis of Parkinson's disease. The client is started on levodopa therapy. This drug will relieve and control symptoms by:
    1. Blocking the effects of acetylcholine
    2. Restoring dopamine levels in the brain
    3. Increasing the production of dopamine
    4. Promoting the production of acetylcholine

972. A client taking levodopa should be taught about the signs of levodopa toxicity. The client and family should be instructed to contact the physician if they note the development of:
    1. Nausea
    2. Dizziness
    3. Twitching
    4. Constipation

973. When teaching a client with severe Parkinson's disease about carbidopa-levodopa (Sinemet), the nurse should include that:
    1. Multivitamins can be taken daily
    2. Alcohol can be used in moderation
    3. The drug should be taken with meals
    4. A high-protein diet should be followed

974. Selegiline (Eldepryl) is prescribed for a client with Parkinson's disease who had had a poor response to levodopa therapy. When teaching the client and family about this drug, the nurse should explain that:
    1. If a severe headache occurs it should be reported to the physician immediately
    2. The side effects of levodopa will decrease when these drugs are taken concurrently
    3. Blood studies should be performed monthly to measure therapeutic blood levels of the drug
    4. The dosage of the drug can be adjusted daily depending on the client's response that day

975. When a client is receiving dexamethasone (Decadron), the nurse should observe for the development of a negative side effect by:
    1. Auscultating for bowel sounds
    2. Measuring blood glucose levels
    3. Culturing respiratory secretions
    4. Monitoring deep tendon reflexes

976. A client is admitted with head trauma after a fall from a ladder. The client is being prepared

for a supratentorial craniotomy with burr holes, and an IV infusion of mannitol is instituted. The nurse is aware that this medication primarily is given to:
1. Lower blood pressure
2. Prevent hypoglycemia
3. Increase cardiac output
4. Decrease fluid in the brain

977. The physician orders mannitol (Osmitrol) for a client with a head injury. The nurse understands that the purpose of this medication is to promote cerebral dehydration by:
1. Decreasing the production of cerebrospinal fluid
2. Limiting the metabolic requirements of the brain
3. Drawing fluid from brain cells into the bloodstream
4. Preventing uncontrolled electrical discharges in the brain

978. Twelve hours after the intravenous administration of mannitol (Osmitrol) to a client with a head injury, the nurse should be alert for:
1. Respiratory failure
2. Cardiac dysrhythmias
3. An increase in the heart rate
4. A rebound increase in intracranial pressure

979. A client is receiving IV mannitol. An assessment specific to the safe administration of mannitol is:
1. Vital signs q2h
2. Body weight daily
3. Urine output hourly
4. Level of consciousness q8h

980. The wife of a client with an intracranial bleed asks why her husband is not receiving anticoagulant therapy. The nurse explains that in her husband's situation anticoagulant therapy:
1. Will be started if necessary to enhance circulation
2. May be necessary to prevent pulmonary thrombosis
3. Is contraindicated because bleeding would be increased
4. Is inadvisable because it would mask signs and symptoms

981. To prevent excessive bruising when administering heparin subcutaneously, the nurse should:
1. Inject the drug into the subcutaneous tissue quickly
2. Avoid rubbing the injection site after the injection

3. Dilute the heparin with 2 mL of sterile normal saline
4. Use the Z-track technique for administering the injection

982. In the event of excessive bleeding in a client who is receiving heparin sodium, the nurse should be prepared to administer:
1. Vitamin K
2. Panheparin
3. Warfarin sodium
4. Protamine sulfate

983. The nurse knows discharge teaching in relation to warfarin sodium (Coumadin) therapy has been understood when the client states, "I will:
1. Take Tylenol for my occasional headaches."
2. Spend most of the day working at my desk."
3. Make an appointment to have a CBC drawn."
4. Ask the doctor for antibiotics before going to the dentist."

984. One month after an endarterectomy the physician instructs the client to take 325 mg of aspirin a day. The nurse evaluates that the reason for taking this drug is understood when the client says, "It will:
1. Limit the inflammation around my incision."
2. Help to prevent further clogging of my arteries."
3. Reduce the discomfort I feel at the surgical site."
4. Lower the slight fever I have had since surgery."

985. Pyridostigmine bromide (Mestinon) therapy is started for a client who has just been diagnosed with myasthenia gravis. The dosage is frequently changed during the first week. While the dosage is being adjusted, it is particularly important for the nurse to:
1. Administer the medication after meals
2. Administer the medication with food or milk
3. Evaluate the client's psychologic responses between doses
4. Evaluate the client's muscle strength hourly after administration

986. A client, newly diagnosed with myasthenia gravis, is started on pyridostigmine (Mestinon), a cholinesterase inhibitor. Two days later, the client develops loose stools and increased salivation. This is indicative of a:
1. Myasthenic crisis
2. Temporary response
3. Cholinergic side effect
4. Toxic effect of the medication

987. A client, who has been experiencing double vision, drooping of eyelids and fatigue, visits the neurologic clinic. A diagnosis of myasthenia gravis is made and the physician prescribes pyridostigmine (Mestinon). The nurse should teach the client that it is important to take this drug:
1. On an empty stomach
2. One hour before meals
3. According to muscle strength
4. At the exact time intervals ordered

988. A client with myasthenia gravis is admitted to the emergency room in crisis. To distinguish between myasthenic crisis and cholinergic crisis, the nurse should expect the physician to administer:
1. Atropine sulfate
2. Protamine sulfate
3. Naloxone (Narcan)
4. Edrophonium chloride (Tensilon)

989. A client with myasthenia gravis improves and is discharged from the hospital. The discharge medications include pyridostigmine bromide (Mestinon) 10 mg every six hours. The nurse would know that the drug regimen was understood when the client says, "I should:
1. Take milk with each dose of Mestinon."
2. Take the Mestinon on an empty stomach."
3. Set my alarm clock to take my medication."
4. Take my pulse and respirations before taking the drug."

990. A client with myasthenia gravis is to receive immunosuppressive therapy. The nurse understands that this therapy is effective because it:
1. Inhibits the breakdown of acetylcholine at the neuromuscular junction
2. Stimulates the production of acetylcholine at the neuromuscular junction
3. Decreases the production of autoantibodies that attack acetylcholine receptors
4. Promotes the removal of autoantibodies that impair the transmission of impulses

991. The physician orders neostigmine (Prostigmin) for a client with myasthenia gravis. The nurse would know that the client understands the teaching about this drug when the client says:
1. "I should keep the drug in a tight container in the refrigerator."
2. "The drug should be taken between meals to promote absorption."
3. "I should take the drug at the exact time specified by my doctor."
4. "The peak action of the drug occurs about three to four hours after ingestion."

992. Trimethoprim sulfamethoxazole (Bactrim) is prescribed for a client with cystitis. When teaching about the medication, the nurse should recommend that the client:
1. Drink 8 to 10 glasses of water daily
2. Increase the acidity of the urine by drinking orange juice
3. Take the medication with meals to avoid gastric irritation
4. Continue to take the medication until symptoms have subsided

993. The physician orders oxacillin sodium (Bactocill) 500 mg every six hours for a client who is to be discharged. The nurse would know that the teaching about the Bactocill is understood when the client says:
1. "I will take the medication with meals."
2. "I should drink a glass of milk with each pill."
3. "I should drink at least six glasses of water every day."
4. "I will take the medication one hour before or two hours after meals."

994. Two days after surgery a client's temperature is normal and the IVPB of gentamicin q8h started earlier is discontinued. The physician orders a clear liquid diet and OOB ad lib. After lunch the client complains of dizziness when walking to the bathroom. The nurse should recognize that the dizziness is probably related to:
1. Bed rest
2. The liquid diet
3. The gentamicin
4. Postanesthesia hypotension

995. The physician orders peak and trough levels of an antibiotic for a client who is receiving the medication IVPB. For peak levels the nurse should have the laboratory obtain a blood sample from the client:
1. Between 30 and 60 minutes after the IVPB
2. Halfway between two IVPB administrations
3. Immediately before administering the IVPB
4. Anytime it is convenient for the client and laboratory

996. Aluminum hydroxide gel is prescribed for a client with phosphatic renal calculi. The nurse should teach this client that aluminum hydroxide gel will decrease the serum phosphorus level by:
1. Dissolving calculi in the urinary tract
2. Preventing absorption of phosphorus in the stomach

3. Promoting excretion of excessive urinary phosphorus

4. Binding with phosphorus in the intestines before excretion

997. The medication that the nurse should crush for a patient who has difficulty swallowing would be:
1. Slow-K
2. Agon SR
3. Tylenol ES
4. Procardia XL

998. When planning discharge teaching for a client who has had a kidney transplant, the nurse should explain the drug regimen that will be needed to prevent rejection of the kidney. The drugs of choice usually include:
1. Ancef, methotrexate, and citric acid
2. Lasix, neomycin, and sirolimus (Rapamune)
3. Methylprednisolone (Solu-Medrol), Dilantin, and insulin

4. Prednisone, tacrolimus (Prograf), and mycophenolate mofetil (CellCept)

999. In relation to a client's treatment with the drug erythropoietin (Epogen), the finding that would be considered significant is an:
1. Elevated liver panel
2. Elevated hematocrit level
3. Increase in the WBC counts
4. Increase in Kaposi's sarcoma lesions

1000. A client who is immunosuppressed is receiving filgrastim (Neupogen). When assessing the client's response to this medication the finding that would be considered significant is an increase in:
1. Platelets
2. Erythrocytes
3. Thrombocytes
4. White blood cells

Medical-Surgical Nursing Answers and Rationales

NURSING PRACTICE (NP)

1. 3 Care provided in the home would be more efficient and cost effective; this couple can manage with assistance from community resources. (2) (SE; MR; PL)

1 There is nothing in the history to demonstrate that a nursing home is necessary.

2 Since the couple appear able to function with assistance at home, it is not necessary to move them to another setting at this time.

4 Same answer as 2.

2. 1 Glucocorticoids are used for their antiinflammatory action, which decreases the development of edema. (2) (PB; CJ; PL)

2 Diuretics may be used in conjunction with steroids; they reduce edema after it is present.

3 Anticonvulsants prevent seizure activity, not cerebral edema.

4 Antihypertensives control hypertension, not cerebral edema.

3. 4 Rapid administration, incorrect positioning, and inadequate solution temperature are common causes of intolerance to tube feedings. (3) (SE; MR; EV)

1 Although this may be done eventually, the feeding technique should be assessed first.

2 Feedings generally are better tolerated if given frequently in small amounts over the entire 24 hours.

3 Same as answer 1.

4. 1 Consent must be acquired when the client is fully oriented and in a clear mental state. (3) (SE; LE; PL)

2 Although important, this can be implemented before surgery even if the client has received medication.

3 Same as answer 2.

4 Same as answer 2.

5. 2 This describes crackles; rhonchi are coarse sounds heard over the larger airways; including rhonchi in the assessment is inaccurate. (3) (PB; CJ; AS)

1 Crackles and rhonchi are client adaptations, not a nursing diagnosis.

3 It is incorrect terminology to refer to fine crackling sounds in a lower lobe of the lung as rhonchi.

4 Crepitus, which indicates subcutaneous emphysema, is a condition unrelated to breath sounds heard on auscultation.

6. 4 The medical history could be obtained during assessment, and a relationship could be established if they were uninterrupted. (3) (SE; MR; IM)

1 Agency information and data could be obtained after the assessment data had been obtained and rapport established.

2 Accepting coffee may be an imposition and is not the best way to develop trust.

3 Assessment of the environment could be less obviously done while obtaining the history and physical data.

7. 4 This includes the client in the problem-solving process. (2) (SE; MR; PL)

1 This does not include the client in the problem-solving process; more data should be obtained from the client before deciding on an intervention, which may or may not be appropriate.

2 Same as answer 1.

3 Same as answer 1.

8. 3 Policies relative to DNR orders vary among hospitals and the nurse must adhere to the policies of the institution. (2) (SE; LE; AN)

1 This is untrue; the wish of the client is the deciding factor.

2 The decision resides with the client.

4 This may not be true for all hospitals or states; the information does not indicate this is so in this situation; these orders are reviewed periodically.

9. 2 Any client who has been sedated, or who is not fully conscious, may not sign the consent for a surgical procedure. (2) (SE; LE; AN)

1 Many clients face contradictory feelings regarding their impending surgery, but their consent is legal unless they withdraw the consent.

3 A second opinion is not required for a consent to be legal.

4 A complete history and physical examination are needed before surgery, but they do not affect the legality of consent.

10. **2** **This response attempts to explore why the client is refusing the procedure; it promotes communication. (3) (SE; LE; IM)**
1 This response is accusatory; the client has the right to withdraw consent at any time.
3 This is a conclusion without appropriate data; it puts the client on the defensive.
4 This is a conclusion without appropriate data; it may raise the client's anxiety level.

11. **1** **The nurse at the scene of an accident should function in a responsible and prudent manner; the use of a soiled cloth on an open wound is not prudent, nor is the independent transfer of an accident victim from the scene. (2) (SE; LE; EV)**
2 Although the Nurse Practice Act defines nursing, it does not provide detailed standards for practice; the nurse's action was not prudent.
3 The nurse's action was not what a reasonably prudent nurse would do and is therefore not protected.
4 The nurse's intervention was not prudent and placed the client in jeopardy; the nurse was not practicing medicine but attempting to provide first aid.

12. **3** **Neurologic aging causes forgetfulness and slower response time; repetition increases learning. (2) (PM; MR; PL)**
1 This is a general principle applicable to all learning.
2 The older adult has no more difficulty learning than a younger person, although it may take longer.
4 Same as answer 1.

13. **4** **A small amount of bile-colored spotting is expected; a moderately large amount is pathologic; this, in conjunction with the presence of pain, needs further assessment. (2) (PB; MR; IM)**
1 Although this would be done eventually, it is not the priority.
2 The client should be on the right side, not the supine position; the right side-lying position compresses the liver capsule against the abdominal wall.
3 Although monitoring of vital signs is important, it is not the priority.

14. **4** **The release of information to an unauthorized person or gossiping about a client's activities constitutes a breach of confidentiality and an invasion of privacy. (1) (SE; LE; AN)**
1 Libel occurs when a person writes false statements about another that may injure the individual's reputation.

2 Slander occurs when a person verbally defames, detracts from, or maligns another's reputation.
3 Negligence is a careless act of omission or commission that results in injury to another.

15. **3** **Before nurses can help others, they must understand feelings about issues that may affect clients; this is the first step toward providing nonjudgmental care. (1) (SE; CJ; AS)**
1 Although it is beneficial for nurses to understand themselves, this does not necessarily mean that the care will be nonjudgmental.
2 Although truthfulness is important in a therapeutic relationship, the nurse should attempt to be nonjudgmental; a nurse who feels uncomfortable should not be caring for the client in the first place.
4 Although this is important for all therapeutic relationships, it follows a thorough self-assessment of attitudes, values, and beliefs.

16. **3** **The bureau of child welfare handles cases of child abuse and neglect, of which the child seems to be a victim. (2) (SE; LE; IM)**
1 The clinic would observe the client medically, but the bureau of child welfare would handle the child abuse and other social problems.
2 The hospital would probably not admit the child unless an immediate medical incident required it.
4 The bureau of the handicapped would be concerned with equipment and supplies required for the individual with a disability.

17. **3** **Palliative measures are aimed at relieving discomfort without curing the problem. (1) (PB; MR; PL)**
1 A cure or recovery is not part of palliative care; with a terminal disease this goal is unrealistic.
2 Same as answer 1.
4 Although support of significant others is indicated, palliative care is directly related to relieving the client's discomfort.

GROWTH AND DEVELOPMENT (GD)

18. **3** **This is the young-adult task associated with intimacy vs isolation. (2) (PM; CJ; AN)**
1 This is a toddler's task associated with autonomy vs shame and doubt.
2 This is a pre-school-age child's task associated with initiative vs guilt.
4 Same as answer 1.

19. **4** **Presbyopia is the decreased accommodative ability of the lens that occurs with aging. (2) (PB; CJ; AN)**

1 Tropia (eye turn) generally occurs at birth.

2 Myopia (nearsightedness) can occur during any developmental level or be congenital.

3 Hyperopia (farsightedness) can occur during any developmental level or be congenital.

20. 1 **Research demonstrates that women past menopause need at least 1500 mg of calcium a day, which is almost impossible to obtain through dietary sources because the average daily consumption of calcium is 300 to 500 mg; vitamin D promotes the deposition of calcium into the bone. (2) (PB; CJ; AN)**

2 These do not contain adequate calcium to meet requirements to prevent osteoporosis; these do not contain vitamin D unless fortified.

3 These do not contain adequate calcium and vitamin D to meet requirements to prevent osteoporosis.

4 If large amounts of magnesium are present, calcium absorption is impeded because magnesium and calcium absorption are competitive; vitamin E is unrelated to osteoporosis.

21. 3 **A common conflict confronting the older adult seems to be between the desire to be taken care of by others and the desire to be in charge of one's own destiny. (1) (PM; CJ; AN)**

1 This may occur but is not common.

2 Same as answer 1.

4 Same as answer 1.

22. 2 **According to Erikson, poor self-concept and feelings of despair are conflicts manifested in the 65-and-older age group. (3) (PM; CJ; EV)**

1 These are conflicts manifested in early childhood between 3 and 6 years of age.

3 These are conflicts manifested during the ages from 6 to 11 years.

4 These are conflicts manifested during middle adulthood, 45 to 65 years of age.

23. 3 **This may cause an older adult to be unaware of a serious illness, thermal extremes, or excessive pressure. (2) (PM; CJ; PL)**

1 There should be no interference with swallowing.

2 Older adults are more sensitive to cold; there seems to be decreased sensitivity to heat with a tendency to be unaware of a burn.

4 There is a decreased response to stimuli in older adults.

24. 4 **A decrease in neuromuscular function slows reaction time. (1) (PM; CJ; IM)**

1 Confusion is not necessarily a process of aging, but it occurs for various reasons such as

multiple stresses, perceptual changes, or medication side effects.

2 The ability to be flexible has less to do with age than with character.

3 The majority of older adults do not have organic mental disease.

25. 4 **For reasons that are still unclear, the thirst reflex diminishes with age and this may lead to a concomitant decline in fluid intake. (1) (PM; MR; IM)**

1 There are no data to support this statement.

2 This would not be true for an alert person who is able to meet the activities of daily living.

3 Research does not support progressive memory loss in normal aging as a contributor to decreased fluid intake.

26. 3 **Vitamin E hinders oxidative breakdown of structural lipid membranes in body tissues caused by free radicals in the cells. (2) (PB; CJ; AN)**

1 This assists in the formation of visual purple needed for night vision.

2 This is used for formation of collagen, which is important for maintaining capillary strength, promoting wound healing, and resisting infection.

4 This is necessary for protein and fat metabolism and normal function of the nervous system.

27. 1 **This increase is a response to the need for oxygen at the cellular level because of the increased metabolic rate associated with exercise. (2) (PB; CJ; EV)**

2 The rate of respiration would increase with mild exercise; because of inflexibility of the chest in the older adult, the depth would increase only minimally.

3 This should not occur with mild exercise, unless the client has cardiac disease.

4 An irregular heart rate would not be an expected response to exercise; it indicates a problem.

28. 3 **Reinforcing strengths promotes self-esteem; reminiscing is a therapeutic tool that provides a life review that assists adaptation and helps achieve the task of integrity associated with older adults. (2) (PM; MR; IM)**

1 Exercise should be encouraged, but naps tend to interfere with adequate sleep at night.

2 Reinforcing ageism would enhance devaluation of the older adult.

4 A well-balanced diet that also includes protein and fiber should be encouraged; the older adult needs to put the past in perspective and a positive self-assessment should be supported.

29. 2 Aging causes a lowering of the physiologic coping reserve of various systems of the body. (3) (PM; CJ; IM)
  1 The pain threshold increases with aging.
  3 There are many etiologies for confusion (e.g., drug intolerance, altered metabolic state, unfamiliar surroundings).
  4 As individuals age they become more entrenched in ideas, environment, and objects that are familiar, and thus do not tolerate change well.

30. 4 During the aging process there is a progressive atrophy of the convolutions of the brain with a decrease in its blood supply, which may produce a tendency to become forgetful, a reduction in short-term memory, and susceptibility to personality changes. (1) (PM; CJ; AS)
  1 Creativity is not affected by aging; many people remain creative until very late in life.
  2 There should be little or no change in judgment.
  3 There is little or no intellectual deterioration; intelligence scores show no decline.

31. 4 With aging, there is some increase in the systolic blood pressure and a slight increase in the diastolic blood pressure; hormone production is decreased with menopause. (3) (SE; MR; IM)
  1 There are no changes in libido with aging; there is a loss of skin elasticity.
  2 Salivary secretions decrease, not increase, causing more difficulty with swallowing; there is some impairment of fat digestion.
  3 There may be a decrease in subcutaneous fat, decreasing body warmth; some swallowing difficulties occur because of decreased secretions.

32. 3 The onset of disabling illness will divert an older person's energies, making it difficult to maintain an optimum level of functioning. (3) (PM; CJ; AN)
  1 This would be an expected response.
  2 This can result from the aging process and the change in environment; it is not as important as the loss of function.
  4 A gradual memory loss and some confusion can be expected; a sudden memory loss would be cause for alarm.

33. 1 A psychosocial task for middle adulthood according to Erikson is generativity; this task is concerned with the sense of productivity and accomplishment. (3) (PM; CJ; PL)
  2 This is not involved in any task of middle adulthood identified by Erikson.
  3 Same as answer 2.
  4 Same as answer 2.

34. 4 Spending time in several short sessions reduces client fatigue and compensates for a shortened attention span, which is common in the elderly. (2) (PM; MR; PL)
  1 The questionnaire may never be completed.
  2 This is degrading to the client; the client should be asked initially and, if necessary, family can be asked to fill in details later.
  3 This may be overwhelming and create feelings of anger and resentment.

EMOTIONAL NEEDS RELATED TO HEALTH PROBLEMS (EH)

35. 2 Lifelong coping styles are most important in how a person will deal with stress. (2) (PI; CJ; AN)
  1 Age may influence defense mechanisms but lifelong coping styles will most significantly affect a person's behavior
  3 This is a factor to be considered, but past coping ability is the most significant factor to predict future coping.
  4 Same as answer 3.

36. 2 This action indicates recognition that the client's reaction is understandable; it creates a climate of acceptance and promotes expression of feelings. (2) (PI; CJ; IM)
  1 This delays the client's use of coping responses.
  3 This suggests that the nurse is unable to deal with the situation; it is not necessary to notify the physician.
  4 This creates a situation in which the client would be hesitant to express any feelings.

37. 3 This provides the opportunity for the client to verbalize the feelings underlying behavior. (2) (PI; CJ; IM)
  1 This has no effect on decreasing the client's anxiety or allowing ventilation.
  2 This explanation will not decrease anxiety so that the client can rest.
  4 Although allowing release of feelings is therapeutic, leaving immediately denies the client the opportunity for verbalization and discussion.

38. 3 This response indicates that the nurse has heard the verbal message and has empathy for the client; it encourages further verbalization. (3) (PI; MR; IM)
  1 This response may increase the client's anxiety.
  2 This response minimizes the client's concerns.
  4 This depersonalizes the client's concerns; it focuses on the tests and the scheduling rather than the client's concern.

39. 1 Projection is the attribution of unacceptable feelings and emotions to others. (2) (PI; CJ; AN)
   2 Sublimation is the substitution of socially acceptable feelings or instincts to replace those that would be threatening to the ego.
   3 Intellectualization is the use of mental reasoning processes to deny facing emotions and feelings involved in a situation.
   4 A reaction formation is the unconscious replacement of feelings or behavior unacceptable to the self-image with the assumption of opposite feelings or behavior.

40. 2 The nurse must identify the client's perception of work before an appropriate response can be made. (1) (PM; CJ; IM)
   1 The client probably can do light work.
   3 This response is vague and demeaning and gives little direction to the client.
   4 The client probably can do light work as well as rest.

41. 2 The client should know there is help available, even though direct supervision is no longer provided. (2) (SE; MR; PL)
   1 This is not the priority at this time.
   3 Same as answer 1.
   4 Ileostomies are not irrigated.

42. 3 Active participation in self care indicates a readiness to learn; it demonstrates that the client is interested in future expectations. (3) (SE; MR; EV)
   1 This may indicate intellectual readiness but not necessarily emotional readiness.
   2 An expected change in body image precipitates the grieving process; a client may be in denial if no concerns are expressed.
   4 The client need not be dependent; this response indicates the need for more teaching and emotional support.

43. 4 Explanation of the underlying mechanism usually helps calm anxiety about an unusual hallucinatory-type experience. (2) (PB; MR; IM)
   1 This is false reassurance because phantom limb sensations may not disappear.
   2 This may distract the client, but does not foster awareness of the cause.
   3 This reinforces the idea that there is something psychologically wrong with the client.

44. 4 The loss of a limb affects the idealized self-image, since it is difficult to deny the body has not been altered. (3) (PI; CJ; PL)
   1 Although sexuality is included in self-image; it is concerned with a variety of other factors not affected by amputation.
   2 Amputation may signify a lack of wholeness, but feelings about it would be influenced by self-image.
   3 Amputation may increase dependency needs, but these needs are influenced by self-image.

45. 3 Intellectualization is the use of reasoning and thought processes to avoid the emotional aspects of a situation; this is a defense against anxiety. (1) (PI; CJ; AN)
   1 Projection is denying unacceptable traits and regarding them as belonging to another person.
   2 Sublimation is a defense wherein the person redirects the energy of unacceptable impulses into socially acceptable behaviors or activities.
   4 Reaction formation is behavior opposite to what the person is feeling.

46. 3 This response encourages the client to review facts and provides an opportunity to talk about feelings. (2) (PI; CJ; IM)
   1 This suggests the nurse does not want to discuss the subject; it abdicates the nurse's responsibility to explore the issue with the client.
   2 Although it is an empathetic answer, it does not encourage the client to explore feelings; it may increase anxiety.
   4 Although the statement is true, the response does not encourage the client to examine feelings.

47. 3 This nonjudgmentally points out the client's behavior. (2) (PI; CJ; IM)
   1 This is too confrontational; the client may not be able to answer the question.
   2 This is too confrontational and an assumption by the nurse.
   4 This is too judgmental, an assumption, and a stereotypic response.

48. 4 It is difficult to work through a loss; however, encouraging the sharing of feelings helps both parties to feel better about having to let go. (1) (PI; CJ; IM)
   1 There is no evidence to suggest that the client cannot deal with these emotions; this is a time for closeness and honesty.
   2 This response impedes the work of acceptance of one's finality and the use of the remaining time to the best advantage.
   3 This response is demeaning, closes off communication, and does not foster the expression of feelings.

49. 4 **Honest discussion with emphasis on functional and psychologic abilities helps promote adjustment. (2) (PM; CJ; IM)**

1 Postoperative depression is not a characteristic feature of thymectomy.

2 This is too soon; it may eventually be necessary if the client has difficulty adjusting to the chronicity of this condition.

3 This provides false reassurance; there is no guarantee the client will feel better on discharge.

50. 4 **This response offers the best combination of factual information and emotional support. (3) (PI; CJ; IM)**

1 This response disregards the client's feelings; it is also inaccurate because, if the bladder is removed, urinary function will not be normal.

2 Although this reflects the client's feelings, further communication is cut off by the second part of the response.

3 This response is factual, but does not answer the question or offer emotional support; it may increase anxiety.

51. 3 **Reflection conveys acceptance and encourages further communication. (2) (PI; CJ; IM)**

1 This is false reassurance that does not help to reduce anxiety.

2 This provides false reassurance and removes the focus from the client's needs.

4 This is unrealistic, and it is too late to suggest this.

52. 1 **The loss of an established lifestyle and the potential for death may result in depression. (1) (PI; CJ; AN)**

2 Paranoia is occasionally seen in the terminal stage of renal failure; this is not known as "post pump psychosis."

3 The superego is not affected by this illness.

4 This is neither a concern nor a common reaction.

53. 4 **The nurse needs to know specifically what the client is asking; this response permits clarification. (2) (PB; CJ; IM)**

1 This assumes that the client is referring to the diabetes in relation to surgery and sidesteps the question.

2 Asking what the physician has said collects more information, but it will not clarify what the client wants to know.

3 The nurse is making an assumption about medical management.

54. 4 **This true statement could be the foundation for developing a positive mental outlook. (2) (PI; CJ; IM)**

1 There is no indication that the client needs drugs to combat depression.

2 This is a patronizing response that does not recognize the despair.

3 Although this is probably true, this response belittles the client's actual concern and physical discomfort.

55. 3 **This is a truthful answer that provides some realistic hope. (1) (PI; CJ; IM)**

1 This provides false reassurance; remissions and exacerbations that may reduce the life span are common.

2 This response avoids the client's question; the family did not ask.

4 This avoids the client's question and transfers responsibility to the physician.

56. 2 **Communication facilitates joint solution of the problem; the nurse must first determine the client's understanding and perceptions before solutions to the problem can be attempted. (2) (SE; MR; AS)**

1 This will not collect data about why the client is leaving the room.

3 This abdicates the responsibility of the primary nurse.

4 This may be done but not until further assessment is done to determine the reason why the client is leaving the room.

57. 4 **Privacy is necessary when the client disrobes; a professional relationship could be established more easily if the nurse and client were uninterrupted. (2) (PI; MR; IM)**

1 Socializing at this time would be an imposition.

2 This would not provide for privacy.

3 This may eventually be necessary, but is not the initial action.

58. 1 **This is a classic sign of denial; by reducing the importance or extent of the problem, the individual is able to cope; not acknowledging that it is really a problem is a form of denial. (2) (PI; CJ; AS)**

2 This indicates repression of affect rather than denial.

3 This usually indicates displacement of anger, not denial.

4 Failure to communicate is insufficient evidence to diagnose denial; the husband/wife relationship may be strained, or the husband may be worried about upsetting the wife.

59. **2 Improved functioning relates most to improved body image, even if the prosthesis is not at all like the original body part. (3) (PB; CJ; AN)**
1 Acceptance by others does not guarantee acceptance by self.
3 While mood may be improved with aggressive rehabilitation, this in itself does not improve body image.
4 An improvement in body image may occur only when the prosthesis is covered with clothing.

60. **4 Anxiety and/or anger associated with other stages of coping interfere with learning. (3) (PI; MR; AN)**
1 This is too late to start preparation for discharge and teaching; many factors influence readiness for learning; planning for teaching must begin on the day of admission.
2 The anxiety associated with mental anguish would interfere with the ability to process new information; mental anguish is associated with an earlier stage.
3 Although clients in the acceptance or adaptation phase are less angry, the reason teaching is most effective is not because of their compliance but because new information can be processed more easily.

61. **2 When a client is anxious and has a decreased ability to cope, minor environmental irritants are magnified; eye contact is avoided to decrease additional stimuli. (3) (PI; CJ; EV)**
1 This would be indicated by complaints of pain, splinting, refusal to move, and alteration in vital signs.
3 If the client were angry, eye contact would be maintained; prolonged eye contact may be used as a form of intimidation or aggression.
4 If this were so, the client would be verbalizing about the need to continue the abduction, not about a variety of other annoyances.

62. **2 The best indicator of acceptance is when the client begins to participate in self care. (3) (PI; CJ; EV)**
1 This does not indicate acceptance and may be an "act."
3 This does not indicate acceptance and may be an attempt to relieve boredom.
4 This does not indicate acceptance and may indicate dependence.

63. **4 Once survival needs are met and pain diminishes, there is a realization of lifestyle alterations in the future. (3) (PI; CJ; AN)**
1 The client is not talking about deformities; she is beginning to realize the implications of going home.
2 Information is not adequate to come to this conclusion.
3 The client is expressing a realistic concern and needs to talk about the future.

64. **1 This reflects the client's feelings and encourages a further exploration of concerns. (3) (PI; CJ; IM)**
2 This response does not reflect the feeling tone of the client's statement; also, the client may not be able to answer this question.
3 This is false reassurance; thyrotoxic crisis is capable of causing death.
4 This could reinforce the client's anxiety and avoids discussing the client's concerns; it cuts off communication.

65. **3 Internal self-stimulation increases as external stimuli decrease. (3) (PB; CJ; AN)**
1 Blindness is an added stress that could increase anxiety, which impairs decision making; lack of visual stimuli limits data for decision making.
2 Lack of visual stimuli would increase restlessness, lethargy, and apathy.
4 Blindness would not precipitate neurotic behavior unless other emotional factors were present.

66. **2 This provides an opportunity for the client to explore concerns with the nurse. (2) (PI; CJ; IM)**
1 The data do not indicate regression; the client is anxious, not regressed.
3 The nurse is basing the response on an incorrect interpretation of the data.
4 The data do not indicate that the client does not understand; the nurse should attempt to provide for consensual validation before coming to this conclusion.

67. **3 Hostility and noncompliance are both forms of anger that are associated with grieving. (2) (PI; CJ; AN)**
1 This is not a conscious attempt to hurt others but a way to relieve and reduce anxiety within the self.
2 This is a self-destructive method of coping, which could result in death.
4 This is an effort to maintain control over a situation that is really controlling the client; it is an unconscious method of coping, and noncompliance may be a form of denial.

68. 1 **This response indicates recognition of the client's need to use denial and opens the way for discussion of feelings. (3) (PI; CJ; IM)**

2 This forces reality on the client and blocks discussion of feelings.

3 This reply focuses on the surgery, which is not the concern expressed by the client.

4 This changes the subject and moves away from the client's feelings.

69. 2 **This identifies the client's feelings and provides an opportunity for further discussion. (2) (PI; CJ; IM)**

1 Although this echoes the client's statement, it does not identify a feeling.

3 This denies the client's feelings and focuses on information; the client may be too emotionally distraught to be able to construct or verbalize questions.

4 This provides false reassurance and cuts off communication.

70. 1 **Communication is a priority; it facilitates interaction, limits anxiety, and promotes safety. (1) (PI; MR; PL)**

2 A nasogastric tube would be traumatic for the suture lines; total parenteral nutrition may be used.

3 This is done postoperatively as the client begins to accept the laryngectomy.

4 After a laryngectomy the client cannot cough; expectoration occurs through the stoma.

71. 1 **The nurse must first explore the client's feelings; an honest discussion with emphasis on concerns helps promote adjustment. (1) (PI; CJ; IM)**

2 This may be necessary if the depression continues.

3 Postoperative depression is not an expected response to surgery.

4 This is false reassurance because there is no guarantee that the depression will lift at home.

72. 2 **Reliving the experience brings back the feelings, such as anxiety and fear, associated with it; the symptoms described reflect sympathetic nervous system activity. (3) (PB; CJ; AN)**

1 The increased pulse and restlessness could indicate bleeding; however, the other data presented support anxiety; additional assessment would be necessary to identify bleeding.

3 Not enough data are present to recognize the client's usual method of seeking sympathy.

4 These symptoms are indicative of a sympathetic, not a parasympathetic, response.

73. 1 **Reflection of the client's statement will enhance further communication. (1) (PI; CJ; IM)**

2 The client did not indicate anxiety concerning the effects of radiotherapy; this is an assumption.

3 This is a conclusion that does not reflect the client's stated concern.

4 This may close the opportunity for further exploration and may reinforce the client's concern.

74. 1 **This meets the client's immediate personal needs and demonstrates respect and concern. (3) (PI; CJ; IM)**

2 This may be explored when planning further support; it is not the priority at this time.

3 This provides false reassurance that may block communication; the nurse, not the wife, should explore this issue with the client.

4 The client's immediate need should be met first; the nurse should explore feelings first before the need for a referral is determined.

75. 3 **These are realistic, productive, and constructive ways of using this time. (1) (PI; CJ; AN)**

1 These are signs of depression.

2 Going from physician to physician demonstrates disbelief, denial, or desperation.

4 This indicates anger and hopelessness, not acceptance.

76. 4 **This is a legal requirement of participating institutions to protect the individuals involved. (1) (SE; LE; AN)**

1 Active euthanasia is a direct act to shorten a person's life and is illegal.

2 No age restrictions exist; a guardian's signature is required.

3 Legal statutes make certain the opposite is true.

77. 2 **Before a teaching plan can be developed, the factors that interfere with learning must be identified. (2) (SE; MR; AS)**

1 Although family members can be helpful, client involvement in care is important for promoting independence and self-esteem.

3 This may be an unrealistic expectation; the client may never accept the change but must learn to manage care.

4 This is premature; assessment comes before intervention; written instructions may not be the most appropriate teaching modality.

78. **4 Sharing concerns and talking about them often releases anxieties; giving the ordered anxiolytic would produce relaxation. (1) (PI; CJ; IM)**
    1 This might relax the client but would do little to reduce the client's level of anxiety.
    2 The client is not in pain at this time but needs to share concerns.
    3 The procedure is over; this might be appropriate before the paracentesis; also, there are no data to support that this is the client's concern.

79. **4 This response identifies the client's feelings and accepts them but also points out the responsibility of the client to take action. (1) (PI; CJ; IM)**
    1 Although this response identifies one of the client's concerns, the identification of the underlying feeling would be more therapeutic.
    2 This response makes the nurse responsible for changing the situation, which is not appropriate or therapeutic.
    3 This response denies the client's feelings and provides false reassurance.

80. **1 Knowing what to expect decreases anxiety. (1) (PB; MR; IM)**
    2 A sedative is not necessary for this test.
    3 A small amount of radiation is emitted during the scan; the client should be assured that the procedure is safe.
    4 Routine medications are not withheld unless ordered by the physician.

81. **1 The client is in the anger or "why me" stage; encouraging the expression of feelings will help the client resolve them and move toward acceptance. (2) (PI; CJ; IM)**
    2 This does not reflect on what the client said.
    3 This abdicates the responsibility of talking with the client; suggesting speaking with a minister ignores the client's present concerns.
    4 This judgmental response may precipitate feelings of guilt and block the nurse-client relationship.

82. **1 Fear of a recurrent myocardial infarction or sudden death is common when the client's environment is to be changed to one that appears less vigilant. (3) (PB; CJ; AN)**
    2 Depression is exhibited by withdrawal, crying, anorexia, and apathy and usually becomes more evident after discharge from the hospital.
    3 Dependency would be exhibited by an unwillingness to increase exercise or perform tasks.

4 Ambivalence is exhibited by contrasting emotions; the client's statement does not demonstrate this.

83. **1 Because vision will be somewhat limited after surgery, it is important to familiarize the client with vital aspects of the environment which would provide for physical and emotional safety. (2) (PB; MR; IM)**
    2 Surgery usually takes approximately two hours followed by a stay in the post anesthesia care unit.
    3 Coughing or other activity that increases intraocular pressure should be avoided.
    4 The physician should discuss the prognosis with the client; an explanation of what will occur during hospitalization will reduce anxiety while hospitalized.

84. **1 Voicing fears often reduces the associated anxiety. (2) (PI; CJ; IM)**
    2 Accepting the client's wishes is not of itself therapeutic.
    3 Encouraging socialization when the client has feelings that need exploration is not therapeutic.
    4 Avoiding the problem is not therapeutic.

85. **3 This is a truthful answer and validates the client's feelings. (2) (PI; MR; IM)**
    1 Although true, this response shuts off communication and further ventilation of feelings.
    2 This response denies the client's fears.
    4 This response denies the client's feelings.

BLOOD AND IMMUNITY (BI)

86. **4 These nutrients stimulate the immune system. (2) (PB; CJ; AN)**
    1 The role of fatty acids in natural defense mechanisms is uncertain.
    2 These have no known effect on natural defense mechanisms.
    3 Same as answer 2.

87. **4 Drains are usually inserted into the splenic bed to facilitate removal of fluid that could lead to abscess formation. (2) (PB; CJ; IM)**
    1 Splenectomy has a low mortality rate (5%) except when multiple injuries are present (15% to 40%).
    2 Bleeding occurs more commonly with splenic repair than with removal.
    3 There is no need to frighten the client unnecessarily, but the operative risk increases with multiple injuries.

88. 3 **With shock the heart rate accelerates to increase blood flow and oxygen to body tissues. (1) (PB; CJ; EV)**
   1 With shock there would be a decreased urinary output because of the lowered glomerular filtration rate.
   2 With shock the respirations would be increased and shallow.
   4 With shock there would be hypotension.

89. 3 **Because of the recumbent position, drainage may flow by gravity under the client and not be noticed unless the bedding is examined. (1) (PB; CJ; EV)**
   1 This assessment would be inaccurate when there is a dressing in place.
   2 In the immediate postoperative period vital signs should be taken more frequently than every four hours; in addition, observation of the site is a more reliable indicator of hemorrhage.
   4 Dressings impede an accurate assessment of the site for ecchymosis.

90. 4 **Hypovolemia results in a decreased cardiac output and a decreased arterial pressure, which are reflected by a feeble, weak peripheral pulse. (3) (PB; CJ; AS)**
   1 The skin would be cool and pale because of vasoconstriction.
   2 These are late signs of shock.
   3 The pulse pressure narrows with decreased cardiac pressure associated with hypovolemic shock.

91. 3 **In shock, arteriolar vasoconstriction occurs, raising the total peripheral vascular resistance and shifting blood to the major organs. (2) (PB; CJ; AN)**
   1 With shock more antidiuretic hormone (ADH) is produced to promote fluid retention, which will elevate the blood pressure.
   2 Although this is a response to hypoxia, peripheral vasoconstriction is a more effective compensatory mechanism.
   4 With shock the mineralocorticoids increase to promote fluid retention, which will elevate the blood pressure.

92. 1 **A decreased intravascular volume results in hypovolemia and hypotension, which is evidenced by a decreased blood pressure and a decreased pulse pressure. (3) (PB; CJ; AN)**
   2 Vasomotor stimulation to the arterial walls is increased with shock.
   3 This is a description of neurogenic shock, which is unlikely in this situation.

   4 Although electrolyte imbalances can precipitate cardiac decompensation, cardiogenic shock is unlikely in this situation.

93. 4 **When an abdominal aneurysm ruptures, shock ensues because fluid volume depletion occurs as the heart continues to pump blood out of the ruptured vessel. (2) (PB; CJ; AN)**
   1 This type of shock results from humoral or toxic substances acting directly on the blood vessels, causing vasodilation.
   2 This type of shock results from decreased neuromuscular tone, causing decreased vasoconstriction.
   3 This type of shock results from a decrease in cardiac output.

94. 2 **Peritonitis and shock are potentially life-threatening complications following abdominal surgery; prompt, rigorous treatment is necessary. (1) (PB; CJ; IM)**
   1 Fluids, not blood, would be needed to expand and maintain the circulating blood volume.
   3 The head of the bed should be flat to increase tissue perfusion and oxygenation to the vital organs.
   4 The physician should be notified; the client is already receiving oxygen and the problem still exists.

95. 1 **This occurs during the progressive stage of shock as a result of accumulated lactic acid. (2) (PB; CJ; AN)**
   2 Metabolic alkalosis cannot occur with the buildup of lactic acid.
   3 Eventually this can result from decreased respiratory function in late shock, further compounding metabolic acidosis.
   4 This may occur as a result of hyperventilation during early shock.

96. 3 **Blood replacement is needed to increase the oxygen-carrying capacity of the blood; the expected hematocrit for women is 37% to 47% and for men is 42% to 52%. (1) (PB; CJ; PL)**
   1 Ringer's lactate does not increase the oxygen-carrying capacity of the blood.
   2 Serum albumin helps maintain volume but does not affect the hematocrit level.
   4 Although dextran does expand blood volume, it decreases the hematocrit because it does not replace red blood cells.

97. 4 **The body attempts to compensate for decreased O_2 to tissues by increasing RBCs, the oxygen carrying component of the blood. (2) (PB; CJ; AS)**

1 With polycythemia the skin, especially the face, appears flushed, not pale.

2 This is not specific to polycythemia; there is more than one cause of dyspnea on exertion.

3 The hematocrit would be increased with polycythemia.

98. 4 **This is absolutely necessary to prevent an acute immunologic reaction if the donated blood is not compatible with the client's blood. (1) (SE; LE; PL)**

1 Although important, this is not the highest priority.

2 This is not the highest priority; these laboratory results were part of the data used to determine the need for the blood.

3 Blood must be kept cool until ready to use; if blood is at room temperature for 30 minutes prior to administration it should be returned to the blood bank; after it is started, blood must be administered within four hours.

99. 3 **Both types are compatible; A negative is the same as the client's blood type and preferred; in an emergency, type O negative blood may be given also. (2) (PB; CJ; PL)**

1 Although type O may be used, it would have to be Rh negative; Rh positive blood is incompatible with the client's and would cause hemolysis.

2 Type AB negative blood is incompatible with the client's blood and would cause hemolysis.

4 Type A negative is compatible with the client's blood but type AB negative is incompatible and would cause hemolysis.

100. 3 **A slow rate provides time to recognize a reaction that is developing before too much blood is administered. (2) (PB; LE; IM)**

1 This is avoided to prevent clotting and hemolysis.

2 Infusion pumps will cause red blood cell damage; blood should flow by gravity through an appropriate filter.

4 This is not necessary.

101. 1 **This is an adaptation associated with a hemolytic transfusion reaction; flank pain is caused by agglutination of red cells in the kidneys and renal vasoconstriction; the infusion must be stopped to prevent further instillation of blood which is being viewed as foreign by the body. (2) (PB; CJ; IM)**

2 Although this will be done eventually, it is not the priority action.

3 Same as answer 2.

4 Same as answer 2.

102. 4 **The blood must be stopped first, and then normal saline should be infused to keep the line patent and maintain blood volume. (2) (PB; CJ; IM)**

1 While the assessment was being made, the client's circulating blood volume would decrease.

2. This would be done later.

3 Same as answer 1.

103. 4 **Fat-soluble vitamin K is essential for synthesis of prothrombin by the liver; a lack results in hypoprothrombinemia, poor coagulation, and hemorrhage. (2) (PB; CJ; EV)**

1 Although cirrhosis may interfere with production of bile, which contains the bilirubin needed for optimum absorption of vitamin K, the best and quickest manner to counteract the bleeding is to provide vitamin K intramuscularly.

2 This is a coenzyme with vitamins B_{12} and C in the formation of nucleic acids and heme; thus a deficiency may lead to anemia, not bleeding.

3 A vitamin A deficiency contributes to development of polyneuritis and beriberi, not hemorrhage.

104. 4 **The length of time a low-grade temperature is present, together with a history of night sweats and other physical findings, is valuable in making a diagnosis. (2) (PM; CJ; AS)**

1 This is not immediately relevant to presenting signs and symptoms; more should be explored about the temperature itself before investigating causes of the temperature.

2 Same as answer 1.

3 Same as answer 1.

105. 2 **Equipment used is disposable; the donor does not come into contact with anyone else's blood. (1) (SE; CJ; AN)**

1 The risk would depend on the spouse's prior behavior.

3 Although condoms do offer protection, they are subject to failure because of condom rupture or improper use; risks of infection are present with any sexual contact.

4 An individual may be infected before testing positive for the antibodies; the individual could still transmit the virus.

106. 1 **These tests confirm the presence of HIV anti-bodies that occur in response to the presence of the human immunodeficiency virus. (1) (PB; CJ; AS)**
   2 This places someone at risk but does not constitute a positive diagnosis.
   3 These do not confirm the presence of HIV; these adaptations are related to many disorders.
   4 An opportunistic infection (included in the CDC surveillance case definition for AIDS) in the presence of HIV antibodies indicates that the individual has AIDS.

107. 1 **The HIV selectively infects helper T cell lymphocytes; therefore 300 or fewer CD4 T cells per cubic millimeter of blood or CD4 cells accounting for less than 20% of lymphocytes is suggestive of AIDS. (1) (PB; CJ; AS)**
   2 The thymic hormones necessary for T cell growth are decreased.
   3 This finding is associated with allergies and parasitic infections.
   4 This finding is associated with drug-induced hemolytic anemia and hemolytic disease of the newborn.

108. 4 **Since this procedure does not involve contact with blood or secretions, additional protection is not indicated. (1) (SE; CJ; IM)**
   1 These are necessary only when there is risk of contact with blood or body fluid.
   2 Same as answer 1.
   3 A mask and gown would be indicated only if there were a danger of secretions or blood splattering on the nurse (for example, during suctioning).

109. 2 **These items prevent contact with feces, sputum, or other body fluids during intimate body care. (2) (SE; CJ; AN)**
   1 Goggles alone would be inadequate because the client is producing copious sputum.
   3 Gloves are not necessary because touching body fluids when giving oral medication is not likely.
   4 Gloves are necessary when assisting the client with a bedpan.

110. 3 *Pneumocystis carinii* **is a protozoan that causes pneumonia in immunosuppressed hosts, which can cause death in 60% of the clients; the client's respiratory status is the priority. (3) (SE; CJ; AN)**
   1 Although this is a concern, the client's respiratory status is the priority.
   2 Same as answer 1.

4 There are no data to support this diagnosis.

111. 3 **Pernicious anemia is caused by the inability to absorb vitamin B_{12} resulting from a lack of intrinsic factor in gastric juices; for the Schilling test, radioactive vitamin B_{12} is administered and its absorption and excretion can be ascertained. (3) (PB; CJ; AS)**
   1 This is not measured by this test.
   2 Same as answer 1.
   4 Vitamin B_{12} is not produced in the body.

112. 3 **IM injections bypass the vitamin B_{12} absorption defect (lack of intrinsic factor, the transport carrier component of gastric juices); a monthly dose is usually sufficient since it is stored in active body tissues such as the liver, kidney, heart, muscles, blood, and bone marrow. (3) (SE; MR; IM)**
   1 The Z-track method need not be used as it is for iron dextran injections; injections once a month are usually sufficient.
   2 Since it is stored and only slowly depleted, it is not necessary to give injections this often.
   4 Vitamin B_{12} cannot be taken by mouth because of the lack of intrinsic factor.

113. 3 **Since the intrinsic factor does not return to gastric secretions even with therapy, B_{12} injections will be required for the remainder of the client's life. (2) (SE; CJ; EV)**
   1 It must be taken on a regular basis for the rest of the client's life.
   2 Same as answer 1.
   4 Same as answer 1.

114. 2 **A protocol consisting of three or four chemotherapeutic agents that attack the dividing cells at various phases of development is the therapy of choice at this stage; alternating courses of different protocols may be used. (3) (PB; CJ; PL)**
   1 Radiation, alone or in combination with chemotherapy, is used in stages IA, IB, IIA, IIB, and IIIA.
   3 This is recommended for use in stage IIIA.
   4 This is not a therapy for Hodgkin's disease at any stage; nodes may be removed for biopsy; nodes may be irradiated as part of therapy.

115. 1 **Women in the childbearing years should be informed of all options available to preserve ovarian function. (3) (SE; MR; AN)**
   2 This is an incorrect statement because radiation can influence or destroy ovarian functioning.
   3 Sterilization could occur; therefore, the ovaries should be protected.

4 Once ova have been destroyed they cannot regenerate.

116. 2 Because of the location of the spleen, postoperative pain will cause splinting and shallow breathing and underaeration of the lung's left lower lobe. (2) (PB; CJ; PL)
1 This would be true of any abdominal surgery and is not specific to a splenectomy.
3 Same as answer 1.
4 Same as answer 1.

117. 2 Moderate leukopenia increases the risk of infection; the client should be taught protective measures. (2) (SE; MR; PL)
1 Leukopenia is a side effect of cyclophosphamide (Cytoxan), not prednisone.
3 The platelet count is not given, so bleeding precautions are not indicated.
4 These are measures to correct anemia; protection from infection takes priority.

118. 4 Thrombocytopenia occurs with most chemotherapy treatment programs; using a soft toothbrush helps prevent bleeding gums. (1) (PB; CJ; IM)
1 While alopecia does occur, it is not related to bone marrow depression.
2 Increasing fluids will neither reverse bone marrow depression nor stimulate hematopoiesis.
3 This is not related to bone marrow depression.

119. 1 Suppression of bone marrow increases bleeding susceptibility associated with decreased platelets. (1) (PB; CJ; IM)
2 This will not affect the bone marrow; citrus juices should be avoided by the client receiving chemotherapy because of the side effects of stomatitis.
3 With bone marrow depression there would be a decrease in red blood cells; rest should be encouraged.
4 With bone marrow suppression the red blood cells are decreased in number and there is a decreased oxygen-carrying capacity of the blood; this position will not increase the number of red blood cells.

120. 2 Myelosuppression involves decreased red blood cells (anemia) resulting in less oxygen-carrying capacity of the blood and fatigue; decreased white blood cells (leukopenia) resulting in potential for infection; and decreased platelets (thrombocytopenia) resulting in potential for bleeding. (2) (PB; MR; IM)

1 Myelosuppression is not directly related to calcium deposition; myelosuppression, a reduction in bone marrow activity, results in decreased numbers of RBCs, WBCs, and platelets.
3 Myelosuppression is not related to these responses.
4 Myelosuppression is related to bone marrow activity, not the nervous system.

121. 1 Brief pressure is generally enough to prevent bleeding. (2) (PB; CJ; IM)
2 Complications are rare; no special positions are required.
3 The site is cleaned prior to aspiration.
4 Complications are rare; frequent monitoring is unnecessary.

122. 3 The hypermetabolic state associated with leukemia causes more urea and uric acid (end products of metabolism) to be produced and to accumulate in the blood. (3) (PB; CJ; AN)
1 Thrombocytopenia causes a decrease in platelets, which causes bleeding.
2 Enlarged lymph nodes would not increase blood urea and uric acid.
4 Hepatic encephalopathy is associated with liver disease, not leukemia.

123. 3 Anemia with petechiae occurs because of bone marrow depression and rapidly proliferating leukocytes; all organs of the body are involved with the development of anorexia. (3) (PB; CJ; AS)
1 While anorexia occurs, the client would more likely be sleeping excessively.
2 There is no change in hair growth in the absence of chemotherapy.
4 Same as answer 2.

124. 4 Thrombocytes are involved in the clotting mechanism; thrombocytopenia is a reduced number of thrombocytes in the blood; hematuria is blood in the urine. (1) (PB; CJ; EV)
1 Fever is a sign of infection; infection results when the white blood cells are reduced (leukopenia).
2 Diarrhea is unrelated to thrombocytopenia; diarrhea may result from the effects of chemotherapy on the rapidly dividing cells of the gastrointestinal system.
3 Headache is unrelated to thrombocytopenia; headache may be caused by the effects of chemotherapy on the central nervous system cells or indicate that the leukemia has invaded the central nervous system.

125. 2 This protein (globulin) results from tumor cell metabolites; it is present in clients with multiple myeloma. (3) (PB; CJ; AN)

1 Hypercalcemia, not hypocalcemia, occurs with multiple myeloma because of bone erosion.

3 This is not specific for the diagnosis of multiple myeloma; it is a late complication of multiple myeloma related to coagulation defects.

4 Multiple myeloma is not caused by a bacterial infection.

126. 1 A definite confirmation of multiple myeloma can only be made through a bone marrow biopsy; this is a plasma cell malignancy with widespread bone destruction. (2) (PB; CJ; AN)

2 While calcium is lost from bone tissue and hypercalcemia results, this is not a confirmation of the disease.

3 While this protein is found in the urine, it does not confirm the disease.

4 X-ray films will show the characteristic "punched-out" areas caused by the increase in the number of plasma cells, which contributes to the making of the diagnosis; the definitive diagnosis is made on biopsy.

127. 4 Because of bone erosion, pathologic fractures are a common complication of multiple myeloma. (2) (PB; CJ; PL)

1 Although this would be done, the priority is to prevent injury.

2 Although this is an adaptation to the associated anemia, it is not life threatening.

3 Although this is important, preventing pathologic fractures is the priority.

128. 4 A variety of drugs affect rapidly dividing cells at different stages of cell division. (3) (PB; CJ; AN)

1 Although this is an acceptable therapy, it is not the first treatment used.

2 This is not a primary approach; it may be used to alleviate pain and treat acute vertebral lesions.

3 Multiple myeloma is a disorder of the bone; there are no lesions that can be removed.

129. 1 Because an elevated temperature increases metabolic demands, the pyrexia must be treated immediately; the physician should be notified because this client is immunodeficient, from both the disease and the chemotherapy; a search for the cause of the pyrexia can then be initiated. (3) (PB; MR; IM)

2 More vigorous intervention is necessary; this client has a disease in which the immunoglobulins are ineffective and the therapy further suppresses the immune system.

3 This is not the immediate priority, although it is important because the cause of the pyrexia must be determined; also, the increased amount of calcium and urates in the urine can cause renal complications if dehydration occurs.

4 This is not the priority, although important because respiratory tract infections are a common occurrence in clients with multiple myeloma.

130. 1 Blood products (packed RBCs or platelets) are administered when warranted. (1) (PB; MR; IM)

2 Renal insufficiency, not infections, may occur due to chronic hypercalcemia, proteinemia, and hyperuricemia.

3 Fluid replacement should be provided in carefully supervised clinical settings because if dehydration occurs it may result in renal shutdown.

4 Ultraviolet rays are not related to exacerbations.

131. 4 These drugs suppress the immune system, decreasing the body's production of antibodies in response to the new organ which acts as an antigen; these drugs decrease the risk of rejection. (3) (PB; CJ; AN)

1 Leukocytosis is inhibited by these drugs.

2 These drugs do not provide immunity; they interfere with natural immune responses.

3 Because these drugs suppress the immune system, they increase the risk of infection.

132. 1 Systemic lupus erythematosus is an autoimmune disease and physical and emotional stresses have been identified as contributing factors to the occurrence of exacerbations. (2) (PB; MR; IM)

2 Although this would be done, inadequate hygiene is not known to produce exacerbations.

3 Although this would be done, nutritional status has not been significantly correlated to exacerbations.

4 Knowledge of the symptoms would not decrease the occurrence of exacerbations.

133. 1 Tetanus antitoxin provides antibodies, which confer immediate passive immunity. (3) (SE; MR; IM)

2 Antitoxin does not stimulate production of plasma cells, the precursors of antibodies.

3 Passive, not active, immunity occurs.

4 Passive immunity, by definition, is not long lasting.

134. 1 It takes this length of time for antibodies to respond to the antigen and form an indurated area. (1) (PM; CJ; AS)
  2 This is longer than necessary; the site will reveal induration in two to three days.
  3 Same as answer 2.
  4 Same as answer 2.

135. 1 Drug hypersensitivity and anaphylaxis are most common with antimicrobial agents. (1) (SE; LE; IM)
  2 This is a dependent function; it is not crucial to starting antibiotic therapy.
  3 This is an important assessment, but it is not crucial to starting antibiotic therapy.
  4 Withholding treatment until culture results are available may extend the infection.

136. 3 Hypersensitivity to a foreign substance can cause an anaphylactic reaction; histamine is released, causing bronchial constriction, increased capillary permeability, and dilation of arterioles; this decreased peripheral resistance is associated with hypotension and inadequate circulation to major organs. (3) (PB; CJ; AN)
  1 These are the problems that result from bronchial constriction and vascular collapse.
  2 Dilation of arterioles occurs.
  4 Arterioles dilate, capillary permeability increases, and eventually vascular collapse occurs.

137. 3 Activity may encourage the dislodgement of more microemboli. (2) (PB; CJ; AN)
  1 Bed rest may enhance platelet aggregation and the formation of thrombi because of venous stasis.
  2 Venous stasis, rather than enhanced circulation, is supported by bed rest.
  4 Bed rest supports venous stasis rather than the circulation of blood to damaged tissues.

138. 4 This is the first screening test done to detect serum antibodies that bind to HIV antigens on test plates. (1) (PB; CJ; AS)
  1 This screening test is not done first; the Western blot is done to validate repeatedly reactive ELISA results.
  2 This is not a screening test; it is done to monitor the progression of HIV infection and response to treatment.
  3 This is not an initial screening test; it is done when there are consistently inconclusive test results with previous screening tests.

139. 4 This test assesses parietal cell function; after radioactive cobalamin is administered, its excretion is measured; if cobalamin cannot be absorbed as in pernicious anemia, very little is excreted in the urine. (2) (PB; CJ; AS)
  1 This test is not affected by medications.
  2 The results of this test are not affected by food; with pernicious anemia there is a deficiency of intrinsic factor, which is necessary for vitamin B_{12} use.
  3 Intake and output records are not necessary with a Shilling test.

CARDIOVASCULAR (CV)

140. 3 The carotid artery is located along the anterior edge of the sternocleidomastoid muscle at the level of the lower margin of the thyroid cartilage. (1) (PB; CJ; AS)
  1 This is not the anatomic landmark for locating the carotid artery.
  2 Same as answer 1.
  4 Same as answer 1.

141. 2 The first heart sound is produced by closure of the mitral and tricuspid valves; it is heard best at the apex of the heart. (2) (PB; CJ; AS)
  1 This is where the second heart sound (S2) is best heard; S2 is produced by closure of the aortic and pulmonic valves.
  3 This border covers a large area; the auscultatory areas that lie near it are the pulmonic and mitral areas.
  4 This border covers a large area; the only auscultatory area near it is the aortic area.

142. 1 Closure of the atrioventricular valves, the mitral and tricuspid, produces the first heart sound (S1). (3) (PB; CJ; AN)
  2 These valves do not close simultaneously.
  3 Same as answer 2.
  4 These are the semilunar valves; closure of these valves produces the second heart sound (S2).

143. 1 Dysrhythmias are abnormal and are associated with acute or chronic pathologic conditions. (1) (PB; CJ; AS)
  2 The normal range in adults is 60 to 100 beats per minute.
  3 This is expected; the radial pulse reflects ventricular contractions.
  4 These are the anatomical landmarks for locating the apex of the heart; they are unaffected by aging.

144. 1 Inactivity causes venous stasis, hypercoagula-bility, and external pressure against the veins, all of which lead to thrombus formation; early ambulation or exercise of the lower extremities reduces the occurrence of this phenomenon. (1) (PB; CJ; IM)
   2 Although this may help, the primary inter-vention is to provide exercise of the extrem-ities until ambulation is permitted.
   3 This will be helpful, but it is not an inde-pendent activity; elastic stockings require a physician's order.
   4 Massaging the client's legs would be con-traindicated because any developing clot could be dislodged.

145. 2 Oxygen is necessary for the production of fire. (1) (SE; CJ; PL)
   1 Oxygen does not burn; it supports combus-tion.
   3 This is irrelevant regarding the need for safety precautions.
   4 Same as answer 3.

146. 3 This is an early typical finding after a myocar-dial infarct because of the altered contractility of the heart. (3) (PB; CJ; AS)
   1 Flattened or depressed T waves indicate hypokalemia.
   2 This occurs in atrial and ventricular fibrilla-tion.
   4 Q waves may become distorted with conduc-tion or rhythm problems, but they do not disappear unless there is cardiac standstill.

147. 4 Pulmonary capillary wedge pressure is an indi-rect measure of left ventricular end diastolic pressure, an indication of ventricular contrac-tility. (2) (PB; CJ; AN)
   1 Right atrial pressure measures only the func-tion of the right side of the heart and indi-rectly its ability to receive blood.
   2 Cardiac output by thermodilution does not measure intracardiac pressures.
   3 Pulmonary artery diastolic pressure may not be as accurate an indicator of left ventricu-lar pressure if COPD or pulmonary hyper-tension exists.

148. 2 This is a radionuclear study that determines viability of myocardial tissue; necrotic or scar tissue does not extract the thallium isotope. (2) (PB; CJ; AN)
   1 This information is available from cardiac catheterization with angiography.
   3 Same as answer 1.
   4 This is determined by a 12-lead ECG.

149. 1 Hypovolemia occurs with decreased cardiac output and the resulting decreased arterial pressure is reflected in weak, thready peripheral pulses. (2) (PB; CJ; AS)
   2 The skin would be cool and pale because of vasoconstriction.
   3 The pulse pressure would be decreased, not increased, with decreased cardiac output associated with hypovolemic shock.
   4 This would occur later as a result of hypov-olemic shock.

150. 1 Sitting maintains alignment of the back and allows the nurses to support the client until ortho-static hypotension subsides. (2) (PB; CJ; IM)
   2 Rapid movement could flex the vertebrae, which would traumatize the spinal cord; taking the blood pressure at this time is not necessary.
   3 This would induce flexion of the vertebrae, which could traumatize the spinal cord.
   4 Same as answer 3.

151. 1 If a closed chest drainage tube becomes obstructed there is increased intrathoracic pres-sure which pushes the heart to the opposite side, thereby reducing venous return and cardiac output. (2) (PB; CJ; IM)
   2 Dyspnea may develop but is not life threat-ening.
   3 A pneumothorax is unrelated to abdominal pressure and if it did occur it is not life threatening.
   4 A hemothorax is not life threatening.

152. 4 This is the recommended allotment of servings from the bread, cereal, rice, and pasta group. (1) (PB; CJ; IM)
   1 An adult should consume 2 to 4 servings of fruit daily.
   2 An adult should consume 3 to 5 servings of vegetables daily.
   3 An adult should consume 2 to 3 servings of meat, poultry, or fish daily.

153. 3 The essential fatty acids, linoleic acid and linolenic acid, are necessary for muscle tissue integrity, especially of the myocardium. (2) (PB; MR; IM)
   1 All fats cannot and should not be elimi-nated from the diet.
   2 Proteins and carbohydrates do not contain the essential fatty acids linoleic acid and linolenic acid.
   4 The body does manufacture cholesterol.

154. 2 Gradual occlusion of the carotid arteries, man-ifested by the transient ischemia attacks, is

caused almost exclusively by atherosclerotic thrombosis. (1) (PB; CJ; AN)

1 Valvular heart disease, whether acquired or congenital, usually causes cerebral emboli, not gradual occlusion of the carotid arteries.

3 Emboli resulting from atrial fibrillation cause complete, not partial, occlusion of the vessels; the occlusion occurs suddenly, not gradually.

4 Developmental defects of the arterial wall are associated with saccular aneurysms.

155. 4 **The fiber component of complex carbohydrates helps bind and eliminate dietary cholesterol and fosters growth of intestinal microorganisms to break down bile salts and release the cholesterol component for excretion. (3) (PB; MR; IM)**

1 It is what the client eats, not when the client eats, that is important.

2 Of the fats in the diet, saturated fats should be decreased.

3 Fat-binding fiber should be increased.

156. 4 **Chocolate has a high caffeine content, which may stimulate catecholamine release and act as a cardiac stimulant. (1) (PB; MR; IM)**

1 Yogurt is not a cardiac stimulant; it aids digestion if lactose intolerance is present.

2 Red meat does not stimulate the myocardium; it may be decreased or eliminated if serum cholesterol levels are elevated.

3 Club soda may contain sodium chloride but does not stimulate the myocardium.

157. 4 **The original myocardial infarct may be extending; the client's symptoms require immediate medical intervention and relief of pain. (3) (PB; CJ; IM)**

1 While this might be done after notification of the physician, notification and pain relief are the priorities.

2 An ECG will provide additional data but will cause a delay in notification of the physician and provision of necessary medical intervention.

3 Nitroglycerin does not relieve the pain associated with a myocardial infarction.

158. 3 **Of all the basic food groups, fresh fruits and juices are the lowest in sodium. (2) (PB; MR; PL)**

1 Most fresh meat or fish contain approximately 50 to 120 mg of sodium per 100 g; processed meats contain approximately 1700 to 2000 mg of sodium per 100 g.

2 Most aged cheeses contain approximately 300 to 1100 mg of sodium per 100 g of cheese.

4 Most dry cereals contain approximately 900 to 1100 mg of sodium per 100 g of cereal.

159. 3 **Angina usually is caused by narrowing of the coronary arteries; the lumen of the arteries can be assessed by cardiac catheterization. (2) (PB; MR; IM)**

1 Although pressures can be obtained, they are not the priority for this client; this assessment is appropriate for those with valvular disease.

2 This is appropriate for infants and young adults with cardiac birth defects.

4 This is appropriate for infants and young children with suspected septal defects.

160. 3 **Bed rest with immobilization of the leg promotes coagulation and healing at the puncture site of the femoral artery. (1) (PB; CJ; AN)**

1 In the absence of bleeding and the presence of adequate fluid replacement, a cardiac catheterization does not cause orthostatic hypotension.

2 These symptoms are not expected after a cardiac catheterization.

4 A small amount of radiopaque dye is injected (via the catheter) directly into the heart, where it is diluted by the blood; it does not create a problem at the puncture site.

161. 3 **Tingling indicates decreased arterial circulation to the extremity; it may be caused by an embolus distal to the arterial insertion site; checking all pulses would help locate an embolus. (3) (PB; CJ; AN)**

1 Tingling sensations of an extremity are not related to bleeding, but rather to lack of circulation.

2 These signs are associated with thrombophlebitis; tingling is associated with arterial obstruction.

4 This would be done if there were systemic responses to compromised heart function; tingling in an extremity is a localized response.

162. 1 **There is increased urinary output as a result of the diuretic affect of the contrast medium. (3) (PB; CJ; EV)**

2 A decrease of 10% to 20% is expected because of the diuretic effect of the contrast medium; a decrease greater than 20% may be pathologic.

3 Respiratory distress may be an indication of a pulmonary embolus from a venous clot and should be reported immediately.

4 Although this may occur during the procedure because of trauma to the conduction system, it usually does not continue after the procedure.

163. **2 An apical pulse is taken to detect dysrhythmias related to cardiac irritability; blood pressure is monitored to detect hypotension, which may indicate bleeding or shock. (1) (PB; CJ; EV)**
   1 This is contraindicated; flexion of the groin may compromise the clot at the femoral insertion site.
   3 This is not necessary; the client did not undergo general anesthesia and will be ambulatory in four to six hours.
   4 A temperature may indicate a bacterial invasion, but this will not be evident during the first few hours after the catheterization.

164. **4 The supine position prevents hip flexion, limiting injury and promoting healing of the catheter insertion site; if the head of the bed is elevated, it should not exceed 20 degrees. (1) (PB; CJ; PL)**
   1 Hip flexion traumatizes the catheter insertion site and should be avoided for at least four hours to promote healing.
   2 This is unnecessary; the gastrointestinal system is not involved and general anesthesia is not used.
   3 This would interfere with rest; the vital signs are measured every 15 minutes until stable, usually for one hour.

165. **3 A warm flushing sensation that lasts approximately 30 seconds will occur when the contrast medium is injected. (1) (PB; MR; IM)**
   1 Medication is given for mild sedation; clients are drowsy but awake enough to follow instructions.
   2 The supine position will be maintained for four to six hours postoperatively; walking may dislodge clots at the catheter insertion site resulting in bleeding.
   4 The supine position is maintained four to six hours postoperatively; the semi-Fowler's position flexes the legs, which may result in bleeding at the femoral insertion site.

166. **4 This is a classic reaction because it dilates coronary arteries, which increases O_2 to the myocardium, thus decreasing pain. (1) (PB; CJ; AN)**
   1 Anginal pain is frequently relieved by immediate rest.
   2 Angina is usually precipitated by exertion, emotion, or a heavy meal.
   3 Angina is usually described as tightness, indigestion, or heaviness.

167. **1 A reclining position would be used to maintain blood supply to vital centers. (2) (PB; CJ; PL)**
   2 This is unsafe; maintaining blood flow to vital centers is essential.
   3 Maintaining blood flow to vital centers, not comfort, is the priority.
   4 While the semi-Fowler's position would facilitate breathing, it would not assist blood flow to vital centers.

168. **3 A sustained diastolic pressure exceeding 90 mm Hg reflects pathology and indicates hypertension. (1) (PM; CJ; AS)**
   1 This is unrelated to hypertension.
   2 This reflects the heart rate, not the pressures within the artery.
   4 Initially hypertension usually is asymptomatic; although headaches can be associated with hypertension, there are other causes of headaches.

169. **3 Further assessment is necessary before the nurse can plan a course of action. (2) (PB; CJ; AS)**
   1 This is not an initial nursing action; further assessment is the priority.
   2 The nurse must gather further data before consulting with the physician.
   4 This is not an expected blood pressure for an older adult; both systolic and diastolic pressures are elevated.

170. **3 Muscle contraction associated with walking prevents edema and pooling of blood in the extremities. (1) (PB; CJ; IM)**
   1 Movement is required, not inactivity.
   2 Same as answer 1.
   4 This does not include movement, which is essential to prevent thrombus formation.

171. **3 The failing left ventricle cannot accept blood returning from the lungs; this results in increased vascular pressure in the lungs. (3) (PB; CJ; AN)**
   1 This is associated with right ventricular failure.
   2 There is no such diagnosis of right atrial failure as a separate entity.
   4 Wheezing and coughing are associated with paroxysmal nocturnal dyspnea and right ventricular failure.

172. **1 Blockage of the myocardial blood supply causes accumulation of unoxidized metabolites that affect nerve endings that generally cause pain. (3) (PB; CJ; AS)**

2 The pain usually is crushing, severe, and of prolonged duration.

3 The pain usually is typically severe.

4 The pain is unrelieved by nitroglycerin.

173. **2 These are classic symptoms of a myocardial infarction; further medical evaluation is needed immediately. (1) (PB; CJ; IM)**

1 This response presumes a dietary problem when a more serious situation may exist; the client needs medical intervention.

3 This response considers only an emotional source of the reported symptoms and ignores a potential medical emergency.

4 This provides false reassurance and ignores a potential medical emergency.

174. **1 Morphine is an opioid analgesic that acts on the central nervous system by a sympathetic mechanism; it decreases systemic vascular resistance, which decreases left ventricular afterload, thus decreasing myocardial oxygen consumption. (2) (PB; CJ; IM)**

2 Oxygen administration elevates arterial oxygen tension with the potential for improving tissue oxygenation; however, oxygen administration does not relieve the pain.

3 Nitroglycerin sublingually is effective in relieving anginal pain but not myocardial infarction pain.

4 Lidocaine is an antidysrhythmic, not an analgesic.

175. **1 Physical activity need not be restricted; clients who have had a myocardial infarction have a cardiovascular rehabilitation exercise program prescribed; exercises should become a part of the client's lifestyle. (2) (SE; MR; IM)**

2 This is desirable because aspirin decreases platelet aggregation.

3 This is desirable because cigarette smoking causes arterial constriction.

4 This is desirable because obesity increases the body's oxygen demands, which increases the work load of the heart.

176. **1 Unrelieved chest pain increases anxiety, fatigue, and myocardial oxygen consumption with the possibility of extending the infarction. (2) (PB; CJ; PL)**

2 The client will not be ready for teaching until the chest pain is relieved.

3 Cardiac monitoring is important, but it does not take priority over relieving the subjective complaint of chest pain.

4 Bed rest is necessary to decrease the workload of the heart, but decreasing the cardiac workload will be difficult to achieve unless the chest pain is relieved.

177. **2 Morphine is a specific central nervous system depressant used to relieve the pain associated with myocardial infarction; it also decreases apprehension and prevents cardiogenic shock. (2) (PB; CJ; IM)**

1 This is not the reason for the use of morphine.

3 This is not the primary reason for the use of morphine.

4 Lidocaine is given intravenously to accomplish this.

178. **3 This response addresses the client's behavior and explains the rationale for bed rest. (2) (PB; CJ; IM)**

1 This is a demeaning response.

2 This identifies feelings but does nothing to reduce the oxygen demands on the heart.

4 This is an authoritarian response, which may precipitate negative feelings in the client.

179. **4 Defecation in the sitting position on a bedside commode uses less energy than walking to the bathroom or getting on and off a bedpan. (2) (PB; CJ; IM)**

1 Defecation is difficult on a bedpan and may cause straining and an increase in oxygen demands.

2 Walking to the bathroom uses more energy than using a bedside commode.

3 Although the use of a fracture pan takes less energy than using a regular bedpan, it takes more energy than using a commode.

180. **3 A decreased urinary output reflects a decreased cardiac output; immediate action is indicated if urinary output decreases. (3) (PB; CJ; AS)**

1 While anxiety may occur, the priority is to monitor urinary output, which reflects cardiac effectiveness.

2 Enzyme results do not reflect effectiveness of cardiac contractions; they reflect tissue damage.

4 While this would be done, urinary output reflects decreased cardiac output; monitoring urinary output is a priority.

181. 3 Troponin I (cTnI) and troponin T (cTnT) are proteins in the striated cells of cardiac tissue and are therefore unique markers for cardiac damage; elevations occur within one hour of a myocardial infarction and persist for 7 to 15 days. (3) (PB; CJ; AS)

1 Serum aspartate aminotransferase (AST) levels begin to rise in 4 to 6 hours, peak at approximately 24 hours, and remain elevated for 3 to 4 days.

2 Myoglobin is the oxygen-binding protein of striated muscle; although it rises within the first few hours after a myocardial infarction, it lacks cardiac specificity.

4 Creatine kinase (CK) isoenzyme levels, especially the MB subunit, begin to rise within 3 to 6 hours, peak in 12 to 18 hours, and are elevated for 48 hours after the occurrence of the infarct.

182. 3 The skin becomes cool and pale as blood shunts from the peripheral blood vessels to the vital organs. (2) (PB; CJ; AS)

1 The heart rate increases in an attempt to meet the oxygen demands of the body.

2 Restlessness occurs because of cerebral hypoxia.

4 The urine output drops to less than 30 mL per hour because of decreased arterial perfusion to the kidneys and the compensatory mechanism of reabsorbing fluid to increase the circulating blood volume.

183. 4 A direct relationship exists between the strength of cardiac contractions and the electrical conductions through the myocardium. (3) (PB; CJ; AN)

1 The heart rate is related to factors such as SA node function, partial pressures of oxygen and carbon dioxide, and emotions.

2 This is the period when the heart is at rest, not when it is contracting.

3 Pulmonary pressure does not influence action potential; it becomes elevated in the presence of left ventricular failure.

184. 3 At least one half of all deaths occur from the life-threatening dysrhythmia of ventricular tachycardia. (2) (SE; CJ; AS)

1 This can occur, but it can be treated aggressively with expectation of recovery.

2 This can occur, but it can be treated so that the client does recover.

4 Failure of the left, not right, ventricle would more likely occur.

185. 3 Dyspnea at night, which usually requires the assumption of the orthopneic position, is a sign of left ventricular failure; orthopnea, a compensatory mechanism, limits venous return, which decreases pulmonary congestion and promotes ventilation, easing the dyspnea. (2) (PB; CJ; AS)

1 This occurs with right ventricular failure because of hypervolemia.

2 Anorexia and nausea occur with right ventricular failure because of venous stasis and venous engorgement of abdominal viscera; weight gain would occur because of fluid retention.

4 This occurs with right ventricular failure because of portal hypertension and liver congestion.

186. 4 A direct relationship exists between the systolic blood pressure and the force of left ventricular contraction. (2) (PB; CJ; AN)

1 An increased blood volume would be indicated by hypertension, not a decreased pulse pressure.

2 Hyperactivity of the heart would be indicated by dysrhythmias and tachycardia.

3 A decreased pulse pressure would indicate decreased cardiac sufficiency.

187.

4 __x__ This is the mitral area at the fifth intercostal space at the left midclavicular line (also called apex of the heart); the S$_1$ heart sound (closure of the mitral and tricuspid valves, the "lub" in the "lub-dub" associated with heart sounds) is heard here; mitral insufficiency produces a high-pitched blowing sound throughout systole. (3) (PB; CJ; AS)

1 ____ This is the aortic area at the second intercostal space to the right of the sternum; this area best reflects closure of the semilunar valves: pulmonic valve between the right ventricle and pulmonary artery; aortic valve between the left ventricle and the aorta; ejection clicks associated with aortic stenosis are heard at this site.

2 ____ This is the pulmonic area at the second intercostal space to the left of the sternum; this area best reflects problems of the pulmonic valve such as pulmonic stenosis.

3 ____ This area is not part of the assessment of the heart; this is the area over the

right main bronchus, which is used to assess bronchovesicular breath sounds.

188. 2 This is the cardinal reason for PVCs. (2) (PB; CJ; AS)
1   This is a type of dysrhythmia, not the cause of PVCs; the source of atrial fibrillation is the atrium, not the ventricles.
3   This type of dysrhythmia is associated with interference with the conduction system.
4   This is a type of dysrhythmia, not the cause of PVCs.

189. 3 This response provides information and reduces anxiety; the nurse should understand that the greater saphenous vein of the leg is used to bypass the diseased coronary artery because one surgical team can obtain the vein while another team performs the chest surgery; this shortens the surgical time and lessens the risks of surgery; the internal mammary arteries are the grafts of choice but the surgery is usually longer because of the procedure of dissecting the arteries from the chest wall. (1) (PB; MR; IM)
1   Cardiopulmonary bypass (extracorporeal circulation) is accomplished by placement of a cannula in the right atrium, vena cava, or femoral vein to withdraw blood from the body; blood is returned to the body via a cannula in the aorta or the femoral artery.
2   This is not done during a coronary artery bypass graft (CABG).
4   Same as answer 2.

190. 4 This addresses the client's request for information; the energy required for sexual intercourse is equivalent to that of climbing one flight of stairs. (3) (PB; MR; IM)
1   Each client is different and may require more or less than six weeks.
2   This avoids the client's question and cuts off communication; the nurse has a responsibility to teach.
3   This answer is too vague and may be dangerous because the client has no basis to make a safe decision.

191. 1 This type of pacemaker synchronizes impulses to the atria and ventricles to more closely simulate the normal action of the heart; it may be a fixed-rate or, most usually, a demand-mode pacemaker and may stimulate the atria, the ventricles, or both. (2) (PB; CJ; IM)
2   The physiologic pacemaker stimulates both the atria and ventricles to contract.
3   It will increase the heartbeat to a more normal rate.

4   It affects the electrical conduction system of the heart, not the anatomic structures.

192. 3 Assessment of the heart's rate and rhythm determines how the newly implanted pacemaker is functioning. (2) (PB; CJ; EV)
1   Unless the client is dehydrated, encouraging fluid would increase the workload of the heart.
2   Although this is an appropriate action, the priority is to assess the functioning of the pacemaker.
4   Same as answer 2.

193. 3 This information will reduce anxiety; milliamps are used, not volts of electricity; higher voltages are needed to electrocute. (1) (SE; MR; IM)
1   This is a patronizing response and minimizes the stated concern.
2   The voltage used in pacemakers can never cause electrocution; technology is not related.
4   The voltage used can never cause electrocution; pacemakers are pretested for accuracy.

194. 3 Heart failure causes a fluid volume excess that results in pulmonary edema and dyspnea in the supine position. (2) (PB; CJ; AS)
1   This is unrelated to the cardiopulmonary system.
2   Same as answer 1.
4   Dependent edema usually occurs after standing or walking; swelling of the ankles would be more evident in the evening, not the morning.

195. 1 Shoes that become too tight indicate pedal edema, which is a sign of fluid retention; 2.2 pounds is equal to 1 liter of fluid. (3) (PB; CJ; AS)
2   Eventually the physician will be notified, but the nurse should have more data before this.
3   With fluid retention the rate is not as significant as a bounding characteristic to the pulse.
4   Although left ventricular failure can proceed to right ventricular failure, the client has given no indication that pulmonary edema may be developing.

196. 4 Dyspnea on exertion occurs with heart failure because of the heart's inability to meet the oxygen needs of body tissues. (1) (PB; CJ; AS)
1   This is not specific to heart failure.
2   Same as answer 1.
3   Same as answer 1.

197. 4 With heart failure the veins distend, not collapse, because of congestion of the cardiopulmonary system. (2) (PB; CJ; AS)

1 This is an expected adaptation in clients with heart failure.

2 Same as answer 1.

3 This is associated with clients who are decompensating or exhibiting early signs of cardiogenic shock.

198. 3 As the heart fails, cardiac output decreases; eventually the decrease will reach a level that prevents tissues from receiving adequate oxygen and nutrients. (2) (PB; CJ; AN)

1 Heart failure is related to an increased, not decreased, circulating blood volume.

2 The condition may be acute or chronic; the pulmonary pressure increases and capillary fluid is forced into the alveoli.

4 The blood pressure usually does not drop; the condition may be acute or chronic.

199. 2 Left-sided heart failure causes fluid accumulation in the capillary network of the lung; fluid eventually enters alveolar spaces and causes crackling sounds at the end of inspiration. (1) (PB; CJ; AS)

1 This is not heard in chronic heart failure; it is associated with tracheal constriction or obstruction.

3 This is not heard in chronic heart failure; it is associated with asthma.

4 This is not heard in chronic heart failure; it is associated with pleurisy.

200. 2 Pulmonary congestion and edema occur because of fluid extravasation from the pulmonary capillary bed, resulting in difficult breathing. (1) (PB; CJ; AS)

1 This is a hallmark of myocardial infarction; it is caused by inadequate oxygen supply to the myocardium.

3 This results from increased pressure in the right atrium associated with right ventricular failure.

4 This is a sign of right, not left, ventricular failure; a weakened right ventricle causes venous congestion in the systemic circulation.

201. 2 Rest decreases demand on the heart and will prevent fatigue. (1) (PB; MR; PL)

1 The client should sleep with the head slightly elevated to facilitate respiration.

3 The client needs potassium; a low-potassium diet when the client is taking digoxin predisposes the client to toxicity and dangerous dysrhythmias.

4 To avoid becoming obsessed with the pulse rate, the client should be taught not to take the pulse so often; once daily is adequate.

202. 4 Crackles are the sound of air passing through fluid in the alveolar spaces; in pulmonary edema, fluid moves from the intravascular compartment into the alveoli. (1) (PB; CJ; AS)

1 The blood pressure would be increased with hypervolemia.

2 This would occur with angina or a myocardial infarction.

3 The pulse would be bounding with hypervolemia.

203. 3 A client's knowledge about the treatment program enhances compliance and reduces stress. (1) (PB; CJ; IM)

1 This response does not answer the client's question and might produce frustration.

2 This response does not answer the client's question.

4 This does not support the treatment regimen; it may cause more stress if the client interprets it as a conflict between the physician and the nurse.

204. 2 This is caused by hypervolemia and pulmonary hypertension. (1) (PB; CJ; AS)

1 The pulse would most likely be rapid and bounding, not slowed.

3 This is present in pleurisy, not heart failure.

4 Hypertension, not hypotension, would occur because of hypervolemia.

205. 3 Stressful situations would increase the body's oxygen demands. (2) (SE; CJ; IM)

1 Clients with low cardiac reserve cannot tolerate extremes of temperature; a hot bath would increase the body's oxygen demands.

2 Hot, humid weather is detrimental for those with heart disease; these individuals should use an air conditioner.

4 The heart of a client with low cardiac reserve cannot tolerate a pulse rate this high.

206. 3 Symptoms of right ventricular heart failure relate to retention of fluid; neck veins become distended because of increased back pressure from the right atrium. (3) (PB; CJ; AS)

1 This is associated with left ventricular heart failure because increased back pressure from the left atrium causes transudation of fluid from the pulmonary capillaries into the alveoli, limiting oxygen exchange.

2 Usually this is associated with left ventricular heart failure because of congestion in the lungs caused by back pressure from the left atrium, which is exaggerated when the client lies down at night.

4 Arterial blood pressure increases because of compensatory mechanisms of the body.

207. **2 This pulse rate increase indicates that activity tolerance is exceeded; rest brings the heart rate back to its preactivity rate. (2) (PM; CJ; IM)**

1 Activity should be stopped, not continued.

3 Though descending the stairs requires less energy than climbing, rest is essential to permit the heart rate to return to normal.

4 This still constitutes activity, which aggravates the cardiac workload.

208. **2 The highest incidence is in people 40 to 70 years of age; it is seen four times more frequently in men than women, with a higher incidence in black, rather than white, men. It occurs most often in the older, hypertensive client. (2) (PM; CJ; AN)**

1 This client is not at as high a risk as a black male.

3 Same as answer 1.

4 Unless the 40-year-old female is pregnant or in labor, she is not at as great a risk as the black male.

209. **4 As the heart contracts, an expanding midline mass can be palpated to the left of the umbilicus. (2) (PB; CJ; AS)**

1 This is not definitive for abdominal aortic aneurysm.

2 These are not definitive for abdominal aortic aneurysm; pallor is associated with shock.

3 There is no problem or pathology in the intestinal tract; this finding is associated with intestinal obstruction.

210. **2 Immediate surgical intervention to clamp the aorta is necessary for survival; the aneurysm has ruptured. (2) (PB; MR; IM)**

1 This may eventually be done, but notifying the physician is the priority.

3 The client is already NPO.

4 Sedatives mask important signs and symptoms.

211. **4 Ambulation is essential to promote venous return and prevent thrombus formation. (1) (PB; CJ; PL)**

1 This causes increased popliteal pressure and impairs venous return.

2 Same as answer 1.

3 This helps prevent atelectasis, not thrombi.

212. **3 When legs are dependent, gravity and incompetent valves promote increased hydrostatic pressure in leg veins; fluid moves into interstitial spaces. (2) (PB; CJ; AS)**

1 This reflects inadequate arterial blood supply; arterial circulation is not affected by varicose veins.

2 Same as answer 1.

4 This pain is referred to as Homans' sign and is associated with thrombophlebitis.

213. **2 To prevent distention of the veins, stockings should be applied before the legs are placed in a dependent position. (1) (SE; MR; IM)**

1 Knee-high stockings should end 2 inches below the knee to avoid popliteal pressure, which limits venous return.

3 Stockings should be used preventively before the discomfort associated with venous pressure and edema occurs.

4 Stockings apply uniform pressure; elastic bandages may slip, creating uneven pressure and constriction; edema may result.

214. **1 Impaired venous return causes increased pressure, with subjective symptoms of fatigue and heaviness. (2) (PB; CJ; AS)**

2 Symptoms of hypoxia are related to impaired arterial, rather than venous, circulation.

3 Homans' sign is indicative of thrombophlebitis.

4 Ecchymosis may occur in some individuals, but there is insufficient bleeding into tissue to cause hematomas.

215. **1 This is the correct description of this surgery; after ligation, the saphenous vein is removed; sclerosing is the treatment of choice. (1) (PB; MR; IM)**

2 Plaque is considered an arterial, rather than a venous, problem.

3 They are normally attached by communicating veins; surgery involves ligation to isolate the saphenous vein.

4 This prevents emboli from traveling to the lung; it is not a vein ligation and stripping.

216. **4 Because of the client's history and the site of the surgery, thrombi are likely to develop; activity is a preventive measure. (2) (PB; CJ; PL)**

1 This alone will not prevent thrombi; activity is necessary.

2 Getting out of bed will provide little exercise if the client only sits in a chair; also, an order is needed.

3 Although body alignment is important for all clients, it will not discourage thrombus formation.

217. 1 **The saphenous vein is ligated at its juncture with the femoral vein; injection sclerotherapy is used as method of choice but, in chronic venous insufficiency and recurrent thrombophlebitis, surgery may be necessary. (2) (PB; MR; IM)**
    2 A bypass is unnecessary; the deep veins compensate for the removed saphenous vein.
    3 Cholesterol plaques are characteristic of atherosclerosis, an arterial disease; not varicose veins.
    4 Tributaries normally exist between the superficial and deep veins; they are ligated to prevent further engorgement and varicosities.

218. 1 **Seeing the exercises demonstrated will reinforce the verbal explanations. (2) (SE; MR; IM)**
    2 This statement is too vague; it does not explain how to move them.
    3 This statement is too vague and thus may be ineffective; the time period should be stipulated.
    4 This response is vague and open to interpretation; nonspecific instructions may be ineffective.

219. 2 **This position supports the leg and promotes venous return by gravity, which reduces edema and pain. (2) (PB; CJ; IM)**
    1 The leg would still be in a position that promotes the development or continuation of edema.
    3 Same as answer 1.
    4 Although this would elevate the foot, it would provide no support under the leg and could cause hyperextension of the knee.

220. 1 **Swelling of the extremity is indicative of thrombophlebitis. (2) (PB; CJ; AS)**
    2 Difficulty with mobility would occur with musculoskeletal or neuromuscular problems.
    3 This is associated with neurologic deficits in the corticospinal tracts.
    4 This assessment would be made to determine the status of the arterial, not venous, system.

221. 3 **Raynaud's phenomenon has unilateral involvement, while Raynaud's disease has bilateral involvement. (3) (PB; CJ; AN)**
    1 Tingling of the fingers, indicating return of blood flow, is characteristic of both Raynaud's phenomenon and Raynaud's disease.
    2 Blanching followed by redness, indicating blood return, is characteristic of both Raynaud's phenomenon and Raynaud's disease.
    4 Coolness of the skin, indicating lack of blood supply, is characteristic of both Raynaud's phenomenon and Raynaud's disease.

222. 3 **Nicotine causes spasms and constriction of the smooth muscles of the arterial vasculature, compromising blood flow to the distal extremities. (2) (PB; CJ; AN)**
    1 Nicotine does not directly cause pain and tingling, although these may occur as consequences of the nicotine-induced vasoconstriction.
    2 Vasoconstriction from nicotine would not result in such severe adaptations.
    4 Smoking raises the carboxyhemoglobin level in the blood; carbon monoxide combines with hemoglobin and occupies the sites on the hemoglobin molecule that binds with oxygen, thus decreasing O_2 content.

223. 3 **Nicotine causes vasoconstriction and spasm of the peripheral arteries. (1) (PB; CJ; AN)**
    1 Alcohol may simulate dilation of the blood vessels.
    2 Lowering the limb enhances flow of blood into the foot by gravity, but does not support the return flow of blood.
    4 This would decrease the viscosity of blood, possibly preventing the formation of thrombi.

224. 4 **Altered quantity and quality of pulses are the earliest indications of increasingly limited circulation. (2) (PB; CJ; IM)**
    1 This could release an embolus into the circulation and cause tissue trauma.
    2 This prevents the use of gravity to carry arterial blood to the legs and feet.
    3 Altered sensation may limit sensitivity to heat, which could result in burns.

225. 3 **An exercise/rest program helps develop collateral circulation which improves well-being and enables clients to increase their ability to walk longer distances. (2) (PB; MR; IM)**
    1 A cool environment favors constriction of peripheral blood vessels and further decreases arterial flow.
    2 Crossing the legs increases local pressure, which tends to occlude blood vessels.
    4 Elevation slows inflow of arterial blood, which leads to further O_2 deprivation and pain.

226. 4 The client's extremities are less sensitive to thermal stress because of peripheral vascular problems, and burns may occur. (1) (SE; MR; PL)
1 Increasing heat of the external environment is an effort to prevent cold, chilling, and further constriction of peripheral vasculature.
2 Applying heat to the abdomen causes reflex dilation of the arteries in the extremities and increases blood flow without untoward effects.
3 Raising the internal temperature by drinking warm fluid prevents vascular constriction and warms the extremities.

227. 3 Intermittent claudication is the pain that occurs during exercise because of a lack of oxygen to muscles in the involved extremities. (2) (SE; MR; AN)
1 It is exercise, not the lack of it, that precipitates the pain.
2 This is related to a venous problem, not an arterial one.
4 Same as answer 2.

228. 2 Decreasing the demand for oxygen by resting will relieve the pain. (1) (PB; CJ; IM)
1 Pain will not resolve as long as exercise and, thus muscle hypoxia, is continued, regardless of whether ASA is taken.
3 This is appropriate for venous insufficiency, not arterial insufficiency.
4 Sublingual nitroglycerin is not indicated for leg cramps.

229. 1 Gravity will assist the flow of blood to the dependent legs and feet. (3) (PB; CJ; IM)
2 An extended knee gatch keeps extremities horizontal, not dependent, and does not facilitate blood flow to the feet.
3 Elevation impedes flow of arterial blood to the extremities; it facilitates venous return.
4 Same answer as 3.

230. 1 Arterial ulcers are painful because of their depth and interruption of the blood supply. (3) (PB; CJ; AN)
2 This is characteristic of venous ulcers.
3 Same as answer 2.
4 Same as answer 2.

231. 3 Pressure promotes coagulation and prevents the complication of bleeding. (2) (PB; CJ; IM)
1 Bending the operative leg may cause decreased perfusion to the leg or bleeding at the catheter insertion site.
2 Elevation would resist gravity flow of arterial blood, reducing oxygen to distal tissue.

4 The client should remain in the supine position for four to six hours to prevent bleeding at the insertion site.

232. 2 This indicates inadequate circulatory status of the left lower extremity. (2) (PB; CJ; AS)
1 This may indicate poor circulation but observation of both extremities for comparison would be necessary.
3 This is subjective and a less significant indication of arterial occlusive disease.
4 This is not as significant as the pulse; it can occur because of poor circulation, aging, or fungal infection.

233. 2 This reassures the client and allays fears of pain. (2) (PB; MR; PL)
1 The contrast medium used is not radioactive.
3 The femoral artery is used.
4 The client will be awake during the procedure.

234. 3 The client is hypertensive, and the intraarterial pressure is elevated; this increased pressure could cause the arterial suture line to rupture. (2) (PB; MR; AN)
1 Hypervolemia would be an assumption; other causes, such as arterial constriction, can precipitate hypertension.
2 This is unlikely because the blood pressure is elevated and the client is at risk for bleeding.
4 Although this could occur, the priority for this client is protecting the graft.

235. 3 Mobility will reduce venous stasis and edema as well as promote arterial perfusion and healing. (3) (PB; CJ; IM)
1 Bed rest is contraindicated because it promotes the development of thrombophlebitis and pulmonary emboli.
2 This is contraindicated; it constricts circulation at the hips and knees.
4 This would limit arterial perfusion.

236. 4 Intermittent claudication is pain that results when the arterial system is unable to provide adequate blood flow to the tissues in the presence of increased demands for oxygen and nutrients during exercise; it is relieved by rest. (2) (SE; MR; PL)
1 Rest pain is not a response to exercise; it occurs in the extremities during rest, especially at night.
2 Phantom limb sensation is the presence of unusual sensations or pain in the missing limb after an amputation.
3 This phenomenon is intermittent episodes of constricted arteries and arterioles in response to extreme cold or emotional stress causing pallor, paresthesias, and pain.

237. 4 Presence of pulses and a normal skin color indicate adequate arterial perfusion and graft viability. (1) (SE; MR; EV)

1 This is contraindicated in peripheral vascular disease because it may traumatize vessels; it could cause a thrombus to become an embolus.
2 This is appropriate for venous, not arterial, problems.
3 The peripheral dilation produced by a hot bath would increase the workload on the heart, which is undesirable in a client with hypertension.

238. 3 Inadequate oxygenation can cause premature ventricular beats. (2) (PB; CJ; AN)

1 While this may be true, it does not explain why adequate oxygenation is important.
2 Hypoxia can precipitate respiratory acidosis; hyperventilation causes respiratory alkalosis.
4 The reverse is true; postoperative pain can increase the respiratory rate.

239. 3 During open heart surgery the conductive system of the heart can be damaged because of trauma during surgery. (3) (PB; CJ; AN)

1 Shock results in a weak, rapid pulse.
2 Hypoxia causes tachycardia.
4 Heart failure causes a rapid pulse rate.

ENDOCRINE (EN)

240. 2 Excessive thirst, excessive hunger, and frequent urination are caused by the body's inability to correctly metabolize glucose. (1) (PB; MR; AS)

1 Lethargy, not irritability, results because of a lack of metabolized glucose for energy.
3 Frequent urination occurs throughout a 24-hour period because glucose in the urine pulls fluid with it; weight loss occurs with type 1 diabetes, not with type 2 diabetes.
4 Diaphoresis occurs with severe hypoglycemia.

241. 3 Protein and lipid catabolism occur because carbohydrates cannot be used by the cells; this results in weight loss and muscle wasting. (2) (PB; CJ; AS)

1 Dehydration, not edema, would be more likely to occur because of the polyuria associated with hyperglycemia.
2 Polyphagia, not anorexia, occurs with diabetes as the client attempts to meet metabolic needs.
4 Hyperglycemia, not hypoglycemia, is present in both type 1 and type 2 diabetes.

242. Answer: 109 g. The equivalent of 2.2 pounds is 1 kilogram; use ratio and proportion to solve this problem.

$$\frac{240 \text{ lbs}}{2.2 \text{ lbs}} = \frac{x \text{ kg}}{1 \text{ kg}}$$
$$2.2x = 240$$
$$x = 240 \div 2.2$$
$$x = 109 \text{ kg}$$

(3) (PB; CJ; AN)

243. 2 This is the normal range for blood glucose. (1) (PB; CJ; AN)

1 This range is indicative of hypoglycemia.
3 This range is indicative of hyperglycemia.
4 Same as answer 3.

244. 3 This will elicit a variety of data such as medications, diet, and other aspects of care. (2) (SE; CJ; AS)

1 Although important, this exploration by the nurse is too narrow and will elicit limited information.
2 Although this information should eventually be obtained, it is not significant at this point.
4 Same as answer 2.

245. 3 The reason for the lack of ketonuria in type 2 diabetes is unknown; one theory is that extremely high hyperglycemia and hyperosmolarity levels block the formation of ketones, stimulating lipogenesis, rather than lipolysis. (2) (PB; CJ; AS)

1 This does not occur with either type of diabetes.
2 This is impossible; if glycosuria is present, there must first be a level of glucose in the blood exceeding the renal threshold of 160 to 180 mg/dl.
4 This is expected in type 1 diabetes.

246. 1 Blood glucose testing is a more direct and accurate measure; urine testing provides an indirect measure that can be influenced by kidney function and the amount of time the urine is retained in the bladder. (1) (PB; CJ; IM)

2 While both blood and urine testing are relatively simple, testing the blood involves additional knowledge.
3 Both procedures can be done by the client.
4 This would not be a factor; while some urine tests are influenced by drugs, there are methods to test urine to bypass this effect.

247. 4 **Knowledge of the signs and treatment for hypoglycemia or hyperglycemia is critical to client health and well-being and essential for survival. (3) (SE; MR; AN)**
    1 Although this is important, it is not the priority.
    2 The client has type 2 diabetes, which usually is controlled by oral hypoglycemics.
    3 Self serum glucose monitoring is more accurate than sugar and acetone (S&A) urine measurements to identify serum glucose levels.

248. 4 **Controlling the diabetes decreases the risk of infection; this is the best prevention. (1) (SE; MR; EV)**
    1 If not completely absorbed, these may provide a warm, moist environment for bacterial growth.
    2 Coexisting neuropathy may result in injury from heat application.
    3 Protein, carbohydrates, and fats must be in an appropriate balance; high carbohydrate intake could provide too many calories.

249. 3 **Insulin facilitates transport of glucose across the cell membrane to meet metabolic needs and prevent fatigue. (2) (PB; MR; IM)**
    1 With diabetes there is decreased cellular metabolism because of the decrease in glucose entering the cells.
    2 Glucose is not absorbed from the intestinal tract by the cells; fatigue would be caused by decreased, not increased, cellular levels of glucose.
    4 Filtration and excretion of glucose by the kidneys do not regulate energy levels; if insulin production is normal, glucose does not spill into the urine.

250. 3 **Exercise increases the metabolic rate, and glucose is needed for cellular metabolism. (2) (PB; CJ; IM)**
    1 Regular vigorous exercise increases cell sensitivity to insulin.
    2 Glucagon action raises blood glucose but does not affect cell uptake or utilization of glucose.
    4 Cellular requirements for glucose increase with exercise.

251. 4 **Exercise improves glucose metabolism; with exercise there is a risk of developing hypoglycemia, not hyperglycemia. (2) (PB; MR; IM)**
    1 Exercise should not be decreased because it improves glucose metabolism.
    2 Control of glucose metabolism is achieved through a balance of diet, exercise, and pharmacologic therapy.

    3 An extra tablet would probably result in hypoglycemia because exercise alone improves glucose metabolism.

252. 4 **Physiologic stress increases gluconeogenesis, requiring continued pharmacologic therapy despite an inability to eat; fluids prevent dehydration; monitoring serum glucose levels permits early intervention if necessary. (1) (PB; MR; IM)**
    1 Food intake should be attempted to prevent acidosis; oral hypoglycemics should be taken, and serum glucose levels should be monitored.
    2 Skipping the oral hypoglycemic could precipitate hyperglycemia; serum glucose levels must be monitored.
    3 These are incomplete instructions; oral hypoglycemics should be taken, and serum glucose levels should be monitored; eating as much as possible could precipitate hyperglycemia.

253. 2 **In the overweight individual with type 2 diabetes, occasional alcohol can be ingested with caloric substitution for equivalent fat exchanges in the diet because it is metabolized like fat. (2) (PB; MR; IM)**
    1 Moderation is vital; these may not be used in unlimited quantities; they must be accounted for in the dietary calculations.
    3 Alcohol can be used as long as it is accounted for in the diet.
    4 This is untrue; regular foods can be used in the ADA diet.

254. 3 **According to the individual's needs, consistency and regularity in the food plan should be maintained; this is a basic principle of dietary management of diabetes. (2) (PB; MR; IM)**
    1 This is not necessary; the client can use the ADA food plan to make selections.
    2 This cannot always be done; it is unnecessary because choices can be made within the ADA diet.
    4 This is unnecessary because the client should be following the food plan.

255. 1 **These vegetables are in the vegetable exchange, as are asparagus, broccoli, and mushrooms. (1) (SE; MR; EV)**
    2 These are starchy vegetables and are listed as bread exchanges.
    3 Same as answer 2.
    4 These food items are from the bread exchange list.

256. 4 Improper foot care can lead to skin breakdown, poor healing, and subsequent infection. (1) (SE; MR; IM)
1 This potentially increases anxiety and reduces the client's ability to learn.
2 This is only one aspect of proper foot care; foot care must be more comprehensive.
3 Same as answer 2.

257. 4 When the head of the pancreas is removed, the client has a greatly reduced number of insulin-producing cells and hyperglycemia will occur; immediate treatment is necessary. (3) (PB; CJ; EV)
1 This is not immediately life threatening and would take time to develop.
2 Same as answer 1.
3 Same as answer 1.

258. 3 The blood glucose level needs to be reduced; regular insulin begins to act in 30 to 60 minutes. (1) (PB; CJ; PL)
1 Oral hypoglycemics are long acting and begin to act about one hour after administration; in addition, the client has type 1, not type 2, diabetes, and an oral hypoglycemic would be ineffective.
2 Blood glucose levels are far more accurate than urine glucose levels.
4 The rate may be increased because polyuria often accompanies hyperglycemia.

259. 3 Emotional and physical stress may cause insulin requirements to remain elevated in the postoperative period. (1) (PB; CJ; PL)
1 Fluctuating insulin requirements are usually associated with noncompliance, not surgery.
2 An increase in the client's insulin requirements could indicate sepsis, but this is not expected.
4 Insulin requirements would remain elevated rather than decrease.

260. 1 Incomplete oxidation of fat results in fatty acids that further break down to ketones. (3) (PB; CJ; AN)
2 Protein metabolism results in nitrogenous waste production, causing an elevated blood urea nitrogen (BUN).
3 Potassium is not oxidized; in hypokalemia or hyperkalemia no ketones are formed.
4 Carbohydrates do not contain fatty acids that are broken down into ketones.

261. 2 Potassium is the principal intracellular cation, and during ketoacidosis it moves out of cells into the extracellular compartment to replace potassium lost as a result of glucose-induced osmotic diuresis; overstimulation of the cardiac muscle results. (3) (PB; CJ; AS)
1 P waves are abnormal because the P-R interval may be prolonged and the P wave may be lost; however, the T wave is peaked, not depressed; the T wave is depressed in hypokalemia.
3 Initially, the QT segment is short, and as the potassium level rises, the QRS complex widens; the ST segment becomes depressed.
4 The P-R interval is prolonged, and the P wave may be lost; QRS complexes and thus T waves become irregular, and the rate does not necessarily change.

262. 3 This is a short-term goal, client-oriented, necessary for the client to control the diabetes, and measurable when the client performs a return demonstration for the nurse. (2) (SE; MR; AN)
1 This is not a short-term goal.
2 This is measurable, but it is a long-term goal.
4 While this is measurable and is a short-term goal, it is not the one with the greatest priority when a client has an insulin pump that must be mastered prior to discharge.

263. 3 The basal infusion rate mimics the low rate of insulin secretion during fasting, and the bolus before meals mimics the high output after meals. (2) (SE; MR; PL)
1 The subcutaneous needle may be left in place for as long as three days.
2 Blood glucose monitoring is done a minimum of four times a day.
4 Most insulin pumps are external to the body and access the body via a subcutaneous needle.

264. 2 Wearing shoes protects the feet; they should fit well and be worn over socks that are wool or cotton to cushion the foot and absorb perspiration. (3) (SE; CJ; IM)
1 Smoking should be avoided, and self-removal of corns can result in injury to the feet.
3 Nylon is not a natural fiber, and it promotes perspiration.
4 Shoes that do not fit well will create friction and cause sores, blisters, and calluses; corn removers should be avoided.

265. 3 The dose of exogenous insulin causes a rapid drop in the blood glucose level, especially if food is not eaten; the oral hypoglycemic acts slowly, and there is time to take evasive measures if hypoglycemia begins to develop. (3) (PB; CJ; AN)
1 This would lead to hyperglycemia.

2 Stress usually contributes to hyperglycemia; the primary reason for this client's precipitous fall in the blood glucose level was because insulin had been taken and the client had not eaten.

4 The use of insulin over long periods neither builds tolerance nor causes blood glucose levels to fluctuate dramatically.

266. 4 **Lipodystrophy is a noninflammatory reaction causing localized atrophy or hypertrophy and a localized increase in collagen deposits. (1) (PB; CJ; AN)**

1 Injections of insulin would not cause a horny growth such as a wart or callus.

2 An allergic response would precipitate a localized or systemic inflammatory response.

3 Hyperthermia and localized heat, erythema, and pain would be associated with an infection.

267. 2 **This occurs with low serum glucose levels because of sympathetic nervous system activity. (2) (PB; CJ; AS)**

1 This is a sign of hyperglycemia and is related to metabolic acidosis and inadequate energy production.

3 This is a sign of hyperglycemia; it is caused by dehydration associated with osmotic diuresis related to glycosuria.

4 This is a sign of hyperglycemia and is related to metabolic acidosis; it is a compensatory response in an attempt to blow off CO_2 and raise the pH level.

268. 1 **These are classic signs of hypokalemia that occur when potassium levels are reduced as potassium reenters cells with glucose. (3) (PB; CJ; EV)**

2 Symptoms of hyponatremia are nausea, malaise, and changes in mental status.

3 Symptoms of hypoglycemia are weakness, nervousness, tachycardia, diaphoresis, irritability, and pallor.

4 Symptoms of hypercalcemia are lethargy, nausea, vomiting, paresthesias, and personality changes.

269. 1 **The suggested treatment of hypoglycemia in a conscious client is a simple sugar (such as two packets of sugar), followed by a complex carbohydrate (such as a slice of bread), and last a protein (such as milk); the simple sugar elevates the blood glucose level rapidly; the complex carbohydrates and protein produce a more sustained response. (2) (PB; MR; EV)**

2 These are fast-acting sugars, and neither of them will provide a sustained response.

3 The fat content of chocolate candy decreases the rate of absorption of glucose.

4 Neither of these is a fast-acting sugar; peanut butter crackers and milk can be used to maintain the glucose level after it has been raised.

270. 3 **An aldosteronoma is an aldosterone-secreting adenoma of the adrenal cortex. (1) (PB; CJ; AN)**

1 An aldosteronoma is not a tumor of the kidney cortex.

2 An aldosteronoma is not a tumor of the thyroid gland.

4 An aldosteronoma is not a tumor of the pituitary gland.

271. 2 **Renal and cardiac complications will occur if hypertension is not arrested. (3) (PB; MR; IM)**

1 An aldosteronoma is a benign tumor; metastasis is not possible.

3 Drugs are not used; the tumor must be removed.

4 This is not true; the tumor must be removed by surgical means.

272. 2 **Once the excessive secretion of aldosterone is stopped, the blood pressure gradually drops to a near normal level. (2) (PB; CJ; EV)**

1 The blood pressure drops gradually; it does not rise.

3 Blood pressure will fluctuate if the hypervolemia is overcorrected; this is not expected.

4 The blood pressure drops gradually in response to decreasing serum corticosteroid levels; a rapid drop immediately following surgery may indicate hemorrhage.

273. 1 **The body has two adrenal glands; an aldosteronoma is a unilateral tumor. (2) (PB; MR; IM)**

2 The prognosis is usually excellent; this is unnecessarily alarming.

3 This is unnecessary; the prognosis is usually excellent.

4 Hormones are not necessary; there is another adrenal gland that will secrete an adequate amount of hormones.

274. 3 **This is a urinary metabolite of steroid hormones that are excreted in large amounts in hyperaldosteronism. (3) (PB; CJ; AS)**

1 With aldosterone hypersecretion sodium is retained and potassium is excreted resulting in hypernatremia and hypokalemia.

2 With Cushing's syndrome, the eosinophil count is decreased, not increased.

4 ACTH levels are usually high in Cushing's syndrome.

275. 3 Increased glucocorticoids cause sodium and water retention, hypertension, and adipose deposition resulting in a "moon-face." (2) (PB; CJ; AS)
  1 These adaptations are associated with hyperthyroidism.
  2 These adaptations are associated with hypothyroidism.
  4 Same as answer 1.

276. 2 Stress and activity increase ACTH and adrenocortical hormones, which would elevate the urine values for these hormonal by-products, invalidating test results. (3) (PB; CJ; PL)
  1 Clients with Addison's disease are chronically dehydrated and do not have edema.
  3 Because of fluid deficits, the client would be hypovolemic and the blood pressure would be decreased.
  4 Adequate fluid intake is necessary for urine production; Addison's disease involves salt wasting and dehydration, which necessitates an increased fluid intake.

277. 2 These tests provide a measure of thyroxine production, a disturbance that is associated with the client's symptoms. (1) (PB; CJ; AS)
  1 Prothrombin time (PT) and partial thromboplastin time (PTT) assess blood coagulation.
  3 The VDRL test is for syphilis; the CBC assesses the hematopoietic system.
  4 This measures the kind and amount of circulating barbiturates; the client's symptoms are not associated with barbiturate intake.

278. 4 Many of these adaptations are associated with hyperthyroidism; palpitations may indicate cardiovascular changes requiring prompt intervention; the increased metabolism associated with hyperthyroidism can lead to heart failure. (2) (SE; MR; AS)
  1 Although a feeling of warmth is an uncomfortable feeling caused by the increased metabolism associated with hyperthyroidism, it is not life threatening.
  2 Although this adaptation can result from catabolism associated with hyperthyroidism, it is not life threatening.
  3 Although an increased appetite becomes a compensatory mechanism for the increased metabolism associated with hyperthyroidism, it is not life threatening.

279. 1 Excessive metabolic activity associated with hyperthyroidism causes fatigue. (1) (PB; CJ; AS)

  2 Warm, moist skin would be expected because of increased peripheral perfusion associated with increased metabolism.
  3 Increased appetite would be expected because of the increased metabolism associated with hyperthyroidism.
  4 Tachycardia would be expected because of the increased metabolism associated with hyperthyroidism.

280. 4 Many radiopaque dyes contain iodine, which would alter the test results. (3) (SE; CJ; AS)
  1 This is important if the client is to be given iodine; the test results would not be affected by these allergies.
  2 This is not specifically related to these studies.
  3 Same as answer 2.

281. 3 These are the classic signs associated with hyperthyroidism; weight loss and restlessness occur because of an increased basal metabolic rate; exophthalmos occurs because of peribulbar edema. (2) (PB; CJ; AS)
  1 These are associated with hypothyroidism because of the decreased metabolic rate.
  2 Lethargy and weight gain are associated with hypothyroidism as a result of a decreased metabolic rate; forgetfulness is not related.
  4 Although weight loss and exophthalmos occur with hyperthyroidism, the client would be hyperactive, not hypoactive.

282. 1 Increased basal metabolic rate, increased circulation, and vasodilation result in warm moist skin. (3) (PB; CJ; AS)
  2 This symptom is associated with hypothyroidism.
  3 Same as answer 2.
  4 Same as answer 2.

283. 4 The mask may irritate or scratch the eye if the client turns and lies on it during the night. (3) (SE; MR; EV)
  1 Blinking of the eyes will bathe the eyes and prevent corneal ulceration.
  2 This will not relieve edema or prevent ulceration of the eyes.
  3 Although this will help reduce periorbital edema, it will not prevent ulceration of the cornea.

284. 3 This relieves tension on the incision and limits the risk of dehiscence. (2) (PB; MR; IM)

1 Coughing should be avoided during the early postoperative period to prevent trauma to the operative site.

2 This should be avoided until advised by the physician, usually after initial healing of the incision occurs.

4 Pressure against the operative area is not necessary to promote the integrity of the incision, and it may act to inhibit swallowing.

285. **2 These beverages contain caffeine, which may increase thyroid activity. (1) (PB; MR; PL)**

1 Hyperactivity is a physiologic response; it is not under conscious control.

3 The increased metabolic rate associated with hyperthyroidism will make the client feel warm; a cool environment is needed.

4 Hyperactivity is a problem, and the client should be encouraged to rest.

286. **2 This thyroid tissue is left because it may provide enough hormone for normal function; if not, supplemental medication may be necessary. (1) (PB; CJ; AN)**

1 This would be a total, not a subtotal, thyroidectomy.

3 The parathyroid glands should not be removed during a thyroidectomy.

4 Same as answer 3.

287. **1 A tracheostomy set should be available in the event there is excessive edema at the surgical site, which can cause tracheal compression. (2) (PB; CJ; PL)**

2 This is not necessary after a thyroidectomy.

3 The head should be kept in anatomical alignment, not flexed or hyperextended.

4 Intermittent suction does not provide the constant suction needed to keep the airway clear.

288. **1 The inflammatory response and trauma of surgery may cause edema, compressing the trachea and compromising the airway. (2) (SE; CJ; IM)**

2 Although this is an important assessment for any postoperative client, it is not the priority.

3 Although deep breathing would be encouraged, coughing this early in the postoperative period would be too traumatic to the operative site.

4 Same as answer 2.

289. **3 If the laryngeal nerve is damaged during surgery, the client will be hoarse and have difficulty speaking. (3) (PB; CJ; EV)**

1 This would not indicate injury to the laryngeal nerve; this is part of the assessment for a compromised airway.

2 This would be an assessment for hypocalcemia resulting from inadvertent removal of the parathyroid glands.

4 This assesses for bleeding and possible hemorrhage, not laryngeal nerve injury.

290. **4 This helps detect complications such as thyrotoxic crisis, hemorrhage, and respiratory obstruction that occur early in the postoperative period. (3) (PB; CJ; EV)**

1 This is contraindicated; humidifiers can contribute to the spread of bacteria and infection.

2 This should not begin until two to four days postoperatively because it can disrupt the suture line.

3 Hoarseness and voice weakness usually are temporary and not life threatening; the priority is to observe for thyroid storm, hemorrhage, and respiratory obstruction.

291. **1 Bleeding may occur, and blood will pool in the back of the neck because the blood will flow via gravity. (1) (PB; CJ; EV)**

2 ROM exercises would increase pain and would put tension on the suture line.

3 Talking should be avoided in the immediate postoperative period except to assess for a change in pitch or tone, which may indicate laryngeal nerve damage.

4 Activity should be gradually resumed and frequent rest periods encouraged.

292. **3 Maintaining airway patency is always the priority. (2) (PB; CJ; PL)**

1 Although important, it does not exceed patency of the airway in priority.

2 Same as answer 1.

4 Same as answer 1.

293. **2 Injury to the parathyroid glands results in a deficiency of parathormone, which decreases calcium levels in the blood. (3) (PB; CJ; EV)**

1 This is characterized by generalized weakness, a decrease in reflexes, shallow respirations, and cardiac dysrhythmias.

3 This is characterized by tachycardia, hyperpyrexia, and an exacerbation of thyroid symptoms.

4 This is characterized by a weak, thready pulse and hypotension.

294. 4 **These symptoms could indicate impending hypocalcemic tetany, a complication after removal of parathyroid tissue during a thyroidectomy. (3) (PB; CJ; AS)**
    1 These symptoms may be related to postoperative anxiety, but the priority is to assess for impending tetany.
    2 This would not be helpful for the complaint made by the client; further assessment for tetany is indicated.
    3 Physical assessment and notification of the physician are the priorities.

295. 4 **Thyrotoxic crisis is severe hyperthyroidism; excessive amounts of thyroxine increase the metabolic rate, thereby raising the pulse and temperature. (2) (PB; CJ; AS)**
    1 During crisis there is usually no increase in the difference between the apical and the peripheral pulse rates (pulse deficit).
    2 The blood pressure will rise to meet the oxygen demand caused by the increased metabolic rate during crisis.
    3 Because of the increased metabolic rate, the pulse and respiratory rates increase to meet the body's oxygen needs.

296. 4 **Thyrotoxic crisis (thyroid storm) is the body's response to excessive circulating thyroid hormones. (3) (PB; CJ; AN)**
    1 A deficiency of iodine results in a deficiency in thyroid hormone production.
    2 A decreased serum calcium causes tetany.
    3 Sodium retention is unrelated to thyrotoxic crisis; thyrotoxic crisis is caused by excessive circulating thyroid hormones.

297. 3 **Dry, sparse hair and cold intolerance are characteristic adaptations to low serum thyroxine. (1) (SE; MR; EV)**
    1 Muscle cramping is associated with hypocalcemia.
    2 Low thyroxine levels reduce the metabolic rate, resulting in fatigue, but do not increase the pulse rate.
    4 Low thyroxine levels reduce the metabolic rate, resulting in weight gain and bradycardia, not tachycardia.

298. 3 **After a subtotal thyroidectomy the thyroxine output may be inadequate to maintain an appropriate metabolic rate. (1) (SE; MR; AN)**
    1 Hypothyroidism is a decrease in thyroid functioning, not a slowing of the entire body's functions.
    2 In hypothyroidism the level of thyroid-stimulating hormone (TSH) from the pituitary is usually increased.

4 Atrophy of the remaining thyroid tissue does not occur.

299.
    1 __x__ **This is a symptom of hypothyroidism that is related to the associated decreased metabolic rate. (2) (PB; MR; EV)**
    2 __x__ **This is a symptom of hypothyroidism that is related to the associated decreased metabolic rate.**
    3 _____ This is a sign of hyperthyroidism, not hypothyroidism.
    4 _____ This is a sign of hyperthyroidism, not hypothyroidism.
    5 __x__ **This is a symptom of hypothyroidism that is related to the associated decreased metabolic rate.**
    6 _____ This is a sign of hyperthyroidism, not hypothyroidism.

FLUIDS AND ELECTROLYTES (FE)

300. 1 **The blood pressure indicates hypovolemia; the increased pulse is an attempt to maintain adequate oxygenation of tissues; the rapid weight loss reflects loss of body fluid. (1) (PB; CJ; AN)**
    2 The problem is an inadequate intake of fluid, not food; also, there are no data to support the presence of altered thought processes.
    3 There are no data to support this diagnosis; the cardiac output is maintained by a compensatory increase in the heartbeat.
    4 The rapid weight loss reflects a loss of fluid, not a loss of body tissue.

301. 2 **Hemodilution has occurred because the 1500 mL of intravenous fluid has lowered the serum sodium level. (2) (PB; CJ; AN)**
    1 This is not the cause of the hyponatremia; in addition, the client has not eaten for several days.
    3 A decreased, not increased, reabsorption of sodium occurs in acute renal failure.
    4 A decreased, not increased, glomerular filtration rate occurs with renal failure.

302. **Answer: +235 mL. The client's intake was 360 (6 oz × 30 mL × 2) and the loss was 125 mL of fluid; 360 − 125 = 235. (1) (PB; CJ; EV)**

303. 3 **One liter of fluid weighs approximately 2.2 pounds; therefore a 4.5-pound weight loss equals approximately 2 liters. (2) (PB; CJ; EV)**
    1 This is approximately a 1-pound weight loss.
    2 This is approximately a 2.2-pound weight loss.

4 This is approximately a 7.5-pound weight loss.

304. **1 With the client's history and the large weight gain, this is the most likely cause of the increase in weight. (1) (PB; CJ; AN)**
2 This occurs in the bladder, not the tissues, and would not account for the large weight gain.
3 This can occur with heart failure, but it is not the primary etiologic factor of the sudden weight gain.
4 Abdominal distention usually is caused by gas and should not contribute to this large a weight gain; if the abdomen is enlarged, assessment by ballottement should be done to determine whether enlargement is caused by fluid.

305. **4 Carbonated beverages are generally high in sodium and should be avoided. (1) (PB; CJ; PL)**
1 Many of these products contain sodium and should be avoided.
2 Steak sauce is high in sodium and should be avoided.
3 Artificial sweeteners do not contain sodium and do not have to be restricted.

306. **3 Hypokalemia is suspected when the T wave on an ECG tracing is depressed or flattened; a serum potassium level less than 3.5 mEq/L indicates hypokalemia. (1) (PB; CJ; AS)**
1 This would have no significance in diagnosing a potassium deficit.
2 Same as answer 1.
4 Same as answer 1.

307. **2 This hypertonic solution should be administered in a continuous and uniform infusion to prevent hyperosmolar diuresis. (2) (PB; CJ; PL)**
1 This is true for any intravenous infusion; this is not unique to total parenteral nutrition; also, infusion pumps can be placed on the bedside table.
3 The tubing set should be appropriate for the type of infusion pump.
4 This is not necessary in total parenteral nutrition; an infusion pump should be used.

308. **2 Potassium is irritating to veins; larger veins can accommodate irritating substances for longer periods than small veins can. (2) (PB; CJ; IM)**
1 Using the antecubital space would restrict client movement unnecessarily because the arm would have to be kept extended to prevent piercing the vein, which could result in an infiltration.
3 The back of the hand does not have veins large enough to accommodate a potassium infusion.
4 Same as answer 3.

309. **1 A rate of 30 mL/hr is considered adequate for perfusion of the kidneys, heart, and brain. (1) (PB; CJ; EV)**
2 A central venous pressure reading of 2 cm H_2O indicates hypovolemia.
3 This indicates improvement but not necessarily adequate tissue perfusion.
4 Same as answer 3.

310. **4 Unless diluted the highly concentrated solution can cause vein irritation or occlusion. (3) (PB; CJ; AN)**
1 Although this is true, the underlying reason is the large amount of blood in the subclavian vein and the superior vena cava, which dilutes the concentrated solution.
2 Although this is true, this is not the primary reason for a central line.
3 This is not the primary reason, although the infusion at this site is more secure than a peripheral site and promotes free use of the arm.

311. **4 Albumin intravenously increases colloid osmotic pressure, resulting in a pull of fluid from the interstitial and intracellular compartments to the intravascular compartment. (3) (PB; CJ; AN)**
1 The interstitial compartment is part of the extracellular compartment.
2 This is opposite to the actual shift of fluids.
3 Same as answer 2.

312. **1 Osmosis is the movement of fluid from an area of lesser solute concentration to an area of greater solute concentration. (3) (PB; CJ; AN)**
2 Filtration is the passage of fluid through a material that prevents the passage of certain constituents; hydrostatic pressure, the pressure exerted within a closed system, is known as filtration force; this force moves fluid by pressure and concentration gradients.
3 Diffusion is the movement of particles across a semipermeable membrane from an area of greater concentration of particles to an area of lesser concentration of particles.
4 In active transport, molecules move against a concentration gradient; this differs from diffusion and osmosis because metabolic energy is expended.

313. 3 Salt substitutes usually contain potassium, which would lead to symptoms of hyperkalemia, such as an abnormal heartbeat. (3) (PB; MR; AN)
  1 Sodium in the diet causes retention of fluid.
  2 Salt substitutes do not contain substances that influence BUN and creatinine levels; these are the result of protein metabolism.
  4 There is no such substance in salt substitutes.

314. 2 Intravenous fluids supply minimal calories; a client on only IV therapy will lose weight and become malnourished. (1) (PB; CJ; EV)
  1 This is not related to weight; lack of bulk in the diet results in constipation.
  3 Vitamins are not related to weight loss.
  4 Intracellular electrolytes are not related to weight loss.

315. 3 Potassium is important for muscle contraction; the heart is a muscle and hypokalemia causes dysrhythmias. (2) (PB; CJ; EV)
  1 Decreased functioning of respiratory muscles may result in hypoventilation.
  2 Decreased functioning of respiratory muscles may result in respiratory acidosis.
  4 A serum potassium level of 5.5 is within the upper range of normal.

316. 1 Blood glucose that exceeds the renal threshold for glucose reabsorption in the kidney tubules (approximately 160 to 180 mg/dL) will cause cellular osmotic diuresis resulting in dehydration. (1) (PB; CJ; EV)
  2 This determines the presence of digested blood in the stool; it is unrelated to total parenteral nutrition.
  3 An altered specific gravity is nonspecific; increases could result from causes other than glycosuria.
  4 This assesses for increased or decreased peristalsis; it is unrelated to total parenteral nutrition.

317. 1 The concentration of glucose (20% to 25%) in the solution is a good culture medium for bacterial and fungal growth. (2) (SE; CJ; AS)
  2 This is not associated with total parenteral nutrition.
  3 Anorexia is often present before the medical decision to begin total parenteral nutrition; it is not a complication.
  4 This is not directly related to total parenteral nutrition but rather to concomitant hypokalemia, which can occur if potassium is not added to the solution.

318. 2 The stomach produces about 3 L of secretions per day; fluid lost through vomiting can produce a fluid volume deficit; the priority is fluid volume deficit, which can lead to dysrhythmias and death. (2) (PB; CJ; AN)
  1 The shallow respirations are not related to a primary respiratory problem or pain; they are a compensatory mechanism to conserve CO_2 to combine with hydrogen to form carbonic acid (H_2CO_3) and lower the plasma pH level.
  3 Although this diagnosis is related, it is not the priority.
  4 This would be true for duodenal ulcer; the gastric acid secretory rate is normal in persons with gastric ulcers; in gastric ulcers there is a decreased resistance of the gastric mucosa to acid-pepsin injury and a reflux of bile-containing duodenal contents back into the stomach.

319. 3 This has a low-sodium content. (3) (PB; CJ; EV)
  1 Shellfish is high in sodium.
  2 Processed meats are high in sodium.
  4 These vegetables are high in sodium.

320. 1 This treats the hyperkalemia associated with renal failure; it moves potassium from the intravascular compartment into the intracellular compartment. (3) (PB; CJ; AN)
  2 This would not increase urinary output.
  3 This is not a treatment for respiratory acidosis.
  4 Insulin and glucose do not decrease serum calcium levels.

321. 2 This is a classic sign of hyponatremia because of its effect on the cerebral cortex; additional symptoms include weakness and apprehension. (3) (PB; CJ; AS)
  1 This is associated with aging and dehydration.
  3 This is associated with hypovolemia.
  4 This is associated with shock and anemia.

322. 1 Fluid and electrolyte replacement is a life-saving strategy; it must be done before surgery is performed. (2) (PB; CJ; IM)
  2 This is not the priority at this time.
  3 The client is neither physically nor cognitively ready for ileostomy education.
  4 The client is not demonstrating a readiness for contact with other persons with ileostomies at this time.

323. 2 **This ensures a well-controlled technique for electrolyte (chloride) replacement. (3) (PB; CJ; AN)**
 1 There is no assurance that adequate chloride will be ingested and absorbed.
 3 Total parenteral nutrition is not necessary at this point, although it may eventually be used.
 4 This is not a well-controlled method to correct electrolyte deficiencies.

324. 2 **The osmotic effect of hyperglycemia pulls fluid from cells, resulting in cellular dehydration. (3) (PB; CJ; AN)**
 1 Hyperglycemia pulls fluid from the interstitial to the intravascular compartment, eventually spilling into the urine.
 3 Interstitial fluid is part of the extracellular compartment; the osmotic pull of glucose exceeds other osmotic forces.
 4 An increase in hydrostatic pressure results in an intravascular to interstitial shift.

325. 1 **A low pH and bicarbonate reflect metabolic acidosis; a low P_{CO_2} indicates compensatory hyperventilation. (3) (PB; CJ; AN)**
 2 A low pH and elevated P_{CO_2} reflect hypoventilation and respiratory acidosis.
 3 An elevated pH and bicarbonate reflect metabolic alkalosis; an elevated P_{CO_2} indicates compensatory hypoventilation.
 4 An elevated pH and low P_{CO_2} reflect hyperventilation and respiratory alkalosis.

326. 2 **This would provide gradual replacement of both fluid and electrolytes without overloading the intravascular compartment. (2) (PB; CJ; PL)**
 1 Water does not supply the necessary electrolytes, and hyponatremia could result.
 3 No data are presented to indicate that the client cannot take fluids orally; an NG tube is not necessary when the client can take fluids by mouth.
 4 Rapid correction of a fluid and electrolyte imbalance is dangerous; therapy should promote a gradual correction.

327. 2 **During the oliguric phase of renal failure the kidneys retain potassium; an elevated potassium level is one of the main indicators of the need for dialysis. (3) (PB; CJ; AS)**
 1 Metabolic acidosis would occur.
 3 Hypercalcemia would occur.
 4 Hyponatremia would occur.

328. 4 **Commercially prepared substitutes are high in potassium. (2) (SE; MR; EV)**
 1 Some complete protein foods must be included in the diet.
 2 Seasoning that contains neither sodium nor potassium, such as lemon juice, pepper, and herbs, can be used to make food more palatable.
 3 These contain high potassium concentrations.

329. 3 **A decreased urinary output will result in the retention of potassium, causing hyperkalemia. (3) (PB; CJ; AS)**
 1 This is a sign of dehydration, which can be corrected with appropriate hydration.
 2 These indicate dehydration, which is probably the rationale for the fluid ordered.
 4 This can precipitate dehydration or compound an existing dehydration and can be prevented by appropriate hydration.

330. 3 **Pyrexia increases fluid loss through the skin; to maintain balance, the body compensates by reducing urinary output. (1) (PB; CJ; AN)**
 1 Blood pressure is not directly affected by antimicrobials, and there are no data to suggest blood pressure is decreasing.
 2 This is unlikely; the client would have to become septic before this could occur.
 4 This represents a possible, but not probable, side effect of antimicrobial agents; also, nephrotoxicity would not be evident so soon.

331. 3 **All the values provided are within normal limits. (3) (PB; CJ; EV)**
 1 The albumin is normal.
 2 The hematocrit is normal; with hemoconcentration the hematocrit would be elevated.
 4 There is no evidence of overload; if the pulmonary arterial wedge pressure were higher, urine output increased, and hematocrit lower, it would indicate possible water intoxication.

332. 3 **Fluids during the first 48 hours are given to replace fluid lost from the intravascular compartment to interstitial spaces. (3) (PB; CJ; AN)**
 1 Administration of fluids treats the fluid shifts, but does not prevent them.
 2 Lactated Ringer's solution and 5% dextrose in saline are not plasma expanders, as is albumin.
 4 Electrolytes are specifically replaced based on serial assessments of serum electrolytes and arterial blood gases.

333. 3 **The pulse rate is one indicator of optimum vascular fluid volume; the pulse rate decreases as intravascular volume normalizes. (3) (PB; CJ; EV)**
1 This indicates inadequate kidney perfusion; if adequate, output should be above 30 mL/hr.
2 This would indicate hypovolemia.
4 This would indicate hemoconcentration resulting from hypovolemia.

334. 2 **Massive amounts of potassium are released from the injured cells into the extracellular fluid compartment; large amounts of sodium are lost in edema. (3) (PB; CJ; AS)**
1 Serum potassium will rise.
3 Serum potassium will rise and a serum sodium deficit will occur.
4 A serum sodium deficit will occur.

335. 1 **Silver nitrate can precipitate electrolyte imbalances; the client's potassium is below the expected range of 3.5 to 5.5 mEq/L and should be supplemented. (3) (PB; CJ; PL)**
2 The client's sodium level is within the expected range of 135 to 145 mEq/L and there is no need to administer additional sodium chloride.
3 This would cause a further depletion of potassium.
4 Same as answer 3.

336. 1 **The blood urea nitrogen (BUN) is above the expected value of 5 to 20 mg/dL; urea nitrogen is the major nitrogenous end product of protein and amino acid catabolism; azotemia is the accumulation of excessive nitrogenous compounds in the blood. (3) (PB; CJ; AN)**
2 The client has hyperkalemia; the expected value for potassium is 3.5 to 5.5 mEq/L.
3 Although the client does have a metabolic acid-base imbalance, it is acidosis not alkalosis because the pH is below the expected range of 7.35 to 7.45.
4 The pH indicates acidosis, not alkalosis, because it is below the expected pH of 7.35 to 7.45; the Po_2 is within the expected range of 80 to 100 mm Hg, which indicates that the problem is metabolic, not respiratory.

337. 2 **The client is hyperkalemic, and potassium intake should be limited; potassium is nonexistent in Jell-O. (3) (PB; CJ; IM)**
1 Milk should be avoided; one cup of milk contains 754 mg of potassium.
3 Orange juice should be avoided; one cup of orange juice contains 496 mg of potassium.
4 This should be avoided; one cup of tomato juice contains 550 mg of potassium

338. 3 **An orange only contains trace amounts of sodium. (3) (PB; CJ; IM)**
1 One cup of ice cream contains approximately 115 mg of sodium.
2 One cup of celery contains approximately 106 mg of sodium.
4 Four peanut butter cookies contain 142 mg of sodium.

339. 2 **Fluid shifts from the intravascular compartment into the abdominal cavity, causing hypovolemia; a rapid, thready pulse is a compensatory response to this shift. (2) (PB; CJ; EV)**
1 Assessing for shock is the priority.
3 After a paracentesis, intravascular fluid shifts into the abdominal cavity, not the lungs.
4 Same as answer 1.

340. 2 **Hypervolemia may precipitate pulmonary edema, which produces symptoms of shortness of breath, wheezing, cough, apprehension, and frothy sputum. (3) (PB; CJ; EV)**
1 Although this could occur, it is not the most serious complication; an altered respiratory status is the priority.
3 This occurs with the IV administration of dye for diagnostic procedures; it does not occur with hydration therapy.
4 Same as answer 1.

341. 3 **Verbalization indicates the client is breathing; elevating the head of the bed facilitates breathing by decreasing pressure against the diaphragm; checking the vital signs after this is the first step in assessing the cause of the distress. (2) (PB; CJ; PL)**
1 There is not enough information to support this option; further assessment is required.
2 Discontinuing the IV access line may cause unnecessary discomfort if it must be restarted; there are too little data to call the physician at this time.
4 There is no information to support this option; assessment for allergies should be done on admission.

342. 2 **The imbalance in intake and output, with a decreasing urinary output, may indicate renal failure with an increase of body fluid and the resulting development of heart failure; assessing breath sounds and vital signs are the first steps when monitoring for these complications. (3) (PB; CJ; EV)**
1 There are no data to support a problem with excretion of urine; the problem is with insufficient production.

3 These are appropriate assessments after respirations and vital signs are evaluated.

4 It is immaterial whether the fluid is given orally or intravenously; if there is hypervolemia, fluid intake would be decreased.

343. **1 This attempts to collect adequate data to plan the most appealing and appropriate diet. (2) (PB; MR; AS)**

2 This alone will not guarantee compliance once the client goes home; the client has the right to accept or reject therapy.

3 Table salt is contraindicated on a 2-g sodium diet.

4 Same as answer 2.

344. **3 Shallow respirations, bronchial tree obstruction, and atelectasis compromise gas exchange in the lungs; an elevated carbon dioxide level leads to acidosis. (1) (PB; CJ; AN)**

1 Metabolic acidosis is seen in diarrhea with loss of base from the lower gastrointestinal tract.

2 Metabolic alkalosis is caused by excessive loss of hydrogen ions from gastric decompression or excessive vomiting.

4 Respiratory alkalosis is caused by increased expiration of carbon dioxide, a component of carbonic acid.

345. **1 This 20 mL must be accounted for in the intake and output, either by including it as intake or by subtracting it from the total gastric drainage. (3) (SE; CJ; AN)**

2 High suction may lead to adherence of mucosa to the tube and potential injury.

3 The surgeon places the tube so that the suture line is not traumatized.

4 Return of 10 mL indicates patency; more frequent irrigations are not indicated.

346.

1 _____ Irritability, as a result of heightened neuromuscular activity, is a sign of hyperkalemia.

2 _x_ **Dysrhythmias are a sign of potassium depletion in cardiac muscle; other cardiovascular effects include irregular, rapid weak pulse, decreased blood pressure, flattened and inverted T waves, prominent U waves, depressed ST segments, peaked P waves, and prolonged QT intervals. (3) (PB; CJ; AS)**

3 _x_ **Muscle weakness is a symptom of potassium depletion in skeletal muscles;**

potassium facilitates the conduction of nerve impulses and muscle activity.

4 _____ Abdominal cramps, as a result of heightened neuromuscular activity, is a symptom of hyperkalemia.

5 _____ Tingling of the fingertips, as a result of a lowered threshold of excitation of peripheral sensory nerve fibers, is a symptom of hypocalcemia.

347. **2 All data are within normal limits; PO_2 is 80 to 100 mm Hg, PCO_2 is 35 to 45 mm Hg, and the pH is 7.35 to 7.45. (1) (PB; CJ; AN)**

1 None of the data are indicators of fluid balance, but of acid-base balance.

3 Oxygen is within normal limits of 80 to 100 mm Hg.

4 The pH would have to be less than 7.35

348. **3 The body fights acidosis by hydrogen exchange, which results in excretion of excess hydrogen in the urine, a compensatory mechanism to raise the serum pH level. (3) (PB; CJ; AN)**

1 In acidosis the pH level of the blood is decreased.

2 Plasma bicarbonates would be decreased.

4 In acidosis the respiratory center in the medulla is stimulated to increase respirations and blow off carbon dioxide, which is carried to the lung as carbonic acid; lowering carbonic acid raises the serum pH level.

349. **2 The client is hyperventilating and blowing off excessive carbon dioxide, which leads to these symptoms; if uninterrupted this could result in respiratory alkalosis. (3) (PB; CJ; AS)**

1 Eupnea is normal, quiet breathing; the client has shallow, rapid breathing.

3 Kussmaul's respirations are deep, gasping respirations associated with diabetic acidosis and coma.

4 These symptoms are related to a decreased carbon dioxide level in the body.

350. **3 Reassurance decreases anxiety and slows respirations; the bag is used so that exhaled carbon dioxide can be rebreathed to resolve respiratory alkalosis and return the client to acid-base balance. (3) (PB; CJ; IM)**

1 This is not necessary because there is no evidence of hypoxia.

2 This is used to prevent atelectasis.

4 The client is already alkalotic; bicarbonate ions would increase the problem.

351. 1 Sodium, which is concerned with the regulation of extracellular fluid volume, is lost with vomiting; chloride, which balances cations in the extracellular compartment, is also lost with vomiting; because sodium and chloride are parallel electrolytes, hyponatremia will accompany hypochloremia. (2) (PB; CJ; PL)
2 These values do not provide significant information in relation to the effects of vomiting.
3 Same as answer 2.
4 Same as answer 2.

352. 4 The normal plasma pH value is 7.35 to 7.45; the client is in alkalosis; the normal plasma bicarbonate value is 23 to 25 mEq/L; the client has an excess of base bicarbonate, indicating a metabolic cause for the alkalosis. (1) (PB; CJ; AS)
1 The normal plasma potassium value is 3.5 to 5.5 mEq/L; the potassium value is within normal limits.
2 The normal plasma sodium value is 135 to 145 mEq/L; the client has hyponatremia.
3 The normal plasma chloride value is 95 to 105 mEq/L; the client has hypochloremia because of vomiting of gastric secretions.

353. 3 Prolonged vomiting results in fluid loss; symptoms reflect dehydration and metabolic alkalosis. (3) (SE; CJ; AN)
1 This is a potential, not actual, problem; the priority must be placed on the actual fluid and electrolyte problem.
2 A duodenal ulcer has not been diagnosed, and it is a medical, not nursing, diagnosis.
4 There is not enough data to support this diagnosis; the priority must be placed on the actual fluid and electrolyte problem.

354. 3 Hyperventilation results in the increased elimination of carbon dioxide from the blood. (2) (PB; CJ; AN)
1 The PO₂ level would not be affected.
2 The pH level will be increased.
4 The carbonic acid level will be decreased.

355. 2 Potassium is plentiful in green leafy vegetables; broccoli provides 207 mg of potassium per one-half cup. (3) (PB; MR; IM)
1 Oatmeal provides 73 mg of potassium per one-half cup.
3 Rice provides 29 mg of potassium per one-half cup.
4 Cooked fresh carrots provide 172 mg of potassium per one-half cup; canned carrots provide only 93 mg of potassium per one-half cup.

356. 2 Decreased oxygen increases the conversion of pyruvic acid to lactic acid, resulting in metabolic acidosis. (3) (PB; CJ; AN)
1 Hyperkalemia would occur because of renal shutdown; hypokalemia could occur in early shock.
3 Respiratory alkalosis could occur in early shock because of rapid, shallow breathing, but in late shock metabolic or respiratory acidosis occurs.
4 The PCO₂ level would be increased in profound shock.

357. 3 The normal range of venous pH is 7.31 to 7.41; any condition that decreases bicarbonate anion concentration in extracellular fluid results in metabolic acidosis. (3) (PB; CJ; AN)
1 This is not an accurate assessment for metabolic acidosis.
2 Same as answer 1.
4 This is within the normal range.

358. 3 Kussmaul's breathing is an abnormally deep, very rapid, sighing type of respiratory pattern that develops as a compensatory response to metabolic acidosis and attempts to raise the pH of the blood by blowing off carbon dioxide. (2) (PB; CJ; AS)
1 Dyspnea is difficult breathing associated with subjective or objective distress in response to oxygen problems.
2 Hyperpnea is a deep, rapid rate of breathing without a subjective sense of extra effort, usually as a response to strenuous effort
4 Cheyne-Stokes respirations are characterized by a waxing and waning of breathing that is usually associated with pathology of the respiratory center in the brain.

359. 3 In respiratory alkalosis the pH level is elevated because of loss of hydrogen ions; the PCO₂ level is low because carbon dioxide is lost through hyperventilation. (3) (PB; CJ; AS)
1 This is partially compensated metabolic alkalosis.
2 This is respiratory acidosis.
4 This is metabolic acidosis with some compensation.

360. 3 The pH of the blood indicates acidosis; CO₂ is the parameter for respiratory function; normal PCO₂ is 40. (3) (PB; CJ; AN)
1 HCO₃ is the parameter for metabolic functions.
2 Same as answer 1.
4 A pH of 7.25 is acidic, indicating acidosis not alkalosis.

361. 3

$$\frac{\text{Amount in mL}}{\text{Amount of hours}} \times \frac{\text{drop factor}}{60 \text{ min}} = \frac{\text{gtt}}{\text{min}}$$

$$\frac{150}{1} \times \frac{15}{60} = \frac{2250}{60} = 37.5 \text{ gtt;}$$

round out and administer 38 gtt/min

(2) (PB; CJ; AN)

1 The client would receive an inadequate amount.
2 Same as answer 1.
4 The client would receive an excessive amount.

362. 3 The client is in respiratory acidosis, probably caused by the depressant effects of an anesthetic or a compromised airway; coughing clears the airway and deep breaths blow off CO_2. (3) (PB; CJ; IM)
1 This is the treatment for respiratory alkalosis; the client is in respiratory acidosis.
2 This will not correct respiratory acidosis and may aggravate hypokalemia if present.
4 This is not necessary if clearing of the airway rectifies the problem.

363. 3 Antidiuretic hormone (ADH) causes water retention, resulting in a decreased urine output and dilution of serum electrolytes. (3) (PB; CJ; AS)
1 Blood volume may increase, causing hypertension; diluting the nitrogenous wastes in the blood decreases rather than increases the BUN.
2 Water retention dilutes electrolytes; the client is overhydrated rather than underhydrated, so turgor is not poor.
4 ADH acts on the nephron to cause water to be reabsorbed from the glomerular filtrate, leading to reduced urine volume; the specific gravity is elevated as a result of increased concentration.

364. 2 The enlarged cirrhotic liver impinges on the portal system causing increased hydrostatic pressure resulting in ascites. (3) (PB; CJ; AN)
1 Bile salts are not responsible for fluid shifts; increased serum bile results from biliary obstruction, not increased secretion.
3 This pressure is unchanged; decreased intravascular osmotic pressure accounts for fluid movement into interstitial spaces.

4 The liver's production of serum albumin is decreased.

365. 4 Albumin is an essential component of the bloodstream that helps maintain both osmotic pressure and fluid and electrolyte balance. (3) (PB; CJ; AN)
1 This is not a cause of hemorrhage; blood components such as platelets, thrombin, and erythrocytes are involved in the prevention of hemorrhage or anemia.
2 This is not directly involved with immunity and resistance; blood components such as T and B lymphocytes are involved in this process; the liver synthesizes specific proteins intrinsic to the function of antibodies.
3 The serum albumin level is not related to nutrition of cells.

366. 2 An elevated serum albumin level increases the osmotic effect and pulls fluid back into the intravascular compartment, decreasing ascites and edema. (3) (PB; CJ; EV)
1 This therapy will increase blood volume and blood flow to the kidney, thereby increasing urinary output.
3 Albumin will not lower the blood ammonia level; an elevated blood ammonia level causes hepatic encephalopathy.
4 Albumin therapy has no effect on blood ammonia levels.

367. 3 This is important in determining whether or not the aspirin has affected the balance of electrolytes. (2) (PB; CJ; AS)
1 A test that requires 24 hours is not helpful in an emergency.
2 The blood glucose level is unrelated to an overdose of aspirin or cold tablets; a serum glucose would be done to confirm diabetic ketoacidosis; the history does not indicate that the client has diabetes mellitus.
4 Toxic hepatic effects of a drug overdose are not apparent soon after ingestion of the drugs.

368. 3 Different infusion sets deliver different preset numbers of drops per milliliter; knowing this is a necessity for calculating the drip rate. (1) (PB; CJ; AN)
1 This does not determine the drip rate.
2 Same as answer 1.
4 This determines the size of the drop, not the drip rate.

369. **3 Air in the secondary line will not enter the vein; fluid from the primary bottle is under pressure and will flow before air from the secondary line could reach the port in the primary line. (1) (PB; CJ; IM)**
   1 This is possibly true, but this answer would increase anxiety.
   2 Gentamicin bypasses the large IV bag because it is piggybacked into the primary line below the drip chamber and check valve.
   4 This is contraindicated; this stops the infusion, which can clog the lumen of the catheter that is inserted into the vein.

370. **1 This position decreases pressure in the vena cava which helps prevent an air embolus when the catheter is disconnected. (3) (PB; CJ; PL)**
   2 Infusion of high concentrations of glucose will cause hypervolemia, not hypovolemia.
   3 No medications or solutions other than the parenteral nutrition should be administered through this line.
   4 The infusion rate is changed only with a physician's order.

371. **1 When blood glucose exceeds the renal threshold for glucose reabsorption in the kidney tubules it acts as an osmotic diuretic resulting in polyuria. (2) (PB; CJ; EV)**
   2 This is not associated with hyperglycemia.
   3 With hyperglycemia there is hyperventilation.
   4 This level is within the expected range.

GASTROINTESTINAL (GI)

372. **1 The mucosa of the mouth and the vomiting center in the brainstem may be affected producing nausea and vomiting. (3) (PB; CJ; EV)**
   2 This is not a side effect of radiation therapy to the oral cavity.
   3 Same as answer 2.
   4 These are not expected responses because of the distance between the radon seeds and the intestines.

373. **3 Gentle sprays are effective in cleaning the mouth and teeth without disturbing the sensitive tissues or radon seeds. (2) (PB; CJ; PL)**
   1 This could dislodge the radon seeds and be traumatic to the compromised oral mucosa.
   2 An antiseptic mouthwash is an astringent that would be too harsh for the sensitive oral mucosa.
   4 Same as answer 1.

374. **1 Cheerios contain 2.64 g of fiber per cup, which is more than the other choices. (3) (PB; MR; EV)**
   2 Corn Flakes contain 0.7 g of fiber per cup.
   3 Froot Loops contain 0.59 g of fiber per cup.
   4 Rice Krispies contain 1.34 g of fiber per cup.

375. **3 Complementary mixtures of essential amino acids in plant proteins provide complete dietary protein equivalents. (3) (PB; MR; IM)**
   1 A total vegetarian does not consume flesh, milk, milk products, or eggs.
   2 Same as answer 1.
   4 Same as answer 1.

376. **4 Increased exercise builds skeletal muscle mass and reduces excess fatty tissue. (3) (PM; MR; EV)**
   1 This is unrelated to weight loss; during aerobic exercise the heart rate should increase, but between periods of exercise the heart rate will decrease because of the development of collateral circulation.
   2 Appetite may be increased.
   3 The metabolic rate will increase.

377. **3 With an inflammatory response the body increases its production of WBCs and fibrinogen, which increases the WBC count and blood sedimentation rate, respectively. (1) (PB; CJ; AN)**
   1 This would not affect the white blood cell count or the sedimentation rate.
   2 Same as answer 1.
   4 Same as answer 1.

378. **2 The stomach is located within the sternal angle and the area is known as the epigastric area. (1) (PM; CJ; AS)**
   1 This is in the area of the iliac bones.
   3 This is the lowest middle abdominal area.
   4 This is the area above the sternum.

379. **2 Barium will harden and may create an impaction; a laxative and increased fluids promote elimination of barium. (2) (PB; CJ; PL)**
   1 Iodine is not used with barium.
   3 The client must be kept NPO.
   4 This is not part of the preparation; feces in the lower GI tract would not interfere with visualization of the upper GI tract.

380. **4 Auscultation must be performed before percussion and palpation because they may influence intestinal peristalsis resulting in inaccurate results. (2) (SE; CJ; AS)**
   1 Percussion or palpation performed before auscultation may result in an inaccurate assessment of bowel sounds.
   2 Same as answer 1.

3 Same as answer 1.

381. 2 Carbohydrates provide 4 kcal/g; therefore 3L × 50 g/L × 4 kcal/g = 600 kcal, only about a third of the basal energy need. (1) (PB; CJ; AN)
  1 This is less than the calories provided by the ordered IV fluid.
  3 This is more than the calories provided by the ordered IV fluid.
  4 Same as answer 3.

382. 3 This diet progresses from the one that makes the least metabolic demand on the client (clear liquid) to a regular diet, requiring the capability of unimpaired digestion. (1) (PB; CJ; AN)
  1 The caloric content is not the focus in a progressive postsurgical diet.
  2 Initially, a progressive diet has very little nutritional value; the focus is to rest the gastrointestinal tract immediately after surgery.
  4 Initially, a limited variety of fluids is presented to rest the gastrointestinal tract; food is not included until later.

383. Answer: 1970 calories. There are 9 calories in each gram of fat and 4 calories in each gram of carbohydrate and protein; this diet contains 1970 calories. (3) (PB; CJ; AN)

384. 2 This serum albumin value indicates severe depletion of visceral protein stores; the normal range for serum albumin is 3.5 to 5.5 g/dl; white meat turkey (two slices 4 × 2 × ¼ inch) contains approximately 28 g of protein. (3) (SE; MR; EV)
  1 A 6-oz serving of mixed fruit contains approximately 0.5 g of protein.
  3 A 3-oz serving of spinach salad contains approximately 9 g of protein.
  4 A 4-oz serving of beef broth contains approximately 2.4 g of protein.

385. 1 The increased osmotic effect of therapy increases the intravascular volume and urinary output; weight loss reflects fluid loss. (1) (PB; CJ; PL)
  2 The vital signs will not change drastically; "frequently" is a nonspecific time frame.
  3 The urinary output is measured hourly; half-hour outputs are insignificant in this instance.
  4 Serum, not urine, albumin levels would be significant; albumin in the urine indicates kidney dysfunction, not liver dysfunction.

386. 3 The RDA requirement for an adult male is 90 mg; smoking accelerates oxidation of tissue vitamin C,

so smokers need an additional 35 mg/day. (3) (PC; CJ; IM)
  1 This is not oxidized more rapidly in the smoker.
  2 Same as answer 1.
  4 Same as answer 1.

387. 1 Tofu products increase protein without increasing vitamin D because, unlike milk products, tofu does not contain vitamin D. (2) (SE; MR; EV)
  2 Eggnog contains milk and should be avoided.
  3 This contains vitamin D and should be avoided.
  4 This contains milk, which has vitamin D, and should be avoided.

388. 3 Vitamin C (ascorbic acid), an antioxidant, is found in vegetables such as broccoli, tomatoes, and potatoes; 1 cup of broccoli has 140 mg of vitamin C. (2) (PB; CJ; AN)
  1 Apples, depending on their size, contain 6 to 8 mg of vitamin C.
  2 An entire head of lettuce contains 13 mg of vitamin C.
  4 Apricots contain 11 mg of vitamin C; they are a source of beta-carotene.

389. 1 The antioxidants vitamin E and beta-carotene, which help inhibit oxidation and therefore tissue breakdown, are found in these foods. (3) (PB; CJ; AN)
  2 These are excellent sources of vitamin E, not beta-carotene.
  3 These are excellent sources of vitamin C, not vitamin E and beta-carotene.
  4 These are excellent sources of beta-carotene, not vitamin E.

390. 3 Stress ulcers are asymptomatic until they produce massive hematemesis and rectal bleeding. (2) (PB; CJ; AS)
  1 Shock is the outcome of massive hemorrhage; it would not be unexplained because the sudden gastrointestinal bleeding would be seen.
  2 Sudden massive bleeding occurs, not the slow oozing that causes melena.
  4 A gradual drop in the hematocrit value indicates slow blood loss.

391. 3 Green vegetables contain fiber, which promotes defecation. (1) (SE; MR; EV)
  1 These have a constipating effect, which would result in straining at stool.
  2 Same as answer 1.
  4 Same as answer 1.

392. 4 This produces bulk, which stimulates defecation; the muscles used in defecation are weak in clients with Parkinson's disease. (2) (PB; CJ; IM)
   1 Bananas are binding and will intensify the problem of constipation.
   2 This will intensify the problem; fluids need to be increased.
   3 Cathartics are irritating to the intestinal mucosa, and their regular administration promotes dependence.

393. 1 Red meat can react with reagents used in the test to cause false-positive results. (2) (PB; CJ; AS)
   2 This may apply for testing for ova and parasites, but not for occult blood.
   3 If the correct procedure is followed, discarding the first specimen is unnecessary.
   4 Random stool testing can be done but must be on three different bowel movements during the screening period.

394. 3 These characteristics describe steatorrhea, which results from impaired fat digestion. (3) (PB; CJ; AS)
   1 This is descriptive of stools resulting from constipation.
   2 This is descriptive of acholic stools occurring with biliary obstruction and resulting from an absence of urobilin.
   4 This would be descriptive of upper and lower gastrointestinal bleeding.

395. 2 Although the central venous catheter remains in situ, total parental nutrition does not have to infuse continuously. (3) (PB; CJ; PL)
   1 Although a feeling of pressure may be experienced, it is not a painful procedure.
   3 Placement of the tube is verified by x-ray.
   4 The subclavian veins are used most often; the jugular vein is too close to hair-growing areas, which increases the possibility of sepsis, and neck movements may interfere with the integrity of the placement of the catheter.

396. 3 The solution is hyperosmolar and a very concentrated source of glucose; too-rapid infusion can cause a shift of fluid into the intravascular compartment, resulting in overload; an infusion device should be used. (3) (PB; CJ; PL)
   1 Although important, it is not the priority.
   2 Same as answer 1.
   4 Same as answer 1.

397. 4 The less disruptive the procedure, the greater the acceptance by the client. (2) (PB; MR; PL)
   1 Most often, total parenteral nutrition is set up to run daily during sleeping hours.
   2 Depending on the type of circulatory access used, it may not need to be changed for weeks.
   3 The client or a significant other can be taught the principles of administration.

398. 2 The *Salmonella* organism thrives in warm, moist environments; washing, cooking, and refrigeration of food limits the growth of or eliminates the organism. (1) (PM; CJ; AS)
   1 Salmonellosis is unrelated to cancer.
   3 Salmonellosis is caused by the *Salmonella* organism, not stress.
   4 The *Salmonella* organism is ingested; it is not an airborne or blood-borne infection.

399. 2 Fluids of dextrose and normal saline and electrolytes are administered to prevent profound dehydration caused by an excessive loss of water and electrolytes through diarrheal output. (3) (PB; CJ; PL)
   1 Salmonellosis is an infection, not a condition caused by hyperacidity.
   3 These are not used when there is a possibility of bacterial infection because slowed peristalsis decreases excretion of the *Salmonella* organism.
   4 Same as answer 3.

400. 1 A cold environment limits growth of microorganisms. (1) (SE; MR; EV)
   2 All food should be refrigerated before and after it is cooked to limit the growth of microorganisms.
   3 This promotes the growth of microorganisms because the stuffing would still be warm for a period before the refrigerator's cold environment cooled the center of the bird; poultry should be stuffed immediately before being cooked.
   4 This promotes the growth of microorganisms because they thrive in warm, moist environments.

401. 4 Gravity facilitates digestion and prevents reflux of stomach contents into the esophagus. (2) (PB; MR; IM)
   1 Exercise immediately after eating may prolong the digestive process.
   2 Water should not be taken with or immediately after meals, since it overdistends the stomach.

3 Lying down immediately after eating facilitates reflux of the stomach contents into the esophagus.

402. 2 **The decreased hemoglobin and hematocrit levels and RBC count may be a result of malnutrition; also, cancer of the esophagus can cause dysphagia and anorexia. (3) (PB; CJ; AN)**
1 There are no data given related to airway obstruction or metastasis.
3 There are no data given related to pressure on surrounding structures producing pain.
4 There are no data given related to airway obstruction or injury.

403. 2 **Because of the trauma of surgery and the proximity of the esophagus to the trachea, respiratory assessments become the priority. (1) (PB; CJ; EV)**
1 Although this is important, an adequate airway is the priority.
3 Same as answer 1.
4 Same as answer 1.

404. 3 **An increased heart rate is related to an autonomic nervous system response; pain is related to the trauma of the perforation and possibly gastric reflux. (3) (PB; CJ; EV)**
1 These are signs of the dumping syndrome.
2 Same as answer 1.
4 An increased blood pressure may occur, but increased output has no relationship to esophageal perforation.

405. 1 **Obesity causes stress on the diaphragmatic musculature, which weakens and allows the stomach to protrude into the thoracic cavity. (1) (PM; CJ; AN)**
2 Inflammation of the bronchi would not weaken the diaphragm.
3 This does not cause a hiatus hernia.
4 This may cause an enlarged liver or pancreatitis but not a hiatus hernia.

406. 2 **Apple juice is not irritating to the gastric mucosa. (2) (PB; MR; PL)**
1 Carbonated beverages distend the stomach and promote regurgitation.
3 Its acidity aggravates the disorder.
4 Most colas should be avoided because they contain caffeine, which causes increased acidity and aggravates the disorder.

407. 3 **Weight reduction decreases intraabdominal pressure, thereby decreasing the tendency to reflux into the esophagus. (3) (PM; MR; IM)**

1 Fats decrease emptying of the stomach, extending the time period that reflux can occur; fats should be decreased.
2 This increases the pressure against the diaphragmatic hernia, increasing symptoms.
4 This would increase pressure; fluid should be discouraged with meals.

408. 3 **Tarry stools indicate upper GI bleeding; hemorrhage can occur if erosion extends to blood vessels. (2) (PB; CJ; AS)**
1 Investigation of bleeding takes priority; later the nurse should help to identify irritating foods that are to be avoided.
2 Nausea is a common symptom of gastritis, but is not life threatening.
4 Attempts to control alcoholism should be supported but this is a long-term goal; assessment of bleeding takes priority.

409. 1 **Classic symptoms include gnawing, boring, or dull pain located in the midepigastrium or back; pain is caused by irritability and erosion of the mucosal lining. (2) (PB; CJ; AS)**
2 This type of pain is more characteristic of cholecystitis.
3 This type of pain is more characteristic of the complication of a perforated ulcer.
4 This type of pain is more characteristic of a hiatal hernia.

410. 2 **Pain occurs after the stomach empties; ingesting food stimulates gastric secretions, which later act on the gastric mucosa of the empty stomach causing the gnawing pain. (1) (PB; CJ; AS)**
1 Vomiting temporarily alleviates pain because acid secretions are removed.
3 There is no intolerance of fats; eating generally alleviates pain.
4 Pain is sharply localized in the epigastrium; it can radiate across the abdomen if an ulcer has perforated.

411. 4 **Abdominal distention, which may be associated with pain, can indicate perforation, a complication that could lead to peritonitis. (3) (PB; CJ; EV)**
1 This, together with cramping, is an expected response.
2 A local inflammatory response to insertion of the fiberoptic tube may result in a sore throat and dysphagia once the anesthesia wears off; this is expected.
3 This is not indicative of any particular problem in this situation.

412. 4 Some medications, such as aspirin, NSAIDs, and prednisone, irritate the stomach lining and may cause bleeding with prolonged use. (2) (PB; CJ; AS)
1 Travel to foreign countries may be related to intestinal irritation, causing diarrhea and intestinal bleeding, not gastric bleeding.
2 This is not the cause of gastric bleeding; it is important to ascertain dietary habits when teaching about diet therapy.
3 Although stress may play a part, the use of some medications has a more direct relationship.

413. 1 These are classic indicators of perforated ulcer, for which immediate surgery is indicated; this should be anticipated. (2) (PB; MR; PL)
2 Tachycardia and tachypnea are related to pain and possible blood loss; keeping the client NPO is the priority.
3 The symptoms are indicative of perforation and the priority is to prepare to surgery.
4 Black, tarry stools or red stools indicate bleeding, not perforation.

414. 3 Without an adequate stomach reservoir, the hypertonic, concentrated food mass "dumps" into the small intestine, drawing fluid from surrounding blood and tissue and causing hypovolemia and typical shock symptoms. (2) (PB; CJ; AN)
1 The opposite is true; the food passes too quickly into the small intestine.
2 The food mass is more concentrated (hypertonic), not dilute.
4 Same as answer 2.

415. 1 After gastric surgery a nasogastric tube is in place for drainage of blood and gastric secretions. (1) (PB; CJ; PL)
2 Oxygen is not required unless the client experiences a complication necessitating its administration.
3 The average client is given about 3500 mL of fluid by IV to meet fluid needs and replace gastric losses.
4 This may or may not be necessary; a nasogastric tube is necessary following gastric surgery.

416. 1 Statistics demonstrate that these are the most likely sites for metastasis of this tumor. (2) (PB; CJ; AN)
2 It is less likely that the tumor will spread to these areas.
3 Same as answer 2.
4 These are routes of metastasis.

417. 3 Large amounts of blood or excessive bloody drainage 12 hours postoperatively must be reported immediately because the client is hemorrhaging. (2) (PB; MR; EV)
1 This must be ordered by the physician; 50 to 100 mL of normal saline at room temperature instilled every 30 to 50 minutes is the usual therapy to prevent lowering the core body temperature.
2 This is contraindicated; accumulation of secretions would cause pressure on the suture line; this prevents further observation of drainage.
4 This is an unsafe intervention at this time; the physician should be notified.

418. 4 Removal of the fundus of the stomach destroys the parietal cells that secrete intrinsic factor (needed to combine with vitamin B_{12} as a preliminary to its absorption in the ileum). (3) (PM; CJ; AS)
1 Hemorrhaging may cause anemia; however, pernicious anemia occurs when the intrinsic factor is not produced.
2 The beta cells of the pancreas are not involved in secretion of intrinsic factor.
3 Dietary intake does not affect the production of intrinsic factor.

419. 1 Intrinsic factor is lost with removal of the stomach, and vitamin B_{12} is needed to maintain the hemoglobin level once the client is stabilized; injections are given monthly for life. (2) (PM; CJ; PL)
2 Adequate diet, fluid intake, and exercise should prevent constipation.
3 This would not be a routine expectation.
4 This surgery does not affect pancreatic enzymes.

420. 4 This cancer is usually asymptomatic in the early stages; the stomach accommodates the mass. (1) (PB; MR; AN)
1 It can be accurately diagnosed by gastric washings or biopsy.
2 This cancer is painless in its early stages.
3 This is typical of Hodgkin's disease, not gastric carcinoma.

421. 1 The thoracic cavity is usually entered for a complete resection, necessitating a chest tube. (2) (PB; MR; PL)
2 Fluids are contraindicated until the suture line has healed and nasogastric suction is no longer being used.
3 There would be no physiologic necessity for this position.

4 The client would ambulate early to minimize the hazards of immobility.

422. **2 Taking fluids with meals causes rapid emptying of the food from the stomach into the jejunum before it has been adequately subjected to the digestive process; the hyperosmolar mixture causes a fluid shift to the jejunum. (1) (PB; MR; IM)**
   1 Rest, not activity, after meals will assist in relieving dumping syndrome.
   3 Small meals with low carbohydrate, moderate fat, and high protein are recommended; these are more readily digested and prevent rapid stomach emptying.
   4 Low-carbohydrate meals are recommended to reduce the osmolarity of chyme as it empties into the jejunum.

423. **2 As a result of the trauma of surgery, some bleeding can be expected for four to five hours. (3) (PB; CJ; EV)**
   1 Clamping the tube would cause increased pressure on the gastric sutures from a buildup of gas and fluid.
   3 Iced saline is rarely used because it causes vasoconstriction, local ischemia, and a reduction in body temperature.
   4 This is not necessary; this is a normal occurrence.

424. **2 Rigidity and pain are hallmarks of bleeding from the suture line and/or of peritonitis; vital signs provide supporting data. (1) (PB; CJ; AS)**
   1 Ambulation would be indicated if pain were the result of flatulence; however, rigidity is clearly associated with bleeding or peritonitis and more data are needed.
   3 An analgesic may mask the symptoms, delaying diagnosis.
   4 This is unrelated to the symptoms presented.

425. **1 Bowel sounds and flatulence indicate the return of intestinal peristalsis; peristalsis is necessary for movement of nutrients through the GI tract. (1) (PB; CJ; EV)**
   2 Incisional pain is unrelated to intestinal peristalsis.
   3 Hematocrit levels indicate blood loss; they are unaffected by GI functioning.
   4 Dumping syndrome occurs after, not before, the ingestion of food and would not be an indication that the client was ready to ingest food.

426. **4 Over-the-counter antacid preparations are taken to neutralize gastric acid and relieve pain. (2) (SE; MR; EV)**
   1 Although eating food initially prevents gastric acid from irritating the gastric walls, it can precipitate acid production and weight gain.
   2 Aspirin is contraindicated because it irritates gastric mucosa and promotes bleeding by preventing platelet aggregation.
   3 Reduction of fluids with meals does not affect pain; it does help control symptoms of dumping syndrome.

427. **1 Treatment with medications, rest, diet, and stress reduction relieves symptoms, heals the ulcer, and prevents complications and recurrence. (2) (PB; CJ; IM)**
   2 Pain occurs 30 minutes to one hour after a meal.
   3 Surgery may be done after multiple recurrences and for treating complications.
   4 Perforation, pyloric obstruction, and hemorrhage, not cancer, are major complications.

428. **4 Dark brown or black stools (melena) could indicate gastrointestinal bleeding. (1) (PB; MR; AS)**
   1 Frothy stools are indicative of poor fat absorption and are associated with sprue.
   2 Ribbon-shaped stools indicate a bowel mass or obstruction.
   3 Clay-colored stools are usually related to problems causing a decrease in bile.

429. **1 Nausea with a nasogastric tube to decompression in place could mean tube displacement or obstruction; checking placement can determine whether it is in the stomach; once placement is verified, then fluid can be instilled to ensure patency. (3) (SE; CJ; IM)**
   2 This may relieve the discomfort but will not determine the cause.
   3 The tube should never be irrigated because it would be too traumatic; if the tube is displaced, it could be in the trachea or bronchi and instillation of fluid would cause respiratory impairment.
   4 The nurse should always assess a situation carefully before notifying the physician.

430. **2 Abdominal distention, nausea, and abdominal pain can be signs of nasogastric tube blockage. (2) (PB; CJ; IM)**
   1 Although opioids are usually ordered postoperatively, they tend to decrease peristalsis and may increase abdominal distention and nausea.
   3 There will be no stools for several days; gastric drainage may contain some blood from surgery.
   4 Bowel sounds are not expected for several days after stomach or intestinal surgery.

431. 4 **Drainage is bright red initially and gradually becomes darker red during the first 24 hours. (2) (PB; CJ; EV)**
  1 If the nasogastric tube is functioning correctly, secretions will be removed and vomiting will not occur.
  2 Since the bowel was emptied before surgery and the client is now npo, there would be no expected intestinal activity.
  3 If the nasogastric tube is functioning correctly, gastric distention will not occur.

432. 3 **Hypertonic food increases osmotic pressure and pulls fluid from the intravascular compartment into the intestine (dumping syndrome). (2) (PB; CJ; AN)**
  1 This is separation of the wound edges, usually accompanied by a gush of pink-tinged fluid; it is not related to the dumping syndrome.
  2 Increased carbohydrates, not fats, are responsible for the increased osmotic pressure often associated with the dumping syndrome.
  4 While peristalsis may be decreased because of surgery, it would not account for the symptoms.

433. 4 **The rapid absorption of sugars from the food mass causes elevation of blood glucose, and the insulin response often causes transient hypoglycemic symptoms. (2) (PB; CJ; AN)**
  1 This is unrelated; usually a bland diet is prescribed following a gastrectomy.
  2 The response is rebound hypoglycemia, not hyperglycemia.
  3 The insulin-adjusting mechanism is not overwhelmed but responds vigorously, causing rebound hypoglycemia.

434. 1 **These characteristics are well-established risk factors for gallbladder disease (female, fat, and 40). (1) (PM; CJ; AS)**
  2 Although these clients usually are over the age of 40, a high fat intake does not predispose one to cholecystitis.
  3 The age is correct, but these clients have an increased serum cholesterol.
  4 Although there is an increased risk with a family history of gallstones, these clients usually are over the age of 40.

435. 1 **Pain is a cardinal symptom; it is helpful to have as much specific information about it as possible, particularly its description and its relationship to foods ingested. (2) (PB; MR; AS)**
  2 It is not necessary to save all urine and stool, although changes in color should be reported.

3 The client should be free to question orders that are not understood or agreed with.
4 This would not add any valuable information.

436. 4 **Cholecystitis is often accompanied by intolerance to fatty foods, including fried foods and butter. (2) (PB; MR; AS)**
  1 These cause flatulence and pain for clients with lower intestinal problems such as diverticulosis.
  2 These foods contain less fat than do fried foods or butter.
  3 Neither chocolate nor boiled seafood has as much fat as fried chicken or butter.

437. 2 **The gallbladder, which concentrates and stores bile, has been removed. (2) (PB; CJ; AN)**
  1 Bile continues to be produced by the liver.
  3 Same as answer 1.
  4 Enough bile is produced to digest some fatty foods.

438. 4 **During the procedure, a sedative is administered intravenously as needed to help the client stay calm. (3) (SE; MR; IM)**
  1 This is not used during this procedure.
  2 Same as answer 1.
  3 Same as answer 1.

439. 1 **Bile promotes the absorption of the fat-soluble vitamins; an obstruction of the common bile duct limits the flow of bile to the duodenum and, thus, the absorption of these vitamins. (3) (PB; CJ; AS)**
  2 This is not relevant to the situation.
  3 This is unnecessary; protein would be desirable for wound healing.
  4 These would be unexpected.

440. 3 **Self-splinting results in shallow breathing, which does not aerate the lungs adequately, particularly the lower right lobe. (1) (PB; CJ; PL)**
  1 The T-tube is never irrigated; it drains by gravity until the edema in the operative area subsides; the tube is then removed by the physician.
  2 The dressing is not changed by the nurse in the immediate postoperative period; the client's respiratory status takes first priority.
  4 The client would be NPO immediately after surgery.

441. 2 **Obstruction of bile flow impairs absorption of fat-soluble vitamin K; prothrombin is not produced and the clotting process is prolonged. (2) (PB; CJ; AN)**
  1 Although deposition of bile salts in the skin leads to pruritus, this is not life threatening.

3 While there may be an increase in flatulence in biliary disease, it is not life threatening.

4 Obstructive jaundice does not affect potassium levels.

442. 3 **The T-tube provides an outlet for bile produced by the liver and is expected to drain 300 to 500 mL in the first day. (3) (PB; CJ; IM)**

1 The rate of fluid administration is prescribed by the physician.

2 Clamping the tube during the early postoperative period may cause a buildup of pressure and leakage of bile into the peritoneum.

4 Drainage from the T-tube is by gravity; negative pressure is not applied.

443. 3 **Maintaining nasogastric tube patency ensures gastric decompression, thus preventing abdominal distension, which would place tension on the incision. (2) (SE; CJ; PL)**

1 Deep breathing should be encouraged to prevent respiratory complications; this places no undue tension on the wound.

2 Maintaining T-tube patency only ensures a portal of exit for bile drainage; the tube is not irrigated and an obstruction would lead to jaundice rather than tension on the surgical wound.

4 The right side-lying position after a cholecystectomy could increase, not decrease, tension in the operative area.

444. 4 **Recovery will be quicker because there is no large abdominal incision. (2) (SE; MR; IM)**

1 Clear liquids may be started as soon as the client is awake and a gag reflex has returned.

2 Carbonated beverages will create gas, which will distend the intestines and increase pain.

3 With a laparoscopic cholecystectomy there will be several puncture wounds, not an incision, on the abdomen.

445. 1 **Vitamin K, a precursor for prothrombin, cannot be absorbed without bile. (2) (PB; CJ; AS)**

2 This is commonly related to electrolyte imbalances, not fat-soluble vitamin deficiency.

3 Jaundice results from a backup of bile, not a deficiency of fat-soluble vitamins.

4 This may be related to electrolyte imbalances or deficiency of B vitamins, which are water soluble.

446. 1 **Biliary colic may occur in the postoperative period as a result of the passage of pulverized fragments of the calculi; this may occur three or more days after the lithotripsy. (3) (PB; CJ; IM)**

2 Fever would indicate pancreatitis, which is a rare occurrence.

3 The delivery of shock waves during the procedure is synchronized with the heartbeat to avoid initiation of dysrhythmias.

4 Light sedation may be used to keep the client comfortable and as still as possible.

447. 3 **Mild shoulder pain is common up to one week after surgery because of diaphragmatic irritation secondary to abdominal stretching or residual carbon dioxide that was used to inflate the abdominal cavity during surgery. (3) (SE; MR; EV)**

1 This is not necessary; the bandages are removed the second day postoperatively.

2 This is not necessary; the client may bathe and shower as usual.

4 This is not necessary; clients generally tolerate food after 24 to 48 hours.

448. 2 **It may take four to six months, but ultimately most people can eat anything they want. (2) (SE; MR; EV)**

1 Although fats may have to be gradually reintroduced, most people can tolerate them after a cholecystectomy.

3 Foods that caused gastric distress before surgery are usually tolerated after surgery.

4 Increased protein is only needed until healing has occurred.

449. 2 **Amylase concentration is high in the pancreas and is elevated in the serum when the pancreas becomes acutely inflamed; this distinguishes pancreatitis from other acute abdominal problems. (3) (PB; CJ; AS)**

1 An elevated blood glucose level is not indicative of pancreatitis, but rather diabetes mellitus; however, hyperglycemia and glycosuria may occur in some people with acute pancreatitis if the islets of Langerhans are affected.

3 This occurs in other disease processes, such as cholecystitis.

4 This is not specific to pancreatitis; white blood cells are elevated in other disease processes.

450. 2 **Pain with pancreatitis is usually severe and is the major symptom; it occurs because of the auto-digestive process in the pancreas and peritoneal irritation. (2) (PB; CJ; AN)**

1 There is no such nursing diagnosis.

3 There are not enough data for this conclusion; additional data such as skin turgor, serum electrolytes, and I&O are needed to make this nursing diagnosis.

4 Although this may be an appropriate nursing diagnosis for this client, it is not the priority at this time.

451. 2 Alcohol increases pancreatic secretions, which cause pancreatic cell destruction. (1) (PB; MR; IM)

1 Spicy foods do not damage the pancreas; spicy foods should be avoided by clients with gastrointestinal problems.

3 A bland diet is not necessary, but large, heavy meals should be avoided.

4 Although this is the desired diet, abstinence from alcohol is more important.

452. 4 A pancreaticoduodenectomy leads to malabsorption because of impaired delivery of bile to the intestine; fat metabolism is interfered with, causing dyspepsia. (3) (PB; MR; IM)

1 These clients are anorexic, require small frequent meals, and should eat high-calorie, high-protein, low-fat diets.

2 High-calorie meals are needed for energy and to promote use of protein for tissue repair.

3 High protein is required for tissue building; there is no problem with the liver in clients with cancer of the pancreas unless direct extension occurs.

453. 4 Polydipsia is characteristic of hypoinsulinism (diabetes mellitus) because of impaired carbohydrate metabolism. (2) (SE; MR; EV)

1 Polyuria, not oliguria, is characteristic of diabetes mellitus because excess fluid is excreted with the glucose by the kidneys.

2 Increased appetite is characteristic of diabetes mellitus because of impaired metabolism.

3 Weight loss characterizes diabetes mellitus because of the use of body mass as a source of energy.

454. 2 Rapid administration can cause glucose overload, leading to osmotic diuresis and dehydration; slowing the infusion decreases glucose overload. (2) (PB; CJ; IM)

1 Stopping the flow would jeopardize the central line; slowing the infusion will give the client's body a chance to handle the excess glucose.

3 Signs of bowel obstruction are not present.

4 The client's headache should disappear with oral fluid replacement; analgesics are not indicated.

455. 4 Formation of lipase necessary for digestion of fats is an exocrine function; the endocrine function is to secrete insulin, which is a hormone essential in carbohydrate metabolism. (3) (PB; CJ; PL)

1 Although it is necessary to avoid alcohol, this is not related to the exocrine functioning of the pancreas.

2 Fluid and electrolyte problems are not related specifically to exocrine or endocrine pancreatic functioning.

3 Deficiencies of both may occur because of poor intake, but these deficiencies are not specifically related to exocrine or endocrine pancreatic functioning.

456. 1 A client's vital signs, especially the pulse and temperature, will rise before the client demonstrates any of the more severe symptoms of withdrawal from alcohol. (3) (PB; CJ; PL)

2 This is contraindicated initially because it may cause cerebral edema.

3 This becomes a priority after the problems of the withdrawal period have subsided.

4 This is not a priority until after the detoxification process.

457. 4 Petechiae are evidence of capillary bleeding; the diseased liver is no longer able to metabolize vitamin K, which is necessary to activate blood clotting factors. (1) (PB; CJ; AN)

1 Although the client may have a deficiency of this vitamin, it is not involved in the clotting process.

2 Same as answer 1.

3 Vitamin A is not involved in clotting, even though the transformation of carotene to vitamin A takes place in the liver.

458. 4 This keeps the bladder in the pelvic area and prevents puncture when the abdominal cavity is entered. (1) (PB; CJ; IM)

1 This is not necessary.

2 This is unsafe; the bladder will rise into the abdominal cavity and may be punctured.

3 Same as answer 1.

459. 1 Hepatitis A is primarily spread via a fecal-oral route; sewage-polluted water may harbor the virus. (3) (PM; CJ; AS)

2 This does not increase the risk of developing the disease but will increase the risk of an infected individual spreading the disease to others.

3 Hepatitis types B, C, and D are more often spread via the blood-borne route; using disposable equipment and proper handling of syringes decreases the risk of spreading the virus.

4 Exposure to arsenic or carbon tetrachloride can cause toxic hepatitis, which is not communicable.

460. 4 Clay-colored stools are indicative of hepatic obstruction. (1) (SE; MR; PL)

1 It is unnecessary to call the physician because this symptom is characteristic of hepatitis from the onset of clinical manifestations.

2 Same as answer 1.

3 This is the normal color of urine.

461. 3 Damage to liver cells affects the ability to remove bilirubin from the blood, with resulting deposition in the skin and sclera. (2) (PB; CJ; AN)

1 With hepatitis, the liver does not secrete excess bile.

2 Destruction of red blood cells does not increase in hepatitis.

4 This is unrelated; decreased prothrombin levels cause spontaneous bleeding, not jaundice.

462. 4 Hepatitis A is spread via the fecal-oral route; transmission is prevented by proper handwashing. (2) (SE; MR; IM)

1 This may increase transmission because no provision is made for the cleaning of equipment or disposal of contaminated wastes.

2 This is untrue; hepatitis can be transmitted via the fecal-oral route and precautions, such as handwashing, must be taken.

3 This is inadequate; transmission is still possible via the roll of toilet tissue unless handwashing is done.

463. 4 Hepatitis A is transmitted via the fecal-oral route; contact precautions must be used when there are articles that have potential fecal and/or urine contamination. (2) (SE; CJ; PL)

1 Neither a private room nor a closed door is required; these are necessary only for respiratory (airborne) infections.

2 Hepatitis A is not transferred via the airborne route and therefore a mask is not necessary; a gown and gloves are required only when handling articles that may be contaminated.

3 This is too limited; a gown and gloves should also be worn when handling other fecally contaminated articles, such as a bedpan or rectal thermometer.

464. 4 This is a vascular lesion associated with cirrhosis thought to be related to elevated estrogen levels. (3) (PB; CJ; AS)

1 This refers to patches of depigmentation resulting from destruction of melanocytes.

2 This is excessive growth of hair; in cirrhosis, endocrine disturbances result in loss of axillary and pubic hair.

3 Dark pigmentary deposits result from a disorder of pigment metabolism.

465. 3 This would indicate that the client has a deficiency in clotting which should be corrected before the biopsy to prevent hemorrhage. (2) (SE; MR; AS)

1 This is not a contraindication; the client would need support and the examiner may need assistance, but the biopsy could be done.

2 A biopsy is not contraindicated in the presence of an infectious disease.

4 Vitamin K is needed for the production of prothrombin; however, this does not guarantee clotting activity.

466. 4 This position exposes the right intercostal space making the large right lobe of the liver accessible. (2) (PB; MR; IM)

1 This position would not provide accessibility to the liver; the small left lobe is not anatomically near the left chest wall.

2 This would not provide accessibility to the liver.

3 In this position the liver would fall away from the chest wall and be less accessible.

467. 3 In this position the liver capsule at the entry site is compressed against the chest wall and escape of blood and/or bile is impeded. (2) (SE; MR; PL)

1 This would be unsafe because no pressure would be applied to the puncture site and the client could bleed.

2 Same as answer 1.

4 Same as answer 1.

468. 1 Pressure applied to the puncture site compresses blood vessels, thereby preventing bleeding. (1) (PB; CJ; IM)

2 This will not restore the circulating blood volume.

3 The semi- or high-Fowler's positions, not the right side-lying position, would be more comfortable because they decrease pressure against the diaphragm.

4 This position will have little or no effect on the biliary ducts.

469. 4 The flow of bile through the puncture site indicates that a biliary vessel was punctured; this is a common complication after a liver biopsy. (2) (PB; CJ; AN)

1 The pancreas does not contain bile; also, it is in the upper left quadrant, not the upper right quadrant.

2 Fluid would leak through the puncture site or into the peritoneum, not the intestine.

3 This is a complication, not an expected outcome.

470. 4 An increased serum ammonia level impairs the CNS, causing an altered level of consciousness; safety is the priority. (3) (PB; CJ; AS)

1 Rising ammonia levels are not related to weight.

2 An alteration in fluid intake will not affect the serum ammonia level.

3 This is not the priority; the priority is to protect the client.

471. 1 The high ammonia levels contribute to deterioration of mental function and then to hepatic encephalopathy and hepatic coma; safety is the priority. (3) (SE; CJ; PL)

2 Although the client may have dyspnea as a result of ascites, it is not life threatening; safety is the priority.

3 Although this is done to monitor ascites, it is not the priority for a confused client; safety is the priority.

4 Providing for client safety is the priority.

472. 3 One lumen inflates the esophageal balloon, the second inflates the gastric balloon, and the third decompresses the stomach. (2) (SE; CJ; AN)

1 It is a triple, not single, lumen tube.

2 It is a triple, not double lumen tube; the stomach, not the intestine, is decompressed.

4 The stomach, not the intestine, is decompressed.

473. 1 Measures must be taken immediately to ensure client safety. (2) (SE; CJ; PL)

2 Although the physician should be notified, the nurse should first take measures to ensure client safety.

3 This is contraindicated because sedatives mask the progressive signs of hepatic encephalopathy.

4 Hepatic encephalopathy is caused by high serum ammonia levels, not hypoxia.

474. 1 The symptoms indicate hepatic coma; protein is reduced according to tolerance, and calories are increased to prevent tissue catabolism. (1) (PB; CJ; PL)

2 This represents a high-protein diet, which is contraindicated in hepatic coma.

3 Same as answer 2.

4 Same as answer 2.

475. 3 With increased intraabdominal pressure, the abdominal wall will become rigid and tender. (2) (PB; CJ; EV)

1 The pulse rate will increase in an effort to compensate for impending septic shock.

2 Hypovolemia and therefore hypotension result because of a loss of fluid, electrolytes, and protein into the peritoneal cavity.

4 Peristalsis and associated bowel sounds will decrease or be absent in the presence of increased intraabdominal pressure.

476. 2 Bowel sounds are the result of peristaltic movements that propel intestinal contents through the alimentary tract and cause characteristic sounds. (2) (PB; CJ; AS)

1 Bowel sounds will be heard before flatus is passed.

3 This has no relationship to the return of peristalsis.

4 Peristalsis will return before the client has a bowel movement.

477. 3 This position promotes localization of purulent material and inflammation and prevents an ascending infection. (1) (SE; CJ; IM)

1 The risk of an ascending infection may be increased in this position because it allows fluid in the abdominal cavity to bathe the entire peritoneum.

2 Same as answer 1.

4 The client would probably prefer a Sims' position, which increases risk of an ascending infection.

478. 1 Decreased motility is associated with serious problems, such as gangrene or toxic megacolon. (3) (PB; CJ; AS)

2 This is an uncomfortable but less serious manifestation.

3 This is an expected response that is not of primary concern at this time.

4 This is a vague symptom of a visceral pathologic condition; a frequent response.

479. 1 Medical treatment is directed toward reducing motility of the inflamed bowel, restoring nutrition, and treating and preventing infection; surgery is used selectively for those who are acutely ill or have excessive exacerbations. (2) (SE; MR; IM)

2 This is untrue; medical treatment is symptomatic, not curative.

3 It is usually performed as a last resort.

4 Although there is an emotional component, the physiologic adaptations determine whether surgery will be necessary.

480. 1 When anxious, in pain, or performing deep-breathing exercises, it is common for air to be swallowed, which can cause gastric distention. (3) (PB; CJ; AN)

2 Preoperative enemas are not given to prevent paralytic ileus postoperatively; they are given to cleanse the lower gastrointestinal tract, decreasing the possibility of peritoneal contamination.

3 A rectal tube does not relieve nausea and vomiting; it facilitates expulsion of gas and some secretions trapped in the large intestines because of lack of peristalsis.

4 Liquids are not given until some peristalsis has returned.

481. 1 **Low-residue foods produce less fecal waste decreasing bowel contents and irritation; protein promotes healing and calories provide energy. (2) (PB; MR; PL)**

2 Bar-B-Q foods are spicy; foods high in fat can increase peristalsis.

3 Fruit and aged, sharp cheese can be irritating to the bowel.

4 Chunky peanut butter and whole wheat bread are high-residue foods.

482. 3 **Decompression removes collected secretions behind the nonfunctioning bowel segment (paralytic ileus), thus reducing pressure on the suture line and allowing healing. (3) (PB; CJ; AN)**

1 Although this is important, the primary concern is decompression of the bowel; the amount of fluid removed will direct fluid and electrolyte replacement therapy.

2 Vomiting will subside as the bowel is decompressed.

4 Same as answer 1.

483. 2 **The client's feelings, knowledge, and skills concerning the ileostomy must be assessed before discharge. (1) (SE; CJ; EV)**

1 People should not be pressured into performing self-care before they are physically and emotionally ready.

3 Often, the client no longer needs a dressing on the incision at the time of discharge; a collection pouch is used over the stoma.

4 After an ileostomy the client is usually encouraged to eat a high-protein diet or a regular diet with supplemental protein; a high-fluid intake should be maintained.

484. 4 **Low-residue foods will not increase motility. (3) (PB; MR; IM)**

1 Warmth and the fiber in the orange juice will increase motility and should be avoided.

2 Wheat cereal contains roughage and should be avoided.

3 Both are high in residue and should be avoided; a western omelet is fried, which also should be avoided.

485. 3 **Constipation, diarrhea, and/or constipation alternating with diarrhea are the most common symptoms of colorectal cancer. (3) (PM; MR; AS)**

1 This is the second most common complaint that results from destruction of the epithelial lining of the intestine.

2 Pain is reported as a symptom in less than 25% of clients; also it is a late sign after other organs are invaded, intestinal obstruction occurs, or tissue necrosis develops.

4 This is a later sign that only becomes evident when the lumen of the intestine narrows as a result of the enlarging mass.

486. 4 **The initiation of the gastrocolic reflex could cause intestinal contents to reach the lower GI tract and interfere with the success of the x-ray series. (2) (PB; MR; PL)**

1 An oil retention enema would interfere with visualization during the GI series and therefore would not be administered.

2 A liquid, not bland, diet should be consumed the night before the test.

3 A cathartic may cause defecation, not diarrhea.

487. 4 **This is an accurate explanation of what the client can expect during the CAT scan. (2) (PB; MR; IM)**

1 It is not necessary to rest in bed for six hours.

2 The procedure causes no physical pain, and an analgesic is not necessary.

3 The client will be awake; neither sedation nor anesthesia is used with a CAT scan.

488. 4 **This diet is low in fiber; after digestion and absorption there is only a small amount of residue to be eliminated. (1) (PB; CJ; AN)**

1 This diet does not influence the flora of the intestine; antimicrobials, such as neomycin, are given to do this.

2 This diet does not promote peristalsis; the products of digestion remain in the intestine longer, and flatus is increased.

3 Although a low-residue diet is less irritating, this is not the primary reason for its use before surgery.

489. 3 Except in an emergency, the client receives an intestinal antibiotic for days preoperatively to reduce the amount of intestinal bacteria. (1) (PB; CJ; PL)

1 Diuretics are not necessary unless they have been prescribed for a preexisting problem.

2 Fluids are not restricted.

4 These are contraindicated initially after surgery because they may cause tension on the suture line and possible dehiscence.

490. 1 When intestinal continuity cannot be restored after removal of the anus, rectum, and adjacent colon, a permanent colostomy is formed. (2) (SE; LE; PL)

2 This segment of colon lies on the right side of the abdomen and has no anatomic proximity to the rectum.

3 This procedure is performed to allow a segment of colon to heal; intestinal continuity can be restored.

4 This procedure is commonly performed for inflammation of the colon when intestinal continuity can be restored.

491. 2 The surface of a stoma is mucous membrane and should be dark pink to red, moist, and shiny; the stoma is usually raised beyond the skin surface. (1) (PB; CJ; EV)

1 The stoma should be moist, not dry; pale pink indicates a low hemoglobin level; although some stomas can be flush with the skin, a raised stoma is more common.

3 The stoma should be moist, not dry; a purple color indicates compromised circulation; a depressed stoma is prolapsed and abnormal.

4 Although the stoma should be moist and dark pink to red, it should not be flush with the skin or painful.

492. 1 There is no need to irrigate before the stool is formed. (2) (PB; MR; PL)

2 The side-lying position is not the position of choice for a colostomy irrigation.

3 If proper technique is used, fecal elimination should flow through the sleeve of the colostomy bag to the commode.

4 The perineal wound may take weeks to heal, and irrigations must be started when the stool is formed.

493. 3 This is caused by the trauma of intestinal manipulation and the depressive effects of anesthetics and analgesics. (1) (PB; CJ; AN)

1 Edema would not totally interfere with peristalsis, which may be less effective but would still result in some output.

2 Any ingested food or fluid initiates the gastrocolic reflex and would therefore result in some output.

4 A nasogastric tube decompresses the stomach; it does not directly influence intestinal motility at this time.

494. 4 The irrigation bag should be hung no higher than 12 to 18 inches above the level of the stoma, and a clothes hook is too high. (1) (SE; MR; EV)

1 Fluid flowing into the intestines can cause distention and discomfort; clamping the tubing is an appropriate intervention.

2 The tip of the catheter should be lubricated to prevent trauma to mucosal tissue and to facilitate insertion.

3 There is not enough information provided to choose this response; the amount of fluid ordered is not included; usually 500 to 1000 mL of water is used.

495. 4 Stoma adhesive protects the skin and helps to keep the bag attached to the skin. (2) (PB; CJ; IM)

1 The bag should be emptied when it is one-third to one-half full.

2 This is too much space between the stoma and the bag; the enzymes in feces can erode the skin.

3 Initially the nurse should change the bag; self-care is usually more gradual.

496. 3 These clients can eat a regular diet; only gas-forming foods that cause distention and discomfort should be avoided. (1) (SE; MR; EV)

1 The amount of stool does not have to be limited; therefore a low-residue diet is not necessary.

2 The affected tissue has been removed, and normal mucosal tissue lines the intestine and forms the stoma; therefore bland foods are not necessary.

4 Nutrients are absorbed by the small, not the large, intestine; a regular diet is usually easily digested and absorbed.

497. 4 Regular irrigation and effective evacuation prevent unexpected bowel movements; generally a drainage pouch is needed only immediately after an irrigation. (3) (PB; MR; PL)

1 Once the colostomy is regulated an appliance will not be necessary except after the irrigation.

2 Appliances collect what is evacuated; they do not control the function of the colostomy; a "special" appliance is not needed.

3 The nurse cannot predict the client's next visit to the physician; this response does not deal with the client's concern.

498. 3 **Pain is wavelike, colicky, and sharp because of obstruction and localized bowel ischemia. (2) (PB; CJ; AS)**
   1 Flatus would be impeded by strangulation.
   2 Vomiting is persistent, not projectile.
   4 This is not an early sign of obstruction; decreased bowel sounds occur after gas and fluid accumulate.

499. 3 **The lowered blood pressure may be caused by pooling of blood in peripheral vessels; this will aid venous return. (2) (PB; CJ; IM)**
   1 This will not increase the blood pressure; this intervention is used for pregnant women to move the gravid uterus off the vena cava, which will increase placental perfusion.
   2 This may be done eventually after initially dealing with the situation and evaluating results.
   4 Opioid analgesics may decrease the blood pressure further.

500. 3 **Because of pain and the proximity of the operative site to the lower urinary tract, voiding problems are common. (3) (PB; CJ; EV)**
   1 This is not a complication of herniorrhaphy.
   2 The abdomen was not entered, and there should be no interference with peristalsis.
   4 This should not be a complication of herniorrhaphy because early ambulation is permitted.

501. **Answer: 258 calories. Carbohydrates yield 4 calories per gram; protein, 4 calories per gram; and fat, 9 calories per gram; the total carbohydrate calories are $32 \times 4 = 128$; the total protein calories are $10 \times 4 = 40$; the total fat calories are $10 \times 9 = 90$; $128 + 40 + 90 = 258$ calories. (2) (PB; CJ; AN)**

INTEGUMENTARY (IT)

502. 4 **Chemotherapy destroys the rapidly dividing cells of the oral mucosa; frequent gentle oral hygiene limits additional trauma. (2) (SE; MR; PL)**
   1 Flossing would disrupt and traumatize the gum surfaces; oral hygiene is needed more than once a day.
   2 Lemon juice would be too caustic to the compromised mucosa.
   3 Vigorous cleansing with hard materials would increase mucosal trauma.

503. 2 **The meat provides proteins and the fruit provides vitamin C; both promote wound healing. (3) (PB; MR; IM)**
   1 Although the meat provides protein, neither of these nutrients provides vitamin C.
   3 These do not meet the client's need for protein or vitamin C.
   4 Same answer as 3.

504. 3 **Brown pigmentation spots (senile lentigines) increase in number, size, and distribution with aging. (2) (PM; CJ; AS)**
   1 Capillary fragility associated with aging contribute to senile purpura; however, ecchymosis indicates ineffective clotting or trauma.
   2 Although sweat glands decrease in size, number, and function, contributing to skin dryness, there should not be marked flaking of skin.
   4 Scaling of the skin is more often associated with psoriasis than aging.

505. 1 **Shearing force occurs when two surfaces move against each other; when the bed is at an angle greater than 30 degrees, the torso tends to slide and cause this phenomenon. (1) (SE; CJ; PL)**
   2 This would raise the head of the bed too high to prevent the client from sliding in bed.
   3 Same as answer 2.
   4 Same as answer 2.

506. 4 **The client who is confined to bed should be encouraged to move in the bed to prevent prolonged pressure on any one skin surface. (2) (SE; CJ; PL)**
   1 This will help promote peripheral circulation, but prolonged pressure must be avoided.
   2 This does not prevent prolonged pressure, although it can help decrease skin breakdown by allowing air to circulate beneath the client.
   3 Range-of-motion exercises move joints to prevent contractures; they do not relieve prolonged pressure.

507. 4 **Exercise would promote extension of the local infection from the leg into the circulation, causing septicemia. (3) (PB; MR; AN)**
   1 This is not accomplished by bed rest.
   2 Although bed rest does this, it is not the purpose for it in this situation.
   3 Same as answer 2.

508. 4 **Because diminished circulation leads to poor healing, early treatment of injuries is essential. (2) (SE; MR; PL)**
1 Toenails should not be too short and should be trimmed straight across.
2 Bath water should be checked with a bath thermometer; toes of persons with PVD may be less sensitive to temperature change and a burn may occur.
3 These clients develop trophic skin changes; the drying action of alcohol would potentiate dryness and skin breakdown.

509. 2 **Pressure on the blister will not allow it to heal; use of the prosthesis should be discontinued until healing occurs. (3) (PB; CJ; IM)**
1 This will neither heal the blister nor alleviate pressure on the blister by the prosthesis.
3 The client should not put the prosthesis back on because it causes pressure and would prevent healing.
4 Changing the type of covering will not help heal the blister.

510. 3 **Bathing removes microorganisms and promotes circulation, which facilitates wound healing; drying prevents maceration of skin and limits moisture, which is conducive to bacterial growth. (2) (SE; CJ; PL)**
1 A sling would interfere with comfort and mobility and could result in elbow or shoulder contractures.
2 Lotion may facilitate adherence of bacteria to wound edges as well as maceration of the skin, which would interfere with wound healing.
4 Soaking may cause maceration of the skin and interfere with wound healing.

511. 1 **Surgical asepsis means that the defined area will contain no microorganisms. (2) (SE; CJ; AN)**
2 This would be true of personal protective equipment.
3 This would apply to medical asepsis.
4 Same as answer 3.

512. 2 **A mask will protect the catheter insertion site from droplet and airborne microorganisms and sterile gloves will protect the insertion site from contact with microorganisms on the nurse's hands. (2) (SE; CJ; PL)**
1 Although sterile gloves will prevent the introduction of microorganisms into the area of the insertion site, they will not protect the client from droplet or airborne microorganism.

3 Although sterile gloves will prevent the introduction of microorganisms into the area of the insertion site, they will not protect the client from droplet or airborne microorganism; a need for a gown depends on institutional protocol.
4 Although a mask and gloves will protect the insertion site from the introduction of microorganisms, the need for a gown depends on institutional protocol.

513. 4 **In the obese individual this helps to inject the medication into subcutaneous tissue rather than adipose tissue, where its absorption would be poor. (2) (PB; MR; IM)**
1 This will result in the drug being injected into adipose tissue, where it will be poorly absorbed.
2 Same as answer 1.
3 Same as answer 1.

514. 2 **An iatrogenic infection is one caused by health care providers or therapy. (1) (SE; CJ; AN)**
1 This is not the cause of an iatrogenic infection.
3 Same as answer 1.
4 Same as answer 1.

515. 2 **A nosocomial infection, by definition, is acquired during hospitalization. (1) (SE; CJ; IM)**
1 Exposure to the pathogen must have occurred after admission to the hospital for classification as a nosocomial infection.
3 It may or may not be highly contagious; protective isolation protects the client from others; in this situation, others need to be protected from the client.
4 This nosocomial infection is a primary, not a secondary, infection.

516. 4 **This creates negative pressure in the portable wound drainage system; a pressure gradient now promotes the flow of drainage from the client to the collection container. (1) (SE; CJ; AN)**
1 This would prevent drainage, not promote it.
2 Negative pressure is increased, not decreased.
3 Negative, not atmospheric, pressure promotes drainage via a portable wound drainage system.

517. 1 **Bile is irritating to the skin; this is a priority. (2) (SE; CJ; IM)**
2 Suction is contraindicated; drainage is via gravity.
3 Repositioning the client is vital but not for facilitating the drainage of bile.

4 The tube is attached to a bag for straight drainage via gravity, not suction that uses negative pressure.

518. 1 **Teaching for the postoperative period should begin as soon as the client is admitted; knowledge of what to expect decreases anxiety and may improve compliance with the treatment regimen. (1) (SE; MR; PL)**
2 This is too late; the client must have time to ask questions and demonstrate the ability to care for the wound; teaching begins preoperatively.
3 At this time the client may be in too much discomfort to concentrate on learning.
4 Same as answer 3.

519. 1 **The nurse epidemiologist acts as a consultant to help devise an infection control strategy. (1) (SE; MR; IM)**
2 This is the role of the laboratory technician or technologist.
3 This usually is done by the nurse.
4 This is the role of the physician.

520. 3 **Barriers reduce the contact of bile with skin and limit excoriation. (2) (SE; CJ; PL)**
1 Dressings should be changed when wet, not reinforced; usually the T-tube drainage empties into a collection chamber.
2 Antiseptics are drying and irritating to excoriated skin, and they sting when applied; this would require a physician's order.
4 This action may help, but the excoriation is probably caused by bile, not adhesive tape.

521. 4 **Sterile NS will soften the dried exudates causing adherence of the dressing to the wound and limit tissue damage when the dressing is removed. (1) (SE; CJ; IM)**
1 The use of hydrogen peroxide requires an order; the action of hydrogen peroxide could be irritating to the tissues.
2 This would be painful and cause unnecessary tissue damage.
3 The use of Betadine requires an order; in addition, it should be diluted and used with caution when large open wounds are present.

522. 3 **Moisture promotes the migration of microorganisms through the dressing to the wound, which could result in an infection. (2) (SE; CJ; IM)**
1 A warm, moist dressing favors growth of microorganisms; a saturated dressing can be uncomfortable or alarming to the client;

it should be changed before saturation occurs.
2 A warm, moist dressing promotes the proliferation of microorganisms; the dressing should be changed.
4 This is a dependent function of the nurse and requires a physician's order.

523. 3 **To make effective decisions, baseline information on the client's condition, extent of injury, and significant past health history are needed. (3) (SE; MR; PL)**
1 This would be unnecessary; hyperimmune antirabies serum is not a preferred treatment because many people are sensitive to horse serum.
2 Notification of authorities is done after the injured person has received basic care.
4 Inoculation for establishment of short-term, passive immunity to rabies would be done after the initial assessment and treatment of the wound.

524. 4 **This is a viral infection that enters the body through a break in the skin and is characterized by convulsions and choking. (3) (SE; CJ; PL)**
1 Rabies is not bacterially caused; its outstanding symptoms are convulsions and choking.
2 Rabies is not associated with a bacterial septicemia; it is caused by a virus.
3 The virus specifically attacks nervous tissue and is carried in the saliva of infected animals.

525. 3 **Melanoma spreads by extension and through cutaneous lymph channels to lymph nodes and ultimately to the bloodstream. (3) (PB; CJ; AN)**
1 Seeding occurs when a body cavity is opened, as in surgery, and cancer cells are carried across the cavity.
2 The initial lesion may be surrounded by satellite lesions, but chains of lesions have not been identified.
4 Melanomas enlarge in size but do not necessarily invade bone tissue.

526. 2 **A radiation dermatitis occurs three to six weeks after the start of treatment. (2) (PB; CJ; IM)**
1 The word burn may increase the client's anxiety and should be avoided.
3 This response does not answer the client's concern.
4 Emollients are contraindicated; they may alter the calculated x-ray route and injure healthy tissue.

527. 2 **Both malignant and healthy cells are affected by radiation; time between courses of treatments allows normal cells to repair. (3) (PB; CJ; IM)**
1 If necessary for treatment protocol, staff would be available; many facilities operate seven days a week.
3 Fatigue occurs in either a five- or seven-day schedule.
4 Some side effects are inevitable, although they vary with each individual.

528. 1 **These should be avoided because they contain alcohol and metals that can exacerbate the skin reaction. (2) (PB; MR; IM)**
2 Gauze and tape may irritate the skin further.
3 This is contraindicated because it can precipitate skin breakdown.
4 This is unnecessary.

529. 3 **The skin is the first line of defense; keeping it dry and safe from injury promotes skin integrity. (1) (SE; MR; PL)**
1 Irradiated skin is fragile; if soap is used, a film left after rinsing can change the angle and intensity of radiation.
2 Irradiated skin is fragile and subject to blistering and sloughing.
4 The skin should be free of emollients because they change the angle or degree of radiation.

530. 1 **Scleroderma causes chronic hardening and shrinking of the connective tissues of any organ of the body including the esophagus and face; pureed foods limit the need to chew and this facilitates swallowing. (2) (PB; CJ; IM)**
2 There is decreased esophageal peristalsis; although liquids are easier to swallow, they are aspirated easily.
3 Same as answer 2.
4 No oral pain is associated with scleroderma.

531. 2 **Raynaud's phenomenon is caused by vasospasm, precipitated by exposure to cold or emotional stress; Raynaud's is commonly associated with scleroderma, a connective tissue disorder. (1) (PB; CJ; PL)**
1 Decreased blood flow would interfere with perception of temperature and increase the risk of burns.
3 Trauma to the hands must be avoided; nerve endings are affected by the diminished blood supply.
4 Vasodilators, not anticoagulants, are prescribed to counteract vasospasm and increase blood flow.

532. 1 **With scleroderma the skin becomes dry because of interference with the underlying sweat glands. (3) (PB; CJ; PL)**
2 Pruritus is not associated with scleroderma.
3 Inflammation is not associated with scleroderma.
4 Skin lesions are not associated with scleroderma.

533. 1 **The changes in connective tissue associated with scleroderma lead to muscle weakness; optimal function must be preserved. (1) (PB; CJ; AN)**
2 Tissue regeneration will not occur; this is a progressive degenerative disorder.
3 Prevention of extension is not possible in this systemic disease, which involves a number of organs.
4 Exercise of stiff and painful joints causes pain, not a sense of well-being.

534. 4 **Because of the recent trauma of surgery, hemorrhage and infection at the operative site are primary problems that can occur. (2) (PB; CJ; PL)**
1 The client will have a nasogastric tube to suction and be kept NPO until peristalsis returns; there should be no oral intake.
2 This is inappropriate at this time; observing for bleeding and infection takes priority during the first 48 hours.
3 This is not the appropriate time for this teaching; an abdominal dressing usually is in place.

535. 4 **This removes microorganisms and irritants and maintains skin integrity. (2) (PB; MR; IM)**
1 Although irritating agents should not be used, soap is the agent of choice to cleanse the skin around the stoma.
2 Hydrogen peroxide may be irritating and is unnecessary; soap and water are adequate.
3 Wiping can cause skin irritation, and a secondary infection caused by bacteria or fungi may develop.

536. 1 **Nerves are the least resistant tissue, followed by blood vessels, skin, muscle, and bone. (3) (PB; CJ; AS)**
2 Alternating electrical current, the most prevalent type in the United States, causes the most severe injuries.
3 Electrical current flows from the point of contact to the point of grounding.
4 It is difficult to track the path of electricity by external visualization; it often requires surgical exploration.

537. 3 This action effectively extinguishes the flames and protects the client from additional injury. (1) (SE; CJ; IM)

　1 This action will not eliminate the oxygen that supports the fire and may in fact fan the flames.

　2 This may protect the client from further injury, but would be dangerous for the rescuer.

　4 This may extinguish the flames, but not as effectively as rolling in the grass.

538. 2 A patent airway is most vital; if the person is not breathing, CPR should be begun. (1) (PB; CJ; AS)

　1 The person should be kept NPO because large burns decrease intestinal peristalsis and the person may vomit and aspirate.

　3 This is not done until the assessment for breathing has been completed.

　4 This is not the priority; this assessment will be done after transfer to a medical facility.

539. 4 A bed sheet is nonfuzzy and nonadhering and will keep the person warm. (2) (SE; MR; PL)

　1 Ice can cause additional tissue damage.

　2 Cream is difficult to remove and may result in additional damage.

　3 This would not meet the individual's immediate needs.

540. 3 In deep partial-thickness burns, destruction of the epidermis and part of the dermis occurs. (3) (PB; CJ; AS)

　1 Eschar, a dry leathery covering of denatured protein, occurs with full-thickness burns.

　2 In full-thickness burns, total destruction of the epidermis, dermis, and some underlying tissue occurs.

　4 In superficial partial-thickness burns, the epidermis is destroyed or injured.

541. 1 This describes a superficial partial-thickness burn. (2) (PB; CJ; IM)

　2 The entire epidermis and part of the dermis are affected with deep partial-thickness burns.

　3 This describes full-thickness burns.

　4 The statement is too vague a description of what is involved; in full-thickness burns the subcutaneous layer, muscle, and bone may or may not be damaged but are rarely destroyed.

542. 3 The percentage of total body surface area burned is 8.5% for each arm (17% for both arms) and 13% for the chest, thus the total body surface area burned is 30%. (1) (SE; CJ; AS)

　1 This percentage is too low.

　2 Same as answer 1.

　4 This percentage is too high.

543. 3 Heat inhalation can cause edema of the respiratory lumina, interfering with oxygenation; evaluation of respiratory status is a priority assessment. (3) (PB; CJ; AS)

　1 This would be done after the client's respiratory status has been evaluated.

　2 Burns should be evaluated by the physician and then the ordered medical therapy should be implemented.

　4 Same as answer 1.

544. 2 Hoarseness is a sign of potential respiratory insufficiency as a result of inhalation burns, which cause edema in the surrounding tissues, including the vocal cords. (3) (PB; CJ; AS)

　1 This would indicate metabolic acidosis, not respiratory insufficiency.

　3 Same as answer 1.

　4 Sputum would be sooty, not frothy; pink-tinged, frothy sputum is associated with pulmonary edema.

545. 2 Massive amounts of potassium are released from the injured cells into the extracellular fluid; large amounts of sodium are lost in edema. (3) (PB; CJ; AS)

　1 Although hyponatremia occurs, the serum potassium level rises.

　3 The serum potassium level rises; the serum sodium level falls.

　4 Although hyperkalemia occurs, the serum sodium level falls.

546. 1 A high caloric diet is needed for the increased metabolic rate associated with burns; the administration of potassium prevents hypokalemia, which can occur after the first 48 hours when potassium moves from the extracellular compartment to the intracellular compartment; protein promotes tissue repair. (2) (PB; MR; PL)

　2 This plan does not meet the body's needs for tissue repair; the calories are too limited.

　3 This plan does not meet the body's needs for tissue repair; the calories, potassium, and protein are too limited.

　4 This plan does not meet the body's needs for tissue repair; the calories and potassium are too limited.

547. 3 Extreme restlessness in a severely burned client usually indicates cerebral hypoxia. (3) (PB; CJ; AS)

1 With renal failure the client would become progressively confused and lethargic, not restless.

2 At this stage the client would be hypovolemic rather than hypervolemic.

4 With metabolic acidosis the client would be lethargic.

548. 2 Pain is from the loss of the protective covering of the nerve endings; blisters and redness occur because of the injury to the dermis and epidermis. (1) (PB; CJ; AS)

1 Because some epithelial cells remain, grafting is not needed with a partial-thickness burn unless it becomes infected and further tissue damage occurs.

3 Partial-thickness burns involve only the superficial layers of skin, unless they become infected.

4 Recovery from partial-thickness burns with no infection occurs in two to three weeks.

549. 2 Topical antibiotics are directly applied to the wound and are effective against many gram-positive and gram-negative organisms found on the skin. (2) (PB; CJ; PL)

1 Although these may be administered, they are most effective for systemic rather than local infections; the vasculature in and around a burn is impaired and the medication may not reach the organisms in the wound.

3 Same as answer 1.

4 Same as answer 1.

550. 3 Adequate intake of protein, carbohydrates, vitamin C, and minerals is necessary for tissue building and wound healing. (1) (PB; CJ; EV)

1 There are no data to come to this conclusion; although the client is not eating, the client may be drinking fluids.

2 This change would take a prolonged period of time; it would not occur during a short period.

4 This is associated with prolonged hypoxia.

551. 4 Care of burns is a painful procedure; pain medication should be administered before care to limit discomfort. (1) (PB; CJ; PL)

1 Surgical asepsis should be used.

2 No dressings are applied when the exposure method is used.

3 Sulfamylon is not hepatotoxic.

552. 3 Isolation precautions are essential for the prevention of infection in clients with burns; policies and procedures include specific interventions related to standard and transmission-based precautions, medical asepsis, surgical asepsis, and room assignments. (2) (SE; CJ; PL)

1 Bathing is done in a large tank tub.

2 Dressings are not used with the exposure method.

4 Clients are more comfortable with a room temperature of 85° F.

553. 2 This gauze is less apt to adhere to the wound; the hand should be maintained in anatomical position of slight flexion with each finger separated. (3) (PB; CJ; IM)

1 Cotton filled or backed gauze should not be used because it may adhere to the wound; the hand should be in anatomical position with fingers slightly flexed.

3 The hand is not anatomically positioned when in full extension or full flexion; the hand should be slightly flexed.

4 Same as answer 1.

554. 2 The first step is to determine what the physician has told the client. (3) (SE; MR; IM)

1 This statement would be inappropriate; grafting begins when the granulation bed is formed.

3 Same as answer 1.

4 Grafting will not be done until the wound is clean and granulation tissue has formed; there are no data to indicate the client has an infection.

555. 1 Clients with burns are sensitive to temperature changes; heat is lost from the burned areas. (2) (PB; CJ; IM)

2 The room temperature should be kept at approximately 85° F because heat is lost from burned areas.

3 A sterile sheet is not necessary; some clients may be treated by the open method and have burns exposed.

4 40% to 50% humidity is needed to maximize the warmth of the room.

556. 1 Mechanical débridement means to physically remove dirt, damaged or dead tissue, and cellular debris from a wound or burn so that infection is prevented and healing is promoted. (2) (PB; CJ; IM)

2 This is not the definition of mechanical débridement; enzymatic preparations are used to débride chemically by dissolving and removing necrotic tissue.

3 This is not the definition of either mechanical or chemical débridement; this refers to grid escharotomy.

4 This is continuous passive range of motion, not débridement.

557. 3 **The graft covers nerve endings, which reduces pain and provides a framework for granulation. (3) (PB; CJ; AN)**

1 The graft promotes epithelialization; enzymatic preparations or surgery débride wounds.

2 Pig skin grafts are not sutured.

4 Topical antimicrobials would soften the graft and impede healing.

558. 1 **An allograft is only a temporary measure; it is expected to come off and the physician should be notified that it is happening at this time. (3) (PB; MR; IM)**

2 This is an unwarranted accusation that places guilt on the client; allografts are temporary.

3 This is inaccurate information that may frighten the client.

4 An allograft is a temporary, not permanent, measure and is expected to fall off.

559. 2 **Range of motion should be instituted as soon as it will not compromise the individual's cardiopulmonary status. (2) (SE; CJ; PL)**

1 Pain will continue for some time, and if ROM is delayed until it subsides, contractures will have already developed.

3 If ROM is delayed until skin grafts heal, contractures will have already developed.

4 Pain and inability to cope may be prolonged; if ROM is delayed, contractures will have already developed.

560. 4 **The negative pressure of a portable wound drainage system exerts a sucking force that pulls fluid toward the collection chamber. (1) (PB; CJ; AN)**

1 Gravity is the environmental force that pulls weight toward the center of the earth; an indwelling urinary catheter allows urine to flow by gravity from the bladder to a collection bag placed below the level of the bladder.

2 Osmosis occurs when solvent moves from a solution of lesser concentration to one of greater solute concentration when the two solutions are separated by a semipermeable membrane; fluid moving from the interstitial compartment into the intracellular compartment uses osmosis.

3 Active transport occurs when ions move across a cell membrane against a concentration gradient with the assistance of metabolic energy; the sodium-potassium pump uses active transport.

561. 2 **Once the drugs that interfere with cell division are stopped, the hair will grow back; sometimes the hair will be a different color or texture. (1) (PB; CJ; IM)**

1 Alopecia is a common side effect of chemotherapy.

3 Hair loss persists while the drugs are being received; once the drugs are withdrawn, the hair grows back.

4 Although ice caps on the head and rubber bands around the scalp have been used to try to limit alopecia, they have not been particularly effective.

NEUROMUSCULAR (NM)

562. 2 **These are used to depress the tongue to observe the pharynx and larynx, and to assess soft palate symmetry and the presence of the gag reflex; the information obtained provides data about cranial nerve X (vagus). (3) (PM; CJ; PL)**

1 This is used to assess cranial nerve VIII (auditory).

3 This is used to assess cranial nerve II (optic).

4 These are used to assess sensory function; that is, light touch and pain.

563. 4 **Having the client swallow or checking the gag reflex is a test of these two cranial nerves. (2) (PB; CJ; AS)**

1 This would test the accessory nerve (cranial nerve XI).

2 This would test the olfactory nerve (cranial nerve I).

3 This would test the facial nerve (cranial nerve VII).

564. 1 **The afferent sensory branch of the trigeminal nerve (cranial nerve V) innervates the cornea. (3) (PM; CJ; AS)**

2 This would test the function of cranial nerve VII.

3 This would test the function of cranial nerves III, IV, and VI.

4 This would test the function of cranial nerve XI.

565. 3 The client should be assured that the symptoms are not caused by a stroke; the majority of clients recover in a few weeks. (2) (PB; CJ; IM)

1 The symptoms are not caused by a TIA; paresis or paralysis of cranial nerve VII occurs; discomfort may or may not be present.

2 Moist heat to increase blood circulation to the nerve would be appropriate.

4 The majority of clients recover without residual effects; occasionally some clients are left with evidence of Bell's palsy; exercises may help to maintain muscle tone; surgery may also be necessary.

566. 4 A nerve block of the trigeminal (fifth cranial) nerve with alcohol is a conservative approach that lasts 6 to 18 months. (2) (PB; CJ; IM)

1 This has been tried but provides little, if any, relief.

2 This is not a conservative approach; this is the most commonly used surgical procedure for trigeminal neuralgia; neuralgia may recur in 30% of clients within six years.

3 Lidocaine is not a treatment used; cranial nerve XI is the spinal accessory nerve, which innervates the sternocleidomastoid and trapezius muscles.

567. 3 This is done to assess electrical activity and determine whether symptoms are primarily musculoskeletal or neurologic. (1) (PB; CJ; IM)

1 No special preparation for an electromyography is required.

2 No special care is required during the procedure.

4 No special care is required after the procedure.

568. 3 Because of the decrease in tone and strength of the respiratory muscles, this is a prominent feature of both crises. (3) (PB; MR; EV)

1 This occurs in cholinergic crisis; it is an effect of an overdose of the medications (anticholinesterases) used to treat myasthenia gravis

2 Same as answer 1.

4 Same as answer 1.

569. 2 Use reduces strength, and rest increases strength; eyelid movement, chewing, swallowing, speech, facial expression, and breathing are often affected and therefore muscle weakness will fluctuate in relation to use and rest. (3) (PB; CJ; EV)

1 Muscle strength decreases, not increases, with activity.

3 Anticholinesterase drugs improve muscle strength.

4 Same as answer 3.

570. 3 Because of the myoneural junction defect, repeated use depletes acetylcholine, elevates cholinesterase, or exhausts acetylcholine receptor sites, resulting in decreased muscle strength. (2) (SE; CJ; PL)

1 Hot baths tend to increase, not decrease, muscle weakness.

2 Muscle weakness increases, not decreases, with muscle use.

4 There is no evidence that eating meals will bring about improvement.

571. 1 Rest will decrease the demands at the synaptic membrane of the neuromuscular junction, reducing fatigue; activity should be paced to prevent fatigue before it begins. (1) (PB; CJ; IM)

2 This will aggravate the fatigue; activity and rest should be delicately balanced to prevent fatigue.

3 Same as answer 1.

4 This cannot be done without a physician's order; rest will usually alleviate the fatigue.

572. 1 These are symptoms of myasthenia gravis and they are aggravated by physical activity. (3) (PB; CJ; AS)

2 Intention tremors are associated with multiple sclerosis.

3 Exercise decreases muscle strength.

4 The proximal muscles are more involved than the distal muscles.

573. 3 Respiratory infections place people with myasthenia gravis at high risk because they do not cough effectively and may develop pneumonia or airway obstruction. (1) (SE; MR; EV)

1 Activity should be conducted earlier in the day before the energy reserve is depleted; periods of activity should be alternated with periods of rest.

2 The client should eat sitting up to prevent aspiration.

4 This is contraindicated; these potentiate weakness because of their effect on the myoneural junction.

574. 4 Increased activity without an increase in medication could precipitate a myasthenic crisis. (2) (PB; MR; EV)

1 Self-medication may result in drug interactions; a change in medical therapy could have serious consequences.

2 A dose should not be skipped because doing so may result in severe respiratory distress.

3 People with myasthenia should avoid crowds and others with colds; they are more prone to respiratory infections because of an ineffective cough and a potential for aspiration.

575. 3 **Tensilon acts systemically to increase muscle strength with a peak effect in 30 seconds; it lasts several minutes. (3) (PB; MR; IM)**
 1 Tensilon produces a brief increase in muscle strength; with a negative response the client would demonstrate no change in symptoms.
 2 The duration of Tensilon's action is about three minutes.
 4 Tensilon acts systemically on all muscles, rather than selectively on the eyelids.

576. 3 **Until the diagnosis is confirmed, the primary goal should be to maintain adequate activity and prevent muscle atrophy. (3) (SE; CJ; AN)**
 1 It is too early to develop a teaching plan; the diagnosis is not yet established.
 2 This is too early; the client cannot adjust if a diagnosis is not yet confirmed.
 4 This is not a goal.

577. 3 **Respiratory failure will require emergency intervention, and inability to swallow may lead to aspiration. (2) (PB; CJ; AS)**
 1 These are symptoms of myasthenia that may occur but are not life threatening.
 2 Same as answer 1.
 4 Although this is important it is not the most significant assessment.

578. 4 **Dysphagia should be minimized during peak effect of Mestinon, thereby decreasing the probability of aspiration. (2) (SE; CJ; IM)**
 1 This is a treatment for, rather than prevention of, aspiration.
 2 This action will not prevent aspiration although it is vital that her respiratory function be monitored.
 3 There are insufficient data to determine whether this is appropriate because liquids are more easily aspirated then semisolids.

579. 4 **Exacerbation of myasthenia may occur temporarily at the beginning of steroid therapy, causing respiratory embarrassment and dysphagia. (2) (PB; CJ; PL)**
 1 Steroids increase sodium retention, and this would be contraindicated.
 2 While clients should avoid contact with persons having upper respiratory infections, protective isolation (neutropenic precautions) is not required.

3 This is unnecessary; adequate fluid intake should be maintained.

580. 1 **Spacing activities will encourage maximum functioning within the limits of the client's strength and endurance. (1) (SE; MR; PL)**
 2 Bed rest and limited activity may lead to muscle atrophy and calcium depletion.
 3 This is necessary for lifelong psychologic adjustment, but does not address the client's concerns at this time.
 4 This should be permitted if requested by the client or family, but does not address the concerns voiced by the client.

581. 3 **Steps are short and dragging; this is seen with basal ganglia defects. (2) (PB; CJ; AS)**
 1 This is a staggering gait often associated with cerebellar damage.
 2 This is associated with unilateral upper motor neuron damage.
 4 This is associated with bilateral spastic paresis of the legs.

582. 3 **Amplitude of the voice is reduced by neuromuscular involvement. (1) (PB; CJ; AS)**
 1 Constipation is a common problem because of a weakness of muscles used in defecation.
 2 The tendency is for the head and neck to be drawn forward because basal ganglia control is lost.
 4 Usually loss of weight occurs because of the embarrassment related to slowness and untidiness when eating.

583. 4 **Bradykinesia is a slowing down in the initiation and execution of movement. (2) (PB; CJ; AS)**
 1 Cogwheel rigidity, not flaccidity, occurs because the disease causes sustained muscle contractions.
 2 Tremors are more prominent at rest and are known as nonintention, not intention, tremors.
 3 The limbs are rigid and move with a jerky quality; the limbs are not paralyzed.

584. 4 **This maintains the range of joint movement with a minimum of energy expenditure by the client. (2) (PB; CJ; PL)**
 1 Ambulation may fatigue the client and does not provide sufficient movement of the upper extremities.
 2 Isometrics do not provide the joint movement necessary to prevent contractures.
 3 This increases the client's metabolic rate and need for oxygen; the client's ability to meet increased O_2 demand is decreased in the presence of pneumonia.

585. 1 Numbness, a sensory deficit, is inconsistent with parkinsonism; further medical evaluation is necessary. (3) (PB; MR; IM)

2 Numbness, even in the absence of other problems, can be indicative of an impending brain attack (CVA).

3 This could cause a delay in the client's receiving immediate medical attention.

4 This symptom is not caused by parkinsonism; increasing the dosage of the anticholinergic medication would not be helpful.

586. 4 Visual disturbances such as diplopia and blurred vision are common initial symptoms of optic nerve lesions. (1) (PB; CJ; AS)

1 Constipation may occur late in the disease because of immobility.

2 Although this is a neuromuscular disorder, headaches are not a common symptom.

3 Pressure ulcers may become infected if they occur late in the disease because of immobility.

587. 4 This is a truthful answer that provides hope for the client. (3) (PB; CJ; IM)

1 This response avoids the client's question and could increase anxiety.

2 Analgesics are not commonly prescribed unless pain results from some other condition.

3 This avoids the client's question; the nurse should respond directly.

588. 3 The client must be flexible and adjust activities to provide for rest when necessary; activity should cease before the point of fatigue. (2) (PB; CJ; IM)

1 While quality time with children is important, it must be done on a flexible schedule to prevent fatigue.

2 Although laudable, it cannot be done if the client is in need of support or if it overtaxes physical resources.

4 This may not be a need at this time; prevention of fatigue is always important.

589. 2 These signs and symptoms result from patchy demyelinization of the peripheral nerves, nerve roots, root ganglia, and spinal cord. (3) (PB; CJ; AS)

1 These symptoms are related to myasthenia gravis.

3 These symptoms are related to amyotrophic lateral sclerosis.

4 These symptoms are related to Parkinson's disease.

590. 2 Muscular weakness with paralysis results from impaired nerve conduction because the motor nerves become demyelinated. (2) (PB; CJ; AS)

1 This usually is not a problem; motor loss is greater than sensory loss, with paresthesia of the extremities being the most frequent sensory loss.

3 Demyelination occurs rapidly early in the disease and the muscles would not have had time to atrophy; this could occur later if rehabilitation is delayed.

4 Only the peripheral nerves are involved; the central nervous system is unaffected.

591. 4 Remyelination usually occurs over several weeks; however, sometimes it may take months or even years. (2) (PB; MR; IM)

1 Recovery is prolonged and progress will not be seen daily.

2 This avoids the client's question and gives no reassurance that there is hope for recovery.

3 Although this response identifies feelings, it avoids the question.

592. 1 An increase in intraocular pressure (IOP) results from a resistance of aqueous humor outflow; open-angle glaucoma, the most common type of glaucoma, results from increased resistance to aqueous humor outflow through the trabecular meshwork, Schlemm's canal, and the episcleral venous system. (1) (PB; MR; IM)

2 This is the description of a cataract.

3 This is the description of astigmatism.

4 This is the description of a detached retina.

593. 4 Increased intraocular pressure damages the optic nerve, interfering with peripheral vision. (1) (PB; CJ; AS)

1 These may be associated with a detached retina.

2 There is difficulty in adjusting to darkness.

3 Same as answer 1.

594. 2 A major objective of early postoperative care is to prevent increased intraocular pressure; lying on the unaffected side or in the supine position will minimize intraocular pressure. (1) (PB; MR; EV)

1 This is contraindicated; this increases intraocular pressure.

3 Same as answer 1.

4 This is not indicated.

595. 4 The eye shield will prevent injury to the newly operated eye. (2) (SE; MR; PL)

1 Only the affected eye will be covered.

2 Coughing is contraindicated in clients who have had cataract surgery.

3 Clients are not kept on bed rest after cataract surgery.

596. 2 **An antiemetic would prevent vomiting; vomiting increases intraocular pressure and should be avoided. (2) (PB; CJ; IM)**

1 Vomiting increases intraocular pressure, and aggressive intervention is required.

3 Same as answer 1.

4 Same as answer 1.

597. 1 **Acute postoperative pain is a sign of increased intraocular pressure and is caused by hemorrhaging; this is a medical emergency. (3) (PB; CJ; AN)**

2 Postoperative discomfort usually is minimal.

3 Isolation and sensory deprivation would not occur because only one eye is patched.

4 The shield may be slightly uncomfortable but would not cause severe discomfort.

598. 4 **Postoperatively the client must check daily for signs of rejection, which include redness, irritation, discomfort, or vision loss; the surgeon should be notified if any of these appear; pain following a cataract extraction may indicate infection or hemorrhage and should be reported to the physician immediately. (3) (PB; MR; EV)**

1 Driving should be avoided until the client is given specific permission to do so by the physician.

2 Soap may irritate the eye, and showers or shampooing the hair should be avoided as instructed, usually for several days to two weeks.

3 This is a symptom of retinal detachment and would not be expected.

599. 1 **To protect against physical injury and infection, the dropper tip should not touch the eye. (1) (SE; MR; EV)**

2 Drops should be placed within the lower lid.

3 The lower lid should be retracted for placement of eyedrops.

4 This would squeeze medication out of the eye.

600. 3 **This subjective symptom is caused by stimulation of retinal cells by ocular movement. (3) (PB; CJ; AS)**

1 This is a disease of the connective tissue, not of the eye.

2 Glaucoma causes the individual to see halos around lights, not flashes of light.

4 Cerebral concussions do not result in this ocular symptom.

601. 4 **This indicates that hemorrhage may be occurring in the eye. (3) (PB; MR; PL)**

1 Four hours is too soon to be concerned that the client has not voided.

2 The eye is patched; in addition, edema of the lid persists for three to four days, which can interfere with opening the eye.

3 This may occur in an unfamiliar environment with the eye patched, especially in older adults.

602. 1 **The medications usually prescribed for clients with retinal detachment reduce the eye's ability to adjust to light. (3) (PB; MR; PL)**

2 Clients should not resume usual activities, such as a return to work, for four to six weeks.

3 The eye movements associated with reading would be too rapid and could cause a redetachment early in the convalescent period.

4 Generally, new lenses will be required in three months or sooner.

603. 3 **This lubricates the eye and prevents drying of the cornea. (2) (PB; CJ; PL)**

1 This is inappropriate; eye irrigations are used to flush foreign matter from the eye.

2 This could lead to corneal abrasion.

4 Taping the eyelids open could cause corneal ulceration or injury.

604. 1 **Decerebrate posturing, limbs hyperextended and arms hyperpronated, indicates upper brainstem damage; this is a grave sign. (3) (PB; CJ; AS)**

2 This is associated with an upper motor neuron disease or lesion.

3 This is associated with decorticate rigidity, which indicates damage to the pyramidal motor tract above the brainstem.

4 This is associated with a lower motor neuron disease or lesion.

605. 1 **The presence of glucose indicates that the drainage is cerebrospinal fluid (CSF); a sterile dressing prevents microbial contamination. (2) (PB; CJ; AS)**

2 This may cause retention of CSF and increase intracranial pressure.

3 Pressure will promote retention of CSF and increase intracranial pressure.

4 Attempts to clean the ear may cause microbial contamination; clean cotton balls are not sterile.

606. 3 This occurs because of the brain's acute sensitivity to hypoxia. (3) (PB; CJ; AN)
  1 The respirations usually are depressed because of brainstem compression.
  2 The systolic pressure increases and the diastolic pressure decreases, resulting in a widening, not narrowing, pulse pressure.
  4 The peripheral vascular resistance is decreased when hypoxia occurs, thereby lowering, not increasing, the diastolic blood pressure.

607. 3 Elevating the head of the bed increases drainage of cerebrospinal fluid and decreases intracranial pressure. (1) (PB; CJ; IM)
  1 This position would not promote cerebral drainage and may lead to increased intracranial pressure.
  2 Same as answer 1.
  4 This would increase retention of cerebrospinal fluid and increase intracranial pressure.

608. 4 This is vital in case of respiratory distress; increased ICP compresses the brainstem, which contains the medulla, the respiratory center. (2) (SE; CJ; PL)
  1 This is important but not of primary urgency; the respiratory status is the priority.
  2 Same as answer 1.
  3 Same as answer 1.

609. 4 A fracture at the base of the cranium can tear meninges with subsequent leakage of cerebrospinal fluid from the nose (rhinorrhea) and bleeding from the ear. (3) (PB; CJ; AN)
  1 A bruise would not cause these responses.
  2 A severe jarring of the brain would not cause these responses.
  3 A nose fracture would not produce a clear drainage, and the ears would not be draining.

610. 3 This indicates a lack of oxygen to the brainstem; it impairs the reticular activating system. (2) (PB; CJ; AS)
  1 The urine output is not related to increased intracranial pressure.
  2 The respiratory rate would decrease.
  4 The pulse would be bradycardic and bounding.

611. 2 This is an appropriate response; a purposeful withdrawal from pain. (1) (PB; CJ; AS)
  1 This response may indicate cortical damage of the brain.
  3 This response may indicate cortical or midbrain compression.
  4 This response to pain indicates decorticate rigidity.

612. 2 Encouraging fluids will hydrate the client and contribute to the restoration of cerebrospinal fluid, which cushions the brain; this should ease the pain. (2) (PB; CJ; IM)
  1 This would increase the pain; the client should be placed in the supine position and kept quiet.
  3 This is contraindicated for a postoperative client; the removal of antiembolism stockings will not influence a post–spinal anesthesia headache.
  4 Same as answer 1.

613. 3 In an attempt to stop the bleeding, adjacent arteries constrict; this in turn contributes to the ischemia responsible for the neurologic deficits. (3) (PB; CJ; AN)
  1 The volume of blood loss is not great enough to significantly alter the oxygen-carrying capability of the remaining blood supply.
  2 While prolonged ischemia may cause necrosis, many of the manifestations of cerebral ischemia are reversed as pressure diminishes, and there may be no permanent damage.
  4 Severe electrolyte imbalance may cause generalized weakness; however, hemiparesis and aphasia are not the result of electrolyte loss.

614. 3 This utilizes the force of gravity to prevent additional intracranial pressure, which would intensify the ischemic manifestations of hemorrhage. (3) (PB; CJ; PL)
  1 This position would not facilitate drainage of cerebral fluid; this position promotes accumulation of fluid, which increases intracranial pressure.
  2 Same as answer 1.
  4 Vomiting can occur with increased intracranial pressure, and placing sandbags to immobilize the head could result in aspiration.

615. 2 Controlled ventilation induces hypocapnia; subsequently it causes vasoconstriction and reduced cerebral blood flow. (3) (PB; CJ; EV)
  1 The fluid may be cerebrospinal fluid; clearing the ear may cause further damage.
  3 Because of manipulation during a craniotomy, anticonvulsants are given prophylactically to prevent seizures.
  4 This would not increase cerebral blood flow.

616. 2 Although this is done to maintain an airway; it is not done routinely because it increases intracranial pressure. (2) (PB; CJ; IM)

1 This keeps the skin from drying, which helps prevent skin breakdown.

3 This allows venous return to the heart and is used to try to limit increased intracranial pressure.

4 The corneal reflex may be absent in the unconscious client; a dry cornea is prone to injury.

617. 4 **Immediate corrective therapy based on current assessments must be implemented. (3) (PB; MR; IM)**

1 Insufficient information is provided to arrive at this conclusion; this is contraindicated with an infratentorial craniotomy.

2 This is a dependent function of the nurse; although it is administered to decrease cerebral edema, it requires a physician's order.

3 Although this is an appropriate action, it is not the priority until the physician has been notified.

618. 4 **This lessens the possibility of hemorrhage, provides for better circulation of cerebrospinal fluid, and promotes venous return. (3) (PB; CJ; IM)**

1 Gatching the knees is contraindicated because it could raise intracranial pressure.

2 This position is appropriate for infratentorial surgery.

3 A low-Fowler's position with the head turned impedes venous return; intracranial pressure could be increased.

619. 2 **Kernig's sign, which is an inability to completely extend the legs, is the classic sign of meningeal irritation. (3) (PB; CJ; AS)**

1 This is associated with hydrocephalus; it occurs when the eyelid falls above the iris, allowing the sclera to show; it occurs only in infants whose cranial bones have not yet fused.

3 This sign indicates the presence of thrombophlebitis; pain is experienced when the foot is flexed because of vascular irritability.

4 This is unrelated to meningeal irritation; it is a typical spinal cord reflex.

620. 2 **Recognition of effort is motivating. (3) (PI; CJ; PL)**

1 This may decrease both self-esteem and motivation.

3 Same as answer 1.

4 The problem is a motor, not a sensory (receptive), problem.

621. 2 **Emboli, occurring from atrial fibrillation, cause complete occlusion of vessels; usually middle**
cerebral arteries are involved; the infarct may cause hemiplegia, aphasia, or spatial perceptual deficits. (3) (PB; CJ; AN)

1 Hypertension may cause spasm of the arteries, but it does not cause anatomic occlusion.

3 Developmental defects of the arterial wall are associated with saccular aneurysms.

4 Seizures are caused by inappropriate paroxysmal discharge.

622. 1 **Narrowing of arteries supplying the brain causes temporary neurologic deficits that last for a short period; between attacks neurologic functioning is normal. (2) (PB; CJ; AN)**

2 Emboli result in a CVA; the damage usually is permanent.

3 This is not the description of a TIA; remissions and exacerbations occur with progressive degenerative neurologic disorders.

4 This occurs with multiple small cerebrovascular accidents; TIAs do not result in permanent damage.

623. 3 **The cause of the hypotension must be evaluated by the physician. (3) (PB; CJ; IM)**

1 This is a dependent function, and the physician must be notified first.

2 This would further decrease blood flow to the brain.

4 This is contraindicated; the physician must be notified first.

624. 3 **Muscles used for swallowing are innervated by the ninth (glossopharyngeal) and tenth (vagus) cranial nerves. (3) (PB; CJ; EV)**

1 This is unrelated to cranial nerves; this is associated with neck edema and potential compromise of the airway.

2 This is unrelated to cranial nerves; some edema is expected because of the inflammatory process at the site of surgery.

4 Alterations in blood pressure may occur but are not caused by cranial nerve dysfunction.

625. 2 **This assessment would indicate whether there is a progression of symptoms or improvement and assist the physician in determining the diagnosis. (2) (PB; CJ; AS)**

1 An elevation in temperature is not an early sign of an extension of a brain attack (CVA).

3 The data indicate the vital signs were normal and do not reflect hypertension; while vital signs would be monitored, the client's motor status in this instance is most significant.

4 This is not the priority assessment.

626. 2 Increasing intracranial pressure is evidenced by an increased pulse pressure and blood pressure and a decreased pulse rate; the physician should be notified. (3) (PB; CJ; AS)

1 The pulse rate has increased and the BP has fallen; these are not signs of increased intracranial pressure.

3 Although the pulse rate is decreased, the BP is not elevated; this is not a sign of increased intracranial pressure.

4 Although the pulse rate has decreased and the BP has risen slightly, the pulse pressure has narrowed; this is not a sign of increased intracranial pressure.

627. 3 This position will neither raise intracranial pressure nor interfere with respirations and will permit oral secretions to drain from the mouth by gravity. (2) (PB; CJ; IM)

1 This could compromise the airway by permitting the tongue to fall to the posterior pharynx and obstruct the airway.

2 Elevating the head of the bed could compromise vital functions by compressing the brainstem.

4 This is contraindicated because it may increase intracranial pressure.

628. 4 Increased intracranial pressure is manifested by a sluggish pupillary reaction and elevation of the systolic blood pressure. (1) (PB; CJ; AN)

1 Spinal shock is manifested by a lowered systolic blood pressure with no pupillary changes.

2 Hypovolemic shock is indicated by a decrease in systolic pressure and tachycardia with no changes in pupillary reaction.

3 Transtentorial herniation is manifested by dilated pupils and severe posturing.

629. 2 This position produces dorsiflexion of the foot and prevents the tendons from shortening, preventing foot drop. (1) (PB; CJ; IM)

1 This would not prevent plantar flexion; it could promote hip and knee flexion contractures.

3 Same as answer 1.

4 The client would not have the ability or strength to perform range-of-motion exercises unassisted at this time.

630. 2 The client has lost vision from the right visual field; scanning compensates for loss. (3) (SE; CJ; IM)

1 This is the approach to be used for apraxia.

3 This is the approach to be used for denial of the right side (unilateral neglect).

4 This aggravates neglect of the affected side.

631. 4 If the client exhibits emotional instability, it is usually caused by lesions affecting the thalamic area—the part of the neural system most responsible for emotions. (1) (PI; MR; IM)

1 The client may have remote memory, but there is no selective process of what events are remembered.

2 This is associated with consistent behavior and cognitive thinking, of which the client is incapable at this time.

3 Same as answer 2.

632. 3 Recovery from aphasia is a continuous process; the amount of recovery cannot be predicted. (1) (PB; CJ; IM)

1 This response abdicates the nurse's responsibility; the physician cannot predict return of function.

2 This gives false reassurance; it may take a year or longer or may never return.

4 Speech return is a continuous process; it may take a year or longer or may never return.

633. 4 In addition to the extent of injury, a factor in relearning speech is the client's motivation and effort; the more the client attempts to talk, the more likely speech will progress to its optimum level; relearning is a slow process. (1) (SE; MR; IM)

1 Clients with aphasia are not deaf.

2 This will create frustration and may infuriate the client.

3 Although the nurse should instruct the family to approve and support the client's efforts to communicate, this support should be for the effort not for correct communication.

634. 3 A weak grasp, pain, and uncoordinated movements could result in the dropping of tools, which could be dangerous. (3) (SE; CJ; AN)

1 Although this could be a problem, safety is the priority.

2 Same as answer 1.

4 Although in the future this could become an issue if the client can no longer work, at this time safety is the priority.

635. 1 Rhythmic contraction and relaxation associated with a tonic-clonic seizure can cause repeated banging of the head. (2) (PB; CJ; IM)

2 This is contraindicated because it can cause broken bones.

3 Moving during a seizure can result in physical injuries; the client should be moved after the seizure.

4 This is contraindicated because damage to the teeth can occur if force is used to insert an airway.

636. **2 The nerves for arm innervation are above the injury level at C4. (3) (PB; CJ; AS)**
1 Innervation of muscles used to move the lower arms is not affected by this injury; these muscles are innervated above C7.
3 Innervation for pain sensation of the hands is not affected by this injury; these muscles are innervated above C7.
4 Diaphragm innervation is not affected by this injury; the diaphragm is innervated above C4.

637. **3 The T6 level is the sympathetic visceral outflow level, and any injury above this level results in autonomic dysreflexia. (3) (PB; CJ; AN)**
1 The reflex arc remains after spinal cord injury.
2 The important point is not that the cord is totally transected but the level at which the injury occurs.
4 This is not related to autonomic dysreflexia; all cord injuries result in flaccid paralysis during the period of spinal shock; as the inflammation subsides, spasticity gradually increases.

638. **4 These signs occur as a result of exaggerated autonomic responses; if autonomic dysreflexia is identified, immediate intervention is necessary to prevent serious complications. (3) (PB; CJ; AS)**
1 Paralysis is related to transection, not dysreflexia; the client will have no sensation below the injury.
2 Profuse diaphoresis occurs.
3 Bradycardia occurs.

639. **4 The client has the capability; this maintains a positive identity and is necessary for progression to long-term goals. (2) (PB; CJ; AN)**
1 This is a long-term goal.
2 Same as answer 1.
3 Same as answer 1.

640. **2 Arm strength is necessary for transfers and activities of daily living and for the use of crutches or a wheelchair. (2) (PB; CJ; IM)**
1 The client does not have neurologic control of this activity.
3 Equilibrium is not a problem.
4 Same as answer 1.

641. **3 Injury and pressure at the nerve roots produce pain. (3) (PB; CJ; AS)**
1 Injury at T6 and T7 is too low to cause paralysis of the respiratory muscles; control of respirations is in the medulla and the cervical plexus (phrenic nerve).

2 With complete crushing at the T6 and T7 level, there is no pain sensation in parts distal to the injury.
4 Initially, paralysis is flaccid; spasticity is a later manifestation.

642. **3 This response offers the realistic assurance that nothing is wrong and also encourages the client to relate information to the nurse. (3) (PB; CJ; IM)**
1 This action will not decrease the numbness; nerve root irritation will lessen only with time.
2 This response tells the client there is a problem when, in reality, there is no reason to call the physician.
4 This provides false reassurance; nerve root numbness will lessen only with time.

643. **4 Elevation of the extremity promotes venous return, which limits edema and the related pressure on nerve endings that causes pain. (2) (SE; CJ; IM)**
1 Vasoconstriction interferes with wound healing and effective circulation, which would limit venous return.
2 A week after surgery the discomfort is probably due to venous congestion related to the limb's dependent position rather than incisional pain.
3 This would be contraindicated because the bandage prevents bleeding and edema and promotes shrinkage of the residual limb.

RESPIRATORY (RE)

644. **4 Oxygen saturation is a measure of the relationship between oxygen and hemoglobin; it measures the amount of oxygen available to tissues and provides a pulmonary assessment for clients at risk for hypoxia; pulse oximetry provides a continuous, noninvasive measurement of an individual's oxygen saturation. (2) (PB; CJ; AS)**
1 PO_2 is a measure of diffusion across the alveolar membrane and this value may be decreased chronically in a heavy smoker; thus it would not be the most accurate measure of this client's postoperative respiratory status; also, it requires an arterial puncture.
2 Although PCO_2 is an accurate measure of alveolar ventilation and is elevated with hypoventilation, which may occur after abdominal surgery because deep breathing often is painful, and it requires an arterial puncture.
3 Hemoglobin is a measure of the blood's capacity to transport oxygen.

645. 3 These are normal respiratory sounds heard on auscultation as inspired air enters and leaves the alveoli. (1) (PB; CJ; AS)

1 These are fine crackling sounds heard at the end of an inspiration; they are associated with pulmonary edema.

2 Adventitious sounds is the general term for all abnormal breath sounds.

4 This is evidence of a reduction in the amount of air entering the alveoli, usually caused by obstruction or consolidation.

646. 2 Oxygen and carbon dioxide exchange is essential for life and is the priority. (1) (PB; CJ; AN)

1 This is not the priority.

3 This is unnecessary with a pneumonectomy because there is no lung to reinflate.

4 Same as answer 1.

647. 2 Rhonchi, particularly on expiration, indicate partial airway obstruction because of bronchiolar alterations associated with COPD. (2) (PB; CJ; AN)

1 Rhonchi sometimes have been described as sonorous-like sounds, but they are more prominent on expiration, not inspiration; snorts are sounds made in the nose.

3 This describes wheezes caused by rapid vibration of bronchial walls.

4 This describes fine crackles, which result when alveoli are partially filled with fluid.

648. 3 Singed nasal hair and nasal discharges that contain carbon are warning signs of respiratory inhalation. (2) (PB; CJ; AS)

1 Changes in chest x-ray findings are a late sign of respiratory problems.

2 This may be a sign of pneumonia or tuberculosis.

4 Changes in arterial blood gases are late signs of respiratory problems.

649. 4 This position promotes lung expansion and gas exchange; it also decreases venous return and cardiac workload. (2) (PB; CJ; IM)

1 This may be done but positioning should be done first because it will have an immediate effect and time will be needed to set up for the delivery of the oxygen.

2 A friction rub is not related to heart failure but to inflammation of the pleura.

3 Maintaining adequate oxygen exchange is the priority; an x-ray film will be obtained, but after breathing is supported.

650. 1 Stridor is a high-pitched, musical sound caused by an obstruction of the trachea or larynx. (2) (PB; CJ; AS)

2 Although coughing and deep breathing are important, they do not help identify stridor.

3 Neck exercises are important for total rehabilitation, but they do not help identify stridor.

4 Auscultating the base of the lungs will determine the presence of vesicular breath sounds or crackles.

651. 4 Abdominal breathing improves lung expansion. (2) (PB; MR; IM)

1 Short breaths do not expand the lungs; deep slow breaths at 16/min should be encouraged.

2 Exhalation with pursed lips promotes expansion of the alveoli.

3 Breathing exercises should be performed at least every two hours.

652. 3 This is secondary to cerebral hypoxia, which accompanies acute respiratory distress syndrome (ARDS); cognition and level of consciousness are reduced. (3) (PB; CJ; AS)

1 Hypotension occurs because of the hypoxia of the heart.

2 The sputum is not tenacious, but it may be frothy if pulmonary edema is present.

4 Breathing will be fast and shallow.

653. 3 The effectiveness of therapy is measured by the client's response. (3) (PB; CJ; EV)

1 This is presumptive; the database is incomplete for the conclusion that surgery is necessary.

2 Endotracheal intubation does not permit verbal communication.

4 This is important but not the priority.

654. 4 Pain causes shallow breathing, which results in carbon dioxide retention. (2) (PB; CJ; AS)

1 Although decreased respiratory functioning could result in an infection, respiratory acidosis is the immediate concern.

2 Blood in vomitus is unrelated to fractured ribs.

3 Fluid in lung tissue is unrelated to a fractured rib; it is associated with heart failure

655. 4 Increased rate and depth of breathing result in excessive elimination of CO_2, and respiratory alkalosis could result. (1) (PB; CJ; EV)

1 Hypoxia is associated with respiratory acidosis, not respiratory alkalosis, which is related to hyperventilation.

2 With hyperventilation, CO_2 levels will be decreased (hypocapnia), not elevated.

3 This results from excess hydrogen ions caused by a metabolic problem, not a respiratory problem.

656. **2 This is necessary to prevent flooding of the trachea with fluid; some systems have receptacles attached to the tubing to collect the fluid and others have to be temporarily disconnected while emptying the fluid. (3) (PB; CJ; IM)**

1 This circumstance does not require assistance from a respiratory therapist.

3 Humidity is necessary to preserve moistness of the respiratory tract and liquefy secretions.

4 The amount of condensation is irrelevant in terms of recording the intake and output.

657. **1 This provides an immediate airway without causing trauma; with assistance, a new tracheostomy tube can be inserted. (3) (PB; LE; IM)**

2 The obturator would obstruct the airway.

3 This tube is contaminated; a sterile tube should be inserted.

4 At the completion of these tasks the airway will have been obstructed too long.

658. **3 This promotes breathing by reducing the pressure of the abdominal organs on the diaphragm and increasing thoracic excursion. (1) (PB; CJ; IM)**

1 This may confirm diminished breath sounds but would not facilitate breathing.

2 This eventually should be done, but it is not the priority.

4 This will impede aeration of the right lung fields.

659. **2 Suctioning also removes oxygen, which can cause cardiac dysrhythmias; the nurse should try to prevent this by hyperoxygenating the client prior to and after suctioning. (2) (PB; CJ; IM)**

1 To prevent trauma to the trachea, suction should be applied only while removing the catheter.

3 This kind of movement could cause tracheal damage.

4 Suction only as needed; excessive suctioning irritates the mucosa, which increases secretion production.

660. **4 This occludes the tracheal lumen around the tracheostomy tube preventing accidental aspiration if regurgitation occurs. (2) (PB; CJ; IM)**

1 This would permit aspiration if regurgitation should occur.

2 The cuff must be inflated during the tube feeding to prevent accidental aspiration, not after the feeding.

3 Same as answer 1.

661. **3 These cuffs do not compress the capillary beds and thus do not cause tracheal damage. (2) (PB; CJ; AN)**

1 A minimal air leak is desirable to ensure the lowest possible pressure in the cuff while still maintaining placement of the tube.

2 Surgical asepsis, not the use of these cuffs, prevents infection.

4 Secretions will be increased because the cuff is a foreign body in the trachea.

662. **2 Internal bleeding after nasal surgery may flow by gravity to the posterior oropharynx where it is swallowed. (2) (PB; CJ; EV)**

1 Facial edema is expected after the trauma of surgery.

3 The edema that results from the trauma of surgery may be perceived as pressure around the eye and is expected.

4 Pink-tinged drainage on the nasal packing and nasal drip dressing is expected for 24 to 48 hours after surgery.

663. **1 Sneezing involves high pressures in the respiratory passageways during the expulsive phase of a sneeze; this can disrupt sutures or alignment of bone and therefore should be avoided. (2) (PB; CJ; IM)**

2 This is not a necessity; the client's regular routine may be followed.

3 This position promotes the accumulation of facial edema and possible aspiration of drainage; the semi- to high Fowler's positions are preferred.

4 Food and fluid that are soothing for the client can be given at any temperature; cool or warm temperatures usually are preferred.

664. **4 Emphysema involves destructive changes in the alveolar walls, leading to dilation of the air sacs; there is subsequent air trapping and difficulty with expiration. (1) (PB; CJ; AN)**

1 Bronchospasm is characteristic of asthma, and it causes narrowing of the airways.

2 The vital capacity is decreased because of restriction of the diaphragm and thoracic movement.

3 Expiration should be slowed by pursed-lip breathing to keep the airways open so there is less air trapping.

665. **2** **This permits more complete exhalation and emptying of carbon dioxide from the lungs. (3) (PB; MR; IM)**

1 This is contraindicated; the client should receive low amounts of oxygen to prevent CO_2 narcosis.

3 These should be part of assessment, but assessment does not decrease dyspnea.

4 This is contraindicated because it increases carbon dioxide retention.

666. **2** **Accessory muscles are used during respiration because of the increased rigidity of the chest. (2) (PB; CJ; AS)**

1 Tachypnea is associated with emphysema; pursed-lip breathing is a technique commonly used by individuals who have COPD.

3 Respiratory acidosis is associated with emphysema because of carbon dioxide retention.

4 Emphysema is accompanied by a prolonged expiratory phase.

667. **3** **With chronically high levels of carbon dioxide, lowered oxygen becomes the stimulus to breathe; high oxygen administration negates this mechanism. (3) (PB; CJ; IM)**

1 This is an appropriate intervention but is not directly related to CO_2 narcosis.

2 This would not bring oxygen into the alveoli for exchange nor would it adequately remove carbon dioxide, because it would increase bronchiolar obstruction.

4 Inhalation should be of regular depth, and expiration should be prolonged to prevent carbon dioxide trapping.

668. **4** **With emphysema the respiratory center no longer responds to elevated carbon dioxide as the stimulus to breathe but rather to lowered oxygen levels; therefore the oxygen being delivered must be lowered to supply enough for oxygenation without being so elevated that it negates the stimulus to breathe. (3) (PB; CJ; IM)**

1 The client is in CO_2 narcosis; increasing oxygen administration will further diminish the respiratory drive until respiratory arrest occurs.

2 A confused client cannot answer questions about the confusion.

3 There are no indications that respiratory secretions have increased.

669. **4** **Pressure from the fluid may cause upward displacement of the diaphragm. (2) (PB; CJ; IM)**

1 Additional fluid would aggravate the problem.

2 The client should already be in the semi-Fowler's position, which would normally relieve dyspnea; however, intraabdominal pressure must be reduced by draining fluid.

3 Auscultation is important, but it does not alleviate the problem.

670. **3** **This pause allows added time for gaseous exchange at the alveolar capillary beds. (3) (SE; MR; EV)**

1 Inhalation should be through the nose to moisten, filter, and warm the air.

2 This decreases the effectiveness of respirations.

4 The expiratory phase should be lengthened, and exhalation should be through pursed lips.

671. **3** **This indicates progressive respiratory failure; ventilatory support is needed when the PCO2 is above 40. (3) (PB; CJ; IM)**

1 This will liquefy secretions but will not correct the respiratory failure.

2 This may dilate bronchi but will not improve respiratory exchange to decrease CO_2.

4 This will not correct respiratory failure.

672. **3** **This aids descent of the diaphragm so that more air can enter and fill the lungs. (2) (PB; MR; IM)**

1 Rapid breathing promotes respiratory alkalosis; diaphragmatic breathing includes slow deep breathing.

2 The hands should be placed lightly on the abdomen to verify abdominal excursion.

4 Diaphragmatic breathing may be performed in any position other than the prone or Trendelenburg; usually the semi-Fowler's position is used.

673. **2** **This is a positive step in reducing smoking; it is the first step toward stopping. (2) (PM; MR; EV)**

1 The client is postponing the decision to quit.

3 The client is rationalizing why quitting smoking will be too difficult.

4 This is unrealistic because giving up smoking is difficult regardless of whether or not the client drinks alcohol.

674. **4** **The enlarged liver is caused by long-term respiratory acidosis with increased pulmonary pressure that eventually causes right ventricular enlargement and failure (cor pulmonale); the elevated pressure causes backup pressure in the hepatic circulation. (3) (PB; CJ; AN)**

1 Liver hypoxia would cause atrophy and necrosis of cells, not enlargement.

2 Right ventricular failure with increased pressure in the ascending vena cava causes increased pressure in the hepatoportal system, resulting in an enlarged liver, not hepatic acidosis.

3 These are the result of hepatic portal hypertension, not the cause of an enlarged liver.

675. 1 **Breath sounds will be decreased in clients with COPD because of reduced air flow, pleural effusion, or lung parenchymal destruction. (3) (PB; CJ; AS)**

2 Crackles indicate fluid in the alveoli which is associated with heart failure or infection; gurgles (rhonchi) signify airway obstruction, not the pathophysiology associated with chronic obstructive lung disease.

3 Expiratory wheezing is associated with asthma or bronchitis.

4 A plural friction rub occurs when one layer of the pleural membrane slides over the other during breathing; this is associated with pleurisy, not chronic obstructive lung disease.

676. 2 **A sudden weight gain is an initial sign of right ventricular failure caused by chronic obstructive pulmonary disease (cor pulmonale). (3) (PB; CJ; AN)**

1 This is associated with polycythemia vera, not chronic obstructive pulmonary disease.

3 A sudden weight gain is not associated with this condition.

4 Right, not left, ventricular failure occurs with chronic obstructive pulmonary disease.

677. 1 **This will help liquefy secretions and promote their expectoration. (2) (PB; MR; IM)**

2 This facilitates breathing; it does not relieve chest congestion.

3 Nonproductive coughing should be avoided because it is irritating and exhausting.

4 This will not help relieve early morning congestion.

678. 1 **Eating small meals will decrease the amount of oxygen necessary for ingestion and digestion at any one time. (1) (PB; MR; IM)**

2 Although fluids do help liquefy secretions, they should not be encouraged in a client with heart failure.

3 Lying down increases intraabdominal pressure, pushing a full stomach against the diaphragm and limiting respiratory excursion.

4 Protein maintains or increases hydrostatic pressure; it does not decrease it.

679. 4 **This technique results in nasal breathing, which negates the effects of aerosol medication. (3) (PB; MR; EV)**

1 The nebulizer tip should be past the lips to deliver the medication.

2 This promotes contact of the medication with the bronchial mucosa.

3 This prolongs and improves delivery of the medication to the respiratory mucosa.

680. 3 **Sitting facilitates breathing by increasing lung expansion; suction clears the airway; 2 liters of oxygen promotes respirations while preventing carbon dioxide narcosis. (3) (PB; CJ; IM)**

1 Five liters of oxygen may cause respiratory depression and carbon dioxide narcosis in a client with COPD.

2 Chest physiotherapy may be done later after the client's condition has improved.

4 Not intervening immediately may result in further respiratory distress.

681. 2 **This should not occur; it is evidence of a leak from the chest tube or the lung into the subcutaneous tissue. (3) (PB; MR; IM)**

1 Clots are expected initially after surgery.

3 This occurs as the lung is expanding; bubbling stops completely when the lung is fully expanded.

4 Bloody drainage is expected immediately after surgery.

682. 4 **The left lung is collapsed; therefore, there are no breath sounds. (3) (PB; CJ; AS)**

1 A tympanic, not a dull, sound would be heard with a pneumothorax.

2 There would be no vocal fremitus because there is no airflow into the left lung as a result of the pneumothorax.

3 These sounds would not be heard because there is no airflow into the left lung as a result of the pneumothorax.

683. 4 **With a pneumothorax, a chest tube attached to a closed chest drainage system removes trapped air and helps to reestablish negative pressure within the pleural space resulting in lung reinflation. (3) (PB; MR; IM)**

1 A closed chest drainage system may be inserted to remove blood related to a hemothorax, not to assess for bleeding.

2 This is not the purpose of inserting chest tubes; the function of the lungs is monitored through the assessment of vital signs, breath sounds, arterial blood gases, and chest x-ray.

3 This is the reason for use of a closed chest drainage system when there is fluid in the pleural space.

684. 2 The return of breath sounds indicates the lung has reinflated. (2) (PB; CJ; EV)

1 A cough that raises sputum (productive cough) may indicate a complication such as infection.

3 The drainage should decrease, not increase.

4 Constant bubbling in the water-seal chamber indicates that there is a leak in the closed chest drainage system; bubbling may occur in this chamber when air exits the pleural space with a cough or forceful expiration; the fluid will rise and fall in this chamber with pleural pressure changes associated with inspiration and expiration (tidaling).

685. 4 This statement indicates understanding of what a lobectomy involves, including closed chest drainage; it shows that the client was given the information needed for an informed consent. (2) (SE; LE; EV)

1 This client's lesion is extensive; laser endoscopic or laser bronchoscopic surgery can be used for some smaller lesions.

2 The right lung has three lobes and the left only two because of the position of the heart.

3 A segmental or wedge resection is used for small tumors near the surface of the lung.

686. 2 There is air in the tissues, and palpation results in a crackling sound referred to as crepitus. (2) (PB; CJ; EV)

1 This is a harsh, vibrating sound usually produced on inspiration because of airway obstruction.

3 This is excessive accumulation of fluid in tissue spaces.

4 The size of the chest is determined by the bony structure; a barrel chest with an increase in the AP diameter is associated with COPD, not cancer of the lung.

687. 2 A mediastinal shift with airway obstruction may occur because pressure builds up on the operative side, causing the trachea to deviate toward the nonoperative side; assessment of the airway takes priority. (3) (PB; CJ; AS)

1 The client needs immediate intervention; the airway is the priority.

3 Same as answer 1.

4 There is no need for a chest tube when a pneumonectomy is performed.

688. 3 This helps to keep the airway patent and prevents atelectasis of the remaining lung by raising intrapleural pressure. (3) (PB; CJ; IM)

1 This is done after the gag reflex returns.

2 Although important, it is not the priority.

4 This would restrict left lung expansion.

689. 3 These positions permit ventilation of the remaining lung and prevent fluid from draining into the sutured bronchial stump. (3) (PB; CJ; PL)

1 Lying on the nonoperative side restricts left lung excursion and may allow fluid to drain into the right bronchial stump.

2 Although the high Fowler's position promotes ventilation, it is extremely tiring.

4 Same as answer 1.

690. 1 Loss of the large vascular lung and/or the presence of a mediastinal shift can result in cardiac overload. (3) (PB; CJ; EV)

2 These signs are associated with hypoxia, which is a common complication of surgery and not unique to a pneumonectomy.

3 These are common complications of thoracic surgeries and are not unique to a pneumonectomy.

4 An elevated BP may be associated with cardiac overload, but the other signs are not unique to a pneumonectomy.

691. 1 Excessive endotracheal secretions after a pneumonectomy require coughing routines that are effective but not exhausting. (3) (PB; CJ; PL)

2 This is not specific for a client who has had a pneumonectomy.

3 This is too exhausting.

4 Same as answer 3.

692. 3 To prevent aspiration during the procedure, clients are required to be NPO for at least 8 to 12 hours prior to the procedure. (2) (PB; CJ; IM)

1 Chest tubes are not required unless the lungs are accidentally punctured; the client will have a small incision near the clavicle.

2 A mediastinoscopy permits visualization of the anterior mediastinum or hilum extrapleurally; a bronchoscopy permits visualization of the main stem bronchus.

4 Fluid is removed from the pleural space during a thoracentesis.

693. 4 This is the lower-lateral chest which is the area of greatest thoracic excursion; with visceral and parietal pleurae inflammation (pleurisy), a low-pitched, coarse, grating sound is heard when the client breathes, particularly when approaching the height of inspiration. (2) (PB; CJ; AS)

1 Bronchial breath sounds are heard over the trachea and at the nape of the neck on either side of the vertebrae; bronchial sounds are loud, high-pitched and hollow, with a short inspiratory phase and long expiratory phase.

2 Bronchovesicular breath sounds are heard on either side of the sternum or between the scapulae; bronchovesicular sounds have a moderate volume and medium pitch, with equal inspiratory and expiratory phases.

3 This is the area where vesicular breath sounds are heard; vesicular sounds are soft and low pitched, with a long inspiratory phase and a short expiratory phase; they are heard over most lung fields.

694. 2 Compression of the lung by fluid that accumulates at the base of the lungs reduces expansion and air exchange. (3) (PB; CJ; AS)

1 There is no fluid in the alveoli, so no crackles are produced.

3 If there is tracheal deviation, it is away from the involved side.

4 Dullness is produced on percussion of the involved area.

695. 3 Tension is placed on the pleura at the height of inspiration and causes pain. (3) (PB; CJ; AS)

1 This is typical of heart failure.

2 This may indicate a pulmonary infection.

4 Same as answer 2.

696. 2 The most significant and life-threatening complication of insertion of a subclavian catheter is a pneumothorax because of the close proximity of the subclavian vein and the apex of the upper lobe of the lung; a client's respiratory status always is a priority. (3) (PB; CJ; EV)

1 A baseline blood glucose level should be obtained before insertion of the catheter; after TPN is started, routine monitoring of blood glucose levels is important.

3 Although this may be done before TPN is begun, it is not the priority immediately after insertion of the catheter.

4 Although this should be done eventually, it is not the priority at this time.

697. 3 The client is in respiratory acidosis probably caused by the depressant effects of anesthesia or a partially obstructed airway; these activities clear the airway and blow off CO_2. (3) (PB; CJ; IM)

1 This is the treatment for respiratory alkalosis; the client is in respiratory acidosis.

2 This will not correct respiratory acidosis and may aggravate it if potassium is depleted.

4 This is not necessary if clearing of the airway rectifies the problem.

698. 4 A general anesthetic is delivered via an endotracheal tube that irritates the posterior pharynx and larynx and causes discomfort when swallowing. (2) (SE; MR; EV)

1 This is not an effect of general anesthesia.

2 Occasionally this may occur; however, it is a systemic, not a local, effect.

3 Same as answer 2.

699. 1 Both sides of the posterior pharynx should be touched to elicit the gag reflex; absence of the reflex indicates the client is at risk for aspiration of secretions or fluid. (1) (SE; CJ; EV)

2 This could happen even in the absence of a gag reflex.

3 If the gag reflex is absent, the client would aspirate.

4 The client might be able to breathe deeply and cough without an adequate gag reflex.

700. 4 There is no respiratory movement in stage 4 of anesthesia; before this stage, respirations are depressed but present. (3) (PB; CJ; AN)

1 The gag reflex is lost in the first phase of stage 3 of anesthesia.

2 The corneal reflex is lost in the second phase of stage 3 of anesthesia.

3 Consciousness is lost in stage 2.

701. 1 To allow for the insertion of the bronchoscope, throat muscles are anesthetized, diminishing the protective gag reflex. (1) (PB; CJ; PL)

2 This does not occur after a bronchoscopy.

3 A general anesthetic usually is not used, therefore paralytic ileus is not a complication.

4 Dysphasia is difficulty in talking and does not occur with a bronchoscopy; dyspepsia is disturbed digestion and is not the reason for withholding food or fluids.

702. 1 This may be indicative of hemorrhage and the physician should be notified. (2) (PB; MR; AS)

2 Overlooking the first signs of hemorrhage may permit the client to go into shock.

3 This is a potentially life-threatening situation; the physician should be notified immediately.

4 This could cause increased bleeding because of an increase in the intrathoracic pressure.

703. 2 This facilitates full expansion of the affected area and promotes drainage by gravity. (3) (SE; MR; IM)

1 This position relieves pain but compromises expansion of the affected lung and therefore should be avoided.

3 Lying on the affected side is most comfortable; lying on the unaffected side promotes expansion and drainage of the affected lung and should be encouraged.

4 This position does not stimulate deep breathing and coughing; gravity keeps secretions lower in the lungs.

704. 4 Increased fluid intake helps to liquefy respiratory secretions, which promotes expectoration. (1) (PB; CJ; IM)

1 Oxygen may dry the mucous membranes, which would thicken secretions; oxygen should be administered only when necessary.

2 Retained secretions are in the bronchi and trachea; gargling lubricates the oropharynx.

3 This position promotes retention of secretions; supine, prone, and Trendelenburg positions promote removal of secretions via gravity.

705. 4 Air is moisturized and warmed as it passes through the nasopharynx; with a laryngectomy this area is bypassed and the tracheobronchial tree compensates by producing copious amounts of secretions. (2) (PB; CJ; AN)

1 This is not a response to bacteria but to the character of the air that is entering the tracheobronchial tract.

2 This occurs regardless of turning and deep breathing.

3 This would produce local irritation and a local response.

706. 2 In this position the tongue does not obstruct the airway so that drainage of secretions and oxygen and carbon dioxide exchange can occur. (2) (PB; CJ; IM)

1 Oxygen may not be necessary; a patent airway takes priority.

3 This assesses ventilation but does not support it.

4 Once the pharyngeal reflex has returned, an in-place airway can cause the client to gag and vomit, and it should be removed; the client may or may not be conscious.

707. 3 A patent airway is the priority; therefore, removal of secretions is necessary. (2) (PB; CJ; PL)

1 This is important, but not the priority immediately after surgery.

2 This is an important postoperative concern, but does not occur immediately.

4 Although important, it is not as important as a patent airway.

708. 4 This is the correct technique; deep inhalation promotes alveolar expansion, holding the breath promotes transfer of gases, and exhalation promotes lung recoil. (2) (SE; MR; EV)

1 The breaths should not be in succession; they should be spaced by several normal breaths to avoid fatigue.

2 Coughing is done after deep breathing.

3 Inhalation should be through the mouthpiece.

709. 2 Oral intake should not be attempted after the procedure until the return of the gag reflex. (1) (PB; MR; AN)

1 Although some slight irritation may occur after the procedure, there is usually no painful sequela.

3 Even an alert person may choke and aspirate if eating or drinking is attempted while the pharyngeal wall is anesthetized.

4 The client should be informed of the need for being npo; anxiety should not be a reason for not providing this information.

710. 3 There is still a pathway from the mouth to the stomach; normal eating patterns are not lost when a laryngectomy is performed. (3) (PB; MR; IM)

1 There is no passage of air from the lungs to the nose; air is expelled through a tracheal stoma.

2 Same as answer 1.

4 Air passes through a tracheal stoma which bypasses the nose and olfactory organs.

711. 3 The client is at risk for airway obstruction, and restlessness and dyspnea indicate hypoxia. (2) (PB; CJ; EV)

1 This is unimportant; the pharyngeal opening is sutured closed and a tracheal stoma is formed; the trachea is anatomically separate from the esophagus.

2 Cloudy drainage may indicate infection, which would not be an immediate postoperative complication.

4 Edema is unlikely to cause dehiscence early in the postoperative period; a patent airway takes priority.

712. 1 Initial attempts at oral feedings may cause a choking feeling, which may produce severe coughing and raise secretions. (2) (SE; CJ; IM)

2 Swallowing does not have an adverse effect on the suture line.

3 Liquids are less obstructive than pureed foods in case aspiration occurs.

4 Pain medication may decrease the respiratory effort and depress the cough reflex.

713. **3 A chest tube drains the leaking chyle from the thoracic area; TPN provides nutrition, boosts immune defenses, and decreases thoracic duct flow; bed rest is recommended because lymphatic flow increases with activity. (3) (PB; CJ; PL)**

1 A gastrostomy tube will not drain fluid from the thoracic area; a high-fat diet is contraindicated, but bed rest is recommended.

2 A rectal tube has no relationship to the drainage of chyle from the thoracic area; a fat-poor diet and bed rest are recommended.

4 The nasogastric tube does not drain fluid from the thoracic area; a low-fat diet and bed rest are recommended; a low-fat diet of medium-chain triglycerides will reduce the production and flow of chyle.

714. **1 After a hemiglossectomy a client will have difficulty swallowing and expectorating oral secretions because of the trauma of surgery. (3) (PB; CJ; PL)**

2 Although this may limit edema or pain, it will not maintain patency of an airway that is compromised by secretions.

3 A side-lying position will better facilitate drainage from the mouth.

4 The client may not be reactive or have energy to cough; the priority is to prevent secretions from entering the respiratory tract.

715. **3 The cardiovascular and nervous systems of older adults are less flexible than when younger; postoperative hypoxia responds to oxygen. (2) (PB; CJ; IM)**

1 This is unnecessary because it is a common reaction of older adults to anesthesia, which may be alleviated by oxygen.

2 Although necessary, it will not help the client adapt.

4 An anxiolytic may increase the agitation.

716. **3 Serosanguineous drainage of 80 to 120 mL is expected during the first 24 hours; drainage more than this should be reported. (3) (PB; CJ; IM)**

1 The negative pressure of a portable drainage system promotes wound drainage, gravity would not.

2 Drainage of 180 mL in six hours is excessive and should be reported.

4 Although this would be done, it is secondary to notifying the physician.

717. **3 During chest surgery, the negative pressure around the lung is disrupted and the lungs do not fill adequately during inspiration; chest tubes are inserted to reestablish negative intrapleural pressure. (3) (PB; CJ; IM)**

1 Atelectasis refers to the collapse of alveoli or a lobule caused by a blockage of small airways; chest tubes do not cause or correct atelectasis.

2 Chest tubes are inserted into the intrapleural space, not the pericardial sac.

4 Although the amount of drainage from chest tubes is measured, the reason for chest tubes is to reestablish negative intrapleural pressure.

718. **3 Fluid in the water-seal chamber should rise and fall as the client breathes in and out (tidaling) until the lungs have expanded completely; a lack of tidaling on the second postoperative day would indicate that the tube is obstructed. (1) (PB; CJ; EV)**

1 This is contraindicated without a physician's order because it could traumatize pleural tissue.

2 The level of the fluid, as long as it covers the tube in the water-seal chamber, does not affect tidaling.

4 While full expansion of the lung will eliminate tidaling, an obstruction of the tube should be ruled out.

719. **3 This allows for measuring the output without interrupting the closed drainage system. (1) (SE; CJ; IM)**

1 This is done only to obtain a specimen for diagnostic procedures.

2 This is done only when the drainage collection chamber is full and the closed chest drainage must continue.

4 Clamping the chest tube is contraindicated because it can precipitate a pneumothorax; opening the system destroys the sterility of the closed drainage system.

720. **1 Excessive bubbling indicates an air leak, which must be eliminated to permit lung expansion. (2) (PB; CJ; IM)**

2 This is contraindicated because it can increase the pressure in the pleural space and cause a pneumothorax.

3 Increased suction pressure results in excessive bubbling in the suction control, not the water-seal chamber.

4 Excessive bubbling in the water-seal chamber is not expected; the system is malfunctioning.

721. 4 **This is ineffective because it exercises the elbow rather than the shoulder joint and muscles. (3) (SE; CJ; EV)**
   1 This is effective because it exercises the trapezius muscle and shoulder joint.
   2 Same as answer 1.
   3 This is effective because it provides circular range of motion to the shoulder joint.

722. 4 **The priority is to stabilize the respiratory status; a chest tube should be inserted. (2) (PB; CJ; PL)**
   1 The client must be stabilized before surgery; this may be necessary later.
   2 To maintain the airway an endotracheal tube would be inserted.
   3 This is secondary to stabilizing respirations.

723. 1 **The chest tube normalizes intrathoracic pressure, drains fluid and air from the pleural space, and improves pulmonary function. (2) (PB; CJ; EV)**
   2 This may be a sign of pain, respiratory obstruction, or bleeding.
   3 This indicates that air has entered the subcutaneous tissue (subcutaneous emphysema).
   4 This indicates a probable leak in the drainage system.

724. 4 **This is an emergency situation and atmospheric air must be prevented from entering the thoracic cavity; the client's respiratory status takes priority over the potential for infection. (3) (PB; CJ; IM)**
   1 This action is useless in this situation and would further impair the client's breathing.
   2 This is unsafe because it would allow atmospheric air to enter the thoracic cavity.
   3 Although an occlusive dressing such as Vaseline gauze is desirable, atmospheric air will enter the thoracic cavity while time is taken to obtain the occlusive dressing.

725. 3 **To prevent further possibility of pneumothorax, the nurse should immediately reconnect the tube. (3) (PB; CJ; IM)**
   1 This is unnecessary.
   2 Clamping is appropriate for changing a broken drainage system or to check for an air leak; it should not be done needlessly.
   4 The high-Fowler's position is appropriate for a client in respiratory distress, but this does not remedy this problem.

726. 2 **This prevents atelectasis and collection of secretions and promotes respiratory exchange. (2) (PB; CJ; IM)**
   1 Observing for dyspnea remains important, but crepitus is unlikely to occur with stabilization of respiratory status.
   3 This is important but not as conducive to improving respiratory status as are coughing and deep breathing.
   4 Activity should be promoted within limits of physical ability; bed rest is unnecessary.

727. 4 **The client's cardiac condition, age, and low socioeconomic status make the client vulnerable to communicable diseases. (3) (PM; MR; EV)**
   1 In the United States, death from tuberculosis has been on the decline because of improved drug therapy.
   2 Children before adolescence have the lowest incidence of tuberculosis.
   3 In the United States, the incidence of tuberculosis has been on the increase, not decrease.

728. 3 **Blood-tinged sputum in the absence of pronounced coughing may be the presenting symptom; diaphoresis at night is a later symptom. (2) (PB; CJ; AS)**
   1 Recurrent fever is present; however, frothy sputum is present with pulmonary edema, not tuberculosis.
   2 The cough would be productive, not dry.
   4 A productive cough may occur, but engorged neck veins are symptomatic of heart failure.

729. 4 **The Mantoux (also known as PPD) is the most accurate skin test for TB because of the testing material and the intradermal method used; no other skin test would be appropriate as a follow-up; further tests are now warranted, including a chest x-ray film. (1) (PM; MR; EV)**
   1 The test result was positive, not negative; further testing is necessary.
   2 The tine test is less accurate than the Mantoux and would not be used as a follow-up test.
   3 More than 10 mm induration is a positive test result, not a doubtful test result.

730. 4 **The tubercle bacilli can be stained with carbolfuchsin, an acid, when the stain is applied with heat; the bacilli resist discoloration when an acid-alcohol wash is applied. (1) (PM; CJ; AS)**
   1 This reflects pulmonary status but does not identify the organism if a lesion is found.

2 This indicates the presence of antibodies but is not diagnostic for the presence of the disease.

3 Same as answer 1.

731. 3 Fresh airflow through the house changes the air and lowers the concentration of microorganisms. (3) (PB; MR; IM)

1 This is not necessary.

2 Only articles contaminated with infected sputum, such as used tissues, should be contained.

4 It is permissible to do this because the extreme heat used to clean the dishes kills the mycobacteria.

732. 3 The directions need further clarification; refrigeration is not necessary; however, the specimen must be taken to the laboratory at the earliest possible time after collection. (1) (PM; MR; EV)

1 The specimen must represent phlegm containing the mycobacterium, which is in the lung, not the oronasopharynx.

2 For the best results the sputum collection should be made when the client awakens in the morning when mucus secretions are more copious.

4 Delivery to the laboratory should be made on the same day as close as possible to the time of collection.

733. 4 Tubercle bacilli are particularly resistant to treatment and can remain dormant for prolonged periods; medication must be taken consistently as ordered for prolonged periods. (1) (PB; CJ; PL)

1 Although this is important, the microorganisms must be eliminated with medication.

2 Same as answer 1.

3 Same as answer 1.

734. 3 The tubercle bacillus is a drug-resistant organism and takes a long time to be eradicated; usually a combination of three medications is used for a minimum of six months and at least six months beyond culture conversion. (2) (PB; CJ; IM)

1 This is too short a time for eradication of this organism.

2 Same as answer 1.

4 Usually, the organism can be eradicated in a shorter period of time, unless a resistant strain of the bacillus has developed.

REPRODUCTIVE AND GENITOURINARY (RG)

735. 4 Laxatives remove feces and flatus, providing better visualization. (2) (PB; CJ; PL)

1 A light supper may be indicated; however, there is no restriction as to fat content.

2 Large amounts of fluids may dilute the dye, impairing visualization.

3 A light dinner and beverage are permitted.

736. 3 The walls of a full bladder are stretched thinner and are more susceptible to rupture when traumatized. (2) (PB; CJ; AN)

1 This predisposes the client to developing infections, not to rupturing the bladder.

2 This might increase the risk of cancer; however, it would not predispose the client to bladder rupture.

4 This would not result in the production of urine large enough to expand the bladder if the client had voided before staring the trip.

737. 1 Frequent position changes are important to ensure proper urinary drainage; gravity promotes flow, which prevents obstruction. (2) (PB; CJ; PL)

2 ROM would be of minimal importance, since the client would be able to move without limitation.

3 Back care is necessary but is not a priority.

4 This is routine care, particularly if the client is sedated; positioning to promote urinary drainage takes priority.

738. 4 This uses gravity to allow urine to exert pressure on the area of the trigone, initiating relaxation of the urinary sphincter and facilitating micturition. (1) (PB; MR; IM)

1 Although this may be important so that urine may be collected to be strained, it will not facilitate micturition.

2 An acid-ash diet may be used to prevent urinary infection and the formation of calcium stones; it will not facilitate micturition.

3 This is important after urination but will not help facilitate micturition.

739. 1 Cranberry juice is excreted as hippuric acid, which helps acidify the urine (decrease the pH) and inhibit bacterial growth. (3) (PM; MR; AN)

2 Although bacterial growth may be inhibited, bacteria are not destroyed.

3 Glomerular filtration is unaffected by cranberry juice.

4 Cranberry juice acidifies the urine and may increase the burning sensation associated with urination when an infection is present.

740. 3 Intercourse may cause urethral inflammation increasing the risk of infection; voiding clears the urinary meatus and urethra of microorganisms. (2) (PM; MR; PL)
   1 Most fruit juices, with the exception of cranberry juice, cause an alkaline urine, which promotes bacterial growth.
   2 Douching is no longer recommended.
   4 Perineal care should be accomplished with wipes from the urinary meatus toward the rectum to prevent microorganisms from the vaginal or rectal areas from reaching the urinary meatus.

741. 2 Cholinergics intensify and prolong the action of acetylcholine, which increases the tone in the genitourinary tract, preventing urinary retention. (3) (PB; CJ; AN)
   1 Cholinergics will not prevent renal calculi.
   3 Anticholinergics are prescribed for the frequency and urgency associated with a spastic bladder.
   4 This would be a secondary gain because cholinergics help prevent urinary retention that can lead to a urinary tract infection, but this is not the primary purpose for administering these drugs.

742. 3 This increases lymphatic drainage, reducing edema and pain. (2) (PB; CJ; IM)
   1 This increases circulation to the area, intensifying edema and pain.
   2 Same as answer 1.
   4 This is not indicated; scrotal swelling is caused by the trauma of surgery, not infection.

743. 3 This method obtains a specimen uncontaminated by environmental organisms. (3) (SE; MR; IM)
   1 This is not as accurate as obtaining the purulent discharge from the site of origin.
   2 This would contaminate the specimen with organisms external to the body.
   4 This would dilute and possibly contaminate the specimen.

744. 2 Anal itching and irritation result from erythema and edema of the anal crypts from the gonococci. (3) (PB; CJ; AS)
   1 Frank rectal bleeding, not upper GI bleeding, occurs.
   3 Diarrhea, not constipation, occurs.
   4 Shape of formed stool does not change; however, diarrhea does occur.

745. 4 The client is in the secondary stage, which begins from six weeks to six months after primary contact; therefore, a six-month history is needed to ensure that all possible contacts and original contacts are located. (3) (SE; MR; IM)
   1 Any time less than six months may miss contacts who could have become infected.
   2 Same as answer 1.
   3 Same as answer 1.

746. 4 Neurotoxicity, as manifested by ataxia, is evidence of tertiary syphilis, which may involve the CNS; other CNS signs include confusion, paralysis, delusions, impaired judgment, and slurred speech. (2) (SE; CJ; AS)
   1 This occurs in the secondary stage.
   2 Same as answer 1.
   3 This is not a sign of late-stage syphilis.

747. 4 Research statistics indicate that hematuria is the most common early sign of cancer of the urinary system, probably because of its rich vascular network. (2) (PB; CJ; AN)
   1 This is not specific for bladder cancer; it is usually associated with an enlarged prostate in the male.
   2 Same as answer 1.
   3 Same as answer 1.

748. 2 This may denote a compromised blood supply to the stoma and impending necrosis. (2) (PB; MR; EV)
   1 This is expected in the early postoperative period following the surgery.
   3 Splinting catheters may be in place in the stoma; pink-tinged urine may be present in the immediate postoperative period.
   4 Same as answer 1.

749. 4 This is expected because mucus is normally secreted by the intestine. (3) (PB; CJ; EV)
   1 This is not necessary; at this point post-surgically the mucus is not an indication of infection; mucus in the urine following ureterostomy may indicate infection.
   2 This is not necessary; mucus is expected with an ileal conduit.
   3 While fluids should be encouraged to maintain urine flow, this will not eliminate mucus, which is continually discharged from the intestinal segment.

750. 2 High fluid intake flushes the ileal conduit and prevents infection and obstruction caused by mucus or uric acid crystals. (3) (PB; MR; IM)
   1 These are not contraindicated with an ileal conduit.
   3 This is expected; as edema decreases the stoma will become smaller.

4 Soap and water on the peristomal area help prevent irritation from waste products.

751. 2 **The headaches occur because of the retention of fluid and hypertension. (3) (PB; CJ; AS)**
1 The client would have oliguria, not nocturia.
3 The client would have a weight gain because of the retention of fluid.
4 The client would have anorexia related to elevated toxic substances in the blood.

752. 2 **Sucking on a hard candy will relieve thirst and increase carbohydrates but does not supply extra fluid. (2) (PB; CJ; IM)**
1 Carbonated beverages contain sodium and provide additional fluid, which must be restricted.
3 A milk shake contains both fluid and protein, which must be restricted.
4 Broth contains sodium, which could increase fluid retention.

753. 3 **A common cause of glomerulonephritis is a streptococcal infection that initiates an antibody formation that damages the glomeruli. (1) (SE; MR; IM)**
1 The alkalinity of bubble baths has been linked to urethritis, not glomerulonephritis.
2 Moderate activity is helpful in preventing urinary stasis, which could precipitate urinary infection.
4 Any fluid restriction is moderated as the client improves; fluid is allowed to prevent urinary stasis.

754. 2 **Infection is responsible for one-third of the traumatic or surgically induced deaths of clients with renal failure, as well as for medically induced acute renal failure (ARF); resistance is reduced in clients with renal failure because of decreased phagocytosis, which makes them very susceptible to microorganisms. (3) (SE; CJ; AS)**
1 Anemia occurs often with ARF, but it is not the most serious complication and should be treated in relation to the client's symptoms; erythropoietin and iron supplements usually are used.
3 Weight loss is not life threatening.
4 Platelet dysfunction does occur because of decreased cell surface adhesiveness, but it is not as serious as infection.

755. 4 **One of the kidney's functions is to excrete nitrogenous waste from protein metabolism; restriction of protein intake decreases the workload of the damaged kidneys. (3) (PB; MR; IM)**

1 The client is encouraged to be as active and independent as possible.
2 Medications are avoided because they may mask symptoms.
3 Iron supplements are not tolerated well by clients in renal failure and reduce the client's own stimulus to produce red blood cells; folate usually is given.

756. 2 **An excessive use of antacids may result in hypercalciuria; most calculi contain calcium combined with phosphate or other substances. (3) (PB; MR; AS)**
1 Cholesterol is unrelated to the formation of renal calculi; cholesterol stones in the gallbladder are the result of increased cholesterol synthesis in the liver.
3 Immobility with the associated demineralization of bone, not exercise, may cause renal calculi.
4 Alcohol intake is unrelated to renal calculi formation.

757. 2 **Hematuria and pain may result from damage to the ureteral lining as the calculus moves down the urinary tract; the urine may become cloudy or pink tinged. (2) (PB; CJ; AS)**
1 Although sharp, severe pain may be present, urgency is not associated with calculi; urgency may be associated with an enlarged prostate, cystitis, or other genitourinary problems.
3 The odor of urine is not foul; the color of urine is not dark, although it may be cloudy, pink, or red from hematuria.
4 Frequency and dysuria occur when the calculus reaches the bladder.

758. 2 **This dilutes the urine and crystals are less likely to coalesce and form calculi. (1) (PB; CJ; PL)**
1 An elevated serum creatinine has no relation to the formation of renal calculi.
3 Calcium restriction is necessary only if calculi have a calcium phosphate or calcium oxalate basis.
4 This is inadequate; urine output should be maintained at 3000 to 4000 mL to limit calculi formation.

759. 1 **Apples are low in phosphate. (3) (PB; MR; PL)**
2 Rye bread contains a higher level of phosphate than apples.
3 Chocolate contains a higher level of phosphate than apples.
4 Cheese is made with milk, which contains phosphate and should be avoided.

760. 3 **Pain with ureteral stones is caused by spasm and is excruciating and intermittent; it follows the path of the ureter to the bladder. (2) (PB; CJ; AS)**
   1 Pain is spasmodic and excruciating, not boring.
   2 Pain intensifies as the stone is caught in the ureter and spasms occur in an attempt to dislodge it.
   4 This is typical of pain caused by a stone in the renal pelvis.

761. 4 **Purines are precursors of uric acid, which crystallizes. (3) (PB; CJ; AN)**
   1 Cystine stones are caused by a rare hereditary defect resulting in inadequate renal tubular reabsorption of cystine (inborn error of cystine metabolism).
   2 A struvite stone is sometimes called a magnesium ammonium phosphate stone and is precipitated by recurrent urinary tract infections with coliform bacteria.
   3 An oxalate stone would be composed of calcium oxalate.

762. 1 **An output of 50 mL/hr is adequate; when urine output drops below 30 mL/hr, it may indicate renal failure and the physician should be notified. (1) (PB; CJ; IM)**
   2 This is contraindicated; the client would probably still be under the influence of anesthesia and the gag reflex might be depressed.
   3 This is unnecessary because the output is adequate.
   4 Same as answer 3.

763. 1 **The tube must be kept patent to prevent urine backup, hydronephrosis, and kidney damage. (3) (PB; CJ; IM)**
   2 This is unnecessary unless the tube is not functioning.
   3 Although this is important, it will not ensure free drainage of urine, which is the priority.
   4 This is a dependent function and requires a physician's order.

764. 2 **Calculi may obstruct the flow of urine to the bladder, allowing the urine to distend the ureter, causing hydroureter. (3) (PB; CJ; AN)**
   1 There is insufficient information to come to this conclusion even though output is less than intake; oliguria is present when the output is between 100 and 500 mL in a 24-hour period.
   3 Calculi do not cause renal shutdown directly; they may obstruct the urinary tract

and cause damage indirectly as a result of pressure from urine buildup.
   4 If the urethra were obstructed, the bladder would be distended.

765. 4 **If the calculus is in the renal pelvis, a percutaneous pyelolithotomy is performed; the stone is removed via a small flank incision. (2) (PB; CJ; AN)**
   1 This is not necessary.
   2 This usually is unnecessary.
   3 This route is used for calculi in the ureters and renal pelvis.

766. 1 **These occur with a urinary tract infection because of bladder irritability; burning on urination and fever are additional signs of a UTI. (1) (SE; MR; EV)**
   2 This is not related to a urinary tract infection.
   3 This is a symptom of a urinary calculus, not infection.
   4 This is not a sign of a urinary tract infection; this may be caused by altering the diet to include foods that form acid ash or alkaline ash.

767. 1 **Cancer of the prostate is rare before age 50 but increases with each decade; Black men develop it twice as often as white men and at an earlier age. (3) (PM; CJ; AS)**
   2 This group of men has a lower incidence of prostatic cancer than white men, as well as a lower mortality rate
   3 Same as answer 2.
   4 White men develop prostatic cancer half as often as Black men, but more commonly than Asian or Hispanic men.

768. 4 **A subjective symptom must be experienced and described by the client; flank pain, pain on the side of the body between the ribs and the ileum, accompanies renal colic and is a subjective symptom. (2) (PB; CJ; AS)**
   1 This is an objective sign that can be verified by observations or measurements.
   2 Same as answer 1.
   3 Same as answer 1.

769. 4 **A full bladder is palpable with urinary retention and distention which are common problems after a cystoscopy because of urethral edema; measures must be taken to relieve discomfort. (2) (PB; CJ; AS)**
   1 Fluids dilute the urine and reduce the chance of infection after cystoscopy and should not be limited.

2 Although true, this response does not relieve the discomfort of urinary retention.

3 More conservative methods such as running water or a sitz bath should be attempted; catheterization carries a risk of infection.

770. **4 This indicates that the bladder is distended with urine and therefore palpable. (2) (PB; CJ; AS)**

1 This is not related to urinary retention and benign prostatic hyperplasia.

2 This may be related to sexually transmitted diseases.

3 This may indicate renal calculi.

771. **1 Ejection of semen into the bladder instead of the urethra is common after a TURP. (3) (PB; CJ; AN)**

2 The surgery will not increase the ability to maintain an erection.

3 The surgery should not make the client permanently impotent; impotence may occur with the retroperitoneal approach.

4 The surgery should not interfere with the sex drive.

772. **2 This will improve bladder tone, which should alleviate dribbling. (2) (PB; CJ; IM)**

1 This identifies feelings but does not actively help the client solve the problem.

3 These interventions do not increase bladder tone; fluids should be increased and bladder volume gradually increased between voidings.

4 Continuous bladder decompression will reduce tone; reduced tone will persist when the indwelling catheter is removed.

773. **2 The pressure of the balloon against the small blood vessels of the prostate causes them to constrict, thereby preventing bleeding. (2) (PB; CJ; AN)**

1 It may do this but is necessary to limit bleeding.

3 Same as answer 1.

4 It is not the balloon but the indwelling catheter that promotes urinary drainage.

774. **4 The amount of irrigant instilled into the bladder must be deducted from the total output to determine the amount of urine produced. (1) (PB; CJ; IM)**

1 Unless irrigant is subtracted from the output, the total would be inaccurate.

2 Specific gravity measures the concentration of urine; this measurement would be inaccurate because the urine is diluted with GU irrigant.

3 This is unnecessary; the bladder is constantly being irrigated with GU irrigant.

775. **4 Retained fluid raises intravesicular pressure, causing discomfort similar to the urge to void. (2) (PB; CJ; EV)**

1 Total intake and output have no relationship to the client's present feeling of the need to void.

2 The client's vital signs are not related to the complaint; the physician should be called only if a blocked drainage tube cannot be corrected.

3 Although this is true, the integrity of the gravity system should be ascertained before determining the cause of the complaint.

776. **3 The urethral mucosa in the prostatic area is affected during surgery, and strictures may form with healing. (3) (SE; MR; EV)**

1 The client should be out of bed ambulating; sitting for several hours is contraindicated because it promotes venous stasis and thrombus formation.

2 The client should void as the need arises; straining can cause pressure in the operative area, precipitating hemorrhage.

4 Although vigorous exercise should be avoided, six months is too long for this restriction.

777. **2 After transurethral surgery, hemorrhage is common because of venous oozing and bleeding from many small arteries in the area. (1) (PB; CJ; EV)**

1 Sepsis is unusual and would occur later in the postoperative course.

3 Leaking around the catheter is not a major complication.

4 Urinary retention is unlikely with an indwelling catheter in place.

778. **4 Laboratory values suggest metastasis to the bone, which results in pain and risk of pathologic fractures; therefore handling must be gentle. (2) (PB; CJ; PL)**

1 Seizure precautions are not necessary; a prostate specific antigen elevation indicates bone, not brain, involvement.

2 Measuring intake and output is necessary for any client with prostatic cancer because of the risk of obstruction.

3 Elevated prostate specific antigen levels do not significantly affect the plasma pH.

779. 4 This action causes the bladder muscle to contract, initiating painful bladder spasms. (2) (PB; MR; IM)

1 Although opiates may dull the pain, they may not limit muscle spasms.

2 Instillation of fluid will not decrease bladder spasms, may be irritating, and can precipitate bladder spasms.

3 Advancing or manipulating the catheter may precipitate bladder spasms.

780. 4 Because of the trauma to the mucous membranes of the urinary tract, burning on urination is an expected response that should gradually subside. (2) (SE; MR; EV)

1 The urine may have a slight pink tinge because of the trauma from the surgery and the presence of the catheter, but it should no longer be dilute once the continuous bladder irrigation is discontinued and removed.

2 This is a sign of hemorrhage that should not occur.

3 This should not occur unless the indwelling catheter is removed too soon and there is still edema of the urethra.

781. 2 A continuous flushing of the bladder dilutes the bloody urine and empties the bladder, preventing clots. (1) (PB; CJ; AN)

1 Only the kidneys form urine; fluid instilled into the bladder does not affect kidney function.

3 Urinary output can be measured regardless of the amount of fluid instilled.

4 This system does not exert any additional pressure within the bladder; it should prevent obstruction.

782. 2 Because venous stasis is the major predisposing factor of pulmonary emboli, venous flow velocity should be increased. (2) (PB; CJ; PL)

1 Increasing the coagulability of the blood would lead to the development of deep vein thrombosis.

3 This would not affect the prevention of deep vein thrombosis.

4 Same as answer 3.

783. 4 This is a classic sign of renal carcinoma; it is due to capillary erosion by the cancerous growth. (1) (PB; CJ; AS)

1 Dull flank pain may occur but not as frequently as bleeding.

2 Weight loss, not weight gain, would occur.

3 This would not occur with renal carcinoma; it might occur with glomerulonephritis.

784. 2 The kidney, an extremely vascular organ, receives a large percentage of the blood flow and hemorrhage from the operative site can occur. (3) (PB; CJ; PL)

1 This may occur, but it would be later in the postoperative period.

3 This can occur but is not acute and develops later.

4 This can occur but is not life threatening.

785. 4 Turning the client prevents respiratory complications. (3) (PB; CJ; PL)

1 Because clients are prone to develop paralytic ileus, they are kept NPO or on clear fluid for at least 24 to 48 hours.

2 There is no need for a nephrostomy tube because the kidney has been removed.

3 The first dressing change is performed by the physician.

786. 2 Digested blood is protein and could increase the BUN. (3) (PB; MR; PL)

1 Renal function already is lost; dialysis performs the function of the kidneys.

3 Although clients with renal failure have problems with bleeding, this does not interfere with identifying the site of bleeding.

4 Renal failure does not affect signs of GI blood loss, hemorrhage, or shock.

787. 2 High-biologic-value (HBV) protein contains essential amino acids needed by the body for tissue building and repair. (1) (PB; MR; EV)

1 A high-calorie diet would provide for weight gain.

3 Less HBV proteins are necessary to meet body needs thereby decreasing nitrogenous wastes.

4 This is not the purpose of high-biologic-value proteins; sodium restrictions would decrease blood pressure.

788. 3 One cup of cottage cheese contains approximately 225 calories, 27 g of protein, 9 g of fat, 30 mg of cholesterol, and 6 g of carbohydrate; proteins of high biologic value (HBV) contain optimal levels of the amino acids essential for life. (1) (PB; MR; EV)

1 Apple juice is a source of vitamins A and C, not protein.

2 Raw carrots are a carbohydrate source and contain beta-carotene.

4 Whole wheat bread is a source of carbohydrates and fiber.

789. 1 Foods high in carbohydrates and low in protein, sodium, and potassium are encouraged for these clients. (2) (PB; MR; IM)

2 This is high in potassium, which is restricted.

3 This is high in sodium, which may be restricted.

4 This is high in protein, sodium, and potassium, which usually are restricted.

790. 2 The accumulation of metabolic wastes in the blood (uremia) can cause pruritus; edema results from fluid overload caused by impaired renal excretion. (1) (PB; CJ; AS)

1 Pallor occurs with chronic renal failure as a result of the related anemia.

3 This is a urinary pattern that is not caused by chronic renal failure; this may occur after prostate surgery.

4 This occurs with an enlarged prostate, not renal insufficiency.

791. 3 An elevation in uremic waste products causes irritation of the nerves, resulting in flapping hand tremors (asterixis, liver flap). (3) (PB; CJ; AS)

1 Hypertension results from kidney failure because of sodium and water retention.

2 The diseased kidney is unable to excrete potassium ions, resulting in hyperkalemia, not hypokalemia.

4 The hematocrit value will be low because of a decreased production of erythropoietin, a hormone synthesized in the kidney; erythropoietin regulates the production of erythrocytes.

792. 4 Insensible losses are 400 to 500 mL in 24 hours; the measured output is about 400 mL in 24 hours based on the available history. (2) (PB; CJ; AN)

1 Based on the history the expected urinary output should be about 400 mL in the next 24 hours, far less than 900 mL.

2 This is an insufficient amount of fluid; at least 2500 mL daily is necessary to help prevent hypostatic pneumonia.

3 Hyperkalemia in acute renal failure is caused by inadequate glomerular filtration and is not related to fluid intake.

793. 3 Vital signs monitor the cardiopulmonary status; the physician must treat this hyperkalemia to prevent cardiac dysrhythmias. (3) (PB; MR; IM)

1 The cardiac arrest team will respond whenever called for a cardiac arrest; there is no sign of arrest in this client.

2 A repeat laboratory test would take time and probably reaffirm the original results; the client needs medical attention.

4 These are correct interventions if available, but the priority is medical attention and the physician should be notified immediately.

794. 1 Insulin causes an increased rate of flow of potassium into the cells, which will then reduce the circulating blood levels of potassium. (3) (PB; MR; IM)

2 This response halts communication and is not supportive.

3 Blood glucose levels usually are not elevated in acute renal failure.

4 Insulin will not lower the metabolic rate.

795. 2 Turning from side to side will change the position of the catheter, thereby freeing the drainage holes, which may have become obstructed. (2) (PB; MR; IM)

1 Taking fluids into the gastrointestinal tract does not influence drainage of dialysate from the peritoneal cavity.

3 This improves pulmonary ventilation but does not improve flow of dialysate from the catheter.

4 The position of the catheter should be changed by the physician.

796. 4 This promotes vasodilation so that urea, a large-molecular substance, can be shifted from the blood vessels into the dialyzing solution. (2) (PB; MR; AN)

1 Heat does not affect the shift of potassium into the cells.

2 The removal of metabolic wastes is affected in renal failure, not the metabolic processes themselves.

3 Excess serum potassium is removed by dialyzing with a potassium-free solution, not by heat.

797. 2 In the diuretic phase fluid retained during the oliguric phase is excreted and may reach 3 to 5 liters daily; hypovolemia may occur and fluids should be replaced. (1) (PB; CJ; AS)

1 Diuresing is an indication of improved renal functioning, not progression into failure.

3 Hyperkalemia develops in the oliguric phase when glomerulofiltration is inadequate.

4 Metabolic acidosis occurs in the oliguric phase.

798. 2 While proteins may be restricted, those eaten should be high-quality proteins to replace proteins lost during the dialysis. (3) (PB; CJ; IM)

1 This client would be encouraged to eat a high-calorie diet.

3 This is inappropriate; there is usually a modest restriction of fluids when the client is on dialysis.

4 This is inappropriate; there is usually a restriction of high-potassium foods when the client is on dialysis.

799. 3 Lack of motivation is the most serious impediment to successful CAPD; CAPD is contraindicated for clients who are blind, have a colostomy, are psychotic, or have PVD. (2) (PI; CJ; AS)
1 These are not a contraindication to CAPD.
2 Same as answer 1.
4 Same as answer 1.

800. 2 The infusion should be at room temperature to lessen abdominal discomfort and allow for dilation of peritoneal vessels. (2) (PB; CJ; IM)
1 The side-lying position may restrict fluid inflow and prevent maximum urea clearance; usually the client is in the semi-Fowler's position.
3 Infusion should be unrestricted, taking approximately 5 to 10 minutes.
4 Medications are added before the infusion of the fluid.

801. 3 Pressure from the fluid may cause upward displacement of the diaphragm. (3) (PB; CJ; IM)
1 Additional fluid would aggravate the problem.
2 Auscultation is important, but it does not alleviate the problem.
4 The client is in the semi-Fowler's position for the dialysis, normally which would relieve dyspnea; however, intraabdominal pressure must be reduced by draining the fluid.

802.
1 ____ Severe itching (pruritus) is caused by metabolic waste products that are deposited in the skin; dialysis removes metabolic waste products preventing this adaptation associated with renal failure.
2 ____ The production of abnormally small amounts of urine (oliguria) is a sign of renal failure, not a complication of peritoneal dialysis.
3 _x_ Tachycardia can be caused by peritonitis, a complication of peritoneal dialysis; the heart rate increases to meet the metabolic demands associated with infection. (3) (PB; CJ; EV)
4 _x_ Cloudy or opaque dialysate outflow (effluent) is the earliest sign of peritonitis; it is caused by the constituents associated with an infectious process.
5 _x_ Abdominal pain is associated with peritonitis, a complication of peritoneal dialysis; pain results from peritoneal inflammation, abdominal distention, and involuntary muscle spasms.

803. 2 The external shunt may come apart; external temperatures make clotting a potential hazard; frequent handling increases risk of infection. (3) (PB; CJ; PL)
1 Neither the shunt nor the fistula will affect the blood pressure reading.
3 Infusion should not be in the extremity with the shunt or the fistula to avoid pressure from the tourniquet and to lessen chance of phlebitis.
4 The ends of the shunt cannula should be left exposed for rapid reconnection in the event of disruption.

804. 3 These are signs and symptoms of the disequilibrium syndrome, which results from rapid changes in composition of the extracellular fluid and cerebral edema; the rate of exchange should be decreased. (3) (PB; CJ; EV)
1 This will not alleviate or reverse the cause of the symptoms, although it will provide relief from the nausea.
2 The cause of the confusion must be reversed, and this intervention will not accomplish this.
4 While these should be assessed, this action will not alleviate the symptoms.

805. 2 Sodium is an electrolyte that can pass through the semipermeable membrane during hemodialysis. (2) (PB; CJ; AN)
1 This does not pass through the semipermeable membrane during hemodialysis.
3 Same as answer 1.
4 Same as answer 1.

806. 1 The recipient's own kidneys are not removed unless a chronic infection is present. (3) (SE; MR; IM)
2 Both kidneys are left in place; the new kidney is placed in the right lower quadrant.
3 Same as answer 2.
4 Same as answer 2.

807. 4 Human leukocyte antigen compatibility provides the most specific predictions of the body's tendency to accept or reject foreign tissue. (2) (PB; CJ; AN)
1 Although ABO compatibility is necessary, the exact blood type is not.
2 This is unsafe unless the family member has matching leukocyte antigen complexes; this may increase the possibility of a match, but there is no guarantee that a family member will match.
3 Differences in body size do not cause rejection.

808. 1 **Output is critical when assessing kidney function; the urinary output should be monitored every 30 to 60 minutes; decreasing urinary output is a sign of rejection. (2) (PB; CJ; EV)**
  2 This is too infrequent to monitor output immediately after transplant; it is essential to monitor output more frequently to evaluate whether the new kidney is working or whether it is being rejected.
  3 Same as answer 2.
  4 It is not necessary to monitor this frequently.

809. 4 **As the transplanted organ functions, nitrogenous wastes are eliminated, lowering the serum creatinine. (2) (PB; CJ; EV)**
  1 As more urine is produced by the transplanted kidney, the specific gravity or concentration of the urine will decrease.
  2 With renal failure, fluid retention causes hypertension; there should be a correction of hypertension, not hypotension.
  3 The serum potassium will correct to a normal level after the transplant.

810. 3 **Hypertension is caused by a return of hypervolemia because of the failure of the new kidney. (2) (PM; MR; EV)**
  1 There will be a weight gain because of fluid retention, which is indicative of failure of the transplanted kidney.
  2 The client will have an elevated temperature exceeding 100° F.
  4 Urine output will be decreased or absent, depending on the degree of failure.

811. 4 **The WBC count can drop precipitously; if leukocytes are less than 3000/mm³, the drug should be stopped to prevent irreversible bone marrow depression. (2) (PB; CJ; EV)**
  1 Leukocytosis, not leukopenia, would occur with an infection.
  2 High creatinine levels are related to kidney failure but do not cause leukopenia.
  3 The WBC count would be elevated, not decreased, if the kidney were being rejected.

SKELETAL (SK)

812. 2 **Weight-bearing and the use of antigravity muscles stimulate bone formation or osteoblastic function. (1) (PB; CJ; AN)**
  1 This will result in bone demineralization, not calcium deposition in the bone.
  3 The aging process contributes to a gradual and progressive demineralization of bone.

  4 Calcium intake has a relationship to osteoclastic mechanisms in that it inhibits the withdrawal of calcium from bone.

813. 3 **These symptoms are consistent with a torn cartilage; this injury is common among basketball players. (1) (PB; CJ; AS)**
  1 A fractured patella would cause pain and usually manifests itself at the time of injury.
  2 A ruptured Achilles tendon is painful and prevents plantar flexion of the foot; symptoms are usually manifested immediately upon injury.
  4 A stress fracture is associated with pain, not with a clicking or locking of the knee.

814. 2 **This describes the procedure in which the physician uses a scope to visualize and operate on the knee. (1) (PB; CJ; IM)**
  1 While this is true, it evades the client's concern and does not describe the procedure.
  3 This is a surgical procedure; the only treatment prescribed would be physiotherapy after surgery.
  4 Arthroscopic surgery is not a radiologic procedure.

815. 4 **A bone scan maps the uptake of a bone-seeking radioactive isotope; an increased uptake is seen in metastatic bone disease, osteosarcoma, osteomyelitis, and certain fractures. (2) (PB; CJ; EV)**
  1 A bone scan measures the uptake of radioactive material, not the absence of calcium, which would be seen in an x-ray examination of bone.
  2 This is a bone marrow aspiration, when a small amount of marrow is examined to determine the presence of abnormal cells in diseases such as leukemia.
  3 A bone scan involves a small diagnostic dosage of a radioactive substance; it is not therapeutic.

816. 2 **Numbness is a neurologic sign that should be reported immediately because it indicates pressure on the nerves and blood vessels. (2) (PB; CJ; EV)**
  1 Warmth is a sign of adequate circulation.
  3 This results from inadequate skin care and can be easily managed with lotion or oil.
  4 Some degree of discomfort is expected following cast application.

817. 2 **This may indicate cast pressure on a nerve and should be investigated further. (2) (SE; MR; AS)**
1 Some swelling is expected after injury to the tissues; it should be noted and monitored further.
3 Some bloody drainage is expected; it should be noted and observed further.
4 The radial pulse of the affected arm could not be assessed because of the placement of the cast; circulation to this extremity would be assessed by briefly compressing a fingernail on the client's affected hand and observing the return of a pink color after releasing the compression.

818. 4 **Damage to the blood vessels may decrease the circulatory perfusion of the toes; this would indicate a lack of blood supply to the extremity. (2) (PB; CJ; EV)**
1 The break is between the knee and the ankle, not in the thigh.
2 Damage to the major blood vessels would more likely cause a decrease in blood pressure from shock.
3 Decreased circulatory perfusion of the foot would cause the skin temperature to decrease, but the foot could also feel cool because of shock.

819. 3 **This indicates tissue hypoxia or breakdown and should be reported to the physician. (1) (SE; MR; IM)**
1 Other data, such as elevated temperature or increased white blood cells, are not present to support the presence of an infection.
2 This is not a typical response to a cast and may indicate a complication.
4 The priority is to notify the physician; this could be done to provide relief to the client after the physician is notified.

820. 3 **Elevation will help control the edema that usually occurs. (3) (PB; CJ; IM)**
1 Because the ankle has been at rest, discomfort and stiffness are expected after the cast is removed.
2 Because the skin has not been exposed, it needs gentle washing to prevent injuring the epidermis.
4 The leg should be put through full range of motion more than once daily.

821. 4 **These movements include all possible ranges of motion for the ankle joint. (1) (PB; CJ; IM)**

1 Although the ankle can be moved in a circular motion, flexion and extension are more specifically called dorsiflexion and plantar flexion in relation to the ankle; also, eversion and inversion should be done when manipulating the ankle.
2 Flexion and extension are more specifically called dorsiflexion and plantar flexion in relation to the ankle; the ankle cannot be abducted or adducted; the ankle can be inverted and everted.
3 These motions refer to the upper extremities.

822. 3 **These sets of muscles will be used in crutch walking and therefore need strengthening. (2) (SE; MR; PL)**
1 Although these muscles keep the person erect, the most important muscles for walking with crutches are the triceps, elbow extensors, finger flexors of the arms, and the muscles in the unaffected leg.
2 This will do nothing to promote crutch walking.
4 A pushing, not a pulling, motion is used with crutches; the triceps, not the biceps, are used.

823. 2 **The palms should bear the client's weight to avoid damage to the nerves in the axilla (brachial plexus). (1) (SE; CJ; EV)**
1 This would be unsafe; pressure on the axillary region could injure the nerves in the brachial plexus.
3 The physician ordered non–weight bearing on the affected leg.
4 Same as answer 1.

824. 2 **In a comminuted fracture, the bone is splintered or crushed. (2) (PB; CJ; AN)**
1 This is a compound fracture.
3 This is a greenstick fracture.
4 This is a complete fracture.

825. 2 **The infected bone is placed at rest and may be in a cast or splint to reduce pain and limit the spread of infection. (2) (SE; CJ; PL)**
1 This would increase pain and spread the infection.
3 Osteomyelitis is usually caused by a microorganism traveling through the bloodstream to the bone, not the reverse; the client is already septic.
4 This is contraindicated; early ambulation may facilitate the spread of infection.

826. 2 Uric acid has a low solubility; it tends to precipitate and form deposits at various sites where blood flow is least active, including cartilaginous tissue such as the ears. (3) (PB; CJ; AS)

1 Urate deposits will not form at this site because the blood flow is ample, and it is not cartilaginous tissue.
3 Same as answer 1.
4 Same as answer 1.

827. 2 Shellfish contains more than 100 mg of purine per 100 g. (2) (SE; MR; EV)

1 This food is low in purine.
3 Same as answer 1.
4 Same as answer 1.

828. 1 Osteoporotic vertebrae collapse under the weight of the upper body or by improper or rapid turning, reaching, or lifting. (2) (PB; CJ; AN)

2 Bones, not the spinal cord, demineralize in osteoporosis.
3 This occurs in osteoarthritis.
4 The spinal cord does not bulge; the nucleus pulposus bulges toward the spinal cord.

829. 3 The antibody called rheumatoid factor is present in 90% of advanced cases of arthritis; it frequently is not found in the early stages of the disease. (3) (PI; CJ; IM)

1 This denies the client's discomfort and does not address the stated confusion.
2 This denies the client's immediate feelings and blocks further communication of feelings.
4 This reinforces the client's confusion over negative test results and felt discomfort.

830. 3 Moist heat increases circulation and decreases muscle tension, which helps relieve chronic stiffness. (1) (PB; CJ; IM)

1 While this is advisable for someone with arthritis, it will not relieve morning stiffness.
2 This is related to muscle fatigue, not to stiffness of joints.
4 Inactivity promotes stiffness.

831. 2 The pathologic process involved with rheumatoid arthritis is accompanied by vascular congestion, fibrin exudate, and cellular infiltrate causing inflammation of the synovium. (1) (PB;CJ; AN)

1 Urate crystals occur with gouty arthritis, not rheumatoid arthritis.
3 This is unrelated to rheumatoid arthritis.
4 Increased interstitial fluid is only one aspect of the inflammatory response.

832. 1 Palpation will elicit tenderness because pressure stimulates nerve endings and causes pain. (1) (PB; MR; IM)

2 Pressure would not increase the swelling of already swollen joints.
3 Nodules associated with rheumatoid arthritis are not caused by pressure; they occur spontaneously in about 25% of individuals with rheumatoid arthritis and are composed of collagen fibers, exudate, and cellular debris.
4 These are present in gout, not arthritis; they are composed of sodium urate.

833. 2 This position provides for extension of joints. (1) (PB; CJ; PL)

1 The side-lying position supports flexion of joints.
3 This creates continued flexion of joints.
4 This does not influence the position of joints.

834. 4 Spacing activity protects joints from overuse, misuse, and stress, limiting inflammation; it provides a balance between rest and activity. (2) (PB; MR; EV)

1 The exercise program should be planned; too much activity can precipitate an exacerbation, and too little may cause contractures.
2 Spaced ROM should be incorporated into daily living activities not just twice a day.
3 This will cause stress at the joints, which may precipitate an exacerbation.

835. 1 Active exercises, alternating extension, flexion, abduction, and adduction, mobilize exudates in the joints and relieve stiffness and pain. (3) (PB; MR; PL)

2 Flexion exercises alone would result in contractures.
3 ROM once a day is not enough to prevent contractures.
4 This would increase stiffness, joint pain, and the occurrence of contractures.

836. 2 This chair allows the hips and shoulders to be against the back of the chair while fully supporting the thighs. (3) (PB; MR; IM)

1 This permits the hips and knees to be flexed greater than 90 degrees, which can cause flexion contractures.
3 The thighs are not fully supported in a wheelchair.
4 This permits the hips to be flexed greater than 90 degrees, which can promote flexion contractures.

837. 1 **Not neglecting joint pain protects the joints, especially if the pain lasts more than one or two hours after a particular activity. (3) (SE; MR; IM)**

  2 The opposite would be true; the client should use large muscles, such as pushing doors open with arms rather than fingers.

  3 This would increase joint stress; heavy and light tasks should be alternated.

  4 When the inflammatory process is active, the joint should be used as little as possible to provide rest.

838. 2 **Flexion contractures of the hips and knees could develop unless some periods of full extension are maintained. (2) (PB; MR; IM)**

  1 The position that usually is assumed is one of flexion, which would lead to contractures.

  3 This may cause flexion contractures of the hips and knees.

  4 This could cause flexion contractures of the hips.

839. 3 **The Valsalva maneuver raises cerebrospinal fluid pressure thereby causing pain. (3) (PB; CJ; AS)**

  1 Calf tenderness is associated with thrombophlebitis.

  2 Dysuria is associated with urinary problems.

  4 This type of pain is not associated with intervertebral disc problems.

840. 3 **Pain results because herniation of a disc into the spinal column irritates the spinal cord or the roots of spinal nerves. (1) (PB; CJ; AN)**

  1 This is not involved; the lamina is that portion of the vertebra removed during surgery to gain access to the disc.

  2 The vertebral bodies themselves are not shifting.

  4 Circulation of cerebrospinal fluid is not affected.

841. 3 **Coughing places strain on the lumbar area, increasing the herniation of the disc. (2) (PB; CJ; IM)**

  1 This does not increase intervertebral pressure.

  2 This will not increase pressure or cause pain; flexed knees are usually a more comfortable position.

  4 This will not increase pressure or increase pain.

842. 4 **This supports vertebral alignment, decreasing trauma to the operative site. (1) (SE; MR; PL)**

  1 This is contraindicated because it will increase intracranial pressure, which is not desirable.

  2 This is contraindicated because it flexes the vertebral column, which can increase intracranial pressure.

  3 Traction is not used after this surgery.

843. 3 **Alteration in circulation and sensation indicates damage to the spinal cord; if these occur the physician must be notified immediately. (2) (PB; CJ; EV)**

  1 After surgery, the physician's order should specify the amount of fluid intake.

  2 This is contraindicated because the prone position will hyperextend the vertebral column; log-rolling from side to side is preferred.

  4 Although this would be done, it is not the priority.

844. 1 **Putting the upper arm and leg toward the side to which the client is turning uses body weight to facilitate turning; the spine is kept straight. (3) (SE; MR; AN)**

  2 This would result in twisting the spinal column.

  3 This could be done if another person were turning the client; when turning alone in this position, the client would have no leverage and turning would probably result in twisting the spinal column.

  4 This would interfere with turning because the bent leg becomes an obstacle and provides a force opposite to the leverage needed to turn.

845. 1 **Sitting maintains alignment of the back and allows the nurses to support the client until orthostatic hypotension subsides. (2) (PB; CJ; IM)**

  2 Rapid movement could flex the vertebrae, which would traumatize the spinal cord; taking the blood pressure at this time is not necessary.

  3 This would induce flexion of the vertebrae, which could traumatize the spinal cord.

  4 Same as answer 3.

846. 2 **Maintaining the sitting position for a prolonged period places excessive body weight and stress on the surgical area. (2) (SE; MR; EV)**

  1 This maintains lordosis of the small of the back and provides proper support.

  3 This relieves pressure on the back and promotes comfort in bed.

  4 This prevents excessive pressure on the musculature and vertebral column.

847. 2 **This is done while in the supine position before the body is subjected to the force of gravity in a vertical position; anatomic landmarks are**

easier to locate for correct application of the brace, and intraabdominal organs have not shifted toward the pelvic floor by gravity. (2) (PB; MR; PL)

1 It should be applied while in the supine position before getting out of bed and should be worn the entire day for support.

3 The brace should be applied while in the supine position, not the sitting position.

4 Twisting exercises are contraindicated because they exert excessive pressure on the operative site.

848. 4 **Phantom limb sensation is a real experience with no known cause or cure. (1) (PB; CJ; AN)**

1 This may be an appropriate diagnosis for the client with an amputation, but it is not the diagnosis related to the phantom limb phenomenon.

2 Same as answer 1.

3 This is not an appropriate diagnosis for the individual with an amputation.

849. 3 **This stretches the flexor muscle and prevents a flexion contraction of the hip. (1) (PB; CJ; IM)**

1 This flexes the hip which may result in a hip flexion contracture; the residual limb is elevated for only 24 to 48 hours.

2 This may result in an abduction deformity; the residual limb should be kept in functional alignment.

4 This type of exercise should be started on a soft surface with a physician's order approximately five days after surgery.

850. 4 **The even distribution of hemosiderin (iron-rich pigment) in the tissue in response to pressure of the prosthesis indicates proper fit. (2) (SE; CJ; EV)**

1 This is not related to a proper fit.

2 This would result in an improper fit.

3 This indicates that the prosthesis is too long or too short.

851. 2 **The client probably has a fat embolus; oxygen reduces surface tension of the fat globules and reduces hypoxia. (3) (PB; CJ; IM)**

1 Oxygen should be administered and the client placed in a semi-Fowler's position before the physician is called.

3 This will cause hip flexion putting stress on the fractured femur; semi-Fowler's is preferred.

4 The client is not in shock resulting from hemorrhage but experiencing a fat embolus; administering oxygen takes priority.

852. 4 **Pressure supports tissue, promotes venous return, and limits edema, thus promoting shrinkage. (2) (PB; CJ; IM)**

1 Although it may limit clot formation, its primary purpose is to promote venous return, prevent edema, and shrink the limb.

2 Activity, not bandaging, usually decreases the occurrence of phantom limb sensation.

3 While pressure may prevent hemorrhage, its primary purpose is to prevent edema and shrink the residual limb.

853. 1 **Preparation for crutch walking includes exercises to strengthen arm and shoulder muscles. (2) (PB; MR; AN)**

2 Position changes are to prevent hip flexion contractures, not to prepare for crutch walking.

3 This is important for healing and as a preparation for the prosthesis, not for crutch walking.

4 The phantom limb phenomenon is a sensation that the absent limb is present; there are no exercises for this.

854. 3 **These indicate that the client has exceeded tolerance for the activity at this time. (1) (SE; CJ; EV)**

1 These are expected adaptations to the activity.

2 Flushed skin is an expected response to activity; respirations would increase in depth rather than become slowed.

4 An increase in blood pressure is an expected response to activity; respirations would increase in depth, not become shallow.

855. 2 **Without the prosthesis, a walker or crutches would be necessary and require the readjustment of weight bearing on one leg. (3) (PB; CJ; AN)**

1 Early use of a prosthesis does not affect the development or presence of phantom limb sensation, which occurs frequently in clients with an amputation.

3 Early use of a prosthesis has no effect on wound infection.

4 While this is true, it is not the major purpose; a prosthesis can easily be fitted after discharge when the residual limb is completely healed and no longer edematous.

856. 3 **The ability to transfer assures mobility and a degree of independence postoperatively. (3) (PB; MR; PL)**

1 Log-rolling is necessary for some spinal surgery but not for amputation.

2 This would not be of prime importance while the surgical wound is healing.

4 Standing on one leg in a weakened condition predisposes one to falling.

857. 3 Gentle intervention reduces pain, shock, and inhibits the release of bone marrow into the system which can cause a fat embolism. (3) (SE; CJ; IM)

1 This will not prevent a fat embolus; it may limit edema and pain, a local effect.

2 This will not prevent a fat embolus; it is not a priority at the scene of an accident.

4 Maintaining alignment will not prevent a fat embolus.

858. 3 A continuous pull on the lower extremity keeps bone fragments from moving and causing further trauma, pain, and edema. (2) (PB; CJ; AN)

1 The fracture will be reduced by surgery; Buck's extension is a temporary measure before surgery.

2 Moving the leg away from the midline would not keep the leg in alignment; it is not the purpose of Buck's extension.

4 External rotation of the femur may still occur with Buck's extension.

859. 1 This provides slight countertraction, which will prevent slipping down in bed. (3) (PB; CJ; IM)

2 This will have no effect.

3 This is unsafe; an interruption in the traction may result in loss of bone alignment.

4 This will not alleviate the cause of the problem; it may be necessary more often than every two hours.

860. 4 A pulmonary embolism is the most common complication of hip surgery because of high vascularity and the release of fat cells from the bone marrow. (3) (PB; CJ; AS)

1 The occurrence of pneumonia is rare because of early activity after surgery; in addition, the operative area is not in close proximity to the diaphragm and lungs, therefore it does not impede deep breathing.

2 Postoperative hemorrhage with hip surgery is rare because bleeding at the operative site is not covert.

3 The incidence of wound infection is no greater than with other postoperative clients.

861. 3 This reduces stress on anatomical structures and maintains the head of the femur in the acetabulum. (2) (PB; CJ; IM)

1 This places stress on the acetabulum and the head of the femur; abduction is essential.

2 Hip flexion may dislodge the head of the femur from the acetabulum.

4 This places stress on the bone, soft tissue, and nail plate; it can cause damage and dislocation of the head of the femur.

862. 4 A complete assessment must be performed to determine the location, characteristics, intensity, and duration of the pain; the pain could be incisional, result from a pulmonary embolus, or be caused by neurovascular trauma to the affected leg, and the intervention for each would be different. (1) (PB; CJ; EV)

1 This may be done after a complete assessment reveals that this would be the appropriate intervention; assessment is the priority.

2 Same as answer 1.

3 Same as answer 1.

863. 2 Compressed air inflates the padded plastic stockings systematically from ankle to calf to thigh and then deflates; this promotes venous return and prevents venous stasis and thromboembolism. (1) (PB; CJ; PL)

1 Turning on the operative side is contraindicated because it places tension on the hip joint and may traumatize the incision.

3 Although this may be ordered to promote muscle strength, the major complication, thromboembolism, is the priority.

4 This is contraindicated immediately after surgery.

864. 2 This position keeps the prosthesis firmly in place; adduction of the extremity could permit the prosthesis to rotate out of position. (2) (PB; CJ; IM)

1 Only partial weight bearing on the affected leg is indicated initially.

3 Flexion to this degree is contraindicated initially to avoid compromising the position of the prosthesis.

4 Full-weight bearing on the unaffected leg and partial weight bearing on the affected leg generally is permitted on the second or third postoperative day.

865. 4 Until the order is written to discontinue the abduction splint, it is only removed for mobility such as physical therapy and hygiene; adduction to or beyond the midline is not permitted for two to three months. (1) (PB; CJ; IM)

1 The splint is needed at this time unless the client can be trusted to maintain abduction; flexing the hip with a prosthesis cannot be beyond 60 degrees for up to 10 days; from then on it cannot be beyond 90 degrees for up to two to three months.

2 This splint helps to maintain position and keep the hip prosthesis in the hip socket.

3 This is inappropriate; this is not the criterion for discontinuing abduction of the affected extremity.

866. 4 **The pelvis is elevated by actions involving the unaffected upper extremities and unaffected leg. (2) (PB; CJ; IM)**
   1 This is not permitted because it causes adduction of the leg and can lead to dislocation of the femoral head.
   2 No pressure is permitted on the operative hip because it can cause dislocation of the femoral head.
   3 Lifting only with the arms requires strength; the use of both heels puts pressure on the operated hip.

867. 4 **These are common signs of a fat embolism. (2) (PB; CJ; AS)**
   1 Chest pain is not a common complaint with a fat embolism; fever may occur later.
   2 This sign occurs with thrombophlebitis; it is not an indication of a fat embolism.
   3 This would indicate neurologic dysfunction; it would not be an indication of a fat embolism.

868. 3 **At the time of a fracture or orthopedic surgery, fat globules may move from the bone marrow into the bloodstream; also, elevated catecholamines cause mobilization of fatty acids and the development of fat globules; in addition to obstructing vessels in the lung, brain, and kidneys with systemic embolization from fat globules, petechiae are noted in the buccal membranes, conjunctival sacs, hard palate, chest, and anterior axillary folds; these adaptations only occur with a fat embolism. (3) (PB; CJ; AS)**
   1 This is a sign of an embolus, but it is not specific to a fat embolus.
   2 Same as answer 1.
   4 Same as answer 1.

869. 3 **Excessive flexion of the hip can cause dislocation of the femoral head. (2) (PB; CJ; PL)**
   1 This should not cause undue strain on the operative site.
   2 This should be encouraged as long as no extremes of positions are used.
   4 This should be encouraged because it prevents hip-flexion contractures.

870. 3 **The client is demonstrating acceptance and is even looking toward the future. (1) (PI; CJ; EV)**
   1 This relates to situational low self-esteem, not body image disturbance.
   2 This response may indicate that the client is trying to lose weight and may not accept present body weight.

   4 While this may indicate adaptability, it is not related to body image.

871. 1 **Effective skeletal traction requires a continuous pull by the weights; the weights should be removed only in an emergency such as cardiac arrest or hospital evacuation. (2) (SE; CJ; IM)**
   2 Removal of the weights would displace the fracture and increase pain.
   3 This problem can be corrected without removing the weights.
   4 Same as answer 3.

DRUG-RELATED RESPONSES (DR)

872. 4 **First convert milligrams (mg) to micrograms (mcg) and then use ratio and proportion (0.2 mg = 200 mcg)**

$$\frac{200 \text{ mcg}}{100 \text{ mcg}} = \frac{x \text{ mL}}{1 \text{ mL}}$$
$$100 \, x = 200$$
$$x = 2 \text{ mL}$$

   (2) (PB; CJ; AN)
   1 This is an inaccurate calculation; this is less than the desired dose.
   2 Same as answer 1.
   3 Same as answer 1.

873. 4 **Total drops per minute divided by total time in minutes:**

$$\frac{50 \text{ mL} \times 60 \text{ gtt/mL}}{30 \text{ min}} = \frac{3000}{30} = 100 \text{ gtt/min}$$

   (3) (PB; CJ; AN)
   1 This is too little; the client would not receive the prescribed medication.
   2 Same as answer 1.
   3 Same as answer 1.

874. 4 **This is the correct flow rate; 500 mg of the drug added to 100 mL of IV fluid produces a solution in which 1 mL contains 5 mg of the drug; the required amount of the drug is contained in 0.3 mL of fluid; to calculate the dosage to be delivered, multiply the amount to be delivered (0.3 mL) by the drop factor (60) and divide the result by the amount of time in minutes (1). (2) (PB; CJ; AN)**
   1 This is too slow; this would not deliver the ordered amount of lidocaine HCl.
   2 Same as answer 1.
   3 Same as answer 1.

875. 3 Use ratio and proportion to calculate:

$$\frac{375 \text{ mg}}{225 \text{ mg}} = \frac{\text{x mL}}{1 \text{ mL}}$$

$$225 \text{ x} = 375$$

$$\text{x} = 1.68 \text{ or } 1.7 \text{ mL}$$

(3) (PB; CJ; AN)
1 This is too little; it would not provide enough drug.
2 Same as answer 1.
4 This is too much; it would provide an excess of drug.

876. 1 250 mg is equal to 0.25 g; therefore,

$$\frac{4 \text{ g}}{0.25 \text{ g}} = \frac{\text{x mL}}{1 \text{ mL}}$$

$$0.25 \text{ x} = 4$$

$$\text{x} = 16 \text{ mL}$$

(2) (PB; CJ; AN)
2 This is an inaccurate calculation; it is too little to provide the ordered amount.
3 Same as answer 2.
4 Same as answer 2.

877. 3 Use ratio and proportion:

$$250 \text{ mg} = 0.25 \text{ g}$$

$$\frac{0.25 \text{ g}}{1 \text{ g}} = \frac{\text{x mL}}{3 \text{ mL}}$$

$$\text{x} = 0.75 \text{ mL or } 0.8 \text{ mL}$$

(2) (PB; CJ; AN)
1 This is an incorrect calculation; too little medication will be administered.
2 Same as answer 1.
4 This is an incorrect calculation; too much medication will be administered.

878. 2 1000 mcg = 1 mg; 500 mg of the drug added to 500 mL of IV fluid results in a solution in which 1 mL contains 1 mg of the drug; the physician's order is for 1 mg/minute, therefore, multiply total solution (1 mL) times the drop factor (60) and divide by total time in minutes (1). **(2) (PT; CJ; AN)**
1 This is an incorrect calculation; this would deliver half the desired dose.
3 This is an incorrect calculation; this would deliver 50% more than the desired dose.
4 This is an incorrect calculation; this would deliver twice the desired dose.

879. 4 1 mg = 2.5 mL; therefore, 14 mg = 35 mL;

$$\frac{\text{Desired 14 mg}}{\text{Have 100 mg}} = \frac{\text{x mL}}{250 \text{ mL}}$$

$$100 \text{ x} = 3500$$

$$\text{x} = 35 \text{ mL}$$

(2) (PB; CJ; PL)
1 This would not deliver the desired dose of morphine.
2 Same as answer 1.
3 Same as answer 1.

880. 4 Morphine is a central nervous system depressant that decreases the respiratory rate, which can lead to respiratory arrest. **(1) (PB; CJ; EV)**
1 Morphine, an opiate, would cause constipation, not diarrhea.
2 Addiction is not a concern for a terminally ill client.
3 Waking the client may assess the degree of sedation, but it will not prevent the side effect of depressed respirations.

881. 1 The transfer of controlled substances from one authorized person to another must occur according to protocol; otherwise the controlled substance must be returned to the pharmacy and delivered at a later time. **(1) (SE; MR; IM)**
2 This individual does not have the authority to receive controlled substances.
3 The nurse cannot delay the securing of controlled substances; if time is not available when the medications are delivered, they must be returned to the pharmacy.
4 Same as answer 2.

882. 2 These signs as well as anemia, irritability, pruritus, and an enlarged spleen occur with vitamin A toxicity. **(3) (PB; CJ; AS)**
1 Excess thiamin is excreted in the urine and rarely, if ever, causes toxicity; excessive doses may elicit an allergic reaction in some individuals.
3 Excess vitamin C (ascorbic acid) does not cause these signs or toxicity; however, vitamin C may cause diarrhea or renal calculi.
4 Pyridoxine (vitamin B_6) is relatively nontoxic, and excess amounts are excreted in the urine.

883. 2 Organism mutation commonly results in drug resistance when treatment is inadequate. **(2) (PB; CJ; IM)**
1 Rifampin decreases tubercle bacillus' replication; pyridoxine (vitamin B_6) is used to prevent neuropathy associated with INH.

3 High concentrations of at least two antitubercular drugs are necessary for an extended period.

4 This may raise anxiety and may not be true; combination drug therapy is always used for tuberculosis.

884. 4 **Rifampin causes the body fluids, such as sweat, tears, and urine, to turn orange. (2) (PB; CJ; EV)**

1 Damage to the eighth cranial nerve is not a side effect of rifampin; it is a side effect of another drug, streptomycin sulfate, sometimes used to treat tuberculosis.

2 It is not necessary to drink large amounts of fluid with this drug; it is not nephrotoxic.

3 This is not a side effect of rifampin.

885. 4 **One of the most common side effects of INH is peripheral neuritis, and vitamin B$_6$ will counteract this problem. (2) (PB; CJ; AN)**

1 It does help nutrition, but that is not the specific reason it is given.

2 It counters the side effects of INH; it does not act to enhance its action.

3 It does not speed the destruction of the causative organism.

886. 1 **This medication causes hyperuricemia, leading to joint swelling and pain; fluids dilute the urine and help remove the uric acid. (2) (SE; MR; EV)**

2 This is not a side effect of this medication.

3 This medication causes GI irritation and should be taken with food.

4 This is a side effect of rifampin (Rifadin), not pyrazinamide.

887. 1 **Antitubercular drugs such as isoniazid (INH), rifampin (Rifadin), and para-aminosalicylic acid (PAS) are hepatotoxic. (3) (PB; CJ; AS)**

2 These are not related to the administration of antitubercular drugs or to their side effects.

3 Same as answer 2.

4 The white blood cell count is expected to be higher in the presence of infection, but with AIDS the WBC count will be less than 2500/cm^3 and helper T cells will be about 400/mm^3; the T4/T8 ratio will be 1:2; these tests will not provide information relative to starting antitubercular therapy or to its side effects.

888. 4 **Pentamidine can cause either hypoglycemia or hyperglycemia even after therapy is discontinued, and therefore blood glucose levels should be monitored. (3) (PB; CJ; PL)**

1 Pentamidine should be mixed with injectable sterile water or 5% dextrose injection and then further diluted before IV administration.

2 Clients should be monitored closely for sudden, severe hypotension; clients should lie flat when receiving the drug.

3 This is too quick; the drug should be given over at least 60 minutes.

889. 4 **This drug relaxes the respiratory muscles; it inhibits transmission of nerve impulses by binding with cholinergic receptor sites and antagonizing the action of acetylcholine; the client will die without mechanical ventilation. (2) (PB; CJ; IM)**

1 This is not the priority.

2 Same as answer 1.

3 Same as answer 1.

890. 3 **Humulin R insulin is the only insulin that acts rapidly and is compatible with intravenous solutions. (1) (PB; CJ; AN)**

1 This insulin is not compatible with intravenous solutions; it is an intermediate-acting insulin.

2 Ultralente insulin is not compatible with intravenous solutions; it is a long-acting insulin.

4 Same as answer 1.

891. 1 **Oral hypoglycemics stimulate endogenous insulin production by the beta cells of the pancreas. (1) (PB; CJ; IM)**

2 This occurs when serum glucose drops below normal levels.

3 This occurs in the presence of insulin and potassium.

4 Beta cells must have some function to enable this drug to be effective.

892. 4 **Oral hypoglycemic agents decrease serum glucose levels. (1) (PB; MR; IM)**

1 This occurs with type 1 diabetes.

2 Weight gain is usually present in type 2 diabetes.

3 Same as answer 1.

893. 2 **Humulin N insulin's onset of action is 1 to 2 hours, peak action is 8 to 12 hours, and duration of action is 18 to 24 hours; if hypoglycemia were to occur, it would happen between 4 PM and 8 PM. (1) (PB; MR; EV)**

1 Semilente insulin peaks in 4 to 7 hours.

3 No insulin peaks in 12 to 14 hours; however, protamine zinc insulin and Ultralente insulin peak in 16 to 18 hours.

4 Humulin R insulin peaks in 2 to 4 hours.

894. 1 These are the most commonly reported signs of hypoglycemia and are related to increased sympathetic nervous system activity. (2) (SE; MR; EV)
  2 These are signs of hyperglycemia.
  3 Same as answer 2.
  4 Same as answer 2.

895. 3 The chemical structure of insulin is altered by gastric secretions, rendering it ineffective. (2) (PB; CJ; IM)
  1 There is no such thing as oral insulin; this comment about the seriousness of the diabetic condition could raise anxiety.
  2 There are no data to support this statement, and insulin is given parenterally, not orally.
  4 Insulin is not absorbed but is destroyed by gastric secretions; there is no po insulin.

896. 2 This drug does not interfere with thyroxine already stored in the gland; symptoms remain until the hormone is depleted. (3) (PB; MR; PL)
  1 Duration of therapy varies depending on the severity of the disease and the client's response to therapy.
  3 This drug is not irritating to mucosal tissue, and no special precautions are necessary.
  4 Absorption is not affected by the presence of food in the stomach.

897. 2 Tapazole blocks thyroid hormone synthesis; the hormone stored in the thyroid gland must be reduced before improvement is seen. (2) (PB; CJ; IM)
  1 There are many common side effects that include nausea, vomiting, diarrhea, rash, urticaria, pruritus, alopecia, hyperpigmentation, drowsiness, headache, vertigo, and fever.
  3 Tapazole should be spaced at regular intervals because blood levels are reduced in approximately eight hours.
  4 Large doses cause toxic side effects that can be life threatening, including nephritis, hepatitis, agranulocytosis, leukopenia, thrombocytopenia, hypothrombinemia, and lymphadenopathy.

898. 2 Ringing in the ears, which interferes with hearing, because of its effect on the eighth cranial nerve, is a classic symptom of aspirin toxicity. (1) (PB; CJ; EV)
  1 This is not a side effect of aspirin; ASA promotes comfort, which may permit rest.
  3 Aspirin may cause diarrhea, nausea, and vomiting.
  4 This is not a side effect of salicylates such as aspirin.

899. 3 This helps to decrease gastric irritation by diluting the acidic substances in the stomach. (2) (PB; CJ; IM)
  1 If aspirin is taken on an empty stomach, gastric irritation is increased.
  2 Although this would limit gastric irritation, it would decrease the effect of aspirin by increasing its renal excretion.
  4 Corticosteroids add to the gastric-irritating and the ulcerogenic effect of aspirin; they should not be taken together.

900. 3 Acetaminophen lacks the antiinflammatory action needed to limit joint inflammation associated with arthritis. (1) (PB; MR; AN)
  1 People with arthritis do not need anticoagulants unless prescribed for a concomitant cardiovascular problem or cardiovascular prophylaxis.
  2 Although they are both analgesics, acetaminophen is not an antiinflammatory agent.
  4 There are fewer side effects with acetaminophen than with aspirin.

901. 4 Dalteparin (Fragmin), a low–molecular-weight heparin, prevents the conversion of fibrin to prothrombin and prothrombin to thrombin by enhancing the inhibitory effects of antithrombin III. (2) (PB; CJ; AN)
  1 Fragmin is not an antipyretic.
  2 Fragmin is not an analgesic.
  3 Fragmin is not an antiinflammatory drug.

902. 2 This is necessary because ibuprofen is nephrotoxic and hepatotoxic and prolongs the bleeding time. (2) (PB; MR; EV)
  1 This is important for all clients with arthritis; it is not related to ibuprofen.
  3 Ibuprofen does not cause postural hypotension.
  4 Ibuprofen causes epigastric distress and occult bleeding; it should be taken with meals or milk to reduce these adverse reactions.

903. 3 Pain is most effectively relieved when the analgesic is administered at the onset of pain, before it becomes intense; this prevents a pain cycle from occurring. (1) (PB; CJ; PL)
  1 Analgesics are least effective when administered as pain is at its peak.
  2 This may or may not be necessary; the medication should be taken when the client begins to feel uncomfortable within the parameters specified by the physician's order.
  4 Same as answer 1.

904. 3 These drugs tend to irritate the gastric mucosa and should be taken with food or milk. (2) (PB; MR; EV)

1 This is an expected side effect; safety precautions are indicated, but the drug should not be discontinued.

2 These drugs should be taken with food or milk to limit GI irritation.

4 This could result in toxicity; the dosage should be prescribed by the physician.

905. 3 This provides for the quickest use of the opioid, so that relief of pain can occur immediately. (3) (PB; CJ; PL)

1 Nausea, vomiting, and paralytic ileus may occur postburn, making oral medication impractical.

2 This route does not provide uniform absorption; also, relief of pain would be delayed.

4 The medication may be sequestered in the tissues and, with fluid shifts, it takes time for the medication to take effect.

906. 2 Anabolic agents are synthetic androgenic steroids, which may produce masculinizing effects in women. (3) (PB; CJ; EV)

1 With an increase in muscle mass and stimulation of erythropoiesis, the client should have an increase in energy.

3 The client may become hypernatremic, not hyponatremic; the client may become hypercalcemic as well.

4 This drug will not cause hyperglycemia; it may cause hypoglycemia in clients with diabetes mellitus.

907. 1 Sulfamylon is effective against a wide variety of gram-positive and gram-negative organisms including anaerobes. (1) (SE; CJ; AN)

2 This is an antimicrobial, not an analgesic; topical application causes pain.

3 It promotes healing and decreases the need for grafting.

4 This medication is an antimicrobial; it does not provide chemical débridement.

908. 1 Silvadene is effective against gram-positive, gram-negative, and fungal organisms; however, it causes agranulocytosis, a serious side effect. (2) (PB; CJ; AN)

2 Sulfamylon is effective against gram-negative and gram-positive organisms, but not fungi; it has serious side effects such as acidosis.

3 Silver nitrate dressings must be kept moist; if they are allowed to dry, silver salts would precipitate into the wound, causing irritation.

4 Neomycin has extremely serious side effects; it is ototoxic, which can cause hearing loss, and it is nephrotoxic, which can cause kidney failure.

909. 1 Aspirin (ASA) is given to this client to prevent platelet aggregation and possible thrombosis and should be given on schedule. (2) (PB; MR; IM)

2 The ASA is not being given for comfort and should not be withheld.

3 The ASA is not being given for comfort, and this should not be implied to the client.

4 Same as answer 3.

910. 3 Sorbitrate dilates the coronary vasculature, improving the supply of oxygen to the hypoxic myocardium. (2) (PB; CJ; IM)

1 This is the action of anticoagulants.

2 This is the action of antidysrhythmics.

4 This is the action of cardiac glycosides.

911. 4 Atenolol (Tenormin) competitively blocks stimulation of β-adrenergic receptors within vascular smooth muscles, which lowers the blood pressure. (2) (PB; MR; PL)

1 This drug does not cause headaches; this drug may be used to relieve vascular headaches.

2 This drug may cause bradycardia, not tachycardia.

3 This drug may cause diarrhea, not constipation.

912. 4 Lasix may cause hypovolemia, which can result in orthostatic hypotension with sudden position changes. (1) (SE; MR; EV)

1 Lasix does not cause photophobia.

2 This has no relationship to Lasix.

3 Citrus fruits, particularly oranges, are high in potassium and should be encouraged when the client is taking Lasix because this medication can cause hypokalemia.

913. 3 Lasix enhances the excretion of potassium, producing symptoms of hypokalemia, such as hyporeflexia. (3) (PB; CJ; EV)

1 This is not a side effect of Lasix.

2 Same as answer 1.

4 Same as answer 1.

914. 4 This drug decreases blood pressure by both of these mechanisms and is used for immediate reduction of blood pressure. (2) (PB; CJ; AN)

1 This drug may increase the heart rate as a response to vasodilation.

2 It decreases cardiac workload by decreasing preload and afterload.

3 It decreases peripheral resistance by dilating peripheral blood vessels.

915. 1 Pruritus is a common side effect of clonidine HCl (Catapres). (3) (PB; MR; EV)

2 This drug causes constipation, not diarrhea.

3 This drug may cause depression, anxiety, fatigue, and drowsiness, not euphoria.

4 This is not a side effect of this medication; photosensitivity occurs with chlorpromazine.

916. 2 Inderal and Lanoxin both exert a negative chronotropic effect resulting in a decreased heart rate. (2) (PB; CJ; AN)

1 Inderal reduces headaches associated with hypertension.

3 These drugs may cause hypotension.

4 These drugs may depress nodal conduction.

917. 4 This is a sign of toxicity. (1) (PB; CJ; EV)

1 Anuria is not caused by toxicity; an increased urinary output is expected with digoxin therapy as cardiac output improves.

2 Constipation is not a sign of toxicity; gastrointestinal signs of toxicity include nausea, vomiting, and diarrhea.

3 Hypokalemia can enhance the effects of digoxin but it is not a sign of toxicity.

918. 1 Coumadin inhibits vitamin K; therefore vitamin K is the antidote for Coumadin. (2) (PB; CJ; PL)

2 This is a blood-clotting factor, not the antidote for Coumadin.

3 Same as answer 2.

4 This is the antidote for heparin.

919. 4 This is the site of action of Lasix. (3) (PB; CJ; AN)

1 Thiazides act here.

2 Potassium-sparing diuretics act here.

3 Plasma expanders and xanthines act here.

920. 4 A cardiac glycoside such as digitalis decreases the conduction speed within the myocardium and slows the heart rate. (2) (PB; CJ; EV)

1 The primary effect of a diuretic is on the kidneys, not the heart; it may reduce the blood pressure, not the heart rate.

2 A vasodilator could cause tachycardia, not bradycardia, which is an adverse effect.

3 This does not drastically reduce the heart rate.

921. 4 "Yellow vision" indicates digitalis toxicity; the medication should be withheld until the physician can assess the client and the digoxin blood level is assessed. (1) (PB; LE; EV)

1 This symptom is related to digoxin.

2 Taking this medication would escalate the digitalis toxicity.

3 This is a sign of toxicity; the medication should be stopped and the physician notified.

922. 4 The most common adverse effect of a tissue plasminogen activator is bleeding because of the thrombolytic action of the drug. (3) (PB; CJ; PL)

1 Although this is important for any client with a decreased cardiac output, it is not specific to the administration of a tissue plasminogen activator.

2 Same as answer 1.

3 Same as answer 1.

923. 4 The major action of intravenous nitroglycerin is venous and then arterial dilation, leading to a decrease in blood pressure. (2) (PB; CJ; EV)

1 This is not a common side effect of intravenous nitroglycerin.

2 This is an infrequent effect when nitroglycerin is given intravenously.

3 Reflex tachycardia may occur with the decrease in blood pressure.

924. 2 Breaking up the tablet increases the surface area of the tablet, which permits it to dissolve faster. (2) (PB; MR; IM)

1 This may slow absorption because the tablet may move away from the absorption site.

3 If taken with water, the tablet is washed away from the site of absorption or may even be swallowed.

4 This would slow absorption because saliva helps to dissolve the tablet.

925. 3 For severe myocardial infarction (MI) morphine sulfate is the drug of choice because it relieves pain quickly and reduces anxiety. (1) (PB; CJ; PL)

1 Alprazolam (Xanax) is an anxiolytic that may be used for its calming effect, but it will not relieve the pain of an MI.

2 Midazolam (Versed) is a sedative/hypnotic that may be used for its calming effect, but it will not relieve the pain of an MI.

4 Gabapentin (Neurontin) is an anticonvulsant and is not the drug of choice to relieve the pain associated with an MI.

926. 4 This response indicates that the client understood the nurse's teaching because taking a nitroglycerin tablet before such an activity is prophylactic use. (2) (SE; MR; EV)

1 This is an example of scheduled administration, not prophylactic use.

2 This indicates avoidance of activity rather than taking medication to prevent angina during the activity.

3 Blood pressure, not pulse, is the parameter most affected by nitroglycerin.

927. 2 The speed of conduction is decreased when digoxin is given, and this can result in premature beats, atrial fibrillation, and first-degree heart block. (1) (PB; CJ; EV)

1 Digoxin does not deplete potassium and therefore orange juice does not need to be given; the orange juice is high in calories and would need to be calculated in the diet.

3 Insulin and digoxin can be given at the same time.

4 The purpose of the drug is to reduce a rapid heart rate.

928. 4 This medication suppresses ventricular activity; therefore, it is used for treatment of PVCs. (3) (PB; CJ; PL)

1 This is used to block vagal stimulation; it increases the heart rate and is used for bradycardia, not PVCs.

2 This increases myocardial contractility and heart rate; therefore it is contraindicated in the treatment of PVCs.

3 This raises the serum pH level; therefore it combats metabolic acidosis.

929. 1 Lidocaine will interrupt the VT before it progresses to ventricular fibrillation. (3) (PB; MR; PL)

2 Epinephrine is not used for VT; it is used for cardiac arrest and may even precipitate ventricular fibrillation.

3 A pacemaker is used for supraventricular tachycardia and bradycardia.

4 CPR is used for cardiac arrest, not VT.

930. 2 A decreased heart rate or sinus bradycardia is the normal response to a beta blocker. (3) (PB; CJ; EV)

1 Anxiety is not related to beta-blocker therapy.

3 Nausea and vomiting may occur as side effects but would not indicate the effectiveness of the medication.

4 Ventricular fibrillation during an electrophysiology study would indicate that the beta blocker was not working effectively.

931. 1 Tremors are a precursor to the major adverse effect of seizures. (3) (PB; MR; EV)

2 Although this can occur, it is not a serious side effect.

3 Bradycardia, which can lead to heart block, occurs, not tachycardia.

4 Hypotension, not hypertension, occurs.

932. 4 Lasix promotes potassium excretion; hypokalemia increases cardiac excitability; digitalis in the presence of low extracellular potassium produces ectopic pacemaker activity. (1) (PB; CJ; AN)

1 Digitalis does not affect potassium excretion; Lasix causes potassium excretion.

2 Lasix causes diuresis and consequent potassium loss regardless of the serum potassium level.

3 Potassium is excreted by the kidneys, not destroyed by the liver.

933. 4 Generalized weakness is a sign of significant hypokalemia, which may be a sequela of diuretic therapy. (1) (PB; MR; EV)

1 Insomnia is not known to be related to hypokalemia or Esidrix therapy.

2 Although this is unrelated to hydrochlorothiazide therapy, it can occur with other antihypertensive drugs.

3 Increased thirst is associated with hypernatremia; because this drug increases excretion of water and sodium in addition to potassium and chloride, hyponatremia, not hypernatremia, may occur.

934. 3 This counteracts the acidosis that occurs secondary to tissue anoxia that accompanies cardiac standstill. (3) (PB; CJ; PL)

1 This medication relaxes smooth muscle of the bronchial airways and pulmonary blood vessels, which is not indicated in this instance.

2 This is a diuretic commonly used for heart failure.

4 This medication is used after resuscitation to counteract seizures if they occur.

935. 4 This medication is contraindicated for an unconscious and neurologically damaged client because it depresses respirations. (3) (PB; LE; AN)

1 This osmotic diuretic is used to reduce increased intracranial pressure.

2 This corticosteroid, antiinflammatory agent, is used to help reduce increased intracranial pressure.

3 This can be given safely to a neurologically damaged client for restlessness.

936. 3 This allows for maximum effectiveness of the preanesthetic medication. (2) (PB; CJ; PL)
1 This is too long a time for maximum effectiveness of the medication.
2 This does not permit sufficient time for maximum effectiveness of the medication.
4 Same as answer 2.

937. 1 This may indicate infection, which must be treated immediately since chemotherapy may lead to pancytopenia and immunosuppression; stomatitis is common with chemotherapy and should be brought to the physician's attention because a swish and swallow anesthetic solution can be ordered to make the client more comfortable. (1) (PB; MR; IM)
2 This low-grade fever does not require immediate medical attention.
3 This is expected and is not a cause for concern unless dehydration results.
4 This is expected but should be reported if it lasts more than 24 hours.

938. 4 Muscle weakness, tingling, and numbness are related to drugs like Oncovin; neuropathies are usually transient if the drug is stopped or reduced. (3) (PB; MR; AN)
1 The client complains of bilateral neuropathy; nodal enlargement would produce vascular rather than neural side effects.
2 This is untrue; neuropathies are a potential side effect of chemotherapy.
3 Tingling and numbness are characteristic of neuropathy, not vascular occlusion.

939. 3 Aspirin has an antiinflammatory action that relieves the inflammation and pain associated with arthritis. (2) (PB; MR; AN)
1 Although both are analgesics, acetaminophen does not have an antiinflammatory action.
2 Acetaminophen does not cause gastritis; this is an effect of aspirin.
4 Although true, this drug does not have the antiinflammatory properties of aspirin.

940. 1 Stomatitis and hyperuricemia are possible complications of therapy; therefore, oral care and hydration are important. (1) (PB; CJ; PL)
2 Abnormal bleeding is a common problem and thus injections are contraindicated; rest is important for increased fatigability.
3 Hot substances are avoided because of the common occurrence of stomatitis.
4 This may be false reassurance; although it accounts for one-fourth of all leukemias in adults it accounts for 85% of acute leukemias with serious bleeding tendencies and infections.

941. 2 Antineoplastic drugs depress bone marrow, which causes leukopenia; the client must be protected from infection, which could be life threatening. (2) (PB; CJ; EV)
1 RBCs diminish slowly and can be replaced with a transfusion of packed cells.
3 These decrease as rapidly as WBCs, but complications can be limited with infusions of platelets.
4 Same as answer 1.

942. 2 Chemotherapy destroys normal erythrocytes, white blood cells, and platelets indiscriminately along with the neoplastic cells because these are all rapidly dividing cells and are most vulnerable to the effects of chemotherapy. (1) (PB; CJ; AN)
1 This is not a true description of the side effects of steroids.
3 This is not the cause for fewer erythrocytes, white blood cells, and platelets.
4 Although true, this does not explain pancytopenia.

943. 4 Alkylating drugs often cause severe bone marrow depression because they affect rapidly dividing cells. (3) (PB; CJ; EV)
1 These are complications that are more common with antimetabolites.
2 These are complications associated with hormonal therapy.
3 These are common side effects with the administration of steroids.

944. 4 Plasma levels will indicate whether therapeutic or toxic levels are present. (3) (PB; CJ; IM)
1 Methotrexate will crystallize in the kidneys if urine becomes acidic.
2 The regimen should include hydration with a minimum of intravenous fluids of 125 mL/hr 6 to 12 hours before and during therapy.
3 The effectiveness of methotrexate, a folic acid antagonist, will be minimized by a diet high in folic acid.

945. 2 Aspirin is contraindicated in the presence of bleeding tendencies, which often occur with ALL because of aspirin's inhibitory effect on platelet aggregation. (2) (SE; MR; IM)
1 An antacid will reduce the gastric irritation common with aspirin but will not alter its effect on platelets.
3 The dosage is within acceptable limits.
4 Action needs to be taken before the temperature is 102° F.

946. 2 Lack of thrombocytes, a factor in blood clotting, causes decreased coagulation of blood. (2) (PB; CJ; EV)

1 Petechiae are tiny hemorrhages, not a sign of nerve trauma.

3 The B cell, a lymphocyte and type of leukocyte, is involved in plasma cell production but leukocytosis is not the cause of the bleeding.

4 Increased blood volume and hypertension are not the cause of bleeding.

947. 4 **Contact with semen of a client taking Proscar can adversely effect a developing male fetus. (3) (PB; CJ; IM)**

1 Finasteride helps prevent male pattern baldness.

2 Results may take 6 to 12 months.

3 This medication can mask the occurrence of prostatic cancer because it decreases the prostatic specific antigen (PSA).

948. 2 **Leucovorin calcium limits toxicity of folic acid antagonists, such as methotrexate sodium, by competing for transport into cells. (3) (PB; CJ; AN)**

1 This is not the action of leucovorin calcium.

3 This is the purpose of antiemetics such as prochlorperazine maleate (Compazine) and ondansetron (Zofran).

4 Leucovorin calcium does not interfere with cell division; this is the purpose of a multiple drug protocol.

949. 4 **THC acts as an antiemetic in some persons and can be absorbed through the gastrointestinal tract or inhaled. (2) (PB; MR; IM)**

1 This does not answer the client's question; also, court permission is not necessary when THC is prescribed.

2 Marijuana is not injected.

3 Marijuana is an effective antiemetic for some clients.

950. 1 **This helps flush the kidneys and prevent nephrotoxicity, especially during the early phase of treatment. (3) (SE; CJ; EV)**

2 Reconstituted solution can be stored in the refrigerator for one month.

3 Confusion, dizziness, and hallucinations are side effects of this drug; the client should avoid hazardous tasks, such as driving or using machinery.

4 Activity may have to be altered because fatigue and other flulike symptoms are common with this drug.

951. 1 **Peripheral paresthesia is an indication of toxicity from a plant alkaloid such as vincristine (Oncovin). (2) (PB; CJ; EV)**

2 This is not a side effect of any of the drugs listed.

3 Same as answer 2.

4 Same as answer 2.

952. 2 **These devices are more accurate because they are easy to use and have improved adherence to insulin regimens by young people because the medication can be administered discreetly. (2) (PB; MR; IM)**

1 One disadvantage of pen-like insulin delivery systems is the longer injection time needed in the tissue to release the medication.

3 Pain and discomfort is decreased because of the use of a larger gauge needle that has a smaller diameter.

4 The insulin cartridges are single use and disposable.

953. 2 **The pancreatic enzymes (amylase, trypsin, and lipase) must be present when food is ingested for digestion to take place. (2) (SE; MR; EV)**

1 At this time the food eaten for dinner has already passed beyond the duodenum; the enzyme would be given too late to aid in digestion.

3 The client would have no chyme in the duodenum for the enzyme to act on.

4 Same as answer 3.

954. 3 **Cisplatin is nephrotoxic and can cause kidney damage unless the client is adequately hydrated to flush the kidneys. (3) (PB; CJ; PL)**

1 This medication, a form of folic acid, is used to combat toxic effects of methotrexate; cisplatin does not interfere with folic acid metabolism.

2 Gentle, not vigorous, oral care is needed to cleanse the mouth without further aggravating the expected stomatitis.

4 This is unnecessary; prolonged gastrointestinal irritation is not the major concern; nausea and vomiting last about 24 hours, and while diarrhea may occur and last longer, it is not the major concern.

955. 3 **Morphine sulfate should be avoided because it causes spasms at the sphincter of Oddi, thereby increasing pain. (3) (SE; MR; IM)**

1 Ranitidine (Zantac) would be useful in reducing gastric acid stimulation of pancreatic enzymes.

2 Cimetidine (Tagamet) is useful in reducing gastric acid stimulation of pancreatic enzymes.

4 Promethazine HCl (Phenergan) is useful as an antiemetic for clients with pancreatitis.

956. 3 It is necessary to clarify the route of administration because Zantac can be given po, IV, or
IM. (2) (SE; MR; IM)
  1 This is the usual dose of ranitidine when
    given twice a day.
  2 Ranitidine is used to decrease gastric acid
    and is helpful for clients with peptic ulcer.
  4 Ranitidine is usually given with meals.

957. 3 Prednisone inhibits phagocytosis and suppresses
other clinical phenomena of inflammation; this
is a symptomatic treatment that is not curative.
(1) (PB; CJ; IM)
  1 The drug suppresses the immune response
    and increases the potential for infection.
  2 The appetite is increased; weight gain may
    result from this or from fluid retention.
  4 Generally, the response is rapid.

958. 3 The GI tract contains numerous bacteria;
antibiotics are given to decrease the number of
microorganisms in the bowel before surgery. (1)
(SE; CJ; IM)
  1 This is a potential complication prevented
    by the use of sterile technique when chang-
    ing the dressing.
  2 This is a potential complication prevented by
    coughing, deep breathing, and ambulation.
  4 This is a potential complication prevented
    by hygiene, meatal care, and adequate
    hydration.

959. 2 Oral corticosteroids should be taken with food
or antacids to prevent gastric irritation and
gastric hemorrhage. (3) (PB; MR; EV)
  1 This is necessary because long-term admin-
    istration of steroids leads to elevated blood
    glucose levels and possible steroid-caused
    diabetes.
  3 Usually a larger dose is given at 8 AM and the
    second dose is given prior to 4 PM to mimic
    the normal hormonal secretion and prevent
    insomnia.
  4 Neurologic and emotional side effects
    include euphoria, mood swings, sleepless-
    ness, and excitement.

960. 4 Neomycin reduces bacterial activity on blood
and wastes in the GI tract, thereby reducing the
level of blood ammonia, a by-product of protein
metabolism; hepatic encephalopathy is a result
of elevated ammonia levels in the blood. (2)
(PB; CJ; AN)
  1 Neomycin interferes with bacterial protein
    synthesis but has little or no effect on intes-
    tinal edema.

  2 Neomycin reduces bacterial action in the
    GI tract but does not reduce abdominal
    distention.
  3 Neomycin is a nonabsorbable intestinal
    tract antibiotic, not a systemic antibiotic.

961. 2 Propylthiouracil may lower the white blood cell
count making the client prone to infection. (2)
(PB; MR; EV)
  1 Propylthiouracil does not cause hypocal-
    cemia; milk does not facilitate absorption of
    the drug.
  3 This would be necessary with iodine prepa-
    rations to prevent staining of the teeth;
    propylthiouracil does not contain iodine.
  4 Propylthiouracil does not cause photo-
    sensitivity.

962. 4 Hormone replacement should stabilize the
metabolic rate and should not interfere with the
client becoming pregnant. (3) (PM; MR; IM)
  1 This may elicit feelings but does not answer
    the client's question.
  2 This ignores the client's request for informa-
    tion and abdicates the nurse's teaching
    responsibility.
  3 If thyroid function remains controlled,
    there is no reason why the client should not
    become pregnant.

963. 4 This detergent action of Colace promotes the
addition of fluid into stool to soften feces. (2)
(PB; CJ; AN)
  1 This is the action of lubricant laxatives such
    as mineral oil.
  2 This is the action of saline laxatives such as
    milk of magnesia.
  3 This is the action of peristaltic stimulants
    such as cascara and castor oil.

964. 4 Dulcolax stimulates nerve endings in the intestinal wall or the intestinal mucosa precipitating
a bowel movement. (2) (PB; CJ; AN)
  1 Dulcolax is not a stool softener; stool sof-
    teners, such as docusate sodium (Colace),
    permit fat and water to penetrate feces
    which softens and delays the drying of the
    feces.
  2 Dulcolax is not a bulk cathartic; bulk-form-
    ing laxatives, such as Metamucil, form soft,
    pliant bulk that promotes physiologic peri-
    stalsis.
  3 Dulcolax is not an emollient; emollient lax-
    atives, such as mineral oil, lubricate the
    feces and decrease absorption of water from
    the intestinal tract.

965. 3 Increased acidity caused by the stress occurring with burns and crushing injuries contributes to the formation of Curling's ulcer; Tagamet, a histamine H_2 antagonist, decreases the formation of gastric acid, and Maalox, an antacid, neutralizes it once it is formed. (1) (PB; CJ; IM)

1 These drugs do not decrease irritability of the bowel; their purpose is to decrease gastrointestinal acidity, not irritation.

2 This does not explain how these drugs work and why they are prescribed for this client.

4 Same as answer 2.

966. 2 Maalox can cause diarrhea and sometimes needs to be given alternately with another more constipating antacid. (2) (PB; CJ; EV)

1 Immobility causes constipation, not diarrhea.

3 Although diet can affect elimination, no data support this conclusion.

4 Esomeprazole (Nexium) may cause constipation, not diarrhea.

967. 3 This is a miotic that constricts the pupil, permitting fluid drainage, which reduces intraocular pressure. (2) (PB; CJ; PL)

1 This is a topical anesthetic; it will not reduce the increased intraocular pressure associated with glaucoma.

2 This is contraindicated because it dilates the pupil and paralyzes ciliary muscles.

4 This mydriatic is contraindicated because it dilates the pupil, obstructing drainage, which increases intraocular pressure.

968. 4 Parenterally administered Valium is a benzodiazepine that has muscle relaxant and anticonvulsant effects that help limit massive muscular spasm. (2) (PB; CJ; PL)

1 Atropine is not used for seizures; it is used for bradycardia resulting from vagal overstimulation but does not reverse bradycardia caused by metabolic changes such as acid-base imbalances or electrolyte imbalances.

2 Epinephrine does not limit seizures; it increases contractility of the heart.

3 Narcan does not limit seizures; it is an opioid antagonist and is used for morphine, meperidine, and methadone overdose.

969. 4 Because of the lethal toxicity of aspirin overdose, hypotensive crisis and cardiac irregularities can occur. (2) (PB; CJ; EV)

1 This is not the priority at this time.

2 The central nervous system is not involved at the reflex level at this time.

3 Central venous pressure readings are not indicated in this situation.

970. 2 Adequate dental hygiene is essential to control or prevent the common side effect of hypertrophy of gums. (1) (PB; MR; PL)

1 This medication should be taken with food or milk to decrease GI side effects.

3 A gradual dosage reduction is recommended; the physician should be consulted before the drug is discontinued or the dosage is adjusted.

4 These are unrelated to phenytoin therapy.

971. 2 Levodopa is a precursor of dopamine, a catecholamine neurotransmitter; it raises dopamine levels in the brain that are depleted in Parkinson's disease. (3) (PB; CJ; AN)

1 This is accomplished by anticholinergic drugs.

3 This would be ineffective because it is believed that the cells that produce dopamine have degenerated in Parkinson's disease.

4 This drug does not affect acetylcholine production.

972. 3 Abnormal involuntary movements (dyskinesias), such as muscle twitching, rapid eye blinking, facial grimacing, head bobbing, and an exaggerated protrusion of the tongue, are signs of toxicity probably resulting from the body's failure to readjust properly to the disappearance of dopamine. (3) (SE; MR; IM)

1 This is a side effect of therapy, not toxicity.

2 Same as answer 1.

4 This is unrelated to levodopa toxicity.

973. 3 This will reduce the nausea and vomiting that can be caused by this drug. (3) (PB; MR; IM)

1 This is contraindicated; vitamins may contain pyridoxine (vitamin B_6) that diminishes the effects of levodopa.

2 Moderate amounts of alcohol would antagonize the drug's effects; a rare, occasional drink would not be harmful.

4 Levodopa is an amino acid and may raise the blood urea nitrogen (BUN) levels; also some proteins contain pyridoxine, which increases peripheral metabolism of levodopa decreasing the amount crossing the brain barrier.

974. 1 This is a sign of an MAOI-induced hypertensive crisis and should be reported to the physician immediately. (3) (SE; MR; IM)

2 The opposite is true because increased amounts of dopamine react with supersensitive postsynaptic receptors.

3 This is unnecessary, but routine medical evaluations of the client should be scheduled.

4 This is unsafe; the recommended daily dose of the drug should not be exceeded.

975. 2 Corticosteroids, such as Decadron, have a hyperglycemic effect. (2) (PB; CJ; EV)

1 Corticosteroids are not known to precipitate cessation of gastrointestinal activity.

3 Corticosteroids would not increase bacterial growth in the lungs.

4 This is required when administering magnesium sulfate.

976. 4 Osmotic diuretics remove excessive cerebral spinal fluid (CSF), reducing intracranial pressure. (2) (PB; CJ; AN)

1 Osmotic diuretics raise, not lower, the blood pressure by increasing the fluid in the intravascular compartment.

2 Osmotic diuretics do not directly influence blood glucose levels.

3 Although this occurs when the vascular bed expands as CSF is removed, it is not the primary purpose for administering the medication.

977. 3 Mannitol, an osmotic diuretic, pulls fluid from the white cells of the brain to relieve cerebral edema. (3) (PB; CJ; AN)

1 Mannitol's diuretic action does not decrease the production of cerebrospinal fluid.

2 Mannitol does not affect brain metabolism; rest and lowered body temperature reduce brain metabolism.

4 This is the action of phenytoin sodium (Dilantin), not mannitol.

978. 4 This client adaptation may occur about 12 hours after mannitol administration. (3) (PB; CJ; EV)

1 Mannitol does not directly affect the respiratory status, although injudicious use can cause heart failure and eventually pulmonary edema; this is not an expected response.

2 Mannitol does not directly affect the heart, although injudicious use can cause electrolyte imbalances and eventually dysrhythmias and heart failure; this is not an expected response.

3 Same as answer 2.

979. 3 The osmotic diuretic mannitol is contraindicated in the presence of inadequate renal function or heart failure because it increases the intravascular volume that must be filtered and excreted by the kidneys. (3) (PB; CJ; EV)

1 This is not specific to mannitol, although vital signs would be monitored.

2 While loss of body fluid is expected with mannitol, a daily weight would be too infrequent to monitor for safe administration of this drug.

4 While level of consciousness would be monitored with a head injury, this is not specific to mannitol and q8h is too infrequent an assessment.

980. 3 Administration of an anticoagulant to a client who is bleeding would interfere with clotting and increase hemorrhage. (2) (SE; MR; IM)

1 Anticoagulants would not be used in this situation because they would increase bleeding; anticoagulants may be used with cerebral thrombosis.

2 Same as answer 1.

4 Although contraindicated, if given, it would increase signs and symptoms.

981. 2 This site should not be rubbed to avoid dispersion of the heparin around the site and subsequent bleeding into the area. (1) (SE; CJ; IM)

1 The drug should be injected deep into the subcutaneous tissue slowly, not quickly.

3 This is not a routine practice; the extra volume would not be advantageous.

4 This technique and the intramuscular route are not used with heparin; subcutaneous injection or intravenous administration is used.

982. 4 This drug binds with heparin sodium to form a physiologically inert complex; it corrects clotting deficits. (3) (PB; CJ; PL)

1 Vitamin K counteracts the effects of drugs like warfarin sodium (Coumadin).

2 This is an alternate name for heparin sodium.

3 This is an oral anticoagulant that interferes with the synthesis of prothrombin.

983. 1 Acetylsalicylic acid (aspirin) should be avoided because it interferes with platelet aggregation; acetaminophen (Tylenol) should be used instead. (2) (SE; MR; EV)

2 This causes venous pooling and could predispose the client to deep vein thrombosis.

3 Prothrombin times, not complete blood counts, need to be done periodically.

4 This is not necessary; this is done when clients have had cardiac problems such as rheumatic fever or cardiac surgery.

984. 2 **Aspirin interferes with platelet aggregation and will impede the formation of thrombi. (2) (SE; MR; EV)**

1 Although aspirin has antiinflammatory properties, one month after the surgery the edema has already subsided.

3 At this point, there should no longer be discomfort at the surgical site.

4 This is not an expected response after surgery, and it would indicate infection; a prescription for antibiotics would be more appropriate.

985. 4 **The peak response occurs one hour after administration and lasts up to eight hours; the response will influence dosage levels. (2) (PB; CJ; EV)**

1 This medication usually is administered before meals to promote mastication.

2 Mestinon should be administered on an empty stomach for better absorption.

3 There are no psychologic side effects associated with Mestinon.

986. 3 **Because this drug inhibits the destruction of acetylcholine, parasympathetic activity may be increased. (3) (PB; CJ; EV)**

1 Myasthenic crisis, like cholinergic crisis, is characterized by increasing muscle weakness.

2 Side effects continue as long as the drug is continued; the dosage may be adjusted or an anticholinergic given to limit the side effects.

4 Toxicity or cholinergic crisis is manifested by increased muscle weakness including muscles of respiration.

987. 4 **This approach promotes even therapeutic blood levels to maintain muscle strength. (2) (PB; MR; IM)**

1 Because of drug-related nausea and gastric irritation, the drug should be taken with crackers or milk.

2 Thirty minutes before meals is recommended for maximum chewing and swallowing function.

3 This is unsafe because it would not maintain constant therapeutic drug levels.

988. 4 **A positive response to the administration of Tensilon indicates myasthenic crisis, whereas an increase in the severity of symptoms indicates cholinergic crisis. (3) (PB; MR; PL)**

1 This is the treatment for cholinergic crisis.

2 This is the antidote for heparin.

3 This is an opioid antagonist.

989. 3 **Mestinon is a vital drug that must be taken on time; missed or late doses can result in severe respiratory and neuromuscular consequences or even death. (3) (PB; MR; EV)**

1 This is unnecessary because it is not a gastric irritant.

2 This is unnecessary because food does not impair absorption of the drug.

4 This is unnecessary.

990. 3 **Steroids decrease the body's immune response thus decreasing the production of antibodies that attack acetylcholine receptors at the neuromuscular junction. (2) (PB; CJ; AN)**

1 This is the action of anticholinergic medications.

2 This is not the action of immunosuppressives.

4 This is the rationale for plasmapheresis.

991. 3 **The drug should be taken as ordered, usually before meals, to limit dysphagia and possible aspiration. (1) (SE; MR; EV)**

1 This is not necessary; it may be kept at room temperature.

2 The drug should be taken with milk to prevent GI irritation; it is usually taken about 30 to 60 minutes before meals.

4 The action of the drug will begin within 30 minutes and start to peak in one hour.

992. 1 **A urinary output of at least 1500 mL daily should be maintained to prevent crystalluria. (1) (PB; MR; IM)**

2 Orange juice produces an alkaline ash, which results in an alkaline urine that supports the growth of bacteria.

3 Bactrim should be taken one hour before meals for maximum absorption.

4 A prescribed course of the medication must be completed to eliminate the infection, which can exist on a subclinical level after symptoms subside.

993. 4 **Oxacillin is a form of penicillin and should be given on an empty stomach; food delays absorption. (2) (SE; MR; EV)**

1 This is incorrect; food or milk delays absorption of this drug.

2 Same as answer 1.

3 This is not necessary; however, it is appropriate with sulfonamides.

994. 3 **Gentamicin can cause ototoxicity, resulting in vertigo, tinnitus, and hearing loss. (3) (PB; CJ; EV)**
  1 This is unlikely; the client has not been on prolonged bed rest.
  2 A liquid diet and IV therapy may cause weakness because of a low-calorie intake, but dizziness does not occur.
  4 This is unrelated; more than 24 hours have passed since an anesthetic was administered.

995. 1 **Because the drug was just administered, the blood level of the drug would be at its highest level. (2) (PB; MR; IM)**
  2 The result would reveal a drug blood level halfway between the peak and trough levels.
  3 This would be done for a trough level when the drug level would be at its lowest.
  4 This would produce inaccurate results; peak and trough levels are measured in relation to the time a drug is administered.

996. 4 **Aluminum hydroxide binds phosphorus in the intestines preventing its absorption, which decreases serum phosphorus. (3) (PB; MR; IM)**
  1 Aluminum hydroxide does not dissolve calculi in the urinary tract.
  2 Phosphorus is not absorbed in the stomach.
  3 Aluminum hydroxide does not promote the excretion of urinary phosphorus.

997. 3 **Tylenol ES is not coated or intended to be released slowly; crushing this medication will not cause a bolus of the medication to be administered to the client. (2) (PB; CJ; IM)**
  1 Crushing of "Slow-K" will cause a bolus of medication to be given at once rather than slowly.
  2 Crushing an "SR" medication will cause a bolus of medication to be administered at once rather than slowly as intended.

  4 Crushing of an "XL" medication will cause a bolus to be given; if crushing is necessary, another form of the medication should be requested of the physician.

998. 4 **Standard triple therapy includes a corticosteroid (Prednisone, Solu-Medrol), an antimetabolite (CellCept), and a calcineurin inhibitor (Prograf, Sandimmune). (3) (PB; MR; IM)**
  1 None of these drugs is used for immunosuppression.
  2 Only sirolimus (Rapamune) is an immunosuppressive; this drug suppresses lymphocytes and inhibits B cells from making antibodies.
  3 Methylprednisolone (Solu-Medrol) in large doses is the only drug in this option that is used to prevent kidney rejection.

999. 2 **Epogen stimulates red blood cell production, thereby elevating hematocrit levels. (3) (PB; CJ; EV)**
  1 An elevated liver panel may signify liver disease; it is not affected by Epogen.
  3 WBC counts are not affected by Epogen.
  4 Increased Kaposi's sarcoma lesions are a sign of AIDS progression and are not affected by Epogen.

1000. 4 **Neupogen, a granulocyte colony-stimulating factor, increases the production of neutrophils with little effect on the production of hematopoietic cells. (3) (PB; CJ; EV)**
  1 The production of these cells is not influenced by Neupogen.
  2 Same as answer 1.
  3 Same as answer 1.

Medical-Surgical Nursing Quiz 1

1. A client with rheumatoid arthritis calls the out-patient clinic to report that the pain lasts for two to three hours after exercise. The nurse's most appropriate initial response would be:
   1. "Stop all exercise for 24 hours."
   2. "Increase the number of repetitions of each exercise."
   3. "Limit progressive resistive exercises to three times a day."
   4. "Decrease the total times and number of repetitions of your exercises."

2. When preparing a client for a liver biopsy, the nurse should instruct the client to:
   1. Turn on the left side after the procedure
   2. Breathe normally throughout the procedure
   3. Hold the breath at the moment of the actual biopsy
   4. Bear down (Valsalva maneuver) during the insertion of the biopsy needle

3. A 40-year-old client visits a neurologist with complaints of blurred or double vision and muscular weakness. After multiple sclerosis is diagnosed the client, visibly upset, reports this diagnosis to a friend who is a nurse. The nurse could best respond:
   1. "Don't worry; early treatment often alleviates symptoms of the disease."
   2. "See another physician. I've heard of several treatments that aid recovery."
   3. "That must have really shocked you. Tell me what the physician told you about it."
   4. "You should see a psychiatrist who will help you cope with this overwhelming news."

4. The major nursing problem when caring for a client with hyperthyroidism would be:
   1. Providing an adequate diet
   2. Keeping the bed linen neat
   3. Modifying hospital routines
   4. Arranging for sufficient rest periods

5. The physician orders propylthiouracil for a client with hyperthyroidism. The nurse explains that this drug:
   1. Increases the uptake of iodine
   2. Causes atrophy of the thyroid gland
   3. Interferes with the synthesis of thyroid hormone
   4. Decreases the secretion of thyroid-stimulating hormone

6. A male client with the diagnosis of multiple myeloma is told that he has a poor prognosis. He and his wife have decided to travel, attend the theater, and go to sporting events. When preparing further teaching for this client, the nurse should take into consideration that:
   1. Travel will cause depletion of his already exhausted energy stores
   2. A positive mental attitude will decrease the effects of stress and improve his prognosis
   3. He is prone to develop infections when exposed to large crowds, which may shorten his life
   4. As long as he does not have an accident causing hemorrhage, his traveling will not affect his prognosis

7. A client who is suspected of having Cushing's syndrome is admitted to the hospital. The nurse should plan to monitor this client for:
   1. Hypokalemia
   2. Hypovolemia
   3. Hypocalcemia
   4. Hyponatremia

8. A person sustains burns of the arms from a barbecue accident in the park. A bystander emerges from the crowd and suggests to a nurse who has come to the person's assistance that butter be applied to the burns. An appropriate response by the nurse would be, "Thanks, but:
   1. We'll just wait for the ambulance."
   2. It is better to use some first aid cream."
   3. I'll just use a tablecloth as a blanket for now."
   4. We should apply ice. Could you go get me some?"

9. The nurse is assigned to a client who has had surgery. Nalbuphine (Nubain) has been ordered for pain. After administering this medication, which side effects/adverse reactions may the nurse expect to occur? Check all that apply.
   1. _____ Oliguria
   2. _____ Depression
   3. _____ Palpitations
   4. _____ Tachycardia
   5. _____ Constipation
   6. _____ Hypertension
   7. _____ Urinary retention

10. A client, who is complaining of severe midsternal pain, is brought to the emergency department. The nurse is aware that the drug of choice utilized to control the pain associated with myocardial infarction would be:
    1. Xanax
    2. Demerol
    3. Morphine
    4. Lidocaine

11. The nurse notes that two weeks after full-thickness burns, a client is losing two pounds of weight daily. The nurse's best action would be to adjust the client's diet by adding:
    1. Low-sodium milk
    2. High-protein drinks
    3. Fruit juices low in potassium
    4. 10% more calories in the form of fats

12. Prior to a total laryngectomy, an important aspect of preoperative nursing care includes:
    1. Having a speech therapist visit the client
    2. Adequate explanation of the nature of the surgery to be performed
    3. Basing instruction on those areas in which the client has questions
    4. Instruction in breathing exercises and/or equipment used postoperatively to prevent complications

13. A client has a tracheostomy tube attached to a tracheostomy collar for the delivery of humidified oxygen. The client will need suctioning primarily because the:
    1. Humidified oxygen is saturated with fluid
    2. Inner cannula of the tracheostomy tube irritates the mucosa
    3. Tracheostomy tube interferes with the ability to cough effectively
    4. Weaning process increases the amount of respiratory secretions

14. A client with ascites is to receive IV albumin to replace each liter of fluid removed via paracentesis. The albumin replacement is expected to decrease:
    1. Capillary perfusion and BP
    2. Ascites and the blood ammonia level
    3. Venous stasis and the blood urea nitrogen level
    4. Tissue fluid accumulation and the hematocrit level

15. A client arrives in the emergency department with multiple crushing wounds of the chest, abdomen, and legs. The assessments that assume the greatest priority are:
    1. Level of consciousness and pupil size
    2. Pain, respiratory rate, and blood pressure
    3. Abdominal contusions and other wounds
    4. Quality of respirations and presence of pulses

16. As the nurse assesses a client's kidney function after surgery, the components of urine will be monitored. Essential to this process is the knowledge that the healthy kidney filters a number of blood components and urine should not contain:
    1. Sodium
    2. Potassium
    3. Urea nitrogen
    4. Large proteins

17. A client with the tentative diagnosis of Hodgkin's disease asks how the physician will know that it is definitely this disease. The nurse explains that the diagnosis is definitively confirmed by:
    1. Bone scan
    2. Lymph node biopsy
    3. Computerized tomography (CT) scan
    4. Radioactive iodine (^{131}I) uptake studies

18. The diet regimen that would be appropriate for a client with a gastric ulcer would be:
    1. A mechanical soft diet
    2. A low-fat, high-protein liquid diet
    3. Hourly feedings of cream and milk
    4. Regular meals that can be tolerated

19. A client with diabetes who has been diagnosed as having peripheral vascular disease tells the nurse that before hospitalization, exercise resulted in severe cramplike pain in both legs. The nurse should include in the teaching plan specific measures the client can use to increase arterial blood flow to the extremities. These measures should include:
    1. Exercises that promote muscular activity
    2. Meticulous care of minor skin breakdown
    3. Elevation of legs above the level of the heart
    4. Daily cleansing of feet by soaking in hot water

20. A client with liver disease is receiving neomycin sulfate (Mycifradin) orally. The purpose of administration of this drug would be to:
    1. Increase urea digestive activity of enteric bacteria
    2. Suppress ammonia-forming bacteria in the intestinal tract
    3. Protect regenerative nodules in the liver from invading bacteria
    4. Prevent the onset of infection while immune mechanisms are deficient

21. Immediately before an abdominal paracentesis, the nurse should ask the client to void because a full bladder:
   1. Decreases the intraabdominal pressure
   2. Decreases the amount of fluid in the abdominal cavity
   3. Increases the danger of puncture during the procedure
   4. Increases the presence of urea in the intraabdominal fluid

22. The nurse should anticipate occasional but serious problems with hypoxia among post-operative clients. In response to a client's report of shortness of breath and chest pain, the nurse should be prepared to initially administer:
   1. Oxygen
   2. Morphine
   3. Sublingual nitroglycerin
   4. Endotracheal medications

23. Two days after a myocardial infarction, a client's temperature is elevated. This indicates:
   1. Pneumonia
   2. Tissue necrosis
   3. Possible infection
   4. Pulmonary infarction

24. The primary responsibility of the nurse when caring for a client with a chest tube attached to a three-chamber underwater seal drainage system would be to:
   1. Maintain the closed system
   2. Encourage deep breathing and coughing
   3. Maintain mechanical suction to the system
   4. Keep the client in the dorsal recumbent position

25. The nurse should teach clients with phosphate calculi that their diets may include:
   1. Pears
   2. Hamburgers
   3. Split pea soup
   4. Cheddar cheese

26. The physician discusses the need for an abdominoperineal resection and a colostomy with a male client. After the physician leaves, the client tells the nurse that he is pleased only minor surgery is necessary. The nurse recognizes that the client's reaction is an example of:
   1. Reflection
   2. Regression
   3. Repudiation
   4. Reconciliation

27. One week after an above-the-knee amputation, a client refuses to go to physical therapy and tells the nurse, "I'll never be a whole person again!" The nurse's best response would be:
   1. "Relax, you're still the same person you've always been."
   2. "You've lost a part of yourself. That must be very difficult for you."
   3. "You may feel that way, but I'm sure your family considers you a whole person."
   4. "You must go to physical therapy every day or you will develop muscle contractures."

28. A 67-year-old client is diagnosed as having a right-sided brain attack (cerebrovascular accident) and is admitted to the hospital. When preparing to care for this client, the nurse should plan to:
   1. Use a bed cradle to prevent dorsiflexion of the feet
   2. Apply elastic stockings to prevent flaccid leg muscles
   3. Do passive range-of-motion exercises to prevent muscle atrophy
   4. Use a hand roll and extend the left upper extremity on a pillow to prevent contractures

29. The nursing assistant assigned to the 7 AM shift has not been coming to work until 8 AM. Nursing care is delayed and assignments are started late. The most appropriate action by the nurse would be to:
   1. Discuss the issue with a friend from another unit
   2. Remind the nursing assistant of the expected start time
   3. Report the problem to the Human Resources Department
   4. Document the information and discuss it with the unit manager

30. A client is diagnosed as having type 2 diabetes, and the physician orders an oral hypoglycemic. The nurse should include in the teaching plan that people taking oral hypoglycemics:
   1. Should not work where food is readily accessible
   2. Are not as threatened by their disease as those taking insulin
   3. Need not be concerned about serious complications
   4. Consciously or unconsciously may tend to relax dietary rules

31. A client is to receive an IV antibiotic in 50 mL to be administered over 20 minutes. At what volume to be infused should the nurse set the infusion device?
   Answer: _____.

32. When discussing immunity with a client who has returned from living in a foreign country for 10 years, the nurse recalls that active immunity occurs when:
    1. Protein antigens are formed in the blood to fight invading antibodies
    2. Protein substances are formed by the body to destroy or neutralize antigens
    3. Blood antigens are aided by phagocytes in defending the body against pathogens
    4. Sensitized lymphocytes from an immune donor act as antibodies against invading pathogens

33. A client with inhalation anthrax has been admitted to the intensive care unit. The most important data that the nurse should gather are related to the client's:
    1. Mental state
    2. Hydration level
    3. Respiratory status
    4. Neurological symptoms

34. After surgery for a parotid tumor, the priority nursing intervention during the immediate postoperative period should be:
    1. Offering psychologic support
    2. Monitoring the client's fluid balance
    3. Keeping the respiratory passages patent
    4. Providing a pad and pencil for writing messages

35. The nurse would expect a client with jaundice to report the presence of:
    1. Pruritus
    2. Diarrhea
    3. Blurred vision
    4. Bleeding tendencies

36. During a teaching session about insulin injections, a client asks the nurse, "Why can't I take the insulin in pills instead of taking shots?" The nurse should respond:
    1. "Insulin cannot be manufactured in pill form."
    2. "Your doctor will order pills when you are ready."
    3. "Insulin is destroyed by gastric juices, rendering it ineffective."
    4. "The route of administration is decided on by the physician."

37. A 50-year-old client is admitted to the hospital with a suspected brain tumor. Based on the history of loss of equilibrium and coordination, the nurse suspects the tumor is located in the:
    1. Cerebellum
    2. Parietal lobe
    3. Basal ganglia
    4. Occipital lobe

38. The nurse checks for hypocalcemia by placing a blood pressure cuff on a client's arm and inflating it. After about three minutes the client develops carpopedal spasm. The nurse records this finding as a positive:
    1. Homans' sign
    2. Romberg's sign
    3. Chvostek's sign
    4. Trousseau's sign

39. A client is admitted for a coronary artery bypass graft. The client states that the physician said that pacemaker wires will be inserted during surgery as a precautionary measure. The nurse explains that the pacemaker is used to:
    1. Prevent a rapid heart rate
    2. Maintain a constant rhythm
    3. Provide access for defibrillation
    4. Manage an abnormally slow rate

40. A male client with a brain attack (cerebrovascular accident) has regained control of bowel movements but is still incontinent of urine. To help reestablish bladder control, the nurse should encourage the client to:
    1. Assume a standing position for voiding
    2. Void every four hours and attempt to hold urine between set times
    3. Attempt to void more frequently in the afternoon than in the morning
    4. Drink a minimum of 4000 mL of fluid equally divided among the hours while awake

41. A client is taken to the emergency department with a stab wound of the left thorax. The nurse should position the client:
    1. In the Trendelenburg position
    2. On the left side with the head elevated
    3. In a high-Fowler's position with the left side supported
    4. On the right side flat in bed with a pillow supporting the left arm

42. When assessing a client with a stab wound of the chest, the nurse should be concerned primarily with the:
    1. Degree and level of pain
    2. Quality and depth of respirations
    3. Amount of serosanguineous drainage
    4. Blood pressure and pupillary response

43. A 35-year-old male who sustained a closed head injury is being monitored for increased intracranial pressure. Arterial blood gases are obtained

and the results include a PCO_2 of 33 mm Hg. It is most important for the nurse to:
1. Encourage the client to slow his breathing rate
2. Auscultate the client's lungs and suction if indicated
3. Advise the physician that the client needs supplemental oxygen
4. Report the results and continue to monitor for signs of increasing intracranial pressure

44. A 42-year-old mentally challenged individual with the mental capacity of a 5-year-old is brought to the emergency department after an accident. The nurse can best assess the client's pain level by:
1. Asking the client's mother
2. Using Wong's "Pain Faces"
3. Marking on a scale of 0 to 10
4. Observing the client's body language

45. To promote independence in a debilitated, older male client with glaucoma who places great value on independence, the nurse should encourage the client to:
1. Prevent stressful events that can increase his symptoms
2. Be able to perform his own household chores and shopping
3. Learn to administer his prescribed eye medications correctly
4. Conserve his eyesight by not reading or watching television

46. A client undergoes removal of a pituitary tumor through a transsphenoidal approach. Postoperatively the nurse should plan to:
1. Provide oral hygiene, including brushing the teeth
2. Encourage the client to deep-breathe and cough frequently
3. Maintain the head of the bed at a 30-degree angle continuously

4. Continue giving nothing by mouth until the nasal packing is removed

47. During preoperative teaching before a transurethral prostatectomy, the nurse tells the client that after the surgery:
1. His urine will be bright red for at least 24 to 48 hours
2. He can expect spasms of the bladder during the first 24 to 48 hours
3. Oral fluids should be avoided because of continuous urinary irrigation
4. He should use the Valsalva maneuver to decrease bladder contractions

48. A 52-year-old engineer is admitted to the hospital with Laënnec's cirrhosis and chronic pancreatitis. Bile salts are ordered, and the client asks why they are needed. The nurse replies that they:
1. Stimulate prothrombin production
2. Promote bilirubin secretion in the urine
3. Aid absorption of vitamins A, D, E, and K
4. Stimulate contraction of the common bile duct

49. Clients are encouraged to perform deep breathing exercises after surgery. The reason for this is that deep breathing exercises help to:
1. Increase blood volume
2. Expand the residual volume
3. Counteract respiratory acidosis
4. Decrease partial pressure of oxygen

50. An older client is hard of hearing and has severe painful rheumatoid arthritis. The client is admitted to a nursing home after becoming incontinent of urine. The primary consideration in the care of this client would be the need for:
1. Control of pain
2. Immobilization of joints
3. Motivation and teaching
4. Bladder control reeducation

Medical-Surgical Nursing Quiz 1
Answers and Rationales

1. 4 **Exercise should be to tolerance only; limiting the amount of exercise should decrease pain. (3) (PB; MR; IM; SK)**
1 This would increase stiffness.
2 Exercises should be decreased, not increased.
3 Resistive exercises usually are not part of the exercise regimen for clients with rheumatoid arthritis.

2. 4 **This ensures that the liver does not move as it does with regular respiratory excursions. (2) (PB; MR; IM; GI)**
1 Lying on the right side after the procedure applies pressure at the insertion site, preventing hemorrhage.
2 Movement or breathing increases the danger of damage to the liver.
3 This instruction is not necessary because the client does not breathe during the Valsalva maneuver.

3. 3 **This acknowledges the impact of this diagnosis on the client and should explore what is known. (1) (PI; CJ; IM; EH)**
1 This statement provides false reassurance.
2 Same as answer 1.
4 There is no evidence of ineffective coping.

4. 4 **Promotion of rest to reduce metabolic demands is a challenging but essential task for a client who has hyperthyroidism. (2) (PB; CJ; PL; EN)**
1 The diet can be increased to meet metabolic demands; the client usually has an excellent appetite.
2 The neatness of linen is not an important aspect of care; the client usually is hyperactive, and it is more important to promote rest.
3 Hospital routines should not be considered a nursing problem; routines should be flexible to meet client needs.

5. 3 **Propylthiouracil (Propyl-Thyracil), used in the treatment of hyperthyroidism, blocks the synthesis of thyroid hormones by preventing iodination of tyrosine. (2) (PB; CJ; IM; DR)**
1 Propylthiouracil does not increase the uptake of iodine.
2 Iodine solutions reduce the size and vascularity of the thyroid gland.

4 Thyroid-stimulating hormone (TSH), secreted by the anterior pituitary, is not affected by propylthiouracil.

6. 3 **The bone marrow is impaired; the effectiveness of white blood cells and immunoglobulins is reduced, which increases susceptibility to bacterial infections. (3) (PB; MR; PL; BI)**
1 Travel can be accomplished with careful planning and adequate rest periods.
2 This will not produce a positive prognosis.
4 Although coagulation is impaired, it is not as life threatening as exposure to infection.

7. 1 **With glucocorticoid excess, aldosterone hypersecretion occurs and sodium is retained, therefore potassium is excreted, leading to hypokalemia. (3) (PB; CJ; PL; EN)**
2 Hypervolemia, not hypovolemia, occurs because sodium and water retention are precipitated by aldosterone.
3 Hypocalcemia is not associated with aldosteronism.
4 Aldosterone hypersecretion causes sodium retention and hypernatremia, not hyponatremia.

8. 3 **A tablecloth is nonfuzzy and nonadhering and will keep the burned person warm. (2) (PB; CJ; IM; IT)**
1 Body heat should be conserved with a nonadhering covering.
2 Cream is difficult to remove and may result in additional damage.
4 This is contraindicated because ice can result in additional tissue damage.

9.
1 ____ The ability to form urine is not affected; an increased urinary output or frequency may occur.
2 ____ Euphoria may occur, not depression.
3 __x__ **Palpitations are a side effect of Nubain. (3) (PB; CJ; EV; DR)**
4 ____ Bradycardia, not tachycardia, is a side effect of Nubain.
5 __x__ **Constipation is a common side effect of Nubain.**
6 ____ Orthostatic hypotension may occur, not hypertension.
7 __x__ **Urinary retention is a severe reaction to Nubain.**

10. 3 **Morphine sulfate is the drug of choice because it reduces severe pain, lowers systemic vascular resistance, and decreases venous return. (1) (PB; CJ; AN; CV)**

1 Alprazolam (Xanax), a benzodiazepine, lowers anxiety, which may reduce some pain but it is not an effective analgesic.

2 Although meperidine (Demerol) is an analgesic, morphine sulfate is the preferred drug in this situation.

4 Lidocaine hydrochloride is used to control ventricular ectopic activity, not pain.

11. 2 **High-protein drinks have twice the calories per volume of other fluids and provide protein for wound healing. (2) (PB; CJ; PL; IT)**

1 Low-sodium milk does not contain adequate calories to help meet the high metabolic rate associated with burns.

3 Fruit juices are comparably low in calories; potassium need not be restricted at this time; potassium is restricted during the first 48 to 72 hours after a burn injury.

4 More fats are not indicated; increased calories in the form of protein and carbohydrates are needed.

12. 3 **Before teaching, the nurse must determine the client's areas of concern; learning increases when anxiety decreases, and it is hoped that knowledge will reduce anxiety. (3) (SE; MR; IM; RE)**

1 This is not beneficial for all preoperative clients.

2 Although this may be part of the information included in preoperative teaching, the teaching should begin at the client's level.

4 The client will be dependent on a respirator postoperatively; breathing exercises are not required.

13. 3 **Because the tracheostomy tube enters the trachea below the glottis, the client is unable to close the glottis to retain air in the lungs and raise the intrathoracic pressure and then open the glottis to expel an explosive cough. (2) (PB; CJ; AN; RE)**

1 This would decrease the need for suctioning because humidified oxygen liquefies secretions, which are then easier to expel.

2 The outer cannula of a tracheostomy tube irritates the mucosa.

4 Weaning begins when the respiratory status improves and the amount of respiratory secretions subsides.

14. 4 **Serum albumin is administered to maintain serum levels and normal oncotic (osmotic) pressures; it does this by pulling fluid from the interstitial**

spaces into the intravascular compartment. (3) (PB; CJ; EV; FE)

1 The administration of albumin results in a shift of fluid from the interstitial to the intravascular compartment, which probably would increase the BP.

2 Serum albumin will not affect blood ammonia levels; fluid accumulated in the abdominal cavity is removed via a paracentesis.

3 Albumin administration does not affect venous stasis or blood urea nitrogen.

15. 4 **These are top priorities in trauma management; basic life functions must be maintained or reestablished. (2) (PB; CJ; PL; RE)**

1 This is an assessment for head injury that follows determination of respiratory and circulatory status.

2 Pain assessment would follow the appraisal of airway, breathing, and circulation.

3 This is an assessment for abdominal injury that follows determination of respiratory and circulatory status.

16. 4 **The glomerulus is not permeable to large proteins such as albumin or red blood cells. (1) (PB; CJ; EV; RG)**

1 The proximal tubules are responsible for regulating water, electrolytes (including sodium and potassium), urea nitrogen, and pH; the by-products of this regulation will appear in normal urine.

2 Same as answer 1.

3 Same as answer 1.

17. 2 **The diagnosis depends on the identification of characteristic histologic features of an excised lymph node. (1) (PB; MR; IM; BI)**

1 This is a diagnostic device to assess bony metastasis of cancers.

3 CT scans identify the extent of the disease in the abdominal and thoracic cavities.

4 These are not indicated for Hodgkin's disease; they are used for radiotherapy or diagnosis of thyroid diseases.

18. 4 **No specific diet is recommended; the client is encouraged to avoid meals that overdistend the stomach and foods that cause GI distress. (3) (PB; CJ; PL; GI)**

1 There is no need for a mechanical soft diet, which would be appropriate for those who have difficulty with chewing and swallowing.

2 The client does not require a liquid diet.

3 High-fat dairy products increase GI secretions and should be avoided.

19. 1 **Exercise causes muscle contractions, which require an increase in arterial circulation to supply oxygen and nutrients for energy being expended. (1) (SE; MR; PL; CV)**

2 This is important for the person with diabetes, but it does not improve arterial blood flow.

3 This would reduce arterial blood flow; the legs should be kept dependent.

4 Hot water is contraindicated because it can burn the skin and/or cause drying; also, individuals with diabetes may have neuropathies, which alter the perception of temperature.

20. 2 **Neomycin aids in reducing the intestinal flora that act on protein substances, causing the production of ammonia; ammonia is detoxified in the liver; when the liver is unable to perform this function adequately, blood ammonia levels rise, causing encephalopathy. (3) (PB; CJ; AN; DR)**

1 Bacteria in the intestines do not digest urea.

3 This does not occur; neomycin controls protein metabolism, a severe problem in liver disease.

4 Although immune mechanisms may be limited in disorders affecting the liver, the neomycin is administered to limit ammonia levels.

21. 3 **When the bladder contains large amounts of urine, it becomes distended and may push upward into the abdominal cavity, where it can be punctured. (1) (SE; CJ; IM; GI)**

1 This is not the rationale for emptying the bladder.

2 The amount of fluid in the bladder has no relationship to ascites.

4 Urea is present in the blood and urine; it is not present in ascitic fluid.

22. 1 **Supplemental oxygen supports the body while the cause of the problem is sought; oxygen support is the first therapy in all cases of hypoxia and can be instituted without a physician's order in an emergency. (1) (PB; CJ; IM; RE)**

2 Morphine is used in the treatment of chest pain, but is not the first therapy and requires a physician's order.

3 Nitroglycerin is available in most client acute care areas and does lessen chest pain if cardiac in origin, but is not the first therapy used and requires the order of the physician.

4 Endotracheal intubation is not an initial treatment; if the client's condition deteriorates, and the client becomes unconscious or experiences respiratory failure or obstruction, intubation is warranted; this procedure would be accomplished by advanced cardiac life support (ACLS) trained personnel or a physician.

23. 2 **The body's inflammatory response to myocardial necrosis causes an elevation of temperature as well as leukocytosis within 24 to 48 hours. (2) (PB; CJ; EV; CV)**

1 This is not an expected finding after tissue damage associated with an infarction.

3 Same as answer 1.

4 This is not a common complication after myocardial infarction; it may be associated with phlebitis or multiple fractures.

24. 1 **An airtight system is needed to reestablish negative pressure and reinflate the lung. (3) (PB; CJ; AN; RE)**

2 This is important, but not the priority.

3 Drainage can be maintained without mechanical suction.

4 Any position is acceptable as long as the tube is not compressed or pulled.

25. 1 **All fresh fruits are low in phosphate. (3) (PB; CJ; PL; RG)**

2 Beef contains phosphate.

3 Split pea soup contains a significant amount of phosphate.

4 This is made with milk, which contains phosphate.

26. 3 **A refusal to recognize anticipated loss in an attempt to protect oneself against the overpowering stress of illness is called repudiation. (2) (PI; CJ; AN; EH)**

1 The data do not suggest that the client has contemplated consequences related to the illness.

2 There are no data to support that the client is demonstrating behavior characteristic of an earlier stage of development.

4 The data do not suggest that the client has made a realistic adjustment to the illness.

27. 2 **This response acknowledges and reflects the client's feelings and encourages further communication. (2) (PI; CJ; IM; EH)**

1 This response negates the client's feelings.

3 The nurse does not know how the client's family feels; this response takes the focus off the client.

4 This is true, but telling the client this serves no therapeutic purpose at this time.

28. 4 These interventions maintain the affected left arm in functional alignment; the left side of the body will be affected with a right-sided brain attack. (2) (PB; CJ; PL; NM)
  1 Plantar flexion (foot drop), not dorsiflexion, may occur with a brain attack; high-top sneakers or splints more appropriately prevent plantar flexion contractures.
  2 Elastic stockings promote venous return rather than prevent flaccid muscles; also, this requires a physician's order.
  3 Passive range-of-motion exercises prevent contractures rather than muscle atrophy; the institution of ROM should be discussed with the physician because activity during the acute phase can increase intracranial pressure; ROM may not be started until after the first 24 hours following the brain attack.

29. 4 This is the best initial response; documentation should include both the missed time and the impact on client care. (2) (SE: MR; IM; NP)
  1 This is not a professional, nor appropriate, response to the problem.
  2 This may be helpful but will not address the issue if the problem continues.
  3 This may be a later response to the problem.

30. 4 Taking a pill may give the client a false sense that the disease is under control, and this can lead to dietary indiscretions. (2) (PM; MR; PL; EN)
  1 A person's ability to follow dietary restrictions is highly individual; the employment setting is not a universal factor in such behaviors.
  2 Having to take any medication for a chronic illness every day can be threatening to some people whether the medication is taken orally or by injection.
  3 Diabetes is a chronic disease, and its complications can affect all individuals with the disease, particularly those who do not comply with the prescribed regimen.

31. Answer: 150 mL per hour; an infusion device delivers a specific volume of fluid to be infused over the period of one hour; calculate the answer by using ratio and proportion:

$$\frac{50 \text{ mL}}{20 \text{ min}} \times \frac{x \text{ mL}}{60 \text{ min}}$$
$$20x = 50 \times 60$$
$$x = 3000 \div 20$$
$$x = 150 \text{ mL}$$

(1) (PB; CJ; AN; DR)

32. 2 Active immunity occurs when the individual's cells produce antibodies in response to an agent or its products; these antibodies will destroy the agent (antigen) should it enter the body again. (3) (PM; CJ; AN; BI)
  1 Antigens do not fight antibodies; they trigger an antibody formation that in turn attacks the antigen.
  3 Antigens are foreign substances that enter the body and trigger antibody formation.
  4 Sensitized lymphocytes do not act as antibodies.

33. 3 Because respiratory collapse is an early sign of inhalation anthrax, a client's respiratory status requires immediate assessment and continued monitoring. (1) (PB; CJ; AS; RE)
  1 Development of anthrax-related meningitis is a late sign of inhalation anthrax.
  2 This is not a nursing assessment specific to this problem.
  4 Same as answer 1.

34. 3 A patent airway is always a priority concern; therefore removal of secretions is imperative. (2) (SE; CJ; PL; RE)
  1 This is an important postoperative intervention but is not the priority immediately after surgery.
  2 Same as answer 1.
  4 Same as answer 1.

35. 1 Itching associated with jaundice is believed to be caused by an accumulation of bile salts in the skin. (1) (PB; CJ; AS; IT)
  2 This is not related to jaundice.
  3 Same as answer 2.
  4 Same as answer 2.

36. 3 Insulin in tablet form would be inactivated by gastric juices; insulin given by injection bypasses the destructive gastric juices. (2) (PM; MR; IM; EN)
  1 Insulin is not given orally at this time because it would be inactivated in the stomach.
  2 This is incorrect information for a client who is currently insulin dependent; this provides false reassurance.
  4 This does not answer the client's question; insulin is administered IV or subcutaneously, and the route depends on the client's needs.

37. 1 The cerebellum is involved in synergistic control of the skeletal muscles and the coordination of voluntary movement. (1) (PM; CJ; AN; NM)
  2 The parietal lobe is concerned with localization and two-point discrimination; tumors here cause motor seizures and sensory function loss.
  3 Basal ganglia are concerned with large subconscious movements and muscle tone; damage here may cause paralysis, as in a brain attack or

involuntary movements and uncontrollable shaking, as in Parkinson's disease.
4 The occipital lobe is concerned with special sensory perception; tumors here cause visual disturbances, visual agnosia, or hallucinations.

38. 4 Peripheral muscular hypoxia precipitates carpopedal spasm in the presence of hypocalcemia. (2) (PB; CJ; AS; FE)
1 This indicates thrombophlebitis when pain results from dorsiflexing the foot.
2 This indicates the loss of position sense; swaying results when the client stands still with the feet close together and the eyes closed.
3 Although this sign indicates hypocalcemia, it is elicited by tapping over the facial nerve.

39. 4 Vagal stimulation during surgery may cause a severe bradycardia; in anticipation, pacemaker wires are inserted into the right atrium to be used to initiate impulses if the natural rate falls below the preset rate of the pacemaker. (3) (PB; MR; IM; CV)
1 This pacemaker initiates an impulse if the heart rate drops below a certain rate; the concept underlying this pacemaker is to speed up the heart, not to slow it down.
2 The rhythm can be irregular; however, if the pause between two beats is too long, the pacemaker will initiate an impulse.
3 The pacemaker wires are not used for defibrillation; defibrillator paddles are placed so that electricity affects the entire heart muscle.

40. 1 Assuming a normal position for voiding reduces tension (physical and psychologic), facilitates the movement of urine into the lower portion of the bladder, and relaxes the external sphincter (increasing pressure and initiating the micturition reflex). (3) (PB; CJ; IM; NM)
2 Bladder training should be instituted by encouraging voiding every one to two hours and progressively increasing the time between attempts.
3 Voiding should be encouraged at regular and frequent intervals during waking hours, not just in the afternoon.
4 This is an extremely large fluid intake and will result in a large volume of urine, probably increasing the frequency of incontinence.

41. 2 When the client lies on the affected side, the unaffected lung can expand to its fullest potential; elevation of the head facilitates respirations by reducing the pressure of the abdominal organs on the diaphragm and allowing the diaphragm to descend with gravity. (3) (PB; CJ; IM; RE)
1 Maximum lung expansion is inhibited when the head is not elevated.

3 It is unclear as to what "left side supported" means; although it facilitates diaphragmatic movement, it does not assist expansion of the right lung.
4 Pressure against the right thorax limits right intercostal expansion and gaseous exchange in the right lung; the supine position allows the abdominal viscera to restrict contraction of the diaphragm and does not permit the diaphragm to drop by gravity.

42. 2 The rate and characteristics of respirations should be assessed so that the amount of exertion required for breathing can be determined; the nurse should evaluate signs such as unilateral chest movements that may indicate pneumothorax and tachypnea, which are associated with hypercapnia and acidosis. (2) (PB; CJ; AS; RE)
1 Although important, pain is not a life-threatening symptom.
3 Drainage may accumulate in the pleural space, which is inaccessible for direct assessment.
4 Excessive blood loss might affect the BP, but such bleeding would be indicated first by respiratory changes, because the blood would accumulate in the pleural space; pupillary response would be unaffected.

43. 4 A lower-than-normal Pco_2 can actually benefit the client because it reduces intracranial pressure by preventing cerebral vasodilation; the results should be reported to the physician and monitoring for signs of increased intracranial pressure should continue. (2) (PB; CJ; PL; NM)
1 Instructing the client to slow the breathing rate is inappropriate because it could elevate the Pco_2, which could increase intracranial pressure.
2 There is no evidence that suction is indicated; suctioning elevates intracranial pressure and therefore should be avoided.
3 There is no evidence that supplemental oxygen is needed; an abnormal PCO_2 does not indicate the need for supplemental oxygen.

44. 2 A 5-year-old may not have the concept of numbers as an indicator of levels of pain; Wong's "Pain Faces" uses pictures to which the individual can relate. (1) (PB; CJ; AS; EH)
1 The client will be able to communicate when appropriate assistance is provided.
3 A client functioning at the level of a 5-year-old may not have the concept of numbers needed to assess pain from 0 to 100.
4 Body language gives some information but may not accurately reflect the client's level of pain.

45. 3 **The responsibility for correctly doing this task will foster independence. (2) (PM; CJ; AN; GD)**
1 This is a laudable goal but it does not relate to independence.
2 This goal is too ambitious for a debilitated, older client.
4 Moderate use of the eyes is not contraindicated in clients with glaucoma.

46. 3 **This decreases pressure on the sella turcica, as well as promoting venous return, thus limiting cerebral edema. (2) (SE; CJ; PL; NM)**
1 Gentle oral hygiene is performed, excluding brushing of teeth to prevent trauma to the surgical site.
2 Although deep breathing is encouraged, initially, coughing is discouraged to prevent increasing intracranial pressure.
4 There is no need to limit oral fluids because of the presence of nasal packing.

47. 2 **Spasms result from irritation of the bladder during surgery; they decrease in intensity and frequency as healing occurs. (3) (PB; CJ; IM; RG)**
1 This is too long; it would indicate hemorrhage; drainage should be dark red and after the first few hours gradually turn pink.
3 The presence of a continuous bladder irrigation is unrelated to the amount of oral fluids that should be consumed; once the CBI is discontinued, oral fluids should be encouraged.
4 The Valsalva maneuver should be avoided because it may initiate prostatic bleeding.

48. 3 **Bile salts are used to aid digestion of fats and absorption of the fat-soluble vitamins A, D, E, and K. (2) (PB; CJ; IM; DR)**
1 Bile salts play no role in prothrombin production.
2 Bile salts are not necessary to stimulate the secretion of bilirubin.
4 Bile salts do not initiate the contraction of the common bile ducts.

49. 3 **Retention of carbon dioxide in the blood lowers the pH, causing respiratory acidosis; deep breathing maximizes gaseous exchange, ridding the body of excess carbon dioxide. (2) (PB; CJ; IM; RE)**
1 Deep breathing improves oxygenation of the blood, but it does not affect volume.
2 Although regular deep breathing improves the vital capacity, residual volume is unaffected.
4 Deep breathing increases the partial pressure of oxygen.

50. 1 **After the need to survive (air, food, water) the need for comfort and freedom from pain closely follow; care should be given in order of the client's basic needs. (2) (PB; CJ; PL; SK)**
2 Joints must be exercised to prevent stiffness, contractures, and muscle atony.
3 Motivation and learning will not occur unless basic needs, such as freedom from pain, are met.
4 Although bladder training should be included in care, it is not a priority when the client is in pain.

Medical-Surgical Nursing Quiz 2

1. A client is admitted with 50% of the body surface area burned following an industrial explosion and fire. The client's serum albumin is 1.5 g/dl, the hematocrit is 30%, the urine specific gravity is 1.025 and the serum globulin is 3.0 g/dl. When evaluating the client's response to fluid replacement, the nurse should prepare to administer a colloid when the:
   1. Globulin is 3.0 g/dl
   2. Albumin is below 2 g/dl
   3. Hematocrit is below 32%
   4. Urine specific gravity is 1.018

2. A common early sign of laryngeal cancer for which the nurse should assess a client would be:
   1. Aphasia
   2. Dyspnea
   3. Dysphagia
   4. Hoarseness

3. At the accident scene, emergency treatment for a client who has sustained partial- and full-thickness burns to the chest, right arm, and upper legs should include:
   1. Covering the client with a blanket
   2. Wrapping the client in a clean dry sheet
   3. Applying sterile dressings to burned areas
   4. Removing clothing from the burned areas

4. A male client with thrombophlebitis is apprehensive about the possibility of a clot reaching his heart and causing sudden death. The nurse's initial intervention should be to:
   1. Clarify his misconception
   2. Explain preventive measures
   3. Encourage discussion of his concern
   4. Teach recognition of early symptoms

5. On entering a client's room, the nurse observes the client vomiting. The nurse had taken a capsule of hydroxyzine (Vistaril) from the stock supply to the client's bedside for administration. The nurse decides the injectable form of the medication should be used rather than the oral form, and calls the physician to change the order. Proper and safe disposal of the oral capsule of hydroxyzine requires the nurse to:
   1. Drop the tablet into a sharps container
   2. Crush the tablet and flush it into the sewer system

   3. Return the tablet to the security of the stock supply
   4. Drop the tablet into a red biohazard bag and tie it shut

6. A client with a history of heavy alcohol use develops portal hypertension and an elevated serum aldosterone level. The nurse should carefully observe the client for:
   1. Chloride depletion and hypovolemia
   2. Potassium retention and dysrhythmias
   3. Sodium retention and fluid accumulation
   4. Calcium depletion and pathologic fractures

7. A female client who is scheduled for a thyroidectomy is concerned that the surgery will interfere with her ability to become pregnant. The nurse bases the response on the knowledge that:
   1. Hyperthyroidism can cause abortions or fetal anomalies
   2. Pregnancy is not advisable for the client with a thyroidectomy
   3. As long as medication is taken as ordered, ovulation will occur
   4. Pregnancy affects metabolism and will require greatly increased thyroid hormone

8. After a thyroidectomy the nurse should carefully observe the client for signs of a thyrotoxic crisis. These include:
   1. Hypothermia
   2. Elevated serum calcium
   3. Sudden drop in pulse rate
   4. Rapid heartbeat and tremors

9. Burns classified as full thickness extend to involve destruction of the:
   1. Hair follicle
   2. Upper dermis
   3. Epidermal layer
   4. Subcutaneous tissue

10. A client with chronic obstructive pulmonary disease is admitted to the hospital with a tentative diagnosis of pleuritis. When caring for this client the nurse should plan to:
   1. Administer opiates frequently
   2. Assess for signs of pneumonia
   3. Administer medication to suppress coughing
   4. Limit fluid intake to prevent pulmonary edema

11. The nurse notes that a client, admitted to the hospital after experiencing an anterior septal myocardial infarction, does not have a prn order for a stool softener. The nurse decides to obtain such an order primarily because the client:
    1. Has poor peripheral perfusion
    2. May be kept npo for several days
    3. Will probably become constipated
    4. Is receiving digoxin, which decreases peristalsis

12. A client has had a right pneumonectomy. The nurse should be vigilant for a specific complication that may occur after this type of surgery which would be:
    1. Hemorrhage
    2. Brain attack
    3. Renal failure
    4. Cardiac overload

13. In a three-chamber underwater drainage system, the main purpose of the third chamber is to:
    1. Act as a drainage container
    2. Provide an airtight water seal
    3. Control the amount of suction
    4. Allow for escape of air bubbles

14. When a client with kidney shutdown complains of thirst, the nurse should offer a:
    1. Hard candy
    2. Glass of milk
    3. Carbonated soda
    4. Bowl of clear soup

15. When a client with severe rheumatoid arthritis reports that pain lasts for two to three hours after exercising, the nurse should teach the client to:
    1. Stop exercising for 24 hours
    2. Substitute isometric exercises for isotonic exercises
    3. Delay doing aerobic exercises until the pain subsides
    4. Decrease the total time and number of repetitions of the exercise

16. Acetylsalicylic acid (Aspirin) is prescribed for a client with rheumatoid arthritis. The nurse recognizes that the major rationale for this treatment would be:
    1. Reduction of fever
    2. Preservation of bone integrity
    3. Reduction of joint inflammation
    4. Prevention of flexion contractures

17. When assessing a client for respiratory involvement during the first two days after a burn injury, the nurse should observe for sputum that is:
    1. Sooty
    2. Frothy
    3. Yellow
    4. Tenacious

18. A client who is receiving multiple medications for a myocardial infarction complains of severe nausea, and the heartbeat is irregular and slow. The nurse should recognize these symptoms as toxic effects of:
    1. Lanoxin
    2. Lidocaine
    3. Morphine
    4. Furosemide

19. A female client with diabetes mellitus tells the nurse that she takes Robitussin (guaifenesin) cough syrup when she has a cold. The nurse should teach her that she:
    1. Can substitute an elixir for the syrup
    2. Must calculate the sugar in her daily carbohydrate allowance
    3. Can increase her fluid intake and humidify her bedroom to control a cough
    4. May take the cough syrup if her serum glucose level remains within an acceptable range

20. A client has laparoscopic surgery to remove a stone from the common bile duct. The nurse is aware that the bile flow into the duodenum has been reestablished after biliary surgery when:
    1. The liver is no longer tender
    2. Stools become brown in color
    3. Colic is absent after ingestion of fats
    4. The serum bilirubin level returns to normal

21. A 59-year-old client, with type 1 diabetes, is admitted to the hospital in ketoacidosis. With medical supervision, the client has been adjusting insulin dosage at home based on blood glucose levels at home. Of the statements made by the client during the health history, the nurse realizes that the best explanation of the etiologic factor of the ketoacidosis is that the client has:
    1. Become a vegetarian
    2. A chronic postnasal drip
    3. Planned to retire next year
    4. Been taking steroids for a rash

22. When receiving chemotherapy for non-Hodgkin's lymphoma, a client states, "I get so sick to my stomach. The medication is useless." The response by the nurse that employs the technique of paraphrasing would be:
    1. "You get sick to your stomach?"
    2. "Tell me more about how you feel."
    3. "I'll get an order for an antiemetic."
    4. "You don't think the medication is helping you?"

23. The nurse is administering vaccine at the local influenza prevention clinic. A client arrives for a vaccination and assessment identifies a current febrile illness with a cough. The nurse should:
    1. Notify the physician
    2. Administer the vaccine
    3. Reschedule the appointment
    4. Administer aspirin and the vaccine

24. A client has fractures of the right tibia and has just had a cast applied. Nursing care that the nurse should plan for this client should include:
    1. Ambulating with full weight bearing
    2. Covering the cast with plastic until dry
    3. Elevating the right leg above the level of the heart
    4. Asking the client to insert a finger inside the cast to check for abrasions

25. When caring for a client who has had a total hip replacement, the nurse should position the client's affected limb in:
    1. Adduction and flexion
    2. Abduction and extension
    3. Adduction and internal rotation
    4. Abduction and external rotation

26. A male client who has had a brain attack (cerebrovascular accident) has varying moods. These moods have ranged from anger to depression and concern his aphasia, hemiparesis, and need for gavage feedings. The behavior observed by the nurse that would indicate the client's acceptance of his physical limitations would be:
    1. Performing his own tube feedings
    2. Smiling and becoming more extroverted
    3. Allowing his wife to participate in his care
    4. Ambulating in the hall and sitting in the lounge

27. A client with type 2 diabetes who is taking an oral hypoglycemic agent is to have a serum glucose test early in the morning. The nurse should instruct the client:
    1. "Eat your usual breakfast."
    2. "Have clear liquids for breakfast."
    3. "Take your medication before the test."
    4. "Do not take any food or fluids before the test."

28. After surgery a client's fever does not respond to antipyretics. The client is placed on a hypothermia blanket. One reaction to hypothermia that should be prevented is:
    1. Shivering
    2. Dehydration
    3. Hypotension
    4. Venous stasis

29. A client has an excision of a thrombosed external hemorrhoid. When cleaning the anus following a bowel movement, the client should be instructed to use:
    1. Betadine pads
    2. Soft facial tissue
    3. Medicated pads (Tucks)
    4. Sterile 4×4-inch gauze pads

30. A client with a rigid and painful abdomen is diagnosed with a perforated peptic ulcer. A nasogastric tube is inserted and surgery is scheduled. Before surgery the nurse should place the client in the:
    1. Sims' position
    2. Supine position
    3. Semi-Fowler's position
    4. Dorsal recumbent position

31. The nurse admitting a client with a myocardial infarction to the cardiac care unit understands that the pain the client is experiencing is a result of:
    1. Compression of the heart muscle
    2. Release of myocardial isoenzymes
    3. Inadequate perfusion of the myocardium
    4. Rapid vasodilation of the coronary arteries

32. A client with Crohn's disease is admitted to the hospital with a history of chronic, bloody diarrhea; weight loss; and signs of general malnutrition. The client has edema, anemia, a low serum albumin level, and symptoms of negative nitrogen balance. The client's health status is related to a major deficiency of:
    1. Iron
    2. Protein
    3. Potassium
    4. Linoleic acid

33. The physician orders IV Ringer's lactate to infuse at the rate of 150 mL/hr. How long will it take a liter bag of this solution to infuse?
    Answer: _____.

34. A 55-year-old mailman is admitted to the hospital with a diagnosis of chronic obstructive pulmonary disease (COPD). He complains of fatigue. To reduce the client's fatigue, the nurse should:
    1. Encourage pursed-lip breathing
    2. Provide small frequent feedings
    3. Schedule nursing activities to allow for rest
    4. Encourage bed rest until energy level improves

35. When assessing a client with a diagnosis of possible myocardial infarction for pain, the nurse would expect the client to describe it as:
    1. Severe, intense chest pain
    2. A burning sensation of short duration
    3. Mild chest pain, radiating down to the fingers
    4. A squeezing chest pain, relieved by nitroglycerin

36. A client who is on a 2 g sodium diet asks for a glass of juice. Since the only kinds of juice available are pear nectar, apple, and tomato, the nurse should:
    1. Suggest that the client drink the tomato juice
    2. Tell the client that juice is not permitted on a low-sodium diet
    3. Offer the apple juice or the pear nectar and ask for the client's preference
    4. Explain that the client cannot have juice between meals but may have a glass of water

37. The nurse is aware that the diagnosis of incarcerated hernia means that:
    1. The bowel has twisted on itself
    2. The protruding hernia cannot be reduced
    3. The blood supply to the intestine has been cut off
    4. An erosion of the involved intestine has occurred

38. To help limit a common complication following the repair of an inguinal hernia, the nurse should:
    1. Apply an abdominal binder
    2. Place a support under the scrotum
    3. Encourage a high-carbohydrate diet
    4. Have the client cough and deep-breathe frequently

39. A client recovering from hepatitis A asks when a return to work will be permitted. The nurse's best response would be:
    1. "As soon as you're feeling less tired, you may go back to work."
    2. "Unfortunately, few people fully recover from hepatitis in less than six months."
    3. "Gradually increase your activities. Relapses may occur in people who return to full activity too soon."
    4. "You cannot return to work for six months because the virus will still be present in your stools for this period."

40. A client newly diagnosed with cancer of the pancreas is scheduled for surgery. When arranging for the next appointment the client says to the nurse, "Wouldn't I be better off with some other treatment instead of surgery?" The nurse's best response would be:
    1. "Why don't you explore the other acceptable treatments for your cancer with the physician?"
    2. "Surgery is the recommended approach, but why don't you discuss this further with the physician?"
    3. "Maybe you would be more confident with a second opinion. Would you like a referral to another physician?"
    4. "With your disease your prognosis will improve if you follow the physician's suggestion and have the recommended surgery."

41. When teaching how to use a nebulizer, the nurse should instruct the client to:
    1. Hold the breath while spraying the medication carefully into each nostril
    2. Instill the medication from the nebulizer while exhaling through the nose
    3. Seal the lips around the mouthpiece taking rapid, shallow breaths through the mouth
    4. Loosely place the lips around the mouthpiece taking a slow, deep breath through the mouth

42. A 60-year-old schoolteacher is admitted to the hospital for a needle biopsy of the liver. The physician suspects cancer of the liver. When teaching about the needle biopsy, the nurse should inform the client that:
    1. A midline abdominal incision will be used
    2. Bed rest must be maintained after the procedure
    3. General anesthesia will be used during the biopsy
    4. The supine position will be maintained after the procedure

43. A client is taught the signs and symptoms of a hypoglycemic reaction. The nurse would be aware that the teaching was effective when the client identifies which of the following signs and symptoms? Check all that apply.
    1. _____ Fatigue
    2. _____ Nausea
    3. _____ Weakness
    4. _____ Nervousness
    5. _____ Increased thirst
    6. _____ Tingling sensations
    7. _____ Increased perspiration

44. A client with Hodgkin's disease, stage III, is started on an MOPP regimen of nitrogen mustard, vincristine (Oncovin), procarbazine, and prednisone. The client wonders why so many drugs have to be used at once. The nurse should explain that:
    1. Using groups of drugs reduces the likelihood of serious side effects

2. Each drug destroys the cancer cell at a different time in the cell cycle

3. The drugs are used to destroy cells that are not susceptible to radiation therapy

4. Since there are stages of Hodgkin's disease, if one drug is ineffective another will work

45. A client develops thrombophlebitis in the right calf. Bed rest is prescribed, and heparin sodium IV is started. When describing the purpose of this drug to the client, the nurse should explain that it:
1. Reduces the size of the thrombus
2. Dissolves the blood clot in the vein
3. Prevents extension of the blood clot
4. Promotes absorption of red blood cells

46. The nurse is preparing a client, who has had a transurethral prostatectomy for benign prostatic hyperplasia. The nurse is aware that the client understands the teaching when he states:
1. "I will drink 8 cups of fluid daily, but none after 9 PM."
2. "I am so glad this is over. Now I don't have to keep going to the doctor."
3. "I will use stool softeners regularly for one to two months after I get home."
4. "I was so worried and now I can hardly wait to get home and have sex with my wife."

47. A client has ear surgery. An early response that may be associated with possible damage to the motor branch of the facial nerve would be:
1. A bitter metallic taste

2. Dryness of the mouth
3. A sensation of pain behind the ear
4. An inability to wrinkle the forehead

48. During the first 36 hours after surgery for cancer of the pancreas, a client complains of severe pain and is medicated with 10 mg of morphine sulfate via IV infusion every four hours. Because the client rests or sleeps between injections, the nurse can conclude that:
1. Pain management is effective
2. The dosage of the drug is excessive
3. Another opiate should be substituted
4. An oral analgesic probably can be started

49. A client is admitted with a diagnosis of atrial fibrillation, and the physician suspects mitral stenosis. When obtaining a health history, it would be most significant if the client presented a history of:
1. Rubella, age 6
2. Cystitis, age 28
3. Pleurisy, age 20
4. Strep throat, age 12

50. A client undergoes a mitral valve replacement. Postoperatively the client's peripheral pulses must be checked frequently. The primary purpose of this is to detect:
1. Atrial fibrillation
2. Postsurgical bleeding
3. Arteriovenous shunting
4. The existence of emboli

Medical-Surgical Nursing Quiz 2
Answers and Rationales

1. 2 Administration of a colloid is indicated when the serum albumin falls below 2 g/dl; then, albumin must be administered to raise the level to the normal 3.5 to 5.5 g/dl; this raises the oncotic pressure and prevents the shift of fluid out of the intravascular compartment. (2) (PB; CJ; PL; FE)

 1 This is within the normal parameters of 2.3 to 3.4 g/dl.
 3 A hematocrit level of 32% is low and indicates overhydration; an administration of a colloid could increase this problem.
 4 This is within the normal limits of 1.010 to 1.030.

2. 4 Hoarseness is caused by the inability of the vocal cords to move adequately during speech when a tumor exists. (2) (PB; CJ; AS; RE)

 1 Aphasia refers to an expressive or receptive communication deficit as a result of cerebral disease; it is not related to laryngeal cancer.
 2 Dyspnea is a late sign, occurring when the tumor is large enough to obstruct air flow.
 3 Dysphagia is a late sign, occurring when the tumor is large enough to compress the esophagus.

3. 2 Covering exposed burned surfaces limits contamination by microorganisms and prevents exposure to air, which increases pain. (2) (SE; MR; IM; IT)

 1 A blanket is not smooth in texture and is more apt to adhere to the burned areas and traumatize the skin when removed.
 3 The decision about open or closed treatment of burns will be made by the physician after the client is transferred to a burn unit.
 4 This is unsafe; it would further traumatize the skin.

4. 1 The client's misconception that the clot can cause sudden death when it reaches the heart must be corrected first; this may reduce the apprehension. (2) (PB; CJ; IM; EH)

 2 This was not the client's question and would not meet the need to explore feelings; this could be done later.
 3 Once the client's understanding is corrected, this may or may not be necessary.
 4 This disregards the client's expressed fears and would increase anxiety.

5. 2 Medication taken from a stock supply cannot be returned; the safest disposal is achieved by rendering it unusable and disposing of it through the sewer system. (3) (SE; MR; IM; NP)

 1 The purpose of sharps containers is for sharp objects; a tablet dropped into a sharps container could be retrieved.
 3 Medications removed from stock supply containers cannot be returned.
 4 Placing the tablet into a biohazard bag does not render it unusable.

6. 3 Aldosterone, a corticosteroid, causes sodium and water retention and potassium excretion by the kidneys. (2) (PB; CJ; AS; FE)

 1 Hypovolemia would not occur with increased aldosterone levels because sodium and water are retained.
 2 Potassium is excreted in the presence of aldosterone and therefore would not accumulate and cause dysrhythmias.
 4 Calcium is unaffected by aldosterone.

7. 3 Medication is regulated to maintain the normal blood levels of thyroxine; therefore ovulation is not affected, and future pregnancy is possible. (3) (PM; CJ; IM; EN)

 1 The client will no longer be hyperthyroid after surgery because the overactive tissue is excised; therefore, this will not affect the fetus.
 2 Pregnancy is not contraindicated after a thyroidectomy.
 4 Thyroid hormones may have to be increased; however, the alterations in dosage are based on individual needs.

8. 4 Thyrotoxic crisis refers to a sudden and excessive release of thyroid hormones, which causes pyrexia, tachycardia, and exaggerated symptoms of thyrotoxicosis; surgery, infection, and ablation therapy can precipitate this life-threatening condition. (3) (PB; CJ; EV; EN)

 1 Temperature and pulse would be elevated in thyroid crisis because of the sudden release of thyrotoxic hormones, which elevate the basal metabolic rate.
 2 Hypercalcemia is not related to thyrotoxic crisis; hypocalcemia may result from accidental removal of the parathyroid glands.
 3 Same as answer 1.

9. 4 Full-thickness burns are those extending into the subcutaneous tissue; they are not painful because of nerve destruction. (3) (PB; CJ; AS; IT)

1 Burns extending through the epidermis and involving part of the dermis are deep partial-thickness burns.
2 Same as answer 1.
3 Burns affecting only the epidermis are superficial partial-thickness burns.

10. 2 Clients with pleuritic disease are prone to develop pneumonia because of impaired lung expansion, air exchange, and drainage. (2) (PB; CJ; AS: RE)

1 This is contraindicated because opiates depress respirations.
3 Coughing should not be suppressed; it enhances lung expansion, air exchange, and lung drainage.
4 Oral fluids are encouraged; pulmonary edema does not develop unless the client has severe cardiovascular disease.

11. 3 Inactivity and opiates decrease peristalsis, which may precipitate constipation; straining at stool should be avoided to prevent the Valsalva maneuver that increases demands on the heart. (2) (SE; MR; PL; GI)

1 This is unrelated to constipation; in addition there is no indication the client has poor peripheral circulation.
2 Being npo is only one small factor that could contribute to constipation; opioid analgesics and bed rest are the primary causes of constipation in this instance.
4 Digoxin is unrelated to intestinal peristalsis; opioid analgesics will decrease peristalsis.

12. 4 This can be caused by the loss of the large vascular lung or a mediastinal shift. (2) (PB; CJ; EV; RE)

1 This is not unique to a pneumonectomy.
2 Same as answer 1.
3 Same as answer 1.

13. 3 The first chamber collects drainage; the second chamber provides for the underwater seal; the third chamber controls the amount of suction. (3) (PB; CJ; AN; RE)

1 The first chamber, not the third chamber, collects drainage.
2 The second chamber, not the third chamber, provides an underwater seal.
4 Although this occurs in a three-chamber system, the purpose of the third chamber is to control suction.

14. 1 Sucking on candy will relieve thirst and provide calories without supplying extra fluid. (3) (PB; CJ; IM; RG)

2 Milk contains both fluids and proteins, which must be restricted.
3 Carbonated beverages may be high in sodium and provide additional fluid; both would be restricted.
4 Soup contains sodium and is a fluid, which can compound the problem of fluid retention and hypernatremia.

15. 4 Exercise should be decreased to a level of tolerance. (2) (PB; MR; IM; SK)

1 Exercise should not be stopped.
2 Isometic exercises promote muscle contraction, not joint movement.
3 The purpose of aerobic exercises is to improve cardiovascular functioning, not joint movement; there is no reason to interrupt aerobic exercises if they are tolerated.

16. 3 The antiinflammatory action of aspirin reduces joint inflammation. (1) (PB; CJ; AN; DR)

1 Aspirin reduces fever but this is not the rationale for prescribing it for clients with rheumatoid arthritis.
2 Aspirin does not preserve bone integrity.
4 Flexion contractures are helped by exercise, not aspirin.

17. 1 The mucous membranes of the respiratory tract may be charred after inhalation burns; this is evidenced by the production of sooty sputum. (2) (PB; CJ; EV; RE)

2 Frothy sputum is usually indicative of pulmonary edema.
3 This finding may indicate respiratory infection.
4 Same as answer 3.

18. 1 Signs of digitalis toxicity include cardiac dysrhythmias, anorexia, nausea, vomiting, and visual disturbances. (2) (PB; CJ; EV; DR)

2 Although nausea and heart block may occur with lidocaine, these symptoms are rarely seen; drowsiness and CNS disturbances are more common side effects of lidocaine.
3 Toxic effects of morphine are slow, deep respirations, stupor, and constricted pupils; nausea is a side effect, not a toxic effect.
4 Toxic effects of furosemide are renal failure, blood dyscrasias, and loss of hearing.

19. 2 Cough syrup contains a sugar base; the client should use a sugar-free product or account for the sugar. (2) (PB; MR; IM; EN)

1 Elixirs have an alcohol base and also contain natural sweeteners.

3 Although this will loosen secretions, it will not suppress a cough.

4 Additional glucose may increase serum glucose levels beyond the desired range; once control is achieved, it is unwise to alter dietary intake or medication without supervision.

20. 2 **The return of brown color to the stool indicates that bile is entering the duodenum and being converted to urobilinogen by bacteria. (2) (PB; CJ; EV; GI)**

1 Liver tenderness is unrelated to bile flow.

3 The absence of biliary colic is related to the removal of the stone, not the flow of bile.

4 The serum bilirubin level is not affected.

21. 4 **Steroids cause gluconeogenesis and glycogenolysis, both of which raise blood glucose levels. (3) (PB; CJ; AN; EN)**

1 An ADA recommended vegetarian diet should not increase blood glucose levels.

2 This is a chronic condition that probably has been incorporated into the client's coping patterns; it would not cause sufficient stress to elevate the serum glucose level to this degree.

3 This event is in the future and would not cause sufficient stress to elevate the serum glucose level to this degree at this time; retirement may be welcomed and may not cause stress.

22. 4 **Rewording of the client's statement is paraphrasing that promotes further verbalization. (2) (PI; CJ; IM; EH)**

1 This is not paraphrasing; this repeats the client's exact words.

2 This is clarifying, a therapeutic technique; it is not paraphrasing.

3 This is not an interviewing technique; it cuts off communication.

23. 3 **The appropriate response is to delay the administration of the vaccine until the client is healthy. (1) (SE; CJ; AS; BI)**

1 This is not necessary with the symptoms presented.

2 Vaccines should not be administered during a febrile illness.

4 Same as answer 2.

24. 3 **This will help to reduce edema formation via the principle of gravity. (1) (PB; CJ; IM; SK)**

1 Full weight bearing should not start until ordered by the physician.

2 This holds moisture and will prevent complete drying of the cast.

4 Nothing should be inserted under the cast; this can cause abrasions.

25. 2 **This reduces stress on the joint capsule incision, preventing the prosthesis from becoming dislocated. (1) (PB; CJ; IM; SK)**

1 Both strain the joint capsule, fostering dislocation.

3 Same as answer 1.

4 External rotation puts strain on the joint capsule, fostering dislocation.

26. 1 **The best indicator of acceptance is when the client begins to participate in self-care. (2) (PI; CJ; EV; EH)**

2 This may be an act and does not indicate acceptance.

3 Allowing others to provide care does not indicate acceptance.

4 This does not indicate acceptance and may be an attempt to relieve boredom.

27. 4 **Fasting prior to the test is indicated for accurate and reliable results; food will elevate the serum glucose levels through metabolism of the nutrients. (2) (PB; CJ; IM; EN)**

1 Food should not be ingested; it will raise the serum glucose level, negating the accuracy of the test.

2 This instruction is inadequate for the client; some clear fluids contain simple carbohydrates, which will increase the serum glucose level.

3 Medications are withheld because of their influence on the serum glucose level.

28. 1 **Shivering should be prevented; peripheral vasoconstriction increases the temperature, the circulatory rate, and oxygen consumption. (2) (SE; CJ; IM; CV)**

2 This is not a response to treatment with hypothermia.

3 Same as answer 2.

4 Same as answer 2.

29. 3 **Witch hazel moistened pads are not irritating and are soothing to the anal mucosa. (2) (PB; CJ; IM; GI)**

1 Betadine may cause excessive drying and irritation; the rectum is always contaminated; external cleansing with Betadine will not appreciably affect the bacteria present.

2 Dry facial tissue is irritating and can cause trauma.

4 Sterile gauze pads are unnecessary; the rectal area is considered contaminated.

30. 3 The semi-Fowler's position will localize the spilled stomach contents in the lower part of the abdominal cavity. (2) (SE; CJ; IM; GI)

1 This position will exert pressure on the abdomen, which may be uncomfortable for the client.

2 This position exerts pressure against the diaphragm, inhibits breathing, and intensifies discomfort.

4 Same as answer 2.

31. 3 Cessation of blood flow to the myocardium results in pain because of ischemia of the tissue, as in angina. (1) (PB; CJ; AN; CV)

1 Neither myocardial infarction nor angina involves compression of the heart.

2 These are not related to pain or relief of pain; isoenzymes are indicators of myocardial damage.

4 Vasodilation would increase perfusion and contribute to pain relief.

32. 2 Protein deficiency causes a low serum albumin level, which permits fluid shifts from the intravascular to the interstitial compartment, causing edema; decreased protein also causes anemia; protein intake must be increased. (2) (PB; CJ; AN; GI)

1 Although a deficiency of iron would result in anemia, it would not cause the other symptoms.

3 Hypokalemia would not cause these symptoms; it causes cramps and weakness.

4 This is unrelated to these symptoms; it is an essential fatty acid.

33. Answer: 6 hours and 40 minutes. The amount of solution (1000 mL) divided by the hourly amount to be infused (150 mL) equals 6.66 hours; the decimal portion of the result must be converted to minutes (0.66 × 60 minutes), which equals 40 minutes; 40 minutes plus the 6 hours equals 6 hours and 40 minutes. (2) (PB; CJ; AN; FE)

34. 3 Rest limits muscle contractions, which diminishes oxygen needs and decreases fatigue. (1) (PB; CJ; PL; RE)

1 Although this helps with gas exchange, it does not diminish the metabolic demand for oxygen.

2 Although this may decrease pressure on the diaphragm, it does not address the client's constant fatigue; rest is of primary importance.

4 Bed rest promotes pooling of pulmonary secretions, which may aggravate respiratory status.

35. 1 Blockage of myocardial blood supply causes accumulation of unoxidized metabolites in the muscle tissue that affect nerve endings and cause pain. (1) (PB; CJ; AS; CV)

2 This is not the type of pain associated with a myocardial infarction.

3 Same as answer 2.

4 Nitroglycerin does not relieve the pain.

36. 3 Apple juice and pear nectar have a low-sodium content and are therefore the better choices for this client. (2) (PM; MR; IM; CV)

1 Tomato juice has a high-sodium content; it should be avoided to prevent fluid retention.

2 Low-sodium juices are not contraindicated.

4 The client is permitted juice between meals.

37. 2 When the intestine cannot be returned to the body cavity, the hernia is incarcerated. (2) (PM; CJ; AN; GI)

1 This is a volvulus.

3 This is a strangulated hernia.

4 Erosion of intestinal tissue may be caused by a variety of conditions; is not related to a hernia.

38. 2 After inguinal hernia repair, the scrotum commonly becomes edematous and painful; drainage is facilitated by elevating the scrotum on rolled linen or using a scrotal support. (3) (PB; CJ; IM; GI)

1 An abdominal binder would not support the operative site; the incision is too low.

3 Obesity is a factor in the development of hernias; high-carbohydrate diets should not be encouraged.

4 Coughing increases intraabdominal pressure and may strain the operative site; deep breathing is encouraged.

39. 3 Relapses are common; they occur after too early ambulation and too much physical activity. (2) (PM; CJ; IM; GI)

1 Fatigue is a cardinal symptom; if the client tires at rest, a return to work must be delayed.

2 The majority of clients recover in 3 to 16 weeks with no further problems.

4 Hepatitis A is most communicable before the onset of symptoms and during the first few days of fever.

40. 2 This response provides needed information and establishes the opportunity for further discussion of surgery. (2) (PI; MR; IM; EH)

1 This implies the other approaches are as effective as surgery; this places doubt in the client's mind that surgery is the most effective option.

3 This is an inappropriate response; the competence of the physician was not questioned, but there exists a need for a further discussion of the treatment; making this type of referral is not the nurse's role.

4 This is false reassurance; it cuts off communication and does not address the need for further discussion.

41. 4 **This permits air to enter through the mouth along with the medication from the nebulizer; slow deep breaths deliver medication deep into the lungs. (1) (SE; MR; IM; RE)**

1 This is a nasal spray that does not deliver medication to the lung.

2 This would not deliver the medication to the lungs but would deposit it in the oral cavity.

3 Shallow breaths are ineffective in delivering medication into the lung.

42. 2 **There is a high risk of bleeding because of hepatic vascularity; bed rest for up to 12 hours supports healing and prevents injury. (2) (SE; CJ; IM; GI)**

1 A needle biopsy requires a stab wound over the liver, not an abdominal incision.

3 The biopsy is done with local anesthesia.

4 The client should lie on the right side for a minimum of two hours after the biopsy.

43.

1 _____ Fatigue is related to hyperglycemia, not hypoglycemia.

2 _____ Nausea is related to hyperglycemia, not hypoglycemia.

3 _x_ **Weakness is related to a decrease in glucose within the central nervous system. (2) (PB; MR; EV; EN)**

4 _x_ **Nervousness is caused by increased adrenergic activity and increased secretion of catecholamines.**

5 _____ Increased thirst with an excessive fluid intake (polydipsia) is one of the cardinal signs of diabetes.

6 _____ Tingling sensation is related to hypocalcemia, not hypoglycemia.

7 _x_ **Increased perspiration is caused by increased adrenergic activity and increased secretion of catecholamines.**

44. 2 **Cells are vulnerable to specific drugs through the stages of mitosis, and a combination bombards the malignant cells at various stages. (1) (PB; CJ; IM; DR)**

1 The side effects of a drug are not ameliorated by a combination with others.

3 Although this is true, it is not the reason for using a combination of drugs.

4 Although there is more than one stage of Hodgkin's, this is not the reason for using a combination of drugs.

45. 3 **Heparin interferes with activation of prothrombin to thrombin and inhibits aggregation of platelets. (2) (PB; CJ; AN; DR)**

1 This is not the action of heparin sodium.

2 Same as answer 1.

4 Same as answer 1.

46. 3 **Straining at stool should be avoided for four to six weeks after surgery, or until permitted by the physician, to permit healing and avoid initiating bleeding. (1) (PM; MR; EV; RG)**

1 This is insufficient fluid; between 2000 to 3000 mL/day should be consumed.

2 The client has carcinoma and needs continued medical supervision.

4 Sexual intercourse should be avoided until permitted by the physician.

47. 4 **The motor fibers of the facial nerve innervate the superficial muscles of the face and scalp. (2) (PM; CJ; AS; NM)**

1 This response usually is not related to damage to the facial nerve but may indicate infection.

2 This is a sensory response that may be manifested when the injury is to the sensory branch of the facial nerve.

3 Same as answer 2.

48. 1 **This behavior indicates that the client is comfortable; therefore the medication regimen is effective. (2) (PB; CJ; EV; NM)**

2 This is the accepted dose; no data exist to indicate it is excessive for this client.

3 This is not necessary; the medication regimen is effective.

4 This is too soon after surgery to institute oral analgesics.

49. 4 **Streptococcal infections occurring in childhood may result in damage to the heart valves; an autoimmune reaction occurs between antibodies made against the bacteria and the heart valves, particularly the mitral. (2) (PB; CJ; AS; CV)**

1 The rubella virus would not affect the valves of the heart.

2 Cystitis usually is caused by *Escherichia coli*, which would not affect the heart valves.

3 Pleurisy usually follows pulmonary problems unrelated to streptococcal infection; it would not result in damage to the heart valve.

50. 4 **Because blood pools in the extremities, there is an increased hazard of peripheral emboli in clients who have received a mitral valve replacement. (3) (PB; CJ; EV; CV)**

1 A peripheral pulse alone will not reveal atrial fibrillation; to detect the presence of a pulse deficit, one must compare a peripheral pulse with the apical pulse.

2 Bleeding is detected by checking the wound dressing and observing for signs of shock (e.g., lowered BP, tachycardia, restlessness).

3 This is not a danger after mitral valve replacement.

Medical-Surgical Nursing Quiz 3

1. The nurse on the medical unit does not administer sufficient, ordered, opioid medication to relieve the intractable pain of a client because the nurse fears the client will become addicted. In this situation the nurse is adhering to the ethical principle of:
   1. Veracity
   2. Autonomy
   3. Paternalism
   4. Beneficence

2. A client has a subtotal thyroidectomy. When discussing ensuing drug therapy, the nurse should tell the client:
   1. To take the iodine daily to increase the formation of thyroid hormone
   2. To report palpitations, nervousness, tremors, or loss of weight that may indicate overdosage
   3. That the need for medication will be temporary until the body adjusts to postsurgical activity
   4. That propylthiouracil may be ordered to stimulate the secretion of the thyroid-stimulating hormone

3. A client has had surgery on the shoulder. The nurse is to obtain a brachial pulse. Use the Figure to the right to determine where the nurse should palpate to best obtain the pulse rate.
   1. a
   2. b
   3. c
   4. d

4. The nurse should recognize that a genitourinary factor that may contribute to urinary incontinence in older adults is:
   1. A sensory deprivation
   2. A urinary tract infection
   3. The frequent use of diuretics
   4. The inaccessibility of a bathroom

5. A 40-year-old client, newly diagnosed with rheumatoid arthritis, is admitted to the hospital with bilateral, painful knee and wrist joints. The nurse identifies the nursing diagnosis of "Impaired physical mobility related to painful, swollen joints." Client education during the acute phase should include directions for:
   1. No exercises to the involved joints
   2. Passive exercises to the involved joints

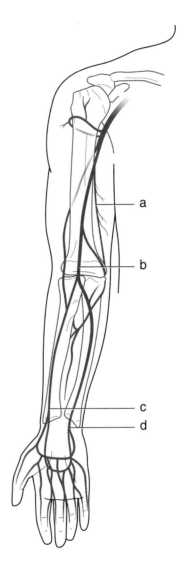

3. Isometric exercises to the involved joints
4. Progressive resistive exercises to the involved joints

6. A client with major burns of the head and chest is admitted to the burn unit. Twenty-four hours after the burn, the client is complaining of severe thirst. The urinary output has been 60 mL/hr for the last 10 hours. No bowel sounds are heard. The nurse's best action would be to:
   1. Increase the IV flow rate
   2. Give 4 oz of water by mouth
   3. Give electrolyte solution orally
   4. Moisten the lips with wet gauze

7. A male client who has had a myocardial infarction asks the nurse, "What's the chance of my having another heart attack if I watch my diet and stress levels carefully?" The most appropriate initial response would be for the nurse to:
   1. Suggest he discuss his feelings of vulnerability with his physician
   2. Tell him that he certainly needs to be especially careful in these areas
   3. Avoid giving him direct information and help him explore his feelings
   4. Recognize that he is frightened and suggest he talk with the psychiatric nurse

8. The key factor in accurately assessing how a client will cope with body image changes is the:
   1. Suddenness of the change
   2. Obviousness of the change
   3. Extent of body change present
   4. Client's perception of the change

9. An obese 42-year-old client has an abdominal cholecystectomy. The client refuses to cough and deep-breathe, saying, "It's too painful." The nurse should:
   1. Give pain medication regularly as soon as possible
   2. Obtain an order to increase the client's pain medication
   3. Medicate the client for pain before coughing and deep breathing
   4. Substitute incentive spirometry for coughing and deep breathing

10. The physician lists a series of orders for a client with less than adequate nutritional intake. The order the nurse should question is:
    1. Provide six small feedings
    2. Have client sit in a chair for meals
    3. Encourage family to bring food from home
    4. Give one can of diet supplement at 8 AM and 4 PM

11. A client with jaundiced skin and acute abdominal pain is refusing all visitors. The most therapeutic nursing intervention would be to:
    1. Listen to the client's fears
    2. Encourage the client to socialize
    3. Grant the client's request about visitors
    4. Darken the client's room by pulling the drapes

12. The nurse discusses resumption of sexual activity with a client who is recovering from a myocardial infarction. The nurse should instruct the client to:
    1. Choose only familiar sexual positions
    2. Return to regular sexual activity after two weeks
    3. Select a quiet, familiar setting for sexual activity
    4. Drink a small glass of wine before engaging in sex

13. A client is transferred to the post anesthesia care unit after abdominal surgery. The client begins vomiting. It is most important for the nurse to:
    1. Turn the client on the side
    2. Measure the amount of vomitus
    3. Check the wound for dehiscence
    4. Administer the prescribed antiemetic to the client

14. When providing preoperative teaching to a client who is scheduled for a cystoscopy, the nurse should include that after the procedure the client should:
    1. Remain flat in bed for the first 24 hours
    2. Increase fluid intake for the next several days
    3. Notify the nurse if there is any drainage on the dressing
    4. Bear down when attempting to void during the first six hours

15. When observing a cardiac monitor, the nurse can ascertain data related to the client's serum potassium level by looking for:
    1. Tall, peaked P waves
    2. A shortened PR interval
    3. Tall or flattened T waves
    4. Runs of trigeminy and bigeminy

16. A 26-year-old client with a history of chronic myelogenous leukemia and splenomegaly is admitted to the hospital. The nurse should expect this client to have:
    1. An increased urinary output
    2. A tender mass in the left upper abdomen
    3. Increased erythrocytes, platelets, and granulocytes
    4. Polydipsia, increased appetite, and urinary frequency

17. When caring for a client who has had chest tubes inserted, the nurse's primary responsibility would be to:
    1. Maintain a closed system
    2. Monitor oxygen saturation levels
    3. Place the client in the supine position
    4. Encourage deep breathing and coughing

18. When teaching older adults how to limit the itching that results from dry skin, the nurse should instruct them to:
    1. Use a moisturizer
    2. Take hot tub baths
    3. Wear warm clothes
    4. Expose skin to the air

19. A 24-year-old college student had a right above-the-knee amputation secondary to trauma sustained in a motor vehicle accident. Six days after surgery the client falls while attempting to transfer to a chair unaided. A fall related to an amputation is most likely the result of:
    1. A loss of balance
    2. Phantom limb sensation
    3. Orthostatic hypotension
    4. Decreased muscle strength

20. The nurse bases a plan of care for a client with Addison's disease on the knowledge that it must include frequent assessments for:
    1. Diarrhea and pyrexia
    2. Edema and hypertension
    3. Moon facies and hirsutism
    4. Hypoglycemia and hypotension

21. Discharge planning for an ambulatory client with Parkinson's disease includes recommending equipment for home use that will help with activities of daily living. The most important equipment to help foster independence would be:
    1. A raised toilet seat
    2. Side rails for the bed
    3. A trapeze above the bed
    4. Crutches for ambulation

22. During a routine clinic visit, an older adult complains to the clinic nurse about being unable to sleep well at night and then feeling sleepy throughout the next day. The care plan for this client should include advising the client to:
    1. Exercise daily
    2. Read in bed prior to sleeping
    3. Avoid naps during the daytime
    4. Have a hot cup of tea prior to bedtime

23. After a client has abdominal surgery, the nurse would suspect impending shock when the client demonstrates:
    1. Diuresis, irritability, and fever
    2. Lethargy, cold skin, and hypertension
    3. Thirst, cool skin, and orthostatic hypotension
    4. Bounding pulse, restlessness, and slurred speech

24. A 78-year-old client's hematocrit and hemoglobin are 32.1% and 11.5 g/dl respectively. Based on these results, the most appropriate nursing intervention would be to:
    1. Conduct a complete nutritional assessment of the client
    2. Advise the client to have the test repeated in three months

3. Nothing because these are normal values for this age adult
4. Understand that mild anemia is a normal response to the aging process

25. A client with hyperthyroidism refuses radioactive iodine therapy and a subtotal thyroidectomy is scheduled. Before having a subtotal thyroidectomy, it is most important that the client be in:
    1. An euthyroid state
    2. A hypotensive state
    3. Normal weight range
    4. Negative nitrogen balance

26. A client is admitted to the hospital for a total hip replacement. The nurse's preoperative teaching plan for the early postoperative period should include instructions related to:
    1. Flexion of the operative hip
    2. Abduction of the operative hip
    3. Turning 45 degrees onto the operative side
    4. Hip flexion of 90 degrees on the operative side

27. A young female client goes to the physician because she has been experiencing fatigue and double vision. The physician suspects myasthenia gravis. When obtaining information from the client, the nurse would expect her to report that:
    1. Her level of fatigue has been constant
    2. The longer she rests, the weaker she feels
    3. Her strength increases with progressive activity
    4. The symptoms seem more severe in the evening

28. When caring for a client with a portable wound drainage system (Hemovac), the nurse understands that the physics principle underlying this drainage system would be:
    1. Gravity causes liquids to flow down a pressure gradient
    2. Siphonage causes fluids to flow from one level to a lower level
    3. The diameter of the lumen will determine the flow rate of fluid
    4. Fluids flow from an area of higher pressure to one of lower pressure

29. A 34-year-old postal worker, who is 5 feet 8 inches tall and weighs 220 pounds, is admitted to the hospital with ureteral colic, blood in the urine, and a blood pressure of 150/90. The immediate objective of nursing care for this client would be to decrease:
    1. Pain
    2. Weight
    3. Hematuria
    4. Hypertension

30. A client with a detached retina is scheduled for surgery to reattach the retina. The nurse explains that the procedure employed involves the use of:
    1. Radiation
    2. Burr holes
    3. Dermabrasion
    4. Laser technique

31. A construction worker falls off the roof of a two-story building and is taken to the hospital unconscious. The nurse would be most concerned if the initial assessment reveals:
    1. Reactive pupils
    2. A depressed fontanel
    3. Bleeding from the ears
    4. An elevated temperature

32. A nurse is assessing clients who are to be given the smallpox vaccination. The client that the nurse should remove from the immunization line for medical counseling would be a:
    1. 20-year-old healthy woman
    2. 45-year-old woman with breast cancer
    3. 50-year-old man with diabetes mellitus
    4. 75-year-old man who has Parkinson's disease

33. When preparing a client with ascites for a paracentesis, the nurse should:
    1. Instruct the client to void
    2. Keep the client npo for four hours
    3. Administer the prescribed analgesic
    4. Position the client on the side in bed

34. The nurse plans to set up emergency equipment at the bedside of a client in the immediate postoperative period following a thyroidectomy. The nurse should include:
    1. A crash cart with bed board
    2. A tracheostomy set and oxygen
    3. An airway and rebreathing mask
    4. Two ampules of sodium bicarbonate

35. The position that would provide for the greatest respiratory capacity for a client with dyspnea would be the:
    1. Sims' position
    2. Supine position
    3. Orthopneic position
    4. Semi-Fowler's position

36. A client with pulmonary tuberculosis is being treated on an outpatient basis. The nurse should expect that the physician will order a diet that:
    1. Includes liquid protein supplements
    2. Has frequent, small, high-calorie meals
    3. Is low in calories but high in carbohydrates
    4. Contains foods high in calories and low in protein

37. An 82-year-old widow with dementia of the Alzheimer's type is admitted to a nursing home. The married son visits and remarks how thin and wrinkled his mother has become. The response by the nurse that would help the son most to understand the aging process would be:
    1. "As we age, we lose the tissue that helps puff out the skin."
    2. "This is typical of the aged; they really don't eat that well."
    3. "At her age, she really shouldn't carry a lot of weight around."
    4. "Her stooped posture is associated with depression, which is common in older adults."

38. When preparing a client for a cardiac catheterization, the nurse should advise the client that:
    1. The procedure will take 15 minutes
    2. The client will be npo six to eight hours before the procedure
    3. Ambulation will be permitted within one hour after the procedure
    4. Complete sedation will be maintained throughout the procedure

39. After taking a client's blood pressure twice, 10 minutes apart, in one arm while the client is seated, the nurse in the blood pressure screening clinic records the two blood pressures of 172/104 and 164/98. The nurse's priority would be to:
    1. Refer the client to a nutritionist after providing health teaching about a low-sodium diet
    2. Place the client in a recumbent position and call the paramedics for transport to the hospital
    3. Talk with the client to assess whether there is stress in the client's life and refer to a counseling service
    4. Take the blood pressure in the other arm and then schedule a physician's appointment for the client as soon as possible

40. During the acute stage of Guillain-Barré syndrome, the most important nursing measure is the frequent assessment of the client's:
    1. Urinary output
    2. Sensation to touch
    3. Neurological status
    4. Respiratory exchange

41. The laboratory data for a client with prolonged vomiting reveal arterial blood gases of pH 7.51, PCO_2 of 50 mm Hg, and HCO_3 58 mEq/L, and a serum potassium level of 3.8 mEq/L. The nurse suspects that the client is exhibiting:
    1. Hypocapnia
    2. Hyperkalemia
    3. Metabolic alkalosis
    4. Respiratory acidosis

42. When the nurse is planning care for a client with abdominal spasms and pain associated with severe diarrhea, the nurse should include monitoring the client's serum levels of:
    1. Calcium
    2. Chloride
    3. Potassium
    4. Creatinine

43. A client is diagnosed as having invasive cancer of the bladder, and radiation therapy is performed prior to surgery. When determining the success of radiation therapy, the nurse should expect the client to demonstrate:
    1. A decrease in urine and feces
    2. An increase in physical strength
    3. A shrinkage of the tumor on scanning
    4. An increase in the quantity of white blood cells

44. A client is admitted to the hospital with a diagnosis of acute pancreatitis. The physician's orders include nothing by mouth and total parenteral nutrition. When the client asks for an explanation for this therapy, the nurse's most accurate response would be:
    1. "It is the easiest method for administering needed nutrition."
    2. "It is the safest method for meeting your nutritional requirements."
    3. "It will satisfy your desire for food without the discomfort associated with eating."
    4. "It will meet your nutritional needs without causing the discomfort associated with eating."

45. A 25-year-old client with a recent history of sinusitis develops meningitis and demonstrates a positive Brudzinski sign. The therapeutic approach by the nurse that has the highest priority would be:
    1. Controlling intracranial pressure
    2. Adding pads to the side of the bed
    3. Administering prescribed antibiotics
    4. Hydrating the client with 0.45% saline

46. A client with recurrent renal disease develops chronic renal failure and is scheduled to begin peritoneal dialysis. When explaining this procedure to the client, the nurse should reiterate that its purpose is to:
    1. Help do some of the work usually done by the kidneys

    2. Prevent the client from developing complicating heart problems
    3. Remove bad chemicals from the body so the disease will not get worse
    4. Speed the client's recovery, since the kidneys are not responding to other therapy

47. After a laparotomy, the nurse can determine that peristalsis has returned when:
    1. Borborygmi are auscultated
    2. The client has a bowel movement
    3. The abdomen is no longer rigid and tender
    4. Nausea is no longer experienced by the client

48. The nurse advises a client receiving furosemide (Lasix) to increase potassium intake. The food that the nurse recommends should be:
    1. Prunes
    2. Apples
    3. Pineapple
    4. Tangerines

49. A client with a history of hypertension is admitted to the hospital immediately after a brain attack (CVA). The client is unconscious and the vital signs are: T 98° F, P 78, R 16, and BP 120/80. The priority nursing diagnosis that would reflect this client's condition would be:
    1. Risk for injury related to seizure activity
    2. Risk for constipation related to immobility
    3. Deficient fluid volume related to inability to swallow
    4. Ineffective airway clearance related to unconscious state

50. A 65-year-old male with squamous cell carcinoma of the tongue is to be treated with interstitially implanted radon seeds. The type of accommodations the nurse should plan for after seed implantation would be:
    1. A room with clients receiving the same therapy
    2. A private room to diminish the radioactivity others receive
    3. A semiprivate room to diminish the risk of sensory deprivation
    4. The same four-bed room so that he will not be in an unfamiliar environment

1. 4 This principle is commonly referred to as "doing of good;" it is related to the nurse's duty to help clients further their legitimate interest within the boundaries of safety. (3) (SE; LE; AN; NP)
  1 Veracity is defined as telling the truth.
  2 Autonomy, as an ethical principle, means that the nurse respects the client and the choices that are made.
  3 Paternalism would occur if the nurse interfered with the individual's autonomy by disregarding the client's choices.

2. 2 Excessive thyroid hormone replacement may lead to the signs and symptoms of hyperthyroidism. (3) (PB; MR; IM; DR)
  1 Iodine may be administered before, not after surgery.
  3 Thyroid hormone replacement will be required for life.
  4 Propylthiouracil blocks thyroid hormone synthesis; this may be administered before, not after, surgery.

3. 2 One of the several pulse points in the body is the brachial artery; it is the main artery of the upper arm and it bifurcates into the radial and ulnar arteries. (2) (SE; CJ; AS; CV)
  1 This is not a major artery of the arm; it is not a pulse point.
  3 This is the radial artery and is where the radial pulse is palpated.
  4 This is the ulnar artery and is where the ulnar pulse is palpated.

4. 2 Urinary tract infections affect the genitourinary tract and interfere with the voluntary control of micturition. (3) (PB; CJ; AN; GD)
  1 This is a neurologic, not a genitourinary, factor.
  3 These are iatrogenic factors.
  4 This is an environmental factor.

5. 1 During the acute phase, immobilization of the joints reduces pain and inflammation. (2) (PB; MR; PL; SK)
  2 These are contraindicated during the acute inflammatory phase.
  3 Isometric exercises involve muscles, not joints.
  4 Same as answer 2.

6. 4 Based on the adequate output, this is the most appropriate intervention; oral fluids are not permitted until bowel sounds have returned. (2) (PB; CJ; IM; FE)
  1 The urinary output indicates adequate fluid replacement; there is no need to increase the IV flow rate.
  2 Oral fluids are not permitted until bowel sounds have returned.
  3 Same as answer 2.

7. 3 The nurse must analyze the feelings that are implied in the client's question and reflect these to help the client verbalize and explore them; the focus is on collecting more data. (1) (PI; CJ; IM; EH)
  1 This is avoiding the responsibility of helping the client explore feelings; it cuts off communication.
  2 Although this may be true, it does not respond to the feelings implicit in the client's comment.
  4 No data presented at this time suggest that such a referral is warranted; this also cuts off communication when the client has expressed a need; the nurse is avoiding responsibility to assist the client.

8. 4 It is not reality, but the client's feeling about the change, that is the most important determinant in the ability to cope. (3) (PI; CJ; AN; EH)
  1 This is not relevant to the client's ability to deal with a change in body image.
  2 Same as answer 1.
  3 The extent of change is not relevant; it is how the client perceives the change.

9. 3 Analgesics limit pain, facilitating effective coughing and deep breathing. (2) (PB; CJ; IM; RE)
  1 Although this may be necessary, it must be coordinated with the deep breathing and coughing exercises.
  2 Large doses of opiates depress the CNS, particularly respirations.
  4 Incentive spirometry will cause pain, and the client may not cooperate if pain is not relieved.

10. 4 **Supplements given before meals would make a client less hungry at meal times; supplements should be given after meals. (3) (PB; MR; EV; GI)**
  1 This would be appropriate; small frequent meals are less overwhelming and generally more appealing for the nutritionally challenged client.
  2 This would be appropriate; this is a more comfortable position vs lying in bed.
  3 This would be appropriate; clients are more likely to eat food familiar to them than institutional food.

11. 1 **Voicing fears often reduces the associated anxiety. (1) (PI; CJ; IM; EH)**
  2 Socialization when feelings need exploration is not therapeutic.
  3 Although this should be done, simply accepting the client's wishes is not by itself therapeutic.
  4 This avoids the problem and is not therapeutic.

12. 3 **An unfamiliar environment increases stress, which will increase cardiac workload. (2) (PB; MR; IM; CV)**
  1 It is advantageous to experiment with positions to find one that is relaxing and permits unrestricted breathing.
  2 Return to sexual activity is determined by the client's recovery; it is usually four to six weeks after a myocardial infarct.
  4 Alcohol dilates blood vessels causing an increase in the workload of the heart

13. 1 **The side-lying position promotes drainage of emesis and secretions from the mouth, reducing the risk of aspiration. (2) (SE; CJ; PL; RE)**
  2 Although accurate assessment of intake and output is important, prevention of aspiration is the priority.
  3 Dehiscence is not probable at this time; it is more common five to seven days after surgery.
  4 Although the antiemetic may prevent additional vomiting, the nurse's priority must be to prevent aspiration.

14. 2 **Increased fluid intake internally irrigates the bladder and helps decrease the risk of infection. (2) (SE; MR; IM; RG)**
  1 This is unnecessary after a cystoscopy.
  3 A cystoscopy is performed through the urethra; a dressing is not used.
  4 Bearing down increases pressure to the area and should be avoided.

15. 3 **T waves reflect serum potassium levels; flattened waves indicate hypokalemia, and tall or peaked waves indicate hyperkalemia. (3) (PB; CJ; AN; FE)**
  1 Changes in P waves reflect atrial activity.
  2 A shortened PR interval is not related to the potassium level.
  4 Trigeminy and bigeminy reflect ventricular irritability, not the serum potassium level.

16. 2 **Splenomegaly usually accompanies chronic myelogenous leukemia; it is usually gross, palpable, and tender and necessitates removal; the spleen is located high in the abdomen on the left side and is not usually palpable unless it is enlarged. (3) (PB; CJ; AS; BI)**
  1 The urinary output is not affected.
  3 With leukemia and splenomegaly there is increased destruction of blood cells; the erythrocyte count will be low.
  4 These signs and symptoms are not associated with leukemia or splenomegaly but rather diabetes.

17. 1 **An airtight system is needed to reestablish negative pressure and reinflate the lung. (2) (PB; CJ; PL; RE)**
  2 Although this would be done, it is not the priority.
  3 A low-Fowler's position, or higher, is preferred to facilitate respirations.
  4 Same as answer 2.

18. 1 **Lubricating the skin with a moisturizer effectively relieves the dryness and thus the pruritus. (1) (PB; CJ; IM; IT)**
  2 Warm or cool, not hot, tub baths would decrease the itching.
  3 This would do nothing to lubricate the skin or relieve the pruritus.
  4 Exposing the skin to air causes further drying and would not relieve the pruritus.

19. 1 **The loss of the limb has eliminated a wide base of support and altered the center of gravity. (1) (PB; CJ; AN; SK)**
  2 This is not related to falls.
  3 This could be a factor in any fall, not specifically one related to an amputation.
  4 While weakness may be a contributory factor in the older adult, it is unlikely in an otherwise healthy young adult.

20. 4 **Adrenocortical insufficiency causes decreased glucocorticoids, resulting in hypoglycemia, and decreased aldosterone, resulting in fluid excretion that leads to hypotension. (3) (PB; CJ; PL; EN)**
  1 Although diarrhea could occur initially, with steroid replacement it should subside; pyrexia would occur only if there were a concomitant infection.

2 These are signs of Cushing's disease, which are related to excessive cortisol and increased aldosterone resulting in fluid and sodium retention.

3 These are related to Cushing's disease; moon facies is caused by adipose tissue deposition, and hirsutism is caused by excessive androgen secretion.

21. 1 **A raised toilet seat will reduce strain on the back muscles and make it easier for the client to rise from the seat without injury. (2) (PB; MR; PL; NM)**

2 This client is not bedridden and would not need this equipment.

3 Same as answer 2.

4 Crutches are never used by clients with Parkinson's disease because of their poor balance and propulsive gait.

22. 1 **Exercise, such as walking or other activity appropriate for the older adult, will be invigorating during the day and prime the client for a better night's sleep. (3) (PB; CJ; PL; GD)**

2 Reading is relaxing before sleeping, but the client should avoid reading in bed; a pattern of going to bed to sleep should be established.

3 Naps should be limited but research has demonstrated that a nap will not affect nighttime sleep.

4 Caffeinated beverages should be avoided before bedtime; tea may contain caffeine.

23. 3 **Extravascular depletion leads to thirst; peripheral vasoconstriction produces cool skin; and poor venous return leads to orthostatic hypotension. (1) (PB; CJ; AN; CV)**

1 Decreased blood flow to the kidney leads to oliguria; the temperature usually decreases.

2 Restlessness, not lethargy, occurs; hypotension, not hypertension, is a sign of shock.

4 With shock, the pulse is thready; subtle changes in sensorium would not result in slurred speech.

24. 1 **A nutritional assessment starts the investigation for a cause of the client's anemia. (3) (PB; CJ; AS; BI)**

2 Treatment should be initiated first and then the test should be repeated to determine the client's response to therapy.

3 These are not normal values; an intervention is indicated.

4 Anemia is not a normal response to the aging process.

25. 1 **Having a normally functioning thyroid (euthyroid) decreases the risk of thyrotoxic crisis after surgery. (2) (PB; CJ; PL; EN)**

2 Ideally the client should be normotensive; some clients are slightly hypertensive because of the increased metabolic rate associated with hyperthyroidism.

3 This may be impossible; the client may be underweight because of the increased metabolic rate associated with hyperthyroidism.

4 The client should be in positive nitrogen balance to promote wound healing.

26. 2 **After surgery, abduction is maintained to reduce the chance of dislocation of the femoral head. (1) (PB; MR; PL; SK)**

1 This can lead to dislocation of the femoral head.

3 This causes adduction, which can lead to dislocation of the femoral head.

4 Same as answer 1.

27. 4 **Increased activity and stress precipitate exacerbation of symptoms because nerve impulses fail to pass to muscles at the myoneural junction; theories include inadequate acetylcholine, excessive cholinesterase, or a nonresponse of the muscle fibers to acetylcholine. (2) (PB; CJ; AS; NM)**

1 Muscle weakness and fatigue come on quickly and disappear rapidly with rest in the initial stages of the disease.

2 Rest promotes a decrease in symptoms because the demand for muscle contraction is reduced.

3 A person's strength decreases with progressive activity.

28. 4 **A portable wound drainage system works via negative pressure; fluid flows down the pressure gradient from the client to the collection chamber. (2) (PB; CJ; AN; IT)**

1 This is Newton's law of gravity; not the physical principle underlying portable wound drainage system functioning.

2 Siphonage is not the principle underlying the functioning of a portable wound drainage system.

3 Although true, the diameter of the tube does not provide the negative pressure that causes the flow of drainage through the tube.

29. 1 **Sharp, severe pain (renal colic) radiating toward the genitalia and thigh is associated with ureteral distention and must be relieved. (1) (PB; CJ; PL; RG)**

2 Weight loss is a long-term goal; reducing pain is the priority.

3 Although this will be addressed, pain reduction is the priority.

4 Same as answer 3.

30. 4 **The thermal inflammatory response, caused by a laser beam, results in a chorioretinal scar that holds the retina in place. (2) (PB; MR; IM; NM)**
  1 Radiation is not used because it destroys retinal tissue.
  2 Burr holes are used in brain surgery.
  3 Dermabrasion is used for acne vulgaris and other disfiguring skin conditions.

31. 3 **Bleeding from the ears occurs with basal skull fractures; this assessment assists with diagnosing the location of the injury. (2) (PB; CJ; AS; NM)**
  1 This would be a positive response; pupils should react to light.
  2 This would occur in an infant in the presence of dehydration.
  4 This occurs with increased intracranial pressure and pressure on the brainstem; it would be an expected response but not an immediate one.

32. 2 **The smallpox vaccine should not be given to individuals with immunologic problems. (2) (SE; CJ; AS; BI)**
  1 There is no contraindication to giving the smallpox vaccination to this client.
  3 Same as answer 1.
  4 Same as answer 1.

33. 1 **The bladder must be emptied to avoid trauma during insertion of the trocar. (2) (PB; CJ; IM; EH)**
  2 This is not necessary; general anesthesia is not used.
  3 Systemic analgesics are not necessary and may mask the symptoms of shock, a potential complication.
  4 A semi-Fowler's position allows fluid to accumulate in the lower abdominal cavity minimizing the risk of damage to vital organs.

34. 2 **Acute respiratory obstruction can result from edema, nerve damage, or tetany. (1) (PB; CJ; PL; EN)**
  1 A cardiac arrest is not an expected response following thyroid surgery.
  3 If the airway were obstructed by postoperative edema, the use of a mechanical airway would be ineffective because it would not reach the point of obstruction; a rebreathing mask would not be used for clients after a thyroidectomy.
  4 Acidosis and cardiac arrest are not expected responses after a thyroidectomy.

35. 3 **The orthopneic position lowers the diaphragm and provides for maximum thoracic expansion. (1) (PB; CJ; PL; RE)**
  1 This would not facilitate thoracic expansion because it permits abdominal organs to press against the diaphragm.
  2 Same as answer 1.
  4 Although this could help, it would not be as beneficial as the orthopneic position.

36. 2 **Clients with tuberculosis tend to have anorexia and lose weight; this diet should encourage food intake and provide calories for weight gain. (1) (PB; CJ; PL; RE)**
  1 This is not necessary; protein and other nutrients can be obtained through natural foods.
  3 This is not possible; carbohydrates contain calories.
  4 Proteins are needed for tissue building.

37. 1 **Collagen tissue, which is the support tissue, decreases with aging. (1) (PM; MR; IM; GD)**
  2 This response stereotypes older adults; some may eat less and lose weight, but not all.
  3 This is not related to aging.
  4 The solidification of the vertebral discs and gravity cause the kyphosis that can occur in older adults; it is not related to depression.

38. 2 **Food and fluids are usually withheld for approximately six to eight hours to prevent vomiting and aspiration. (1) (PB; MR; PL; CV)**
  1 The procedure takes approximately two hours.
  3 The client remains on bed rest with legs extended for four to six hours after the femoral method of entry.
  4 A mild sedative is used because the client must be alert enough during the procedure to follow directions.

39. 4 **According to the U.S. Department of Health and Human Services, both of these readings indicate hypertension and, thus, require further evaluation by a physician; having a baseline for both arms can assist the physician with the medical diagnosis. (2) (PM; CJ; AS; CV)**
  1 There are insufficient data to support this intervention; the priority is control of the hypertension to help prevent a crisis.
  2 Same as answer 1.
  3 Although emotional stress can precipitate hypertension, physical causes should be ruled out first.

40. 4 **The respiratory center in the medulla oblongata can be affected, which can lead to death from respiratory failure. (1) (PB; CJ; PL; NM)**
  1 Although this is important, it is not the priority.
  2 Same as answer 1.
  3 Same as answer 1.

41. 3 Elevated plasma pH and elevated bicarbonate levels support metabolic alkalosis. (2) (PB; CJ; AN; FE)

    1 The arterial carbon dioxide level of 50 mm Hg is elevated above the normal value of 35 to 45 mm Hg; hypercapnia, not hypocapnia, is present.
    2 Normal potassium levels are 3.5 to 5.0 mEq/L.
    4 In respiratory acidosis the pH will be below 7.35.

42. 3 Potassium, a gastrointestinal (GI) constituent, moves quickly through the GI tract of a client with diarrhea and is not absorbed; therefore serum potassium can become dangerously low and cause dysrhythmias. (3) (PB; CJ; AS; FE)

    1 Calcium is unaffected by diarrhea; with diarrhea there is a loss of potassium, sodium, and water.
    2 Diarrhea does not affect chloride levels; excessive vomiting results in a loss of chloride.
    4 Creatinine reflects muscle and renal function and would remain stable, unless the client was extremely hemoconcentrated.

43. 3 Radiation interferes with cell multiplication, which should control the growth and metastasis of cancerous tumors. (2) (PB; CJ; EV; RG)

    1 Radiation affects normal as well as abnormal cells; frequency and diarrhea could result.
    2 Malaise is a side effect of radiation therapy.
    4 Bone marrow sites may be affected by the radiation, resulting in a reduction of WBCs.

44. 4 Providing nutrients by the intravenous route eliminates pancreatic stimulation, therefore reducing the pain experienced with pancreatitis. (1) (PB; MR; IM; GI)

    1 TPN is used to meet the client's needs, not the nurse's needs.
    2 TPN creates many safety risks for the client.
    3 Hunger can be experienced with total parenteral nutrition therapy.

45. 3 The Brudzinski sign indicates bacterial meningitis, a complication of sinusitis; the client's greatest need is a regimen of antibiotics to which the causative agent is sensitive. (3) (SE; CJ: PL; NM)

    1 Bacterial meningitis causes increased intracranial pressure and it is important for the nurse to monitor for manifestations of increased intracranial pressure; however, in this circumstance, it is not the highest priority.

    2 Because of the risk for seizures in bacterial meningitis, padded side rails are an important nursing intervention, however this intervention does not have priority over instituting the appropriate antibiotic therapy to eradicate the cause of the meningitis.
    4 The data do not indicate the use of a hypotonic solution for hydrating the client.

46. 1 Dialysis removes chemicals, wastes, and fluids usually removed from the body by the kidneys. (3) (PB; MR; IM; RG)

    2 The mention of heart problems is a response that may cause increased fear or anxiety.
    3 This response can cause an increase in the level of anxiety.
    4 Dialysis does not speed recovery; it helps maintain fluid and electrolyte balance.

47. 1 The nurse should auscultate the abdomen and listen for bowel sounds (borborygmi), which signify the passage of flatus. (2) (PB; CJ; AN; GI)

    2 The first bowel movement occurs after peristalsis returns and after food is eaten.
    3 Peristalsis should return before tenderness of the abdomen subsides.
    4 Nausea may be present, even though peristalsis has begun.

48. 1 Prunes contain 262 mg of potassium per 100 g, more than the other choices. (3) (PB; MR; IM; GI)

    2 Apples contain 110 mg of potassium per 100 g.
    3 Pineapple contains 146 mg of potassium per 100 g.
    4 Tangerines contain 126 mg of potassium per 100 g.

49. 4 An obstructed airway is a top priority when a client is unconscious; reduced O_2 intake may lead to serious complications. (3) (PB; CJ; AN; RE)

    1 This is not as immediately life threatening; the priority is airway clearance.
    2 Same as answer 1.
    3 Same as answer 1.

50. 2 Radon seeds emit radiation; the client should be isolated in a private room to decrease radiation to others. (2) (SE; LE; PL; NP)

    1 This is contraindicated because this would expose other clients and staff to radiation.
    3 Same as answer 1.
    4 Same as answer 1.

Chapter 6

Comprehensive Examination I

1. The hypertonicity of the muscles in an infant with cerebral palsy causes scissoring of the legs. The nurse should suggest to the infant's mother that the best way to carry the baby is in a sitting position:
   1. Astride one of her hips
   2. Strapped in an infant seat
   3. Wrapped tightly in a blanket
   4. Under the arm using a football hold

2. A client with portal hypertension and ascites is given 2 units of salt-poor albumin IV. The purpose of salt-poor albumin is to:
   1. Provide parenteral nutrients
   2. Increase the client's protein stores
   3. Elevate the client's circulating blood volume
   4. Temporarily divert blood flow away from the liver

3. When obtaining the health history from a client who is seeking contraceptive information, the nurse should consider that oral contraceptives are contraindicated for a client who:
   1. Is older than 30 years
   2. Smokes a pack of cigarettes per day
   3. Has had at least one multiple pregnancy
   4. Has a history of borderline hypertension

4. A 37-year-old female comes to the fertility clinic with a history of being unable to conceive after four years of unprotected intercourse. The client complains of recurring headaches with pain radiating down the neck. The physical examination reveals a blood pressure of 170/100 mm Hg. The client is advised to limit salt intake and to take her basal temperature for three months. The health professionals are:
   1. Not helping the client
   2. Avoiding the major problem
   3. Overlooking the hypertension
   4. Encouraging self-responsibility

5. After a mastectomy, a client returns from surgery with a portable suction unit in place and a dry sterile dressing covering the site of the incision. When observing this client for signs of bleeding, the nurse should:
   1. Empty and measure the output in the portable suction unit hourly
   2. Inspect the bedclothes under the client's axillary area for signs of drainage
   3. Turn the client on the affected side to inspect for blood that may flow backward
   4. Reinforce the operative site with a pressure dressing if any drainage appears on the dressing

6. The nurse empties a portable wound suction device when it is half full because:
   1. It is easier and safer to empty the unit when it is half full
   2. This facilitates a more accurate measurement of drainage output
   3. The negative pressure in the unit lessens as fluid accumulates in it, interfering with further drainage
   4. As fluid collects in the unit, it exerts positive pressure, forcing drainage to back up in the tubing and into the wound

7. Before discharge after a myocardial infarction, a male client asks the nurse how long he should wait before having sexual relations with his wife. The nurse's best reply would be:
   1. "It depends on how you are feeling."
   2. "Two weeks is the usual waiting time."
   3. "You should wait until your heart feels stronger."
   4. "Have you discussed this with your physician?"

8. The laboratory report of a client receiving lithium carbonate indicates a level of 1.5 mEq/L. The nurse should:
   1. Observe for signs of lithium toxicity
   2. Expect an increase in manic behavior
   3. Administer the next dose of lithium as ordered
   4. Decide that the lithium level is within the therapeutic range

9. The glossopharyngeal (ninth), the vagus (tenth), and the hypoglossal (twelfth) cranial nerves frequently are involved in Guillain-Barré syndrome. The nurse is aware that the signs and symptoms that would be unrelated to the function of these nerves would be:
   1. Diminished corneal reflex
   2. Fluctuation in blood pressure
   3. Regurgitation of food and fluids
   4. Difficulty or inability to swallow

10. A 37-year-old male cocaine addict, remanded for rehabilitation by the court, is very angry at being hospitalized. When his wife comes to visit, he is furious and curses at her. He refuses to visit with her and tells her to go home. After the wife leaves in tears, the nurse should approach the client and say:
    1. "Are you very angry right now?"
    2. "Let's go to your next scheduled activity."
    3. "I think we should talk about what just happened."
    4. "You should go to the gym and use the punching bag."

11. After the administration of epinephrine to a child with asthma, the nurse would carefully monitor for the common side effect of:
    1. Flushing
    2. Dyspnea
    3. Tachycardia
    4. Hypotension

12. A 22-year-old client with an antisocial personality disorder is being discharged after a suicide attempt and is to continue psychotherapy on an outpatient basis. When evaluating chances for improvement, the nurse recognizes that the:
    1. Client's prognosis for adjusting to a limited lifestyle is excellent
    2. Client will not change unless the client's parents are willing to set and keep firm limits
    3. Client requires intensive psychotherapy along with an anxiolytic drug to produce a remission

4. Client's ability to change will be limited unless there is a readiness to accept the uncertainty associated with change

13. A factor learned while obtaining the nursing history that probably predisposed a client to type 2 diabetes would be:
    1. Having diabetes insipidus
    2. Eating low-cholesterol foods
    3. Being 20 pounds overweight
    4. Drinking a daily alcoholic beverage

14. The tentative diagnosis for a client with neuropathy is Guillain-Barré syndrome. When collecting a nursing history from this client, the nurse can elicit information that would support this diagnosis by asking:
    1. "Did you receive a head injury during the past year?"
    2. "Is there a history of this disorder in your family?"
    3. "Have you experienced an infection recently?"
    4. "What medications have you taken in the last three months?"

15. The nurse tells a laboring client that she must avoid lying on her back during labor. The nurse bases this instruction on the knowledge that the supine position most significantly can:
    1. Prolong labor
    2. Cause decreased placental perfusion
    3. Lead to transient episodes of hypertension
    4. Interfere with free movement of the coccyx

16. When planning care for a child with leukemia, the nurse must keep in mind that the prognosis of a child with acute lymphocytic leukemia who is receiving therapy is:
    1. Very poor, but the therapy keeps them pain free
    2. Limited to a few months in 70% of the children affected
    3. Extended to at least five years in over 60% of the children treated
    4. Very positive, with a probable cure in 90% of the children affected

17. The nurse arrives at the scene of an accident in which a 5-month-old infant is found unconscious. After performing the initial steps of cardiopulmonary resuscitation, the nurse plans to locate the infant's pulse. Identify the pulse site in the Figure on p. 633 that should be palpated:

1. a
2. b
3. c
4. d

18. A subclavian catheter is inserted and the client is started on total parenteral nutrition (TPN). To prevent the most common complication of TPN, the nurse should plan to teach the client to:
1. Avoid disturbing the dressing
2. Keep the head as still as possible whenever moving
3. Regulate the flow rate on the infusion pump as necessary
4. Weigh daily at the same time, wearing the same clothing

19. During the first session of a therapy group one of the clients asks, "What is supposed to happen in this group?" The most appropriate response by the nurse leader would be:
1. "Before I answer that, I'd like for you to tell me what you want to happen."
2. "This is your group and your participation will largely determine what happens."

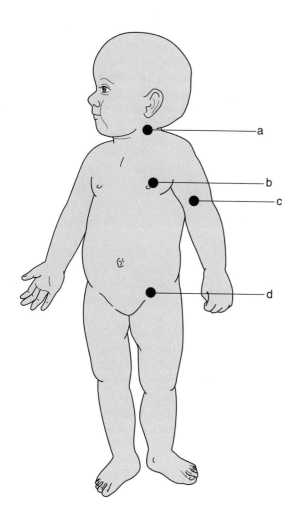

3. "The purpose of this group is to examine the way each of you interacts with the other."
4. "You and the others are supposed to discuss any reality-based concerns you have about your illness."

20. To relieve the symptoms of parkinsonism, the nurse would expect the physician to order:
1. Levodopa
2. Dopamine
3. Vitamin B_6
4. Isocarboxazid

21. After a transurethral prostatectomy, a client returns to the recovery room with a three-way indwelling catheter with continuous bladder irrigation. An initial nursing priority in the client's care plan would be to:
1. Monitor for signs of confusion and agitation
2. Observe the suprapubic dressing for drainage
3. Maintain the client in a semi-Fowler's position
4. Encourage fluids by mouth as soon as the gag reflex returns

22. Five days after resection of the colon the nurse assesses the client's incision site for signs of dehiscence by observing for:
1. Increased bowel sounds
2. Loosening of the sutures
3. Serosanguineous drainage
4. Purplish color of the incision

23. While doing a newborn assessment, the nurse suspects that the infant has a talipes equino-varus when the infant's toes are:
1. Lower than the heel with the foot pointing inward
2. Higher than the heel with the foot pointing inward
3. Lower than the heel with the foot pointing outward
4. Higher than the heel with the foot pointing outward

24. A 40-year-old client, scheduled for a hemicolectomy because of ulcerative colitis, asks if having a hemicolectomy means wearing a pouch and having bowel movements in an abnormal way. The best answer by the nurse would be:
1. "Yes, hemicolectomy is the same as a colostomy."
2. "No, that is necessary when a tumor is blocking the rectum."
3. "Yes, but it will only be temporary until the colitis is healed."
4. "No, only part of the colon is removed, and the rest reattached."

25. A nursing care plan for a client with implanted radon seeds in the oral cavity should include:
    1. Providing a regular diet within two days
    2. Administering nursing care in a short period of time
    3. Giving frequent mouth care to prevent mucosal drying
    4. Having a member of the nursing staff or family with the client continuously

26. A client with a diagnosis of bipolar I disorder, with a single manic episode, is receiving tiagabine hydrochloride (Gabitril). The nurse would be aware that the drug has been effective when the client becomes:
    1. More high-spirited
    2. Able to laugh off criticism
    3. More willing to care for activities of daily living
    4. Able to spend the morning entertaining several quiet clients

27. Immediately after a child is admitted to the hospital with acute bacterial meningitis, the nurse should plan to:
    1. Give oral antibiotic medications as ordered
    2. Assess the child's vital signs every four hours
    3. Check the child's level of consciousness every hour
    4. Restrict parental visiting until isolation precautions are discontinued

28. A neonate develops hyperbilirubinemia, and phototherapy is begun. The care plan for an infant during phototherapy should include:
    1. Taking vital signs q1h
    2. Giving additional fluids q2h
    3. Drawing blood for a Guthrie test q.d.
    4. Dressing the neonate in a light shirt and diaper

29. An 8-year-old child is admitted with a tentative diagnosis of acute glomerulonephritis. Diagnostic tests are ordered. The nurse knows that the tests should include:
    1. Routine urinalysis, complete blood chemistry, nasopharyngeal culture, ASO titer
    2. Electrocardiogram, heterophil antibody test, urinalysis, chest x-ray examination
    3. Routine urinalysis, chest x-ray examination, blood glucose levels, intravenous pyelogram
    4. Upper GI series, 24-hour urine collection, complete blood chemistry, nasopharyngeal culture

30. A male client on the psychiatric unit asks one of the female staff members for a date. It is most likely that the:
    1. Staff member may have led the client on
    2. Client misinterpreted the staff member's friendliness
    3. Client may be trying to protect a threatened sexual identity
    4. Staff member may have been acting unprofessionally toward the client

31. A pediatric client is receiving busulfan (Myleran). The child's blood tests should be monitored for side effects, which include:
    1. Polycythemia
    2. Hyperuricemia
    3. Aplastic anemia
    4. Hypoalbuminemia

32. The physician prescribes a low-fat, 2-gram sodium diet for a client with hypertension. The nurse understands that a low-sodium diet will:
    1. Chemically stimulate the loop of Henle
    2. Diminish the thirst response of the client
    3. Prevent reabsorption of water in the distal tubules
    4. Cause fluid to move toward the interstitial compartment

33. A client, who has had an open reduction and insertion of a prosthesis for a fracture of the femoral neck, tolerates the surgery well and is returned to the surgical unit. When positioning this client, the nurse must be careful to:
    1. Maintain both legs in abduction
    2. Keep both legs in functional body alignment
    3. Avoid placing the client in the supine position
    4. Prevent adduction and external rotation of the affected leg

34. A client with mild preeclampsia is instructed to rest at home. She asks the nurse, "What do you mean by rest?" The most appropriate response would be:
    1. "Take three to four naps each day."
    2. "What do you consider to be rest?"
    3. "Stay off your feet as much as possible."
    4. "Would you like to know what I think it means?"

35. A client is admitted in active labor. She complains of back pain. The nurse should suggest that her coach try to comfort her by:
    1. Positioning her with her legs elevated
    2. Having her perform a panting-breathing pattern
    3. Applying pressure to the sacrum during contractions
    4. Encouraging her to do Kegel exercises between contractions

36. After an infant has the cast that was used to correct a talipes equinovarus (clubfoot) removed, the nurse teaches the mother how to exercise the baby's foot. The nurse would know that the mother understood the instructions when she says that she will exercise the foot:
1. With each diaper change
2. Every four hours without fail
3. Once a day, after the baby naps
4. Twice a day, morning and evening

37. A child is about to receive chelation therapy for lead poisoning. The nurse should be aware that a condition that can be attributed to lead toxicity is:
1. Heart failure
2. Hypocalcemia
3. Gastrointestinal bleeding
4. Increased intracranial pressure

38. Six hours after a herniorrhaphy, a male client complains of severe abdominal pain, is pale and perspiring, has a thready, rapid pulse, and states he feels faint. The nurse checks the chart and notes that the client can receive another injection for pain in an hour. The most appropriate action by the nurse would be to:
1. Explain to the client that it is too early to have an injection for pain
2. Call the physician, report the client's symptoms, and obtain further orders
3. Reposition the client for greater comfort and turn on the television as a distraction
4. Prepare the injection and administer it to the client early because of the severe pain

39. A client returns from surgery after a total laryngectomy with a laryngectomy tube in the permanent stoma. To facilitate respirations and promote comfort, the client should be placed in the:
1. Side-lying position
2. Orthopneic position
3. High Fowler's position
4. Semi-Fowler's position

40. A 20-year-old client at 38-weeks' gestation comes to the prenatal clinic for the first time. She is accompanied by her 21-year-old boyfriend, who is the father of the baby. When they are in the waiting room the nurse observes that they are sneezing, yawning, and have teary eyes. The nurse becomes concerned because these signs are associated with withdrawal from:
1. LSD
2. Heroin

3. Morphine
4. Phenobarbital

41. An infant born with a cleft lip is to have a surgical repair of the lip at about 2½ months of age. In preparation for the postoperative period, the nurse should instruct the infant's mother to:
1. Teach the infant to drink from a cup
2. Burp the infant as little as possible after feeding
3. Keep the infant's arms in restraints for long periods
4. Place the infant in the supine position for extended periods

42. A couple interested in delaying the start of a family discuss the various methods of family planning. Together, they decide to use the basal body temperature method. Before they begin using this method they should understand that the fertility period surrounding ovulation usually extends from:
1. 12 hours before to 24 hours after ovulation
2. 72 hours before to 24 hours after ovulation
3. 24 to 48 hours before to 48 hours after ovulation
4. 72 to 80 hours before to 72 hours after ovulation

43. When the parents visit their young hospitalized child, the child continues to play and ignores their presence. The parents are extremely disturbed by the child's reaction to them. The nurse informs them that this behavior is common among hospitalized children and tells them this is called:
1. Denial
2. Undoing
3. Repression
4. Sublimation

44. When the second (acute) phase of burn recovery is beginning, the nurse should anticipate:
1. A rise in serum potassium
2. An increased urinary output
3. An elevated hematocrit level
4. A fall in central venous pressure

45. A client with a history of chronic obstructive pulmonary disease develops a pneumothorax, and a chest tube is inserted. The primary purpose of the chest tube is to:
1. Lessen the client's chest pain and discomfort
2. Restore negative pressure in the pleural space
3. Drain accumulated fluid from the pleural cavity
4. Prevent subcutaneous emphysema in the chest wall

46. The nurse understands that the major cause of right ventricular failure, unrelated to cardiac disease, would be:
    1. Renal disease
    2. Hypovolemic shock
    3. Severe systemic infection
    4. Chronic obstructive pulmonary disease

47. After gastrointestinal surgery, a client's condition improves and a regular diet is ordered. The food that will most likely be tolerated with little discomfort is:
    1. Fresh fruit
    2. Baked fish
    3. Bran cereal
    4. Whole milk

48. A pregnant client's last menstrual period was on February 11. By July 18, a physical assessment of the client should indicate that the top of the fundus is:
    1. Even with the umbilicus
    2. Just above the symphysis pubis
    3. Two fingerbreadths above the umbilicus
    4. Halfway between the symphysis and umbilicus

49. A 2-year-old requires close supervision to protect against potential accidents, because at this age the child's learning occurs primarily from:
    1. Playmates
    2. The parents
    3. Older siblings
    4. Trial and error

50. When talking with a client in crisis, the crisis intervention nurse should:
    1. Restate the problem, putting it in the proper perspective
    2. Respect the client and involve the client in deciding what will be done and how it will be done
    3. Explain to the client that the center has helped many other people with the same problem
    4. Explore the client's religious and cultural beliefs so the instructions are within the client's value system

51. A client at 39-weeks gestation arrives in the birthing suite stating she is having regular contractions. A vaginal examination identifies that the presentation is a double footling breech. A decision is made to proceed to a cesarean birth. An important nursing intervention to prevent postoperative complications would include:
    1. Providing scrupulous skin care
    2. Maintaining adequate hydration
    3. Notifying the neonatal intensive care unit

    4. Monitoring the maternal vital signs frequently

52. An obese 45-year-old adult develops an abscess after abdominal surgery. The wound is healing by secondary intention and requires repacking and redressing every four hours. To best meet this client's immediate nutritional needs, the daily diet should be:
    1. High in calories and fiber
    2. Low in residue and bland
    3. Low in fat and vitamin D
    4. High in protein and vitamin C

53. A client has a colon resection with an anastomosis. What assessments by the nurse would support a suspicion of impending shock? Check all that apply.
    1. _____ Fever
    2. _____ Oliguria
    3. _____ Lethargy
    4. _____ Irritability
    5. _____ Hypotension
    6. _____ Slurred speech
    7. _____ Bounding pulse
    8. _____ Cold, clammy skin

54. A client with newly diagnosed hyperthyroidism is treated with propylthiouracil, an antithyroid drug, along with potassium iodide. The nurse teaches the client about these medications with the knowledge that:
    1. Iodide solutions such as these must be taken on an empty stomach and diluted in water
    2. The use of these drugs prior to thyroidectomy will increase the risk of postoperative hemorrhage
    3. The client should carefully observe for signs of infection or bleeding while on this therapy
    4. These drugs will be discontinued as soon as the client's temperature and pulse rate return to normal

55. During a well-baby visit the nurse recognizes that an 18-month-old's growth and development is within the normal range when the child:
    1. Climbs up the stairs
    2. Pedals a tricycle easily
    3. Says 150 different words
    4. Builds a tower of 8 blocks

56. A young adolescent is diagnosed as having anorexia nervosa. The nurse is aware that anorexia nervosa is usually precipitated by:
    1. The acting out of aggressive impulses, which results in feelings of hopelessness
    2. An unconscious wish to punish a parent who tries to dominate the adolescent's life

3. The inability to deal with being the center of attention in the family and a desire for independence
4. An inaccurate perception of hunger stimuli and a struggle between dependence and independence

57. Shortly after an amniotomy, the nurse determines that the fetal heart rate has decreased from 140 to 80 beats per minute. The most urgent nursing action should be to:
1. Inspect the vagina
2. Notify the physician
3. Administer oxygen via nasal cannula
4. Place the client in the knee-chest position

58. When planning interventions to help a client with bipolar I disorder, manic episode meet needs for rest and sleep, the nurse should remember that the manic client:
1. Is easily stimulated by the environment
2. Experiences few sleep pattern disturbances
3. Requires less sleep than the average person
4. Needs to expend energy to be tired enough to sleep

59. The nurse understands that the primary goal of treatment for a child with developmental dysplasia of the hip would be to achieve:
1. Flexion of the hip
2. Extension of the hip
3. Adduction of the hip
4. Abduction of the hip

60. Many clients with schizophrenia experience opposing emotions simultaneously. The nurse recognizes this phenomenon as:
1. Double bind
2. Ambivalence
3. Loose association
4. Inappropriate affect

61. When the pediatric nurse practitioner examines the genital area of a 5-year-old child suspected of being sexually abused, the primary nurse can be most therapeutic by:
1. Explaining the procedure and remaining with the child during the examination
2. Telling the child that the practitioner wants to see if there is "anything wrong down there."
3. Helping the mother explain the examination and the findings in terms the child will understand
4. Asking whether the child would prefer the nurse or the mother to be present during the examination

62. A client in preterm labor is to receive a tocolytic medication, and bed rest is ordered. The nurse is aware that the most therapeutic position for the client would be the:
1. Supine
2. Lateral
3. Fowler's
4. Semi-Fowler's

63. A nurse is called upon to assist with an emergency home birth. To facilitate uterine contractions after the baby is born, the nurse should:
1. Have the mother breastfeed the baby
2. Push down vigorously on the fundus
3. Place gentle continuous tension on the cord
4. Encourage the mother to vigorously bear down

64. A client is diagnosed with an ectopic pregnancy. The nurse prepares the client for an immediate:
1. Hysterotomy
2. Myomectomy
3. Salpingostomy
4. Dilation and curettage

65. The nurse is caring for a client with dysuria. Urinary tract infection is the presumed diagnosis and a urine analysis is completed. The nurse is aware that the results exclusively indicating the development of infection would include the presence of:
1. Nitrate
2. Protein
3. Bilirubin
4. Erythrocytes

66. A 42-year-old female teacher has been admitted to the psychiatric unit with the diagnosis of bipolar I disorder, manic episode. Her physician has prescribed tiagabine hydrochloride (Gabatril). The side effects from this medication that the nurse can expect would be:
1. Dizziness, lethargy, and generalized weakness
2. Sensitivity to the sun, agitation, and restlessness
3. Abdominal cramps, tremors, and muscular weakness
4. Weight gain, drowsiness, and decreased concentration

67. When caring for a child with cystic fibrosis, the nurse plans to include times for postural drainage in the child's care plan. This therapy should be scheduled:
1. Once a day, after breakfast
2. Three times a day, before meals
3. Three times a day, halfway between meals
4. Two times a day, on awakening and at bedtime

68. When giving discharge instructions to the parents of a child with cystic fibrosis, the nurse realizes that further explanation about the problems caused by cystic fibrosis is needed when the parents state, "We will:
1. Keep our child in an air-conditioned room."
2. Give our child the pancreatic enzymes with meals."
3. Move to Florida where the climate is better for our child."
4. Provide our child skin care after each bowel movement."

69. A client who is to begin continuous peritoneal dialysis (CAPD) asks the nurse what this entails. The nurse's explanation includes information that:
1. There is a continuous hemodialysis and peritoneal dialysis
2. Peritoneal dialysis is performed in an ambulatory care clinic
3. There is continuous contact of dialysate with the peritoneal membrane
4. About a quarter of a liter of dialysate is maintained in the peritoneal cavity

70. A malnourished client with a history of cirrhosis is admitted to the hospital with nausea, ascites, and gastrointestinal bleeding. The nurse recognizes that the ascites primarily is a result of the client's malnourished state, especially the lack of adequate:
1. Iron to prevent proper hemoglobin synthesis
2. Vitamins to maintain cell coenzyme functions
3. Sodium to maintain its proper concentration in tissue fluid
4. Plasma protein to maintain proper capillary-tissue circulation

71. A client, at 38-weeks' gestation, is experiencing painless bleeding and has been diagnosed as having placenta previa. The client is concerned that she may have done something to cause the bleeding. Recognizing that the client appears worried, it would be most therapeutic for the nurse to say:
1. "You probably have a weak uterus."
2. "It's not your fault; these things happen."
3. "Don't worry; it's just a sign of beginning labor."
4. "The placenta is lying low and separates when you dilate."

72. When planning activities for a withdrawn, hallucinatory client, the nurse should recognize that it would be most therapeutic for the client to:
1. Go for a walk with the nurse
2. Watch a movie with other clients
3. Play cards with a group of clients
4. Play solitaire alone in the dayroom

73. A client with type 1 diabetes develops ketoacidosis. The laboratory value that would support a diagnosis of diabetic ketoacidosis would be:
1. A normal BUN
2. Elevated serum lipids
3. Low serum-calcium levels
4. A decreased hematocrit level

74. A client returns from surgery after a right below-the-knee amputation with the residual limb elevated on a pillow to prevent edema. After the first day, this client should be positioned:
1. Prone for short periods of time
2. With the residual limb immobilized
3. In the same position for two more days
4. On the right side, alternating with the low-Fowler's position

75. The nursing action most likely to reduce the pancreatic and gastric secretions of a client with pancreatitis would be:
1. Encouraging clear liquids
2. Obtaining an order for morphine sulfate
3. Administering anticholinergic medications
4. Assisting the client into a semi-Fowler's position

Part B Questions

76. A 66-year-old woman, whose history indicates a 30-pound weight loss in three months, as well as periods of constipation and diarrhea, has been diagnosed with cancer of the colon. The nurse is aware that malignant tumors of the colon and rectum are.
   1. Easily detected
   2. Usually localized
   3. Occur more frequently in women than in men
   4. The third most common cause of cancer in women

77. A 35-year-old client, who has type 1 diabetes and has been maintaining glycemic control, is pregnant for the third time. Her first child is 4 years old, and her second pregnancy resulted in a stillbirth. She is seen in the Antepartum Testing Unit for a non-stress test (NST) at 33-weeks' gestation. The nurse is aware that the client's history indicates that she is a candidate for an NST primarily because:
   1. The client is 35 years old
   2. The client is maintaining glycemic control
   3. An NST is indicated for high-risk clients with possible placental insufficiency
   4. An NST measures plasma levels of maternal estriols, which may indicate fetal distress

78. A client is worried about what to expect after having a pancreatoduodenectomy (Whipple procedure) for cancer of the pancreas. When assisting the client to plan, it would be most important for the nurse to know:
   1. Any history of alcohol or tobacco use
   2. The state and grade of the client's cancer
   3. Any previous exposure to known carcinogens
   4. The survival rate for individuals with pancreatic cancer

79. After a modified radical mastectomy, the nurse recognizes that a 36-year-old female client understands the schedule for self-examination of her remaining breast when she states she will carry out the procedure:
   1. Seven days after each menstrual period
   2. Several days before an expected menstrual period
   3. Halfway between menstrual periods, preferably after taking a shower
   4. The same date every month, regardless of when menstruation occurs

80. When assessing a child with leukemia, the nurse would expect:
   1. Epistaxis
   2. Tachycardia
   3. Flushing of the skin
   4. An elevated temperature

81. During the administration of total parenteral nutrition (TPN), an assessment of the client reveals a bounding pulse, distended jugular veins, dyspnea, and cough. The nurse should:
   1. Restart the infusion at another site
   2. Slow the rate of infusion of the TPN
   3. Interrupt the infusion and notify the physician
   4. Obtain the vital signs and continue monitoring the client's status

82. A client with pulmonary tuberculosis is to receive more than one anti-tubercular medication. Of the first-line medications being considered, the drug that could damage the eighth cranial nerve would be:
   1. Isoniazid (INH)
   2. Rifampin (Rifadin)
   3. Ethambutol (Myambutol)
   4. Streptomycin (Streptomycin)

83. The nurse should be aware that the defense mechanism a client with the diagnosis of schizophrenia, undifferentiated type, would most probably exhibit is:
   1. Projection
   2. Repression
   3. Regression
   4. Rationalization

84. After an automobile accident, a client who sustained multiple injuries is oriented as to person and place but is confused as to time. The client complains of a headache and drowsiness, but assessment reveals that the pupils are equal and reactive. A significant nursing intervention would be to:
   1. Keep the client alert and responsive
   2. Prevent unnecessary movement by the client
   3. Prepare the client for the administration of mannitol
   4. Monitor the client for symptoms of increased intracranial pressure

85. In discussions with the nurse, a school-age child recently diagnosed with type 1 diabetes learns that insulin acts by:
    1. Preventing the glucose from being stored in the liver
    2. Helping to carry glucose into cells where it is burned for energy
    3. Helping to break down protein and fat to provide needed glucose
    4. Preventing the wasting of blood glucose by converting it to glycogen

86. After an uneventful pregnancy, a client gives birth to a baby with a meningomyelocele. The baby has an Apgar score of 9/10. An immediate priority nursing care for this newborn would be:
    1. Administering oxygen by nasal catheter
    2. Protecting the sac with sterile, moist gauze
    3. Transferring the infant to the intensive care nursery
    4. Placing a name bracelet on the ankle and taking footprints

87. A depressed, suicidal client is placed on one-to-one observation. A short-term goal specific for this client's nursing care needs is that within:
    1. Two days the client will go for a walk on the grounds with others
    2. Two days the client will understand why there was a desire for suicide
    3. Three days the client will verbally accept responsibility for own actions
    4. Three days the client will understand the continued presence of a staff member

88. The physician orders a fetal scalp pH sample because of persistent abnormal fetal heart rate patterns. The nurse recognizes that the fetus may be compromised when the fetal pH is:
    1. 7.18
    2. 7.26
    3. 7.31
    4. 7.35

89. A client who is scheduled for a muscle biopsy tells the nurse, "They better give me a general anesthetic. I don't want to feel anything." The most therapeutic response by the nurse would be:
    1. "You seem to be worried about the test."
    2. "This test is done under local anesthesia."
    3. "Tell them when you have pain, and they'll take care of it."
    4. "Try not to think about it. I doubt that you will have any pain."

90. The nurse recognizes that a chelating agent used for lead poisoning would be:
    1. Calcium gluconate
    2. Lomustine (CCNU)
    3. Sodium bicarbonate
    4. Calcium disodium edetate (EDTA)

91. The condition of a child dying from leukemia deteriorates and the child becomes comatose. The parents state that a relative said they should not allow the child to be resuscitated, but that they are unsure about this. The response by the nurse that would best demonstrate a recognition of the ethical issues involved is:
    1. "Let me tell you about the implications of a DNR order, then you decide."
    2. "Have you talked to your physician about this yet? I'll be happy to page him."
    3. "You should discuss this thoroughly with your physician and with your religious adviser."
    4. "The final decision must be made by you and your physician, but it is important to talk about it."

92. Before a postpartum client is discharged, the nurse advises her about problems that should be reported to the physician. One of the problems the client should report would be:
    1. An increase in the quantity of lochia following activity
    2. Feelings of urgency, frequency, and burning on urination
    3. Development of breast engorgement and feelings of fullness
    4. Inadequate lubrication and some tenderness when intercourse is first resumed

93. In response to a client's question concerning the cause of polyarteritis nodosa, the nurse should state that:
    1. The disease affects both males and females in equal numbers
    2. With current therapy, clients with this disease have an excellent prognosis
    3. Arteriolar pathology of the disease affects only the kidneys and the retina of the eyes
    4. The disease is considered one of hypersensitivity, but the exact cause is unknown

94. A slightly overweight client is to be discharged from the hospital after a cholecystectomy. When teaching the client about nutrition, the priority intervention should be:
    1. Listing those fatty foods that may be included in the diet
    2. Explaining that fatty foods may not be tolerated for several weeks
    3. Teaching the importance of a low-calorie diet to promote weight reduction
    4. Encouraging the client to join a weight reduction program in the local community

95. A client is admitted to the hospital for acute gastritis and ascites secondary to alcoholism and cirrhosis. It is important for the nurse to assess this client routinely for:
1. Obstipation
2. Blood in the stool
3. Complaints of nausea
4. Any food intolerances

96. A client is at high risk for developing ascites. To assess for this condition the nurse should:
1. Observe for signs of respiratory distress
2. Percuss the abdomen, listening for dull sounds
3. Palpate the lower extremities over the tibia and observe for edema
4. Auscultate the abdomen, listening for decreased or absent bowel sounds

97. To further develop trust among members in a therapy group, the nurse plans to:
1. Reveal some personal data as a role model for trusting behavior
2. Remind group members about the need for confidentiality in the group
3. Have group members reveal some personal information about themselves
4. Bring up for discussion the need for and the importance of trusting each other

98. A male client with advanced AIDS tells the nurse that all he wants is to pass his high school equivalency test before he dies. He asks the nurse whether this is possible. The nurse's best approach would be to:
1. Refocus the conversation on the things the client has already accomplished in his life
2. Attempt to get the client to understand that his wish is too taxing and slightly unrealistic
3. Suggest to the client that he use this energy to work through his unexpressed anger at dying
4. Set up a study schedule with the client and offer to work with him in preparing for the test

99. The nurse understands that a 4-year-old child's greatest fear related to hospitalization usually is the fear of:
1. Bodily harm
2. Loss of control
3. Loss of independence
4. Separation from the mother

100. Nursing care for a child admitted to the hospital with acute glomerulonephritis should be directed toward:
1. Encouraging fluids
2. Promoting diuresis
3. Enforcing strict bed rest
4. Eliminating sodium from the diet

101. A 5-month-old is brought to the pediatric clinic because of probable exposure to an adolescent sibling with measles. The infant's mother anxiously asks the clinic nurse whether the baby can be vaccinated against measles at this age. The nurse's reply should take into consideration the history of:
1. Immunization of this baby
2. Previous viral illnesses of this baby
3. Maternal diseases and immunizations
4. Preexisting tuberculosis of the mother

102. A client has an open reduction and internal fixation of the hip. The client is to be transferred to a chair on the second postoperative day for a half hour. Before the transfer, the nurse should:
1. Assess the strength of the affected leg
2. Explain how the transfer will be accomplished
3. Encourage the client to keep the affected leg elevated
4. Instruct the client to bear weight evenly on both legs

103. A 2-year-old child, previously diagnosed with hemophilia, has been admitted to the hospital unit for observation after a motor vehicle accident. The child has a few bruises but no other apparent injuries. The most specific appropriate nursing diagnosis for this child would be Risk for:
1. Falls
2. Injury
3. Infection
4. Deficient fluid volume

104. A client who has been on IV magnesium sulfate therapy for preeclampsia gives birth to an infant weighing 4 lb in the 37th week of gestation. The nurse is aware that a finding in the newborn that may indicate magnesium sulfate toxicity would be:
1. Pallor
2. Tremors
4. Hypotonia
3. A pulse of 200 beats/min

105. A teenager, hospitalized with preeclampsia, is anorectic and appears depressed. The nurse plans to further explore the client's emotional status when the client comments:
1. "I'm tired of feeling so clumsy."
2. "I'll be glad when I can sleep all night."
3. "I dreamed my baby had only one arm."
4. "I was really happy before I got pregnant."

106. A client who has been diagnosed with atherosclerosis and hypertension always has been an active individual. The client is interested in measures that would help maintain health. The nurse explains that maintenance of vessel patency can be promoted by:
    1. Practicing relaxation techniques
    2. Leading a more sedentary lifestyle
    3. Decreasing the amount of exercise
    4. Increasing saturated fats in the diet

107. The nurse teaches a client with hypertension to reduce dietary sodium. The nurse should emphasize that:
    1. Salt-free natural seasonings can be used and taste the same as salt
    2. The taste for salt is inherent but it can be overcome with practice
    3. The taste for table salt is learned and increases over time, but it is not a biologic necessity
    4. Salt substitutes with potassium chloride bases can be used freely with foods to provide the same taste

108. The nurse in the birthing room when assessing a newborn knows that an Apgar value of 2 should be assigned to:
    1. A strong, lusty cry
    2. Body pink, extremities blue
    3. Arms and legs slightly flexed
    4. Heart rate of 90 beats per minute

109. When preparing a toddler with celiac disease for discharge, the nurse should caution the parents that a typical characteristic that would make their child most susceptible to a celiac crisis is:
    1. Invention
    2. Autonomy
    3. Narcissism
    4. Negativism

110. The nurse is aware that 60% of brain tumors in children result in symptoms of increased intracranial pressure and are most commonly found in the:
    1. Cortex
    2. Cerebellum
    3. Temporal lobe
    4. Subarachnoid space

111. The mother of a preschooler with acute glomerulonephritis asks the nurse whether her child will have to stay in bed. The nurse should tell the mother that bed rest:
    1. Is no longer part of the usual treatment no longer during the acute phase

    2. Is limited to 72 hours after the institution of antihypertensive drug therapy
    3. Will be necessary for three to four weeks, regardless of the response to therapy
    4. Is needed until the child's blood pressure decreases and the hematuria has lessened

112. Cor pulmonale is a common complication of COPD. The sign that would lead the nurse to suspect that the client is developing cor pulmonale would be:
    1. Peripheral edema
    2. A productive cough
    3. Twitching of the extremities
    4. Lethargy progressing to coma

113. A client has chest tubes inserted to treat a hemopneumothorax that resulted from a crushing chest injury. When connecting the water-seal drainage system ordered, the nurse must understand that the chamber attached to the chest tube provides the:
    1. Suction
    2. Water seal
    3. Seal and suction
    4. Drainage receptacle

114. The nurse should plan to involve a client with anorexia nervosa in activities that will:
    1. Save the client's depleted energy
    2. Force the client into decision making
    3. Focus the client on sexual attractiveness
    4. Provide the client with peer group involvement

115. A client with the diagnosis of obsessive-compulsive disorder who has a need to wash the hands about 50 to 60 times a day tearfully tells the nurse, "I know my hands are not dirty, but I just can't stop washing them." The nurse's best response would be:
    1. "Let's talk about why you feel you must wash your hands."
    2. "I think you're getting better; you're beginning to understand your problem."
    3. "Don't worry about it; these actions are part of your illness, and these feelings will pass."
    4. "I understand that, but maybe we can work together to limit the number of times you wash them."

116. An 18-month-old child is visiting the clinic for scheduled immunizations. The vaccine that the nurse would expect to administer is the:
    1. First pneumococcal (PCV) vaccine
    2. Second hepatitis B (HepB) vaccine

3. Fifth inactivated polio (IPV) vaccine

4. Fourth diphtheria, tetanus, pertussis (DTaP) vaccine

117. When performing the initial assessment of a client in ketoacidosis the nurse notes:
    1. Nervousness and cool, pale skin
    2. Erythema toxicum rash and pruritus
    3. Deep respirations and fruity odor to the breath
    4. Diaphoresis and instability as with intoxication

118. The nurse would be aware that a therapy group had reached the working stage when the members:
    1. Appear happy in their group interactions
    2. Focus on a wide variety of needs and concerns
    3. Show concern for the feelings of the group leaders
    4. Say and do what is expected and wanted by the others

119. A client, pregnant for the first time, questions the nurse about all the changes in her body. The nurse, when explaining these changes, is aware that the most profound change of all during pregnancy occurs in the:
    1. Urinary system
    2. Endocrine system
    3. Cardiovascular system
    4. Gastrointestinal system

120. Without knocking, the nurse enters the room of a young male client with the diagnosis of panic disorder and observes him masturbating. The nurse should:
    1. Say, "Excuse me," and leave the room
    2. Tactfully assess why he needs to masturbate
    3. Pretend nothing was seen and carry out whatever task needs to be done
    4. Explain in a calm, quiet manner that his behavior is inappropriate in the hospital

121. After a modified radical mastectomy a female client tells the nurse, "This diagnosis is as good as a death sentence, and I would rather go now than to suffer." At this time it would be most important for the nurse to:
    1. Recommend that the client admit herself to the psychiatric unit of the hospital
    2. Determine whether the client has experienced self-destructive or suicidal thoughts
    3. Explore the possibility of a vacation after hospitalization to reduce the client's stress level

4. Encourage the client to think positively and to try and focus on the good things in her life

122. A client with Crohn's disease is to have an upper gastrointestinal series. The nurse understands that an upper GI series with barium would be contraindicated if the client had:
    1. Hemorrhoids
    2. A perforation
    3. Hyperkalemia
    4. An inflamed colon

123. While obtaining a health history from a client newly diagnosed with cervical cancer, it would be most important for the nurse to determine the client's:
    1. Sexual history
    2. Support system
    3. Obstetrical history
    4. Elimination patterns

124. A client's contraction stress test (CST) is positive and identifies potential problems. The nurse understands that a positive test:
    1. Indicates the need to perform a nonstress test
    2. Indicates the need for an immediate cesarean birth
    3. Showed a fetal heart rate of 110 to 140 beats per minute
    4. Showed late decelerations of the fetal heart rate with contractions

125. A male client with the diagnosis of schizophrenia, paranoid type, often displays overt sexual behavior toward female clients and nurses. The nurses can best respond to the client's behavior by:
    1. Refusing to speak with the client until he stops this behavior
    2. Sending the client to his room when the behavior is observed
    3. Matter-of-factly telling the client that his behavior is unacceptable
    4. Ignoring this behavior until the client is more in control of his responses

126. A client develops bronchopneumonia. To help determine the effectiveness of therapy, the nurse should refer to the results of the client's:
    1. Lung scan
    2. Bronchoscopy
    3. Pulmonary function studies
    4. Culture and sensitivity tests of sputum

127. During the administration of an enema prior to gastrointestinal surgery, a client complains of cramps. The nurse should:
    1. Discontinue the enema and try again at a later time
    2. Lower the container to the floor to decrease intestinal pressure
    3. Close the lumen of the tubing until the client's cramps subside
    4. Administer the enema rapidly to permit a quicker evacuation of fluid

128. A mother, whose infant was diagnosed with cerebral palsy at 6 months of age, asks why she was not told that her baby had cerebral palsy when the infant was born. The nurse should reply:
    1. "Joint deformities of cerebral palsy appear only after 6 months of age."
    2. "The health care personnel in the clinic did not want to alarm you until it was necessary."
    3. "Neurologic lesions responsible for this condition may have changed as your baby matured."
    4. "Early diagnosis of cerebral palsy is difficult in infants until they develop control of voluntary movements."

129. A 2-year-old child is admitted with gastroenteritis and dehydration. The physician orders peripheral intravenous fluids. The most appropriate site for the first intravenous insertion would be the:
    1. Scalp veins
    2. Venous arch on the top of the foot
    3. Basilic vein at the antecubital fossa
    4. Dorsal metacarpals on the back of the hand

130. A grand multigravida at 34-weeks' gestation is brought to the emergency department by her husband because she is experiencing vaginal bleeding. The nurse would suspect that the client had a placenta previa if the bleeding were:
    1. Painful vaginal bleeding in the first trimester
    2. Painful vaginal bleeding in the third trimester
    3. Painless vaginal bleeding in the first trimester
    4. Painless vaginal bleeding in the third trimester

131. A female client who has been delusional is found staring at the television set, which is on. The client suddenly rises and shouts, "Stop saying that. Who do you think you are?" It would be most therapeutic for the nurse to:
    1. Point out to her the inappropriateness of her behavior
    2. Attempt to distract the client by taking her for a walk
    3. Take the client to her room so she can have a quiet place to think
    4. Tell her that the voices she hears are coming from the television set

132. A female client has terminal cancer. Her family is concerned because she appears to be accepting less and less responsibility for her own care. To help family members plan for her care, the nurse should:
    1. Point out that denial is a normal response and will be temporary
    2. Assist them to identify methods to give her more control over the situation
    3. Encourage them to accept her regression until she can cope more effectively
    4. Explain that her anger is normal and identify ways for the family to deal with it

133. A client has a paracentesis, and the physician removes 1500 mL of fluid. It is essential that the nurse observe the client for:
    1. A hypertensive crisis
    2. Abdominal distention
    3. An increased pulse rate
    4. Dry mucous membranes

134. A client is scheduled for an amniocentesis. Before the procedure, the nurse should:
    1. Remind the client to empty her bladder
    2. Instruct the client to take nothing by mouth
    3. Give the client the ordered sedation to minimize fetal movement
    4. Administer a Fleet enema to the client to prevent contamination

135. An episiotomy is performed to facilitate a vaginal birth and prevent tearing of maternal tissues. The physician orders sitz baths three times a day after the first 24 hours. The nurse should include in the teaching plan that sitz baths promote healing by:
    1. Promoting vasodilation
    2. Softening the incision site
    3. Cleansing the perineal area
    4. Tightening the rectal sphincter

136. A client with osteoporosis is encouraged to drink milk. The client refuses the milk, explaining that it causes gassiness and bloating. A food rich in calcium that may be digested easily by clients who do not tolerate milk would be:
    1. Eggs
    2. Yogurt
    3. Potatoes
    4. Bananas

137. A client receiving steroid therapy states, "I have had difficulty controlling my temper, which is so unlike me, and I don't know why this is happening." The nurse's best response would be to:
1. Tell the client it is nothing to worry about
2. Encourage the client to talk further about these findings
3. Instruct the client to attempt to avoid situations that cause irritation
4. Try to determine whether the client has been experiencing other mood swings

138. A client has a femoral-popliteal bypass graft. Four hours after surgery the client's blood pressure is 200/110. The nurse should notify the physician immediately because the:
1. Graft could rupture
2. Client is anaphylactic
3. Client is hypervolemic
4. Graft may be occluded

139. The nurse has been working for the past three months with a 10-year-old client who has a diagnosis of conduct disorder. The evaluative statement that would show a resolution of expected problems for this child would be, the child has:
1. Verbalized ten alternative methods to address anger
2. Avoided verbally aggressive behavior for three months
3. Been sent to the principal's office three times in five weeks
4. Had no physically aggressive episodes during the last three months

140. When assessing a client who has a history of several myocardial infarctions, the nurse is aware that the most common early indication of right ventricular failure would be:
1. Bradypnea
2. Chest pain
3. Bradycardia
4. Peripheral edema

141. A biopsy of a brain tumor removed from a child identifies the tumor as a cerebellar astrocytoma. The nurse is aware that this tumor is:
1. Fast growing and highly malignant
2. Benign and associated with a high rate of cure
3. A cause of pituitary malfunction as the child grows
4. Close to vital centers and only partial excision is possible

142. A 9-year-old is admitted to the hospital with a diagnosis of possible infratentorial brain tumor. The nurse identifies the common presenting sign of this type of tumor when the child demonstrates:
1. Ataxia
2. Seizures
3. Papilledema
4. Cranial enlargement

143. One morning a male client, whose thought processes are marked by ideas of reference and persecutory ideation, appears very upset. The client tells the nurse that the reporter on television told everyone that the client is "a queer." The most therapeutic response by the nurse would be:
1. "It sounds to me like you're having some frightening feelings."
2. "I will call the station and ask why the reporter said that about you."
3. "You seem upset by this. Why do you think the reporter said that about you?"
4. "Sometimes when we are unsure of ourselves we project our feelings on others."

144. When preparing a teaching plan for the parents of a child with celiac disease, the nurse recalls that the basic problem in celiac disease is the:
1. Presence of meconium stool
2. Clumping of the intestinal villi
3. Absence of the enzyme peptidase
4. Susceptibility to profound dehydration

145. The nurse is caring for an observant Jewish client one day after surgery. The diet has been increased from full liquid to a general diet as tolerated. The nurse should remember that:
1. Eating fish with scales is prohibited
2. The use of beef and veal is prohibited
3. A combination of meat and milk is prohibited
4. Consuming alcohol, coffee, and tea are prohibited

146. The best nursing action to prevent heat loss in the neonate would be to:
1. Administer oxygen to prevent shivering
2. Dress the baby in a shirt and gown immediately
3. Bathe the infant in warm water as soon as possible after birth
4. Maintain skin-to-skin contact between mother and baby under a cover

147. A client at 20-weeks' gestation visits the prenatal clinic for the first time. Assessment reveals T, 98.8°F; P, 80; BP, 128/80; weight, 142 pounds (prepregnancy weight was 132 pounds); FHR, 140 beats per minute; urine negative for protein; and a fasting blood glucose of 92 mg/dL. After making these assessments the nurse should:
    1. Report the findings because the client needs immediate intervention
    2. Document the observations because they are expected at 20-weeks' gestation
    3. Record and report these findings, since they are not within the norm but are not critical
    4. Prepare the client for an emergency admission, since these findings may jeopardize the mother and fetus

148. A male client, accompanied by his wife, is admitted to the psychiatric unit with a diagnosis of schizophrenia. The nurse's priority intervention should be to:
    1. Observe and evaluate his behavior
    2. Obtain a copy of the admission history
    3. Write a plan of care for the health team
    4. Meet with his wife and explore why he was admitted

149. A young pregnant client, who has been noncompliant with her prenatal visits, is admitted to the birthing unit complaining of contractions. Assessment of the client reveals a nutritional deficit. A physical finding that can be related to inadequate protein intake would be:
    1. Petechiae
    2. Bradycardia
    3. Bleeding gums
    4. Significant nondependent edema

150. The nurse caring for a 32-week appropriate-for-gestational age (AGA) neonate establishes a list of potential interventions for the infant. The intervention that is the priority would be:
    1. Promoting bonding
    2. Preventing infection
    3. Maintaining respirations
    4. Supporting body temperature

151. After several days on bed rest, a preschooler with the diagnosis of acute glomerulonephritis becomes demanding and will not listen to the nurses. The child was found in the playroom twice on the previous shift. To best meet the needs of this child the nurse should:
    1. Ask the child not to get up again and explain the reason for bed rest

    2. Place soft restraints on the child when family members cannot be present
    3. Have a color television set moved into the child's room as soon as possible
    4. Move the child into a room with another preschooler who has a liver laceration

152. When assessing a client after a thyroidectomy, the nurse should understand that:
    1. Hypercalcemia could result from parathyroid damage
    2. Hypotension and bradycardia could result from thyroid crisis
    3. Tetany could result from underdosage of thyroid hormone replacement
    4. Hoarseness and airway obstruction could result from laryngeal nerve damage

153. A client returns from the post-anesthesia care unit after a radical neck dissection. To facilitate respirations and promote comfort the client should be placed in the:
    1. Sims' position
    2. Side-lying position
    3. Orthopneic position
    4. Semi-Fowler's position

154. A client with cancer of the stomach is scheduled for a subtotal gastrectomy. Nursing intervention directed toward minimizing the postoperative complication of dumping syndrome includes teaching the client to:
    1. Ambulate after every meal
    2. Remain on a diet low in fat
    3. Eat in a semirecumbent position
    4. Increase the fluid intake with meals

155. When teaching the parents of an 8-year-old with newly diagnosed type 1 diabetes, the nurse should tell them that with type 1 diabetes, it is common to develop:
    1. Obesity
    2. Ketoacidosis
    3. Resistance to treatment
    4. Hypersensitivity to other drugs

156. An 11-year-old has just been diagnosed with type 1 diabetes. The child, who likes sweets, asks about sugar and sugar substitutes in the diet. The nurse and the dietitian should tell the child that:
    1. Honey can be used as a natural sugar substitute
    2. Simple sugars such as sucrose or fructose should be avoided

3. The sweet taste habit can be broken by eliminating sweets altogether
4. Sugar substitutes such as saccharin, aspartame, or sucralose can be used

157. The parents of a child who recently has been diagnosed with leukemia ask the nurse why the physician said that their child had too many white blood cells. The nurse's best response would be:
    1. "You seem to be focusing on your child's white blood cells."
    2. "Your doctor is the best one to answer that question for you."
    3. "It sounds like you really do not understand what occurs in leukemia."
    4. "The bone marrow isn't working properly and makes too many white blood cells."

158. A full-term neonate born with a meningomyelocele is scheduled for surgery. The priority preoperative nursing goal is to make certain that this baby:
    1. Remains sedated
    2. Gains 1 ounce per day
    3. Continues infection-free
    4. Develops a strong sucking reflex

159. The nurse manager of the unit comes to work obviously drunk. The staff nurse's ethical obligation is to:
    1. Call the security guard
    2. Tell the nurse manager to go home
    3. Have the supervisor validate the observation
    4. Walk the nurse manager around and offer coffee

160. The nurse is concerned with a client's mothering ability when on the first postpartum day she refuses to:
    1. Breastfeed the newborn
    2. Undress and inspect the infant
    3. Attend classes for new mothers
    4. Look at the face when holding the baby

161. After head and neck surgery, hyperextension of the neck for the first few postoperative days may cause:
    1. Cervical trauma
    2. Laryngeal spasm
    3. Laryngeal edema
    4. Wound dehiscence

162. When checking the cervical dilation of a client in labor, the nurse notices that the umbilical cord has prolapsed. The nurse's first action should be to:
    1. Take the fetal heart rate
    2. Turn the client on her side
    3. Cover the cord with sterile saline soaks
    4. Put the client in the Trendelenburg position

163. After abdominal surgery a goal is to have the client achieve alveolar expansion. This goal would be most effectively achieved by:
    1. Postural drainage
    2. Pursed-lip breathing
    3. Incentive spirometry
    4. Prolonged exhalation

164. A young woman comes to the mental health clinic because she has lost her job and does not know what to do. The history reveals that the client lives alone and her family lives in another state. The client states she feels like a failure. An appropriate nursing diagnosis for this client probably would be:
    1. Risk for self-directed violence related to panic state
    2. Disturbed thought processes related to impaired judgment
    3. Social isolation related to absence of satisfying personal relationships
    4. Disturbed personal identity related to inability to distinguish self from nonself

165. A client with advanced cancer of the bladder is scheduled for a cystectomy and ileal conduit. Physical preparation for the surgery should include:
    1. Instillation of urinary antiseptics
    2. Insertion of an indwelling catheter
    3. A well-balanced diet with vitamins
    4. Administration of neomycin sulfate

166. A hospitalized client, diagnosed with an obsessive-compulsive disorder, tells the nurse that co-workers and roommates get upset because at least 30 minutes are spent in the bathroom six times a day. The client states, "This prevents me from getting nervous." The nurse's most appropriate response would be:
    1. "That is not a problem now because you have your own bathroom here."
    2. "Explain how spending time in the bathroom helps you avoid becoming nervous."
    3. "Tell me more about what you do in the bathroom during those 30-minute periods."
    4. "We can compromise. Let's start by cutting down the time you spend in the bathroom to 20 minutes three times a day."

167. After an automobile accident in which a child sustained a fractured femur, the laboratory blood tests of the child indicate a slight decrease in hemoglobin and hematocrit levels. The most appropriate nursing action would be to:
    1. Order a type and crossmatch
    2. Notify the physician immediately
    3. Provide additional meat for dinner
    4. Assess the child's abdomen for internal bleeding

168. In her eighth month of gestation, a client's membranes spontaneously rupture but she does not have contractions. Specific nursing care for clients with ruptured membranes should include:
    1. Monitoring temperature frequently
    2. Observing for signs of preeclampsia
    3. Assessing for heavy vaginal bleeding
    4. Preparing for fetal scalp pH sampling

169. The physician prescribes the drug cholestyramine (Questran), an anion exchange resin used to treat a client's persistent diarrhea. This drug reduces the absorption of fat, which may produce a deficiency of:
    1. Thiamine
    2. Vitamin A
    3. Riboflavin
    4. Vitamin B_6

170. A client is diagnosed with acute lymphoid leukemia and is receiving chemotherapy. The nurse must monitor the client for the thrombocytopenic side effects associated with chemotherapy. Check all those that must be considered.
    1. _____ Fever
    2. _____ Nausea
    3. _____ Melena
    4. _____ Purpura
    5. _____ Diarrhea
    6. _____ Hematuria

171. When reviewing the breast self-examination procedure with a client, the comment by the client that the nurse should consider significant is, "My:
    1. Bra feels tight when I am menstruating."
    2. Breasts feel lumpy just before menstruation."
    3. Left breast was always slightly larger than my right."
    4. Right breast feels and looks thicker than my left breast."

172. A terminally ill client is furious with one of the staff nurses. Over the next several days the client refuses the nurse's care and insists on doing self-care. A different nurse is assigned to care for the client. The nurse's initial step in revising the nursing care plan to meet the client's needs would be to:
    1. Get a full report from the first nurse and adjust the plan accordingly
    2. Ask the physician for a report on the client's condition and plan accordingly
    3. Tell the client about the change in staff responsibilities and assess the client's reaction
    4. Assess the client's present status and capabilities and include the client in a discussion of revisions of the care plan

173. A client who has been admitted with the diagnosis of severe preeclampsia is now receiving an intravenous infusion of magnesium sulfate. The nurse is aware that this medication is classified as:
    1. A diuretic
    2. An oxytocic
    3. An antihypertensive
    4. A central nervous system depressant

174. The nursing care plan for a client who is being admitted to the hospital with a diagnosis of abruptio placentae should include careful assessment for signs and symptoms of:
    1. Jaundice
    2. Hypertension
    3. Impending seizures
    4. Hypovolemic shock

175. When developing a plan of care for an older client with a diagnosis of dementia, the nurse should:
    1. Explain to the client the details of the therapeutic regimen
    2. Demonstrate interest in the client's various likes and dislikes
    3. Be firm when dealing with the client's attitudes and behaviors
    4. Provide consistency in carrying out nursing activities for the client

176. While supervising a smallpox vaccination program, the nurse manager observes a nurse cleansing the arm of a client with an alcohol swab before giving the vaccination. The nurse manager's first reaction would be to:
    1. Continue observing the vaccination clinic
    2. Give the nurse a povidone swab to use instead
    3. Stop the nurse from giving the vaccination to the client

4. Notify all members of the vaccination team about the use of swabs

177. A child with a puncture wound, whose history of immunizations is uncertain, is given tetanus immune human globulin. The nurse knows that the chief reason for using tetanus immune human globulin instead of tetanus antitoxin is that it is:
   1. As effective as the antitoxin
   2. More convenient to administer
   3. Not likely to cause anaphylaxis
   4. Safe to give to everyone who needs it

178. A 2½-year-old is admitted to the hospital with a fever of 103° F, stiffness of the neck, and generalized malaise. The child is diagnosed as having acute bacterial meningitis. Priority nursing care for this child would include:
   1. Increasing fluids
   2. Administering oxygen
   3. Instituting droplet precautions
   4. Giving the child a tepid sponge bath

179. A client with a fractured tibia and fibula is to be discharged with a right leg cast and crutches. In addition to teaching the technical aspects of crutch walking, the nurse plans to advise the client to:
   1. Increase intake of vitamin C to enhance healing
   2. Avoid taking showers until the cast is removed
   3. Gradually increase weight bearing on the injured leg
   4. Remove loose rugs and rearrange furniture as necessary

180. X-ray films reveal that a client has closed fractures of the right femur and tibia. Multiple soft-tissue contusions also are present. An important short-term intervention would be to:
   1. Prepare the client for application of skeletal traction
   2. Reassure the client that these injuries are not that serious
   3. Prepare the client for operative reduction of the injured extremity
   4. Assess the circulatory, motor, and sensory status of the client's injured extremity

181. A client with bilateral varicose veins of the lower extremities questions the nurse about the brownish discoloration of the lower legs. The nurse should explain that this is probably the result of:
   1. An inadequate arterial blood supply

2. Delayed healing of tissues after an injury
3. Leakage of RBCs through the vascular wall
4. Increased production of melanin in the area

182. The nurse evaluates that the mother of a 10-week-old infant is demonstrating an understanding of her infant's postoperative needs after a cleft lip repair when she:
   1. Allows the infant to cry for short periods
   2. Cleanses the suture line after each feeding
   3. Offers a pacifier when the infant becomes restless
   4. Gives the feeding while the infant is in a side-lying position

183. A pregnant client is classified as a having Class II cardiac disease. To best plan her care, the nurse should understand that the client:
   1. Can participate in as much activity as she desires
   2. Should be hospitalized if there is evidence of cardiac decompensation
   3. Will have to be on bed rest for most of the day during her pregnancy
   4. May have to consider a therapeutic abortion because her life is in danger

184. A client comes into the emergency department with neurologic deficits after falling from a ladder while painting a house. The nurse uses the Glasgow coma scale to assess the client. The responses the nurse would assess are:
   1. Pupil response to light, verbal response to speech, and tendon reflexes
   2. Eye accommodation to light, tendon reflexes, and breathing pattern
   3. Motor response to verbal command, eye opening in response to speech, and breathing pattern
   4. Eye opening in response to speech, motor response to verbal command, and verbal response to speech

185. A client presents to the medical clinic with a history of headaches. The nurse measures the blood pressure at 172/114. The nurse should:
   1. Page the on-call physician and monitor the blood pressure
   2. Administer Motrin and have the client rest quietly for twenty minute
   3. Elevate the head of the bed, provide reassurance, and reassess the blood pressure
   4. Place the client in the supine position, administer oxygen, and notify the physician

186. The results of a biopsy indicate a client has a malignant sarcoma of the liver, and chemotherapy via regional perfusion is the treatment of choice. This method of drug administration probably was selected for this client because:
    1. The drug therapy can be continued at home with little difficulty
    2. Larger doses of drugs can be delivered to the actual site of the tumor
    3. Combinations of drugs can be used to attack neoplastic cells at various stages of the cell cycle
    4. The toxic effects of the chemotherapeutic drugs will be confined to the area of the tumor

187. When caring for a child in acute respiratory distress from laryngotracheobronchitis who has a temperature of 103° F the nurse should give priority to:
    1. Delivering 40% humidified oxygen
    2. Initiating measures to reduce the fever
    3. Constantly assessing the child's respiratory status
    4. Providing support to reduce the child's apprehension

188. When assessing a client for the development of increased intracranial pressure, an early sign of this complication for which the nurse should observe would be:
    1. Nausea
    2. Lethargy
    3. Sunset eyes
    4. Hyperthermia

189. After an open reduction and internal fixation of a hip fracture in an older individual, the assessment that requires immediate nursing intervention would be:
    1. Complaints of pain in the chest six days postoperatively
    2. A rectal temperature of 100.2° F three days postoperatively
    3. An inability to cough productively two days postoperatively
    4. Fatigue in the leg on the unaffected side five days postoperatively

190. A client scheduled for surgery has a history of methicillin-resistant staphylococcus aureus (MRSA) since developing an infection in a surgical site nine months ago. The site is healed and the client reports having received antibiotics for the infection. To determine if the infecting organism is present the nurse should:
    1. Notify the infection control officer

2. Inform the operating room of the MRSA
    3. Obtain an order to culture the client's blood
    4. Call the surgeon for an infectious disease consultation

191. A 13-year-old child in vaso-occlusive sickle-cell crisis has a hematocrit of 23.2%, hemoglobin of 8.1 g/dL, and pulse oximetry of 92% on room air. The intervention that has the highest priority in the initial care of this child would be the administration of:
    1. An analgesic
    2. Oxygen therapy
    3. Intravenous fluids
    4. A blood transfusion

192. The nurse is concerned when an 11-month-old girl is brought to the clinic weighing 9 pounds, 3 ounces. The 17-year-old mother appears very jittery and never looks directly at her baby or provides any comforting. The priority nursing intervention would be to:
    1. Determine if the mother had been physically abused as a child
    2. Request that the mother give a description of the infant's behavior
    3. Ascertain how the mother copes with stress and the availability of a support system
    4. Inform the mother that her child would gain weight if stimulation, affection, and food were adequate

193. When auscultating the lungs of a client admitted with severe preeclampsia, the nurse notices the presence of crackles and is aware that this can be an indication that:
    1. A seizure is imminent
    2. Pulmonary edema has developed
    3. The stress of pregnancy precipitated bronchial constriction
    4. Her enlarged uterus has impaired diaphragmatic functioning

194. After surgery for repair of a myelomeningocele, the nurse places the newborn in a side-lying position with the head slightly elevated because it:
    1. Prevents aspiration
    2. Promotes respiration
    3. Keeps the suture site clean
    4. Reduces intracranial pressure

195. A 44-year-old client has been unable to function since her husband asked for a divorce two weeks ago. She is brought to the crisis intervention center by a friend. The nurse would identify this client's crisis as:
    1. Social

2. Situational
3. Maturational
4. Developmental

196. A client develops subcutaneous emphysema after a laryngectomy. This is most readily detected by:
1. Palpating the neck or face
2. Evaluating the blood gases
3. Auscultating the lung fields
4. Reviewing the chest x-ray film

197. A client who complains of memory loss, nervousness, insomnia, and fear of going out of the house is admitted to the hospital after several days of increasing incapacitation. Initially, considering this client's history, the nurse should give priority to:
1. Evaluating the client's adjustment to the unit
2. Providing the client with a sense of security and safety
3. Exploring the client's memory loss and fear of going out
4. Assessing the precipitating factors for the client's hospitalization

198. After gastric surgery a client has a nasogastric tube in place. The nurse should plan to:
1. Change the tube at least once every 48 hours
2. Monitor the client for signs of electrolyte imbalance
3. Connect the nasogastric tube to high continuous suction
4. Assess placement by injecting 10 mL of water into the tube

199. A 9-year-old, recently diagnosed as having type 2 diabetes, attends the center for diabetic teaching with the parents. The nurse notes that the child's concerns about the illness center on:
1. How the parents will react to the diagnosis of the disease
2. How much school might have to be missed because of the disease
3. Whether or not the physician will be successful in controlling the diabetes
4. Whether having diabetes means it will be impossible to have children as an adult

200. A client comes to the clinic complaining of a productive cough with copious yellow sputum, fever, and chills for the past two days. The first thing the nurse should do when caring for this client is to:
1. Administer oxygen
2. Begin to push fluids

3. Collect a sputum specimen
4. Take the client's temperature

201. The nurse admits a client with a diagnosis of cholelithiasis for scheduled surgery. The client asks many questions about the postoperative course after laparoscopic surgery. Teaching should include:
1. Long-term dietary restrictions
2. Postoperative abdominal exercises
3. Surgical incisions and wound care
4. Explanation of abdominal and scapular pain

202. Twenty-four hours after a client is admitted with partial-thickness burns over 30% of the body surface, the client, who has an IV of 5% dextrose in saline running, shows signs of tremors, twitching, and disorientation. During the last hour, the urinary output was 110 mL. The nurse should:
1. Slow the IV rate and notify the physician
2. Slow the IV rate and check the last chest x-ray film
3. Increase the IV rate and assess the arterial blood gases
4. Increase the IV rate and request an order for calcium gluconate

203. When planning for a client's care during the detoxification phase of acute alcohol withdrawal, the nurse should anticipate the need to:
1. Supervise the client continuously
2. Keep the client's room lights dim
3. Speak to the client in a loud, clear voice
4. Restrain the client during periods of agitation

204. A client with Hodgkin's disease is to receive the cyclic antineoplastic vincristine (Oncovin) as part of a therapy protocol. The nurse understands that Oncovin helps destroy the malignant cells by:
1. Arresting mitosis in metaphase
2. Inhibiting the synthesis of pyrimidine
3. Alkylating nucleic acids needed for mitosis
4. Inactivating DNA and inhibiting RNA synthesis

205. During the postoperative period after a craniotomy for the removal of an astrocytoma, a child develops a sudden right pupillary dilation. The nurse recognizes this as a sign of:
1. Severe pain
2. Intense fear
3. Uncal herniation
4. Reduced intracranial pressure

206. A primigravida who is in the active phase of labor demonstrates irritability, an increased bloody show, moderate to intense contractions every two minutes that last 60 to 90 seconds, and complains of nausea. The nurse determines that the client is in the phase of labor known as:
1. Early first
2. Transition
3. Early third
4. Late second

207. A young mother, who brings a 9-month-old infant with developmental lags significantly below the expected to the clinic, appears very nervous and avoids eye contact with the infant. The nurse should be alert for signs of stress between the mother and child as well as the level of anxiety in the mother because:
1. The pediatric history may have incomplete or incorrect information.
2. The birthing experience may not have been conducive to parent-child bonding
3. Consideration should be given to the needs of the mother in her child-rearing role
4. The present findings have little relationship to the mother's past history or present health

208. A 16-year-old girl with sickle-cell disease is now in vaso-occlusive crisis and has a patient-controlled analgesia (PCA) pump. She complains of severe pain (10 on a scale of 1-10) in her right elbow. The nurse observes that the pump is "locked out" for another 10 minutes. The nurse should:
1. Turn on the television for a diversion
2. Place a warm wet compress on the elbow
3. Call the physician for another analgesic order
4. Gently tell the client that she must wait another 10 minutes

209. When lithium therapy is instituted, the nurse should teach the client to maintain an adequate daily intake of:
1. Iron
2. Sodium
3. Potassium
4. Magnesium

210. To meet the needs of a client who has a seizure disorder and who has recently had a generalized seizure, the nurse should plan to:
1. Outline ways to prevent physical trauma from occurring during a seizure
2. Teach that anticonvulsant medications should be taken on an empty stomach
3. Explain that the client need not tell others of the illness because the medication will be increased
4. Teach the client that the symptoms and treatment of seizure disorders are similar, regardless of the cause

211. After surgery for a meningomyelocele, an infant is being fed by gavage. When checking placement of the feeding tube, the nurse is unable to hear the air injected because of noisy breath sounds. The nurse should:
1. Notify the physician
2. Advance the tube 1 to 2 cm
3. Carefully insert 1 mL of formula
4. Attempt to aspirate the stomach contents

212. The physician orders 10 mL of a 10% solution of calcium gluconate for a client with a severely depressed serum calcium level. The client also is receiving an IV solution of D_5W and digoxin (Lanoxin) 0.25 mg daily. The nurse should be aware that calcium gluconate:
1. Can be added to any IV solution
2. Is nonirritating to surrounding tissues
3. Potentiates the action of digitalis preparations
4. Cannot be added to the IV of 1000 mL D_5W

213. The nurse is aware that after a thyroidectomy the client should be observed carefully for symptoms indicating:
1. Perforation of the lung
2. Laceration of the esophagus
3. Fracture of the laryngeal cartilage
4. Accidental removal of the parathyroids

214. A 7-lb baby is born and admitted to the newborn nursery with an order for phytonadione (vitamin K) (AquaMEPHYTON) 1 mg IM. The nurse is aware that this treatment is administered to:
1. Facilitate bilirubin excretion
2. Increase liver glycogen stores
3. Promote clotting of the blood
4. Stimulate the growth of bowel flora

215. After surgery to create an ileal conduit, a client awakens and asks for a sip of water. The nurse informs the client that water by mouth cannot be given until the:
1. Ileal loop begins to drain
2. Intestinal anastomosis heals

3. Nasogastric suction is discontinued
4. Client leaves the post-anesthesia care unit

216. A 20-year-old male college student tells the nurse at the college health clinic that he has become increasingly anxious, cannot sleep, and has lost his appetite. He also states that he cannot concentrate and his grades have dropped considerably. An appropriate question by the nurse would be:
    1. "With whom have you shared your feelings of anxiety?"
    2. "What have you identified as the cause of your anxiety?"
    3. "It must be difficult for you. How long has this been going on?"
    4. "Sounds like you're having problems adjusting; shall we talk about it?"

217. The mother of a 17-year-old boy, who is going to be a foreign exchange student, asks the nurse why he must have a tetanus toxoid immunization instead of the immune globulin. The nurse should respond that the toxoid confers:
    1. Life-long passive immunity
    2. Longer-lasting active immunity
    3. Life-long active natural immunity
    4. Temporary passive natural immunity

218. A client with active genital herpes has a cesarean birth. The nurse teaches the mother how to limit transmission of the virus to her newborn. The nurse would evaluate that the instructions were understood when the mother states, "I:
    1. "Should avoid kissing my baby on the lips."
    2. "Must wear gloves when I'm holding my baby."
    3. "Must wash my clothes and my baby's clothes separately."
    4. "Should wash my hands thoroughly with soap and water before handling the baby."

219. The son of a terminally ill client is concerned about his mother's condition. He asks the nurse, "Will she get better?" The nurse's most appropriate response would be:
    1. "Her vital signs are stable, so she is holding her own."
    2. "Of course she will. You can't give up. You must hope for the best."
    3. "Her condition is very serious. It might help to discuss your concerns with me?"
    4. "I don't know. You'll have to ask the physician. I'll leave a note that you are here."

220. The nurse encourages a terminally ill client to make decisions about daily activities and care. The nurse would know that the client, who had been extremely angry with everything and everybody, had resolved some of the anger when the client states:
    1. "You've got a busy morning ahead of you! I'm really a mess."
    2. "What are you going to let me do this morning? You know I can help."
    3. "It's so hard to let someone do so much for me. It just doesn't seem right."
    4. "I can do my face, hands, arms, and chest today, but I think you'd better do the rest."

221. A nurse was just hired to work in a facility where the nurse assumes responsibility for a number of clients' needs. Implementation of this care is recognized as:
    1. Team nursing
    2. Modular nursing
    3. Functional nursing
    4. Primary care nursing

222. An IV of 800 mL/24 hours is ordered for a 2½-year-old child. At how many milliliters per hour should the nurse set the volume control device?
    Answer: _____.

223. A client is admitted to the emergency department with head and chest injuries received in an automobile accident. When evaluating the client's responses to treatment, the assessments that indicate that the client is ready to be transferred to a critical care unit would be:
    1. Alert but restless, stable vital signs, cyanosis
    2. Stable vital signs, apprehension, complaints of pain
    3. Drowsy but easily roused, improving tissue perfusion, fluctuating vital signs
    4. Elevated temperature, slowing pulse and respirations, pain in the injured areas

224. A 26-year-old client recently diagnosed with HIV needs an update on immunizations. The nurse plans a schedule which includes:
    1. Influenza, MMR, varicella and hepatitis A vaccines
    2. Diphtheria, tetanus, hepatitis A and C vaccines
    3. Pneumococcal, MMR, influenza and varicella vaccines
    4. Tetanus, diphtheria, hepatitis B and pneumococcal vaccines

225. A client has had a suction curettage for the removal of a hydatidiform mole. When planning for the client's discharge, the nurse should emphasize the:
    1. Need for follow-up care for six weeks
    2. Risk factors for developing another hydatidiform mole
    3. Reason for postponing another pregnancy for a whole year
    4. Justification for chemotherapy if the human chorionic gonadotropin hormone (hCG) level decreases slowly

226. Several hours after admission to the hospital with laryngotracheobronchitis (viral croup), the nurse notes the child has developed tachypnea and tachycardia, accompanied by intercostal and substernal retractions and increased restlessness. The nurse should immediately:
    1. Suction secretions from the child's trachea
    2. Dislodge mucus by striking the child on the back
    3. Report the child's respiratory status to the pediatrician
    4. Increase the level of oxygen being delivered to the child

227. After surgery for a fractured hip, a client is restless and appears anxious. When the nurse and nursing assistant enter the room to provide evening care, the client becomes upset. The nurse should:
    1. Explain that hip fractures are not life threatening
    2. Reassure the client that they will be very careful
    3. Describe the need for various personnel at this time
    4. Suggest that the client can turn on the television for diversion

228. When planning the development of a nurse-client relationship, the nurse is aware that the most important aspect of this relationship during the early phase of its development would be:
    1. Trust
    2. Empathy
    3. Personal rapport
    4. Open communication

229. A 28-year-old male client is admitted to the hospital for confirmation of the diagnosis of Hodgkin's disease. The client and his wife are concerned that he may have cancer. The wife states, "Wouldn't it be unlikely for someone like my husband to have cancer?" Before responding to the emotional aspects of the question, the nurse should recall that:
    1. It is impossible to predict who will develop cancer or when
    2. Cancer is typically a disease of older rather than younger adults
    3. Women rather then men are more likely to have Hodgkin's disease
    4. Hodgkin's disease in males frequently occurs during their third decade of life

230. A primigravida is concerned about her "blotchy skin on her face," her "dark nipples," and the "dark line" from her navel to her pubis. The nurse should explain that these adaptations are caused by hypersecretion of the:
    1. Adrenal gland
    2. Thyroid gland
    3. Anterior pituitary gland
    4. Posterior pituitary gland

231. A client who is formula feeding her infant complains of discomfort from her engorged breasts. The measure most appropriate to relieve the engorgement would be:
    1. Expression of breast milk to relieve pressure
    2. Application of ice packs and a binder to her breasts
    3. Use of hot, moist towels as compresses on the breasts
    4. Restriction of oral fluid intake to less than 1000 mL daily

232. The physician prescribes propylthiouracil for a client with hyperthyroidism. Two months after being started on the antithyroid medication, the client calls the nurse and complains of feeling tired and looking pale. The nurse should:
    1. Advise the client to get more rest
    2. Schedule an appointment for the client
    3. Instruct the client to skip one dose daily
    4. Tell the client to increase the medication

233. A client who is suspected of having had a silent myocardial infarction and is to have an electrocardiogram (ECG) asks the nurse, "Why are they doing this test?" The best reply by the nurse would be: "This test will:
    1. Detect your heart sounds."
    2. Reflect any heart damage."
    3. Help us change your heart's rhythm."
    4. Tell us how much stress you can tolerate."

234. Twelve hours after sustaining full-thickness burns to the chest and thighs, a client is complaining

of severe thirst. The client's urinary output has been 60 mL/hr for the past 10 hours. No bowel sounds are heard. The nurse should:
1. Increase the client's IV flow rate
2. Give the client orange juice by mouth
3. Offer the client 4 oz of water by mouth
4. Moisten the client's lips with wet gauze

235. The nursing diagnosis that takes priority when planning care for a client who has sustained partial- and full-thickness burns of the chest in a fire would be:
1. Risk for infection related to burn trauma
2. Impaired physical mobility related to bed rest
3. Impaired gas exchange related to smoke inhalation
4. Risk for deficient fluid volume related to decreased intake

236. When considering the family's role in discharge planning for an adult client who has been in a psychiatric facility, if the client agrees, it would be most therapeutic for the nurse to:
1. Include the family when making specific discharge plans
2. Inform the family in advance when discharge will occur
3. Answer family members' questions about the client's illness
4. Have family members help assess the client's readiness for discharge

237. Eight days after a client starts antidepressant medication therapy, the nurse notices that the client, who has been severely depressed, is neatly dressed and well groomed. The client smiles at the nurse and states, "Things sure look better today." Based on an awareness of depressed behavior, the nurse should:
1. Begin preparing the client for discharge
2. Increase the client's privileges as a reward
3. Compliment both the client's appearance and smile
4. Assign a staff member to provide constant surveillance of the client

238. On the morning of a scheduled outing the parents of a client hospitalized for incapacitating obsessive behavior call to say that they cannot come because of problems with the accountant for their small business. The client appears upset and goes into elaborate detail about the parents' business and the monthly visit of the accountant. The nurse's best response would be:
1. "It's disappointing to have plans change at the last minute."
2. "Would you like to talk about what you had planned to do today?"
3. "Would you like to make new plans now that they are not coming?"
4. "It's good that you can recognize that your parents are sometimes busy."

239. A young female client comes to the trauma center stating that she had been raped. She is disheveled, pale, and staring blankly. Taking what has occurred into consideration, the nurse asks the client to describe in detail what happened because:
1. It will help the nursing staff in giving legal advice and providing counseling
2. Talking about what led to the assault will help her see what may have precipitated it
3. The victim can put the event in better perspective, and it helps begin the resolution process
4. Discussing details will keep the victim from covering up the intimate happenings in the assault situation

240. A client's respiratory status may be affected after abdominal surgery. When planning care to provide for this problem, the behavioral objective for this client should be:
1. Demonstrates the technique of coughing and deep breathing
2. Respirations will improve with coughing and deep breathing
3. Coughing and deep breathing will facilitate output of secretions
4. Will cough and deep breathe five or six times every hour while awake

241. An older, noncommunicative client is being maintained in the home on percutaneous endoscopic gastrostomy (PEG) feedings. An adult child of the client is the primary caregiver. On several home visits, the nurse has been told by the adult child that the PEG feeding was stopped because of vomiting or diarrhea. On other occasions, the nurse observes that the ordered feeding has been diluted or is running behind schedule. The nurse suspects elder abuse. The nurse should:
1. Discuss the situation with the adult child
2. Ask the client if the adult child is abusive
3. Report the suspected abuse to adult protective services
4. Avoid reporting the situation to prevent alienation of the adult child

242. During the assessment of a client who was admitted to the hospital because of a productive cough, fever, and chills, the nurse percusses an area of dullness over the right posterior lower lobe of the lung. Considering the presenting signs and symptoms, the nurse is aware that this finding may be indicative of:
    1. Pleurisy
    2. Bronchitis
    3. Pneumonia
    4. Emphysema

243. A male client with aortic stenosis is scheduled for a valve replacement in two days. He tells the nurse, "I told my wife all she needs to know if I don't make it." The response by the nurse that would be the most therapeutic would be:
    1. "Men your age do very well."
    2. "You are worried about dying."
    3. "I know you are concerned, but your physician is excellent."
    4. "I'll get you a sleeping pill tonight. I know you will need it."

244. To decrease or control the sensory and cognitive disturbances that can occur after a client has open heart surgery, the nurse should:
    1. Restrict family visits
    2. Withhold analgesic medications
    3. Plan for maximum periods of rest
    4. Keep the room light on most of the time

245. Four hours after a liver biopsy, the client complains of pain, and the nurse notes that there is a leakage of a moderately large amount of bile on the dressing. Based on these findings, the nurse should:
    1. Medicate the client for pain as ordered
    2. Tell the client to remain flat on the back
    3. Notify the client's physician immediately
    4. Monitor the client's vital signs every 10 minutes

246. The first child of adolescent parents is brought to the pediatric unit with a diagnosis of nonorganic failure to thrive (NFTT). In light of this diagnosis and the family structure, the priority nursing diagnosis for this family would be:
    1. Impaired parenting related to knowledge deficit
    2. Risk for injury related to mothering failure
    3. Disturbed sensory perception related to infant deprivation
    4. Imbalanced nutrition: less than body requirements related to child abuse

247. A client is admitted for induction of labor. An IV with oxytocin via an infusion pump is started. The client's contractions begin and they are 1½ to 2 minutes in duration. While the nurse is in the room, one contraction occurs that is 3 minutes in length. The first action to be taken would be to:
    1. Administer oxygen
    2. Turn off the oxytocin infusion
    3. Place a call light next to the client
    4. Reposition the monitoring belts for a better reading

248. A client with heart failure is digitalized and placed on a maintenance dose of digoxin 0.25 mg qd. If a therapeutic effect is achieved, the nurse would expect to observe:
    1. Diuresis, decreased pulse rate, decreased edema
    2. Increased blood pressure, decreased pulse pressure, weight loss
    3. Lowered pulse rate, reduced heart murmur, increased blood pressure
    4. Regular pulse rhythm, stable fluid balance, decreased blood pressure

249. A child with acute spasmodic bronchitis who is receiving humidified air removes the face mask. During the bath, the nurse observes that the child has increased respiratory distress. The nurse should:
    1. Do postural drainage and clap the child's chest
    2. Discontinue the bath and replace the face mask
    3. Suction the child's nasal passages to clear the airway
    4. Put the child in the orthopneic position and call the physician

250. The nurse on the community's terrorism response team is reviewing the triage protocols. In contrast to triage policies in local emergency situations, triage in mass casualty events would not give care to clients who have:
    1. Multiple fractures
    2. Closed head injuries
    3. Closed abdominal wounds
    4. Chemical/radiation exposures

251. A client has a permanent colostomy. During the first 24 hours, there is no drainage from the colostomy. The nurse should realize that this is a result of the:
    1. Edema after the surgery
    2. Absence of intestinal peristalsis
    3. Decrease in fluid intake prior to surgery
    4. Proper functioning of the nasogastric tube

252. A client is admitted to the hospital for surgery for colon cancer. The client complains of malaise, constipation, and stomach rumbling. When obtaining a health history, the nurse should expect the client to report changes in the:
1. Shape of stools
2. Ability to digest fat
3. Amount of fluid intake
4. Use of spices in the diet

253. An infant who had been receiving humidified oxygen because of dyspnea caused by acute spasmodic laryngitis is being discharged. The parents ask the nurse about caring for their baby at home. The nurse's best response would be:
1. "Give 2 ounces of water after the feeding of formula."
2. "No one should be allowed to visit the baby for a while."
3. "All allergen producers such as animals should be avoided."
4. "No specific restrictions are necessary after your baby goes home."

254. A priority of care for a client with dementia of the Alzheimer's type would be:
1. Planning for remotivational therapy
2. Arranging for long-term custodial care
3. Structuring the environment for safety
4. Stimulating thinking with new experiences

255. An emergency tracheotomy is performed on a toddler in acute respiratory distress from laryngotracheobronchitis (viral croup). In addition to routine suctioning of the tracheotomy, the nurse should also suction if the toddler:
1. Becomes diaphoretic and cyanotic
2. Verbalizes an increased difficulty in breathing
3. Has severe substernal retractions and stridor
4. Becomes restless or pale or has an increased pulse rate

256. The nurse is instructing a client on foods appropriate for a low sodium diet. The food group lowest in sodium is:
1. Meat
2. Dairy
3. Fresh fruit
4. Fresh vegetables

257. The nurse is aware that group therapy with abusive parents should be designed to help these parents to first:
1. Confront their own rage
2. Admit publicly and to themselves that they are child abusers
3. Recognize the long-range psychologic effects of child abuse
4. Share information about their parenting techniques and skills

258. The African-American parents of a newborn ask the nurse about several areas of deep blue coloring on their baby's lower back and buttocks. The nurse's response is based on the knowledge that these:
1. Areas are usually found on dark-skinned newborns
2. Color changes represent transient mottling that occurs when the baby is cold
3. Are characteristic of the harlequin color change that occurs when the baby lies on the side
4. Discolorations are probably bruises and the baby will be observed for the development of jaundice

259. A male client who had a brain attack (CVA) frequently cries when his family visits. The family members are obviously upset by the crying. The nurse should explain to the family that the client is:
1. Mourning his obvious loss of function
2. Having difficulty controlling his emotions
3. Conveying his unhappiness about the situation
4. Demonstrating his usual premorbid personality

260. A client is admitted to the hospital with a diagnosis of left ventricular failure secondary to rheumatic heart disease. The nurse should be aware that the symptoms of heart failure occur because the:
1. Excessive blood volume increases the workload of the heart muscles
2. Heart can no longer pump blood adequately in relation to venous return
3. Arterial system is less flexible because of hypertension or arteriosclerosis
4. Valves in the heart have become stenotic or regurgitant and impede blood flow

261. After a basal cell carcinoma is removed by fulguration, a client is given a topical steroid to apply to the surgical site. The nurse would recognize that the teaching regarding steroids and skin lesions was effective when the client states that the purpose of the medication is to:
1. Prevent infection of the wound
2. Increase fluid loss from the skin
3. Reduce inflammation at the surgical site
4. Limit itching around the area of the lesion

262. The nurse is reviewing a list of current medications with an 80-year-old client who has developed gastrointestinal bleeding. The medication that should be questioned would be:
1. Ibuprofen (Advil)
2. Digoxin (Lanoxin)
3. Furosemide (Lasix)
4. Spironolactone (Aldactone)

263. Considering the fact that a client with a right-sided brain attack (CVA) is right-handed, the task that probably will present the most difficulty would be:
1. Eating meals
2. Writing letters
3. Combing the hair
4. Dressing every morning

264. A client with diabetes mellitus was diagnosed with diabetic ketoacidosis and initially treated with intravenous fluids followed by an IV bolus of regular insulin. The nurse anticipates that the physician probably will order a continuous infusion of:
1. Humulin N insulin
2. Humulin R insulin
3. Prompt zinc suspension insulin (Semilente)
4. Extended zinc suspension insulin (Ultralente)

265. When caring for a client with catatonic schizophrenia, the nurse should expect that the client would exhibit:
1. Self-mutilation
2. Sadness with crying
3. Repetitious activities
4. Immobile posturing behavior

Part A Answers and Rationales

1. 1 **Straddling the hip would prevent scissoring by keeping the infant's legs abducted. (2) (PB; CJ; IM; PE; NM)**
2 An infant seat would not prevent scissoring.
3 Tight wrapping would maintain the infant's legs in a scissored position.
4 When the football hold is used, the infant is carried in a supine position with the legs adducted, which promotes scissoring.

2. 3 **This increases oncotic pressure, which pulls interstitial fluid into the blood vessels, restoring blood volume and limiting ascites. (3) (PB; CJ; AN; MS; FE)**
1 Nutrients are provided by total parenteral nutrition, not salt-poor albumin.
2 Salt-poor albumin is not given to increase protein stores.
4 Salt-poor albumin has no effect on diverting blood flow away from the liver.

3. 4 **Oral contraceptives may cause hypertension and place the client at risk for the development of a brain attack (CVA). (2) (PB; CJ; AN; CW; RC)**
1 Oral contraceptives are not contraindicated for women older than 30 years of age if there are no known risk factors.
2 Clients should be strongly cautioned about smoking even 15 cigarettes a day; if this client were over 35 years of age, oral contraceptives would be contraindicated.
3 There is no relationship between oral contraceptives and multiple births.

4. 2 **Only superficial attention has been directed to hypertension; ongoing health supervision is needed. (2) (PB; CJ; AN; CW; NP)**
1 Teaching and encouraging the client to engage in self-care is helping the client.
3 This is untrue; however, limiting sodium intake is too superficial.
4 Involving the client is important, but professional supervision is required.

5. 2 **Drainage will flow with the force of gravity; therefore the dependent area should be checked for bleeding. (2) (SE; CJ; EV; CW; WH)**
1 The drainage is assessed for amount and characteristics; it is not emptied hourly, but either once per shift or when necessary.

3 Turning the client on the affected side could be painful and should be avoided; the client should turn to the unaffected side.
4 If the drainage on the dressing is excessive, the physician should be notified.

6. 3 **As drainage collects and occupies space, the original level of negative pressure decreases; the lower the negative pressure, the less effective the drainage. (1) (SE; CJ; AN; MS; IT)**
1 It is easy and safe to empty, regardless of the amount of drainage in the unit.
2 Drainage can be measured accurately by the calibrations on the unit or in a calibrated container after emptying.
4 A one-way valve between the tubing and the collection chamber prevents drainage from entering the tubing and causing trauma to the wound.

7. 4 **The physician should be consulted because the decision depends on the amount of damage and extent of healing. (3) (SE; MR; IM; MS; EH)**
1 This is a medical decision that depends on the amount of damage, not how the client feels.
2 It would be false reassurance to determine an exact time and date; this would be too early.
3 Same as answer 1.

8. 1 **A lithium plasma level of 0.8 to 1.2 mEq/L is appropriate for prophylaxis; the client's level is above that recommended. (3) (PB; CJ; IM; MH; DR)**
2 This would be unexpected; the client should be monitored for signs and symptoms of toxicity such as nausea, vomiting, diarrhea, increased tremor, vertigo, and blurred vision.
3 This would cause a further increase in the plasma level of lithium which is already elevated beyond the therapeutic range.
4 The plasma level of lithium is beyond the therapeutic range of 0.8 to 1.2 mEq/L.

9. 1 **The corneal reflex is related to the fifth cranial nerve. (3) (PB; CJ; AS; MS; NM)**
2 Involvement of the sympathetic fibers of the vagus nerve causes the orthostatic hypotension seen in this syndrome.
3 The ninth cranial nerve innervates the pharynx, the tenth cranial nerve innervates the palate, pharynx, and larynx, and the twelfth cranial nerve innervates the tongue.
4 Same as answer 3.

10. **3 This does not allow the client to escape responsibility for the behavior, a common characteristic of the addicted person. (2) (PI; MR; IM; MH; SA)**
    1 This leads the client to believe the behavior was an acceptable response to feelings of anger.
    2 Ignoring the client's behavior can be interpreted as approval of the behavior.
    4 Although this may provide an outlet for the anger, it supports acting out rather than control of feelings.

11. **3 Epinephrine produces sympathetic nervous system side effects such as tachycardia and hypertension. (2) (PB; CJ; EV; PE; DR)**
    1 Pallor, not flushing, is a common side effect.
    2 This is not a common side effect; this medication is given to decrease respiratory difficulty.
    4 Hypertension, not hypotension, is a common side effect.

12. **4 Change is always accompanied by anxiety and uncertainty; without motivation, change will not occur. (2) (PI; CJ; EV; MH; PR)**
    1 The lifestyle of these individuals is rarely limited because they tend to be rather gregarious and outgoing; in reality, they attempt to live by their guile.
    2 The reactions of the client's parents would be of little influence at this age.
    3 These usually do not work unless the individual is motivated to change; there is no need for an anxiolytic to reduce anxiety.

13. **3 Obesity is a known predisposing factor to type 2 diabetes; the exact relationship is unknown. (2) (PM; CJ; AS; MS; EN)**
    1 Diabetes insipidus is caused by too little ADH and has no relationship to type 2 diabetes.
    2 High-cholesterol diets and atherosclerotic heart disease are associated with type 2 diabetes.
    4 Alcohol intake is not known to predispose a person to type 2 diabetes, and alcohol lowers the blood glucose level.

14. **3 Symptoms usually appear one to three weeks after an acute infection; this syndrome may be linked to diseases such as HIV, viral hepatitis, the Epstein-Barr virus, and infectious mononucleosis.(2) (PB; CJ; AS; MS; NM)**
    1 This syndrome is unrelated to head trauma.
    2 There is no known familial tendency that exists in the development of Guillain-Barré syndrome.
    4 Drug therapy has not been implicated as a contributing factor in Guillain-Barré syndrome.

15. **2 In this position the gravid uterus impedes venous return; this causes decreased cardiac output and results in reduced placental circulation. (1) (SE; CJ; AN; CW; HC)**
    1 Although this may be partially true, it is not the most significant reason for avoiding the supine position while in labor.
    3 This is false; it can lead to supine hypotension.
    4 Same as answer 1.

16. **3 Long-term disease-free survival rates for children with acute lymphocytic leukemia approach 75%. (3) (PB; CJ; AN; PE; BI)**
    1 This projected prognosis is too fatalistic.
    2 Same as answer 1.
    4 This projected prognosis is too favorable.

17. **3 The brachial pulse is recommended for infants and can be palpated on the inner aspect of the arm midway between the elbow and the shoulder; this site is most readily accessible for this age group. (2) (SE; MR; PL; PE; CV)**
    1 The carotid artery is difficult to palpate in infants because of their short fat necks; the carotid artery is the most accessible and central site for individuals over 1 year of age.
    2 Obtaining a pulse at this site during CPR is not recommended for any age group.
    4 Same as answer 2.

18. **1 Infection is the most common complication; sterile technique at the catheter insertion site must be maintained. (2) (SE; MR; PL; MS; IT)**
    2 This is not necessary; the catheter is sutured in place, and reasonable movement is permitted.
    3 The client should be taught to leave the infusion pump as set and to call the nurse if the alarm rings.
    4 Excessive weight gain or loss is not a complication of total parenteral nutrition.

19. **1 To achieve the greatest therapeutic value from a group session, the members must be involved in deciding what will be discussed. (3) (SE; MR; PL; MH; TR)**
    2 By this response the nurse leader abdicates the leadership role and places the entire responsibility for the success of the group on its members.
    3 This response presents an extremely structured view of the purpose of a therapy group; the members must be involved in the selection of the topics to be discussed.
    4 Same as answer 3.

20. 1 Levodopa can cross the blood-brain barrier and be converted to dopamine, a substance depleted in Parkinson's disease. (2) (PB; MR; PL; MS; DR)

    2 Dopamine is not given because it does not cross the blood-brain barrier.

    3 Vitamin B_6 can reverse the effects of some anti-Parkinson's disease medications and is contraindicated.

    4 Isocarboxazid (Marplan) is an MAO inhibitor used for the treatment of severe depression, not symptoms of parkinsonism.

21. 1 Clients may develop cerebral edema caused by excessive absorption of irrigating solution by the venous sinusoids during surgery. (3) (PB; CJ; EV; MS; RG)

    2 The surgery is performed through the urinary meatus and urethra; there is no suprapubic incision.

    3 It is unnecessary to keep the client in this position.

    4 The client is initially npo and then advanced to a regular diet as tolerated; continuous irrigation supplies enough fluid to flush the bladder.

22. 3 Serosanguineous drainage from the wound or on the dressing forewarns separation of the wound edges (dehiscence) and movement of abdominal organs outside of the abdominal cavity (evisceration). (3) (PB;CJ; EV; MS; GI)

    1 Bowel sounds have no relationship to wound status; bowel sounds are expected around the third or fourth postoperative day as intestinal peristalsis returns.

    2 Loosening of sutures may occur after the initial wound edema subsides but would not be a sign of failure of the suture line.

    4 This is the expected coloration of a healing wound.

23. 1 This is a correct description of talipes equinovarus. (2) (PB; CJ; AS; PE; SK)

    2 This describes talipes calcaneovarus.

    3 This describes talipes equinovalgus, also known as rocker-bottom foot.

    4 Same as answer 2.

24. 4 Hemicolectomy is removal of part of the colon with an anastomosis between the ileum and transverse colon; a colostomy is not necessary. (2) (PB; MR; IM; MS; GI)

    1 With a colostomy the intestine opens on the abdomen, whereas in a hemicolectomy a portion of the intestine is resected and the ends connected.

    2 A colostomy is done for reasons other than a tumor; a colectomy with a colostomy is only one intervention that may be used to treat a tumor.

    3 This is the description of a temporary colostomy.

25. 2 Nursing care should be organized and administered efficiently so that exposure can be kept to a minimum. (1) (SE; CJ; PL; MS; NP)

    1 This is contraindicated until the radon seeds are removed because chewing can dislodge them.

    3 This is contraindicated because it could dislodge the seeds; drying cannot be prevented.

    4 This would expose the provider of care to excessive radiation.

26. 3 The client will be able to attend to the activities of daily living because tiagabine hydrochloride effectively controls and reduces grandiosity, poor judgment, and psychomotor hyperactivity. (2) (PI; CJ; EV; MH; DR)

    1 This would not reflect an effective response to Gabatril.

    2 Same as answer 1.

    4 Same as answer 1.

27. 3 This measure assesses for increasing intracranial pressure, which may occur if drainage channels are obstructed by the bacterial infection. (2) (PB; CJ; PL; PE; NM)

    1 Antibiotics are administered intravenously throughout the course of treatment.

    2 This is insufficient monitoring; many changes could occur in this time span.

    4 Parents can visit if they are taught how to carry out isolation precautions.

28. 2 Insensible and intestinal fluid losses are increased during phototherapy; extra fluid prevents dehydration. (3) (PB; CJ; PL; CW; HN)

    1 This is unnecessary unless changes from the baseline occur.

    3 A Guthrie test is done for PKU screening.

    4 The total body needs to be exposed to light.

29. 1 These tests would confirm glomerulonephritis because they identify the causative organism and its pathologic effects. (3) (PB; CJ; AN; PE; RG)

    2 Although a urinalysis would be done, the other tests are not specific for glomerulonephritis.

    3 Same as answer 2.

    4 Although a blood chemistry and nasopharyngeal culture would be done, the other tests are not specific for glomerulonephritis.

30. 3 **Clients commonly respond in this manner when they feel their sexual identity is threatened; this behavior supports the client's ego integrity. (2) (PM; CJ; AN; MH; BA)**
   1 Staff members' actions play only a minor role in these situations.
   2 The client's feelings, not the situation, precipitated this response.
   4 Same as answer 1.

31. 3 **A serious side effect of busulfan is aplastic anemia, a common reaction to the drug; blood studies would monitor RBCs, as well as WBCs and thrombocytes. (3) (PB; CJ; EV; PE; DR)**
   1 A decrease, not an increase, in RBCs occurs.
   2 This is unrelated to busulfan.
   4 Same as answer 2.

32. 3 **Sodium absorbs water in the kidney's renal tubules; when dietary intake of sodium is decreased, water is not reabsorbed and edema is reduced. (2) (PB; CJ; AN; MS; FE)**
   1 This is untrue; a decrease in sodium will prevent the reabsorption of water; furosemide stimulates the loop of Henle.
   2 Adequate hydration is the major factor that diminishes the thirst response.
   4 This will not be caused by a low-sodium diet; a low-sodium diet will cause fluid to enter the intravascular compartment.

33. 4 **Adduction may cause dislocation of the new prosthesis, and external rotation increases tension on the suture line. (2) (SE; CJ; IM; MS; SK)**
   1 Only the operated leg needs to be kept abducted.
   2 This position adducts the affected leg and increases the danger of hip dislocation.
   3 The supine position is permitted as long as the affected leg is abducted and external rotation avoided, which help keep the prosthesis firmly in the acetabulum.

34. 2 **This reflects the client's statement and permits clarification, which provides information that can be used in future planning. (3) (PM; CJ; IM; CW; NP)**
   1 This is too specific an interpretation of a rest requirement; there is more to maintaining rest than this.
   3 This is a vague interpretation of a rest requirement; there is more to maintaining rest than this.
   4 What the nurse thinks it means does not give a clear picture of what the client interprets as rest.

35. 3 **Counterpressure helps alleviate some discomfort. (1) (PM; MR; IM; CW; HC)**
   1 This will increase tension and discomfort.
   2 Panting may lead to hyperventilation, which could cause maternal respiratory alkalosis and fetal acidosis; if performed, this technique should be monitored by the nurse.
   4 Kegel exercises do not help relieve back pain, they tone the pelvic musculature.

36. 1 **Exercising should be done often; association with a specific activity makes it easier to incorporate it into the lifestyle, leading to increased compliance. (2) (SE; MR; EV; PE; SK)**
   2 Although this is frequent enough, such a rigid schedule is difficult to follow with an infant, and compliance becomes more difficult.
   3 This is not frequent enough.
   4 Same as answer 3.

37. 4 **Lead encephalopathy causes serious elevation of intracranial pressure; this is not related to Ca EDTA. (3) (PB; CJ; EV; PE; RG)**
   1 This does not occur with lead toxicity, nor is it likely to occur with the Ca EDTA preparation, which replaces calcium.
   2 Same as answer 1.
   3 Same as answer 1.

38. 2 **The client's signs and symptoms suggest the possibility of shock; the physician must be alerted to this possible life-threatening condition. (1) (PB; CJ; IM; MS; CV)**
   1 The client has unmet needs that must be addressed first.
   3 Distraction is effective with mild, not severe, pain.
   4 This is outside the scope of nursing practice; drug orders must be followed as prescribed or the physician notified.

39. 4 **The semi-Fowler's position helps to maintain the head in proper body alignment and facilitates respiration. (2) (PB; CJ; PL; MS; RE)**
   1 The side-lying position inhibits respiratory excursion.
   2 This position may cause flexion of the neck, which would inhibit respirations and place pressure on the suture line.
   3 Same as answer 2.

40. 2 **Research indicates that these are the first physical signs that accompany withdrawal from heroin. (3) (PB; CJ; AS; CW; DR)**
   1 Depression is a sign of withdrawal from LSD.

3 Restlessness, shakiness, hallucinations, and possibly coma are signs of withdrawal from morphine.

4 Insomnia, convulsions, weakness, sweating, and anxiety are signs of withdrawal from phenobarbital.

41. **4 Because the infant will be kept supine after surgery to prevent irritation to the lips, using this position early, even when awake, prepares the infant for its use later. (2) (PM; MR; IM; PE; GI)**

1 The baby is too young and will miss out on some oral gratification with this method.

2 Babies with a cleft lip need increased burping time because they tend to swallow large amounts of air during feeding.

3 Restraint of the arms could be injurious; the infant needs to move about.

42. **3 The ovum is fertilizable for 12 to 24 hours, and sperm remain motile for about 72 hours. (1) (PM; CJ; PL; CW; RC)**

1 The fertility period is longer than this.

2 This time period is too long before ovulation and too short after ovulation.

4 The period of fertility is shorter than this.

43. **1 Children commonly use denial of parents as a stage of coping with separation; they avoid the fact that separation is real. (1) (PI; CJ; IM; MH; CS)**

2 Undoing is a behavior or communication technique calculated to neutralize earlier behavior or communication.

3 Repression is the involuntary exclusion of painful thoughts, impulses, or memories; this child's behavior is voluntary.

4 Sublimation is the act of substituting socially acceptable behavior for an unacceptable feeling or drive.

44. **2 As fluid returns to the vascular system, increased renal flow and diuresis occur. (3) (PB; CJ; PL; MS; FE)**

1 During the second phase, potassium moves back into the cells, decreasing serum potassium.

3 This would indicate hemoconcentration and hypovolemia; in the second phase hemodilution and hypervolemia occur.

4 As fluid returns to the vascular system, the central venous pressure rises and hypervolemia may occur.

45. **2 Negative pressure is exerted by gravity drainage or by suction through the closed system. (1) (PB; CJ; AN; MS; RE)**

1 Though the discomfort may be lessened, this is not the primary purpose.

3 In a pneumothorax associated with COPD, there is an accumulation of air, not fluid.

4 Subcutaneous emphysema in the chest wall is most commonly associated with clients receiving air under pressure, such as that received from a ventilator.

46. **4 COPD causes destruction of capillary beds around the alveoli, interfering with blood flow to the lungs from the right side of the heart; as the heart continues to strain against this resistance, heart failure eventually results. (2) (PB; CJ; AN; MS; RE)**

1 This would cause stress on the left side of the heart.

2 This would not cause stress on the right side of the heart.

3 This probably would produce greater stress on the left side of heart.

47. **2 Baked fish is a low-residue, low-fat, high-protein, and non-gas-producing food that usually is well tolerated. (2) (PB; CJ; EV; MS; GI)**

1 This has fiber and irritates the gastrointestinal tract.

3 Same as answer 1.

4 This irritates the gastrointestinal tract and stimulates mucous production.

48. **1 At about the 22nd week of gestation, the top of the fundus is at the level of the umbilicus. (3) (PM; CJ; AS; CW; HC)**

2 This would be too low for a pregnancy between the fifth and sixth months.

3 In a normal pregnancy, this would be too high for 20 to 22 weeks of gestation.

4 Same as answer 2.

49. **4 The child is developing autonomy, is curious, and learns from experience. (1) (PM; CJ; AN; PE; GD)**

1 The toddler is still learning from experiences, not from others; this is the level of parallel, not interactive, play.

2 The toddler is still attempting to distinguish self as separate from the parents; the struggle for autonomy limits learning from parents.

3 The struggle for autonomy at this age limits learning from older siblings, even though the toddler attempts to copy their behaviors.

50. 2 Behavior that reflects the recognition of the intrinsic worth of each individual is essential in all supportive relationships; problem-solving potential is increased when clients are involved in exploring alternatives that will affect the direction of their own lives. (1) (PI; CJ; PL; MH; CS)

1 The client, not the worker, is encouraged to identify the problem.

3 This is useless; the client is unable to empathize with others at this time.

4 This is impossible during the immediate intervention period; the client needs to find direction immediately.

51. 2 Because of the administration of regional anesthesia and the potential for blood loss associated with a cesarean birth, the client should be well hydrated before surgery to maintain adequate blood volume. (3) (PB; CJ; PL; CW; HP)

1 This is not relevant; just before surgery the skin will be cleansed.

3 Unless the fetus is known to be preterm or compromised, there is no reason for notifying the neonatal intensive care unit.

4 Only routine monitoring of vital signs is necessary unless there has been some indication of infection or preeclampsia

52. 4 Protein and vitamin C promote wound healing; this is a postoperative priority. (2) (PB; CJ; PL; MS; IT)

1 A high-calorie diet could increase obesity, and there is no indication that this client is at risk for constipation.

2 This could cause constipation; the priority is for nutrients to promote healing.

3 Although a low-fat diet is preferred for an obese client, vitamin D, as well as other vitamins, should not be limited.

53.

1. _____ The temperature usually decreases.

2. __x__ **Decreased blood flow to the kidneys leads to oliguria or anuria. (2) (PB; CJ; AS; MS; CV)**

3. _____ Restlessness usually occurs because of decreased cerebral blood flow.

4. __x__ **Irritability, along with restlessness and anxiety, occurs because of a decrease in oxygen to the brain.**

5. __x__ **Hypotension and a narrowing of the pulse pressure occur because of declining blood volume.**

6. _____ There are various changes in sensorium, but slurred speech is not a manifestation of shock.

7. _____ The pulse is rapid and thready; the heart rate increases in an attempt to meet the oxygen demands of the body; a thready quality to the pulse occurs because peripheral vessels constrict, conserving blood to the vital centers.

8. __x__ **The peripheral vessels constrict, shunting blood to the vital centers; and as a result the skin becomes cold and clammy.**

54. 3 Propylthiouracil can cause a depression of leukocytes and platelets. (3) (PB; CJ; EV; MS; DR)

1 They are given with milk, juice, or food to prevent gastric irritation.

2 Drug therapy decreases the risk of postoperative hemorrhage because it decreases the size and vascularity of the thyroid gland.

4 Therapy will be continued for at least six to eight weeks, even if the client's temperature and pulse return to normal.

55. 1 This is expected developmental behavior for 18-month-olds; however, they may have trouble coming down the stairs. (2) (PM; CJ; EV; PE; GD)

2 This is above the level of an 18-month-old child.

3 Same as answer 2.

4 Same as answer 2.

56. 4 This is a theoretical explanation for the development of anorexia nervosa. (2) (PI; CJ; AN; MH; ES)

1 This does not play a role in the development of anorexia nervosa.

2 Same as answer 1.

3 The basis is the struggle between dependence and independence, not a desire for independence alone.

57. 1 Inspection seeks to identify the cause for the decreased fetal heart rate; the cord may have prolapsed. (2) (PB; CJ; EV; CW; HP)

2 The physician should be notified after a further assessment of the client when there is more information.

3 This may be done later, but it is not the priority.

4 This is the intervention if the cord is prolapsed; it relieves pressure on the cord, which increases the flow of oxygen and nutrients to the fetus.

58. 1 These individuals readily respond to environmental cues; increased stimulation increases activity; decreased stimulation decreases activity. (2) (PB; CJ; PL; MH; MO)

2 Sleep pattern disturbances characteristically occur because of psychomotor activity.

3 All individuals require adequate rest and sleep; hyperactive clients may become exhausted because of their high activity level.

4 Expending energy only increases the tendency to remain awake.

59. 4 **Abduction will enable the head of the femur to fit into the acetabulum, thereby correcting the dysplasia. (2) (PM; CJ; AN; PE; SK)**

1 This would cause the head of the femur to move away from the acetabulum.

2 Same as answer 1

3 Same as answer 1.

60. 2 **Ambivalence describes the existence of two conflicting emotions, impulses, or desires. (2) (PI; CJ; AN; MH; SD)**

1 Double bind is two conflicting messages, not emotions, in a single communication.

3 Loose associations are not two conflicting emotions but the loosening of connections between thoughts.

4 Inappropriate affect is not two conflicting emotions but the inappropriate expression of emotions.

61. 1 **This would provide reassurance and support for the child. (2) (SE; MR; IM; MH; CS)**

2 Using the phrase "anything wrong down there" could cause the child to have negative feelings about the self.

3 Depending on the mother's involvement, this might be threatening rather than supportive to the child.

4 Asking the child to make this decision at this time would be nontherapeutic and may be threatening.

62. 2 **The lateral position removes pressure on the vena cava thus promoting venous return and increasing placental perfusion. (1) (PB; CJ; AN; CW; HP)**

1 This would promote hypotension because it interferes with the return of blood from the lower extremities.

3 Same as answer 1.

4 This position inhibits cardiac output and respirations because of the pressure of the visceral organs against the diaphragm.

63. 1 **Suckling will induce neural stimulation of the posterior pituitary gland, which in turn will release oxytocin and cause uterine contractions. (2) (PM; CJ; IM; CW; HC)**

2 Vigorous fundal pressure should never be utilized; this could cause a uterine prolapse.

3 If the placenta is still attached to the uterine wall, this may disconnect the cord from the placenta or cause uterine prolapse

4 This could cause a uterine prolapse.

64. 3 **The portion of the tube containing the ectopic pregnancy is removed and any residual tissue is treated with methotrexate. (2) (PB; CJ; PL; CW; RP)**

1 The uterus usually is uninvolved in a tubal pregnancy; there is no reason to incise the uterus.

2 This is the procedure for removing myomas (fibroids) from the uterus and is unrelated to an ectopic pregnancy.

4 The fertilized ovum was in the fallopian tube not the uterus; a D&C cleans the uterine cavity.

65. 1 **The presence of nitrate in the urine is characteristic of infection. (3) (PB; CJ; AS; MS; RG)**

2 This may occur for a variety of reasons; it is not specific to infection.

3 This is abnormal, but it is not related to infection.

4 This may occur with various problems, including infection; it is not exclusive to infection.

66. 1 **These are side effects during initial therapy; Gabatril causes the typical symptoms of CNS depression. (2) (PB; CJ; AS; MH; DR)**

2 These are common side effects of the phenothiazines.

3 This indicates lithium toxicity, not side effects.

4 These are common side effects of tricyclic antidepressants.

67. 3 **Treatment is done several hours after meals to avoid regurgitation and several hours before meals so that the unpleasant odor and taste do not affect the appetite. (2) (PB; CJ; PL; PE; RE)**

1 Treatment is done more frequently than this.

2 Postural drainage should not be done before meals because the unpleasant odor and taste will interfere with eating.

4 Same as answer 1.

68. 3 **Hot climates are contraindicated for children with cystic fibrosis because sweating brings about excessive loss of sodium chloride. (3) (PB; CJ; EV; PE; EN)**

1 This is advisable because it will keep the child from sweating.

2 Pancreatic enzymes are essential to help in the digestion of nutrients so that they can be absorbed by the intestinal mucosa.

4 After passage of the feces associated with this disorder, the rectum may become inflamed if not adequately cleaned.

69. 3 Dialysate is introduced into the peritoneal cavity where fluids, electrolytes, and wastes are exchanged through the peritoneal membrane. (2) (PB; MR; IM; MS; RG)

1 Hemodialysis is not necessary with CAPD.
2 The client can dialyze alone in any location without the need for continuous technical supervision.
4 About 2 liters of dialysate are maintained intraperitoneally and can be instilled and drained by the client.

70. 4 Malnutrition and liver damage lead to a reduced serum albumin level and failure of the capillary fluid shift mechanism, resulting in ascites. (2) (PB; CJ; AN; MS; FE)

1 Iron promotes hemoglobin synthesis; this is unrelated to cirrhosis.
2 Vitamins are unrelated to ascites.
3 The sodium level usually is excessive with cirrhosis.

71. 4 This response presents facts that help to reduce anxiety. (2) (PI; CJ; IM; CW; EC)

1 This is not reassuring, as well as incorrect, because placenta previa can occur in a woman with a normal uterus.
2 This is an inadequate explanation and gives the client no idea of what is happening.
3 This is untrue, and labor may not be beginning at this time.

72. 1 This would facilitate a one-to-one interaction and the development of a trusting relationship. (3) (PI; CJ; PL; MH; SD)

2 This activity would allow the client to withdraw.
3 This activity would foster competition and could increase anxiety.

4 Same as answer 2.

73. 2 With diabetic ketoacidosis, serum lipid levels can go so high that the serum appears opalescent and creamy. (3) (PB; CJ; AS; MS; EN)

1 With diabetic ketoacidosis, the BUN is generally elevated because of dehydration.
3 This is unrelated to diabetic ketoacidosis.
4 With diabetic ketoacidosis, the hematocrit level generally is elevated because of dehydration.

74. 1 This position prevents hip flexion contractures. (2) (SE; CJ; PL; MS; SK)

2 Exercises to prevent contractures are begun as soon as possible.
3 The residual limb should not be elevated for more than 48 hours because hip flexion contractures can result.
4 Lying on the residual limb can cause trauma to the incision site and should be avoided.

75. 3 Anticholinergic drugs block the neural impulses that stimulate pancreatic and gastric secretions; they inhibit the action of acetylcholine at postganglionic cholinergic nerve fibers. (3) (PB; CJ; IM; MS; GI)

1 Oral fluids would stimulate pancreatic secretion.
2 Morphine sulfate is an analgesic and therefore does not decrease gastric secretions; morphine would be contraindicated because it precipitates spasms of the smooth musculature of the pancreatic ducts and the sphincter of Oddi; meperidine hydrochloride (Demerol) is the preferred analgesic.
4 This position decreases pressure against the diaphragm; it will not decrease pancreatic secretions.

How to Use Worksheet 1: Errors in Processing Information

Common errors in processing information are listed in the left hand column of this worksheet. At the top of the worksheet is a row of blank spaces for inserting the number of the question missed. Directly below each number, check any errors you made in answering that question. You may have made more than one type of error in an answer.

Worksheet 1: Errors in Processing Information

Question number																						
Did not read situation/ question carefully																						
Missed important details																						
Confused major and minor points																						
Defined problem incorrectly																						
Could not remember terms/ facts/concepts/principles																						
Defined terms incorrectly																						
Focused on incomplete/incorrect data in assessing situation																						
Interpreted data incorrectly																						
Applied wrong concepts/ principles in situations																						
Drew incorrect conclusions																						
Identified wrong goals																						
Identified priorities incorrectly																						
Carried out plan incorrectly/ incompletely																						
Was unclear about criteria for evaluating success in achieving goals																						

How to Use Worksheet 2: Knowledge Gaps

Types of common knowledge gaps are listed along the top of this worksheet. Write a brief description of topics you want to review in the spaces provided. For example, if you missed a question on administration of a particular drug, write the drug name and problem (e.g., dosage) in the appropriate space under the column labeled *Pharmacology*.

Worksheet 2: Knowledge Gaps

Basic science	Skills/ procedures	Basic human needs	Growth and development	Normal nutrition	Psychosocial factors	Clinical area/ topic	Stressors/ coping mechanisms	Patho-physiology	Pharma-cology	Therapeutic nutrition	Legal implications	Other

Part B Answers and Rationales

76. 4 Colorectal cancer in women is common in the United States; approximately 68,000 women are diagnosed each year. (1) (PB; CJ; AN; MS; GI)

1 In the early stages, symptoms of cancer of the colon are vague or absent.

2 Malignancy means a tendency to progress in virulence; a localized tumor usually is benign.

3 Colorectal cancer is more common in men than women.

77. 3 Pregnant women with diabetes have a tendency for developing placental insufficiency, which can threaten fetal well-being. (3) (PB; CJ; AN; CW; HP)

1 Advanced maternal age alone is not an indication for an NST.

2 The pregnant woman with diabetes requires fetal monitoring (NST) regardless of glycemic control.

4 The NST does not measure plasma levels.

78. 2 This individualized information would be the best basis for predicting the outcome of therapy. (2) (PB; CJ; PL; MS; EH)

1 This knowledge would not be helpful in understanding the likelihood of additional problems associated with the current cancer.

3 Same as answer 1.

4 This would be useful, but it is not specific for this client.

79. 1 At this time breast engorgement is minimal, and this provides a regular examination cycle. (1) (PM; MR; EV; CW; WH)

2 Premenstrual breast engorgement may cause the breast to feel lumpy.

3 Ovulation is occurring, and hormones may influence breast consistency.

4 Breast consistency is altered by the menstrual cycle; the same date each month would fall in a different stage of the cycle; this method is recommended for women who do not menstruate.

80. 1 Nosebleeds (epistaxis) would be expected in a child with leukemia because of a decrease in platelets from the bone marrow. (3) (PB; CJ; AS; PE; BI)

2 Tachycardia would not be expected unless there was severe anemia.

3 Usually children with leukemia have a pale skin tone.

4 An elevated temperature would occur only if there were an infection secondary to the leukemia.

81. 3 The client is experiencing pulmonary edema because of a fluid volume excess; the high concentration of the TPN precipitates a fluid shift from the interstitial compartment into the intravascular compartment. (2) (PB; CJ; IM; MS; FE)

1 Fluid would continue to be infused, which would continue to increase the intravascular volume.

2 Same as answer 1.

4 Same as answer 1.

82. 4 This medication is ototoxic and causes damage to the eighth cranial nerve, resulting in deafness; assessment for ringing or roaring in the ears, vertigo, and hearing should be made before, during, and after treatment. (3) (PB; CJ; EV; MS; DR)

1 This medication does not affect the ear; blurred vision and optic neuritis, as well as peripheral neuropathy, may occur.

2 This medication does not affect hearing, visual disturbances may occur.

3 Same as answer 2.

83. 3 Regression is the defense mechanism commonly used by clients with schizophrenia to reduce anxiety by returning to earlier behavior. (2) (PI; CJ; AN; MH; SD)

1 This organized defense is used by clients with schizophrenia, paranoid type, in which the delusions are well systematized.

2 This unconscious forgetting is not a major defense used by clients with schizophrenia; if it were, they would not need to break with reality.

4 Rationalization, in which the individual blames others for problems and attempts to justify actions, is seldom used by clients with schizophrenia.

84. 4 Limitation of increased intracranial pressure and resultant brain damage depend on frequent, systematic observations. (3) (PB; CJ; AS; MS; NM)

1 This is unrealistic; the state of consciousness should be observed, but otherwise rest is not contraindicated.

2 There is no indication that movement should be restricted.

3 Mannitol is administered to reduce cerebral edema; there is no indication yet that this will be needed.

85. 2 Specialized insulin receptors on insulin-sensitive cells transport glucose through cell membranes, making it available for use. (1) (SE; MR; AN; PE; DR)

1 This is not the action of insulin.

3 Same as answer 1.

4 Same as answer 1.

86. 2 Preventing infection and trauma are the priorities; rupture of the sac may lead to meningitis. (1) (SE; MR; IM; CW; HN)

1 The Apgar is 9/10; there is no respiratory complication.

3 The sac must be protected before this is done.

4 This can be done before the infant leaves the birthing room; the priority is care of the sac.

87. 4 In three days the client should understand that the staff cares enough to prevent suicidal acting out. (3) (PI; CJ; PL; MH; MO)

1 This is unrealistic within the stated time period.

2 Same as answer 1.

3 Same as answer 1.

88. 1 A pH of 7.18 indicates fetal hypoxia; any reading under 7.2 is dangerous and the fetus should be delivered immediately. (3) (PB; CJ; AN; CW; HP)

2 Any reading above 7.2 is not considered life threatening.

3 Same as answer 2.

4 Same as answer 2.

89. 1 This acknowledges the client's apprehension and encourages further communication. (1) (PI; CJ; IM; MS; EH)

2 This does not address the client's feelings and may cause more anxiety.

3 This is perhaps true, but it does not foster communication; the client may focus on the word "pain."

4 This negates the client's feelings and promotes false reassurance

90. 4 Calcium in EDTA is displaced by the lead to form a stable compound that is excreted in the urine. (1) (PB; CJ; AN; PE; DR)

1 This is a calcium salt; it is used as an antidote for magnesium sulfate toxicity.

2 This is an antineoplastic drug used in cancer therapy

3 This is used as an antidote for aspirin poisoning.

91. 4 This ethically sound response clearly defines who is involved in decision making and allows for parental expression of ideas and thoughts. (2) (SE; MR; AN; MH; NP)

1 Discussion of the implication of a DNR order should not take place until after the family has spoken with the physician.

2 Although the answer promotes the physician-client relationship, it stops the nurse-client interaction.

3 This answer could be interpreted as negative; it also abdicates nursing responsibility.

92. 2 These adaptations are indicative of a urinary tract infection and should be reported immediately. (2) (PB; MR; EV; CW; HP)

1 An increase in lochial flow or reappearance of lochia after it has ceased is an indication that the activity may have been too demanding; the client should have been advised that this can occur; it need not be reported.

3 Engorgement is expected and should subside in a few days.

4 This is expected; the client may find it helpful to use a water-soluble lubricant initially.

93. 4 An autoimmune response plays a role in the development of polyarteritis, although drugs and infections may precipitate it. (3) (PB; CJ; IM; MS; CV)

1 Men are affected three times more often than women.

2 The disease is often fatal, usually as a result of heart or renal failure.

3 Arteriolar pathology can affect any organ or system.

94. 2 Bile, which aids in fat digestion, is not as concentrated as before surgery; once the body adapts to the absence of the gallbladder, the client should be able to tolerate a regular diet that contains fat. (2) (SE; MR; IM; MS; GI)

1 Initially, the client should avoid fatty foods unless the physician indicates otherwise.

3 This is inappropriate at this time; a temporary avoidance of fatty foods with the

gradual resumption of a regular diet is the priority.

4 Same as answer 3.

95. **2 Erosion of blood vessels may lead to hemorrhage, a life-threatening situation further complicated by decreased prothrombin production which occurs with cirrhosis. (3) (PB; CJ; AS; MS; GI)**

   1 Although increased intra-abdominal pressure may cause this, there is no immediate threat to life; assessment for bleeding takes priority.

   3 Same as answer 1.

   4 Although this may cause gastritis, there is no immediate threat to life; assessment for bleeding takes priority.

96. **2 Percussing over fluid produces a dull sound, not the expected tympanic sound. (3) (PB; CJ; AS; MS; GI)**

   1 Respiratory distress occurs with ascites but is not an early sign.

   3 This would assess for dependent edema, not ascites.

   4 Bowel sounds may be heard with developing ascites; when ascites is extensive, bowel sounds may diminish.

97. **2 Members must feel comfortable to discuss things in the group; there must be an awareness that what is discussed in the group will remain in the group. (2) (PI; CJ; PL; MH; TR)**

   1 This will not establish trust and will increase anxiety because the members will feel their turn for exposure will come whether they want it or not.

   3 Same as answer 1.

   4 Talking about trust does little to foster it.

98. **4 This is the client's desire, and the nurse should do everything possible to assist the client to achieve it. (2) (PB; MR; PL; MH; TR)**

   1 This would not be therapeutic; the client has an unmet need, and the nurse should not try to refocus the client away from the objective.

   2 The client should be encouraged, not discouraged; mental activity should not be too taxing and it is not unrealistic if the client wishes to do it.

   3 No data support the conclusion that the client needs to work through anger.

99. **1 The psychosexual development of a preschooler focuses on the fear of invasive procedures. (2) (PM; CJ; AN; PE; GD)**

   2 Hospitalization threatens the toddler's autonomy.

   3 The adolescent may be threatened with the loss of independence when hospitalized.

   4 Separation from the mother is most critical during infancy and toddlerhood.

100. **2 With the reduction of edema the child's health improves, the appetite increases, and the blood pressure normalizes. (2) (PB; CJ; PL; PE; RG)**

   1 Fluids should not be encouraged because the kidneys are inflamed and cannot tolerate large amounts.

   3 Ambulation does not have an adverse effect on this disorder; most children voluntarily restrict their activities during the acute phase.

   4 Sodium is lowered, not eliminated; sodium restriction is not tolerated well by children and may further decrease their appetite.

101. **3 This is important in determining whether the baby has maternally transmitted antibodies against measles. (2) (PM; CJ; AS; PE; BI)**

   1 Vaccination against measles is not done until the infant is between 12 and 15 months of age.

   2 This has no relationship to the present exposure to measles.

   4 Same as answer 2.

102. **2 The client needs to know details of transfer to assist appropriately and avoid injury. (1) (SE; MR; IM; MS; SK)**

   1 This is not advisable because this could disrupt the repair of the affected hip.

   3 This is unnecessary; the client may touch the floor with the foot but may not bear weight on this extremity.

   4 More commonly, no weight-bearing is permitted on the operative leg at first.

103. **2 Although the child has no apparent injuries, internal bleeding may have occurred; the child should be monitored for adaptations indicating internal bleeding, which is a priority in this situation. (3) (PB; CJ; AS; PE; BI)**

   1 Although all two-year-olds are at risk for falls, falls are not the greatest danger for this child in this situation.

   3 A child with hemophilia is at no greater risk for infection than any other child; the skin is intact, so this diagnosis is not a priority.

   4 Although all toddlers are at risk for fluid imbalances because of their larger percentage of body fluid to body mass, this nursing diagnosis is not a priority in this situation.

104. 3 Hypotonia occurs in magnesium sulfate toxicity because of skeletal and smooth muscle relaxation. (3) (PB; CJ; EV; CW; DR)
   1 This is not a sign of magnesium sulfate toxicity.
   2 Same as answer 1.
   4 Same as answer 1.

105. 4 This indicates failure to resolve conflicting feelings about pregnancy that commonly occur in the first trimester. (3) (PI; CJ; PL; CW; EC)
   1 This is a normal feeling in the third trimester.
   2 Same as answer 1.
   3 Concerns about the expected baby having physical abnormalities are common in the third trimester.

106. 1 Research has shown that decreasing stress will slow the rate of atherosclerotic development. (1) (PM; CJ; PL; MS; CV)
   2 Exercise is thought to decrease atherosclerosis and the formation of lipid plaques.
   3 Same as answer 2.
   4 Saturated fats in the diet increase atherosclerosis.

107. 3 The taste for salt is learned from habitual use and can be unlearned or reduced with health improvement motivation and creative salt-free food preparation. (3) (PB; CJ; IM; MS; FE)
   1 This is untrue; substitutes may have a metallic taste and do not taste like salt.
   2 The taste for salt is learned.
   4 This is unsafe; abnormally high potassium levels can result.

108. 1 A strong cry indicates effective respiratory function and is assigned a value of 2. (1) (PM; CJ; AS; PA; NN)
   2 A value of 1 is assigned when the body is pink and the extremities are blue.
   3 If the flexion of the arms and legs is only slight and movement is diminished, the value assigned is 1.
   4 The heart rate should be more than 100 per minute and therefore is assigned a value of 1.

109. 2 Autonomy leads to exploring and self-feeding; the child may eat food not on the diet. (2) (PM; CJ; AS; PE; GD)
   1 Although this is a common characteristic of a toddler, it would not lead to the child's eating restricted foods.
   3 Same as answer 1.
   4 Same as answer 1.

110. 2 The cerebellum is the most common area; symptoms of increased intracranial pressure result from obstruction of cerebrospinal fluid flow. (2) (PB; CJ; AN; PE; NM)
   1 This is an uncommon site in children.
   3 Same as answer 1.
   4 Same as answer 1.

111. 4 Bed rest promotes decreased cardiac output; it also decreases tissue catabolism, which lowers the workload of the kidneys, eventually increasing filtration by the renal glomeruli; limiting activity helps lower the blood pressure. (2) (PB; CJ; PL; PE; RG)
   1 Bed rest is necessary during the initial acute phase of this illness.
   2 The activity level depends on the response to therapy.
   3 Same as answer 2.

112. 1 Cor pulmonale is right ventricular failure caused by pulmonary congestion; edema results from increasing venous pressure. (3) (PB; CJ; AS; MS; CV)
   2 A productive cough is symptomatic of the original condition, COPD.
   3 This is caused by alterations in oxygen and hydrogen ion levels and their effects on the central nervous system.
   4 Same as answer 3.

113. 4 The chamber closest to the client collects drainage, and the second chamber acts as the water seal. (3) (PB; CJ; AN; MS; RE)
   1 Suction requires the addition of a third chamber or a modified system.
   2 The water seal in a two-chamber system is provided by the second chamber.
   3 In a one-chamber system the seal and drainage are combined, and there is no suction chamber.

114. 4 These individuals need peer group relations to validate their feelings and to experience peer group pressures. (3) (PI; MR; PL; MH; ES)
   1 These individuals have a remarkable store of energy that does not reflect their malnourished state.
   2 These individuals rarely have trouble making decisions, so they do not have to be forced into the role.
   3 These individuals totally relate their attractiveness to thinness; they have diminished libido, and in addition, females have amenorrhea.

115. 4 The nurse shows an understanding of the client's needs by not totally restricting the handwashing. (3) (PI; CJ; IM; MH; PR)

1 At this time, the client is still too anxious and is incapable of dealing with the reasons for handwashing.
2 Continued handwashing does not reveal an understanding of the underlying problem or a sign of progress.
3 This denies the client's feelings, is untrue, and will close off communication.

116. 4 **The recommended age for the fourth dose of DTaP is 12 to 18 months. (3) (PM; CJ; AN; PE; BI)**
1 The recommended age for the initial dose of PCV is 2 months.
2 The recommended age for the second dose of HepB is 1 to 4 months.
3 The recommended age for the fifth dose of IPV is 4 to 6 years.

117. 3 **These are classic signs of ketoacidosis because of the respiratory system's attempt to compensate by blowing off excess carbon dioxide, a component of carbonic acid. (2) (PB; CJ; AS; MS; EN)**
1 This is indicative of an insulin reaction (diabetic hypoglycemia).
2 This is a hypersensitivity reaction; it is unrelated to diabetes.
4 Diaphoresis is associated with an insulin reaction, not diabetic ketoacidosis.

118. 2 **This behavior is typical of the working stage of the group; trust has been established, and a willingness to discuss any problems or needs is present. (2) (SE; MR; EV; MH; TR)**
1 This can occur at any stage; it occurs in social, as well as therapeutic, relationships.
3 This would occur in the early phase of the group before trust is established and when everyone is trying to adapt.
4 Same as answer 3.

119. 3 **Total blood volume increases 50%, which necessitates the heart pumping harder and working more to accommodate this increase. (2) (PM; CJ; AN; CW; HC)**
1 Although the renal threshold is lowered, the major changes occur in the cardiovascular system.
2 Changes in hormone levels occur but are not as profound as changes in the cardiovascular system.
4 There are few changes in this system, but pressure from the growing uterus can result in digestive discomfort and altered patterns of elimination.

120. 1 **The client has the right to privacy; the behavior is acceptable in the privacy of his room. (3) (SE; CJ; IM; MH; NP)**
2 Masturbation is a normal sexual outlet; assessment is unnecessary unless the act is practiced to excess or in public.
3 This can cause needless embarrassment to the client and may close off further communication.
4 The behavior is not inappropriate because the client was in the privacy of his own room.

121. 2 **When clients in obvious crisis appear depressed, anxious, and desperate, the nurse should question them regarding the presence of suicidal thoughts. (2) (PI; CJ; IM; CW; EC)**
1 Further assessment and exploration are needed before encouraging clients to admit themselves to a psychiatric facility.
3 Running away from problems does not help solve them, nor will escaping bring lasting relief.
4 When clients are overwhelmed with problems, it is difficult for them to think positively.

122. 2 **When a client has perforated viscera, barium could leak out of the intestinal tract and cause inflammation and/or an abscess. (2) (SE; CJ; AN; MS; GI)**
1 Although it may be irritating, this does not contraindicate barium studies.
3 Barium studies are not contraindicated and are useful in diagnosing ulcerative colitis and Crohn's disease.
4 Serum potassium would be unaffected; barium is insoluble and would not affect blood content.

123. 2 **During a health crisis, the client will need support from significant others. (2) (PI; CJ; PL; CW; NP)**
1 This information is an expected part of a complete health history for a female client; this particular client needs emotional support.
3 Same as answer 1.
4 This information is an expected part of a complete health history for all clients.

124. 4 **This is the definition of a positive CST result. (3) (PB; CJ; AN; CW; HP)**
1 A CST is performed after an NST is nonreactive or equivocal, not before.
2 A positive CST result does not dictate a cesarean birth; an expeditious vaginal birth may be attempted.
3 This fetal heart rate is expected in a healthy fetus.

125. 3 **This rejects the behavior, not the client; it helps separate the client from the behavior. (3) (PI; CJ; IM; MH; SD)**
    1 This does not help the client learn self-control; it rejects both the client and the behavior.
    2 Isolating this client limits learning more acceptable responses.
    4 Part of recovery is learning acceptable behavior; ignoring inappropriate behavior does not help.

126. 4 **The aim of therapy is to eliminate the causative agent, which can be determined from culture and sensitivity tests of sputum. (1) (PB; CJ; EV; MS; RE)**
    1 A lung scan permits visualization of lung vasculature but does not provide data on the condition of the lung tissue itself.
    2 Bronchoscopy shows the appearance of the bronchi but does not indicate the presence or absence of microorganisms.
    3 Pulmonary function studies indicate air volume that may fall within the expected range despite the presence of bronchopneumonia.

127. 3 **Stopping the flow reduces cramping caused by distention. (1) (PB; CJ; IM; MS; GI)**
    1 There is no need to discontinue the enema; flow should be interrupted temporarily until discomfort subsides; an effective enema must be administered before this surgery.
    2 This would result in the administration of a Harris flush; the purpose of the preoperative enema is to evacuate the bowel of feces, not flatus.
    4 This would increase the discomfort.

128. 4 **Cortical control of voluntary muscles occurs between 2 and 4 months. (3) (PM; CJ; IM; PE; NM)**
    1 Cerebral palsy is not diagnosed by the presence of joint deformities; these may develop later because of spastic muscle imbalance.
    2 Parents have a right to be informed of their child's diagnosis as soon as possible.
    3 The neurologic lesions are fixed and will neither progress nor regress.

129. 4 **The first insertion site should be distal (low) on the periphery of an extremity and progress proximally (upward) toward the trunk; the upper extremities are the most appropriate sites for intravenous insertions for adults and children older than 1 year. (2) (PB; CJ; PL; PE; BI)**
    1 The scalp veins are used only for infants.
    2 Foot veins should not be used once a child is walking.
    3 This site should be avoided because the arm would have to be immobilized to stabilize the intravenous insertion site to prevent an infiltration.

130. 4 **As the lower uterine segment stretches and thins, tearing and bleeding occur at the low implantation site. (2) (PM; CJ; AS; CW; HP)**
    1 First trimester bleeding is associated with spontaneous abortion or inadequate implantation, not placenta previa.
    2 This is usually associated with abruptio placentae rather than placenta previa.
    3 Same as answer 1.

131. 4 **This presents the reality of the situation and helps support the client during a threatening hallucination. (2) (PI; CJ; IM; MH; SD)**
    1 This would have little effect on the client's behavior and would not stop the hallucination.
    2 Clients cannot be distracted from hallucinations without competing stimuli.
    3 This would encourage withdrawal and isolation and would not stop the hallucination.

132. 3 **Regression to a more immature, helpless developmental level is expected and should be supported at this time. (2) (PI; MR; PL; MS; EH)**
    1 Denial is not the response described.
    2 The client's behavior is inconsistent with the need for more control.
    4 The client's behavior does not indicate anger.

133. 3 **Fluid may shift from the intravascular space to the abdomen as fluid is removed leading to hypovolemia and compensatory tachycardia. (3) (PB; CJ; EV; MS; GI)**
    1 The fluid shift can cause hypovolemia with resulting hypotension, not hypertension.
    2 A paracentesis should decrease the degree of abdominal distention.
    4 This sign of dehydration may occur, but it is not as vital or immediate as signs of shock.

134. 1 **This reduces the possibility of bladder puncture. (1) (SE; CJ; IM; CW; HP)**
    2 The mother may eat and drink before the test.
    3 Sedation is unnecessary and is not given.
    4 This procedure is not done via the colon, so fecal material does not have to be expelled.

135. 1 Heat causes vasodilation and an increased blood supply to the area. (2) (PB; CJ; PL; CW; HC)

   2 This is not the purpose of the sitz baths.

   3 Cleansing is done immediately after voiding and defecating usually with a squeeze bottle filled with cleansing solution or water.

   4 Relaxation of the rectal sphincter is promoted by the sitz bath; this will provide comfort but will not increase healing.

136. 2 Yogurt, which contains calcium, is more easily digested because it contains the enzyme lactase, which breaks down milk sugar. (1) (PB; CJ; AN; MS; GI)

   1 These are deficient in calcium.

   3 Same as answer 1.

   4 Same as answer 1.

137. 4 Mood changes can occur as a side effect of steroid therapy. (3) (PI; CJ; EV; MS; DR)

   1 This denies the value of the client's statement and offers false reassurance.

   2 The client has already stated the problem and does not know why this is happening.

   3 This is difficult to do because the mood swings may occur without an overt cause.

138. 1 Hypertension increases pressure on the suture lines of the graft. (2) (PB; CJ; IM; MS; CV)

   2 Signs of anaphylactic shock, including a drop in BP, would be associated with a severe allergic reaction.

   3 An increased BP does not necessarily mean the client is hypervolemic.

   4 This would be indicated by absent pedal pulses.

139. 4 A child with a conduct disorder is physically aggressive; no physical aggression in three months demonstrates that treatment has been successful; the physical aggression differentiates it from oppositional defiant disorder. (3) (PI; CJ; EV; MH; BA)

   1 This is an appropriate short-term, not long-term, goal for this child.

   2 Controlling verbal aggression alone would not be appropriate for this child; this outcome would more correctly address the problems of a child with oppositional defiant disorder.

   3 This statement would show a negative outcome for this child.

140. 4 Increased venous pressure resulting from backup of blood, as the right ventricle of the heart fails, forces capillary fluid to seep into interstitial spaces resulting in peripheral edema. (2) (PB; CJ; AN; MS; CV)

   1 Tachypnea and dyspnea occur.

   2 Chest pain may be present with a myocardial infarction or cardiovascular insufficiency, not heart failure.

   3 Bradycardia does not occur; the heartbeats may vary in intensity, a pulse deficit may be present, or a bounding pulse may be felt.

141. 2 Cerebellar astrocytomas, unlike those in the cerebrum, are slow growing and benign, with a cure rate of 70% to 90% after surgery. (2) (PM; CJ; IM; PE; NM)

   1 Other infratentorial tumors, such as medulloblastomas, are rapid growing and highly malignant.

   3 This is not true of a cerebellar astrocytoma.

   4 Same as answer 3.

142. 1 This commonly begins with what parents describe as clumsiness that becomes progressively worse; the cerebellum controls coordination. (2) (PM; CJ; AS; PE; NM)

   2 Seizures usually occur with cerebral or supratentorial tumors.

   3 This is a very late sign of tumor involvement.

   4 At this age, sutures are completely closed and the cranium does not get larger.

143. 4 Sexual anxiety and conflict can occur with schizophrenia; projection is an ego defense mechanism. (2) (PI; CJ; IM; MH; SD)

   1 This avoids the issue and is a threatening response; this could increase anxiety.

   2 This validates ideas of reference and is an inappropriate response.

   3 The anxious client may not be able to handle being confronted with feelings; this may precipitate a panic reaction.

144. 3 Absence of peptidase results in an inability to metabolize the gliadin component of grains; this results in excessive glutamine that is toxic to the mucosal cells. (1) (PI; CJ; AN; PE; GI)

   1 Meconium is present in the bowel of a newborn.

   2 This does not occur.

   4 Fluid balance is not the basic problem with celiac disease; however, dehydration can occur in celiac crisis.

145. 3 Jewish dietary laws prohibit any combination of milk and meat. (3) (SE; MR; AN; MS; NP)

1 Fish that have scales and fins are considered clean, therefore allowable.

2 The Hindu religion prohibits the ingestion of beef and veal; many believe the cow is sacred.

4 Seventh Day Adventists, Baptists, Mormons, and Muslims prohibit some or all of these beverages.

146. 4 Skin-to-skin contact between mother and infant is most effective in maintaining the infant's body temperature; heat is transferred by conduction. (1) (PM; CJ; IM; CW; NN)

1 Oxygen is not administered unless the infant is experiencing respiratory and cardiac difficulties; oxygen has a cooling effect.

2 This is not very effective and leaves much of the baby exposed; a blanket and warmer also would be necessary.

3 Bathing the infant should be delayed until the body temperature is stabilized.

147. 2 All data presented are within the norm for a client at 20-weeks' gestation and should be recorded. (1) (PM; CJ; AS; CW; HC)

1 Since all data are within the norm, there is no need to report them.

3 Same as answer 1.

4 There is no evidence to suggest the need for an emergency admission; all findings are within the norm.

148. 1 The client and his needs are the priority, and assessment is the first step of the nursing process. (2) (PI; CJ; AS; MH; SD)

2 The nurse must deal with the present, not the past.

3 This is not the priority; it would be done later.

4 Same as answer 3.

149. 4 Inadequate protein decreases colloidal osmotic pressure within the vascular space, allowing fluid to shift into the interstitial spaces. (2) (PB; CJ; AS; CW; HP)

1 Petechiae result from an abnormality in the clotting mechanism, such as thrombocytopenia.

2 A protein deficit does not affect heart rate unless it is severe.

3 Bleeding gums result from a deficiency in vitamin C or platelets, not protein.

150. 3 If the airway is not patent and gas exchange is inadequate, life cannot be sustained; thus, this must be the top priority. (3) (PB; CJ; PL; CW; HN)

1 Although bonding is important to the parent-child relationship, without oxygen life could not be sustained.

2 Although preventing infection is important, without oxygen life could not be sustained.

4 Although body temperature is important because the baby is lacking brown fat and other defense mechanisms needed to maintain temperature, without oxygen life could not be sustained.

151. 4 Preschoolers are active, sociable individuals who enjoy the company of peers and become bored when isolated. (3) (PM; CJ; IM; PE; GD)

1 Preschoolers have a limited ability to understand complex explanations of cause and effect; they employ concrete thinking.

2 This will increase agitation, and it is punitive.

3 Although this would provide some distraction, it is better to permit peer contacts.

152. 4 Laryngeal nerve injury can cause laryngeal spasms resulting in airway obstruction. (2) (PB; MR; IM; MS; EN)

1 Parathyroid damage would result in hypocalcemia, not hypercalcemia.

2 Thyrotoxic crisis (thyroid storm) increases vital signs resulting in hypertension, tachycardia, and tachypnea.

3 Tetany is caused by decreased parathormone, a parathyroid hormone not a thyroid hormone.

153. 4 This position helps maintain the head and neck in functional alignment and facilitates respirations because the abdominal organs are not pressing against the diaphragm, which allows the thoracic cavity to expand without resistance. (2) (PB; CJ; PL; MS; RE)

1 This position would place tension on the operative site because the head must be turned to the side.

2 This position inhibits respiratory excursion because the abdominal organs press against the diaphragm, and full expansion of the lung on the side on which the client is lying is inhibited.

3 This may cause flexion of the neck, which may place tension on the suture line.

154. 3 Eating in a semirecumbent position slows gastric emptying, thereby preventing premature gastric dumping of contents. (3) (PM; CJ; PL; MS; GI)

1 This would speed gastric emptying and should be avoided.

2 Same as answer 1.

4 Same as answer 1.

155. **2 Children, because of the demands of growth and their dietary indiscretions, have a fragile glucose balance. (1) (PB; CJ; IM; PE; EN)**

1 Obesity is more often associated with type 2 diabetes.

3 Resistance to treatment is not common; problems are related to the changing requirements associated with growth.

4 Hypersensitivity is unrelated to either type of diabetes.

156. **4 Saccharin (Sweet and Low), aspartame (Neutrasweet), and sucralose (Splenda) are non-nutritive sweeteners recommended for clients with diabetes. (2) (PB; MR; IM; PE; EN)**

1 Honey, a fructose, provides 1.3 times as many kilocalories as does table sugar and must be calculated into the diet.

2 Simple sugars may be used in controlled amounts and must be calculated into the diet.

3 Foods do not have to taste sweet to contain sugar; individuals who enjoy sweetened foods do not break the sweet-taste habit.

157. **4 This accurately responds to the parents' question, reinforcing what the physician explained. (2) (PI; CJ; IM; PE; BI)**

1 This is an insensitive response that places the parents on the defensive.

2 This would abdicate the nurse's teaching responsibilities.

3 This statement reinforces parental insecurity about the information they have recently received from the physician; this may increase anxiety.

158. **3 Prevention of infection continues as a priority both before and after the repair of the sac. (2) (SE; CJ; PL; PE; NM)**

1 A neurologically impaired infant would not be given sedatives because they would interfere with accurate assessment.

2 This is unrealistic; newborns lose weight in the first few days of life.

4 This is not the priority at this time.

159. **3 The staff nurse should call the supervisor to confirm and deal with the problem. (2) (SE; LE; IM; MS; NP)**

1 The security guard has no authority in this situation.

2 Although this removes the nurse manager from the clinical setting, it does not provide for documentation of the situation; also, the nurse manager may be in no condition to go home independently.

4 Walking about and drinking coffee do not make a person less intoxicated; the nurse manager's condition needs to be confirmed and dealt with by a supervisor.

160. **4 Looking at the face or seeking eye-to-eye contact with the infant is an early sign of the beginning of bonding with the infant. (3) (PM; CJ; EV; CW; EC)**

1 This may indicate that the mother is worried that she does not have enough milk, a common concern.

2 Mothers may feel inept or worry about upsetting the nurse by undressing their infant; new mothers need encouragement to undress their infant.

3 Mother's classes usually are given during the prenatal period; if refused at this time, there should be no cause for concern.

161. **4 Hyperextension of the neck places tension on the suture line. (2) (PB; CJ; AN; MS; RE)**

1 The cervical vertebrae are designed to flex and hyperextend; there should be no ill effects.

2 Hyperextension would not cause this.

3 Same as answer 2.

162. **4 This position may prevent further prolapse and relieves pressure on the cord. (1) (SE; CJ; IM; CW; HP)**

1 Although this will be done later, the priority is to relieve pressure on the cord.

2 This promotes placental perfusion but would not relieve pressure on the cord.

3 Same as answer 1.

163. **3 This expands collapsed alveoli and enhances surfactant activity, thereby preventing atelectasis. (3) (PB; CJ; PL; MS; RE)**

1 This helps clear accumulated secretions from the pulmonary tree; it does not directly promote alveolar expansion.

2 This promotes sustained exhalation, not inhalation.

4 This promotes collapse of, not expansion of, alveoli.

164. **3 The lack of a social support system can precipitate feelings of isolation. (1) (PI; CJ; AN; MH; AX)**

1 The data do not support this nursing diagnosis.

2 Same as answer 1.

4 Same as answer 1.

165. 4 Intestinal antibiotics and a complete cleansing of the bowel with enemas until returns are clear are necessary to reduce the possibility of fecal contamination when the bowel is resected. (1) (SE; CJ; PL; MS; GI)
  1 This is not necessary; there is no evidence of urinary infection.
  2 The bladder will be removed, so there is no need for an indwelling catheter.
  3 A clear liquid diet usually is prescribed for several days with npo for at least eight hours before surgery.

166. 2 This response encourages the client to explore the defenses employed to cope with anxiety. (2) (PI; CJ; IM; MH; AX)
  1 This is a nontherapeutic response that denies the importance of a problematic area of behavior.
  3 This focuses on tasks rather than feelings; also, it may be perceived as threatening or judgmental.
  4 This is a nontherapeutic response; the client has not expressed a desire to modify or change this behavior.

167. 3 This is an iron-rich food appropriate for mild anemia, which probably has occurred from blood loss into the tissues at the site of the injury. (2) (PB; CJ; IM; PE; BI)
  1 This is not necessary unless there is a marked decrease.
  2 Same as answer 1.
  4 If internal bleeding occurred, there would have been earlier signs other than a slight reduction in hemoglobin and hematocrit levels.

168. 1 The possibility of ascending infection increases when membranes are ruptured and birth is not imminent; the client must be monitored for signs of infection. (2) (SE; CJ; AS; CW; HP)
  2 This is unrelated to spontaneous rupture of the membranes.
  3 This would be a sign of placenta previa, which would have been diagnosed before the membranes ruptured.
  4 This is not indicated with spontaneous rupture of membranes; it is indicated if persistent late decelerations are observed on the fetal monitor during labor.

169. 2 This fat-binding agent would also bind and eliminate other fat-soluble vitamins such as vitamins D, E, and K. (2) (PB; CJ; EV; MS; DR)
  1 This is not a fat-soluble vitamin and would be unaffected.

3 Same as answer 1.
4 Same as answer 1.

170.
  1 _____ Fever may indicate the presence of an infection, which is associated with a reduction in white blood cells (leukopenia).
  2 _____ Nausea and vomiting are side effects of chemotherapy because of the effect of chemotherapy on the rapidly dividing cells of the mucous membranes of the gastrointestinal system.
  3 _x_ **Black, tarry feces due to the action of intestinal secretions on blood are associated with bleeding in the gastrointestinal tract; bleeding is related to a reduced number of thrombocytes, which are part of the coagulation process. (3) (PB; CJ; EV; MS; BI)**
  4 _x_ **Hemorrhages into the skin and mucous membranes (purpura) may occur with reduced numbers of thrombocytes, which are part of the coagulation process.**
  5 _____ Diarrhea may be a side effect of chemotherapy, but it is not a thrombocytopenic side effect.
  6 _x_ **Blood in the urine (hematuria) may occur with reduced number of thrombocytes, which are part of the coagulation process.**

171. 4 Together, lack of symmetry and palpation of a thickening are abnormal findings. (1) (PB; CJ; EV; CW; WH)
  1 Engorgement is an expected response to menstrual hormones.
  2 Premenstrual engorgement may cause the breast to feel lumpy.
  3 This is a common deviation that is within normal limits.

172. 4 Because the client is feeling a loss of control, it is most important to include the client in revision of the plan. (2) (SE; MR; PL; MH; NP)
  1 This does not consider changes in the client or the client's feelings.
  2 Planning nursing care is within the nurse's function and judgment, not the physician's; the client should be included.
  3 This is very authoritarian and places total control with the nurse.

173. 4 Magnesium sulfate is a central nervous system depressant; it decreases cerebral irritability thus preventing seizures. (2) (PB; CJ; AN; CW; DR)

1 Magnesium sulfate is not a diuretic; adequate kidney function is necessary to promote its excretion, otherwise toxicity will result.

2 Magnesium sulfate is not an oxytocic; oxytocin is used to promote uterine contractions and can cause an increased BP.

3 Magnesium sulfate is not an antihypertensive; however, it may cause a transient decrease in BP because of the drug's peripheral dilating effect.

174. 4 **In abruptio placentae there is uterine bleeding that can result in massive internal hemorrhage, causing hypovolemic shock. (2) (PB; CJ; AS; CW; HP)**

1 Jaundice occurs only when there is a deposition of bilirubin into subcutaneous tissues and skin; this is not associated with abruptio placentae.

2 It is more likely that with internal bleeding, blood pressure will fall rather than increase.

3 Seizures are associated with preeclampsia; there is no information indicating the presence of this condition.

175. 4 **Familiarity with situations and continuity add to the client's sense of security and foster trust in the relationship. (2) (PI; CJ; PL; MH; DD)**

1 Detailed explanations will be forgotten; instructions should be simple and to the point and given when needed.

2 Although this helps individualize care, continuity is the priority.

3 Some degree of flexibility by the nurse would help to individualize care.

176. 3 **Alcohol deactivates the smallpox vaccine; cleansing of the arm should not to be done before the immunization is given unless the arm is dirty; if dirty, only water should be used to cleanse the site. (3) (SE; MR; IM; MS; BI)**

1 Observation is insufficient; the nurse manager must intervene to make sure that the vaccine is given using the correct technique.

2 Povidone will deactivate the smallpox vaccine.

4 Cleansing of the arm is unnecessary unless the arm is dirty; if so, only water should be used to cleanse the site.

177. 3 **Tetanus immune human globulin should not cause anaphylaxis because it is derived from human serum. (2) (SE; CJ; AN; PE; BI)**

1 Tetanus immune human globulin is not as effective as the antitoxin, but it is not derived from horse serum and should not cause anaphylaxis.

2 It is necessary to perform skin tests for both types of medications to determine the presence of sensitivity.

4 These medications always carry the risk of hypersensitivity; it cannot be assumed they can be given safely to everyone.

178. 3 **This prevents the spread of infection to others; isolation is a priority that should be implemented immediately. (1) (SE; MR; IM; PE; NM)**

1 There is no indication that the child is dehydrated; fluid maintenance is a continuing goal.

2 There is no indication that the child needs oxygen, and it would not be given routinely.

4 This would not be given because these children are sensitive to stimuli, and movement causes increased discomfort.

179. 4 **Furniture and loose rugs can interfere with crutch walking and should be removed to prevent further injury. (1) (SE; MR; PL; MS; SK)**

1 Calcium, rather than vitamin C, would be encouraged to enhance bone healing; vitamin C prevents capillary fragility.

2 The client may shower if the cast is protected from becoming wet or is water proof.

3 This is a medical, not a nursing, decision.

180. 4 **Nerve and vascular injury and significant blood loss may be present. (2) (SE; CJ; AS; MS; SK)**

1 This is a medical decision that has not yet been made; closed fractures generally are reduced by manipulation.

2 False reassurance is never appropriate.

3 Closed fractures generally do not require operative reduction; they are usually reduced by manipulation.

181. 3 **Increased venous pressure alters the permeability of the veins allowing extravasation of RBCs; lysis of RBCs causes the brownish discoloration. (2) (SE; MR; IM; MS; CV)**

1 The arterial circulation is not affected by the pathology of varicose veins.

2 Although tissue healing may be delayed, the brownish discoloration results from lysis of RBCs, not trauma.

4 There is no increase in melanocyte activity in the skin surrounding varicose veins.

182. 2 **Cleansing after feeding keeps the suture line from becoming infected. (2) (SE; CJ; EV; PE; IT)**

1 This exerts pressure on the suture line and may cause wound separation.

3 Same as answer 1.

4 The baby should be held and cuddled during feedings.

183. 2 **Clients with cardiac disease should be taught the signs and symptoms of cardiac decompensation; if they occur, the client should stop the activity that precipitated them and notify the health care provider. (3) (PB; MR; PL; CW; HP)**

   1 This is acceptable for a client with Class I cardiac disease.
   3 This is the treatment for a client with Class III cardiac disease.
   4 This is the recommendation for a client with Class IV cardiac disease.

184. 4 **The three areas of assessment to determine level of consciousness using the Glasgow Coma Scale are eye-opening in response to speech, motor response to verbal commands, and verbal response to speech. (3) (PB; CJ; AS; MS; NM)**

   1 Response to light and tendon reflexes are not included in the Glasgow Coma Scale.
   2 These responses are not included in the Glasgow Coma Scale.
   3 Breathing pattern is not included in the Glasgow Coma Scale.

185. 3 **Blood pressure increases with pain and stress; reevaluation is critical before determining if the physician should be notified. (3) (PB; CJ; AS; MS; CV)**

   1 Assessment should be completed before notifying the physician.
   2 Medication should not be administered until the cause of the headache is determined.
   4 Oxygen is not indicated; the physician should be notified if a second blood pressure reading remains elevated.

186. 2 **This therapy permits relative isolation of the tumor area and saturation with the drug(s) selected. (2) (PB; CJ; AN; MS; GI)**

   1 This is not true; this procedure requires medical and nursing supervision.
   3 Combinations of drugs can be administered via IV or oral routes as well.
   4 These effects cannot be confined completely to the treated area; some migration still occurs.

187. 3 **Laryngeal spasms can occur abruptly; patency of the airway is determined by constant assessment for signs of respiratory distress. (1) (PB; CJ; PL; PE; RE)**

   1 This is important, but maintenance of respiration has priority.
   2 The fever should be treated, but it is not critical at 103° F; maintenance of respiration has priority.
   4 Same as answer 1.

188. 2 **This is an early sign of a changing level of consciousness; it is one of the first signs of increased intracranial pressure. (3) (PB; CJ; AS; MS; NM)**

   1 This is a subjective symptom that may or may not be present with increasing intracranial pressure.
   3 This is a late sign that occurs in children with hydrocephalus.
   4 This is a late sign that occurs as compression of the brainstem increases.

189. 1 **This is a prime time for symptoms of a pulmonary embolus to appear. (2) (PB; CJ; EV; MS; SK)**

   2 This could result from the inflammatory process; the temperature-regulating mechanisms in older adults may be compromised slightly, and they may show a slight elevation in body temperature for a longer period of time after surgery.
   3 This would not require nursing intervention; a productive cough would indicate a respiratory infection.
   4 Weight-bearing is being done by the affected leg at this time, and fatigue may be expected.

190. 3 **Obtaining cultures is the most reliable method of determining the presence of an infecting agent. (1) (PM; MR; AS; MS; BI)**

   1 Although this may be done, the presence of an infecting agent should be identified first.
   2 This is usual when an infecting organism is present; it is not yet confirmed that the infecting microorganism is present.
   4 Same as answer 1.

191. 1 **The pain caused by vascular occlusion is often described as excruciating, and analgesics should be administered immediately after a pain assessment. (3) (PB; CJ; PL; PE; BI)**

   2 Oxygen is not helpful in reversing the sickling which is causing the pain.
   3 Although this is important, it is not the priority; pain relief is the priority.
   4 Although this might be done to treat the anemia and reduce the viscosity of the sickled blood, it would be done after analgesic administration.

192. 3 **To plan intervention, the nurse must be aware of how the mother has handled stress and if she has someone she can rely on for support. (3) (PI; CJ; IM; MH; CS)**

   1 It is too early to deal with sensitive areas; these are introduced after a relationship has been developed.
   2 This serves no purpose; it is more important to know past coping mechanisms and the present support system.

4 The implications of this response will hinder further communication; it is too early to determine the cause of the infant's failure to thrive.

193. 2 **Pulmonary edema is associated with severe preeclampsia; as vasospasms worsen, capillary endothelial damage results in capillary leakage. (3) (PB; CJ; AN; CW; HP)**
1 Crackles are not an indication of an impending seizure; signs of an impending seizure include hyperreflexia, developing or worsening clonus, severe headache, visual disturbances, and epigastric pain.
3 Pregnancy does not precipitate bronchial constriction; the hormones associated with pregnancy can cause nasal congestion.
4 This is a discomfort associated with pregnancy that may result in shortness of breath or dyspnea, not crackles.

194. 4 **This position promotes venous return by gravity, which helps reduce intracranial pressure, a problem after myelomeningocele repair (2) (PB; CJ; AN; CW; HN)**
1 Although this is important, minimizing intracranial pressure is the priority.
2 Same answer as 1.
3 Same answer as 1.

195. 2 **Situational crises involve an unanticipated loss, such as a divorce that is threatening to the client. (1) (PI; CJ; AN; MH; CS)**
1 Social crises involve multiple losses such as those occurring during major disasters.
3 Maturational crises occur in response to stress experienced as one struggles with developmental tasks.
4 Developmental (maturational) crises are associated with developmental tasks; divorce is not a developmental task.

196. 1 **Subcutaneous emphysema refers to the presence of air in the tissue that surrounds an opening in the normally closed respiratory tract; the tissue appears puffy, and a crackling sensation is detected under the fingertips because trapped air is compressed between the tissue. (2) (PB; CJ; AS; MS; RE)**
2 Gas exchange, and thus blood gases, are not affected.
3 The lungs are not affected.
4 Same as answer 3.

197. 2 **The client is anxious and afraid of leaving home; the priority is provision for safety and security needs. (3) (PI; CJ; PL; MH; AX)**

1 Unless the client is provided with a sense of security, adjustment probably will be unsatisfactory because the anxiety will most likely escalate.
3 This cannot be done until anxiety is reduced.
4 The client is experiencing memory loss and may not be able to remember what precipitated admission to the hospital; some memory loss may be a result of high anxiety and thought blocking.

198. 2 **Gastric secretions, which are electrolyte rich, are lost through the NG tube; the imbalances that result could prove life threatening. (1) (PB; CJ; EV; MS; FE)**
1 This is unnecessary and could damage the suture line.
3 This could result in suture line disruption.
4 This is unsafe; if respiratory intubation has occurred, aspiration will result.

199. 2 **School-age children are most concerned about school, if not for the academics, for the social aspects. (2) (PM; MR; AS; PE; GD)**
1 This may be of some concern, but not as much as school is.
3 School-age children generally look at physicians as authority figures and do not doubt their competence.
4 School-age children generally are not this future oriented.

200. 4 **Baseline vital signs are extremely important; physical assessment precedes diagnostic measures and intervention. (2) (SE; CJ; AS; MS; RE)**
1 This might be done after it is determined whether a specimen for blood gases is needed; this is not usually an independent function of the nurse; oxygen is administered independently by the nurse only in an emergency situation.
2 This would be done after the physician makes a medical diagnosis; this is not an independent function of the nurse.
3 A sputum specimen should be obtained after vital signs and before administration of antibiotics.

201. 4 **Knowing what to expect allows the client to have control and decreases fear. (3) (PB; MR; IM; MS; EH)**
1 Usually there are no long-term dietary restrictions.
2 Routine exercises would not be prescribed.
3 There are no incisions with laparoscopic surgery.

202. 1 **These are signs of water intoxication, which may proceed to pulmonary edema; the physician should be notified. (3) (PB; CJ; IM; MS; FE)**
    2 Chest x-ray findings lag behind clinical manifestations; the last chest x-ray film does not reflect current status.
    3 Increasing the IV rate should never be done, particularly if water intoxication is suspected.
    4 Same as answer 3.

203. 1 **During detoxification this provides safety and prevents suicide, which is a real threat. (2) (PI; MR; PL; MH; SA)**
    2 Bright light is preferable to dim light, which creates shadows and increases illusions and misinterpretations.
    3 This type of client does not usually lose the sense of hearing, so there is no need to shout.
    4 Restraints may upset the client further; if at all possible, they should not be used.

204. 1 **This is a plant alkaloid that is cell-cycle specific; it affects cell division during metaphase by interfering with spindle formation and causing cell death. (3) (PB; CJ; IM; MS; DR)**
    2 This is typical of antimetabolites such as fluorouracil.
    3 Alkylating agents such as nitrogen mustard act in this way.
    4 Antibiotics such as dactinomycin act in this way.

205. 3 **This is an emergency situation; sudden pressure is exerted on the third cranial nerve on the affected side caused by displacement of the tentorium or uncus. (3) (PB; CJ; AN; PE; NM)**
    1 Response to severe pain would not result in this reaction.
    2 An autonomic response to fear would affect both pupils equally.
    4 Reduced pressure would not cause one pupil to dilate; more likely, increasing pressure would cause this response.

206. 2 **The signs and symptoms described, in conjunction with the longest and strongest contractions, occur in the transition phase of the first stage of labor. (1) (PM; CJ; AS; CW; HC)**
    1 In this stage the contractions are well spaced, with more time to relax in between.
    3 This is the period after the birth of the infant to the birth of the placenta.
    4 In this stage the fetal head begins to crown and would be seen at the perineum.

207. 3 **Respect and concern for both child and mother are necessary because both respond according to the message they receive. (2) (PI; CJ; AS; MH; CS)**
    1 The pediatric history is not so important a variable as the relationship between mother and child.
    2 This may be true, but the nurse should deal with the present relationship.
    4 The present findings may indeed be influenced by the mother's past history and present health.

208. 2 **Vasodilation should help reduce pain from cellular clumping; this will address the pain until the pump can be activated. (3) (PB; CJ; IM; PE; BI)**
    1 The pain can be excruciating; television may be an adequate distractor for mild pain, not severe pain.
    3 Nursing measures should be used before calling the physician.
    4 This does not address the problem and provides no comfort for a person with severe pain.

209. 2 **Decreased sodium intake can accelerate lithium retention, with subsequent toxicity. (2) (PB; MR; IM; MH; DR)**
    1 This is unrelated to the administration of lithium.
    3 Same as answer 1.
    4 Same as answer 1.

210. 1 **The client may become injured in many ways during a seizure, and trauma prevention is a priority. (2) (SE; CJ; PL; MS; NM)**
    2 Anticonvulsants can cause GI disturbances, especially early in therapy; they should be taken with food.
    3 Others should be aware of the condition and taught how to help in case of a seizure.
    4 This is untrue; symptoms and treatment of seizure disorders vary greatly.

211. 4 **Gastric returns would indicate correct placement. (1) (SE; CJ; IM; PE; GI)**
    1 Further assessment is necessary.
    2 This could cause undue trauma regardless of where the tube is located.
    3 This is unsafe until correct placement is verified; feeding could enter the lung if the tube is not in the stomach.

212. 3 **Toxicity can result because the action of calcium ions is similar to that of digitalis. (3) (PB; CJ; AN; MS; DR)**
    1 Calcium gluconate cannot be added to a solution containing carbonate or phosphate because a dangerous precipitation will occur.

2 If calcium infiltrates, sloughing of tissue will result.

4 Calcium can be added to this solution.

213. 4 **Because of the anatomic position of the parathyroids, they may be accidentally removed during surgery. (3) (PB; CJ; EV; MS; EN)**
  1 The thoracic cavity is not entered.
  2 The thyroid is nearer to the trachea.
  3 Usually this results from a blunt blow.

214. 3 **The newborn's intestinal tract is sterile and therefore does not have intestinal flora to synthesize vitamin K, a precursor to prothrombin that is necessary for clotting. (2) (PB; CJ; AN; CW; NN)**
  1 This is not affected by vitamin K.
  2 Same as answer 1.
  4 Same as answer 1.

215. 3 **Nasogastric suction is maintained to prevent pressure on the intestinal anastomosis; no oral fluids are permitted until peristalsis resumes and nasogastric suction is stopped. (3) (PB; CJ; IM; MS; RG)**
  1 This drains immediately unless it is a continent conduit; this has no bearing on when oral fluids can be started.
  2 This would be too long to wait; sips of water are permitted when peristalsis returns and the nasogastric tube is removed.
  4 The return of peristalsis and removal of the nasogastric tube are determinants.

216. 3 **This response recognizes the client's feelings and attempts to collect data about the duration of the problem. (3) (PI; CJ; AS; MH; AX)**
  1 This is irrelevant and will not elicit data about the extent of the anxiety.
  2 Anxiety is most often a response to a vague, nonspecific threat; the client may not be able to answer this question.
  4 It is too early to identify the cause of the anxiety; crisis intervention with anxious clients requires a more structured approach than "shall we talk."

217. 2 **Toxoids are modified toxins that stimulate the body to form antibodies that can last up to 10 years against the specific disease; because the child will be in a foreign country, the toxoid is given prophylactically. (2) (PM; CJ; IM; PE; BI)**
  1 It provides active, not passive immunity; all passive immunity is short acting.
  3 Only by having the disease can lifelong natural immunity become possible.
  4 Toxoids confer lifelong active, not temporary passive, immunity.

218. 4 **The virus disintegrates rapidly on contact with soap. (2) (SE; MR; EV; CW; HP)**
  1 The lesion is in the genital area, not on the lips; kissing will not affect the infant.
  2 This is unnecessary; meticulous handwashing is required.
  3 This is not necessary because soap effectively disintegrates the virus.

219. 3 **This provides the family member with an opportunity to express feelings. (1) (PI; CJ; IM; MH; CS)**
  1 This statement does not address the family members' concerns.
  2 This is false reassurance and cuts off communication.
  4 This shuts off communication and abdicates nursing responsibility toward the client.

220. 4 **This demonstrates the client's diminished anger and is a realistic assessment and acceptance of present capabilities and limitations. (2) (PI; CJ; EV; MH; CS)**
  1 This shows dependency; the client either has given up or is being sarcastic.
  2 Anger is still apparent at loss of decision making; there is no evidence of sharing.
  3 This shows dependency and suggests the client has given up.

221. 4 **This is the definition of primary care nursing. (2) (SE; MR; AN; MS; NP)**
  1 In team nursing a mix of staff members provide care with a team leader who usually is a registered nurse.
  2 In modular nursing clients are assigned according to geographic location and a variety of professionals are involved; this is similar to team nursing, but the teams are smaller.
  3 In functional nursing the nurse manager makes work assignments with specific tasks for each nurse.

222. **Answer: 33 mL per hour; 800 mL divided by 24 hours equals 33 mL per hour. (1) (PB; CJ; AN; PE; FE)**

223. 2 **Stable vital signs are the major indicators that transfer will not jeopardize the client's condition; apprehension and complaints of pain do not place the client in jeopardy. (2) (SE; MR; AS; MS; CV)**
  1 Restlessness may be an early sign of shock; the client needs further assessment.
  3 The vital signs are not stabilized, and transfer at this time is contraindicated.
  4 These are signs of increased intracranial pressure, and the client should not be transferred at this time.

224. 4 According to recent Centers for Disease Control recommendations, adults with HIV should receive tetanus, diphtheria, influenza, hepatitis B and pneumococcal vaccines. (2) (SE; CJ; PL; MS; BI)

1 The varicella vaccine is contraindicated for individuals who are immunosuppressed.
2 Currently, there is no immunization for hepatitis C.
3 Same as answer 1.

225. 3 The client is monitored for beta-hCG levels twice a week until they return to normal and remain so for three weeks; monthly measurements are taken for up to six months and then are done bimonthly for the remainder of the year; if at any time during the year there is a rising titer, choriocarcinoma is suspected; if measurements remain normal for a year, another pregnancy may be attempted. (2) (PB; MR; PL; CW; RP)

1 This could be dangerous; follow-up care should continue for at least one year.
2 This is not a priority because attempting a pregnancy should not be considered for one year.
4 Chemotherapy for choriocarcinoma is given only if titers rise.

226. 3 These are signs of increasing hypoxia; a tracheotomy may be necessary to maintain an open airway. (2) (SE; MR; IM; PE; RE)

1 The signs and symptoms are not indicative of increased secretions; suctioning can precipitate sudden laryngospasm.
2 This is ineffective for laryngeal spasms.
4 Further assessment is warranted before increasing oxygen therapy.

227. 2 The client's major concern at this time is pain caused by inappropriate handling. (2) (SE; MR; IM; MS; EH)

1 This is not the major concern, and false reassurance should not be given.
3 The number of personnel will not ensure careful handling; this does not address the client's primary concern.
4 Diversion at this time would not be an appropriate response to the client's primary concern.

228. 1 Without trust, the nurse-client relationship will achieve nothing. (1) (PI; CJ; AN; MH; TR)

2 Although this is important, trust must be developed first.
3 Same as answer 2.

4 Open communication occurs after trust is developed.

229. 4 The disease occurs most often between the ages of 15 and 35 and older than 50. (2) (PI; CJ; AN; MS; BI)

1 This is not completely accurate; sometimes it is possible to predict this.
2 Incidence is not limited to any age group.
3 It is twice as prevalent in men as in women.

230. 3 Hypersecretion of melanocyte-stimulating hormone (MSH) from the anterior pituitary causes darkened pigmentations. (3) (PM; MR; IM; CW; HC)

1 This gland does not secrete this hormone.
2 Same as answer 1.
4 Same as answer 1.

231. 2 Application of cold relieves discomfort, and the binder provides support and aids in pressure atrophy of acini cells so that milk production is suppressed. (3) (PB; CJ; IM; CW; HC)

1 This is suitable for the engorged breastfeeding mother because it promotes comfort and stimulates milk production.
3 Same as answer 1.
4 Restriction of fluids will not prevent engorgement and might cause dehydration.

232. 2 Anemia may result because of the bone marrow depressant effect of this drug. (1) (SE; MR; IM; MS; DR)

1 A physical examination and blood studies are necessary to determine the cause of the client's symptoms.
3 This is unsafe; this is not the role of the nurse.
4 Same as answer 3.

233. 2 Changes in an ECG will reflect the area of the heart that has been damaged because of hypoxia. (1) (PB; CJ; AN; MS; CV)

1 A stethoscope is used to detect heart sounds.
3 Medical interventions such as cardioversion or cardiac medications, not an ECG, can alter heart rhythm; an ECG will reflect heart rhythm, not change it.
4 This is accomplished through a stress test; this uses an ECG in conjunction with physical exercise.

234. 4 No bowel sounds are present; therefore the client must remain NPO. (2) (PB; CJ; IM; MS; IT)

1 The urinary output is adequate; there is no need to increase IV fluids.

2 This is unsafe; the client must be kept NPO until bowel sounds are present.

3 Same as answer 2.

235. 3 **Maintaining a patent airway is the priority; inhalation burns may have occurred. (1) (PB; CJ; PL; MS; RE)**

1 This is important but not the first priority.

2 Same as answer 1.

4 Same as answer 1.

236. 1 **Involving the family in the decision-making process usually helps them become more committed to making plans work. (3) (PI; MR; PL; MH; TR)**

2 If the family is included in discharge planning, informing them of the discharge date and time will not be necessary.

3 If the family is included in discharge planning, they should understand the client's illness long before discharge is being considered.

4 The family should have been included in the planning for discharge long before this.

237. 4 **A change in behavior may indicate the client has worked out a plan for suicide; the potential for acting out on suicide increases when physical energy returns. (2) (PI; MR; IM; MH; MO)**

1 The client should not be considered for discharge simply because of a change in behavior.

2 This is not indicated at this time.

3 This may increase the client's feelings of inadequacy, because it implies the client did not look good before.

238. 1 **This intervention recognizes and supports justified feelings and provides an opportunity to ventilate further. (2) (PI; CJ; IM; MH; TR)**

2 This response ignores the client's feelings and directs communication away from the emotionally charged area.

3 Same as answer 2.

4 Same as answer 2.

239. 3 **Talking about what actually happened helps the client sort out the truth from confused thoughts and begins to help the client accept what happened as a part of the history. (2) (PI; CJ; IM; MH; CS)**

1 The victim should be told of the legal services available; legal counsel should come from a legal authority.

2 Sexual assaults often are planned in advance and are violent acts of the perpetrators who are responsible for their behavior; nevertheless, the victim often feels unjustified guilt related to the incident.

4 If the client does not want to discuss intimate details, this should be respected.

240. 4 **This objective includes observable client behavior, which is specified by amount and time and therefore is measurable. (2) (PB; CJ; AN; MS; RE)**

1 This objective is not stated in measurable terms.

2 Same as answer 1.

3 This is a statement, not an objective.

241. 3 **The nurse has a legal responsibility to report suspicions of abuse to adult protective services, and failure to do so could result in charges being brought against the nurse. (2) (SE; LE; IM; MS; NP)**

1 Although the nurse can address concerns with the caregiver, the nurse has a legal responsibility to report suspicions of abuse.

2 The client is noncommunicative and would not be able to respond.

4 Although this is a concern for the home health nurse, the nurse legally must report the situation.

242. 3 **The data presented indicate an infectious process within the lung. (1) (PB; CJ; AN; MS; RE)**

1 The cardinal signs would be pain in the lower lobe at the height of inspiration and a pleural friction rub.

2 Although fever and chills can occur later in the disease, the cardinal signs are irritating cough, chest pain, and shortness of breath.

4 The cardinal signs would be barrel chest; resonance on percussion; and thick, tenacious sputum.

243. 2 **This is a reflective statement that conveys acceptance and encourages further communication. (2) (PI; CJ; IM; MS; EH)**

1 This is false reassurance that does not lessen anxiety.

3 This is too direct; this statement does not encourage the client to discuss feelings.

4 The reliance on a pill to help the client in this instance evades the problem and cuts off further communication.

244. 3 **Sleep deprivation alone can cause these disturbances. (2) (PB; CJ; IM; MS; NM)**

1 Lack of contact with significant others increases anxiety and feelings of isolation and can lead to disturbances in rest.

2 Pain limits or interrupts periods of sleep and rest.

4 Constant light limits sleep.

245. 3 A small amount of bile-colored spotting is expected, but a moderately large amount is abnormal; the physician should be notified. (2) (PB; MR; IM; MS; GI)
   1 The findings need further assessment; this intervention treats only the pain and disregards the need for medical evaluation of the complication.
   2 The client should be on the right side to compress the liver capsule against the chest wall.
   4 Although this is important, the priority is to notify the physician.

246. 1 This is the most appropriate nursing diagnosis because it is the impaired parenting that forms the basis for the other problems experienced by the child and family. (3) (PM; CJ; AN; PE; EH)
   2 Risk for injury is not an actual problem at this time because there is no history or evidence of physical abuse.
   3 Disturbed sensory perception is a diagnosis that is related most specifically to the infant; the problem may be resolved by addressing the parenting problems.
   4 Imbalanced nutrition is a problem for the child but only indirectly for the family; the history does not support child abuse.

247. 2 This is a hypertonic contraction; the oxytocin must be stopped before another contraction occurs to prevent uterine rupture and/or fetal hypoxia. (2) (PB; LE; IM; CW; HP)
   1 Although this is important and eventually should be done, it is not the priority.
   3 This is unnecessary; the client receiving oxytocin for induction of labor should be attended constantly.
   4 Although this may be necessary, it is not the priority.

248. 1 Digoxin slows the heart rate, which is reflected in a slowing of the pulse; it also increases kidney perfusion, which promotes urine formation, resulting in diuresis and decreased edema. (2) (PB; CJ; EV; MS; DR)
   2 Digoxin does not decrease the pulse pressure or directly influence the blood pressure; diuresis will lower the weight and blood pressure.
   3 Although digoxin will decrease the pulse rate, it will not increase the blood pressure or reduce a heart murmur.
   4 Digoxin does not regulate an irregular pulse; it produces diuresis as a result of improved cardiac output, which may result in a decreased blood pressure.

249. 2 This reduces energy requirements, allows for rest, and lessens the demand for oxygen. (2) (PB; CJ; IM; PE; RE)
   1 Although this loosens secretions in the lungs, it should not be used when the child is in distress.
   3 This is not done unless respiratory distress is severe; it increases restlessness and energy demands.
   4 This position change will not reduce energy and oxygen demands.

250. 2 Clients with serious head injuries would not be cared for immediately in mass casualty events because the need is to care for the largest number of people who have the least severe injuries. (2) (SE; MR; IM; MS; NP)
   1 Persons with fractures would be cared for in mass casualty events.
   3 Persons needing uncomplicated abdominal surgeries would be cared for in mass casualty events.
   4 Persons with survivable radiation or chemical exposures would be cared for in mass casualty events.

251. 2 This is caused by manipulation of abdominal contents and the depressant effects of anesthetics and analgesics. (1) (PB; CJ; AN; MS; GI)
   1 Edema would not interfere with peristalsis; edema may cause peristalsis to be less effective, but some output would result.
   3 An absence of fiber has a greater effect on decreasing peristalsis than does decreasing fluids.
   4 A nasogastric tube decompresses the stomach; it does not cause cessation of peristalsis.

252. 1 A cancerous mass can grow into the lumen of the intestines, altering the shape of the stool; stools may be ribbon-like or pencil thin. (1) (PB; CJ; AS; MS; GI)
   2 This is not specific to colon cancer.
   3 Same as answer 2.
   4 Same as answer 2.

253. 4 Care for an infant after croup should be directed toward personal care, proper nutrition, and stimulation. (1) (PM; CJ; PL; PE; RE)
   1 The infant does not require additional fluids if all feedings are consumed.
   2 Young infants need environmental stimuli.
   3 Croup is not directly related to antigen-antibody responses.

254. 3 This action supports the client's ability to function. (3) (PI; CJ; PL; MH; DD)

1 The priority should be directed toward cognitive maintenance rather than trying to remotivate the client, which is not always possible with organic damage.
2 There are no data to indicate the client needs "custodial care" at this time.
4 Structure and routines will decrease anxiety and increase performance of activities of daily living.

255. 4 **These are some of the first signs of hypoxia; the airway must be kept patent to promote oxygenation. (2) (PB; CJ; AS; PE; RE)**
1 These are late signs of hypoxia; suctioning should have been done before this time.
2 The child will not be able to communicate verbally after a tracheotomy.
3 These are late signs of respiratory difficulty; suctioning and other measures should have been done before this time.

256. 3 **Fresh fruit has the overall lowest sodium content. (2) (PB; CJ; AN; MS; GI)**
1 This is higher in sodium than fruit.
2 Same as answer 1.
4 Same as answer 1.

257. 1 **Most child abusers have been abused themselves; they do not know how to deal with the rage they feel. (2) (PI; CJ; PL; MH; CS)**
2 Parents in abusing parent groups have already admitted and begun to seek help for their problem.
3 This type of presentation usually alienates individuals who are struggling with their present problems.
4 Therapy should focus on and encourage the sharing of feelings, not personal parenting information.

258. 1 **They are called Mongolian spots, and they are a variation within the norm and disappear in the first year. (1) (PM; CJ; AN; CW; NN)**
2 Mottling caused by cold would cover the entire body.
3 The harlequin color change is not purple or blue and involves entire halves of the body.
4 In this newborn these are expected findings; if the baby were light skinned, the possibility of bruises would be investigated.

259. 2 **A common complication of a brain attack (cerebrovascular accident) is an inability to control emotional affect; clients may be depressed or apathetic and have a lability of mood. (2) (PI; CJ; IM; MS; NM)**

1 There are no data to support this conclusion.
3 Same as answer 1.
4 Same as answer 1.

260. 2 **The heart muscle begins to fail and does not contract with enough strength to pump sufficient blood to meet the body's metabolic needs. (3) (PB; CJ; AN; MS; CV)**
1 Hypervolemia can precipitate heart failure in individuals with a diseased heart, but it is not specific to rheumatic heart disease.
3 Hypertension and arteriosclerosis can add stress to this situation, but they are not the reason for this client's heart failure.
4 Heart valves can become stenotic or regurgitant as a result of rheumatic fever; however, left ventricular failure will occur only when the heart can no longer pump an adequate amount of blood to maintain cardiac output.

261. 3 **Steroids are used for their antiinflammatory, vasoconstrictive, and antipruritic effects. (2) (SE; MR; EV; MS; DR)**
1 Steroids increase the incidence of infections by masking symptoms.
2 Steroids increase fluid retention.
4 Although steroid ointments have an antipruritic effect, their major purpose after surgery is the antiinflammatory effect.

262. 1 **Advil is a nonsteroidal anti-inflammatory drug (NSAID) that can cause bleeding in the GI tract; clients with a history of gastrointestinal (GI) bleeding should not take NSAIDS. (1) (SE; MR; IM; MS; DR)**
2 Lanoxin is an antidysrhythmic used to slow the heart rate; it does not contribute to GI bleeding.
3 Lasix, a commonly used diuretic, is not contraindicated with GI bleeding.
4 Aldactone is a diuretic which often causes potassium retention; it does not cause GI bleeding.

263. 4 **Many closures require the use of two hands, and some clothing requires movement of both sides of the body when dressing. (1) (PB; CJ; AN; MS; NM)**
1 The client can continue to use the right hand to perform this activity.
2 Same as answer 1.
3 Same as answer 1.

264. 2 **Regular insulin is the only insulin that can be administered by IV. (2) (PB; CJ; PL; MS; DR)**
   1 This insulin cannot be administered by IV.
   3 Same as answer 1.
   4 Same as answer 1.

265. 4 **Catatonic clients exhibit rigidity and posturing behaviors (1) (PI; CJ; AS; MH; SD)**

   1 Self-mutilation is associated with depression.
   2 Most clients with catatonic schizophrenia are unable to express feelings.
   3 Repetitious activities are associated with obsessive-compulsive disorders.

How to Use Worksheet 1: Errors in Processing Information

Common errors in processing information are listed in the left hand column of this worksheet. At the top of the worksheet is a row of blank spaces for inserting the number of the question missed. Directly below each number, check any errors you made in answering that question. You may have made more than one type of error in an answer.

Worksheet 1: Errors in Processing Information

Question number																								
Did not read situation/ question carefully																								
Missed important details																								
Confused major and minor points																								
Defined problem incorrectly																								
Could not remember terms/ facts/concepts/principles																								
Defined terms incorrectly																								
Focused on incomplete/incorrect data in assessing situation																								
Interpreted data incorrectly																								
Applied wrong concepts/ principles in situations																								
Drew incorrect conclusions																								
Identified wrong goals																								
Identified priorities incorrectly																								
Carried out plan incorrectly/ incompletely																								
Was unclear about criteria for evaluating success in achieving goals																								

How to Use Worksheet 2: Knowledge Gaps

Types of common knowledge gaps are listed along the top of this worksheet. Write a brief description of topics you want to review in the spaces provided. For example, if you missed a question on administration of a particular drug, write the drug name and problem (e.g., dosage) in the appropriate space under the column labeled *Pharmacology*.

Worksheet 2: Knowledge Gaps

Basic science	Skills/ procedures	Basic human needs	Growth and development	Normal nutrition	Psychosocial factors	Clinical area/ topic	Stressors/ coping mechanisms	Patho- physiology	Pharma- cology	Therapeutic nutrition	Legal implications	Other

Chapter 7

Comprehensive Examination 2

PART A QUESTIONS

1. A 10-year-old boy who has sustained a head injury is brought to the emergency department by his mother. A diagnosis of a mild concussion is made. At the time of discharge, the nurse should instruct the mother to:
   1. Withhold food and fluids for 24 hours
   2. Allow him to play outdoors with his friends
   3. Arrange for a follow-up visit with the child's primary care provider in one week
   4. Check for any change in responsiveness every two hours until the follow-up visit

2. A client who has been in a motor vehicle accident is now in hypovolemic shock. The nurse should frequently assess the client's vital signs during the compensatory stage of shock, because:
   1. Arteriolar constriction occurs
   2. The cardiac workload decreases
   3. Decreased contractility of the heart occurs
   4. The parasympathetic nervous system is triggered

3. A paranoid male client with schizophrenia is losing weight, reluctant to eat, and voicing concerns about being poisoned. The best intervention by the nurse would be to:
   1. Allow the client to open canned or pre-packaged food
   2. Restrict the client to his room until 2 lbs are gained
   3. Have a staff member personally taste all of the client's food
   4. Tell the client the food has been x-rayed by the staff and is safe

4. One day the mother of a young adult confides to the nurse that she is very troubled by her child's emotional illness. The nurse's most therapeutic initial response would be:
   1. "You may be able to lessen your feelings of guilt by seeking counseling."
   2. "It would be helpful if you become involved in volunteer work at this time."
   3. "I recognize it's hard to deal with this, but try to remember that this too shall pass."
   4. "Joining a support group of parents who are coping with this problem can be quite helpful."

5. To check for wound hemorrhage after a client has had surgery for the removal of a tumor in the neck, the nurse should:
   1. Loosen an edge of the dressing and lift it to see the wound
   2. Observe the dressing at the back of the neck for the presence of blood
   3. Outline the blood as it appears on the dressing to observe any progression
   4. Press gently around the incision to express accumulated blood from the wound

6. A 16-year-old primigravida arrives at the labor and birthing unit in her 38th week of gestation and states that she is in labor. To verify that the client is in true labor the nurse should:
   1. Obtain slides for a fern test
   2. Time any uterine contractions
   3. Prepare her for a pelvic examination
   4. Apply nitrazine paper to moist vaginal tissue

7. As part of a diagnostic workup for pulmonic stenosis, a child has a cardiac catheterization. The nurse is aware that children with pulmonic stenosis have increased pressure:
   1. In the pulmonary vein
   2. In the pulmonary artery
   3. On the left side of the heart
   4. On the right side of the heart

8. An obese client asks the nurse how to lose weight. Before answering, the nurse should remember that long-term weight loss occurs best when:
   1. Eating patterns are altered
   2. Fats are limited in the diet
   3. Carbohydrates are regulated
   4. Exercise is a major component

9. As a very anxious female client is talking to the nurse, she starts crying. She appears to be so upset that she cannot control her crying. The most appropriate response by the nurse would be:
   1. "Is talking about your problem upsetting you?"
   2. "It is OK to cry; I'll just stay with you for now."
   3. "You look upset; let's talk about why you are crying."
   4. "Sometimes it helps to get it out of your system."

10. The nurse is planning to obtain a blood specimen from a newborn to assess the glucose level. Using the Figure below, identify the appropriate site on the sole of the infant's foot where the nurse should place the spring-loaded automatic puncture device:
    1. a
    2. b
    3. c
    4. d

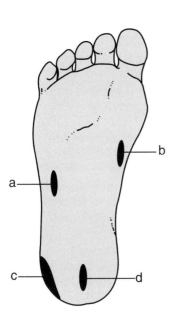

11. The nurse is aware that the most reliable indicator of pain in a 4-year-old child would be:
    1. Crying and sobbing
    2. Decreased heart rate
    3. Changes in behavior
    4. Verbal reports of pain

12. During the first 48 hours after a severe burn of 40% of a client's body surface, the nurse's assessment should include observations for water intoxication. Associated adaptations include:
    1. Sooty-colored sputum
    2. Frothy pink-tinged sputum
    3. Twitching and disorientation
    4. Urine output below 30 mL per hour

13. After a muscle biopsy, the nurse should teach the client to:
    1. Change the dressing as needed
    2. Resume the usual diet as soon as desired
    3. Bathe or shower according to preference
    4. Expect a rise in body temperature for 48 hours

14. Before a client whose left hand has been amputated can be fitted for a prosthesis, the nurse is aware that:
    1. Arm and shoulder muscles must be developed
    2. Shrinkage of the residual limb must be completed
    3. Dexterity in the other extremity must be achieved
    4. Full adjustment to the altered body image must have occurred

15. The nurse applies a fetal monitor to the abdomen of a client in active labor. When the client has contractions, the nurse notes a 15-beat-per-minute deceleration of the fetal heart rate below the baseline lasting 15 seconds. The nurse should:
    1. Change the maternal position
    2. Prepare for an immediate birth
    3. Call the physician immediately
    4. Obtain the client's blood pressure

16. A male client receiving prolonged steroid therapy complains of always being thirsty and urinating frequently. The best initial action by the nurse would be to:
    1. Perform a finger stick to test the client's blood glucose level
    2. Have the physician assess the client for an enlarged prostate
    3. Obtain a urine specimen from the client for screening purposes
    4. Assess the client's lower extremities for the presence of pitting edema

17. The nurse recognizes that a pacemaker is indicated when a client is experiencing:
    1. Angina
    2. Chest pain
    3. Heart block
    4. Tachycardia

18. When administering pancrelipase (Pancrease capsules) to a child with cystic fibrosis, the nurse knows they should be given:
    1. With meals and snacks

2. Every three hours while awake
3. On awakening, following meals, and at bedtime
4. After each bowel movement and after postural drainage

19. A preterm neonate is receiving oxygen by an overhead hood. During the time the infant is under the hood, it would be appropriate for the nurse to:
   1. Hydrate the infant q15 min
   2. Put a hat on the infant's head
   3. Keep the oxygen concentration consistent
   4. Remove the infant q15 min for stimulation

20. A 2-month-old infant, who had surgery for hypertrophic pyloric stenosis (HPS), is ready to be discharged. The nurse, knowing that the infant is being bottle-fed, instructs the mother to:
   1. Hold her baby during all feedings, continue the regular formula, feed slowly, and bubble frequently
   2. Feed her baby half of the formula thickened with cereal and finish the feeding with the regular formula
   3. Position her baby on the right side in a crib, continue the regular formula, and handle as little as possible for two hours after feeding
   4. Give her baby about 1 ounce of regular formula per hour for the next two weeks and progress slowly to larger amounts as tolerated

21. A client's sputum smears for acid-fast bacilli (AFB) are positive, and transmission-based airborne precautions are ordered. The nurse should instruct visitors to:
   1. Limit contact with nonexposed family members
   2. Avoid contact with any objects present in the client's room
   3. Wear an Ultra-Filter mask when they are in the client's room
   4. Put on a gown and gloves before going into the client's room

22. A client with a head injury has a fixed, dilated right pupil; responds only to painful stimuli; and exhibits decorticate posturing. The nurse should recognize that these are signs of:
   1. Meningeal irritation
   2. Subdural hemorrhage
   3. Medullary compression
   4. Cerebral cortex compression

23. After a lateral crushing chest injury, obvious right-sided paradoxic motion of a client's chest demonstrates multiple rib fractures, resulting in a flail chest. The complication the nurse should carefully observe for would be:
   1. Mediastinal shift
   2. Tracheal laceration
   3. Open pneumothorax
   4. Pericardial tamponade

24. A 7-year-old boy is attending a new school. The teacher observes his behavior over six months and then discusses this with the school nurse who suspects he may be showing behaviors associated with attention deficit hyperactivity disorder (ADHD). These adaptations would include:
   1. Anger and hostility
   2. Excellent testing ability
   3. Positive peer relationships
   4. Restlessness and impulsivity

25. When planning care for a client at 30-weeks' gestation, admitted to the hospital after vaginal bleeding secondary to placenta previa, the nurse's primary objective would be to:
   1. Provide a calm, quiet environment
   2. Prepare the client for an immediate cesarean birth
   3. Prevent situations that may stimulate the cervix or uterus
   4. Ensure that the client has regular cervical examinations to assess for labor

26. A mother, exceedingly upset about her child being diagnosed as having a pinworm infestation, is taught by the public health nurse how the pinworm infestation is transmitted. The nurse evaluates that the teaching was effective when the mother states, "I'll:
   1. Need to be sure the cat stays off my child's bed at night."
   2. Have to reinforce my child's handwashing, especially before eating or handling food."
   3. Be sure to disinfect the toilet seat after my child's bowel movements for the next few days."
   4. Report to the school nurse the school's dirty toilet seats caused my child to contract this infestation."

27. When planning discharge teaching for a young female client who has had a pneumothorax, it is important that the nurse include the signs and symptoms of a pneumothorax and teach the client to seek medical assistance if she experiences:
   1. Substernal chest pain
   2. Episodes of palpitation
   3. Severe shortness of breath
   4. Dizziness when standing up

28. After a laryngectomy, the most important equipment to place at the client's bedside would be:
    1. Suction equipment
    2. Humidified oxygen
    3. A nonelectric call bell
    4. A cold-steam vaporizer

29. The nurse interviews a young female client with anorexia nervosa to obtain information for the nursing history. The client's history is likely to reveal a:
    1. Strong desire to improve her body image
    2. Close, supportive mother-daughter relationship
    3. Satisfaction with and desire to maintain her present weight
    4. Low level of achievement in school, with little concern for grades

30. The nurse should plan to assist a client with an obsessive-compulsive disorder to control the use of ritualistic behavior by:
    1. Providing repetitive activities that require little thought
    2. Attempting to reduce or limit situations that increase anxiety
    3. Getting the client involved with activities that will provide distraction
    4. Suggesting that the client perform menial tasks to expiate feelings of guilt

31. A 2½-year-old child undergoes a ventriculoperitoneal shunt revision. Before discharge, the nurse, knowing the expected developmental behaviors for this age group, should tell the parents to call the physician if the child:
    1. Tries to copy all of the father's mannerisms
    2. Talks incessantly regardless of the presence of others
    3. Becomes fussy when frustrated and displays a shortened attention span
    4. Frequently starts arguments with playmates by claiming all toys are "mine"

32. A client with the diagnosis of otosclerosis undergoes a stapedectomy with insertion of a middle-ear prosthesis. A few days after the operation, the client is discouraged because there is no improvement in hearing. The nurse should base the response on the knowledge that this probably is a result of:
    1. Swelling within the ear canal
    2. Damage to the organ of Corti
    3. Perforation of the tympanic membrane
    4. The graft having slipped out of position

33. A urinary tract infection is a potential danger with an indwelling catheter. The nurse can best plan to avoid this complication by:
    1. Assessing urine specific gravity
    2. Maintaining the ordered hydration
    3. Collecting a weekly urine specimen
    4. Emptying the drainage bag frequently

34. A client has sustained a fractured right femur in a fall on the ice. The nurse with the emergency response team assesses for signs of circulatory impairment by:
    1. Turning the client to the side-lying position
    2. Asking the client to cough and deep breathe
    3. Taking the client's pedal pulse in the affected limb
    4. Instructing the client to wiggle the toes of the right foot

35. To assess orientation to place in a client suspected of having dementia of the Alzheimer's type, the nurse should ask:
    1. "Where are you?"
    2. "Who brought you here?"
    3. "Do you know where you are?"
    4. "How long have you been here?"

36. The nurse assesses a postpartum client who had an abruptio placentae and suspects that disseminated intravascular coagulation (DIC) is occurring when assessments demonstrate:
    1. A boggy uterus
    2. Multiple vaginal clots
    3. Hypotension and tachycardia
    4. Bleeding from the venipuncture site

37. When a client in labor experiences the urge to push at 9 cm dilation, the breathing pattern that the nurse should instruct the client to use is the:
    1. Expulsion pattern
    2. Slow-paced pattern
    3. Shallow-chest pattern
    4. Panting-blowing pattern

38. The nurse is caring for a client with type 1 diabetes. For which signs or symptoms of insulin reaction should the nurse particularly be observant? Check all that apply.
    1. _____ Lethargy
    2. _____ Headache
    3. _____ Diaphoresis
    4. _____ Excessive thirst
    5. _____ Deep respirations
    6. _____ Increased appetite

39. The nurse should explain that the most beneficial between-meal snack for a client who is

recovering from full-thickness burns would be a:
1. Cheeseburger and a malted
2. Piece of blueberry pie and milk
3. Bacon and tomato sandwich and tea
4. Chicken salad sandwich and soft drink

40. A client with a fractured right head of the femur and osteoporosis is placed in Buck's extension before surgical repair. Until surgery is performed, the nurse should plan to:
    1. Remove the weights from the traction every two hours to promote comfort
    2. Raise and maintain the knee gatch on the bed to limit the shearing force of traction
    3. Assess the circulation of the affected leg at least every four hours to prevent trauma
    4. Turn the client from side to side every four hours to prevent pressure on the coccyx

41. The nurse recognizes that failure of a newborn to make the appropriate adaptation to extrauterine life would be indicated by:
    1. Flexed extremities
    2. Cyanotic lips and face
    3. A heart rate of 130 beats per minute
    4. A respiratory rate of 40 breaths per minute

42. When taking the health history and assessing a 6-year-old child with celiac disease, the nurse would expect to find:
    1. Diarrhea, malnutrition, rickets, anemia, steatorrhea
    2. Constipation, abdominal distention, flatulence, rickets
    3. Diarrhea, muscle wasting, anemia, osteomalacia, steatorrhea
    4. Constipation, abdominal distention, peripheral edema, decreased clotting time

43. The laboratory calls to state that a client's lithium level is 1.9 mEq/L after 10 days of lithium therapy. The nurse should:
    1. Notify the physician of the findings because the level is dangerously high
    2. Monitor the client closely because the level of lithium in the blood is slightly elevated
    3. Continue to administer the medication as ordered because the level is within the therapeutic range
    4. Report the findings to the physician so the dosage can be increased because the level is below the therapeutic range

44. A 3-year-old boy in respiratory distress is treated in the emergency department. A diagnosis of croup is made. At the time of discharge the mother asks how to handle another croup attack at home. The nurse's response should be to:
    1. Give him warm tea sweetened with honey to soothe his larynx
    2. Keep him quiet and give him cough syrup to interrupt the laryngeal spasm
    3. Bring him to the emergency department whenever a croup attack occurs
    4. Take him to the bathroom where a hot shower has filled the room with steam

45. A client has regular 30-day menstrual cycles. When teaching about the rhythm method, which the client and her husband have chosen to use for family planning, the nurse should emphasize that the client's most fertile days are:
    1. Days 9 to 11
    2. Days 12 to 14
    3. Days 15 to 17
    4. Days 18 to 20

46. Increased socialization and verbalization of reality-based concerns is the nurse's primary goal for clients with a diagnosis of schizophrenia who are in group therapy. At the first session of the group, after introductions, the nurse could best begin by:
    1. Allowing the clients to discuss anything they wish to bring up
    2. Asking the clients what they hope to gain from the meetings
    3. Having each of the clients identify a specific concern to be discussed
    4. Sharing with the clients the purpose of the meetings and explaining the rules of behavior

47. Before an amniocentesis, the nurse should:
    1. Initiate the intravenous therapy as ordered by the physician
    2. Inform the client that the procedure could precipitate an infection
    3. Assure that informed consent has been obtained from the client
    4. Perform a vaginal examination on the client to assess cervical dilation

48. While a client is on intravenous magnesium sulfate therapy for preeclampsia, it is essential for the nurse to monitor the client's deep tendon reflexes to:
    1. Determine her level of consciousness
    2. Evaluate the mobility of the extremities
    3. Determine her response to painful stimuli
    4. Prevent development of respiratory depression

49. When assessing a client who has been immobilized since her husband has requested a divorce and moved out, the nurse in the crisis intervention center should first attempt to determine:
    1. If she is receptive to suggestions
    2. What divorce means to the client
    3. Her relationship with her husband
    4. How she plans to support herself financially

50. A preschooler is admitted to the hospital with a diagnosis of acute glomerulonephritis. The child's history reveals a 5-pound weight gain in one week and periorbital edema. For the most accurate information on the status of the child's edema, nursing intervention should include:
    1. Obtaining the child's daily weight
    2. Doing a visual inspection of the child
    3. Measuring the child's intake and output
    4. Monitoring the child's electrolyte values

51. The nurse is administering dexamethasone (Decadron) for the early management of a client's cerebral edema. This treatment is effective because it:
    1. Acts as a hyperosmotic diuretic
    2. Increases tissue resistance to infection
    3. Reduces the inflammatory response of tissues
    4. Decreases the formation of cerebrospinal fluid

52. During a newborn nursing assessment, a positive Ortolani's sign would be indicated by:
    1. A unilateral droop of the hip
    2. A broadening of the perineum
    3. An apparent shortening of one leg
    4. An audible click on hip manipulation

53. When caring for a dying client who is in the denial stage of grief, the best nursing approach would be to:
    1. Agree with and encourage the client's denial
    2. Allow the denial but be available to discuss death
    3. Reassure the client that everything will be OK
    4. Leave the client alone to confront feelings of impending loss

54. To decrease the symptoms of gastroesophageal reflux disease (GERD), the physician orders dietary and medication management. The nurse should teach the client that the meal alteration that would be most appropriate would be:
    1. Ingest foods while they are hot
    2. Divide food into four to six meals a day
    3. Eat the last of three meals daily by 8 PM
    4. Suck a peppermint candy after each meal

55. After surgery the physician orders an antibiotic IVPB q6h and daily peak and trough levels. This is done primarily so that:
    1. A drop in the client's fever may be correlated with the peak level
    2. Any allergy that the client might have to the drug would be detected early
    3. The presence of an adequate therapeutic level of the drug can be determined
    4. The blood specimen can be obtained when the antibiotic is at its lowest level

56. When entering a depressed client's room one morning, the nurse finds the client still in bed. The client states, "I am unable to get dressed and go to breakfast." The nurse's best response would be:
    1. "You cannot just lie in bed. You must get up now and go to breakfast."
    2. "I'll get you dressed. I recognize that you have difficulty helping yourself."
    3. "Take your time. It is not necessary to hurry. I'll help you if you need me to."
    4. "You can lie there for awhile if you promise me you'll get dressed for lunch."

57. A mother, newly diagnosed with ovarian cancer, knows she must tell her 5-year-old child about the diagnosis and how her upcoming treatment will impact on their family life. She asks the nurse how she should answer if her child asks, "Are you going to die?" The nurse suggests she could respond by saying:
    1. "No, but why do you ask that?"
    2. "I might, but we'll talk about this later."
    3. "Everyone dies, but I'll be around a long time."
    4. "I don't know, but I will do everything I can to stay with you."

58. After helping a neighborhood family through a crisis situation, a male executive asks the nurse to come to his business to discuss with the employees the principles of maintaining mental health in today's world. A primary consideration before deciding the approach or content for the discussion would be to:
    1. Involve the employees in the initial planning for the session
    2. Explore the available physical facilities and audiovisual equipment
    3. Plan for employees to share personal experiences related to avoiding mental illness
    4. Assess the mental health of the employees through the use of a mental status examination

59. After a mastectomy or hysterectomy, clients may feel incomplete as women. The statement that

should alert the nurse to this feeling would be:
1. "I can't wait to see all my friends again."
2. "I feel washed out; there isn't much left."
3. "I can't wait to get home to see my grandchild."
4. "My husband plans for me to recuperate at our daughter's home."

60. A client with obstruction of the common bile duct may show a prolonged bleeding and clotting time because:
1. Vitamin K is not absorbed
2. The ionized calcium level falls
3. The extrinsic factor is not absorbed
4. Bilirubin accumulates in the plasma

61. Realizing that hypokalemia is a side effect of steroid therapy, the nurse should monitor a client taking steroid medication for:
1. Hyperactive reflexes
2. An increased pulse rate
3. Nausea, vomiting, and diarrhea
4. Leg weakness with muscle cramps

62. When assessing a newborn suspected of having Down syndrome, the nurse would expect to observe:
1. Long, thin fingers
2. Large, protruding ears
3. Hypertonic neck muscles
4. Simian lines on the hands

63. A 10-year-old girl is admitted to the pediatric unit for recurrent pain and swelling of her joints, particularly her knees and ankles. Her diagnosis is juvenile rheumatoid arthritis. The nurse recognizes that besides joint inflammation, a unique manifestation of the rheumatoid process involves the:
1. Ears
2. Eyes
3. Liver
4. Brain

64. A disturbed client is scheduled to begin group therapy. The client refuses to attend. The nurse should:
1. Accept the client's decision without discussion
2. Have another client ask the client to reconsider
3. Tell the client that attendance at the meeting is required
4. Insist that the client join the group to help the socialization process

65. Because a severely depressed client has not responded to any of the antidepressant medications, the psychiatrist decides to try electroconvulsive therapy (ECT). Before the treatment the nurse should:
1. Have the client speak with other clients receiving ECT

2. Give the client a detailed explanation of the entire procedure
3. Limit the client's intake to a light breakfast on the days of the treatment
4. Provide a simple explanation of the procedure and continue to reassure the client

66. The nurse is aware that teaching about colostomy care is understood when the client states, "I will contact my physician and report:
1. If I notice a loss of sensation to touch in the stoma tissue."
2. When mucus is passed from the stoma between irrigations."
3. The expulsion of flatus while the irrigating fluid is running out."
4. If I have any difficulty in inserting the irrigating tube into the stoma."

67. The client's history that alerts the nurse to assess closely for signs of postpartum infection would be:
1. Three spontaneous abortions
2. B negative maternal blood type
3. Blood loss of 850 mL after a vaginal birth
4. Maternal temperature of 99.9° F 12 hours after delivery

68. A client is experiencing stomatitis as a result of chemotherapy. An appropriate nursing intervention related to this condition would be to:
1. Provide frequent saline mouthwashes
2. Use karaya powder to decrease irritation
3. Increase fluid intake to compensate for the diarrhea
4. Provide meticulous skin care of the abdomen with Betadine

69. During a group therapy session, one of the clients asks a male client with the diagnosis of antisocial personality disorder why he is in the hospital. Considering this client's type of personality disorder, the nurse might expect him to respond:
1. "I need a lot of help with my troubles."
2. "Society makes people react in odd ways."
3. "I decided that it's time I own up to my problems."
4. "My life needs straightening out and this might help."

70. A child visits the clinic for a 6-week checkup after a tonsillectomy and adenoidectomy. In addition to assessing hearing, the nurse should include an assessment of the child's:
1. Taste and smell
2. Taste and speech
3. Swallowing and smell
4. Swallowing and speech

71. A client is diagnosed with cancer of the jaw. A course of radiation therapy is to be followed by surgery. The client is concerned about the side effects related to the radiation treatments. The nurse should explain that the major side effect that will be experienced is:
    1. Fatigue
    2. Alopecia
    3. Vomiting
    4. Leukopenia

72. As the nurse prepares an older-adult client for sleep, actions are taken to help reduce the likelihood of a fall during the night. Targeting the most frequent cause of falls, the nurse should:
    1. Offer the client assistance to the bathroom
    2. Move the bedside table closer to the client's bed
    3. Encourage the client to take an available sedative
    4. Assist the client to telephone the spouse to say "goodnight"

73. When evaluating growth and development of a 6-month-old infant, the nurse would expect the infant to be able to:
    1. Sit alone, display pincer grasp, wave bye-bye
    2. Pull self to a standing position, release a toy by choice, play peek-a-boo
    3. Crawl, transfer toy from one hand to the other, display fear of strangers
    4. Turn completely over, sit momentarily without support, reach to be picked up

74. A breastfeeding mother asks the nurse what she can do to ease the discomfort caused by a cracked nipple. The nurse should instruct the client to:
    1. Manually express milk and feed it to the baby in a bottle
    2. Stop breastfeeding for two days to allow the nipple to heal
    3. Use a breast shield to keep the baby from direct contact with the nipple
    4. Feed the baby on the unaffected breast first until the affected breast heals

75. The nurse observes that there is blood coming from the client's ear after a head injury. The nurse should:
    1. Turn the client to the unaffected side
    2. Cleanse the client's ear with sterile gauze
    3. Test the drainage from the client's ear with Dextrostix
    4. Place sterile cotton loosely in the external ear of the client

76. The nurse plans long-term care for parents of children with sickle-cell anemia, which includes periodic group conferences. Some of the discussions should be directed towards:
    1. Finding special school facilities for the child
    2. Making plans for moving to a more therapeutic climate
    3. Choosing a means of birth control to avoid future pregnancies
    4. Airing their feelings regarding the transmission of the disease to the child

77. It is lunchtime at a mental health facility and a 27-year-old female client is unable to open her door because she has used up all the paper towels she uses to avoid touching the doorknob. The priority intervention by the nurse would be to:
    1. Hold her tray and instruct her to ask for it when she is ready to eat
    2. Explore the feelings that triggered her use of the ritual for opening doors
    3. Give her a supply of paper towels and then send her to the dining room
    4. Open the door for her and tell her that the staff will attempt to find more towels

78. A client has been diagnosed with preeclampsia, and bed rest at home has been prescribed. It is doubtful that this client will be able to comply with this order because she has two preschool children. To help promote compliance, plans for her care should include a:
    1. Suggestion to find a housekeeper
    2. Description as to why bed rest is necessary
    3. Warning of the risks involved in noncompliance
    4. Contract that four hours of nap time will be taken each day

79. The central problem the nurse might face with a disturbed schizophrenic client is the client's:
    1. Suspicious feelings
    2. Continuous pacing
    3. Relationship with the family
    4. Concern about working with others

80. When planning care with a client during the postoperative recovery period following an abdominal hysterectomy and bilateral salpingo-oophorectomy, the nurse should include the explanation that:
    1. Surgical menopause will occur
    2. Urinary retention is a common problem
    3. Weight gain is expected, and dietary plans are needed
    4. Depression is normal and should be expected

81. The nurse prepares a client who has had coronary artery bypass surgery for discharge by teaching that there will be:
    1. No further drainage from the incisions after hospitalization
    2. A mild fever and extreme fatigue for several weeks after surgery
    3. Little incisional pain and tenderness three to four weeks after surgery
    4. Increased edema in the leg used for the donor graft with progressive activity

82. An adolescent client with anorexia nervosa refuses to eat, stating, "I'll get too fat." The nurse can best respond to this behavior initially by:
    1. Not talking about the fact that the client is not eating
    2. Stopping all of the client's privileges until food is eaten
    3. Telling the client that tube feedings will eventually be necessary
    4. Pointing out to the client that death can occur with malnutrition

83. A pain scale is used to assess the degree of pain. The client rates the pain as an 8 on a scale of 10 before medication and a 7 on a scale of 10 after being medicated. The nurse determines that the:
    1. Client has a low pain tolerance
    2. Medication is not adequately effective
    3. Medication has sufficiently decreased the pain level
    4. Client needs more education about the use of the pain scale

84. To enhance a neonate's behavioral development, therapeutic nursing measures should include:
    1. Keeping the baby awake for longer periods of time before each feeding
    2. Assisting the parents to stimulate their baby through touch, sound, and sight
    3. Encouraging parental contact for at least one 15-minute period every four hours
    4. Touching and talking to the baby at least hourly, beginning within two to four hours after birth

85. Before formulating a plan of care for a 6-year-old boy with attention deficit hyperactivity disorder (ADHD), the nurse is aware that the initial aim of therapy is to help the child to:
    1. Develop language skills
    2. Avoid his own regressive behavior
    3. Mainstream into a regular class in school
    4. Recognize himself as an independent person of worth

86. The nurse knows that the most important aspect of the preoperative care for a child with Wilms' tumor would be:
    1. Checking the size of the child's liver
    2. Monitoring the child's blood pressure
    3. Maintaining the child in a prone position
    4. Collecting the child's urine for culture and sensitivity

87. At 11:00 PM the count of hydrocodone (Vicodin) is incorrect. After several minutes of searching the medication cart and medication administration records, no explanation can be found. The primary nurse should notify the:
    1. Nursing unit manager
    2. Hospital administrator
    3. Quality control manager
    4. Physician ordering the medication

88. When caring for a client with a pneumothorax, who has a chest tube in place, the nurse should plan to:
    1. Administer cough suppressants at appropriate intervals as ordered
    2. Empty and measure the drainage in the collection chamber each shift
    3. Apply clamps below the insertion site whenever getting the client out of bed
    4. Encourage coughing, deep breathing, and range of motion to the arm on the affected side

89. Fourteen months after the traumatic death of a spouse, a client comes to the mental health clinic complaining of continuing depression. The client states, "I have not been seeing any of my friends or attending any of the activities I previously enjoyed. My married children live in another state, and I rarely have any contact with them." The most accurate nursing diagnosis for this client would be:
    1. Impaired verbal communication related to social isolation
    2. Compromised family coping related to separation from children
    3. Ineffective coping related to low motivation to resume activities of daily living
    4. Dysfunctional grieving related to difficulty reestablishing lifestyle following the death of a spouse

90. The nurse plans to administer vitamin K to a newborn. The muscle that the nurse should use for the injection would be the:
    1. Deltoid
    2. Quadriceps
    3. Vastus lateralis
    4. Gluteus maximus

91. A depressed client is admitted to the hospital after being found bleeding from a self-inflicted superficial gunshot wound. The client does not respond to any of the nurse's questions. To assess the client's current potential for suicide, the nurse should:
    1. Ask the client why suicide was attempted
    2. Determine whether there is a family history of suicide
    3. Ask the family about any previous suicide attempts or threats by the client
    4. Observe the client for scars on the wrists or other signs of previous suicide attempts

92. When talking with a depressed client, the statement that would give the nurse a clue that the client may attempt suicide would be:
    1. "I don't feel too good today."
    2. "I feel much better; today is a lovely day."
    3. "I'm very tired today, and I'd like to be alone."
    4. "I feel a little better, but it probably will not last."

93. While receiving a blood transfusion, a client develops flank pain, chills, fever, and hematuria. The nurse recognizes that the client is probably experiencing:
    1. An allergic transfusion reaction
    2. A pyrogenic transfusion reaction
    3. A hemolytic transfusion reaction
    4. An anaphylactic transfusion reaction

94. The wife of a client who is dying tells the nurse that, although she wants to visit her husband

daily, she can visit only twice a week because she works and has to take care of the house and their cat and dog. The nurse assesses that the wife's statement demonstrates the use of the defense mechanism known as:
1. Projection
2. Sublimation
3. Compensation
4. Rationalization

95. After surgery a client is to receive an antibiotic by IV piggyback in 50 mL of D$_5$W. The piggyback is to infuse in 20 minutes. The drop factor of the IV set is 15 gtt/mL. The nurse should set the piggyback to flow at:
Answer: _____ gtt/mL.

96. When administering digitalis, the nurse must be observant for signs of digitalis toxicity. The sign that would be an early indication of toxicity would be:
1. Nausea
2. Urticaria
3. Photophobia
4. Yellow vision

97. After a craniotomy for the removal of a hematoma sustained in a fall, a child is returned to the postanesthesia care unit. The nurse places the child in a semi-Fowler position to:
1. Increase cranial drainage and prevent accumulation of fluid
2. Decrease pressure on diaphragm and increase thoracic expansion
3. Reduce subdural pressure and promote reaction from the anesthetic
4. Decrease the cardiac workload and facilitate oxygenation after surgery

98. Immediately after abdominal surgery a client begins to hemorrhage. The nurse should observe the client for signs of progressive hypovolemia, which include:
1. Oliguria
2. Bradypnea
3. Pulse deficit
4. Hyperkalemia

99. A preterm infant born at 30-weeks' gestation is receiving an electrolyte solution at a rate of 20 mL per hour via an umbilical arterial line. At the hourly intake measurement, the nurse finds that 40 mL have infused in the last hour. The nurse's first intervention should be to:
1. Administer a diuretic
2. Take the infant's vital signs
3. Check the physician's orders

4. Compare the intake to the output

100. The supervised activity that would be most therapeutic for a client during the early phase of hospitalization for a manic episode of a bipolar I disorder would be:
1. Joining a brief swimming competition
2. Writing letters and doing a needlepoint
3. Playing a board game with another client
4. Walking around the hospital grounds with one of the nurses

101. A nurse overhears a psychiatric client talking on the unit telephone. The conversation concerns ordering a "fix" to be brought to the unit during visiting hours. The nurse knows that the client, who has a history of drug use, has a contract with the attending psychiatrist that states the client is not to use street drugs while being treated in the inpatient unit. The nurse should now:
1. Telephone the client's psychiatrist and ask how the situation should be handled
2. Call security to make certain hospital policies are enforced to maintain a safe environment
3. Bring the information to the daily staff meeting for a treatment modification and action plan
4. Confront the client regarding the telephone conversation, then report the incident to the attending psychiatrist

102. After abdominal surgery a client has a nasogastric tube attached to low continuous suction. The nurse should monitor the client for indications of hypokalemia such as:
1. Tingling of fingertips and toes
2. Dry, sticky mucous membranes
3. Abdominal cramps and irritability
4. Muscle weakness and dysrhythmias

103. A female adolescent is concerned about her body image after amputation of a leg for bone cancer. The most appropriate nursing intervention would be to:
1. Limit visitors to the family
2. Encourage her peers to visit
3. Put her in a room by herself
4. Cover her lower body before visitors arrive

104. A client underwent pelvic surgery 24 hours ago. The finding that is most suggestive of a pulmonary embolus that should be reported to the physician would be:
1. Flushed face
2. Elevation of temperature
3. Pain rating increase from 2 to 8
4. Sudden onset of shortness of breath

105. When developing a plan of care for a female client with an obsessive-compulsive personality disorder, the nurse should be aware that the client's anxiety level would be increased if the staff:
    1. Helped her to understand the nature of her anxiety
    2. Provided a nonjudgmental and accepting environment
    3. Involved her in establishing and implementing the therapeutic plan
    4. Permitted her ritualistic behaviors to be carried out at three set times during the day

106. A window washer falls 25 feet and develops cardiopulmonary arrest. The nursing intervention with the highest priority would be to:
    1. Maintain an open airway
    2. Begin chest compressions
    3. Check for the brachial pulse
    4. Perform the abdominal thrust maneuver

107. The nurse is aware that the therapy of primary importance for a client with a basilar head injury, which results in rhinorrhea and bleeding from the ear, would be:
    1. Physical
    2. Antibiotic
    3. Nutritional
    4. Psychosocial

108. A newborn is circumcised before discharge from the hospital. Immediate postoperative care should include:
    1. Encouraging the mother to cuddle her baby
    2. Changing the dressing frequently using dry, sterile gauze
    3. Providing alkaline fluids to reduce the acidity of the urine
    4. Keeping the baby fasting for four hours to avoid vomiting

109. A client with type 1 diabetes is found unconscious having Kussmaul respirations, a fruity odor to the breath, and dry, hot, flushed skin. The nurse suspects that the client is experiencing:
    1. Diabetic ketoacidosis
    2. A hypoglycemic reaction
    3. The Somogyi phenomenon
    4. Hyperosmolar nonketotic coma

110. A client has had a subtotal thyroidectomy. To prevent thyrotoxic crisis, nursing care for this client should include:
    1. Providing a high-calorie diet
    2. Maintaining a quiet, relaxing environment
    3. Describing postoperative breathing exercises
    4. Demonstrating how to support the neck after surgery

111. The nurse is aware that the phase of the nurse-client relationship in which most of the problem solving occurs is called the:
    1. Initial stage
    2. Working stage
    3. Planning stage
    4. Evaluation/termination stage

112. A client, who has participated in caring for her infant in the neonatal intensive care unit for several days in preparation for the baby's discharge, comes to the unit on the last hospital day with an alcohol odor on her breath and slurred speech. The nurse's most appropriate action would be to:
    1. Talk with the mother about her condition and assess her willingness to participate in an alternate plan for discharge
    2. Speak openly to the mother about her condition and have her see a social worker about discharge to a foster home
    3. Avoid confrontation by asking the mother to wait in the hospital lobby and calling the physician to cancel the discharge order
    4. Continue with the discharge procedure, alerting the home health nurse that immediate follow-up is needed for the mother

113. After six weeks, a female client who was hospitalized for a bipolar mood disorder, manic phase, is to be discharged. She and her husband have agreed to have outpatient counseling. As the client is about to have the last interview with the nurse, the client says, "I've told you a lot about my life and my problems, but there are a few things that bother me that I've told no one." The nurse's best response would be:
    1. "Let's work on those during the few minutes we have left."
    2. "The purpose of us getting together is to discuss your problems."
    3. "Out-patient counseling is to allow you to discuss things that bother you."
    4. "What kind of problem have you not shared with me during our times together?"

114. A client with 36% of the body surface burned is receiving hydrotherapy. The best approach to wound care would be to:
    1. Use a consistent approach to care and encourage the client's participation
    2. Prepare equipment while doing the procedure and explain interventions to the client

3. Change staff every four to five days and have the client select the time for the procedure to be done

4. Heat the water to 102° F to prevent loss of body temperature and prepare the equipment before starting

115. On admission to the mental health unit, a client with the diagnosis of schizophrenia, paranoid type, says, "They all are trying to kill me. They all are." The nurse's best response would be:
1. "No one wants to hurt you."
2. "We are here to protect you."
3. "You are having very frightening thoughts."
4. "Tell me more about their wanting to kill you."

116. A client in active labor turns to the supine position. When fetal heart rate tracing abnormalities are noted on the fetal monitor, the action by the nurse that would be most beneficial would be to:
1. Help the client change her position
2. Begin oxygen by mask at 2 liters/minute
3. Inform the client of the problem with the fetus
4. Readjust the fetal monitor to determine if there was an error

117. A major complication of hypertensive disease associated with pregnancy that the nurse should anticipate would be:
1. Placenta previa
2. Polyhydramnios
3. Isoimmunization
4. Abruptio placentae

118. A 2-year-old child with cerebral palsy is admitted to the hospital for orthopedic surgery. During the admission interview, the nurse should:
1. Tell the mother that her child will be put in a private room
2. Let the mother know at what hours she will be permitted to visit
3. Explain to the mother that the hospital will provide a pureed diet
4. Ask the mother about the therapy program used by the family at home

119. While a client with a parotid tumor and enlarged lymph nodes in the neck is undergoing radiotherapy, the nurse should monitor for the development of:
1. Ataxia
2. Hypoxia
3. Arthralgia
4. Dysphagia

120. A 4-year-old child is admitted for surgery to correct strabismus. When taking the admission history, the nurse learns that the mother had her child examined when she first noticed:
1. Bloodshot sclera
2. Excessive blinking
3. Frequent squinting
4. Continuous tearing

121. Sterile warm saline soaks tid are ordered for a client with cellulitis from a puncture wound. The primary nurse has placed a clean basin, washcloth, and protective pad at the bedside in preparation for the soak but is unable to continue the procedure. The nurse assigned to complete the soak should:
1. Continue the procedure as started
2. Collect new supplies before starting
3. Report the primary nurse to the supervisor
4. Discuss the type of soak with the physician

122. A client was hospitalized because of an inability to walk. After a physiologic basis for the problem was ruled out, a diagnosis of somatoform disorder, conversion type, was made. The nurse realizes that the client's paralysis is a:
1. Nondisabling illness
2. Way of getting attention
3. Loss of contact with reality
4. Result of intrapsychic conflict

123. The diagnosis of placenta previa indicates to the nurse that the placenta is:
1. Infarcted
2. Low-lying
3. Immaturely developed
4. Separating prematurely

124. When the nurse is caring for a client with a severe head injury, the nursing priority would be to:
1. Prevent contractures and deformities
2. Position the client in a supine position
3. Monitor the blood pressure every 15 minutes
4. Maintain respiratory exchange and ventilation

125. An early sign that the nurse may observe in newborns, who are later diagnosed as having cystic fibrosis, would be:
1. Meconium ileus
2. Imperforate anus
3. Elevated bilirubin level
4. Necrotizing enterocolitis

126. The verbalizations of a client with schizophrenia contain many words that sound like the client is speaking a different language. The nurse recognizes that this communication is an example of:
    1. Clanging
    2. Echolalia
    3. Echopraxia
    4. Neologisms

127. The physician prescribes ofloxacin (Floxin) for a woman who has been experiencing frequency and burning during urination for 24 hours. The nurse knows the teaching about this medication was understood when the client says she should:
    1. Limit her fluid intake
    2. Strain all urine for calculi
    3. Expect that her urine will become orange in color
    4. Delay taking mineral supplements within two hours of each dose

128. During a precipitous labor, the nurse remembers that a complication associated with rapid descent of the fetus would be:
    1. Microcephaly
    2. Fetal head trauma
    3. Fracture of the maternal coccyx
    4. Prolonged retention of the placenta

129. Postoperatively, a client asks, "Can't I have a pillow under my knees? My legs feel stretched." The nurse can best reinforce the client's preoperative teaching by responding:
    1. "I'll get pillows for you. I want you to be as rested as possible."
    2. "It's not a good idea, but you do look uncomfortable. I'll get one."
    3. "A pillow under the knees slows blood flow and can cause clot formation."
    4. "We don't allow pillows under the legs because it will put you out of alignment."

130. The nurse is aware that compulsive behavior usually incorporates the defense mechanism of:
    1. Regression
    2. Sublimation
    3. Displacement
    4. Rationalization

131. A client with a history of binge eating and purging is admitted to the eating disorder unit with a diagnosis of bulimia nervosa. The nurse is aware that bulimia nervosa can best be defined as the:
    1. Uncontrollable pilfering and hoarding of food for later consumption
    2. Refusal to eat in public and engaging in private, excessive overeating
    3. Mood swings, ranging from euphoria to depression, associated with food
    4. Uncontrollable ingestion of large quantities of food in a short period with subsequent purging

132. A child, recently diagnosed with idiopathic scoliosis, has a mild structural curve. The child's mother asks whether the problem can be corrected with exercise and is told by the nurse that an exercise program will be:
    1. Used in conjunction with a Milwaukee brace
    2. Avoided because it can exaggerate the curvature
    3. The only intervention needed to correct the curvature
    4. Employed if the child appears highly motivated

133. A client with an acute exacerbation of rheumatoid arthritis is in severe pain and tells the nurse, "The only time I am pain free is when I lie perfectly still." The nurse should explain that the client needs to exercise every day to prevent:
    1. Paresthesias of the feet
    2. Osteoblastic development
    3. Shortening of the muscles
    4. Loss of muscular coordination

134. By the third day of life an infant weighs 5% less than at birth. The nurse is aware that the weight loss most likely results from:
    1. The development of sepsis
    2. An obstructive gastrointestinal anomaly
    3. Generalized muscle response to stimulation
    4. An imbalance between nutrient intake and fluid loss

135. A client at 40-weeks' gestation awakens at 8 AM in early labor. Her last full meal was eaten at about 6 PM the preceding evening. She did not eat breakfast. During labor the nurse should monitor the client for:
    1. A blood pressure of 130/70
    2. Urinary protein excretion of 3+
    3. Increased levels of serum electrolytes
    4. Signs of decreased blood glucose levels

136. A laboring client's membranes rupture. The nurse assesses the fetal heart rate, which is being monitored electronically. A severe variable deceleration that lasts over 90 seconds followed by bradycardia is noted. The nurse suspects that this may be happening because of:
    1. Fetal acidosis

2. A prolapsed cord
3. Head compression
4. Uteroplacental insufficiency

137. A visitor in the waiting room has a syncopal episode and collapses on the floor. The event is witnessed by a nurse who provides initial care. In addition to assessing the client, maintaining safety of the environment, and giving a report to the emergency department nurse, the nurse who witnessed the event should:
    1. Call the family
    2. Document the incident
    3. Report to the nurse manager
    4. Escort the client to radiology

138. The nurse is aware that a preschool child views death:
    1. As permanent and irreversible
    2. In a frightening and horrible way
    3. Without comprehending its meaning in any way
    4. As a departure from which the person returns

139. When caring for a child with acute glomerulonephritis the nurse plans to:
    1. Maintain bed rest, use isolation techniques, encourage fluids, and provide meticulous skin care
    2. Maintain bed rest, provide a low-sodium diet, monitor blood pressure hourly, and monitor IV therapy
    3. Prevent chilling, monitor vital signs every two hours, provide a no-sodium diet, and get the child up in a chair
    4. Promote rest, monitor the child's intake and output, weigh the child daily, and provide a regular diet with no added salt

140. A client is diagnosed with gastric cancer and a subtotal gastrectomy is performed. After surgery, the client begins to hemorrhage. The nurse should observe for signs of progressive hypovolemia which include:
    1. Oliguria
    2. Dizziness
    3. Bradypnea
    4. Hypertension

141. During a therapy session with a recently-formed group, two members who like to talk want the floor at once. Another member interrupts and says angrily, "I wish both of you would shut up. I'm tired of listening to you." The response by the nurse leader that would be most beneficial for the group would be to:
    1. Discuss the behavior and feelings observed in the group
    2. Plan to discuss this problem at the next group session
    3. Make no comment and allow the group to deal with the situation
    4. Ask a fourth group member to divulge thoughts about what is happening in the group

142. When assessing a child with glomerulonephritis, the nurse should expect to find:
    1. A decrease in joint mobility
    2. An increase in urine volume
    3. The presence of periorbital edema
    4. The occurrence of an intermittent fever

143. If a 5½-month-old infant's immunizations are on schedule, the nurse can assume that the baby has already received:
    1. Measles, mumps, and rubella vaccine
    2. A booster dose of inactivated polio vaccine
    3. Two doses of diphtheria, tetanus, and pertussis vaccine
    4. The first booster dose of diphtheria, tetanus, and pertussis vaccine

144. A client is placed on a 2-gram sodium diet. When discussing discharge plans with the client, the nurse teaches the client that the foods with the lowest sodium content would be:
    1. Orange and apple juice
    2. Dried apricots and peas
    3. Carrot and celery sticks
    4. Tomato and grape juice

145. A postpartum client who had been receiving an IV infusion of oxytocin to stimulate labor asks the nurse why it has not been discontinued now that the baby has been born. The nurse should respond that it:
    1. Promotes the flow of lochia
    2. Contracts the uterine musculature
    3. Enhances tissue healing in the uterus
    4. Decreases the discomfort of involution

146. A 23-year-old male is admitted to the surgical unit with superficial wounds of both wrists as the result of a suicide attempt. When the nurse enters the client's room, he states, "I suppose you're going to ask me about my suicide attempt!" The nurse's best response would be:
    1. "Do you want to talk about it?"
    2. "Tell me how you feel about it."
    3. "It's best not to dwell on it right now."
    4. "Why do you think I'd ask you about it?"

147. A client is placed on a 1500-calorie diet. The client should be taught that 1 gram of carbohydrate contains:
    1. 2 calories
    2. 4 calories
    3. 9 calories
    4. 12 calories

148. The nurse understands that clients with a long history of alcohol abuse ingest alcohol primarily because they:
    1. Are dependent on it
    2. Lack the motivation to stop
    3. Enjoy the associated socialization
    4. Have no other coping mechanism

149. After an uneventful vaginal birth, the nurse should plan the postpartum care of a Class I cardiac client based on the knowledge that:
    1. Fluids should be increased, particularly if she is breastfeeding
    2. The client is out of immediate danger because the stress of pregnancy is over
    3. The first 24 hours postpartum places the most stress on the cardiopulmonary system
    4. Clients with cardiac problems should be kept on bed rest for a minimum of four days

150. A child is receiving vincristine (Oncovin) as a part of the chemotherapy protocol. The nurse should monitor the child for untoward reactions affecting the:
    1. Emotional status
    2. Neurologic status
    3. Respiratory status
    4. Cardiovascular status

151. A client with lymphosarcoma is receiving allopurinol (Zyloprim) and methotrexate. The nurse can help the client prevent complications related to uric acid nephropathy by administering the:
    1. Methotrexate after providing an antacid
    2. Allopurinol and promoting urine acidity
    3. Methotrexate and restricting the intake of fluid
    4. Allopurinol and encouraging the intake of fluid

152. A client who had an above-the-knee amputation has an elastic bandage around the residual limb. The physician's orders include bathing the residual limb daily and rewrapping the elastic bandage prn. In regard to the bandage, the nurse should:
    1. Reapply it only if it slips off
    2. Apply it tightly so that it does not slip off
    3. Apply it smoothly without wrinkles or creases
    4. Reapply it while the residual limb is in the dependent position

153. A client receiving benztropine mesylate (Cogentin) experiences orthostatic hypotension, a side effect of this medication. Based on the physician's orders, the nurse should:
    1. Initiate gait training
    2. Apply elastic stockings
    3. Withhold the next dose
    4. Increase the fluid intake

154. A 22-year-old primigravida is admitted to the hospital in labor. A vaginal examination determines that she is 2 cm dilated, 80% effaced, and the presenting part is at 0 station. The nurse knows that the presenting part is:
    1. Below the ischial spines
    2. At the level of the ischial spines
    3. Above the level of the ischial spines
    4. Still floating and not near the ischial spines

155. Before irrigating a client's nasogastric tube, the nurse must first:
    1. Assess breath sounds
    2. Auscultate for bowel sounds
    3. Instill 15 mL of normal saline
    4. Check the tube for placement

156. When assessing a client with osteoporosis, the nurse should recognize that most observable changes will occur in:
    1. Facial bones
    2. The long bones
    3. The vertebral column
    4. Joints of the hands and feet

157. While caring for a client during a manic episode of a bipolar I disorder, the priority when planning care would be:
    1. Arranging for the client to participate in a daily discussion group
    2. Encouraging frequent close contact with the staff and a few selected clients
    3. Reducing the number of people interacting with the client during any given day
    4. Varying the staff members assigned to care for the client to reduce the opportunity for manipulation

158. When assessing the rate of involution of a client's uterus on the second postpartum day,

the nurse palpating the fundus would expect it to be:
1. At the level of the umbilicus
2. One fingerbreadth above the umbilicus
3. One to two fingerbreadths below the umbilicus
4. Three to four fingerbreadths below the umbilicus

159. When evaluating the appropriateness of a response by a family member in the developing awareness stage of grief, the nurse must be aware of the family's:
1. Personality traits
2. Educational levels
3. Cultural background
4. Socioeconomic class

160. A single teenage mother brings her 5-year-old daughter to the emergency department with a broken arm and contusions. Because of the type of injury and a history of conflict, the staff determines that the injury was not accidental. In addition, the nurse suspects abuse because of the mother's:
1. Effective use of defense mechanisms
2. Assertive and dominating personality
3. Isolation and lack of emotional support
4. Lack of knowledge about child development

161. Several days after a client has had a total laryngectomy, the physician orders a progressive diet as tolerated. The nurse should:
1. Keep a suction apparatus readily available in case aspiration occurs
2. Administer the diet through a nasogastric tube until the suture line heals
3. Encourage intake of pureed foods because they promote the swallowing reflex
4. Administer pain medication as ordered 30 minutes before meals to limit discomfort

162. An adolescent with allergies has been using oxymetazoline (Afrin) nasal spray. The nurse explains that if more than the recommended dose is taken, the client may develop:
1. Nasal polyps
2. Ringing in the ears
3. Bleeding tendencies
4. Increased nasal congestion

163. The nurse suspects that a preterm neonate, who is receiving gastric feedings, may be developing necrotizing enterocolitis (NEC) when the infant:
1. Develops persistent diarrhea

2. Vomits 5 mL after a feeding of 1 ounce or more
3. Exhibits a decreasing abdominal circumference
4. Has increasing nasogastric residual from prior feedings

164. An older adult is hospitalized with the diagnosis of dementia. Considering the client's diagnosis, the behavior that the nurse would most likely observe would be an:
1. Increased attention span and perceptual disturbances
2. Inability to learn new things and a disturbance in thinking
3. Acceptance of personality and social changes due to declining years
4. Expanded capacity for adaptation to the environment based on past life experiences

165. Gamma globulin and aspirin are ordered for a 3-year-old with Kawasaki disease. When administering the aspirin to the child, the nurse should:
1. Let the child decide how the medication will be taken
2. Disguise the medication in the child's favorite food
3. Offer the child a reward for taking the prescribed medication
4. Not respond to questions about the taste of the drug to avoid lying

166. Immediate postpartum care for a client with Class II cardiac disease would be based on the fact that:
1. The cardiac status improves rapidly after delivery
2. Cardiac output decreases rapidly in the first three postpartum days
3. Cardiac output increases rapidly in the immediate postpartum period
4. The first postpartum hour is hazardous, but after that routine care is possible

167. A 50-year-old male client has difficulty communicating because of expressive aphasia after a brain attack (cerebrovascular accident). When the nurse asks the client how he is feeling, his wife answers for him. The nurse should:
1. Ask the wife how she knows how the client feels
2. Instruct the wife to let the client answer for himself
3. Acknowledge the wife but look at the client for a response
4. Return later to speak to the client after the wife has gone home

168. A 26-year-old homosexual client is diagnosed with AIDS. The primary nurse reports to the nursing team that the client wept when told of the diagnosis. One of the nursing assistants responds, "I don't feel sorry for him. He made his bed, and now he can lie in it." To best help the nursing assistant, the nurse manager should recognize that this comment is most likely a result of the nursing assistant's:
    1. Values and beliefs about sexual lifestyles
    2. Anger and mistrust of homosexual males in general
    3. Discomfort with men who are unable to control their emotions
    4. Hostility over having to care for someone with a sexually transmitted disease

169. The physician orders aspirin therapy to be continued at home for a client with severe arthritis. When teaching regarding aspirin intake, the nurse should emphasize that the client should:
    1. Switch to Tylenol if tinnitus occurs
    2. See the dentist if bleeding gums develop
    3. Take the medicine on a full stomach or with meals
    4. Avoid spicy foods while taking the medication

170. A 10-year-old child who has head lice tells the school nurse, "My mother said I got lice because I don't keep myself clean." The nurse's best reply to this statement would be:
    1. "You have problems getting along with your mother?"
    2. "Do you feel that your mother is putting you down?"
    3. "There is no relationship between cleanliness and lice."
    4. "Lice are more common if you have poor personal hygiene."

171. A female client with nodular poorly differentiated lymphocytic lymphoma, who has been treated with multiple chemotherapeutic agents, comes for her first radiation treatment. As the nurse prepares her for the therapy, the client states, "I'm so discouraged" and starts to cry. The nurse should:
    1. Leave her alone so that she can regain her composure
    2. State, "It's difficult to deal with your diagnosis and treatment."
    3. Explain the therapy and reiterate that it will cause only a little discomfort
    4. Complete the preparation and tell her, "We can talk about this later."

172. The nurse recognizes that a tachycardic fetal heart rate pattern frequently is associated with:
    1. Fetal head compression
    2. Umbilical cord compression
    3. Increased maternal metabolism
    4. Administration of pudendal anesthesia

173. A client is admitted to the hospital with severe flank pain, nausea, and hematuria caused by a ureteral calculus. A lithotripsy is scheduled. The initial nursing action should be to:
    1. Strain all urine output
    2. Increase the oral fluid intake
    3. Administer the prescribed analgesic
    4. Obtain a urine specimen for culture

174. The nurse is aware that the toy that would be most appropriate for a 3-year-old child would be a:
    1. Fuzzy stuffed animal
    2. Seven-piece jigsaw puzzle
    3. Lunch box filled with plastic figures
    4. Blunt scissors and pictures to cut out

175. A client with cirrhosis of the liver and ascites fails to respond to chlorothiazide. Spironolactone (Aldactone) is prescribed in addition to the chlorothiazide. The advantage of Aldactone is that it:
    1. Promotes water excretion
    2. Stimulates sodium excretion
    3. Helps prevent potassium loss
    4. Reduces arterial blood pressure

176. After her 6-week-old infant's surgery for hypertrophic pyloric stenosis, the mother is reluctant to resume feeding the baby but readily assists with all other aspects of infant care. The care plan for this infant specifically states that the mother should be encouraged to participate in the oral feedings. The rationale for the focus of this nursing care is that the mother is:
    1. Unaware that family involvement in care is permitted
    2. Uncertain how the thickened oral feedings are administered
    3. Reluctant to feed the baby because of the present need to use a special nipple
    4. Probably afraid to resume feedings because of the frequent vomiting before surgery

177. The nurse can best initially prepare a client for the termination of their relationship by:
    1. Periodically summarizing the client's progress during the working phase
    2. Stating that, if the client feels it is necessary, their meetings could be extended

3. Telling the client how long they will be working together during their first meeting
4. Waiting until the termination phase, then reminding the client periodically of the duration of their meetings

178. The nurse would know that a client who had a mastectomy understands the discharge teaching when she states she will report to the physician any:
1. Persistent itching around the incision
2. Swelling and erythema around the incision
3. Decreased sensations in the area around the incision
4. Slightly irregular-appearing skin around the incision

179. A client with a history of Crohn's disease develops an intestinal obstruction. An enteric catheter is inserted and connected to low continuous suction. When assessing for a fluid volume deficit the nurse should monitor this client for:
1. Oliguria
2. Restlessness
3. Constipation
4. Hypertension

180. An 8-year-old child is admitted with acute glomerulonephritis. When planning care, the nurse realizes that the priority need of this child would be:
1. Cortisone therapy
2. Rest and symptomatic care
3. A high protein and high fluid intake
4. Treatment of the underlying infection

181. A 24-year-old client who has had type 1 diabetes for the past 6 years is concerned about how her pregnancy will affect her diabetes, especially her diet and insulin needs. The nurse should inform the client that pregnancy:
1. Decreases the need for insulin because the excess glucose will be used by the fetus for growth
2. Is a normal state, and that a revised diet and her usual insulin regimen will meet her and the fetus' needs
3. Increases the need for protein, and adjustments have to be made to meet the need for increasing doses of insulin
4. Will affect her diet and insulin needs, and she will have to monitor her blood glucose more often to make appropriate adjustments

182. The mother of a child recently diagnosed with type 1 diabetes asks why her child cannot be given an oral medication instead of insulin. The nurse explains that oral hypoglycemic drugs

would not work for her child because they:
1. Promote the transport of glucose into the cell
2. Promote the release of glycogen from the liver
3. Stimulate the beta cells of the pancreas to produce and release insulin
4. Stimulate the release of glucagon from the pancreas to produce insulin

183. The primary difficulty for the nurse in establishing long-range goals for clients with antisocial personality disorders is related to the fact that such clients usually are:
1. Reluctant to change their lifestyle
2. Unwilling to accept their need for help
3. Unable to deal with their feelings of guilt
4. Resistant to any demonstration of feeling

184. Three days after a below-the-knee amputation, a client is refusing to eat, talk, or perform any rehabilitative activities. The best initial nursing approach would be to:
1. Frequently explain why there is a need to quickly increase activity
2. Emphasize that with a prosthesis there will be a return to the previous lifestyle
3. Appear cheerful and noncritical regardless of the client's response to attempts at intervention
4. Accept and acknowledge that the client's withdrawal is a normal and necessary part of initial grieving

185. A newborn boy is placed on his mother's abdomen immediately after birth and starts to suck on his fist. His mother asks, "Why is he doing that?" The most appropriate response by the nurse would be:
1. "He's telling us he's insecure outside the uterus."
2. "He's hungry. He needs to nurse as soon as possible."
3. "His sucking indicates that he is tired from being born."
4. "His sucking prepares him for when he starts to nurse later."

186. A 5-year-old boy with a tentative diagnosis of leukemia is to have a bone marrow aspiration. Before the procedure the child should be told that he will:
1. Be put to sleep and will not feel anything
2. Have to stay in bed for three hours after the test
3. Be given medication to relax him, and he will feel a little pressure
4. Have a few stitches at the site, but he can get up and go to the playroom

187. A client is scheduled for an ileostomy. Preoperative teaching should include a statement that:
    1. Skin irritation at the stoma site can occur easily
    2. Fecal matter from the stoma can be controlled by daily irrigation
    3. Regular bowel habits can be established within a few weeks postoperatively
    4. Effluent discharge from the stoma will be formed fecal matter if the diet is regulated

188. A client with a seizure disorder is receiving phenytoin (Dilantin) and phenobarbital. The nurse is confident that the instructions regarding the medications are understood when the client states:
    1. "I will not have any seizures with these medications."
    2. "These medicines must be continued to prevent falls and injury."
    3. "Stopping the drugs can cause continuous seizures, and I may die."
    4. "By my staying on the medicines I will prevent postseizure confusion."

189. A client with a history of ulcerative colitis has an ileostomy. After this surgery, an appropriate nursing diagnosis related to a potential life-threatening complication would be:
    1. Risk for infection related to fecal excretion
    2. Risk for injury related to exposed intestinal mucosa
    3. Disturbed body image related to altered bowel elimination
    4. Deficient fluid volume related to limited water reabsorption

190. While undergoing chemotherapy with doxorubicin (Adriamycin) for Hodgkin's disease, it is essential for the client to report immediately the presence of:
    1. Nausea
    2. Constipation
    3. A sore throat
    4. A loss of hair

191. A client with a chest tube is to be transported via a stretcher. When transporting the client, the nurse should keep the:
    1. Collection device attached to mechanical suction
    2. Collection device below the level of the client's chest
    3. Chest tube end covered with sterile 4 × 4s securely taped
    4. Chest tube clamped between the water-seal chamber and the client

192. After a client with hyperthyroidism is treated with radioactive iodine to ablate thyroid tissue, the nurse should instruct the client:
    1. Not to leave the house for two weeks
    2. Not to hold an infant near the neck for three days
    3. To continue taking propylthiouracil for six weeks
    4. To use a separate bathroom than other family members for three weeks

193. A nurse assesses a client who is experiencing a crisis and formulates a nursing diagnosis. The nursing diagnosis that is made could be defined as a statement:
    1. To explain the client's present needs
    2. That describes the client's health status and related factors
    3. Of the client's responses that are within the scope of nursing
    4. That rewords the client's medical diagnosis in nursing terminology

194. A primipara has a right mediolateral episiotomy after a vaginal birth of an 8 lb baby. When inspecting the client's perineum, the nurse recalls that a mediolateral episiotomy is associated with:
    1. Less edema
    2. Less bleeding
    3. More comfort
    4. More infections

195. A couple interested in family planning ask the nurse about the cervical mucus method of family planning. The nurse explains that with this method the couple who do not wish to become pregnant must avoid intercourse when and a few days after the cervical mucus is:
    1. Clear and thick
    2. Yellow and thin
    3. Cloudy and viscid
    4. Clear and stretchable

196. A client who has been forced into early retirement is admitted to the psychiatric unit with severe depression. The client states, "I feel useless and have nothing to do." The best initial response by the nurse would be:
    1. "Tell me what you would like to do."
    2. "Your illness is adding to your feelings."
    3. "Have you thought about volunteering?"
    4. "You feel useless; tell me more about that."

197. When caring for clients who are at risk for suicide, the nurse should be aware that:
    1. A client who fails in a suicide attempt will probably not try again

2. It is best not to talk to clients about suicide because it may give them the idea

3. The more formalized the plan, the greater the possibility that the client will attempt suicide

4. Clients who talk about suicide do not commit suicide; they just use the threat to gain attention

198. A 65-year-old retiree with benign prostatic hyperplasia is scheduled for a transurethral prostatectomy. As he is being admitted to the surgical unit, he tells the nurse he is concerned that his operation will result in impotence. The nurse's best reply would be:
1. "It's understandable that you are worried; it is a very real possibility."
2. "Most men worry about their ability to function. You should speak with your physician."
3. "I can understand your concern, but this operation usually does not cause impotence."
4. "You may be impotent for a while, but normal functioning will probably return within five months."

199. A client with Parkinson's disease begins bromocriptine mesylate (Parlodel). A nursing priority should be to:
1. Observe sleeping patterns weekly
2. Perform a physical assessment daily
3. Assess the vital signs every four hours
4. Monitor the intake and output every eight hours

200. In a client's 10th week of pregnancy, the presumptive signs of pregnancy that might be assessed by the nurse include:
1. Abdominal enlargement, urinary frequency, and nausea
2. Fatigue, abdominal enlargement, and hCG in her urine
3. Nausea and vomiting, urinary frequency, and amenorrhea
4. Breast changes, abdominal enlargement, and urinary frequency

201. A 59-year-old teacher with coronary artery disease is scheduled for a cardiac catheterization. The nurse's preoperative teaching would be considered effective if the client can describe:
1. What will occur if an emergency occurs
2. What will be experienced during the procedure
3. The risks associated with this invasive procedure

4. The importance of immediate postoperative exercises

202. Morphine sulfate is ordered for pain for a client just admitted with burns to the anterior trunk, entire right arm and anterior right leg. The preferred method of administering pain medication to this client would be:
1. Orally
2. Intravenously
3. Subcutaneously
4. Intramuscularly

203. The nurse is aware that a high level of lead in the blood of children with lead poisoning (plumbism) can lead to:
1. Liver damage
2. Marked anemia
3. Increased urination
4. Severe malnutrition

204. The nurse is preparing to counsel a client whose two previous pregnancies were uneventful with term vaginal births of healthy children. The nurse demonstrates an understanding of this client by recognizing that:
1. Multiparas cope more successfully with pregnancy than do primigravidas
2. Each pregnancy is a unique experience; therefore, this pregnancy is stressful
3. This pregnancy creates a crisis because the client has two children to take care of at home
4. Support persons are less important because the mother has gone through similar experiences before

205. When working with clients who have spontaneously aborted a pregnancy, it is important for nurses to first deal with their own feelings about abortion, death, and loss so that they can:
1. Share personal grief with the clients
2. Allow the clients to express grief fully
3. Teach the clients to cope more effectively
4. Maintain complete control of the situation

206. The nurse assists a client who has had a brain attack (cerebrovascular accident) with lunch. The nurse suspects left hemianopia when the client:
1. Asks to have all food moved to the left side of the tray
2. Drops the coffee cup when trying to use the right hand
3. Ignores the food on the left side of the tray when eating
4. Complains about not being able to use the left arm to help eat

207. An initial nursing assessment of a 9-month-old infant with severe dehydration probably will reveal:
    1. Stools that are frothy
    2. Bulging of the fontanels
    3. A weak, decreased pulse
    4. An elevated urine specific gravity

208. After treatment for a bladder infection, a female client asks whether there is anything she can do to prevent cystitis in the future. The nurse tells her to plan to:
    1. Avoid the regular use of tampons
    2. Decrease her intake of prune juice
    3. Increase her daily fluid consumption
    4. Cleanse from vaginal orifice to urethra

209. On her first visit to the neonatal intensive care unit to see her preterm newborn daughter, the mother stands two feet away and does not touch the infant. The mother's only comment to the nurse is, "She looks so fragile. Do you think she'll make it?" The most appropriate comment for the nurse to make would be:
    1. "The staff is confident because all preterm babies look like this at first."
    2. "Your baby is small, but many infants born as small as she is have done just fine."
    3. "I can understand that she looks fragile to you. What have you learned about her condition?"
    4. "She's not as fragile as she might appear. You need to get used to her, and then it won't be so frightening."

210. A client who has an adenocarcinoma of the descending colon with a partial obstruction is receiving doxorubicin (Adriamycin) IV to reduce the tumor mass. The nurse should assess for signs of toxicity, which include:
    1. A minor skin rash
    2. A blue tinge to the urine
    3. An alteration in cardiac rhythm
    4. An increased feeling of nervousness

211. Understanding that there is a need to protect susceptible persons from exposure to chickenpox during the acute phase, the nurse should question the mother of a child with chickenpox about relatives or friends who are receiving:
    1. Long-term anticonvulsant therapy
    2. Prolonged topical antibiotic therapy
    3. High doses of systemic steroid therapy
    4. Therapeutic doses of vitamins and minerals

212. The nurse, when assessing the adequacy of a client's fluid replacement during the first two to three days after full-thickness burns to the trunk and right thigh, would be aware that the most significant data would be obtained from recording:
    1. Weights every day
    2. Urinary output every hour
    3. Blood pressure every 15 minutes
    4. Extent of peripheral edema every four hours

213. Formulating a nursing diagnosis for all clients, including clients experiencing a crisis, occurs during the stage of the nursing process known as:
    1. Analysis
    2. Planning
    3. Evaluation
    4. Assessment

214. A client with an abdominal aortic aneurysm being prepared for surgery complains of feeling light-headed. The client is pale and has a very rapid pulse. The nurse assesses that the client may be:
    1. Hyperventilating
    2. Going into shock
    3. Extremely anxious
    4. Developing an infection

215. After a cleft lip repair, the nurse places elbow restraints on the infant. The mother questions the nurse about the reason for the restraints. The nurse's best response would be:
    1. "They are used routinely on all children with lip surgery."
    2. "The surgeon insists that all postoperative infants have them on."
    3. "By keeping the arms straight, it is difficult for the hands to touch the mouth."
    4. "We can't be with your child all the time to watch that the hands do not touch the mouth."

216. A 25-day-old infant is admitted to the hospital after three days of vomiting, and hypertrophic pyloric stenosis is diagnosed. The most important nursing assessment at the time of admission is the:
    1. Amount of formula taken at the last feeding
    2. Character, amount, and times when the baby vomited
    3. Presence of an olive-shaped mass in the lower abdomen
    4. Amount and color of last voiding, skin turgor, and respiratory status

217. According to the ANA Standards of Clinical Nursing, expected outcomes are:
    1. Client focused, measurable, attainable and realistic
    2. Interventions to help the client change behaviors

3. Provided by the nurse to encourage the client to change lifestyle
4. Specific broad-based criteria focusing on family interactions

218. After a cardiac catheterization is completed, a client is most likely to complain of:
1. A fear of dying
2. Feelings of warmth
3. Skipped heartbeats
4. Pain at the insertion site

219. During labor a client receives epidural anesthesia. The nurse should assess the client for a frequent side effect of this anesthesia, which is:
1. Urinary frequency
2. Respiratory distress
3. Maternal tachycardia
4. Hypotensive episodes

220. Bed rest is ordered for a client with rheumatoid arthritis. To prevent flexion deformities during the acute phase, a positioning schedule should include:
1. Sims' position
2. Supine position
3. Contour position
4. Side-lying position

221. A nursing care plan for a client who has just been placed on benazepril hydrochloride (Lotensin) for hypertension would include:
1. Monitoring the client's EEG
2. Observing the client for dizziness
3. Administering the drug after meals
4. Varying the time of administration each day

222. The nurse assesses a 3-month-old infant who has been hospitalized for dehydration caused by vomiting. The nurse should expect:
1. Weight loss
2. Dilute urine
3. Flushed skin
4. Bulging fontanels

223. At a therapy group session, a female client tearfully tells the other members that she lost her job as a receptionist during the past week. It would be most appropriate for the nurse to:
1. Ask her to look at the reasons this may have occurred
2. Quietly observe how the group responds to her statement
3. Suggest she check the help-wanted advertisements in the local paper
4. Request that the group help her see how she may have precipitated the dismissal

224. The mother of a young man suspected of having Cushing's syndrome expresses anxiety about her son's condition. To help the mother better understand the illness, the nurse should inform her that:
1. He will need to take exogenous steroids for several months
2. His condition is improving as demonstrated by his weight gain
3. His physical changes are permanent but will improve with therapy
4. He may have mood swings or depression as a result of his disease

225. It has been three days since a client's surgical above-the-knee amputation. To prevent contractures, it would be most appropriate for the nurse to place the client:
1. Lying on the abdomen
2. Sitting in the high-Fowler's position
3. Supine with pillows between the thighs
4. Flat with a pillow under the residual limb

226. At 5 AM, two hours after a long labor and vaginal delivery, a client is transferred to the post-partum unit. When planning morning care for this client, the nurse's highest priority would be:
1. Arranging an individual session in which the client can learn all that is necessary about successful breastfeeding
2. Preparing for the probability of hemorrhage and assessing the client's uterus every 15 minutes for firmness and position
3. Anticipating possible safety needs and instructing the client to remain in bed and call for assistance before attempting to ambulate
4. Planning activities so that the client has time to rest and providing mild analgesics as needed and other comfort measures to facilitate this rest

227. When making rounds, a nurse finds a client experiencing a seizure. The nurse should:
1. Hyperextend the client's neck
2. Move obstacles away from the client
3. Restrain the client's head and limb movements
4. Attempt to place an airway in the client's mouth

228. A child with meningitis suddenly assumes an opisthotonic position. The nurse should place the child in a:
1. Side-lying position
2. Knee-chest position
3. High-Fowler's position
4. Trendelenburg position

229. A client returns from surgery after an abdominal cholecystectomy for a gangrenous gallbladder. The location of the surgical site high in the abdominal cavity places the client at risk for the postoperative complication of:
    1. Atelectasis
    2. Hemorrhage
    3. Paralytic ileus
    4. Wound infection

230. A client with malabsorption syndrome develops signs of tetany. The nurse is aware that this is caused by inadequate absorption of:
    1. Sodium
    2. Calcium
    3. Potassium
    4. Phosphorus

231. The physician decides to treat a client with a history of chronic renal failure with continuous ambulatory peritoneal dialysis (CAPD). When assessing the client before the institution of CAPD, the nurse should be alert for the presence of:
    1. Motivation
    2. Dysrhythmias
    3. Emotional lability
    4. Pulmonary problems

232. The ritual of a female client with an obsessive-compulsive personality disorder focuses on checking her pocketbook for her keys and other belongings every four minutes. If prevented from doing this, she becomes upset. The nurse should:
    1. Permit her to continue to check her pocketbook for as long as she wants and wait for her to get tired
    2. Keep her actively involved in projects to distract her so she will forget about checking her pocketbook
    3. Lock her pocketbook in a safe place in the morning, thereby relieving the client of the necessity to check it
    4. Allow the behavior, but with the client's agreement, set limits on the amount of time and the frequency of the checks

233. When caring for a client after an ileostomy, the nurse should expect drainage from the ileostomy in the first 24 to 48 postoperative hours to be:
    1. Fecal with flatus
    2. Bloody with clots
    3. Clear with mucoid shreds
    4. Mucoid and serosanguineous

234. A client with chronic obstructive pulmonary disease (COPD) continues to smoke and does not perform the prescribed chest physiotherapy exercises because they cause fatigue. The most appropriate nursing diagnosis for this client would be:
    1. Self-care deficit related to fatigue
    2. Disturbed thought processes related to cerebral hypoxia
    3. Noncompliance with therapeutic regimen related to indifference
    4. Knowledge deficit related to causal relationship of smoking to lung disease

235. Discharge planning for a 5-year-old girl who has had a myringotomy should include teaching the parents to:
    1. Clean the ears with Q-tips four times a day
    2. Keep the child out of day care for at least a week
    3. Put ear plugs in their child's ears when she takes a bath
    4. Place a cotton swab in their child's external ear canal until drainage subsides

236. While observing a mother visiting her preterm infant son in the neonatal intensive care nursery, the nurse recognizes that the mother has not yet begun the bonding process when the mother says:
    1. "It looks like such a tiny baby."
    2. "Do you think he will make it?"
    3. "He looks so much like my husband."
    4. "Why does he need to be in an incubator?"

237. Clinical manifestations of Cushing's syndrome that the nurse might observe in a client who is suspected of having a pituitary tumor include:
    1. Retention of sodium and water
    2. Hypotension and a rapid, thready pulse
    3. Increased fatty deposition in the extremities
    4. Hypoglycemic episodes in the early morning

238. An older adult, whose conformance to social norms, hygiene, and dress requirements have deteriorated over the last three months, is admitted to the psychiatric unit. The nurse notes the client seems quite anxious, frequently paces about, has a short attention span, and is very forgetful. The nurse can best cope with these behaviors associated with dementia by:
    1. Having staff members reinforce reality with each client contact
    2. Providing a restrictive environment, including restraints, to prevent self-injury
    3. Ignoring instances when confabulation is used to substitute for memory lapses

4. Focusing on the client's positive coping skills to prevent precipitating feelings of inadequacy

239. An adolescent male who has had a leg amputated for bone cancer begins to experience a phantom limb sensation. When he complains of this pain the nurse should:
    1. Withhold pain medication to avoid possible addiction
    2. Acknowledge that the pain is real and give medication to relieve it
    3. Explain that the limb has been removed and why the pain is psychological
    4. Describe phantom limb sensation, explain it will disappear over time, and give a backrub

240. A client who has had a severe weight loss is told by the physician that more protein foods must be eaten to provide the needed essential amino acids. The client asks the nurse why these substances in protein foods are "essential." The nurse should respond, "They:
    1. Will give you the added energy you need."
    2. Are essential for rebuilding your body tissue protein."
    3. Contain the necessary nitrogen you need for healing."
    4. Must come from your food because your body cannot make them."

241. The most beneficial lifestyle modification for the nurse to teach the client diagnosed with peripheral arterial disease would be:
    1. Stop smoking
    2. Control blood glucose
    3. Start a walking program
    4. Eat a low-fat, low-cholesterol diet

242. The intervention the nurse should include when planning care for a client with dementia would be:
    1. Schedule varied activities that will keep the client occupied
    2. Provide familiar activities that the client can successfully complete
    3. Ensure that the client actively participates in the unit's daily activities
    4. Offer challenging activities to maintain the client's contact with reality

243. A 3-year-old is admitted to the pediatric unit with a diagnosis of acute asthma. The child is short of breath, the respirations are 56, the pulse is 102, and there is a nonproductive cough. The nurse would expect the child's blood gas values to indicate a:
    1. pH of 7.32

    2. PO_2 of 95 mm Hg
    3. PCO_2 of 40 mm Hg
    4. HCO_3 of 26 mEq/L

244. A client is burned on the anterior part of both legs, from the knees to the feet. Using the Lund-Browder Chart, the nurse determines what percentage of total body surface area is burned?
    Answer: _____ %.

245. When working in a psychiatric setting, it is imperative that the nurse prevent clients from:
    1. Breaking contracts
    2. Using delusional thinking
    3. Harming themselves or others
    4. Increasing hallucinatory behaviors

246. The nurse evaluates that a client's placenta has separated during the third stage of labor when:
    1. There is a gush of blood
    2. The uterus becomes boggy
    3. The uterus decreases in size
    4. There is an abrupt drop in BP

247. On the first postoperative day after a mastectomy, the nurse encourages the client to perform exercises such as flexion and extension of the fingers and pronation and supination of the hand. These interventions are done primarily to:
    1. Preserve muscle tone
    2. Prevent joint contractures
    3. Assess extent of lymphedema
    4. Stimulate peripheral circulation

248. Rehabilitation of a client with chronic obstructive pulmonary disease (COPD) involves teaching techniques and principles to decrease hospital admissions and to live a more active life. Therefore the nurse would teach the client to:
    1. Implement activities to eliminate infection
    2. Inhale during movements that require energy
    3. Incorporate humidification into the home environment
    4. Implement breathing that uses the abdominal and neck muscles

249. A client with a chronic progressive disease repeatedly expresses the fear of becoming a burden and states, "I want to die." The client asks the nurse for help. Before responding, the nurse recognizes that a nurse actively or passively aiding a client with euthanasia is:
    1. Liable to be tried for a crime
    2. Acting within the law in most states
    3. Practicing medicine without a license
    4. Negligent in performing nursing duties

250. A client comes to the infertility clinic for a workup and is told by the nurse to prepare for a Papanicolaou test. The client states, "I do not want this test. I want to speak to the doctor." The nurse should:
    1. Recognize that the client is uncooperative
    2. Inform the physician of the client's request
    3. Encourage the client to comply with clinic procedures
    4. Remind the client of the importance of cancer detection

251. An older adult with a chronic degenerative disease progresses to the stage where self-care is no longer possible, and admission to a nursing home becomes necessary. According to Erikson, the major developmental conflict for this client would be:
    1. Intimacy vs isolation
    2. Ego integrity vs despair
    3. Identity vs role diffusion
    4. Generativity vs stagnation

252. A 13-year-old girl with recently diagnosed idiopathic scoliosis is upset about the treatment regimen and is worried about being different from her friends. To help the child develop a positive self-image during treatment, the nurse should:
    1. Help the child select appropriate clothing to improve her appearance
    2. Refer the child for psychologic counseling until the treatment program is over
    3. Remind the child how crooked the back would be if treatment were not started
    4. Instruct the mother to focus on the child's positive attributes and avoid focusing on negative attributes

253. While walking to the examination room with the nurse, a toddler with autism suddenly runs over and begins head-banging on the wall. The nurse's initial action should be to:
    1. Allow the toddler to act out feelings
    2. Ask the toddler to stop this behavior
    3. Restrain the toddler to prevent head injury
    4. Tell the toddler that the behavior is unacceptable

254. During the first six to eight hours after a thyroidectomy, the nurse should:
    1. Place two pillows behind the client's head and neck
    2. Assess the sides and back of the neck of the client for evidence of bleeding
    3. Encourage the client to perform deep breathing and coughing exercises
    4. Monitor the client for the complication of tetany resulting from hypocalcemia

255. The physician has ordered digoxin (Lanoxin) and furosemide (Lasix) for a client with pulmonary edema. The nurse's evaluation that indicates the client may continue with the present dosage of digoxin would be:
    1. Nausea
    2. Pulse of 64
    3. Dysrhythmia
    4. Yellow vision

256. A client is admitted in active labor. The nurse, performing Leopold's maneuvers, assesses that the fetus is in the left occiput anterior (LOA) position. To best monitor the fetal heart, the nurse should place the transducer of the electronic fetal monitor on the client's:
    1. Left lower quadrant
    2. Left upper quadrant
    3. Right lower midline
    4. Right upper quadrant

257. The nurse should expect the physician's orders for a pregnant woman admitted to the hospital with mild preeclampsia to include:
    1. Diuretics, low-salt diet, intake and output
    2. Complete bed rest, intake and output, diuretics
    3. Daily weights, glucose monitoring, side-lying bed rest
    4. A 24-hour urine collection, daily weights, side-lying bed rest

258. During a generalized tonic-clonic seizure a child becomes cyanotic. The nurse should:
    1. Insert an oral airway
    2. Administer oxygen by mask
    3. Continue to observe the seizure
    4. Notify the physician immediately

259. The nurse is aware that the genotypic makeup of the parents of a child with sickle-cell disease is:
    1. Mother-homozygous (no sickle trait); father-heterozygous (sickle trait)
    2. Mother-heterozygous (sickle trait); father-heterozygous (sickle trait)
    3. Mother-heterozygous (sickle trait); father-homozygous (no sickle trait)
    4. Mother-homozygous (has sickle cell disease); father-homozygous (no sickle trait)

260. A client with type 2 diabetes is admitted to the hospital for elective surgery. The client is now being given regular insulin, even though oral hypoglycemics were adequate prior to

hospitalization. The nurse recognizes that regular insulin is now needed because the:
1. Client will need a higher serum glucose level while on bed rest
2. Possibility of acidosis is greater when a client is on oral hypoglycemics
3. Dosage can be adjusted to changing needs during recovery from surgery
4. Surgery may result in complications and regular insulin must be available

261. A client with an antisocial personality disorder continually uses manipulative behavior. The nurse is aware that this behavior can best be controlled by having the staff:
1. Avoid focusing on this aspect of the client's behavior
2. Develop and use a unified approach in response to this behavior
3. Designate one staff member to approach the client about this behavior
4. Assign staff members who are not easily manipulated to care for the client

262. A client with Crohn's disease, being treated with steroids, is admitted to the hospital during an exacerbation. The most appropriate roommate for this client would be a client with a diagnosis of:
1. Hepatitis
2. Pharyngitis
3. Conjunctivitis
4. Thrombophlebitis

263. The nurse is reinforcing previous learning about cystic fibrosis and its treatment with a 9-year-old with the disease. The most suitable information for this child's stage of development would be:
1. "The postural drainage will help you feel better."
2. "The dietitian says this meal schedule is best for you."
3. "Your medication is scheduled at this time because your doctor has prescribed it this way."
4. "Your mucus is thick because cystic fibrosis interferes with how your mucous glands work."

264. A 19-year-old college sophomore is admitted to the hospital with schizophrenia, undifferentiated type. The client sits in a corner for long periods rocking and responds to voices using words that the staff cannot understand. When developing the plan of care for this client, the nurse should:
1. Arrange to spend short periods with the client
2. Include the client in a discussion group on the unit
3. Encourage the client to talk to other clients during the day
4. Allow the client to be alone, but maintain observation from a distance

265. After surgical repair of a cystocele, the nurse teaches the client how to cleanse her perineal area after using the toilet. The nurse should focus on the importance of:
1. Bathing the perineum in a sitz bath
2. Spraying the perineum with Betadine
3. Using a wiping motion from meatus to anus
4. Employing a patting motion from the vagina to the anus

Part A Answers and Rationales

1. 4 **Signs of an epidural hematoma in children usually do not appear for 24 or more hours; a follow-up visit usually is arranged for one to two days after the injury. (2) (SE; MR; IM; PE; NM)**
   1 If there is no nausea, food and fluids are not restricted.
   2 The child should be encouraged to rest and should be with an adult so that responsiveness can be monitored.
   3 The child should be seen by the primary care provider within one to two days after the injury.

2. 1 **The early compensation of shock is cardiovascular and is seen in changes in pulse, BP, and pulse pressure; blood is shunted to vital centers, particularly the heart and brain. (2) (PB; CJ; AS; MS; CV)**
   2 The cardiac workload will increase, not decrease.
   3 The heart compensates by increasing contractility, which will increase, not decrease, cardiac output.
   4 The sympathetic, not parasympathetic, nervous system is triggered to produce vasoconstriction.

3. 1 **The client's comfort, safety, and nutritional status are the priorities; the client may feel comfortable to eat if the food has been sealed before reaching the mental health facility. (1) (PI; CJ; IM; MH; SD)**
   2 This would increase the client's isolation and paranoid thoughts.
   3 This is unrealistic and reinforces the client's delusions.
   4 This is a dishonest statement and reinforces the client's delusions.

4. 4 **Talking with others in similar circumstances provides support and allows for sharing of experiences. (1) (PI; CJ; IM; MH; TR)**
   1 The feeling of guilt has not been expressed.
   2 This avoids the mother's concerns and cuts off communication.
   3 This offers false reassurance.

5. 2 **Drainage flows by gravity. (3) (SE; CJ; EV; MS; BI)**
   1 Lifting and replacing a dressing would contaminate the surgical site.
   3 Although this might be done, it does not take into consideration that drainage flows by gravity.

   4 This is unsafe because it would interfere with the healing process.

6. 3 **Pelvic examination would reveal dilation and effacement. (3) (PM; CJ; AS; CW; HC)**
   1 Ferning is the characteristic frond-like pattern of crystallization in amniotic fluid when it dries. This test assesses for the rupture of membranes.
   2 Contractions can be present with false labor and are called preparatory contractions.
   4 This test differentiates between amniotic fluid and urine; the onset of true labor can occur with or without the rupture of membranes.

7. 4 **Pulmonic stenosis increases resistance to blood flow, causing right ventricular hypertrophy; with right ventricular failure there is an increase in pressure on the right side of the heart. (3) (PB; CJ; AN; PE; CV)**
   1 The pressure would be decreased in pulmonic stenosis.
   2 Same as answer 1.
   3 Same as answer 1.

8. 1 **A new dietary regimen, with a balance of foods from the food pyramid, must be established and continued for weight reduction to occur and be maintained. (3) (PB; CJ; AN; MS; GI)**
   2 Although this is true in a weight reduction diet, this response does not address this nutrient's relationship to the other food groups.
   3 Same as answer 2.
   4 This is one part of a weight reduction regimen; usually an obese individual's caloric intake exceeds energy expenditure; lifestyle changes are required.

9. 2 **This portrays a nonjudgmental attitude that recognizes the client's needs. (2) (PM; CJ; IM; MH; AX)**
   1 The client is upset that she cannot control her crying.
   3 This is unrealistic; the anxiety level must be lowered and the crying stopped before a discussion can begin.
   4 This implies that crying will make the client feel better.

10. 3 A puncture in the lateral aspects of the heel provides enough capillary blood for screening blood tests; these locations will prevent the accidental puncturing of an artery or penetrating a bone of the heel. (2) (SE; CJ; IM; PE; BI)

1 Performing a puncture in this area could injure the lateral plantar nerve or penetrate the lateral plantar artery.
2 Performing a puncture in this area could injure the medial plantar nerve or penetrate the medial plantar artery.
4 Performing a puncture in this area could injure the medial calcaneal nerves or penetrate the bone of the heel.

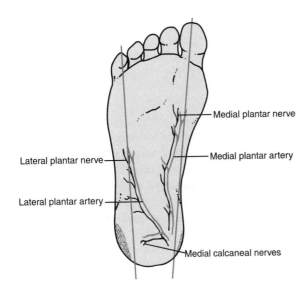

11. 3 Although there are several indicators of pain in children, a change in behavior is the one that occurs most often. (2) (PM; CJ; AS; PE; NM)

1 Many things can cause crying, including pain, fear, separation, and unhappiness; crying does not always indicate pain.
2 Vital signs are often normal in children, even in the presence of pain.
4 Children often hide their pain; they may perceive it as punishment, or they may fear the treatment that would be given to relieve the pain.

12. 3 Excess extracellular fluid moves into cells (water intoxication); intracellular fluid excess in sensitive brain cells causes altered mental status; other signs include anorexia, nausea, vomiting, twitching, sleepiness, and convulsions. (3) (PB; CJ; AS; MS; FE)

1 Sooty sputum indicates inhalation of smoke or flames.

2 Frothy, pink-tinged sputum is associated with pulmonary edema.
4 Decreased urinary output indicates insufficient fluid replacement or dehydration.

13. 2 As long as the client has no nausea or vomiting, there are no dietary restrictions. (2) (PB; CJ; IM; MS; IT)

1 The client should not disturb the dressing; it should be changed by the physician on a follow-up visit.
3 The biopsy site will be sutured and should not get wet.
4 Temperature elevation is not a usual response and may indicate infection.

14. 2 Shrinkage of the residual limb, resulting from reduction of subcutaneous fat and interstitial fluid, must occur for an adequate fit between the limb and the prosthesis. (2) (PB; CJ; AN; MS; SK)

1 Although desirable, it is the condition of the residual limb itself that is the priority factor in the fitting of a prosthesis.
3 Same as answer 1.
4 The prosthesis probably will facilitate an improved body image.

15. 1 Stimulation of the sympathetic nervous system is an initial response to mild hypoxia that accompanies partial cord compression (umbilical vein) during contractions; changing the maternal position can alleviate the compression. (3) (PM; CJ; EV; CW; HC)

2 Variable decelerations are not indicative of the need for an imminent birth.
3 This is a compensatory physiologic response by a healthy fetus; the nurse should intervene to assist by alleviating cord compression.
4 This would delay nursing intervention to help the fetus.

16. 1 The client has signs of diabetes, which may result from steroid therapy; testing the blood glucose level is a method of screening for diabetes, thus gathering more data. (2) (PB; CJ; AS; MS; EN)

2 The symptoms are not those of benign prostatic hyperplasia.
3 Assessing the urine for glucose and ketones is not as accurate as a blood glucose level.
4 The symptoms presented are not those of fluid retention but of diabetes.

17. 3 This is the primary indication for a pacemaker because there is an interference with the electrical conduction system of the heart. (1) (PB; CJ; AN; MS; CV)

1 The primary treatment for this disorder is medication; this is not an indication for a pacemaker.
2 Same as answer 1.
4 Same as answer 1.

18. 1 **Pancrease must be taken with food and snacks because it acts on the nutrients and readies them for absorption. (3) (PB; CJ; PL: PE; DR)**
2 The enzyme is useless when taken without food.
3 Same as answer 2.
4 The enzyme is needed only when food is eaten.

19. 2 **Oxygen has a cooling effect, and the baby should be kept warm so that metabolic activity and oxygen demands are not increased. (1) (PB; CJ; IM; CW; HN)**
1 This could produce fluid overload, which would lead to increased cardiac output, an undesired outcome especially for an infant with respiratory distress.
3 Oxygen concentration is determined by blood gas levels and is changed accordingly.
4 This would tire the baby and increase the need for oxygen.

20. 1 **Without complications, the infant usually is ready to resume regular feedings within 24 to 48 hours after surgery; the infant would not be discharged from the hospital if not tolerating feedings. (2) (PB; MR; IM; PE; GI)**
2 This is unnecessary; regular formula should be tolerated by the time of discharge.
3 Although limited handling for several hours after the feeding is advised, the infant should be held during the feeding because, not only does it enhance the flow of fluid by gravity, but it is an important part of the mother-child relationship at this age.
4 Same as answer 2.

21. 3 **Tubercle bacilli are transmitted through air currents; therefore personal protective equipment such as an Ultra-Filter mask is necessary. (1) (SE; MR; IM; MS; RE)**
1 This is unnecessary as long as appropriate precautions are followed.
2 This would not be necessary unless objects are contaminated by respiratory secretions.
4 This is not necessary; tuberculosis is spread by airborne microorganisms; gloves are necessary only when touching articles contaminated by respiratory secretions.

22. 4 **Cerebral compression affects pyramidal tracts, resulting in decorticate rigidity and cranial nerve**
injury, which cause pupil dilation. (3) (PB; CJ; AN; MS; NM)
1 Meningeal irritation will not produce postural or pupillary changes without cerebral compression.
2 Collection of blood between the dura and arachnoid will not cause postural or pupillary changes without cerebral compression.
3 This will result in alterations in vital signs.

23. 1 **Mediastinal structures move toward the uninjured lung, reducing oxygenation and venous return. (3) (PB; CJ; AS; MS; RE)**
2 This is unusual with a crushing chest injury.
3 Flail chest is a closed chest injury; open pneumothorax results from a penetrating injury to the chest wall.
4 This is a result of cardiac contusion and usually occurs from sternal, not lateral, compression.

24. 4 **Criteria for attention deficit hyperactivity disorder include maladaptive behavior for at least six months' duration characterized by inattention, impulsiveness, and overactivity. (1) (PI; CJ; AS; MH; BA)**
1 These behaviors are more characteristic of oppositional defiant disorder.
2 This would be unexpected; inattention to detail, careless mistakes, difficulty organizing work, and a strong dislike for mental effort—which are associated with ADHD—would hinder one's test-taking ability.
3 Peer relationships usually are strained and of short duration.

25. 3 **Stimulation of the cervix or uterus may cause bleeding or hemorrhage and should be avoided. (2) (PM; CJ; PL; CW; HP)**
1 This is desired for all clients, not just those with placenta previa.
2 If bleeding is under control and the client is stable, delivery can be delayed.
4 This is contraindicated for clients with placenta previa.

26. 2 **This infestation is transferred by the anal-oral route, and handwashing is the most effective method to prevent transmission. (1) (SE; MR; EV; PE; GI)**
1 Cats do not transmit this parasite.
3 This is unnecessary; pinworms are found in the rectum or colon and travel to the perianal area only when the person sleeps.
4 This is not the usual mode of transmission.

27. 3 **This could indicate a recurrence of the pneumothorax as one side of the lung is inadequate to meet the oxygen demands of the body. (1) (PB; MR; PL; MS; RE)**
   1 A pneumothorax causes sharp chest pain on the involved side.
   2 Usually this reflects a cardiac, not a respiratory, problem.
   4 This is not specific to a pneumothorax; this is orthostatic hypotension, which may be related to a variety of medical problems.

28. 1 **Respiratory complications can occur because of edema of the glottis or injury to the recurrent laryngeal nerve. (1) (PB; CJ; PL; MS; RE)**
   2 Oxygen may not be necessary unless there is a complication.
   3 This is unnecessary because oxygen usually is not required; the call bell can be electric.
   4 Although this may promote moist mucous membranes, it usually is unnecessary.

29. 1 **Clients with anorexia nervosa have a disturbed self-image and always see themselves as fat and needing further reducing. (2) (PI; CJ; AS; MH; ES)**
   2 The relationship usually is not supportive; it is disturbed.
   3 Usually there is dissatisfaction with weight and a desire to lose weight.
   4 Usually there is high achievement and great concern about grades.

30. 2 **Persons with high anxiety levels develop various behaviors to relieve their anxiety; by reducing anxiety, the need for these obsessive-compulsive actions is reduced. (3) (PI; CJ; PL; MH; AX)**
   1 Simple repetitive activities are not therapeutic for this client and could increase anxiety.
   3 This is a temporary action that does not address the feelings that cause anxiety.
   4 These individuals do not have a need to expiate guilt; their problem relates to anxiety.

31. 3 **Shortened attention span and fussy behavior may indicate a change in intracranial pressure and/or shunt malfunction. (2) (PM; MR; EV; PE; NM)**
   1 This is expected behavior for a 2½-year-old child.
   2 Same as answer 1.
   4 Same as answer 1.

32. 1 **Edema associated with the inflammatory reaction after surgery limits the conduction of sound. (3) (PB; CJ; AN; MS; NM)**
   2 This should not happen because the inner ear is not involved in this surgery.

3 This is unlikely.
4 If the graft slips out, the hearing loss would be worse than before surgery.

33. 2 **Promoting hydration maintains urine production at a higher rate, which flushes the bladder and prevents urinary stasis and possible infection. (2) (SE; CJ; PL; MS; RG)**
   1 Although this could help identify a urinary tract infection, it would not prevent it.
   3 Same as answer 1.
   4 The drainage bag is emptied once every shift unless it fills before then; changing the bag periodically, not emptying it, would help prevent infection.

34. 3 **Monitoring a pedal pulse will assess circulation to the foot. (1) (PB; CJ; AS; MS; SK)**
   1 This would be contraindicated if a fracture of the femur were suspected; moving this client could cause further trauma.
   2 This is associated with assessment of the respiratory system.
   4 The inability to wiggle toes indicates neurologic impairment.

35. 1 **"Where are you?" is the best question to elicit information about the client's orientation to place because it encourages a response that can be assessed. (3) (PI; CJ; AS; MH; DD)**
   2 This question focuses on recent memory; it does not assess orientation to place.
   3 This question would probably be answered by "yes" or "no"; this could not objectively determine the client's orientation.
   4 This question focuses on orientation to time, not place.

36. 4 **This indicates afibrinogenemia; massive clotting in the area of the separation has resulted in a lowered circulating fibrinogen level. (2) (PB; CJ; AS; CW; HP)**
   1 A boggy uterus indicates uterine atony.
   2 Blood clots indicate adequate fibrinogen levels; vaginal clots may indicate a failure of the uterus to contract and should be explored further.
   3 These findings may be indicative of hypovolemic shock, which may occur after DIC; these findings are not unique to only DIC.

37. 4 **Clients should use a panting or blowing pattern to overcome the premature urge to push. (2) (PM; MR; IM; CW; HC)**
   1 Expulsion breathing should not be used at this time because the cervix is not fully

dilated, and cervical edema and lacerations can occur.

2 This pattern would be ineffective during the transition phase of labor; this would be used during early labor.

3 Same as answer 2.

38.

1 _____ Lethargy is associated with hyperglycemia because glucose is not being utilized for cellular metabolism.

2 _x_ **Hypoglycemia affects the central nervous system causing headache. (2) (PB; CJ; EV; MS; EN)**

3 _x_ **Hypoglycemia affects the sympathetic nervous system causing diaphoresis.**

4 _____ Excessive thirst is associated with hyperglycemia because fluid shifts with the excessive glucose being excreted by the kidneys, resulting in polyuria.

5 _____ Deep respirations (Kussmaul respirations) are associated with hyperglycemia because the body is attempting to blow off carbon dioxide to compensate for the metabolic acidosis.

6 _x_ **Hypoglycemia affects the sympathetic nervous system causing hunger.**

39. 1 **Of the selections offered, this is the highest in calories and protein, which are needed for the increased basal metabolic rate and for tissue repair. (3) (PB; CJ; PL; MS; IT)**

2 These foods do not provide as high an amount of calories and protein as the correct choice.

3 Same as answer 2.

4 Same as answer 2.

40. 3 **Arterial perfusion and the presence of hemorrhage must be assessed at least every four hours to prevent complications or to identify problems early. (1) (PB; CJ; PL; MS; SK)**

1 This is unsafe; this will interfere with the pull of traction.

2 Same as answer 1.

4 Same as answer 1.

41. 2 **Central cyanosis (blue lips and face) indicates lowered oxygenation of the blood, caused by either decreased lung expansion or right-to-left shunting of blood. (2) (PI; CJ; AS; CW; HN)**

1 This is expected in the healthy newborn.

3 Same as answer 1.

4 Same as answer 1.

42. 3 **These are classic signs of celiac disease caused by pathologic mucous cells and atrophy of intestinal villi, which result in poor absorption of nutrients and increased stools. (2) (PB; CJ; AS; PE; GI)**

1 Rickets is not seen because bone growth is arrested in celiac disease; the remaining signs do occur.

2 Constipation is not expected, although this may occur because of decreased peristalsis; rickets is not seen.

4 There is an inability of the villi to absorb vitamin K, with a tendency toward inadequate or prolonged blood coagulation.

43. 1 **Levels close to 2 mEq/L are dangerously close to the toxic level; immediate action must be taken. (3) (SE; MR; EV; MH; DR)**

2 The level is dangerously high, and the priority is the immediate notification of the physician rather than continued monitoring.

3 Same as answer 2.

4 The level is dangerously high; the therapeutic range for lithium is 0.6 to 1.2 mEq/L.

44. 4 **During a croup attack, a fast home remedy is to provide humidified air to relieve the laryngeal spasms. (2) (SE; MR; IM; PE; RE)**

1 This is ineffective in treating croup.

2 Cough syrup would be ineffective because it does not relieve the laryngeal spasms.

3 An attempt should be made to interrupt the attack at home first.

45. 3 **Ovulation occurs approximately 14 days before the next menses, about the 16th day in a 30-day cycle; the 15th to 17th days would be the best time to avoid sexual intercourse. (2) (PM; CJ; IM; CW; RP)**

1 This is too early; ovulation occurs 14 days before the next menstrual period.

2 Same as answer 1.

4 This is too late; ovulation occurs 14 days before the next menstrual period.

46. 4 **This action by the leader would be most therapeutic because it sets both the parameters of discussion and limits on behavior. (2) (SE; MR; IM; MH; TR)**

1 This would not be therapeutic for a group of clients with the diagnosis of schizophrenia; because of the disruption of cognitive processes, these clients would be unable to make this contribution.

2 Same as answer 1.

3 Same as answer 1.

47. 3 An invasive procedure such as amniocentesis requires informed consent. (1) (SE; LE; IM; CW; NP)
    1 Intravenous therapy is unnecessary.
    2 The infection rate is 1%; this is not an appropriate nursing intervention.
    4 A vaginal examination is not done before amniocentesis.

48. 4 Respiratory distress or arrest may occur when the serum level of magnesium sulfate reaches 12 to 15 mg/dl; deep tendon reflexes disappear when the serum level is 10 to 12 mg/dl; the drug is withheld in the absence of deep tendon reflexes; the therapeutic serum level is 5 to 8 mg/dl. (3) (PB; CJ; EV; CW; DR)
    1 This is an inappropriate assessment to determine client response to magnesium sulfate; deep tendon reflexes need to be assessed.
    2 Same as answer 1.
    3 Same as answer 1.

49. 2 Determining the significance of the divorce to the client is a method of identifying the client's perception of the event; it is critical to adequate assessment and appropriate intervention. (2) (PI; CJ; AS; MH; CS)
    1 Receptivity to suggestions would be explored later in therapy, as in the planning stage.
    3 These data are secondary in importance and may divert attention from the problem.
    4 Although financial concerns are important, they should not be the first factor addressed.

50. 1 Weight monitoring is the most useful means of assessing fluid balance and changes in the edematous state; 1 liter of fluid weighs about 2.2 pounds. (2) (PB; CJ; PL; PE; FE)
    2 This would be subjective and probably inaccurate.
    3 This is not as accurate as daily weights; fluid can be trapped in the third compartment with no alteration in intake and output.
    4 This is unreliable; these may or may not be altered with fluid shifts.

51. 3 Corticosteroids act to decrease inflammation, which decreases edema. (2) (PB; CJ; AN; MS; DR)
    1 This is an anti-inflammatory agent, not a diuretic; it does not cause diuresis by action on the kidney.
    2 Resistance to infection is decreased, but this is not pertinent in this situation.
    4 The problem is not with increased cerebrospinal fluid.

52. 4 With specific manipulation, an audible click may be heard or felt as the femoral head slips into the acetabulum. (1) (PM; CJ; AS; PE; SK)
    1 This is Trendelenburg's sign; it is associated with weight bearing.
    2 This is not Ortolani's sign; this is associated with bilateral dislocation.
    3 This is Allis' sign.

53. 2 This does not remove the client's only way of coping, and it permits future movement through the grieving process when the client is ready. (2) (PI; CJ; PL; MS; EH)
    1 The client's denial should be neither supported nor removed; encouraging denial is a form of false reassurance.
    3 This is false reassurance.
    4 The client must not be abandoned; the nurse's presence is a form of emotional support.

54. 2 The volume of food in the stomach should be kept small to limit pressure on the cardiac sphincter. (2) (PB; MR; IM; MS; GI)
    1 Foods should be neither cold nor hot; foods should be tepid when ingested.
    3 The last meal should be eaten at least three hours before bedtime; individual bedtimes vary.
    4 Peppermint promotes reflux because it relaxes the esophagastric sphincter allowing food to be regurgitated into the esophagus.

55. 3 Drug dose and frequency are adjusted according to these results to enhance efficacy by maintaining therapeutic levels. (1) (PB; CJ; EV; MS; DR)
    1 A sustained drop in fever is the desired outcome, not reduction just at peak serum levels of the drug.
    2 Peak and trough levels reveal nothing about allergic reactions.
    4 Blood cultures are obtained when the client spikes a temperature; they are not related to peak and trough levels for an antibiotic.

56. 3 This response recognizes capability without adding stress or increasing dependency. (3) (PI; CJ; IM; MH; MO)
    1 This does not address the client's needs and is punitive.
    2 This increases dependency, which is not therapeutic.
    4 This attempts to manipulate compliance; the client cannot accept responsibility for the future.

57. 4 In the first discussion the mother should convey some facts, but not overload the child with details, and offer hope; honest answers are important for the child's sense of security and well being. (1) (PI; MR; IM; PE; EH)

1 A 5-year-old child may not be able to respond to the "why" and become anxious, overwhelmed, and defensive.

2 This response is not therapeutic because it closes off communication, which may increase feelings of uncertainty and anxiety.

3 This is not an honest response; it is false reassurance because the mother's prognosis is uncertain at this time.

58. 1 **Beginning at the learner's level of understanding and including the learner in the planning fosters acceptance and stimulates motivation. (3) (SE; MR; PL; MH; NP)**

2 Although desirable, including the participants in the planning is more vital for success.

3 This may be helpful; however, it is more important that participants be included in the initial planning.

4 This is not a prerequisite to teaching mental health principles.

59. 2 **The client's statement infers an emptiness with an associated loss. (1) (PI; CJ; EV; CW; EC)**

1 Resumption of social activities indicates an acceptance of her condition and a willingness to move on with life.

3 This is a typical response of a grandparent anxious to resume life.

4 The client is planning for rehabilitation, not expressing a sense of loss.

60. 1 **Vitamin K, a fat-soluble vitamin, is not absorbed from the GI tract in the absence of bile; bile enters the duodenum via the common bile duct. (1) (PB; CJ; AN; MS; GI)**

2 Calcium is related to rhythmic muscle contraction, not coagulation.

3 The extrinsic factor (cyanocobalamin) is a water-soluble vitamin; bile is not necessary for its absorption.

4 Bilirubin is formed by the breakdown of hemoglobin and RBCs and is not related to coagulation.

61. 4 **Impulse conduction of skeletal muscles is impaired with decreased potassium levels; muscular weakness and cramps may occur with hypokalemia. (2) (PB; CJ; EV; MS; FE)**

1 Hyperactive reflexes indicate hyperkalemia, not hypokalemia.

2 The pulse would be weak and irregular with hypokalemia because of an impaired conduction system in the cardiac muscle.

3 Diarrhea is caused by hyperkalemia, not hypokalemia.

62. 4 **This is a characteristic finding in newborns with Down syndrome. (1) (PM; CJ; AS; CW; HN)**

1 Stubby fingers commonly are found in children with Down syndrome.

2 Small ears commonly are found in newborns with Down syndrome.

3 Newborns with Down syndrome have hypotonic muscles.

63. 2 **Rheumatoid arthritis can cause inflammation of the iris and ciliary body of the eyes which may lead to blindness. (3) (PB; CJ; AN; PE; SK)**

1 The ears are not affected.

3 The liver is not affected.

4 The brain is not affected.

64. 1 **This is all the nurse can do until trust is established; forcing the client to attend will disrupt the group. (2) (PI; CJ; IM; MH; TR)**

2 This will create a confrontation between clients.

3 This will serve little purpose and will result in a confrontation; behavior cannot be altered by arguing.

4 Same as answer 3.

65. 4 **The nurse should offer support and use clear, simple terms to allay the client's anxiety. (1) (PI; CJ; IM; MH; MO)**

1 This may be too frightening or confusing to the client.

2 When severely depressed, the client cannot retain details.

3 The client generally is kept NPO before ECT to prevent aspiration during the treatment.

66. 4 **This occurs with stenosis of the stoma; forcing insertion of the tube could cause injury. (2) (SE; MR; EV; MS; GI)**

1 This is an expected response.

2 Same as answer 1.

3 This is expected; feces and flatus accompany fluid expulsion.

67. 3 **Excessive blood loss predisposes the client to an increased risk of infection because of decreased maternal resistance; the expected blood loss is 350 to 500 mL. (3) (PB; CJ; EV; CW; HP)**

1 A history of habitual abortions does not predispose the client to postpartum infection.

2 B negative blood type does not predispose the client to a postpartum infection.

4 This is an acceptable temperature because a maternal temperature up to 100.4° F may occur in response to the exertion and dehydration associated with labor.

68. 1 **This is soothing to the oral mucosa and helps prevent infection. (1) (PB; CJ; IM; MS; IT)**

  2 Stomatitis refers to the oral cavity; karaya is used to protect the skin around a stoma created on the abdomen.

  3 There is no diarrhea or fluid loss caused by stomatitis.

  4 The abdomen is not involved; stomatitis is an inflammation of the oral mucosa.

69. 2 **The client is incapable of accepting responsibility for self-created problems and blames society for the behavior. (2) (PI; CJ; AS; MH; PR)**

  1 This response demonstrates insight, and these individuals rarely develop insight into their problems.

  3 Same as answer 1.

  4 Same as answer 1.

70. 1 **Swelling can obstruct nasal breathing, interfering with the senses of taste and smell. (2) (SE; MR; EV; PE; RE)**

  2 Speech should not be affected because the vocal cords are not within the operative area.

  3 The operative site should be healed and not cause discomfort when swallowing.

  4 The vocal cords are outside the operative area; the site should be healed and not cause discomfort when swallowing.

71. 1 **Fatigue is a major problem caused by an increase in waste products because of catabolic processes. (2) (PB; MR; IM; MS; GI)**

  2 This can occur when the hair on the head is in the field of radiation, but it is not a major side effect.

  3 This is not common unless the stomach or intestine receives radiation.

  4 This is not a problem unless 25 percent or more of the bone marrow is in the treatment field.

72. 1 **Statistics indicate that the most frequent cause of falls by hospitalized clients is getting up or attempting to get up to the bathroom unassisted. (1) (SE; CJ; PL; MS; NP)**

  2 Moving the bedside table closer to the bed is helpful in reducing falls, but is not the primary intervention.

  3 Sedatives contribute to the risk for falls.

  4 Although talking to the spouse may calm the client and contribute to sleep; it does not reduce the incidence of falls.

73. 4 **These abilities are age-appropriate for the 6-month-old child. (2) (PM; CJ; PL; PE; GD)**

  1 These abilities should be developed by 10 months of age.

  2 Same as answer 1.

  3 Same as answer 1.

74. 4 **The most vigorous sucking will occur during the first few minutes of breastfeeding when the infant would be on the unaffected breast; later suckling is less traumatic. (3) (PB; CJ; IM; CW; HC)**

  1 Manual expression may not completely empty the breast, interfering with lactation.

  2 Stopping nursing for two days is unnecessary and would interfere with lactation.

  3 A breast shield confuses an infant because it is necessary to use a different sucking pattern to obtain milk.

75. 4 **This would absorb the drainage without causing further trauma. (2) (PB; CJ; IM; MS; NM)**

  1 This would allow fluid to collect in the ear.

  2 Manipulation of the ear could cause further injury.

  3 This might be done if the drainage were serous, to determine if it was cerebrospinal fluid.

How to Use Worksheet 1: Errors in Processing Information

Common errors in processing information are listed in the left hand column of this worksheet. At the top of the worksheet is a row of blank spaces for inserting the number of the question missed. Directly below each number, check any errors you made in answering that question. You may have made more than one type of error in an answer.

Worksheet 1: Errors in Processing Information

Question number																										
Did not read situation/ question carefully																										
Missed important details																										
Confused major and minor points																										
Defined problem incorrectly																										
Could not remember terms/ facts/concepts/principles																										
Defined terms incorrectly																										
Focused on incomplete/incorrect data in assessing situation																										
Interpreted data incorrectly																										
Applied wrong concepts/ principles in situations																										
Drew incorrect conclusions																										
Identified wrong goals																										
Identified priorities incorrectly																										
Carried out plan incorrectly/ incompletely																										
Was unclear about criteria for evaluating success in achieving goals																										

How to Use Worksheet 2: Knowledge Gaps

Types of common knowledge gaps are listed along the top of this worksheet. Write a brief description of topics you want to review in the spaces provided. For example, if you missed a question on administration of a particular drug, write the drug name and problem (e.g., dosage) in the appropriate space under the column labeled *Pharmacology*.

Worksheet 2: Knowledge Gaps

Basic science	Skills/ procedures	Basic human needs	Growth and development	Normal nutrition	Psychosocial factors	Clinical area/ topic	Stressors/ coping mechanisms	Patho-physiology	Pharma-cology	Therapeutic nutrition	Legal implications	Other

Part B Answers and Rationales

76. 4 Discussion with parents who have children with similar problems helps to reduce some of their discomfort and guilt. (2) (SE; MR; PL; PE; EH)
1 When not in crisis, the child should be allowed to attend school and should not be exposed to developmental damage by social isolation.
2 There is no recommended therapeutic climate for these children, and moving may not be beneficial to the child or the family.
3 Some parents do not choose to avoid future pregnancies and should not be encouraged to do so.

77. 3 This action takes into consideration that the client's anxiety will increase if the ritual is interrupted; this allows the client to complete the ritual and encourages going to the dining room for lunch. (2) (PI; CJ; IM; MH; AX)
1 This denies the ritual which will result in an increase in anxiety; this client's priority is for towels to complete the ritual, not going to lunch.
2 This is an inappropriate time for this discussion because it would increase anxiety and result in the client's missing a meal.
4 This action would precipitate a conflict between completing the ritual and going to the dining room, and conflict would increase anxiety.

78. 2 Clients who understand the "why" of treatment are more likely to comply. (3) (PB; CJ; PL; CW; HP)
1 This may be an unrealistic suggestion; more data are needed to see if this is feasible.
3 This is a negative approach; the benefits, rather than the risks, of compliance should be discussed.
4 This does not meet the requirement of bed rest.

79. 1 The nurse must deal with these feelings and establish basic trust to promote a therapeutic milieu. (2) (PI; CJ; PL; MH; SD)
2 Continuous pacing is not a problem because the nurse can walk back and forth with the client.
3 This may be of long-range importance but has little influence on the nurse's response to the client.

4 Same as answer 3.

80. 1 When a bilateral oophorectomy is performed, both ovaries are excised, eliminating ovarian hormones and initiating menopause. (1) (PM; MR; PL; CW; WH)
2 This is more often associated with vaginal hysterectomy.
3 There is no physiologic reason for weight gain following a hysterectomy; overeating is sometimes associated with depression.
4 Although depression may occur, it should not be expected; if it does occur, it requires intervention.

81. 4 Because the client is up more at home, edema usually increases. (3) (SE; MR; IM; MS; CV)
1 Serosanguineous drainage may persist after discharge.
2 These should not be expected and are in fact signs of post-pericardiotomy syndrome.
3 These symptoms may persist longer because it takes 6 to 12 weeks for the sternum to heal.

82. 1 The client expects the nurse to focus on eating, but the emphasis should be placed on feelings rather than actions. (2) (PM; CJ; IM; MH; ES)
2 This is a threat that will not convince the client to eat; privileges are associated with a contracted weight gain.
3 Threats will not convince the client to eat; this response sets up a challenge that the nurse will not win.
4 This is a threat that will not convince the client to eat; the client is not concerned about the effects of malnutrition.

83. 2 The expected effect should be more than a one-point decrease in the pain level. (1) (PB; CJ; EV; MS; NM)
1 This cannot be determined with the data available.
3 The medication has not achieved an adequate response; pain is generally considered to be tolerable if it is 4 or below on a pain scale of 1 to 10.
4 Same as answer 1.

84. 2 Stimuli are provided via all the senses; since the infant's behavioral development is enhanced through parent-infant interactions, these interactions should be encouraged. (2) (PM; CJ; PL; CW; EC)

1 Infants require interactions soon after birth and consistently thereafter, but interactions should occur during the infant's regular waking periods.

3 Infants have various awake and sleep states; touching and talking should coincide with these states and should not be scheduled.

4 Same as answer 3.

85. 4 Academic deficits, an inability to function within constraints required of certain settings, and negative peer attitudes often lead to low self-esteem. (3) (PI; CJ; AN; MH; BA)

1 These children usually are very verbal; children with autism need assistance with language development.

2 When the child receives therapy, regressive behavior is expected because it is a strategy to reduce anxiety.

3 This would be a long-term goal; the immediate goal is to increase the child's self-esteem.

86. 2 Because the tumor is of renal origin, the renin-angiotensin mechanism can be involved, and blood pressure monitoring is important. (3) (PB; CJ; PL; PE; RG)

1 This could put pressure on the involved area, possibly causing rupture of the tumor and seeding of cancer cells.

3 Same as answer 1.

4 This is unnecessary; no infection is present.

87. 1 Controlled substance issues for a particular nursing unit are the responsibility of that unit's nurse manager. (1) (SE; MR; IM; MS; NP)

2 Responsibility flows directly from the staff of a nursing unit to the nurse manager; the nurse manager would report to a nurse administrator.

3 There is no direct flow of accountability from the primary nurse to the quality control manager.

4 Physicians are responsible for medical management issues, not issues associated with management of a nursing unit.

88. 4 All these interventions promote aeration of the re-expanding lung and maintenance of function in the arm and shoulder on the affected side. (3) (PB; CJ; PL; MS; RE)

1 Cough suppressants would not be indicated because coughing and deep breathing are to be encouraged.

2 Drainage is marked with time tapes on the side of the device; the closed system is not entered for emptying; when full, the entire device is replaced.

3 Clamps are not necessary and should be avoided in almost all instances because of the danger of tension pneumothorax.

89. 4 The client's grieving process is severe and extended, indicating dysfunction. (2) (PI; CJ; AN; MH; CS)

1 The data do not support this; the client is communicating effectively with the nurse.

2 There are not enough data to support this conclusion.

3 This is not as specific as identifying grieving; also, low motivation is not the reason for the client's inability to cope.

90. 3 The vastus lateralis is the most appropriate muscle for injection in a newborn because it is well developed and there is little danger of causing nerve injury. (1) (PM; CJ; PL; CW; DR)

1 This muscle is too small for an IM injection in a newborn.

2 The vastus lateralis is one of the muscles of the quadriceps; it is the safest to use.

4 The sciatic nerve in the newborn is near the outer aspect of the gluteus maximus; there is a danger that it might be injured.

91. 3 Because the client refuses to talk, pertinent data must be obtained from the family. (2) (SE; MR; AS; MH; MO)

1 The client is not responding to questions; the client may not know the reason.

2 This may or may not have influenced current behavior.

4 The presence of scars may or may not be an accurate way to determine past behavior; family information would be more accurate.

92. 2 A rapid mood upswing and psychomotor change commonly signals that the client has made a decision and has developed a plan for suicide. (2) (PI; CJ; EV; MH; MO)

1 This statement is typical of the depressed client; it does not signal a change in mood.

3 Same as answer 1.

4 Same as answer 1.

93. 3 This results from a recipient's antibodies that are incompatible with transfused red blood cells; it is called a type II hypersensitivity; these signs result from RBC hemolysis, agglutination, and capillary plugging. (3) (PB; CJ; EV; MS; BI)

1 This results from an immune sensitivity to foreign serum protein; it is called a type I

hypersensitivity; signs include urticaria, wheezing, dyspnea, and shock.

2 Bacterial pyrogens are present in contaminated blood and can cause a febrile transfusion reaction; signs include fever and chills.

4 There is no transfusion reaction called by this name, although anaphylaxis occurs with an allergic transfusion reaction.

94. **4 Rationalization is offering a socially acceptable or logical explanation to justify an unacceptable feeling or behavior. (1) (PI; CJ; AS; MH; CS)**

1 Projection is the denial of emotionally unacceptable feelings and the attribution of the traits to another person.

2 Sublimation is the substitution of a socially acceptable behavior for an unacceptable feeling or drive.

3 Compensation is making up for a perceived deficiency by emphasizing another feature perceived as an asset.

95. **Answer: 38 gtts/minute; solve the problem by dividing the total number of drops by the total number of minutes; because ½ drop cannot be administered, the answer must be rounded up to the next number.**

$$\frac{50 \text{ mL} \times 15 \text{ gtt/mL}}{20 \text{ minutes}}$$

$$\frac{750}{20} = 37.5$$

(2) (PB; CJ; AN; MS; FE)

96. **1 The first indication of toxicity in approximately 50% of clients who take a cardiac glycoside, such as digoxin, is nausea and loss of appetite. (2) (PB; CJ; EV; MS; DR)**

2 This is a rare manifestation of digitalis toxicity.

3 This may occur later.

4 Same as answer 3.

97. **1 This position utilizes gravity to drain fluid from the head, which helps prevent cerebral edema. (1) (PB; CJ; IM; PE; NM)**

2 This is true, but it is done primarily to prevent cerebral edema.

3 The semi-Fowler's position has no effect on chemicals, but it does reduce subdural pressure.

4 Although the cardiac workload is decreased in the semi-Fowler's position, when compared to the supine position, and the semi-Fowler's position does facilitate oxygenation when compared to the supine position, these are not the reasons for placing the child in the semi-Fowler's position; the priority is to prevent cerebral edema.

98. **1 A decreased blood volume leads to decreased glomerular filtration; compensatory ADH and aldosterone secretion cause sodium and water retention. (2) (PB; CJ; EV; MS; BI)**

2 The respirations become rapid and shallow to compensate for decreased cellular oxygenation.

3 The peripheral pulse rate may be rapid and thready, but it is the same rate as the apical rate.

4 Hypokalemia occurs because as sodium is retained potassium is excreted.

99. **2 The priority action is to assess for circulatory overload; changes in the vital signs would indicate a problem that must be addressed quickly. (2) (PB; LE; EV; CW; NP)**

1 This is a dependent function and requires a physician's order.

3 This would waste valuable time that should be spent assessing the infant's response.

4 Same as answer 3.

100. **4 This involves no element of competition and still allows for channeling of excessive energy. (2) (PI; CJ; PL; MH; MO)**

1 The sense of competition and increased stimulation may raise the client's anxiety.

2 This requires fine motor skill from a client who is hyperactive and whose attention span is limited.

3 The client is too hyperactive to complete this task and may respond with distractibility or aggressiveness toward others.

101. **3 The nurse must bring this information to the attention of the treatment staff for their information and action; a team approach is necessary. (3) (SE; MR; IM; MH; NP)**

1 This may be done but after the staff is made aware of the situation and the treatment plan has been modified.

2 This would be premature before the staff can develop a plan of action; this may or may not be necessary.

4 Confronting the client eventually will occur, but a plan of how and when this will take place needs to be developed; safety is an issue that must be considered.

102. **4 These are related to potassium depletion in the skeletal and cardiac muscles; potassium facilitates conduction of nerve impulses and muscle activity. (3) (PB; CJ; AS; MS; FE)**

1 These are related to hypocalcemia.

2 This is related to hypernatremia.

3 These are related to hyperkalemia.

103. 2 Peer acceptance is crucial during this period; they must have the opportunity to accept her with one leg. (3) (PI; CJ; PL; PE; EH)
1 An adolescent needs to relate to and be accepted by peers as well as family.
3 Isolating the client will increase feelings of alienation and being different.
4 Concealing the loss does not help the adolescent or others with acceptance.

104. 4 Because capillary perfusion is blocked by the embolus, oxygen saturation drops and the client becomes short of breath. (3) (PB; CJ; AS; MS; RE)
1 A flushed face is not recognized as a sign of a pulmonary embolus.
2 An elevation of temperature may occur for many reasons; it is not an early sign of a pulmonary embolus.
3 Many pulmonary emboli do not produce chest pain; if present it can be mild to severe.

105. 4 This sets an unrealistic limit that would increase anxiety by removing a defense the client needs at this time; rituals cannot be this controlled until other defenses are developed to replace them. (2) (PI; CJ; EV; MH; PR)
1 This is done in therapy as the client's condition improves; insight must be developed slowly to minimize anxiety.
2 This would reduce, not increase, anxiety because the client would feel free to express feelings.
3 This would increase self-esteem and self-control, not increase anxiety.

106. 1 Opening and maintaining the airway is always the highest priority; maintaining oxygenation is the priority. (1) (PB; CJ; PL; MS; RE)
2 Chest compressions may be initiated after the airway is open.
3 The carotid pulse is palpated to evaluate for the presence of a heartbeat.
4 The abdominal thrust (Heimlich) maneuver is used to relieve airway obstruction and is not appropriate in this instance.

107. 2 Tearing the meninges could have introduced infectious organisms. (2) (SE; CJ; AS; MS; NM)
1 Physical therapy begun too early can raise intracranial pressure; preventing infection takes priority.
3 Prevention of infection takes priority over nutrition at this time.
4 Although psychosocial support is important, it is unrelated to leakage from the nose and ear; preventing infection takes priority.

108. 1 This is comforting for the mother and baby and provides an opportunity to teach circumcision care. (2) (PM; CJ; AN; CW; EC)
2 Dry gauze removal would cause bleeding; sterile petrolatum gauze is used and changed with each diaper change.
3 This is inappropriate and can lead to fluid and electrolyte imbalance.
4 There is no contraindication to feeding the baby after the circumcision; nutrition may be withheld before, not after the circumcision.

109. 1 Ketoacidosis occurs when insulin is lacking and carbohydrates cannot be used for energy; this increases the breakdown of protein and fat, causing Kussmaul respirations, decreased alertness, decreased circulatory volume, metabolic acidosis, and an acetone breath. (1) (PB; CJ; EV; MS; EN)
2 Hypoglycemia is manifested by cool, moist skin, not hot, dry skin or Kussmaul respirations.
3 The Somogyi phenomenon is a rebound hyperglycemia induced by severe hypoglycemia; there are not enough data to determine whether this occurred.
4 Hyperosmolar nonketotic coma usually occurs in clients with type 2 diabetes because available insulin prevents the breakdown of fat.

110. 2 Unnecessary stimuli contribute to the metabolic demands of the body and can precipitate thyrotoxic crisis. (3) (PB; CJ; PL; MS; EN)
1 This does not prevent crisis; a high-calorie diet restores glycogen reserves depleted by an increased metabolic rate.
3 This prevents respiratory complications, not crisis.
4 This limits tension on the suture line, thereby decreasing the risk of hemorrhage, not crisis.

111. 2 During the working stage, goals are met, problems are resolved, and changes in behavior occur. (1) (SE; CJ; AN; MH; NP)
1 During the initial stage, trust is the primary focus, goals and contracts are set, and problems are identified.
3 There is no such stage in the nurse-client relationship; this is a step in the nursing process.
4 The evaluation/termination stage focuses on accomplishments, reinforces new behaviors, and closes the relationship.

112. 1 Confrontation about the active substance abuse and the mother's diminished ability to safely care for the infant at this time is necessary to protect the baby and also to refer the mother for help. (2) (PI; LE; IM; CW; NP)

2 Although the nurse should speak openly with the mother, making arrangements for discharge to a foster home would be premature.

3 Decisions should not be made without input from the mother.

4 This would be unsafe; the mother may not be capable of caring for the infant.

113. 3 Clients may introduce new topics during the last session to avoid termination; the nurse can encourage the client to discuss the problem as an out-patient. (2) (PI; MR; IM; MH; TR)

1 The last few minutes of the last interview is not the appropriate time to introduce new problems.

2 The purposes of the last interview are to summarize and terminate, not to begin discussion of new problems.

4 It is best not to introduce new subjects during the final interview because there is not enough time to explore the issues.

114. 1 Client participation provides for a sense of control, and a consistent approach provides a routine with no surprises; these approaches may limit pain and promote compliance with the regimen. (2) (PM; CJ; PL; MS; IT)

2 Preparation of the equipment and explanation of the procedure should be performed before the procedure; when performed during the procedure, it wastes time, which can prolong pain.

3 Changing staff disrupts the client's routine and sense of trust.

4 This is too hot; the water should be approximately 100° F.

115. 3 This response is a reflection of the client's feelings; it leaves communication lines open. (3) (PI; CJ; IM; MH; SD)

1 This response discounts the client's thoughts and may increase agitation.

2 This does not provide security because the client may believe the nurse is one of those involved in the plot to kill.

4 This supports the client's delusional system.

116. 1 Changing the maternal position is the most beneficial action, especially with late- and variable-deceleration patterns, because it will increase placental perfusion. (1) (PM; CJ; IM; CW; HP)

2 If oxygen were to be used, a greater concentration than 2 L per minute should be used.

3 Although the client should be kept informed of the fetus' condition, this can be done during or immediately after the position change; the priority is to meet the needs of the fetus.

4 Although this may be done after the position change, the priority is to meet the immediate needs of the fetus.

117. 4 Vasospasms of placental vessels occur because of elevated blood pressure, and the placenta may separate prematurely (abruptio placentae). (2) (PB; CJ; PL; CW; HP)

1 Placenta previa is an abnormal placental implantation and is not related to hypertension.

2 This is an excessive amount of amniotic fluid and is not associated with hypertensive disorders of pregnancy.

3 Isoimmunization in pregnancy is associated with Rh incompatability, not hypertension.

118. 4 The therapy program in use in the home should be incorporated into the care plan to maintain continuity. (1) (SE; MR; PL; PE; SK)

1 The child has social needs, and interaction should be promoted; there is no need for a private room.

2 The parents should be encouraged to stay with the child and actively participate in care.

3 The child should have a regular diet appropriate for the developmental age.

119. 4 The proximity of the parotid gland to the esophagus necessitates assessment of swallowing because dysphagia may be a side effect. (2) (PB; CJ; PL; MS; GI)

1 This is not a side effect of radiotherapy unless the central nervous system is involved.

2 The lungs are not being radiated; hypoxia should not result.

3 This is not a side effect of radiotherapy.

120. 3 Squinting, a classic sign of strabismus, occurs because of the malalignment of the eyes. (2) (PM; CJ; AS; PE; NM)

1 This is associated with conjunctivitis, not strabismus.

2 This may indicate an affectation or nervous tic, not strabismus.

4 This may indicate blockage of the tear ducts, not strabismus.

121. 2 An open wound requires sterile technique; the supplies at the bedside are not sterile and the physician ordered sterile soaks. (2) (SE; MR; IM; MS; NP)
    1 This is unsafe; a clean basin and washcloth are not sterile.
    3 Client safety is the priority at this time.
    4 This is unnecessary; the physician has already indicated the type of soak desired.

122. 4 When action on either side of a conflict creates anxiety, a physical reason for not acting at all may unconsciously be used. (3) (PI; CJ; AN; MH; AX)
    1 These disorders are disabling; the client truly believes the symptoms are real.
    2 These individuals do not enjoy their illness; their anxiety is relieved by it.
    3 These individuals are in contact with reality.

123. 2 Because normal implantation occurs in the upper third of the uterus, a low-lying placenta would indicate placenta previa. (2) (PB; CJ; EV; CW; HP)
    1 Infarctions may appear on a placenta because of some interference with the blood supply; this is not related to its position.
    3 Placenta previa indicates where the placenta has implanted and has no relationship to placental aging.
    4 Abruptio placentae is the premature separation of a normally implanted placenta.

124. 4 The brain requires continuous and large quantities of oxygen to function; maintaining the airway is the priority. (2) (SE; CJ; PL; MS; RE)
    1 This is true for all clients but is not the priority.
    2 The supine position does not facilitate respirations; the semi-Fowler's position promotes venous return, prevents venous stasis, and aids ventilation.
    3 Although a widening pulse pressure may indicate increasing intracranial pressure, maintaining respiration is always the priority.

125. 1 The intestine is obstructed by thick, tenacious, pasty meconium. (2) (PB; CJ; AS; PE; GI)
    2 Imperforate anus is a congenital malformation in which the anal opening is obliterated; it is not associated with cystic fibrosis.
    3 This occurs in most newborns because of destruction of immature erythrocytes; it may be physiologic or pathologic.
    4 Preterm, high-risk infants are prone to this disorder.

126. 4 Neologisms are newly coined words with personal meanings to the client with schizophrenia. (2) (PI; CJ; AN; MH; SD)
    1 Clanging is the association of words by sound rather than meaning.
    2 Echolalia is parrot-like echoing of spoken words or sounds.
    3 Echopraxia is mimicking the movements of others.

127. 4 Mineral substances taken within two hours of a dose decreases the medication's effectiveness. (2) (SE; MR; EV; CW; WH)
    1 Fluid intake should be increased to prevent crystalluria.
    2 Although the urine should be observed for crystals, straining is not necessary.
    3 The urine will not turn orange with this medication; if bloody or smoky urine were present before treatment, it would become the typical color once treatment was initiated.

128. 2 If there is any bony or soft tissue resistance to descent and delivery, trauma to the fetal head may occur. (3) (SE; CJ; AN; CW; HP)
    1 This is not associated with a birth event.
    3 This is not associated with a precipitous labor.
    4 Although this could occur, the placenta usually is expelled shortly after the fetus.

129. 3 This explanation is short and easily understood by most clients; the information is accurate regarding the pathophysiology of clot development and is included in preoperative teaching. (1) (PM; CJ; IM; MS; CV)
    1 Although positioning with pillows does increase the client's comfort, their placement under the knees is contraindicated in the care of postoperative clients.
    2 To say an action is not good and then carry it out confuses the client; a pillow or any object that impedes venous flow is contraindicated in the care of postoperative clients.
    4 Pillows under the knees causes flexion of the knees, which is within the capability of this joint; however, pillows are contraindicated because they can slow blood flow contributing to clot formation in the postoperative client.

130. 3 Displacement is the unconscious redirection of an emotion from a threatening source to a non-threatening source. (3) (PI; CJ; AN; MH; PD)

1 Regression is the return to an earlier, more comfortable level of behavior; it is a retreat from the present.

2 Sublimation channels forbidden impulses into acceptable activities; usually it is constructive, not destructive.

4 Rationalization is the attempt to make unacceptable behavior or feelings acceptable by justification of the reasons for them.

131. 4 **This is the most complete definition of bulimia. (2) (PI; CJ; AN; MH; ES)**

1 This may occur with bulimia, but it is not the definition.

2 Although clients with bulimia do consume large amounts of food in private, they do eat in public.

3 Same as answer 1.

132. 1 **An exercise program and the Milwaukee brace are the treatments of choice for mild structural scoliosis. (2) (PM; CJ; IM; PE; SK)**

2 Exercises are to be encouraged, regardless of the type or extent of scoliosis.

3 Exercises alone are used only with scoliosis that is related to posture, not structure.

4 Although compliance will affect the ultimate outcome of treatment, exercises alone are not helpful in this type of scoliosis.

133. 3 **Flexion and extension prevent tightening of muscles and tendons. (2) (PB; CJ; PL; MS; SK)**

1 These are abnormal sensations and are related to neurologic, not musculoskeletal, alterations.

2 Weight-bearing, not exercise, would promote the development of osteoblasts.

4 This is the result of cerebellar changes; it is not related to immobility.

134. 4 **The newborn's intake of milk is gradual and small, and, at the same time, there is loss of extracellular fluid primarily in the form of stool and urine. (2) (PM; CJ; AN; CW; NN)**

1 This is untrue; slight weight loss after birth is an expected physiologic response.

2 Same as answer 1.

3 Same as answer 1.

135. 4 **Labor is hard work and can cause a pregnant woman in labor to deplete her glucose stores, especially if she had not eaten for over 14 hours. (1) (PM; CJ; EV; CW; HC)**

1 This blood pressure is within expected limits and would not indicate a problem.

2 Excretion of protein in the urine generally is related to chronic hypertension or preeclampsia; there is no indication of an elevated blood pressure.

3 Electrolyte losses occur because of vomiting, diarrhea, and intense labor and there is no indication that any of these have occurred.

136. 2 **This variable pattern with bradycardia is an ominous sign; it is indicative of cord compression, which can cause fetal hypoxia. (2) (PB; CJ; EV; CW; HP)**

1 Fetal acidosis can occur with uteroplacental insufficiency.

3 Early decelerations are associated with head compression and are not dangerous.

4 Late decelerations and tachycardia are associated with uteroplacental insufficiency.

137. 2 **Documentation on an incident report provides a legal record and is critical in providing appropriate care and follow up. (1) (SE; LE; IM; MS; NP)**

1 This is the responsibility of the physician and nurse providing ongoing care.

3 This will be done but is not as critical as documentation of the incident.

4 This is not the responsibility of the witnessing nurse after transferring care to another nurse who would provide the ongoing care.

138. 4 **Between the ages of 3 and 5 years, death is viewed as a departure or sleep, which is reversible. (3) (PM; CJ; AN; PE; GD)**

1 This is the concept of death held by children 9 or 10 years of age; death is viewed as reversible by the preschooler.

2 The early school-age child of 6 or 7 years personifies death and sees it as horrible and frightening; this is consistent with the concrete thinking present at this age.

3 Children of all ages, except infants, have some concept of death.

139. 4 **Bed rest conserves energy; a diet with no added salt is permitted; the other care monitors the response to therapy. (2) (PB; CJ; PL; PE; RG)**

1 Isolation is unnecessary because the illness is not communicable; fluids would not be encouraged but limited or permitted as desired.

2 The blood pressure is not monitored every hour, and IV therapy is not used unless there is no oral intake or seizures occur.

3 Vital signs do not need to be monitored every two hours, a no-sodium diet is not possible, and bed rest is maintained to conserve energy.

140. 1 Decreased blood volume leads to decreased glomerular filtration; compensatory ADH and aldosterone secretion cause sodium and water retention. (2) (PB; CJ; AS; MS; FE)

2 Dizziness is an earlier sign; oliguria occurs as hypovolemia progresses.

3 Respirations become rapid and shallow to compensate for decreased oxygenation.

4 Hypotension, not hypertension, is the response to hypovolemia and shock as a result of hemorrhage.

141. 1 Discussing behaviors and feelings in the group assists members to learn new ways to behave that are more constructive. (2) (PI; MR; IM; MH; TR)

2 An emotionally charged situation should not be left until the next group session.

3 Since the group has just formed, they probably are not yet able to handle problems constructively without a leader.

4 Selecting members to participate in the group discussion decreases spontaneity and hinders group responsibility for its members.

142. 3 Because of glomerular dysfunction, there is decreased filtration of plasma, leading to excessive water accumulation and sodium retention; this leads to congestion and edema. (3) (PB; CJ; AS; PE; RG)

1 This does not occur with glomerulonephritis.

2 There is a decrease in urine volume.

4 Same as answer 1.

143. 3 The schedule for active immunization is three doses of DTaP at 2-month intervals beginning at 2 months of age. (2) (PM; CJ; AN; PE; BI)

1 Measles vaccine is not given until 12 to 15 months because maternal antibodies block the formation of the infant's antibodies.

2 IPV booster is due at 18 months; it is given at the same time as the DTaP booster dose.

4 This is given at 18 months, or approximately one year after the third dose that is given at 6 months of age.

144. 1 These juices each contain 1 mg of sodium per 100 grams. (2) (PB; CJ; IM; MS; GI)

2 Dried apricots contain 8 mg of sodium per 100 grams; peas contain 35 mg of sodium per 100 grams.

3 Carrots contain 47 mg of sodium per 100 grams; celery contains 126 mg of sodium per 100 grams.

4 Tomato juice contains 200 mg of sodium per 100 grams; grape juice contains 2 mg of sodium per 100 grams.

145. 2 Oxytocin increases contractions of the uterus and promotes return of the uterus to its prepregnant state. (2) (PM; CJ; IM; CW; HC)

1 As the uterus contracts, the flow of lochia decreases.

3 Oxytocin does not promote tissue healing.

4 Oxytocin tends to increase discomfort; the client may have pain as the uterus contracts.

146. 2 This moves the emphasis from facts to feelings; it focuses on the client without setting the direction for communication. (3) (PI; CJ; IM; MH; MO)

1 This is a rhetorical question because the client has already brought up the topic.

3 This denies the client's feelings and cuts off further communication.

4 This asks a direct question that the client will probably be unable to answer.

147. 2 This is an accurate statement; each gram of carbohydrate contains 4 calories. (1) (PB; MR; PL; MS; GI)

1 This provides too few calories; carbohydrates contain 4 calories per gram.

3 This provides too many calories; fat contains 9 calories per gram.

4 This provides too many calories; no nutrient contains this many calories per gram.

148. 1 Alcohol causes both physical and psychologic dependence; the individual needs and depends on the alcohol to function. (2) (PI; CJ; AN; MH; SA)

2 Alcoholism is a disorder that entails physical and psychologic dependence.

3 People with alcoholism usually drink alone or feel alone in a crowd; this is not the prime reason for their drinking.

4 This is a myth often associated with alcoholism; the individual needs to learn how to use other coping mechanisms more consistently and effectively.

149. 3 During the first 24 postpartum hours there is a rapid fluid shift, which causes an increase in cardiac output and blood volume; this taxes an already compromised heart. (2) (PB; CJ; PL; CW; HP)

1 This is not recommended because this will further increase circulating blood volume and necessitate an increase in cardiac workload.

2 This is false; the first 24 hours are crucial because of the rapid fluid shift and the stress

of increased cardiac output on a compromised heart.

4 Progressive ambulation starting during the first 24 hours postpartum is recommended because it decreases the risk of thromboembolic events.

150. 2 **Vincristine is neurotoxic; therefore, clients should be monitored for paresthesias, foot drop, bowel and bladder problems, and alterations of function of cranial nerves. (3) (PB; CJ; EV; PE; DR)**

1 Emotional states may be altered by corticosteroid therapy; vincristine (Oncovin) does not affect the emotional status.

3 Respiratory problems are not associated with vincristine (Oncovin) therapy.

4 Problems such as anemia, thrombocytopenia, and leukopenia occur with drugs such as cyclophosphamide (Cytoxan) and doxorubicin hydrochloride (Adriamycin), not with vincristine (Oncovin).

151. 4 **Allopurinol decreases serum uric acid levels before and during chemotherapy; increased fluid intake aids in the increased excretion of uric acid; allopurinol and increased fluids help prevent renal tubular impairment and kidney failure because of hyperuricemia. (3) (PB; CJ; PL; MS; DR)**

1 If the oral route is used, this will limit gastric irritation, not uric acid nephropathy.

2 The client should be encouraged to follow a diet that promotes urine alkalinity.

3 Fluid intake should be increased to 2 to 3 liters per day to prevent urate deposits and calculus formation.

152. 3 **The elastic bandage must be applied smoothly without wrinkles, folds, or creases because these can cause excessive pressure or irritation. (2) (SE; CJ; PL; MS; SK)**

1 The bandage should be reapplied whenever necessary; this may be necessary if it slips off, if it is too tight or too loose, or if it has wrinkles or creases.

2 This would be unsafe because it could impede circulation; the bandage should be snug, not tight.

4 This would be unsafe because the dependent position allows the blood vessels to become engorged; the bandage should be applied with the residual limb level with the heart.

153. 2 **Elastic stockings help decrease venous pooling of blood and help maintain systemic blood pressure when the client stands up. (2) (PB; CJ; IM; MS; CV)**

1 Orthostatic hypotension occurs on rising to an upright position; gait training will not affect this.

3 An alteration in dosage may be ordered by the physician, but sudden withdrawal is dangerous and unwarranted.

4 This may increase the intravascular fluid volume temporarily but will not affect reflexes involved in orthostatic hypotension.

154. 2 **The ischial spines are an important landmark in relation to the fetus' head because they reflect the progression of labor; 0 station indicates that the presenting part is at the ischial spines. (2) (PM; CJ; AN; CW; HC)**

1 Below the ischial spines is designated by positive numbers, for example +1.

3 Above the ischial spines is designated by a minus number; for example, −1.

4 When the presenting part is floating, the fetus is at −5 station.

155. 4 **This reduces the risk of introducing the irrigant into the lungs. (1) (SE; CJ; AS; MS; GI)**

1 This is irrelevant to nasogastric tube irrigation.

2 Same as answer 1.

3 This increases the risk of introducing irrigant into the lungs if tube placement is not checked first.

156. 3 **Compression fractures of the vertebrae are the most common fractures in clients with osteoporosis; a gradual collapse of vertebrae may be asymptomatic and observed as kyphosis. (1) (PM; CJ; AS; MS; SK)**

1 This is not observable to the naked eye.

2 Same as answer 1.

4 Arthritis is observable in the joints as inflammation and changes in the natural alignment of the bones.

157. 3 **This will help decrease irritability and impulsiveness caused by the client's increased responsiveness to changing stimuli. (2) (PI; CJ; PL; MH; MO)**

1 This is not helpful because of the client's easy distractibility and minimal attention span.

2 At this time, the client may misidentify this approach as threatening and may retaliate with aggression.

4 A strange environment and new caregivers tend to increase the anxiety level, not reduce manipulation.

158. 3 The fundus tends to stay at or slightly above the umbilicus for about 24 hours, then decreases in size about 1 fingerbreadth per day. (1) (PM; CJ; EV; CW; HC)

1 This would be the position in the first 24 hours postpartum.

2 Same as answer 1.

4 This would be the position on the fourth or fifth day postpartum.

159. 3 In this stage the degree of anguish experienced or expressed is most often set or imposed by the cultural background of the individual. (2) (PI; CJ; EV; MH; NP)

1 Although this factor does enter into the grief process, it is not as important in the developing awareness stage as is cultural background.

2 Educational level has no relationship to the grieving process

4 Socioeconomic class has no relationship to the grieving process.

160. 3 Studies have shown that parental role support and contact with other adults is very important in parenting. (2) (PI; CJ; AS; MH; CS)

1 Present defenses are ineffective when an adult engages in child abuse.

2 No personality type is specifically associated with abusive behavior.

4 Although lack of knowledge may lead to unrealistic expectations of the child, this factor alone does not significantly contribute to abusive behavior; inconsistency between the history and accident should alert the staff.

161. 1 Initial attempts at oral feeding may cause a choking feeling that may produce severe coughing and raise secretions. (3) (PB; CJ; IM; MS; RE)

2 Swallowing does not have an adverse effect on the suture line; a nasogastric tube would not be used because it could traumatize the suture line.

3 A progressive diet is started with liquids, not pureed foods.

4 Administering pain medication is not the priority.

162. 4 With frequent and continued use, Afrin can cause rebound congestion of mucous membranes. (2) (PB; CJ; IM; PE; RE)

1 Nasal polyps may be associated with allergies, but are unrelated to Afrin.

2 Ringing in the ears (tinnitus) is unrelated to this drug; Afrin may cause hypotension, tachycardia, and dizziness.

3 Bleeding tendencies are related to inadequate clotting mechanisms, which are not related to allergies; nasal bleeding may be associated with dry mucous membranes, but with rebound congestion the tissues are filled with fluid.

163. 4 An increasing residual without increasing intake indicates that absorption is decreasing, a sign of NEC. (3) (PB; CJ; EV; CW; HN)

1 Diarrhea may or may not be related to NEC.

2 Small amounts of vomitus (spitting up) are common in the neonate because the cardiac sphincter is weak.

3 The abdominal circumference increases with NEC.

164. 2 Dementia is a global intellectual impairment that decreases cognitive abilities, and learning and thinking are compromised. (2) (PI; CJ; AS; MH; DD)

1 The attention span would be decreased.

3 This is not specific to dementia or aging; it depends on the individual.

4 Psychologic stress and changes caused by aging result in a decreased capability to adapt to the environment; familiar routines provide security.

165. 1 When children are allowed to have some control in their care, their cooperation and willingness to tolerate procedures and medications are enhanced. (2) (PB; CJ; PL; PE; EH)

2 A child's favorite food should never be used to disguise medication because it may cause an aversion to that food and affect the child nutritionally.

3 Bribing sets up a nontherapeutic relationship between the child and the nurse and should not be used.

4 The nurse should be truthful about the taste of medication so that the child can have an opportunity to suggest ways to deal with the taste.

166. 3 After the birth of the fetus and placenta, the additional circulating fluid remains in the mother's intravascular compartment; cardiac output increases and remains elevated for at least 48 hours. (3) (PB; CJ; AN; CW; HP)

1 The immediate postpartum period remains critical because of the increased cardiac output.

2 Cardiac output increases in the early postpartum period; after the first 48 hours there is a rapid decrease for two weeks, and it

returns to the pre-pregnancy state within 24 weeks.

4 Cardiac decompensation may last up to six days postpartum.

167. **3 The opportunity must be provided for the client to practice language skills; family participation must be accepted and recognized. (1) (PI; CJ; IM; MS; NM)**
1 This demeans the spouse and cuts off communication.
2 Same as answer 1.
4 The spouse should be included and involved in the client's care.

168. **1 This statement reflects values and beliefs regarding homosexuality as being bad and deserving of punishment. (2) (SE; MR; AN; MS; NP)**
2 There is not enough evidence presented to justify drawing this conclusion.
3 Same as answer 2.
4 Although this may be true, no information is given to suggest that the nursing assistant has been assigned to care for this client.

169. **3 ASA is irritating to the stomach lining and can cause ulceration; the presence of food, fluid, or antacids decreases this response. (1) (PB; CJ; IM; MS; DR)**
1 Tylenol does not contain the anti-inflammatory properties present in aspirin; tinnitus should be reported to the physician.
2 This should be reported to the physician, not the dentist.
4 This is unnecessary as long as aspirin is taken with food.

170. **2 This statement focuses on the child's perceptions and promotes further communication. (3) (PI; CJ; IM; PE; EH)**
1 This reads too much into the client's statement and may be too emotionally charged.
3 This is untrue; there is a higher incidence of lice in people with inadequate personal hygiene.
4 Although this statement may be valid, it is accusatory; it discourages further communication.

171. **2 This response focuses on the client's feelings of despair and provides the opportunity to talk about them. (1) (PI; CJ; IM; MS; EH)**
1 This abandons the client and leaves the client with no support.
3 This focuses on the nurse's interpretation of the problem, not the client's.

4 This response avoids a pressing problem and misses an opportunity for discussion of feelings.

172. **3 A rapid fetal heart rate occurs when the maternal metabolism is accelerated; this can be a result of maternal fever. (3) (PB; CJ; AN; CW; HP)**
1 Fetal head compression causes early decelerations of the fetal heart rate, not fetal tachycardia.
2 Umbilical cord compression is most commonly associated with variable decelerations.
4 Pudendal anesthesia does not affect the fetal heart rate.

173. **3 The pain of renal colic is excruciating and should be relieved. (3) (PB; CJ; AN; MS; RG)**
1 Any urine can be saved and strained after the client's priority need is met.
2 Increasing fluid intake helps mobilize the stone, but a client who has severe pain may be nauseated and unable to drink.
4 Although a culture generally is ordered, it is not a priority when a client has severe pain.

174. **3 A child this age loves to collect and manipulate; this meets the need to develop fine motor skills. (2) (PM; CJ; IM; PE; GD)**
1 This is more appropriate for an older infant.
2 This would be frustrating for this child's developmental level.
4 The child is too young for scissors and fragile toys.

175. **3 Aldactone is a potassium-sparing diuretic often used in conjunction with thiazide diuretics. (1) (PB; CJ; AN; MS; DR)**
1 Both diuretics do this, so it is not a particular advantage of Aldactone.
2 Same as answer 1.
4 Same as answer 1.

176. **4 Previous experiences with projectile vomiting are frightening; an explanation that surgery has eliminated this problem will provide support for and encouragement of the parents as they resume care of their infant. (1) (SE; MR; EV; PE; EH)**
1 The data indicate the mother is eager to assist with other aspects of care.
2 These are not used initially; oral feedings are reinstituted with clear liquids and electrolytes and progress to formula as tolerated.
3 No special nipple is required.

177. 3 A first step in any therapeutic relationship should include setting parameters of meetings, such as time, frequency, and duration. (3) (PI; CJ; PL; MH; TR)

1 This is part of the working phase of a therapeutic relationship and therefore not an initial intervention.

2 The nurse should not deviate from the original contract.

4 Duration of meetings should be set when setting the initial ground rules during the first stage of the nurse/client relationship.

178. 2 These would be signs of infection and should be reported to the physician. (1) (SE; MR; EV; CW; WH)

1 This is a sign of healing that is expected.

3 This results from severance of nerves and formation of scar tissue, which are expected.

4 There is little subcutaneous fat in the thoracic area, and the skin may be taut at the operative site, appearing irregular; this commonly occurs.

179. 1 When there is decreased plasma volume flowing through the kidneys, the kidneys attempt to conserve water and oliguria will occur. (2) (PB; CJ; EV; MS; FE)

2 Lethargy and fatigue, not restlessness, are expected with dehydration.

3 When there is an intestinal obstruction, there would be an absence of bowel movements (obstipation); clients with Crohn's disease frequently have watery stools.

4 Hypotension, not hypertension, is associated with hypovolemia.

180. 2 Bed rest is important, and treatment is symptomatic; early recognition and treatment of complications are important. (2) (PB; CJ; PL; PE; RG)

1 Steroids are given to children with nephrotic syndrome, not acute glomerulonephritis.

3 Proteins and fluids may be limited if the child is hypertensive and has oliguria.

4 Acute glomerulonephritis is a noninfectious, immune-complex renal disease that occurs 10 to 21 days after a streptococcal infection.

181. 4 Insulin requirements may decrease in early pregnancy because of increased fetal needs for nutrients and the possibility of maternal nausea and vomiting; insulin requirements increase in the second and third trimesters as a resistance to insulin develops; the blood glucose level is monitored to prevent ketoacidosis and harm to both the mother and fetus. (1) (PB; CJ; IM; CW; HP)

1 This is true only during early pregnancy; during the second and third trimesters of pregnancy, there is a resistance to insulin and more insulin is required.

2 Even the nondiabetic woman makes a dietary adjustment to keep pace with the increased demands of pregnancy; in addition, insulin requirements increase in the second and third trimesters.

3 Most nutrient requirements, not just protein, increase in pregnancy.

182. 3 Oral hypoglycemics stimulate pancreatic beta cells to synthesize and release insulin; functional beta cells are usually not present in children with type 1 diabetes, and they are dependent on exogenous insulin. (1) (PB; CJ; IM; PE; DR)

1 This is the action of insulin, which is a hormone.

2 Glucagon from the pancreas promotes the release of glycogen from the liver; this raises blood glucose while hypoglycemics lower blood glucose.

4 Pancreatic alpha cells secrete glucagon, which stimulates the liver to release glycogen, raising blood glucose.

183. 2 Anxiety about the behavior is absent, as is motivation for change; these persons usually are unwilling to accept help. (2) (PI; CJ; AN; MH; PR)

1 More than lifestyle needs to change; the client's entire view of life and interpersonal responses are involved.

3 These individuals do not experience feelings of guilt about their behavior.

4 It is not a resistance to demonstrating feelings but a lack of feeling for others.

184. 4 The withdrawal provides time for the client to assimilate what has occurred and integrate the change in body image. (2) (PI; CJ; IM; MS; EH)

1 The client is not ready to hear these explanations until assimilation of the surgery has occurred.

2 This does not acknowledge that the client must grieve; it also does not allow the client to express any feelings that may be present that life will never be the same again.

3 The client might feel that the nurse has no comprehension of the situation or understanding of feelings.

185. 4 An active sucking reflex is a typical response in a full-term newborn, especially after an uneventful birth. (1) (PM; MR; IM; CW; NN)

1 Newborns show distress by vigorous crying, not through thumbsucking.

2 A baby sucks at various times; sucking is a reflex in the newborn and is not the sole indicator of hunger.

3 Sucking is not related to fatigue in the newborn.

186. **3 The child should know that he will remain awake; he should be prepared to experience the pressure of the aspiration or the biopsy needle entry. (2) (SE; MR; IM; PE; BI)**

1 False statements must be avoided, or the child will not trust what is said in the future.

2 The child will be permitted to ambulate freely.

4 A bone marrow specimen is obtained through a puncture wound; sutures are not necessary.

187. **1 Drainage from the small intestine contains residual digestive enzymes that can cause the skin to break down. (1) (SE; MR; PL; MS; GI)**

2 An ileostomy is not irrigated; the stool is liquid and drains unassisted.

3 An ileostomy will continually drain liquid stool; control of fecal elimination is impossible.

4 An ileostomy will continually drain liquid stool; this is unrelated to diet; the stool is excreted before fluid can be reabsorbed in the large intestine.

188. **3 Sudden withdrawal of antiepileptic medication can cause status epilepticus. (2) (PB; CJ; EV; MS; DR)**

1 It is important to take medication as prescribed to lessen the frequency of seizures; medication may or may not eliminate the seizures; stress may cause a seizure to occur.

2 This is not why antiepileptics are prescribed.

4 Same as answer 2.

189. **4 The continuous excretion of liquid feces may deplete the body of fluid and electrolytes resulting in a life-threatening fluid deficit and electrolyte imbalance. (2) (PB; CJ; AN; MS; FE)**

1 Although the irritation of the skin by fecal material may result in an infection, this usually is not a life-threatening complication.

2 Although the stoma should be protected from injury, this is not a life-threatening complication.

3 Although this is a concern, it is not a life-threatening complication.

190. **3 Respiratory tract infection may be the first clinical sign of bone marrow suppression. (2) (PB; CJ; EV; MS; DR)**

1 This is an expected side effect that is not life threatening.

2 Same as answer 1.

4 This is not a side effect of doxorubicin.

191. **2 The collection device must be kept below the level of the chest to prevent backflow of fluid into the pleural space. (1) (PB; CJ; IM; MS; RE)**

1 For transport, suction should be turned off and the suction tubing disconnected distal to the water-seal connection.

3 There is no reason to disconnect the chest tube from the water-seal system; this would allow atmospheric air to enter the pleural space.

4 The chest tube should not be clamped because it may precipitate a tension pneumothorax.

192. **2 Infants are particularly sensitive to radioactivity; even the small amount emitted during the first few days after treatment may affect them. (3) (PB; MR; IM; MS; DR)**

1 This is not necessary.

3 The recommended medication to be taken until the radioactive iodine destroys thyroid tissue is propranolol.

4 The bathroom may be used by the entire family.

193. **2 The nursing diagnosis consists of two parts: the statement of the client's health status (health problem) and the related factors (probable causes). (3) (SE; CJ; AN; MH; NP)**

1 The nursing diagnosis includes a statement of the problem; the client's needs are addressed in the plan of care.

3 Although the client's responses may reflect health status, this is only one part of the diagnosis.

4 A medical diagnosis describes a disease process; a nursing diagnosis describes a person's response to a disease process, condition, or situation.

194. **4 There is a greater chance for infection to occur with this type of episiotomy because there is more tissue damage and healing is slower. (2) (SE; CJ; AN; CW; HC)**

1 There is more tissue damage so there would be more edema.

2 More blood vessels are injured, so there is more bleeding and bruising.

3 The mediolateral episiotomy cuts large muscles used in ambulation, so there is more discomfort with movement.

195. 4 **The cervical mucus is clear and stretchable (spinnbarkeit) at ovulation because of maximum estrogen stimulation. (3) (PM; MR; IM; CW; RC)**
   1 These characteristics do not occur at any specific point during the cycle.
   2 Same as answer 1.
   3 Same as answer 1.

196. 4 **This open-ended response encourages further discussion and allows for an exploration of feelings. (2) (PI; CJ; IM; MH; MO)**
   1 This response ignores the client's feelings expressed in the statement.
   2 The depression is not adding to the feelings, the feelings are causing the depression.
   3 Same as answer 1.

197. 3 **A formal plan demonstrates determination, concentration, and effort, with conclusions already thought out. (2) (PI; CJ; AS; MH; MO)**
   1 Failure to successfully complete the suicidal act can add to feelings of worthlessness and stimulate further acts.
   2 Talking about suicide does not give clients the idea; verbalizing feelings may help reduce clients' need to act out.
   4 Many clients verbalize their suicidal thoughts as they are working on their decision and plan of action; suicide may not be attempted just for the attention it achieves.

198. 3 **This response recognizes the concern and provides accurate information that may reduce anxiety. (2) (PI; MR; IM; MS; EH)**
   1 This is inaccurate information; impotence usually does not result.
   2 This reply closes off communication and transfers responsibility to the physician.
   4 This does not recognize feelings and provides inaccurate information; impotence rarely, if ever, occurs with this operation.

199. 2 **Because of the adverse effects of Parlodel, a thorough daily nursing assessment is a priority. (3) (PB; CJ; PL; MS; DR)**
   1 This is only one part of a thorough nursing assessment.
   3 Vital signs would be a priority if there were an additional abnormality or indication beyond the drug therapy.
   4 Isolating this as a priority would be indicated if there were a fluid imbalance.

200. 3 **These are all presumptive of pregnancy; they can be caused by other conditions and cannot be considered proof of pregnancy. (2) (PM; CJ; AS; CW; HC)**
   1 Abdominal enlargement is a probable sign; urinary frequency and nausea are presumptive signs.
   2 Abdominal enlargement and hCG in the urine are probable signs; their presence does not offer a definite diagnosis of pregnancy.
   4 Urinary frequency and breast changes, such as tingling and enlargement, are presumptive signs; abdominal changes are probable signs of pregnancy.

201. 2 **Knowing what to expect reduces fear of the unknown. (2) (SE; CJ; EV; MS; EH)**
   1 This increases fears associated with the experience.
   3 This is the physician's responsibility; the nurse does not give this information; the nurse determines the client's awareness.
   4 Exercise is not immediate; bed rest is prescribed with operative site immobilization for several hours.

202. 2 **The intravenous route is the preferred route for medication for a client with impaired peripheral circulation. (2) (PB; CJ; PL; MS; DR)**
   1 Oral medications usually are not given to burn clients because of the frequent occurrence of paralytic ileus; oral analgesics take too long to provide immediate relief from pain.
   3 Impaired peripheral circulation does not permit accurate prediction of the dose absorbed.
   4 Same as answer 3.

203. 2 **Lead blocks the formation of RBCs because it is very toxic to the biosynthesis of heme; this leads to anemia. (2) (PB; CJ; AN; PE; BI)**
   1 This does not occur; the child usually has anemia and CNS disturbances.
   3 Same as answer 1.
   4 Same as answer 1.

204. 2 **Each pregnancy creates a stress situation and is a developmental crisis. (3) (PM; CJ; AN; CW; EC)**
   1 It has not been determined that multigravidas are more successful in coping with pregnancy than primigravidas.
   3 Each pregnancy is unique, and this pregnancy may or may not be more stressful than the others.
   4 Support persons are important during any crisis or stressful situation.

205. 2 **The nurse can be more sensitive to the needs of the client by addressing personal emotions first. (3) (PI; CJ; AS; CW; EC)**
   1 The focus should be on the client's feelings, not the nurse's.
   3 A time of crisis is not the time to teach; the client is not ready to learn.
   4 Complete control is not, and should not be, the goal of the nurse.

206. 3 **Clients with left hemianopia ignore whatever is in the left field of vision. (3) (PI; CJ; EV; MS; NM)**
   1 This would occur if the client had right hemianopia and wished to see better when eating.
   2 This would occur with right hemiparesis, not with hemianopia.
   4 This indicates hemiplegia, not hemianopia.

207. 4 **This is an expected adaptation to a state of dehydration; the urine will be concentrated. (2) (PB; CJ; AS; PE; FE)**
   1 There is no indication of celiac disease.
   2 One of the signs of dehydration in an infant is a sunken, not a bulging, fontanelle.
   3 The initial response to decreased circulating fluids would be an increased pulse rate.

208. 3 **Increasing fluids flushes the urinary tract of microorganisms. (3) (SE; CJ; PL; CW; WH)**
   1 Tampons do not increase the risk of cystitis.
   2 Fluids should be increased, not decreased; prune juice promotes an acidic urine.
   4 This promotes the transfer of microorganisms to the urethra, where they could ascend to the bladder.

209. 3 **This statement conveys acceptance by the nurse and encourages the mother to verbalize additional concerns; it also explores the mother's understanding of the physician's explanation. (2) (PI; CJ; IM; CW; EC)**
   1 This reply belittles the mother's concern and cuts off further communication.
   2 Although this response does acknowledge part of the mother's concerns, it denies her the opportunity of further exploration of her fears that her infant may not respond to therapy.
   4 Same as answer 1.

210. 3 **Doxorubicin is cardiotoxic and causes dysrhythmias. (2) (PB; CJ; EV; MS; DR)**
   1 Toxicity causes severe, not minor, dermatitis.
   2 This is a side effect of doxorubicin, not a toxic effect.

4 Same as answer 2.

211. 3 **Individuals taking steroids have lowered resistance and may become fatally ill if exposed to the varicella virus. (1) (SE; CJ; IM; PE; BI)**
   1 This does not lower body resistance; therefore it does not increase susceptibility.
   2 This does not affect body resistance because topical antibiotics do not have a systemic effect.
   4 This may increase resistance rather than decrease it.

212. 2 **Urinary output reflects circulating blood volume; it is the most reliable, immediately available information to assess fluid needs. (1) (PB; CJ; EV; MS; FE)**
   1 Although daily weights reflect fluid retention or loss, they are not as immediately accurate as hourly urine measurements.
   3 This may indicate hypervolemia or hypovolemia but is not as accurate an indicator of insufficient fluid replacement as hourly urine output.
   4 Peripheral edema may have many causes; it is not an effective indicator of fluid balance.

213. 1 **During this stage the nurse reaches a conclusion about the collected data and makes a nursing diagnosis. (3) (SE; MR; AN; MH; NP)**
   2 During this stage, the nurse sets priorities, establishes goals, identifies outcome criteria, and develops a nursing care plan.
   3 The client's response to nursing care is assessed in relation to the stated outcome criteria to determine whether goals have been met.
   4 The nurse gathers and clusters data during this stage of the nursing process.

214. 2 **These are early signs of shock; shock ensues rapidly after a ruptured aortic aneurysm because of profound hemorrhage; this is a surgical emergency. (3) (PB; CJ; EV; MS; CV)**
   1 The nurse can observe hyperventilation by watching the client's breathing patterns; rapid respirations, rather than a rapid pulse, would be expected.
   3 Extreme anxiety is not usually associated with light-headedness unless there is hyperventilation.
   4 The signs and symptoms are not inclusive enough to indicate infection; there is no indication of fever or a rising white blood cell count.

215. 3 **An explanation of how the restraints work and why may reassure the mother. (2) (PM; CJ; AN; PE; GI)**
   1 This does not explain why the restraints are being used now.
   2 This implies strict adherence to the physician's wishes without apparent independent thought.
   4 This response gives the mother the feeling that her baby's needs are not being met.

216. 4 **When a baby has scanty dark urine, poor skin turgor, and increased depth of respirations, it is likely that dehydration and metabolic alkalosis are present; these occur because of the fluid and hydrochloric acid loss and the potassium depletion; immediate intervention is necessary. (2) (PB; CJ; AS; PE; FE)**
   1 These are not indicators of immediate needs; assessment for signs of dehydration and metabolic alkalosis are more important.
   2 This would be difficult to determine accurately; it is far more important to assess the infant for signs of dehydration and metabolic alkalosis.
   3 The olive-shaped mass is in the epigastric area, not the lower abdomen.

217. 1 **This gives the client, the nurse, and other caregivers a goal that is achievable and measurable. (1) (SE; MR; PL; MS; NP)**
   2 Interventions help achieve expectations; change may not be necessary.
   3 The client and nurse must both be involved in determining goals.
   4 This is vague and may not be achievable.

218. 4 **Pain at the arterial puncture site is attributable to entry and cannulation of the artery. (2) (PB; CJ; AN; MS; CV)**
   1 This might occur during the pre-catheterization period.
   2 This occurs during the procedure when the contrast medium is injected.
   3 Although this may occur during the procedure because of trauma to the conduction system, it usually does not continue after the procedure.

219. 4 **This anesthesia creates a sympathetic block that causes loss of peripheral resistance and a decrease in venous return; this leads to a reduced cardiac output and results in lowered BP. (2) (PB; CJ; EV; CW; DR)**
   1 The urge to void is diminished with this kind of anesthesia; the client should be encouraged to void to prevent distention.
   2 This is not a frequent side effect of this anesthesia; it may occur if an accidental high placement of anesthetic occurs or excessive amount of anesthesia is used.
   3 Bradycardia, not tachycardia, may result.

220. 2 **This position permits the hip, knee, and elbow joints to extend rather than flex. (2) (PB; CJ; PL; MS; SK)**
   1 This position requires that one or more of the hip, knee, and elbow joints be flexed.
   3 Same as answer 1.
   4 Same as answer 1.

221. 2 **Dizziness may occur during the first few weeks of therapy until the client adapts physiologically to the medication. (1) (PB; CJ; EV; MS; DR)**
   1 Cardiac monitoring may be instituted because of possible dysrhythmias; however, an electroencephalogram would not be necessary.
   3 Ordinarily, this is not necessary, but if nausea occurs, the medication may be taken with food or at bedtime.
   4 The medication should be taken at the same time each day to maintain a constant effect on blood pressure.

222. 1 **Vomiting leads to weight loss, a sign of dehydration; weighing daily is an accurate assessment measure. (1) (PB; CJ; AS; PE; FE)**
   2 Concentrated, not dilute, urine is associated with dehydration.
   3 The skin would be pale and gray with dehydration.
   4 Depressed fontanelles are associated with dehydration.

223. 2 **The leader should not intervene at this point; the client addressed the statement to the group, and the group response should be fostered. (2) (SE; MR; IM; MH; TR)**
   1 This response may be viewed as aggressive and would make other members fearful of contributing because they might be confronted.
   3 This denies the client's feelings.
   4 Same as answer 1.

224. 4 **High levels of steroids result in emotional changes; the actual cause is unknown, but knowing the response may help the mother to better cope with her son's behavior. (2) (SE; CJ; IM; MS; EN)**
   1 This is unnecessary; the problem has been excessive production of steroids.

2 Weight loss, not weight gain, would indicate an improving condition.

3 The changes are not permanent with adequate therapy.

225. 1 **Lying prone will prevent flexion contractures of the hip because it keeps the hip in extension. (1) (PB; CJ; IM; MS; SK)**

2 Sitting will promote the development of a flexion contracture, especially when prolonged, and should be avoided.

3 Lying supine with pillows between the thighs will promote external rotation and hip abduction and should be avoided.

4 Elevating the residual limb with pillows could cause a flexion contracture.

226. 4 **After laboring all night the client is tired. (3) (PB; CJ; PL; CW; HC)**

1 This would be premature; the client is not ready to learn.

2 This assessment would be too frequent and would interfere with the client's rest.

3 This is necessary only the first time the client ambulates; otherwise the client can ambulate ad lib.

227. 2 **This helps the client avoid hitting objects and thus prevents trauma during the tonic-clonic phase of the seizure. (1) (SE; MR; IM; MS; NM)**

1 This is contraindicated; it could injure the client.

3 Same as answer 1.

4 If done during the tonic-clonic phase of the seizure, it could cause injury; if necessary, this is done immediately after the seizure to establish an airway.

228. 1 **The position of maximum safety and comfort is side-lying because the child's neck and back are hyperextended. (2) (SE; CJ; IM; PE; NM)**

2 This would be impossible because the child is in a rigid opisthotonic position.

3 Same as answer 2.

4 This would increase intracranial pressure.

229. 1 **Subcostal incisional pain causes the client to splint and avoid deep breathing, which impedes air exchange in the alveoli. (3) (PB; CJ; AN; MS; GI)**

2 The location of the incision does not increase the risk of hemorrhage.

3 This can be a postoperative problem, but it is unrelated to the site of the incision.

4 The site is not specifically vulnerable to infection.

230. 2 **The muscle contraction-relaxation cycle requires a normal serum calcium-phosphorus ratio; the reduction of the ionized serum calcium level associated with malabsorption syndrome causes tetany (spastic muscle spasms). (2) (SE; CJ; AN; MS; FE)**

1 Sodium is the major extracellular cation; the major route of excretion is the kidneys, under the control of aldosterone; although it plays a part in neuromuscular transmission, it is not related to the development of tetany.

3 Potassium is the major intracellular cation; it is part of the sodium-potassium pump and helps to balance the response of nerves to stimulation; it is not related to the development of tetany.

4 Although phosphorus is closely related to calcium because they exist in a definite ratio, phosphorus is not related to the development of tetany.

231. 1 **Lack of motivation is the most serious impediment to successful continuous ambulatory peritoneal dialysis (CAPD); CAPD is contraindicated for clients who are blind or have a colostomy, a psychosis, or PVD. (3) (PB; CJ; AS; MS; RG)**

2 This is not a contraindication if the client is receiving medical supervision.

3 Same as answer 2.

4 Same as answer 2.

232. 4 **It is important to set limits on behavior, but it is also important to involve the client in decision making. (2) (PI; MR; IM; MH; PR)**

1 Some limits must be set by the client and the nurse together.

2 Rarely can a client be distracted from a ritual.

3 This would increase anxiety because the client uses the ritual as a defense against anxiety.

233. 4 **The stoma secretes mucus immediately following surgery and continues to secrete mucus mixed with serum and blood because of surgical trauma; fecal drainage begins in about 72 hours. (2) (PB; CJ; EV; MS; GI)**

1 This would not occur until about 72 hours after surgery.

2 Drainage that is bloody with clots would indicate hemorrhage; the expected drainage is mucoid and serosanguineous.

3 Drainage will not be clear; it will be serosanguineous because of the trauma of surgery.

234. 3 The client's behaviors are contrary to the medical regimen and are not conducive to positive self-interest. (2) (PI; CJ; AN; MS; RE)
  1 The behavior does not indicate a self-care deficit.
  2 The client's behavior does not indicate disturbed thought processes.
  4 There are no data to support this conclusion.

235. 3 Water in the ears after myringotomy may be a source of an infection. (2) (SE; MR; PL; PE; NM)
  1 This is contraindicated because it can cause trauma.
  2 There is no reason to keep the child isolated.
  4 The ear should be kept open to the air and allowed to drain naturally.

236. 1 By failing to acknowledge the baby as a person, the client indicates that she has not released her fantasy baby and accepted the real one. (1) (PM; CJ; AN; CW; EC)
  2 The mother has acknowledged the infant by using "he," and her question denotes a relationship.
  3 The mother has incorporated the infant into the family by this statement.
  4 Same as answer 2.

237. 1 Increased levels of steroids and aldosterone cause sodium and water retention. (3) (PB; CJ; AS; MS; EN)
  2 Hypertension, not hypotension, would be expected because of sodium and water retention.
  3 The extremities would be thin; subcutaneous fat deposits occur in the upper trunk, especially the back between the scapulae.
  4 Hyperglycemia, not hypoglycemia, occurs because of increased secretion of glucocorticoids; hyperglycemia is sustained and not restricted to the morning hours.

238. 1 This will help to decrease the client's anxiety, provide a safe environment, and compensate for impaired cognition. (2) (PI; CJ; PL; MH; DD)
  2 Restraints may increase confusion and agitation; they should be used only when absolutely unavoidable.
  3 Confabulation should be accepted; reality orientation should be employed when necessary.
  4 Focusing on coping skills would not be realistic; it would not help the client to adjust or address activities of daily living that have deteriorated.

239. 2 Pain medication may be required for a few days along with intensive supportive nursing care. (2) (PB; CJ; IM; PE; EH)

  1 To the client, the pain is real requiring pain medication; addiction is not a concern at this time.
  3 Explanation does not suffice to relieve the pain; medication and constant emotional support are required.
  4 This offers false reassurance; the pain will not recede; a backrub may help to divert attention but pain medication should be administered

240. 4 All amino acids are needed for the synthesis of various proteins, but the term "essential" refers to those amino acids the body cannot make, which are thus essential in the diet. (2) (PB; CJ; IM; MS; GI)
  1 All amino acids in a protein contribute the same number of calories for energy.
  2 All amino acids, not just essential amino acids, are necessary for rebuilding body tissue.
  3 All amino acids, not just essential amino acids, contain nitrogen.

241. 1 Smoking is the single most important risk factor for peripheral arterial disease (PAD), and cessation should be encouraged. (2) (SE; MR; IM; MS; CV)
  2 While hyperglycemia is a contributory factor, it is not the primary risk factor for PAD.
  3 While a sedentary lifestyle is a contributory factor, it is not the primary risk factor for PAD.
  4 While a high-fat/high-cholesterol diet is a contributory factor, it is not the primary risk factor for peripheral arterial disease.

242. 2 Routines tend to provide a sense of security, and successful completion of activities supports self-esteem and limits frustration. (1) (PI; CJ; PL; MH; DD)
  1 Varying routines increases stress and frustration.
  3 Decreased physical capacity and attention limit the ability to participate actively.
  4 Challenging activities can be frustrating and lead to hostility or withdrawal.

243. 1 This is less than the normal range of 7.35 to 7.45; hypoxia causes hypercapnia, resulting in a fall in the pH. (3) (PB; CJ; AS)
  2 This is within the normal range of 80 to 100 mm Hg.
  3 This is within the normal range of 35 to 45 mm Hg.
  4 This is within the normal range of 21 to 28 mEq/L.

244. Answer: 7%; the anterior part of each lower leg from knee to foot is 3.5%, which equals 7%. (2) (PB; CJ; AS; MS; IT)

245. 3 **Physical safety of the client and others is the priority. (1) (SE; MR; PL; MH; NP)**
    1 Although it is important for the clients to live up to contracts, it is not imperative.
    2 The nurse cannot prevent or control clients' use of defensive behavior.
    4 Same as answer 2.

246. 1 **A gush of blood occurs when the placenta separates from the uterine wall before the normal physiologic clamping off of the vessels at this site. (2) (PM; CJ; AS; CW; HC)**
    2 The uterus contracts and becomes firm when the placenta separates.
    3 The uterus appears to increase in size when the placenta separates.
    4 The blood pressure returns to prenatal status shortly after birth; the decrease is gradual and unrelated to placental separation.

247. 4 **These movements require muscle contraction, putting pressure on blood vessels, increasing tissue oxygen, and thus promoting circulation. (3) (SE; MR; AN; CW; WH)**
    1 Muscle atrophy is not a common complication following a mastectomy.
    2 Contractures are a rare complication following a mastectomy.
    3 Lymphedema is assessed by measuring the circumference of the extremity, not by having the client exercise.

248. 3 **Humidification of the environment helps to liquefy respiratory secretions, which will then be easier to expectorate. (3) (PB; MR; IM; MS; RE)**
    1 Measures to prevent infection are essential; however, infections are impossible to eliminate.
    2 Exhaling requires less energy than inhaling; therefore movements that utilize energy should be done during exhalation.
    4 The use of diaphragmatic muscles rather than abdominal and neck muscles improves the client's breathing

249. 1 **Euthanasia is a crime and is against the law in the United States. (1) (SE; LE; AN; MS; NP)**
    2 Euthanasia is against the law in the United States.
    3 Neither physicians nor nurses have the legal authority to perform acts of euthanasia.
    4 This is not negligence; it is a crime.

250. 2 **The client has the right to refuse the Papanicolaou test; the nurse must accept the client's need to talk with the physician first. (2) (PI; LE; IM; CW; EC)**
    1 This is a subjective conclusion; the client has the right to refuse the test.
    3 This is inappropriate; this action is not client centered.
    4 The client's need must be recognized first.

251. 2 **The need for acceptance of life as fulfilling and meaningful is the major task of the older adult. (2) (PM; CJ; AN; MH; GD)**
    1 This is the task of young adulthood (18 to 25 years); it involves establishment of an intimate relationship and occupation.
    3 The task of the adolescent (12 to 20 years) is establishing identity through work and development of relationships and an occupation.
    4 This is the task of adulthood (21 to 45 years); it involves establishment of a family and guiding of the next generation.

252. 1 **Properly chosen clothes can minimize the appearance of a brace, especially if an effort is made to keep up with the current styles. (1) (PM; CJ; IM; PE; EH)**
    2 There are no data to indicate that the child will not adjust to the treatment regimen.
    3 This has a negative connotation that emphasizes the child's problem.
    4 This may be misinterpreted as false praise, which can cause mother/child conflict.

253. 3 **The autistic child needs protection from self-injury. (2) (PI; CJ; IM; MH; BA)**
    1 This can be permitted only if it does not place the child in jeopardy.
    2 The autistic child has difficulty following directions, especially when out of control.
    4 The autistic child cannot separate self from behavior; a punitive approach will decrease the child's self-esteem.

254. 2 **In a back-lying (dorsal) position blood will flow with gravity down the sides of the neck and not be seen. (2) (PB; CJ; IM; MS; EN)**
    1 This flexes the neck excessively, which increases tension on the suture line and may inhibit the passage of gases through the oral, pharyngeal, and tracheal areas; a small pillow behind the head keeps the head and neck in functional alignment and limits tension on the suture line.
    3 Coughing should not be encouraged during the first 24 to 48 hours to limit stress on the suture line.
    4 Tetany will not occur during the first eight hours after surgery.

255. 2 This heart rate is acceptable when the client is receiving digoxin; digoxin lengthens the atrioventricular conduction time, which slows the heart rate; toxicity may be present if the heart rate drops below 60. (2) (PB; CJ; EV; MS; DR)

1 This is a symptom of toxicity; nausea and vomiting can occur because of gastric irritation and its action at central nervous system sites

3 This is a sign of toxicity; premature nodal or ventricular impulses and varying degrees of heart block can occur because of slowed transmission of impulses through the AV node.

4 This is a symptom of toxicity; xanthopsia (yellow vision) is caused by digoxin's effect on visual cones.

256. 1 The LOA position indicates that the fetus is on the left side of the mother and is in a head presentation with the occiput anterior; therefore, fetal heart sounds are best found in the laboring woman's left lower quadrant. (2) (PM; CJ; AS; CW; HC)

2 The fetus would have to be in the breech presentation on the left side of the mother to find the fetal heartbeat in the left upper quadrant.

3 For the fetal heartbeat to be found toward the right lower midline of the mother, the fetus probably would be in a shoulder presentation, in the right scapular anterior (RScA) position.

4 The fetus would have to be in the breech presentation on the right side of the mother to find the fetal heartbeat in the right upper quadrant.

257. 4 Rapid weight gain may indicate an edematous state; while the client is on bed rest, the blood pressure decreases and interstitial fluid is mobilized into the intravascular space, enhancing flow to the uterus and kidneys; a 24-hour collection of urine for protein and creatinine clearance is reflective of true renal status. (2) (PB; CJ; PL; CW; HP)

1 Diuretics and low-salt diets will gradually decrease circulating fluid, creating hypovolemia, which decreases placental circulation.

2 Diuretics are contraindicated in pregnancy because they decrease circulating fluids and may impair fluid supply to the placenta; side-lying bed rest and intake and output would be ordered.

3 Elevated serum glucose levels are unrelated to preeclampsia; daily weights and side-lying bed rest would be ordered.

258. 3 The child's status and the progression of the seizure should be monitored; the child will not breathe until the seizure is over, and cyanosis should subside at that time. (1) (SE; CJ; IM; PE; NM)

1 Attempting to open clenched jaws could result in injury to the child.

2 Oxygen will be useless until the child breathes when the seizure is over.

4 The physician can be notified later; provision of safety and observation are the priorities.

259. 2 This is an autosomal recessive disorder; each parent contributes one affected gene. (2) (PM; CJ; AN; PE; BI)

1 There is only a 50% chance that a child will have the sickle-cell trait, not sickle-cell disease.

3 Same as answer 1.

4 All of the children from these parents will have the sickle-cell trait but not sickle-cell disease.

260. 3 There is better control with short-acting (regular) insulin. (3) (PB; CJ; AN; MS; EN)

1 The level of glucose must be maintained as close to normal as possible.

2 The occurrence is greater when the client is receiving exogenous insulin.

4 This is not the reason for using regular insulin; both oral hypoglycemics and insulin are available.

261. 2 Limit-setting must be consistent for a client who is using manipulative behavior; a unified approach is vital because the client will play staff members against each other. (1) (SE; MR; IM; MH; PR)

1 Limit-setting is required to control inappropriate behavior.

3 This must be a group decision, not the responsibility of one staff member alone; the client is unable to set self-limits.

4 The most important concept is unity of approach, not the ability of a few to resist manipulation.

262. 4 Because steroids decrease the body's defenses against infection, a person with thrombophlebitis, a noninfectious process, would be the best selection for a roommate. (2) (SE; MR; AN; MS; NP)

1 This would be unsafe because this is a communicable disease.

2 Same as answer 1.

3 Same as answer 1.

263. **4 This explanation illustrates that the child can understand cause-effect relationships and offers information to increase the child's understanding of the illness. (2) (PM; MR; IM; PE; GD)**
    1 This is too general and does not explain why the child will feel better.
    2 This is too authoritarian; the child needs information that will increase understanding and compliance with the regimen.
    3 Same as answer 2.

264. **1 Withdrawn clients can tolerate personal contact only for short periods. (2) (PI; CJ; PL; MH; SD)**
    2 The client could not function in this type of group.
    3 The client has a problem with interpersonal relations; therefore, this would be counter productive.

4 Allowing the client to be alone would not relieve anxiety; it would foster further withdrawal.

265. **3 Cleansing the perianal area from "clean to dirty" protects the surgical site from microorganisms that can cause infection. (2) (SE; MR; IM; CW; WH)**
    1 This is not practical after each voiding; cleaning the perineum from clean to dirty is more hygienic and limits the risk of vaginal and urinary infections.
    2 This is not a routine method of cleansing; it would have to be prescribed.
    4 Repetitive patting can be traumatic; this technique does not include the urinary meatus.

How to Use Worksheet 1: Errors in Processing Information

Common errors in processing information are listed in the left hand column of this worksheet. At the top of the worksheet is a row of blank spaces for inserting the number of the question missed. Directly below each number, check any errors you made in answering that question. You may have made more than one type of error in an answer.

Worksheet 1: Errors in Processing Information

Question number																							
Did not read situation/ question carefully																							
Missed important details																							
Confused major and minor points																							
Defined problem incorrectly																							
Could not remember terms/ facts/concepts/principles																							
Defined terms incorrectly																							
Focused on incomplete/incorrect data in assessing situation																							
Interpreted data incorrectly																							
Applied wrong concepts/ principles in situations																							
Drew incorrect conclusions																							
Identified wrong goals																							
Identified priorities incorrectly																							
Carried out plan incorrectly/ incompletely																							
Was unclear about criteria for evaluating success in achieving goals																							

How to Use Worksheet 2: Knowledge Gaps

Types of common knowledge gaps are listed along the top of this worksheet. Write a brief description of topics you want to review in the spaces provided. For example, if you missed a question on administration of a particular drug, write the drug name and problem (e.g., dosage) in the appropriate space under the column labeled *Pharmacology*.

Worksheet 2: Knowledge Gaps

Basic science	Skills/ procedures	Basic human needs	Growth and development	Normal nutrition	Psychosocial factors	Clinical area/ topic	Stressors/ coping mechanisms	Patho- physiology	Pharma- cology	Therapeutic nutrition	Legal implications	Other